ANTIEPILEPTIC DRUGS

Second Edition

ANTIEPILEPTIC DRUGS

Second Edition

Editors

Dixon M. Woodbury, Ph.D.

Professor of Pharmacology
Division of Neuropharmacology and Epileptology
University of Utah College of Medicine
Salt Lake City, Utah

J. Kiffin Penry, M.D.

Professor of Neurology
Bowman Gray School of Medicine
of Wake Forest University
Winston-Salem, North Carolina

C. E. Pippenger, Ph.D.

Associate Professor of Neuropharmacology
Columbia University College
of Physicians and Surgeons
New York, New York

Assistant Editor

B. J. Hessie

Rockville, Maryland

The Joseph W. England Library
Philadelphia College of Pharmacy & Science
42nd & Woodland Avenue
Philadelphia, Pa. 19104
RELEASED

Raven Press ∎ New York

Raven Press, 1140 Avenue of the Americas, New York, New York 10036

Made in the United States of America

International Standard Book Number 0-89004-498-8
Library of Congress Catalog Card Number 79-5501

Great care has been taken to maintain the accuracy of the information contained in the volume. However, Raven Press cannot be held responsible for errors or for any consequences arising from the use of the information contained herein.

Materials appearing in this book prepared by individuals as part of their official duties as U.S. Government employees are not covered by the above-mentioned copyright.

Preface

When *Antiepileptic Drugs* was first published a decade ago, as a compilation of the available information concerning all aspects of drug therapy for the epilepsies, it was obvious that our knowledge of the mechanisms of action of antiepileptic drugs was incomplete and that the therapeutic application of the existing information was inadequate.

During the past 10 years, however, many of the gaps in our knowledge of the antiepileptic drugs have been filled and the clinical management of the epilepsies has improved. Many factors are responsible for these advances. Improved techniques of video monitoring and telemetered electroencephalography allowed better determination of the seizure type. Rapid technological developments in the quantification of antiepileptic drugs in biological fluids by gas-liquid chromatography, high-pressure liquid chromatography, and homogeneous enzyme immunoassay permitted the correlation of drug concentration with clinical response. With this information, it was then possible to establish the pharmacokinetic profiles of individual patients in various clinical situations.

Simultaneously with the clinical studies, basic research on the epilepsies provided new insights into the mechanisms that cause and regulate seizure activity in the central nervous system and into the ways that antiepileptic drugs alter these mechanisms. Such basic studies are exemplified by exploration of the role of neurotransmitters in the regulation of neuronal activity and investigation of ionic channels, the gating process, and ion transport across neuronal membranes.

Without a doubt, however, the key factor in the advances in our knowledge and use of the antiepileptic drugs is the dedicated efforts of investigators throughout the world to provide better care for patients with epilepsy. It is impossible to cite each individual who has contributed to these advances, but special recognition should be given to the National Institute of Neurological and Communicative Disorders and Stroke, the Epilepsy Foundation of America, the International League Against Epilepsy, and the organizers of the Workshops on the Determination of Antiepileptic Drugs in Body Fluids.

The aim of this second edition duplicates that of the original work, namely, to "present in a single source all of the recent advances in knowledge concerning the antiepileptic drugs as well as an in-depth review of basic pharmacologic data from both animals and man." With an up-to-date presentation of this information on both old and new drugs and the addition of current findings on the mechanisms of action of antiepileptic drugs, this new volume offers a thorough treatment of the pharmacological approach to the epilepsies.

Notwithstanding the recent advances mentioned above, the drug therapy of epilepsy is still wanting. It is our hope that this book will enhance our basic and clinical understanding of the antiepileptic drugs for the good of patients with epilepsy. We hope, too, that it will serve to stimulate future investigations in this field.

The Editors

Acknowledgments

We are grateful, first of all, to the many contributors, whose cooperation, enthusiasm, and patience made this work possible. Special thanks and gratitude are extended to B. J. Hessie, without whose devotion and sustained effort this new edition would not have been prepared. Finally, we thank Raven Press, and particularly Ann Berlin and Virginia B. Martin, for the careful production of this book.

Contents

Contributors

AGOSTINO BARUZZI, M.D.
Neurological Clinic, University of Bologna School of Medicine, 40123 Bologna, Italy

DANIEL L. BIUS
Department of Pharmacology, Epilepsy and Anticonvulsant Drug Research Laboratory, University of North Carolina School of Medicine, Chapel Hill, North Carolina 27514

HAROLD E. BOOKER, M.D.
Director, Neurology Service, Veterans Administration Central Office, Washington, D.C. 20420

LAURA BOSSI, M.D.
Department of Clinical Research, Synthelabo—L.E.R.S., 75013 Paris, France

JAMES J. CEREGHINO, M.D.
Epilepsy Branch, Neurological Disorders Program, National Institute of Neurological and Communicative Disorders and Stroke, Bethesda, Maryland 20205

TSUN CHANG, M.S.
Research Associate, Warner-Lambert/Parke-Davis, Pharmaceutical Research, Ann Arbor, Michigan 48105

JAMES C. CLOYD, Pharm.D.
Assistant Professor, University of Minnesota College of Pharmacy, St. Paul–Ramsey Medical Center, St. Paul, Minnesota 55101

JOYCE A. CRAMER
Epilepsy Center, Veterans Administration Medical Center, West Haven, Connecticut 06516

MOGENS DAM, M.D.
Consultant Neurologist, University Clinic of Neurology, Hvidovre Hospital, DK-2650 Hvidovre, Denmark

F. E. DREIFUSS, M.B., M.R.C.P., F.R.A.C.P.
Professor of Neurology, University of Virginia Medical Center, Charlottesville, Virginia 22901

KENNETH H. DUDLEY, Ph.D.
Department of Pharmacology, Epilepsy and Anticonvulsant Drug Research Laboratory, University of North Carolina School of Medicine, Chapel Hill, North Carolina 27514

MERVYN J. EADIE, M.D., Ph.D., F.R.A.C.P.
Professor of Clinical Neurology and Neuropharmacology, University of Queensland; and Department of Medicine, Royal Brisbane Hospital, Brisbane, Australia 4029

J. W. FAIGLE, Ph.D.
Senior Research Associate, Research Department, Pharmaceuticals Division, CIBA-GEIGY Limited, CH-4002 Basle, Switzerland

K. F. FELDMANN, PH.D.
Senior Staff Scientist, Research Department, Pharmaceuticals Division, CIBA-GEIGY Limited, CH-4002 Basle, Switzerland

JAMES A. FERRENDELLI, M.D.
Professor of Pharmacology and Neurology, Washington University School of Medicine, St. Louis, Missouri 63110

R. W. FINCHAM, M.D.
Department of Neurology, University of Iowa College of Medicine, Iowa City, Iowa 52242

ANTHONY J. GLAZKO, PH.D.
Director, Drug Metabolism, Warner-Lambert/Parke-Davis, Pharmaceutical Research, Ann Arbor, Michigan 48105

MARK A. GOLDBERG, PH.D., M.D.
Professor of Neurology and Pharmacology, University of California, Los Angeles, School of Medicine, Harbor–UCLA Medical Center, Torrance, California 90509

PIETER J. M. GUELEN
ABL Drug Studies Unit, Applied Bioresearch Laboratories, Assen, The Netherlands

PETER M. JEAVONS, M.A., F.R.C.P., F.R.C.PSYCH.
Honorary Visiting Professor, The University of Aston in Birmingham, Birmingham B4 7ET, England

SVEIN I. JOHANNESSEN, PH.D.
Head, Department of Clinical Chemistry, The National Center for Epilepsy, N-1301 Sandvika, Norway

DANIEL JOHNSTON, PH.D.
Department of Neurology, Baylor College of Medicine, Houston, Texas 77030

GARY L. JONES, PH.D.
Department of Pharmacology, Texas College of Osteopathic Medicine, Fort Worth, Texas 76107

ROBERT M. JULIEN, M.D., PH.D.
University of Oregon Health Sciences Center, Portland, Oregon 97201

BARRY J. KARAS, PHARM.D.
Postdoctoral Fellow, Neurology Service, Veterans Administration Medical Center, Gainesville, Florida 32602

JOHN W. KEMP, PH.D.
Division of Neuropharmacology and Epileptology, University of Utah College of Medicine, Salt Lake City, Utah 84132

BETSY T. KING
Department of Pharmacology, Epilepsy and Anticonvulsant Drug Research Laboratory, University of North Carolina School of Medicine, Chapel Hill, North Carolina 27514

WILLIAM E. KLUNK
Department of Pharmacology, Washington University School of Medicine, St. Louis, Missouri 63110

HARVEY J. KUPFERBERG, Ph.D.
Epilepsy Branch, Neurological Disorders Program, National Institute of Neurological and Communicative Disorders and Stroke, Bethesda, Maryland 20205

HENN KUTT, M.D.
Associate Professor of Neurology and Pharmacology, The New York Hospital—Cornell Medical Center, New York, New York 10021

ALLEN A. LAI, Ph.D.
Department of Clinical Research, Medical Division, Burroughs Wellcome Company, Research Triangle Park, North Carolina 27709

ILO E. LEPPIK, M.D.
Assistant Professor of Neurology, University of Minnesota, St. Paul–Ramsey Medical Center, St. Paul, Minnesota 55101

RENÉ H. LEVY, Ph.D.
Professor and Chairman, Department of Pharmaceutics, University of Washington School of Pharmacy, Seattle, Washington 98195

KENNETH G. LLOYD, Ph.D.
Department of Clinical Research, Synthelabo—L.E.R.S., 75013 Paris, France

JOAN S. LOCKARD, Ph.D.
Professor, Department of Neurological Surgery, University of Washington School of Medicine, Seattle, Washington 98195

RICHARD L. MASLAND, M.D.
Emeritus Professor of Neurology, Columbia University College of Physicians and Surgeons, New York, New York 10032

RICHARD H. MATTSON, M.D.
Clinical Professor of Neurology, Yale University School of Medicine, New Haven, Connecticut 06510; and Director, Epilepsy Center, Veterans Administration Medical Center, West Haven, Connecticut 06516

E. W. MAYNERT, M.D., Ph.D.
Professor of Pharmacology, University of Illinois College of Medicine, Chicago, Illinois 60680

ROBERTO MICHELUCCI, M.D.
Neurological Clinic, University of Bologna School of Medicine, 40123 Bologna, Italy

PAOLO L. MORSELLI, M.D.
Director of Clinical Research, Synthelabo—L.E.R.S., 75013 Paris, France

HELGA PARIS-KUTT, M.D.
Staff Associate in Neurology, Columbia University College of Physicians and Surgeons, New York, New York 10032

J. KIFFIN PENRY, M.D.
Professor of Neurology and Associate Dean for Neurosciences Development, Bowman Gray School of Medicine of Wake Forest University, Winston-Salem, North Carolina 27103

ROBERT J. PERCHALSKI, M.S.
Research Chemist, Medical Research Service, Veterans Administration Medical Center, and Adjunct Assistant Professor, University of Florida College of Pharmacy, Gainesville, Florida 32602

E. PERUCCA, Ph.D.
Department of Pharmacology, Unit of Clinical Pharmacology, Piazza Botta, 10, Pavia, Italy

C. E. PIPPENGER, Ph.D.
Associate Professor of Neuropharmacology, Columbia University College of Physicians and Surgeons, New York, New York 10032

ANTHONY V. PISCIOTTA, M.D.
Professor of Medicine, Blood Research Laboratory, Department of Medicine, The Medical College of Wisconsin, Milwaukee County Medical Complex, Milwaukee, Wisconsin 53226

WILLIAM H. PITLICK, Ph.D.
Epilepsy Branch, Neurological Disorders Program, National Institute of Neurological and Communicative Disorders and Stroke, Bethesda, Maryland 20205

GABRIEL L. PLAA, Ph.D.
Professor and Chairman, Department of Pharmacology, University of Montreal Faculty of Medicine, Montreal, P.Q. H3C 3J7, Canada

ROGER J. PORTER, M.D.
Chief, Epilepsy Branch, Neurological Disorders Program, National Institute of Neurological and Communicative Disorders and Stroke, Bethesda, Maryland 20205

JAMES W. PRICHARD, M.D.
Professor of Neurology, Yale University School of Medicine, New Haven, Connecticut 06510

A. RICHENS, Ph.D., F.R.C.P.
Clinical Pharmacology Unit, Department of Clinical Neurology, Institute of Neurology, The National Hospital, Queen Square, London WC1N 3BG, England

SUSUMU SATO, M.D.
Epilepsy Branch, Neurological Disorders Program, National Institute of Neurological and Communicative Disorders and Stroke, Bethesda, Maryland 20205

Dr. rer. nat. HELMUT R. SCHÄFER
Research Department, Desitin-Werk Carl Klinke GmbH, 2000 Hamburg 63, Federal Republic of Germany

Asst. Prof. Dr. DIETER SCHMIDT
Free University of Berlin, University Clinic Charlottenburg, 1000 Berlin 19, Federal Republic of Germany

FRED SCHOBBEN, Ph.D.
Apotheek Academisch Ziekenhuis Utrecht, 3500 CG Utrecht, The Netherlands

DOROTHY D. SCHOTTELIUS, Ph.D.
Department of Neurology, University of Iowa College of Medicine, Iowa City, Iowa 52242

ALLAN L. SHERWIN, M.D., PH.D.
Professor of Neurology, Montreal Neurological Institute, Montreal, P.Q. H3A 2B4, Canada

GERALD E. SLATER, M.D.
Departments of Neurology and Pediatrics, Hennepin County Medical Center, University of Minnesota, Minneapolis, Minnesota 55415

EWART A. SWINYARD, PH.D.
Emeritus Professor of Pharmacology and Former Dean, College of Pharmacy, University of Utah Colleges of Medicine and Pharmacy, Salt Lake City, Utah 84112

CARLO ALBERTO TASSINARI, M.D.
Professor, Neurological Clinic, University of Bologna School of Medicine, 40123 Bologna, Italy

EPPO VAN DER KLEIJN, PH.D.
Department of Clinical Pharmacy, St. Radboud Hospital, University of Nijmegen, 6525 GA Nijmegen, The Netherlands

B. G. WHITE, PH.D.
Epilepsy Branch, Neurological Disorders Program, National Institute of Neurological and Communicative Disorders and Stroke, Bethesda, Maryland 20205

B. J. WILDER, M.D.
Chief, Neurology Service, Veterans Administration Medical Center, and Professor of Neurology and Neuroscience, University of Florida College of Medicine, Gainesville, Florida 32602

C. D. WITHROW, PH.D.
Associate Professor of Pharmacology, University of Utah College of Medicine, Salt Lake City, Utah 84132

DIXON M. WOODBURY, PH.D.
Professor of Pharmacology, Division of Neuropharmacology and Epileptology, University of Utah College of Medicine, Salt Lake City, Utah 84132

JOSE H. WOODHEAD
Research Specialist, Department of Biochemical Pharmacology and Toxicology, University of Utah College of Pharmacy, Salt Lake City, Utah 84112

Antiepileptic Drugs, edited by D. M. Woodbury, J. K. Penry, and C. E. Pippenger. Raven Press, New York © 1982.

1

Introduction

Ewart A. Swinyard

Contemporary antiepileptic drug therapy emerged only after millennia of treatment based on ignorance, superstition, and antique remedies. The first effective anticonvulsant drugs were the direct result of advances in synthetic chemistry, neuropathology, and experimental pharmacology. The discovery of bromine in the waters of the Mediterranean Sea by A. J. Balard in 1826 and the synthesis of urea by F. Wöhler in 1828 marked the beginning of synthetic chemistry and led to the laboratory synthesis of the first drugs demonstrated to be useful in the treatment of epilepsy. As a consequence of the isolation of bromine, potassium bromide was synthesized and soon widely used as a sedative. This prompted Sir Charles Locock in 1857 (42) to use potassium bromide in the treatment of hysterical and menstrual epilepsies in women; all but one of 14 such cases responded favorably to therapy. As a result of the synthesis of urea, phenobarbital was synthesized in 1911 and introduced by Hauptmann in 1912 (29) for the treatment of epilepsy. The barbituric acid moiety was easily modified in the chemical laboratory, and numerous synthetic congeners appeared during the next 25 years. One of these, mephobarbital, was reported by Weese in 1932 (68) to be clinically useful in epilepsy.

Meanwhile, John Hughlings Jackson (1825–1911), often referred to as the "father of the modern concepts of epilepsy," proposed that seizures are caused by "occasional, sudden, excessive, rapid and local discharges of gray matter in the brain"; this established a neuropathological basis for the disease. Within this same time frame, several workers demonstrated that the obvious symptom of epilepsy, the seizure, could be replicated in laboratory animals by electroshock and a variety of naturally occurring chemicals. In 1864, Marcé (44) induced convulsions in dogs and rabbits by the administration of absinthe; in 1870, Fritsch and Hitzig (18) evoked seizures in animals by the excessive electrical stimulation of the brain; in 1875, Browne (4) described the convulsive effects induced in animals by the administration of picrotoxin. These early studies in experimental pharmacology prompted Albertoni, in 1882, to test bromides, atropine, and cinchona alkaloids against electrically induced seizures in dogs (1). Pentylenetetrazol was synthesized in 1924, and its convulsant action was demonstrated by Hildebrant (30) in 1926. Although it soon replaced other chemical convulsants, its use for evaluating potential antiepileptic drugs was not considered reliable (46,58).

If any of the above-mentioned areas of investigation had not been pursued, the most significant antiepileptic drug discovery of this century could have been delayed by many years.

In 1937, Putnam and Merritt (56) described a technique in which seizures were induced in cats by interrupted (80/sec) direct current delivered to the brain for 10 sec through mouth–occipital electrodes. By means of this procedure, Putnam and Merritt discovered diphenylhydantoin (now known as phenytoin) and reported that in cats, doses minimally depressive to spontaneous

1

motor activity increased convulsive thresholds to such an extent that a "fit" could not be induced with current intensities four times the control levels. The clinical efficacy of phenytoin in epilepsy, especially grand mal and psychomotor attacks, was reported by Merritt and Putnam in 1938 (47). It is worthy of note that it required only 1 year and little expense to get phenytoin from the laboratory to market. In 1976, it required a minimum of 8 years and approximately 54 million dollars to take a drug from the laboratory to market (28).

The discovery of diphenylhydantoin by Merritt and Putnam was important for several reasons: it established the fact that an antiepileptic drug need not be a sedative or impair consciousness; it demonstrated the value of systematic laboratory testing for new antiepileptics; it encouraged the search for drugs with selective anticonvulsant action, that is, drugs effective in different types of epilepsy; it opened a new era for the study of structure–activity relations; and it provided a new tool for the study of the neurophysiological and neurochemical basis of seizures.

As a result, the search for new anticonvulsant drugs was intensified: pharmaceutical firms initiated anticonvulsant screening programs, academic institutions studied the physiology and pharmacology of experimental seizures with the objective of developing better methods for "sorting out" drugs with antiepileptic potential, and medicinal chemists set about trying to improve or alter the activity of phenytoin by structural modification.

In 1944, Richards and Everett (57) reported that the oxazolidinedione trimethadione, a potent analgesic agent (60), prevented pentylenetetrazol (Metrazol®)-induced threshold seizures in rats. Subsequently, Everett and Richards (16) demonstrated that these seizures were also prevented by phenobarbital but not by phenytoin. Goodman and co-workers (20, 21,23) confirmed these findings and also reported that the electroshock seizure threshold is moderately increased by trimethadione, less so by phenobarbital, and not at all by phenytoin. Moreover, these investigators reported that phenytoin and phenobarbital modified the pattern of maximal electroshock seizures to a much greater extent than did trimethadione. These laboratory observations suggested that there are significant differences in the anticonvulsant actions of phenytoin, trimethadione, and phenobarbital and a qualitative difference between threshold and maximal seizures. Meanwhile, Lennox (38) reported that trimethadione decreased the frequency or stopped petit mal attacks but failed to control, or even exacerbated, grand mal attacks. Subsequent confirmation of this unique action (14,24,39) established the selectivity of trimethadione in the treatment of absence seizures. This was an important advance for a number of reasons. It reemphasized the value of a systematic search for new anticonvulsant drugs by means of laboratory tests; it provided the first clear indication that drugs could be selective for various types of epilepsies; and it provided another tool for probing the physiology and pharmacology of experimental seizures. Trimethadione was marketed in 1946 and soon became the drug of choice for absence (petit mal) seizures.

In 1944, Goodman and co-workers (22,65) began an intensive study of the "physiology and therapy of experimental convulsive disorders." Initial efforts were directed toward the duplication of the Putnam and Merritt model (56). This study revealed that phenytoin effectively shortened the duration of the seizure produced by long stimulation; consequently, the seizure was over well before the termination of the 10-sec stimulus. Hence, the discovery of phenytoin was totally unrelated to its ability to elevate seizure threshold. This fact must be remembered when one evaluates the report by Merritt and Putnam (48) on the anticonvulsant properties of over 700 compounds tested by their procedure. Goodman and associates (21,25,61,64,65) standardized the maximal electroshock seizure pattern, the minimal electroshock threshold, and the subcutaneous pentylenetetrazol (Metrazol®) threshold tests. In addition, they developed the "psychomotor" seizure test (64) and the hyponatremic electroshock threshold test (21,61). The "psychomotor" seizure test (now known as the low-frequency electroshock threshold test) produces seizures characterized by abnormal behavior, stunning, and automatisms. The hyponatremic electroshock threshold test lowers the seizure threshold of the test animal by 50% (24). The former is a very sensitive test for normal minimal threshold; the latter produces an exquisitely sensitive animal with an abnormally lower threshold. These studies led to the development of a battery of electrical and chemical methods for the evaluation of candidate antiepileptic drugs (25,61,62).

The test batteries developed by Goodman and co-workers measured the ability of the candidate substance to prevent the hindleg tonic extensor component of maximal electroshock seizures and/or to increase the threshold for minimal seizures induced by electroshock and chemoshock. When the maximal electroshock seizure (MES) pattern test is used to identify anticonvulsant activity, one determines the dose of the candidate substance that will prevent the tonic extensor component in 50% of animals (ED_{50} against MES). Drugs with marked activity by this test are thought to prevent seizure spread. When a threshold test (such as the s.c. pentylenetetrazol test) is used to identify anticonvulsant activity, one determines the dose of the candidate substance that will prevent even a minimal threshold seizure in 50% of animals (ED_{50} against s.c. pentylenetetrazol). Drugs with marked activity by this test are thought to elevate seizure threshold.

The results obtained with these two simple tests, maximal electroshock seizure pattern and pentylenetetrazol seizure threshold tests, were soon shown to delineate profiles of anticonvulsant activity that correlated well with the clinical efficacy and specificity of candidate agents. As shown in Table 1, phenytoin and phenobarbital, the only substances at that time useful in grand mal and psychomotor epilepsy (now known as generalized tonic–clonic and complex partial seizures, respectively), were characterized in the laboratory by marked ability to modify seizure pattern; however, only phenobarbital had the ability to elevate seizure threshold. Consequently, it was speculated that drugs useful in grand mal and psychomotor seizures must have the ability to modify maximal seizure pattern but may or may not elevate seizure threshold. In contrast, trimethadione, the only drug at that time useful in petit mal epilepsy (now known as absence seizures), was characterized in the laboratory by marked ability to elevate threshold and had little or no ability to modify maximal seizure pattern. Thus, it was theorized that drugs useful in petit mal epilepsy must have the ability to increase the seizure threshold but may or may not modify seizure pattern. These basic tests or modifications of them were soon widely used in virtually all laboratories engaged in the search for new antiepileptic drugs. As indicated in Chapter 7, they are still among the most useful laboratory tests for screening large numbers of chemicals for anticonvulsant potential.

The impetus generated by the discovery of phenytoin and trimethadione and the availability of methods for "sorting out" active agents resulted in the laboratory screening of thousands of candidate agents and the introduction of a spate of new antiepileptic agents during the next 15-year period ending in 1960. For example, two new hydantoins, mephenytoin (32,43) and

TABLE 1. *Clinical and experimental profiles of phenytoin, phenobarbital, and trimethadione*

Drug (clinical use)	Maximal seizure[a] pattern test	Minimal seizure[a] threshold test
Phenytoin		
Phenobarbital	+ +	±
(grand mal and psychomotor)		
Trimethadione	±	+ +
(petit mal)		

[a]Induced by various agents.

ethotoin (40,59), another barbiturate, metharbital (51), and the deoxybarbiturate, primidone (27) were marketed for the treatment of generalized tonic–clonic (grand mal) and complex partial (temporal lobe or psychomotor) seizures. Another oxazolidinedione, paramethadione (14), and three new succinimides, phensuximide (12), methsuximide (70), and ethosuximide (5,71), were introduced for the management of absence (petit mal) seizures. Other agents introduced during this period included phenacemide, a noncyclic ureide primarily effective for temporal lobe seizures (19), and acetazolamide, a carbonic anhydrase inhibitor effective in absence seizures (3); the clinical usefulness of the former is limited by its toxicity, and that of the latter by the development of tolerance. A complete list of antiepileptic drugs marketed in the United States is shown in Table 2.

Thirteen new agents were introduced between 1946 and 1960 (Table 2). Surprisingly and unfortunately, this kind of interest and activity did not continue; not one new agent was introduced between 1960 and 1974 specifically for the treatment of epilepsy. Fortunately, the National Institute of Neurological and Communicative Disorders and Stroke (NINCDS) established the Epilepsy Branch and an Epilepsy Advisory Committee in 1966 (33). Available space will not permit a detailed account of the many significant accomplishments of the Epilepsy Branch. However, not the least of these were the survey completed in 1967 on the status of antiepileptic drug development in the United States (54), the epidemiological studies reported in 1972 and 1973 (2,6,58), and the evaluation in 1971 of the clinical efficacy of available drugs as revealed by a careful study of all clinical literature (13). The results of these studies brought the following five points into sharp focus: not one new antiepileptic drug had been introduced since 1960; there were no antiepileptic drugs under development by the pharma-

TABLE 2. *Antiepileptic drugs marketed in the United States*

Year introduced	International nonproprietary name	U.S. trade name	Company
1912	phenobarbital	Luminal	Winthrop
1935	mephobarbital	Mebaral	Winthrop
1938	phenytoin	Dilantin	Parke-Davis
1946	trimethadione	Tridione	Abbott
1947	mephenytoin	Mesantoin	Sandoz
1949	paramethadione	Paradione	Abbott
1950	phenthenylate[a]	Thiantin	Lilly
1951	phenacemide	Phenurone	Abbott
1952	metharbital	Gemonil	Abbott
1952	benzchlorpropamide[b]	Hibicon	Lederle
1953	phensuximide	Milontin	Parke-Davis
1954	primidone	Mysoline	Ayerst
1957	methsuximide	Celontin	Parke-Davis
1957	ethotoin	Peganone	Abbott
1960	aminoglutethimide[c]	Elipten	Ciba
1960	ethosuximide	Zarontin	Parke-Davis
1968	diazepam[d]	Valium	Roche
1974	carbamazepine	Tegretol	Geigy
1975	clonazepam	Clonopin	Roche
1978	valproic acid	Depakene	Abbott

[a]Withdrawn, 1952.
[b]Withdrawn, 1955.
[c]Withdrawn, 1966.
[d]Approved by FDA as adjunct.

ceutical industry; in marked contrast to statements in the textbooks, available drugs effectively controlled seizures in only 50% of the patients; the experimental literature had not been critically reviewed since 1960; and there was little evidence that advances in related scientific fields were being applied either to antiepileptic drug development or to a better understanding of this disorder.

These observations made it abundantly clear that Federal intervention was necessary if advances in the neurosciences were to be brought to bear on the problems of the epilepsies. Consequently, the Epilepsy Branch moved positively to review the neuroscience literature related to this disorder, to identify new substances that may be more effective and/or less toxic than those presently available, to improve the therapeutic effectiveness of presently available antiepileptic agents, to enhance the quality of care available to the epileptic patient, and to establish clinical research centers capable of doing in-depth studies on the etiology, treatment, and rehabilitation of the epileptic patient. The steps taken to accomplish these objectives are briefly summarized below.

By means of workshops and symposia, the neuroscience and clinical literature of importance to epilepsy was reviewed and published in monograph and book form. The following titles are representative of this effort: *Symposium on Laboratory Evaluation of Anticonvulsant Drugs* (67), *Basic Mechanisms of the Epilepsies* (31), *Experimental Models of Epilepsy* (55), and *Antiepileptic Drugs* (69).

In 1969, an Antiepileptic Drug Development Program was initiated. Clinical testing facilities were obtained by contract at various universities and a state hospital for epileptic patients. At about this time, the development of a primate epilepsy model came under Epilepsy Branch support (41). This model provides an excellent resource for the pharmacokinetic and efficacy testing of candidate antiepileptic agents. In addition, it has the capability of identifying drug effects that should be monitored during clinical trials. Working in close collaboration with investigators associated with these facilities, the

Epilepsy Branch supported controlled laboratory and/or clinical trials of four drugs that needed definitive proof of efficacy for marketing approval. Support of these trials not only facilitated the development of these drugs at reduced cost but also provided an environment within which the Epilepsy Branch could develop the methodology and standards to conduct controlled clinical evaluations of candidate drugs (9).

The data collected eventually supported the new drug applications of the iminostilbene carbamazepine (8) and the benzodiazepine clonazepam (15), which were marketed in 1974 and 1975, respectively. However, trials on sulthiame (26) and albutoin (7) failed to support clinical efficacy; consequently, these drugs have not been marketed in the United States. In 1978, valproate was approved for use in the United States for the treatment of absence seizures. Although this unsaturated fatty acid was synthesized in 1881, its anticonvulsant properties remained unrecognized until 1963, at which time it was serendipitously discovered by Meunier and co-workers (49). Three years later it was marketed in France. By 1973, valproate was widely used in Europe, and reports of its clinical efficacy prompted the Epilepsy Branch to urge its use in the United States. The New Drug Application, filed in 1977, included data from a controlled clinical trial supported by the Epilepsy Branch. The following year, with evidence from clinical studies supported by the Epilepsy Branch, valproate was approved for use in absence and myoclonic seizures.

In the early 1970s, with few new drugs approaching clinical trial, the Epilepsy Branch turned its attention to other ways it could facilitate antiepileptic drug development, particularly in the laboratory identification of new chemical substances with anticonvulsant potential. In 1975, the Epilepsy Branch established an anticonvulsant drug screening project (34). The objective of this program is to "sort out" those chemicals with anticonvulsant properties and evaluate their potential to the point where their development into antiepileptic drugs might become more feasible and to extend the methodology of drug screening so that it might become more predictive of clinical usefulness. To date, more than 5,000 chemical substances have been evaluated in rodents for anticonvulsant activity, and several have been scheduled for preclinical toxicity studies. In 1979, research grants were awarded to 10 medicinal chemists to synthesize substances for evaluation in the "screening" program. The Antiepileptic Drug Development Program is a classical example of how academia, the pharmaceutical industry, and a federal agency can cooperatively seek solutions to a health care problem.

In 1971, the Epilepsy Branch organized a pharmacology laboratory to develop reliable analytical methods for the determination of blood levels of antiepileptic drugs and to promote the routine clinical determination of serum antiepileptic drug levels to individualize antiepileptic drug dosage. In 1974, a blind survey of laboratories in the United States that routinely analyze antiepileptic drugs revealed that more than half were reporting unacceptable results (53). Consequently, a voluntary Antiepileptic Drug Levels Quality Control Program was instituted under the auspices of the Epilepsy Foundation of America. This was followed by a symposium on the reliable quantification of antiepileptic drugs under the cosponsorship of the Epilepsy Branch and Epilepsy Foundation of America (52). As a result, the importance of reliable antiepileptic drug level determinations and their clinical application to the successful management of the epilepsies was brought into sharp focus. In 1979, the American Epilepsy Society sponsored the publication of a *Voluntary Directory of Antiepileptic Drug Laboratories* in order to help physicians throughout the United States and Canada obtain this vital service for their epileptic patients.

In response to the advice and recommendations of the Epilepsy Advisory Committee, initial steps were taken in 1973 for the development of several comprehensive epilepsy programs. The core aspects of these programs include clinical epilepsy research and the diagnosis, treatment, and rehabilitation of epileptic patients, as well as coordination of the programs with community resources.

The Clinical Epilepsy Section of the Experimental Therapeutics Branch, NINCDS, was established in July 1976. This center provides a facility capable of doing in-depth studies on the etiology, monitoring, and treatment of seizures and rehabilitation of the epileptic patient.

This considerable historical detail is intended to direct attention to the carefully conceived programs that have been developed during the decade since the publication of the first edition of *Antiepileptic Drugs*. These programs had an enormous impact on neuroscience research, antiepileptic drug development, basic and applied pharmacokinetics and pharmacodynamics of antiepileptic drugs, and on the quality of care available to the epileptic patient. With respect to research in the neurosciences, a quantum-sized advance has been made in the understanding of brain chemistry, including the isolation and quantification of several neurotransmitters, the identification of specific receptors for the benzodiazepines (63), the development of methods for revealing when these sites are occupied (receptor binding studies), and the possibility of a direct correlation between drug potency and the tenacity of drug binding. The demonstration that the newest antiepileptic drug, valproate, significantly increases the brain levels of γ-aminobutyric acid (GABA) focused attention on the inhibitory role of this neurotransmitter in the central nervous system. This observation tempts one to speculate that valproate may exert its anticonvulsant activity via the GABA mechanism. Despite the obvious importance of GABA in CNS transmission, there is still no unequivocal evidence that the antiepileptic effectiveness of valproate, or of any other clinically effective antiepileptic drug, is specifically related to its action on GABA transmission. There is also substantial evidence that other neurotransmitters, such as the indoleamine 5-hydroxytryptamine (11), and the neuropeptide endorphin (17,66), may be involved in seizure mechanisms. However, the precise role of these neurotransmitters has not been established.

Perhaps the most significant advance in antiepileptic drug development will evolve from the demonstration of the remarkable antipentylenetetrazol potency of the benzodiazepines (50).

Many studies under way suggest that the 1,5-benzodiazepines may exhibit a more favorable profile of anticonvulsant action than the 1,4-benzodiazepines (10). Such investigations coupled with continued search for structures that bind tightly to benzodiazepine receptor sites could lead to the discovery of a new series of highly selective antiepileptic drugs.

The development of rapid, accurate, analytical methods for the determination of antiepileptic drug concentrations in any body fluid or tissue is largely responsible for dramatic advances in the pharmacokinetics and pharmacodynamics of antiepileptic drugs. The sites and rates of absorption, the distribution and biotransformation, and the excretion patterns are known for virtually all of the clinically useful antiepileptic drugs. Information on the effect of genetic defects and multiple-drug therapy on drug biotransformation, therapeutic efficacy, and duration of action has accumulated at an accelerated pace.

The relationships between plasma levels of antiepileptic drugs and seizure control or drug-induced toxicity are well documented for all clinically useful agents. These developments all have a direct application in the therapeutic management of the epileptic patient. For example, it is generally agreed that the optimal plasma phenytoin levels for seizure control in most patients range from 10 to 20 μg/ml; efficacy is sometimes attained at plasma levels as low as 8 μg/ml, and nystagmus may be present at concentrations as low as 15 μg/ml (45). Kutt (35) has shown that the majority of patients are capable of metabolizing up to 10 mg/kg of phenytoin per day, as indicated by the maintenance of stable blood levels and the absence of accumulation of the unmetabolized drug. However, an occasional patient given the conventional adult daily dose of 4 to 5 mg/kg of phenytoin may have an excessive accumulation of unmetabolized drug and exhibit symptoms of drug toxicity (37), whereas others on the same dose may have very low phenytoin levels (0 to 2 μg/ml) and no seizure control (36). It is not clear whether the former is due to a qualitative difference in the metabolizing enzyme or to its limited total synthesis and whether the latter results from a qualitatively different enzyme or to its unusually high inducibility. Nevertheless, with available analytical techniques and careful monitoring of antiepileptic drug levels, the physician can now determine whether failure to achieve seizure control is due to genetic, pharmacological, or physiological factors that alter the absorption, distribution, metabolism, or excretion of the drug, to faulty patient compliance, or to lack of drug effectiveness in a particular patient or seizure type. The important point, according to Pippenger et al. (52), is that with the routine use of these analytical techniques and careful adjustment of drug dosage 80% of all epileptic patients could become seizure free with the currently available drugs.

The above example emphasizes the major objective of this volume: to decrease the time lag between the development of new pharmacological information and the application of this information to the care of the epileptic patient. It has now been 10 years since the first edition of this book was published. Hence, it is time once again to close the gap between the accumulated new pharmacological knowledge of antiepileptic drugs and the application of this knowledge to the management of the epilepsies. It is hopefully anticipated that the information presented herein will not only enable a significantly larger number of epileptic patients to experience the joy that comes from seizure control but will also stimulate research scientists and clinical investigators to seek still more insight into the pharmacology of antiepileptic drugs.

REFERENCES

1. Albertoni, P. (1882): Untersuchung über die Wirkung einiger Arzneimittel auf die Erregbarkest des Grosshirns nebst Beiträgen zur Therapie der Epilepsie. *Arch. Exp. Pathol. Pharmackol.*, 15:248–288.
2. Alter, M., and Hauser, W. A. (1972): *The Epidemiology of Epilepsy: A Workshop.* U.S.D.H.E.W. Publication No. (NIH)73-390, Bethesda.
3. Bergstrom, W. H., Cerzoli, R. F., Lombroso, C., Davidson, D. T., and Wallace, W. M. (1952): Observations on the metabolic and clinical effects of carbonic-anhydrase inhibitors in epilepsy. *Am. J. Dis. Child.*, 84:771–772.
4. Browne, J. C. (1875): On the actions of picrotoxin and the antagonism between picrotoxin and chloral hydrate. *Br. Med. J.*, 1:409–411.
5. Browne, R. T., Dreifuss, F. E., Dyken, P. R., Goode,

D. J., Penry, J. K., Porter, R. J., White, B. G., and White, P. T. (1975): Ethosuximide in the treatment of absence (petit mal) seizures. *Neurology (Minneap.)*, 25:515–524.

6. Cereghino, J. J. (1973): Epidemiology of epilepsy. *Public Health Rev.*, 3:92–100.

7. Cereghino, J. J., Brock, J. T., Van Meter, J. C., Penry, J. K., Smith, L. D., Fisher, P., and Ellenberg, J. (1974): Evaluation of albutoin as an antiepileptic drug. *Clin. Pharmacol. Ther.*, 15:406–416.

8. Cereghino, J. J., Brock, J. T., Van Meter, J. C., Penry, J. K., Smith, L. D., and White, B. G. (1974): Carbamazepine for epilepsy. A controlled prospective evaluation. *Neurology (Minneap.)*, 24:401–410.

9. Cereghino, J. J., and Penry, J. K. (1972): General Principles. Testing of anticonvulsants in man. In: *Antiepileptic Drugs*, edited by D. M. Woodbury, J. K. Penry, and R. P. Schmidt, pp. 63–73. Raven Press, New York.

10. Chapman, A. G., Horton, R. W., and Meldrum, B. S. (1978): Anticonvulsant action of a 1,5-benzodiazepine, clobazam, in reflex epilepsy. *Epilepsia*, 19:293–299.

11. Chase, T. N., and Murphy, D. L. (1973): Serotonin and central nervous system function. *Annu. Rev. Pharmacol.*, 13:181–197.

12. Chen, G., Portman, R., Ensor, C. R., and Bratton, A. C., Jr. (1951): The anticonvulsant activity of α-phenyl succinimides. *J. Pharmacol. Exp. Ther.*, 103:54–61.

13. Coatsworth, J. J. (1971): *Studies on the Clinical Efficacy of Marketed Antiepileptic Drugs.* NINDS Monograph No. 12, HEW Publication No. (NIH) 73-51, Bethesda.

14. Davis, J. P., and Lennox, W. G. (1947): The effect of trimethyloxazolidinedione and of dimethylethyloxazolidinedione on seizures and on the blood. *Res. Publ. Assoc. Res. Nerv. Ment. Dis.*, 26:423–426.

15. Dreifuss, F. E., Penry, J. K., Rose, S. W., Kupferberg, H. J., Dyken, P., and Sato, S. (1975): Serum clonazepam concentrations in children with absense seizures. *Neurology (Minneap.)*, 25:255–258.

16. Everett, G. M., and Richards, R. K. (1944): Comparative anticonvulsive action of 3,5,5-trimethyloxazolidine-2,4-dione (Tridione), Dilantin and phenobarbital. *J. Pharmacol. Exp. Ther.*, 81:402–407.

17. Frenk, H., McCarty, B. C., and Liebeskind, S. C. (1978): Different brain areas mediate the analgesic and epileptic properties of enkephalin. *Science*, 200:335–336.

18. Fritsch, G., and Hitzig, E. (1870): Ueber die elecktrische Erregbarkeit des Grosshirns. *Arch. Anat. Physiol. Wissenseh. Med.*, 37:300–332.

19. Gibbs, F. A., Everett, G. M., and Richards, R. K. (1949): Phenurone in epilepsy. *Dis. Nerv. Syst.*, 10:47–49.

20. Goodman, L., and Manuel, C. (1945): The anticonvulsant properties of dimethyl-*N*-methyl barbituric acid and 3,5,5,trimethyloxazolidine-2,4-dione (Tridione). *Fed. Proc.*, 4:119.

21. Goodman, L. S., Swinyard, E. A., and Toman, J. E. P. (1945): Laboratory technics for the identification and evaluation of potentially antiepileptic drugs. *Proc. Am. Fed. Clin. Res.*, 2:100–101.

22. Goodman, L. S., Swinyard, E. A., and Toman, J. E. P. (1946): Studies on the anticonvulsant properties of diphenylhydantoin. *Fed. Proc.*, 5:180.

23. Goodman, L., and Toman, J. E. P. (1945): Experimental indices for comparing the efficacy of compounds with anticonvulsant and antiepileptic properties. *Fed. Proc.*, 4:120.

24. Goodman, L. S., Toman, J. E. P., and Swinyard, E. A. (1946): The anticonvulsant properties of Tridione: Laboratory and clinical investigations. *Am. J. Med.*, 1:213–228.

25. Goodman, L. S., Toman, J. E. P., and Swinyard, E. A. (1949): Anticonvulsant drugs: Mechanisms of action and methods of assay. *Arch. Int. Pharmacodyn. Ther.*, 78:144–162.

26. Green, J. R., Troupin, A. S., Halpern, L. M., Friel, P., and Kanarek, P. (1974): Sulthiame: Evaluation as an anticonvulsant. *Epilepsia*, 15:329–349.

27. Handley, R., and Stewart, A. S. R. (1952): Mysoline: A new drug in the treatment of epilepsy. *Lancet*, 1:742–744.

28. Hansen, R. W. (1979): *The Pharmaceutical Development Process: Estimate of Development Costs and Times and the Effects of Regulatory Changes.* The Center for the Study of Drug Development, University of Rochester Medical Center, Rochester.

29. Hauptmann, A. (1912): Luminal bei Epilepsie. *Munch. Med. Wochenschr.*, 59:1907–1909.

30. Hildebrandt, F. (1926): Pentamethylenetetrazol (Cardiazol) I. Mitteilung. *Naunyn Schmiedebergs Arch. Pharmacol.*, 1168:100–116.

31. Jasper, H. H., Ward, A. A., and Pope, A. (1969): *Basic Mechanisms of the Epilepsies.* Little, Brown, Boston.

32. Kozol, H. L. (1946): Epilepsy. Treatment with a new drug: 3-Methyl 5,5-phenyl-ethyl-hydantoin (phenantoin). *Am. J. Psychiatry*, 103:154–158.

33. Krall, R. L., Penry, J. K., Kupferberg, H. J., and Swinyard, E. A. (1978): Antiepileptic drug development. I. Background and program. *Epilepsia*, 19:393–408.

34. Krall, R. L., Penry, J. K., White, B. G., Kupferberg, H. J., and Swinyard, E. A. (1978): Antiepileptic drug development: II. Anticonvulsant drug screening. *Epilepsia*, 19:409–428.

35. Kutt, H. (1971): Biochemical and genetic factors regulating Dilantin metabolism in man. *Ann. N. Y. Acad. Sci.*, 179:704–722.

36. Kutt, H., Haynes, J., and McDowell, F. (1966): Some causes of ineffectiveness of diphenylhydantoin. *Arch. Neurol.*, 14:489–492.

37. Kutt, H., Wolk, M., Scherman, R., and McDowell, F. (1964): Insufficient parahydroxylation as a cause of diphenylhydantoin toxicity. *Neurology (Minneap.)*, 14:542–548.

38. Lennox, W. G. (1945): The petit mal epilepsies. Their treatment with Tridione. *J.A.M.A.*, 129:1069–1074.

39. Lennox, W. G. (1947): Tridione in the treatment of epilepsy. *J.A.M.A.*, 134:138–143.

40. Livingston, S. (1956): The use of Peganone (AC 695) in the treatment of epilepsy. *J. Pediatr.*, 49:728–732.

41. Lockard, J. S., and Barensten, R. I. (1967): Behavioral experimental epilepsy in monkeys. I. Clinical

seizure recording apparatus and initial data. *Electroencephalogr. Clin. Neurophysiol.*, 22:482–486.

42. Locock, C. (1857): Discussion of paper by E. H. Sieveking, Analysis of 52 cases of epilepsy observed by author. *Lancet*, 1:527.

43. Loscalzo, A. E. (1945): Treatment of epileptic patients with a combination of 3-methyl 5,5-phenylethyl-hydantoin and phenobarbital (preliminary report). *J. Nerv. Ment. Dis.*, 101:537–544.

44. Marcé, M. (1864): Sur l'action toxique de l'essence d'absinthe. *C. R. Acad. Sci. [D] (Paris)*, 58:628–629.

45. *Medical Letter* (1976): Drugs for epilepsy. *Med. Lett.*, 18:25–28.

46. Merritt, H. H., and Brenner, C. (1947): Studies in new anticonvulsants. *Bull. N. Y. Acad. Sci.*, 23:292–301.

47. Merritt, H. H., and Putnam, T. J. (1938): Sodium diphenylhydantoinate in treatment of convulsive disorders. *J.A.M.A.*, 111:1068–1073.

48. Merritt, H. H., and Putnam, T. J. (1945): Experimental determination of anticonvulsive activity of chemical compounds. *Epilepsia*, 3:51–75.

49. Meunier, G., Carraz, G., Meunier, Y., Eyrnard, P., and Amard, M. (1963): Propriétés pharmacodynamiques de l'acide *n*-dipropylacetique. *Thérapie*, 18:435–438.

50. Paul, S. M., Syapin, P. J., Paugh, B. A., Moncada, V., and Skolnick, P. (1979): Correlation between benzodiazepine receptor occupation and anticonvulsant effects of diazepam. *Nature*, 281:688–689.

51. Perlstein, M. A. (1950): Gemonil (5,5-diethyl 1-methyl barbituric acid): New drug for convulsive and related disorders. *Pediatrics*, 5:448–451.

52. Pippenger, C. E., Penry, J. K., and Kutt, H. (1978): *Antiepileptic Drugs: Quantitative Analysis and Interpretation.* Raven Press, New York.

53. Pippenger, C. E., Penry, J. K., White, B. G., Daly, D. D., and Buddington, R. (1976): Interlaboratory variability in determination of plasma antiepileptic drug concentrations. *Arch. Neurol.*, 33:351–355.

54. Public Health Service Advisory Committee on the Epilepsies (1967): *Minutes of Meeting, February 9, 1967.* National Institutes of Health, Bethesda.

55. Purpura, D. P., Penry, J. K., Tower, D., Woodbury, D. M., and Walter, R. (1972): *Experimental Models of Epilepsy—A Manual for the Laboratory Worker.* Raven Press, New York.

56. Putnam, T. J., and Merritt, H. H. (1937): Experi-

mental determination of the anticonvulsant properties of some phenyl derivatives. *Science*, 85:525–526.

57. Richards, R. K. and Everett, G. M. (1944): Analgesic and anticonvulsive properties of 3,5,5-trimethyloxazolidine-2,4-dione (Tridione). *Fed. Proc.*, 3:39.

58. Rose, S. W., Penry, J. K., Markush, R. E., Radloff, L. A., and Putnam, P. L. (1973): Prevalence of epilepsy in children. *Epilepsia*, 14:133–152.

59. Schwade, E. D., Richards, R. K., and Everett, G. M. (1956): Peganone, a new antiepileptic drug. *Dis. Nerv. Syst.*, 17:155–158.

60. Spielman, M. A. (1944): Some analgesic agents derived from oxazolidine-2,4-dione. *J. Am. Chem. Soc.*, 66:1244–1245.

61. Swinyard, E. A. (1949): Laboratory assay of clinically effective antiepileptic drugs. *J. Am. Pharm. Assoc.*, 38:201–204.

62. Swinyard, E. A., Brown, W. C., and Goodman, L. S. (1952): Comparative assays of clincially effective antiepileptic drugs in mice and rats. *J. Pharmacol. Exp. Ther.*, 106:319–330.

63. Tallman, J. F., Paul, S. M., Skolnick, P., and Gallager, D. W. (1980): Receptors for the age of anxiety: Pharmacology of the benzodiazepines. *Science*, 207:274–281.

64. Toman, J. E. P., Everett, G. M., and Richards, R. K. (1952): The search for new drugs against epilepsy. *Tex. Rep. Biol. Med.*, 10:96–104.

65. Toman, J. E. P., and Goodman, L. S. (1946): Conditions modifying convulsions in animals. *Proc. Assoc. Res. Nerv. Ment. Dis.*, 26:141–163.

66. Tortella, F. C., Moreton, J. E., Khazan, N. (1978): Electroencephalographic and behavioral effects of *d*-ala²-methionine-enkephalinamide and morphine in the rat. *J. Pharmacol. Exp. Ther.*, 206:636–642.

67. U.S. Public Health Service, National Institute of Neurological Diseases (1969): Symposium on Laboratory Evaluation of Antiepileptic Drugs. *Epilepsia*, 10:101–336.

68. Weese, H. (1932): Pharmacologie des Prominal. *Dtsch. Med. Wochenschr.*, 58:696.

69. Woodbury, D. M., Penry, J. K., and Schmidt, R. P. (1972): *Antiepileptic Drugs.* Raven Press, New York.

70. Zimmerman, F. T. (1953): New drugs in the treatment of petit mal epilepsy. *Am. J. Psychiatry*, 109:766–773.

71. Zimmerman, F. T., and Burgemeister, B. B. (1958): A new drug for petit mal epilepsy. *Neurology (Minneap.)*, 8:769–775.

Antiepileptic Drugs, edited by D. M. Woodbury,
J. K. Penry, and C. E. Pippenger. Raven Press,
New York © 1982.

2

General Principles

Drug Absorption, Distribution, and Elimination

René H. Levy

The discipline of pharmacokinetics has undergone a great deal of evolution in the last decade. For a number of drugs, evidence has accumulated documenting a close relationship between disposition kinetics and efficacy and toxicity. Application of some of the principles of pharmacokinetics in therapeutic monitoring has given birth to the field of clinical pharmacokinetics. In parallel with these developments, progress was made in our understanding of the basic determinants of drug disposition in the body. Simultaneously, the emphasis in pharmacokinetics has shifted from mathematics to physiology. Recently, mathematical models have been developed that include concepts of perfusion and blood flow. Volumes of distribution, originally conceived as mathematical (nonanatomical) quantities, have been related to anatomical volumes such as plasma volume and total body water. The effects of various disease states (e.g., renal, hepatic disease) on the processes of drug distribution and elimination are better understood. This chapter presents a modern overview of the principles of pharmacokinetics with an emphasis on newer concepts. The approach selected emphasizes mechanisms of pharmacokinetic phenomena rather than their mathematical description. Wherever possible, references to textbooks or review articles are given to avoid detailed derivations. Also, an attempt was made to select examples from the literature on antiepileptic drugs.

DEFINITIONS AND TERMINOLOGY

Several definitions of pharmacokinetics have been proposed. Some definitions are quite broad in that they include not only the kinetics of absorption, distribution, and elimination but also the kinetics of pharmacological response, sometimes referred to as pharmacodynamics. This chapter will focus mainly on the principles of drug disposition. Elimination is understood as referring to drug disappearance by all routes and includes metabolism (or biotransformation) as well as excretion of drug in its unchanged form by any route.

The growth of knowledge in pharmacokinetics has enabled a clearer distinction to be made between linear and nonlinear pharmacokinetic phenomena. Nonlinearities exist with respect to dose and time. Kinetic linearity with respect to dose has been defined as direct proportionality of transfer (e.g., elimination rate) to concentrations. This definition implies that all distribution and elimination processes are first order. Kinetic linearity with respect to time includes the notion of constancy of all rate constants and pharmacokinetic parameters with respect to time.

One of the main objectives of pharmacokinetics is to describe and interpret quantitatively the time course of drug and metabolite(s) levels. To do so, it is necessary to use mathematical representations or models. These models vary in degree of complexity depending on the characteristics of the system they emphasize and involve one or more compartments. Traditionally, the fate of drugs in the body was conceived of in terms of compartmentalized systems in which compartments are theoretical concepts resulting from specific kinetic behaviors. Such examples are the classical one- and two-compartment models in which each compartment represents an average, rather than an exact, state. Recently, multicompartment models have appeared that emphasize the physiological and anatomical bases of individual compartments. The parameters used in these models are blood flow through organs, tissue-to-plasma distribution coefficients, and extracellular spaces. Such multicompartment physiological models enable a description of tissue concentrations and have been applied to a few drugs, in particular, antineoplastic agents.

LINEAR PHARMACOKINETICS

Kinetics After Intravenous Administration

Although few drugs are commonly administered intravenously, an examination of this route of administration makes possible a logical presentation of the concepts of clearance, extraction ratio, volume of distribution, and biological half-life. This is so because administration of an intravenous bolus dose is equivalent to instantaneous absorption and, consequently, intravenous kinetics essentially reflect the processes of distribution and elimination.

One Compartment Model

The one-compartment model is applicable to drugs for which the kinetics of distribution are rapid compared with the kinetics of elimination

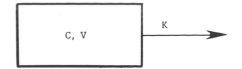

FIG. 1. The one-compartment model for determining the kinetics of a drug given intravenously. *K:* first order elimination rate constant; *C:* drug concentration at any time; *V:* single compartment of volume to represent the body.

from the body.[1] In this model, the body is represented as a single compartment of volume V (Fig. 1). Distribution is so rapid that there is no visible distribution phase. However, rapid distribution does not imply uniform distribution (as explained below). The first-order rate constant, K, is equal to the sum of several rate constants corresponding to individual processes of elimination (metabolism and excretion). C and A represent drug concentration and amount, respectively, at any time, t, and D refers to the dose of drug injected as a bolus at $t = 0$. In quantitative terms, first-order elimination means that at any time $t > 0$, drug concentration decreases in a monoexponential fashion according to

$$C = C_0 \, e^{-Kt} \qquad [1]$$

Several notions are contained in this relationship: at time zero, C has a value C_0; the decrease in concentration is largest at the beginning, when concentrations are high, and smaller as time increases and concentrations decrease (Fig. 2); what is constant in an exponential process is the relative rate of decrease of concentration (it is equal to K.)

A semilogarithmic ($\log_{10}$) plot of concentration versus time is linear (intercept = C_0 and slope = $K/2.3$). In the special case where

---

[1]The gastrointestinal tract, as well as the urine, sweat, and expired air, are considered to be outside the body in a pharmacokinetic sense.

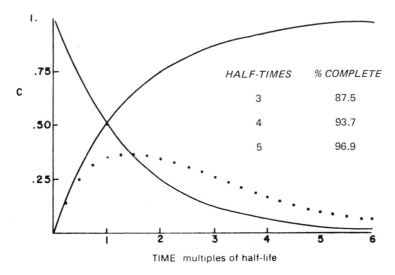

HALF-TIMES	% COMPLETE
3	87.5
4	93.7
5	96.9

FIG. 2. Time course of decrease (i.v. bolus) and increase (i.v. infusion) in blood levels as a function of drug half-life (*smooth curves*). The *filled circles* represent the time course of blood concentration following a single oral dose. (From ref. 10, with permission.)

$C = \frac{1}{2}C_0$, equation 1 yields a relationship useful in defining the biological half-life, $T_{1/2}$

$$T_{1/2} = \frac{0.693}{K} \qquad [2]$$

$T_{1/2}$ is the time required for blood concentration of the drug to decrease by one-half. This relationship shows that the larger the elimination rate constant, the smaller the half-life.

Physiological Basis for Drug Distribution and Elimination

Volume of distribution.

At time zero, immediately after injection of the dose of drug, the amount of drug in the body A_0 is equal to the administered dose. Similarly, at that time, the concentration has a value C_0 (which is also apparent in equation 1 when $t = 0$). The volume of distribution can then be determined from the ratio:

$$V = \frac{D}{C_0} = \frac{A}{C} \qquad [3]$$

For drugs exhibiting one-compartment behavior, the volume of distribution is the ratio of amount of drug in the body to blood drug concentration at any time. It is defined as an apparent volume of body fluids in which the drug would be distributed at a concentration equal to that of blood. Although it was traditionally emphasized that this volume is apparent and lacks physiological meaning, it was shown by Gillette (13) that this volume can be related to real body spaces. It can be defined in terms of plasma volume, V_P, and extravascular space (plus erythrocyte volume), V_T, as given by

$$V = V_P + V_T \frac{f}{f_t} \qquad [4]$$

where f represents the fraction of drug unbound in plasma and f_t the fraction of drug unbound in tissues. This approach to volume of distribution has several ramifications. Qualitatively, it shows that the volume of distribution is a function of the drug's affinity for binding to plasma proteins as well as to tissue constituents. Consequently, intersubject variability in volume of distribution can be attributed to individual variation in body size and composition as well as variation in drug binding. This approach is especially useful to explain changes in drug distribution in pathophysiological states where drug binding might be altered, such as in hypoalbuminemia and in uremia. For example, an increase in f (or decrease in binding) should produce an increase in V as long as the other variable, f_t, is not affected. This is, in fact, the case for phenytoin in uremia. However, the decrease in V of digoxin in uremia is attributed to an increase in f_t larger than the increase in f.

Clearance concepts.[2]

Clearance is one of the basic determinants of drug disposition, and, therefore, an understanding of clearance concepts is of paramount importance. Clearance emerges as a pharmacokinetic parameter not simply because it represents a mathematical quantity but primarily because it reflects a physiological (and, in some cases, an anatomical) reality. There exist several clearance terms and, in order to analyze them in a relatively simple fashion, a few assumptions become necessary. In particular, let us assume that drug elimination occurs only by metabolism through the liver and that the latter behaves as a "well-stirred" organ, such that free drug concentration in the liver is equal to that in the hepatic venous blood. The pharmacokinetic description of clearance takes into consideration the following anatomical and physiological facts: drug is brought to the liver by the portal vein and the hepatic artery and leaves the organ by the hepatic vein. It diffuses from plasma water to reach metabolic enzymes in the smooth endoplasmic reticulum. Therefore, *a priori*, there are at least three major parameters to consider in quantifying drug elimination by the liver: (a) blood flow through the organ, Q, which reflects transport of drug to the organ; (b) degree of protein binding expressed as free fraction of drug in blood, f, which affects access of the drug to the metabolic enzymes; (c) intrinsic ability of

hepatic enzymes to metabolize the drug once it has reached the metabolic enzymes.

The ability of liver enzymes to metabolize a drug, independent of the limitations of liver blood flow and drug binding in blood, is mea-sured as a clearance term, the intrinsic clearance, Cl'. It is defined as the volume of liver water cleared of drug per unit time. Its relationship to enzyme parameters (maximum velocity, V_{max}, and Michaelis constant, K_m) is a direct one, as seen from the Michaelis–Menten equation under first-order conditions (substrate concentration much smaller than K_m):

$$Cl' = \frac{V_{max}}{K_m} \qquad [5]$$

V_{max} has units of amount per time, and K_m has units of concentration; the ratio has units of volume per time. The net organ clearance or hepatic clearance, Cl_H, is a resultant of the interplay among these three parameters, as shown in the following relationship:

$$Cl_H = \frac{Q \cdot f \cdot Cl'}{Q + f \cdot Cl'} \qquad [6]$$

The terms Cl_H, Q, and Cl' have units of flow or volume per time, whereas f is a fraction and is therefore unitless. Cl_H is the apparent volume of blood cleared of drug per unit time. Intuitively, it should be apparent that the maximum clearance that a drug could have should be equal to the total volume of blood reaching that organ per unit time, i.e., blood flow through the organ.

Thus, it is reasonable to compare the actual hepatic clearance of a drug to hepatic flow. In fact, the ratio of Cl_H to Q is an important drug parameter and is called the extraction ratio, E. Its minimum value is 0 for a drug that is not metabolized in the liver, and its maximum value is 1 when $Cl_H = Q$. The above relationship shows that E is equal to zero when $f \cdot Cl'$ is 0. When $f \cdot Cl'$ is very small relative to Q, hepatic clearance becomes equal to $f \cdot Cl'$, and all flow terms disappear from equation 6 (Fig. 3). In such

---

[2]For additional information on clearance concepts, consult Pang and Rowland (24,25), Rowland et al. (28), and Wilkinson and Shand (37).

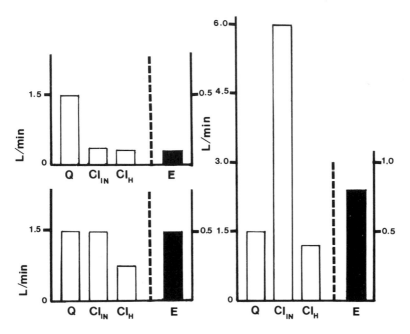

FIG. 3. Relationship between intrinsic clearance (Cl_{in}) and blood flow (Q) and its consequences on hepatic clearance (Cl_H) and extraction ratio (E). The three cases presented illustrate drugs with extraction ratios of 0.10, 0.50, and 0.80.

a case, clearance is called flow independent. It is also referred to as restrictive clearance because it is limited by the free fraction of drug in blood. The product $f \cdot Cl'$ is also a clearance term. Its relationship to Cl' is as follows: whereas Cl' refers to elimination of drug from plasma water in free form, $f \cdot Cl'$ refers to elimination of drug in the free plus bound form. When $f \cdot Cl'$ is much larger than Q (intrinsic ability of liver enzymes is very large), the extraction ratio ($f \cdot Cl'/Q + f \cdot Cl'$) approaches unity, and hepatic clearance approaches hepatic flow. In such a case, clearance is called flow dependent or flow limited (Fig. 3).

Thus, to each drug molecule metabolized by the liver, we can attach an extraction ratio. Drugs can be compared to one another and classified according to their extraction ratios. Most of the antiepileptic drugs in clinical use belong to the low-extraction-ratio category, $E < 0.2$. Examples of drugs with medium or high extraction ratios are lidocaine, propranolol, and meperidine.

When the liver is not the sole organ responsible for drug elimination from the body, overall elimination is dependent on the drug systemic clearance, Cl_s, which is defined as the volume of blood cleared of drug from the systemic circulation per unit time. Clearance terms are additive. For example, when a drug is eliminated by hepatic metabolism and renal excretion of unchanged drug, Cl_s is given by:

$$Cl_s = Cl_H + Cl_R \qquad [7]$$

where Cl_R is the renal clearance.

The determination of Cl_s is linked to the calculation of area under the curve (AUC). When a dose, D, of drug is administered intravenously, and blood samples are measured for several half-lives, the area under the blood concentration–time curve, AUC_{iv}, can easily be calculated. Systemic clearance is equal to the ratio D_{iv}/AUC_{iv}. Systemic clearance and AUC_{iv} are inversely proportional to each other: although AUC is a measure of drug presence in the body, it also reflects the inability of the eliminating organs to remove a drug; a large AUC is a direct consequence of a low ability of the body to remove a drug.

Relationship among clearance, volume of distribution, and half-life.

In the early pharmacokinetic literature, the half-life of a drug was often used as an index of the body's ability to remove a drug. However, for the majority of drugs, half-life and clearance cannot be used interchangeably for that purpose. Relative to clearance and volume of distribution, half-life is a dependent parameter. Individual organ clearances constitute direct measures of the abilities of those organs to eliminate a drug. Independently, a particular value of volume of distribution results from a binding interaction between the drug molecule and tissue constituents and plasma proteins. The more extensive the tissue binding (the lower the f_t in equation 4), the larger the volume of distribution. Half-life is a resultant of all these phenomena of distribution and elimination and therefore reflects both processes.[3] Quantitatively, the relationship among these three parameters is:

$$T_{1/2} = \frac{0.693\ V}{Cl_s} \qquad [8]$$

This relationship shows that the larger the volume of distribution, the longer the half-life. Independently, the larger the clearance, the smaller the half-life. Half-life is dependent on systemic clearance and volume of distribution, whereas clearance and volume are independent of each other and independent of half-life. This approach to the relationship among these three parameters is essential to the understanding of changes in kinetic parameters in disease states.

---

[3]It appears that the confusion in the early literature arose from the fact that clearance was calculated as the product $K \times V$. Clearance was erroneously interpreted as being dependent on K and V.

Kinetics After Oral Administration

Qualitative Aspects

The oral route represents the most frequent mode of drug administration, especially since it enables the use of solid dosage forms (tablets, capsules). A number of reviews in the field of biopharmaceutics have discussed the factors that affect drug absorption from the gastrointestinal tract (3,26). Each dosage form should be considered as a drug delivery system which releases the drug in a definite pattern, eventually determining the rate and extent of absorption or bioavailability. Drug must be in solution before it can cross the gastrointestinal membranes and be absorbed. A tablet, for example, must first disintegrate into small particles in order to increase the surface area of drug exposed to gastrointestinal fluids and enhance the dissolution rate. For certain drugs, the processes of disintegration and/or dissolution can become rate limiting. These processes are affected by physicochemical variables, such as salt and crystalline form, and manufacturing variables, such as nature of lubricants and binders and compression pressure. Physiological variables such as gastric emptying time can also become significant. From the stomach to the duodenum and jejunum, there is an increase in pH and a very large increase in surface area of contact for absorption. Gastric emptying and the accompanying increase in pH are especially significant for drug absorption from enteric-coated tablets. Once in solution, drug molecules are absorbed, mostly by passive diffusion and, less frequently, by facilitated diffusion. When the drug is ionizable, absorption of drug in solution is governed by the pH partition hypothesis and diffusion of the un-ionized species.

Quantitative Aspects

Rate of absorption.

The data accumulated to date on gastrointestinal absorption indicate that, for many drugs, absorption behaves like a first-order process in spite of the fact that a number of variables influence this process. The gastrointestinal tract behaves as a single compartment in which the amount of drug decreases at a rate controlled by a first-order absorption rate constant, k_a. A typical oral curve is shown in Fig. 2. The shape of this curve is a direct consequence of the fact that absorption and elimination are first-order processes and can be explained by following the changes in absorption and elimination rates over time. The rate of change of amount of drug in the body at any time is equal to the absorption rate minus the elimination rate. At time zero, all of the initial dose, D, is in the gastrointestinal tract. The absorption rate (which is equal to the product of k_a and the amount of drug in the gastrointestinal tract) is at its maximum, since that amount is equal to the total dose. In the body, the elimination rate is equal to the product of the elimination rate constant, K, and the amount of drug in the body, A. At time zero, there is no drug in the body, and, consequently, the elimination rate is equal to zero and is at its minimum. Thus, the amount of drug in the body increases rapidly at first since the absorption rate is much larger than the elimination rate. As time increases, the amount of drug in the gastrointestinal tract decreases, and, therefore, the absorption rate decreases. Simultaneously, in the body, the amount of drug increases, and the elimination rate (which is proportional to that amount) increases. There comes a time when the elimination rate reaches a value equal to the absorption rate. At that time, the amount of drug in the body is at its maximum (peak time). At times longer than peak time, the absorption rate continues its decrease toward zero, and the elimination rate also decreases. For the majority of drugs, k_a is larger than K, and the absorption rate becomes negligible shortly after peak time. In this latter phase, drug disappearance in the body reflects only the kinetics of elimination. Consequently, a semilogarithmic plot of concentration versus time is linear in its terminal phase, and the elimination half-life can be determined from that portion of the curve.

In some cases, k_a is smaller than K, and absorption becomes the rate-limiting step during the apparent "elimination" phase. This situation results from the fact that, absorption being slow, the majority of the dose is still in the gastrointestinal tract at peak time. The half-life determined in the terminal phase is the half-life of absorption. This phenomenon is encountered with drugs with slow dissolution rate characteristics and is taken advantage of in the design of sustained-release formulations. The time course of drug amount (or concentration) can be described quantitatively by a biexponential equation (see Appendix). Dose, k_a, and K are three independent variables which determine the value of A at any time. Increasing dose yields increasing peak concentrations (in a proportional fashion), with no change in time course of absorption, k_a, or in elimination half-life. Decreasing the absorption rate constant results in lower peak height and longer peak time. Decreasing the elimination rate constant produces higher peak concentration and delayed peak times.

Extent of absorption.

The fraction of a dose of drug reaching the systemic circulation, or availability (also called bioavailability), is an important pharmacokinetic parameter (30). Before appearing in the systemic circulation, a drug must cross three different barriers: the gastrointestinal lumen, the intestinal wall, and the liver. Each of these barriers tends to decrease the systemic availability. In the gastrointestinal tract, the dosage form must release the drug (i.e., in the case of a tablet, the processes of disintegration and dissolution must leave the total dose dissolved in the gastrointestinal fluids). Loss of drug can occur through a number of degradation reactions, enzymatic and nonenzymatic (acid hydrolysis), and complexations. The relationship between drug permeability through the intestinal membrane and gastrointestinal transit time must be optimal to enable drug transfer on the mucosal side. Metabolism by enzymes in the intestinal wall must also be avoided. The fraction of dose appearing in the portal circulation, F_G, must then cross the liver where it is subject to the so-called "first-pass effect." The fraction of F_G that is lost by metabolism during the first pass through the liver is equal to the extraction ratio, E. The fraction $F_L = 1 - E$ represents the metabolic availability across the liver. The systemic availability, F, is equal to the product $F_G \cdot F_L$ since F_L can only operate on the fraction of the dose, F_G, that reaches the liver.

$$F = F_G \cdot F_L \qquad [9]$$

The component F_L of bioavailability is metabolic in nature and cannot be altered by modifications of the dosage form. A drug with an extraction ratio of 0.4 has a maximum bioavailability of 0.6. If 10% of the administered dose is lost prior to appearance in the portal vein, the systemic availability is $F = 0.9 \times 0.6 = 0.54$. Loss of drug by first-pass metabolism is not of consequence among antiepileptic drugs, since they have low extraction ratios. On the other hand, drugs such as aspirin, lidocaine, propranolol, and propoxyphene exhibit significant first-pass effects. The bioavailability, F, is determined by comparison of areas under the curve following oral [$(AUC)_o$] and intravenous [$(AUC)_{iv}$] administration of drug (with dose correction, if the intravenous and oral doses are different).

$$F = \frac{(AUC)_o}{(AUC)_{iv}} \times \frac{D_{iv}}{D_o} \qquad [10]$$

This determination is based on the rationale that it is the same systemic clearance that operates on the dose, D_{iv}, to yield AUC_{iv}, and on the amount, FD_o, to yield AUC_o. The constancy of clearance between the two experiments is an assumption. This assumption can be avoided by using newer methods of determination of bioavailability involving the use of stable isotopically labeled species. Both studies are performed simultaneously, but each route involves a different isotopic label. This approach is not widespread because blood samples have to be assayed by mass spectrometry to distinguish between the two isotopic masses.

Oral clearance.

The relationship between the determinants of hepatic elimination (blood flow, intrinsic clearance) and the rate and extent of drug bioavailability requires further elaboration. The determination of bioavailability is based on the relationship

$$AUC_o = \frac{FD_o}{Cl_s} \qquad [11]$$

Another clearance term, the apparent oral clearance, Cl_o, which relates D_o and AUC_o is defined such that

$$AUC_o = \frac{D_o}{Cl_o} \qquad [12]$$

Assuming that the total dose reaches the portal circulation (i.e., $F = F_L = 1 - E$), the term Cl_o can be written as

$$Cl_o = \frac{Cl_s}{F} = \frac{QE}{1 - E} \qquad [13]$$

From the relationship that defines hepatic clearance as a function of Q and Cl' (equation 6), it can be shown that

$$f \cdot Cl' = \frac{QE}{1 - E} \qquad [14]$$

and therefore, $Cl_o = f \cdot Cl'$. Thus, the apparent oral clearance of a drug is its intrinsic clearance. This finding has several consequences, especially in assessing the effects of disease states on drug kinetics.

Kinetics of Urinary Excretion

Since the kidney, like the liver, is an organ of drug elimination, mass balance considerations show that renal clearance, Cl_R, is the ratio of urinary excretion rate (dA_e/dt where A_e refers to amount of drug in urine) and plasma concentration:

$$Cl_R = \frac{dA_e/dt}{C} = \frac{k_eA}{C} = k_eV \qquad [15]$$

where k_e is the rate constant for urinary excretion.

From a knowledge of the value of renal clearance of a drug, inferences can be made as to the mechanisms of renal excretion. Since the value of glomerular filtration rate is equal to 120 ml/min, a renal clearance of 60 ml/min indicates that tubular reabsorption is prevalent. Similarly, a renal clearance larger than 120 ml/min reflects the presence of active secretion.

The proportionality between excretion rate and blood concentration indicates that the excretion rate of a drug will also be governed by the drug's biological half-life. For example, a semilogarithmic plot of excretion rate versus time will be linear with a slope equal to $-K/2.3$. Another consequence of the constancy of renal clearance is the fact that the fraction of a dose excreted unchanged in urine is constant and represents a property of the drug. It is equal to the ratio of excretion rate constant to elimination rate constant (k_e/K).

Urinary excretion studies present some practical advantages over blood-level studies. Foremost, they are noninvasive. Also, urinary concentrations are much higher than plasma concentrations and thus easier to assay analytically. However, little use has been made of urinary excretion data in therapeutic drug monitoring.

Multiple-Dose Kinetics

Plateau Principle: Constant-Rate Intravenous Infusion

This principle can be stated in general terms as follows: if the rate of input into a system is constant (zero order), and the rate of output is exponential (first order), the content of the system will accumulate until a steady state is reached. In pharmacokinetics, when a drug is infused at a constant rate, it will eventually reach a steady-state or plateau level in blood and tissues. As long as the infusion is maintained, the plateau level is maintained.

Why is a steady state achieved? This question is best answered by comparing the elimination rate to the infusion rate, R, as time increases. At time zero, the amount of drug in the body, A, is equal to zero, and the elimination rate, KA, which is proportional to A, is also equal to zero. Since the infusion rate has a finite value, A begins to increase rapidly. As A increases, the elimination rate, KA, increases. Eventually, KA approaches the value of R, and when KA equals R, A cannot increase further, and a steady state is achieved (A_{ss}). What factors control the value of the steady state? The answer to this question emerges after equating infusion and elimination rates, i.e.,

$$R = KA_{ss} \qquad [16]$$

The amount and concentration at steady state, C_{ss}, are given by:

$$A_{ss} = \frac{R}{K} \qquad [17]$$

$$C_{ss} = \frac{R}{KV} = \frac{R}{Cl_s} \qquad [18]$$

Steady-state drug concentration is directly proportional to the infusion rate, and the constant of proportionality between C_{ss} and R is the reciprocal of clearance. If R is doubled, C_{ss} is also doubled, but, as will be explained further, this does not imply that steady state is reached sooner. Although it is apparent that C_{ss} is also inversely proportional to Cl_s, this notion is not emphasized, since Cl_s is not a parameter that can be varied for a given drug.

When is steady state achieved? The rate at which steady state is achieved is determined solely by the elimination rate constant of the drug as shown in the following relationship:

$$C = C_{ss} (1 - e^{-Kt}) \qquad [19]$$

By simple substitutions of values of t equal to multiples of the half-life, we find that $C = 0.5$ C_{ss} at $t = T_{1/2}$; $C = 0.75 C_{ss}$ at $t = 2T_{1/2}$, and $C = 0.875 C_{ss}$ at $t = 3T_{1/2}$ (Fig. 2). Steady state is practically achieved (97%) after five biological half-lives. Thus, when the infusion rate is doubled, drug concentration at any time is also doubled, but the rate at which steady state is achieved is unchanged. In one half-life, concentration is equal to half of the new steady state.

These notions have several applications in the therapeutic management of patients receiving drugs such as lidocaine which are commonly administered by prolonged constant-rate intravenous infusion. In particular, it is relatively simple to calculate an infusion rate by multiplying the desired steady-state concentration with the value of clearance ($R_0 = C_{ss} \cdot Cl_s$). Also, when it is necessary to achieve a steady state rapidly, it is possible to combine the constant rate infusion with an intravenous bolus dose.

Multiple Dosing

The plateau principle described above is also applicable in the case of a discontinuous mode of administration as long as elimination is first order and the rate of drug administration is constant. The latter is the case with a fixed-dose, fixed-time schedule in which the administered dose, D, and the dosing interval, τ, are constant. The dosing rate is equal to the ratio D/τ in the case of intravenous administration and FD/τ for oral dosing. Since drug administration is discontinuous, the steady-state situation is characterized by a maximum, a minimum, and an average drug amount or concentration ($\overline{C}_{ss}$). The relationship that defines $\overline{C}_{ss}$ is essentially the same as that derived for the infusion case:

$$\overline{C}_{ss} = \frac{FD}{Cl_s \tau} \qquad [20]$$

$\overline{C}_{ss}$ is proportional to the dose (also called maintenance dose) and inversely proportional to the dosing interval. The rate of rise of drug concentration toward the steady state is governed by the drug's biological half-life (consistent with the plateau principle). In one half-life, $\overline{C} = 0.5$ $\overline{C}_{ss}$, and in five half-lives, $\overline{C} = 0.97 \overline{C}_{ss}$. A number of complex equations have been derived to describe drug concentration at any time during the period of drug accumulation (12,35). However, such concentrations can be simply determined by addition; i.e., the concentration at any time is equal to the sum of the remaining concentrations from all previous doses.

If steady state needs to be achieved rapidly, a loading dose (D_L) can be administered at the first dose. D_L can be obtained by multiplying D by the multiple dose factor [$1/(1 - e^{K\tau})$ for intravenous dosing and $1/(1 - e^{-K\tau})(1 - e^{-K\tau})$ for oral dosing]. Alternatively, it can be approximated from the product of the desired steady-state concentration and the volume of distributon ($\overline{C}_{ss} \cdot V$).

The above notions can be used to derive dosage regimens for new drugs or to understand the rationale behind established dosing schedules for old drugs. The frequency of drug administration depends on two parameters: the width of the therapeutic range of the drug and the value of the biological half-life. In cases in which the therapeutic range is narrow (digoxin, phenytoin), there are at least two possibilities: (a) if the half-life is long (longer than 24 hr, digoxin), the dosing interval will be shorter than the half-life ($\tau = 24$ hr or 12 hr or even 8 hr), and oscillations will be less than 50% (the amount of drug in the body at steady state is much larger than the maintenance dose); (b) if the half-life is short (less than 6 hr, lidocaine), the oscillations associated with dosing intervals of 6 to 8 hr are not tolerable (in light of the therapeutic range), and the drug is best administered by constant-rate intravenous infusion. In cases in which the therapeutic range is wide (antibiotics), oscillations are of less concern, and a convenient dosing interval can be selected almost independently of the drug's half-life. If the half-life is short (less than 6 hr), a significant fraction of the dose will be eliminated between doses (A_{ss} is only slightly larger than D). If the half-life is relatively long (over 24 hr), the oscillations between maximum and minimum during the dosing interval would be minimal (A_{ss} is much larger than D). In this latter case, it would take several days to achieve steady state, and a loading dose would be indicated.

Multicompartment Models

For the majority of drugs, the assumption of instantaneous distribution is unrealistic. Drug distribution requires a finite time during which drug elimination also takes place. This is seen clearly after intravenous bolus injection. Drug disappearance from blood (or plasma) is rapid at first, mostly because drug is leaving plasma to enter tissues. This first phase is often referred to as the distributive phase, whereas the slower phase is called the elimination phase. The most commonly used multicompartment model is the two-compartment model which distinguishes between accessible body fluids and highly perfused organs (heart, liver, kidney, brain) and poorly perfused tissues (fat, muscle). Several types of two-compartment models have been derived. Also, three- and four-compartment models have been used. These models generally contain first-order transfer or elimination (input is variable) rate constants. Such models yield differential equations that, when integrated, are of a polyexponential nature (35). The mathematical complexity of such systems is beyond the scope of this chapter, and the reader is referred to several textbooks in which multicompartment systems have been adequately described (11). However, it is important to retain the notion that there are model-dependent and model-independent pharmacokinetic parameters. For example, the relationship between clearance and area under the curve is model independent. Therefore, independently from the polyexponential nature of a given curve, the area under that curve can be determined by the trapezoidal rule, and clearance can be determined. Similarly, the volume of distribution can

be determined in a model-independent fashion (2). These basic parameters have the same properties as described previously in the case of a one-compartment model.

Kinetics of Drug Metabolites

In humans, the majority of therapeutically useful drugs are eliminated, at least in part, by biotransformation. A given molecule can lead to many (in some cases 50 or more) metabolites. From a clinical point of view, only the efficacious and/or toxic metabolites are of interest. Examples of parent–metabolite pairs among antiepileptic drugs are primidone–phenobarbital and diazepam–nordiazepam. Also, some metabolites devoid of efficacy or toxicity can influence the therapeutic outcome of a drug by interacting pharmacokinetically with the parent drug (e.g., inhibition of phenytoin metabolism by its hydroxy metabolite in the rat). From a drug disposition point of view, it is important to describe all the metabolic conversions that take place once a drug enters the body. In spite of the relevance of this topic, the literature on the kinetics of genesis and elimination of metabolites is relatively limited. As pointed out by Gillette (14), urinary profiles of metabolites do not reflect the "past history" of metabolism in blood or plasma. This section emphasizes the time course of metabolites in blood.

The following discussion is based on a number of assumptions: (a) metabolism of the parent drug occurs only in the liver; (b) the liver behaves as a homogeneous, well-stirred compartment; (c) parent drug and metabolite have low hepatic extraction ratios; (d) all processes are first order. The basic model considered is shown in Fig. 4.

Area and Steady-State Relationships

The following mass balance relationship holds at all times:

Rate of change of amount of metabolite
= Formation rate − Elimination rate [21]
= $C \cdot Cl_f - C_m \cdot Cl_m$

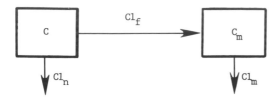

FIG. 4. The basic model for determining the kinetics of drug metabolites in the blood. C and C_m represent parent drug and metabolite concentrations; Cl_f is the formation clearance (intrinsic) of the metabolite considered; Cl_m is the elimination clearance (intrinsic) of the metabolite and Cl_n is the clearance of parent drug by all other routes.

where C and C_m represent parent drug and metabolite blood concentrations; Cl_f is the formation clearance (intrinsic) of the metabolite considered; and Cl_m is the elimination clearance (intrinsic) of the metabolite. Integration of this relationship from time 0 to infinity yields a relationship between areas under the curve of parent drug (AUC) and metabolite ($\mathrm{AUC_m}$):

$$\frac{\mathrm{AUC_m}}{\mathrm{AUC}} = \frac{Cl_f}{Cl_m} \qquad [22]$$

Since, by definition, the sum of $Cl_f + Cl_R$ is equal to the total clearance of parent drug, Cl_s, it follows that the fraction of dose metabolized, f_m, is equal to the ratio of Cl_f/Cl_s. Therefore, the area ratio above can also be expressed as

$$\frac{\mathrm{AUC_m}}{\mathrm{AUC}} = f_m \frac{Cl_s}{Cl_m} \qquad [23]$$

It has been shown that the same relationships hold with average steady-state concentrations of parent drug ($\overline{C}_{ss}$) and metabolite ($\overline{C}_{mss}$) (18).

$$\frac{\overline{C}_{mss}}{\overline{C}_{ss}} = \frac{f_m Cl_s}{Cl_m} \qquad [24]$$

These relationships indicate that when a parent drug yields a polar metabolite with a clearance larger than that of its precursor ($Cl_m > Cl_s$), that metabolite will yield an area under the curve smaller than that of the parent drug. Also, its steady-state concentration will be lower than that of its precursor. Conversely, a metabolite with a clearance lower than that of its precursor ($Cl_m < Cl_s$) will tend to accumulate, yielding high metabolite-to-parent-drug concentration ratios. Thus, a high metabolite-to-parent-drug concentration ratio does not simply reflect a high fraction metabolized. The above relationships also show that in order to determine the fraction of dose of a drug metabolized to a particular metabolite, a knowledge of the clearance of this metabolite is needed. This, in turn, requires administration of the metabolite by a systemic route. The above principles and relationships are independent of the number of metabolites formed.

Kinetic Relationships

The time course of metabolite concentration following a single intravenous dose of parent drug (monoexponential decay) is analogous to that of an oral dose of a drug. The relationship of concentration of metabolite as a function of time is also biexponential (see Appendix), depending on the elimination rate constants of the parent drug (K) and metabolite (K_m). When the half-life of the metabolite is shorter than that of the parent drug ($K_m > K$), the disappearance of the metabolite is rate-limited by that of the parent drug (the slower). In such a case, the true metabolite half-life cannot be obtained (unless the metabolite is administered separately). When the half-life of the metabolite is longer than that of the parent drug ($K_m < K$), the disappearance of the metabolite is slower than that of parent drug. The half-life of the metabolite can be determined from data on metabolite concentration following administration of the parent drug (after several half-lives of decay of the parent drug).

Pharmacokinetics in Disease States[4]

Many of the developments in the field of clinical pharmacokinetics have been based on the finding that the pharmacokinetic properties of

---

[4]The volumes edited by Benet (1) and Evans et al. (9) are recommended reading on this subject.

several drugs are altered in specific pathological states involving the two main organs responsible for drug elimination, the kidney and liver. This section includes the mechanisms of modifications in pharmacokinetic parameters in renal and hepatic disease.

Drug Kinetics in Renal Disease

The early contributions in this area were made by Kunin (17) and Dettli (7,8). The effects of renal disease on the pharmacokinetic behavior of a given drug are related to the drug class to which it belongs. There are three drug classes: type A, drugs eliminated completely by renal excretion; type B, drugs eliminated by hepatic or other nonrenal routes; and type C, drugs eliminated by both renal and nonrenal routes.

Dettli (7) proposed a linear relationship between the elimination rate constant, K, and a measure of glomerular filtration rate such as the clearance of creatinine, Cl_{cr}

$$K = R\ Cl_{cr} + k_{nr} \qquad [25]$$

where k_{nr} is the rate constant for drug elimination by nonrenal routes. The latter is equal to zero for type A drugs.

When such a relationship has been established for a given drug, a new dosing regimen can be calculated as a function of the degree of renal failure using the computed value of K. The new maintenance dose is reduced proportionately to the reduction in K. Alternatively, a new dosing interval (inversely proportional to the elimination rate constant) can be used. Dosing nomograms have been developed for a number of drugs, including gentamicin, kanamycin, and digoxin.

However, the approach of Dettli does not take into consideration that renal failure can affect drug elimination by nonrenal routes, as is the case with procainamide. Elimination of metabolites with efficacious or toxic properties is also affected. For example, N-acetyl procainamide, a metabolite of procainamide with antiarrhythmic properties, is eliminated primarily by renal excretion. Finally, renal disease has been associated with a reduction in the plasma protein binding of many drugs. An increase in plasma free fraction[5] is expected to produce an increase in plasma clearance (with no change in intrinsic clearance) (equation 6) and an increase in volume of distribution (equation 4). An example that has been extensively studied is phenytoin. Phenytoin free fraction, which is normally around 6 to 10%, increases in uremic patients to reach values as high as 30%. Gugler et al. (15) compared phenytoin steady-state concentrations (C_{ss}), total clearance (Cl_s), and free concentration (Cf_{ss}) in a group of normal subjects (N) and in hypoalbuminemic patients (P) with the nephrotic syndrome: C_{ss} values were 6.8 and 2.9 µg/ml in groups N and P, respectively; corresponding Cl_s values were 0.022 and 0.048 liter/kg·hr; Cf_{ss} values were not significantly different at 0.69 and 0.59 µg/ml, respectively; f values were 0.10 and 0.19 in the two groups. These findings were reanalyzed and explained by pharmacokinetic theory (19). The latter predicts that if the free fraction of a drug with low extraction ratio is increased, the C_{ss} will decrease, but Cf_{ss} will remain unchanged:

$$C_{ss} = \frac{R}{Cl_s} = \frac{R}{f \cdot Cl'} \qquad [26]$$

When f increases, total clearance increases (proportionately), and C_{ss} decreases accordingly. But since $Cf_{ss} = f\ C_{ss}$, it can be seen that Cf_{ss} is independent of a change in f

$$Cf_{ss} = \frac{R}{Cl'} \qquad [27]$$

This is in fact the case for phenytoin in patients with the nephrotic syndrome. The increase in clearance in accordance with the increase in free fraction is seen by computing the intrinsic clearance for both groups: 0.22 and 0.25 liter/kg·hr for the N and P groups, respectively. The decrease in C_{ss} with the lack of difference in Cf_{ss}

---

[5]Although the same symbol is used for plasma and blood free fractions, it should be noted that they are related by the blood/plasma concentration ratio: free fraction in blood = free fraction in plasma/(blood concentration/plasma concentration).

is compatible with the pharmacokinetic rationale provided. These findings suggest that, in such instances, monitoring of free drug levels would be indicated.

Drug Kinetics in Hepatic Disease

There are at least five categories of liver disease that have been examined with respect to their effects on drug disposition: (a) chronic liver disease, (b) acute hepatitis, (c) drug-induced hepatotoxicity, (d) cholestasis, and (e) hepatic neoplastic disease. The most significant alterations in drug disposition occur in chronic liver disease. A rational understanding of these alterations must be based on physiological models of hepatic elimination that identify the basic determinants of clearance as free fraction in blood (or plasma), intrinsic clearance, and blood flow (5,29,36,39).

In cirrhotic patients, albumin levels are frequently lower than normal. For several drugs that are highly bound to albumin (diazepam, phenytoin, phenylbutazone, propanolol), the low albumin levels result in a decrease in extent of binding and an increase in free fraction in plasma. As explained previously in the section on hepatic clearance, the consequences of an increase in free fraction in plasma depend on the extraction ratio of the drug. If the latter is high, clearance is independent of free fraction and limited mostly by blood flow. If the extraction ratio is low, an increase in free fraction should result in a concomitant increase in hepatic clearance. This is the case for tolbutamide, amobarbital, and phenytoin. However, intrinsic clearance of free drug may also be affected by the disease state, and the effect on the total clearance is a resultant of the effects of hepatic disease on its components.

In the discussion on volume of distribution, it was pointed out that an increase in plasma free fraction is expected to result in an increase in volume of distribution if tissue binding remains unaltered. This has been shown to be the case for several drugs (diazepam, clorazepam, chlordiazepoxide, and valproic acid). In the cases of phenytoin and tolbutamide in viral hepatitis, it was also suggested that tissue binding was

decreased. Consequently, the volume of distribution remained unchanged.

The ultimate effect on drug half-life is a resultant of the changes in clearance and volume of distribution (as shown by equation 8). This is illustrated in the case of tolbutamide. It was found that tolbutamide half-life was decreased in acute viral hepatitis (38). This was totally explained by an increase in plasma clearance, since volume of distribution was unchanged. However, the intrinsic ability of the liver to eliminate the drug was not significantly altered, since all the increase in clearance could be accounted for by an increase in free fraction in plasma.

Although decreases in intrinsic clearance of free drug would be expected in hepatic disease, such occurrences are not systematically found. For example, the intrinsic clearances (free) of theophylline and diazepam were decreased in cirrhotic patients, whereas those of lorazepam and oxazepam were not affected. Similarly, in viral hepatitis, the intrinsic clearances of phenytoin, tolbutamide, warfarin, oxazepam, and lorazepam are not affected, whereas those of antipyrine, diazepam, chlordiazepoxide, and hexobarbital are decreased. As was the case for free fraction, decreases in intrinsic clearances of free drug will primarily influence the clearances of drugs with low extraction ratios. In addition, decreases in intrinsic clearance are expected to yield higher oral bioavailabilities for drugs with medium and high extraction ratios (examples are chlormethiazole, labetalol, and pentazocine).

Hepatic blood flow appears to be decreased in chronic liver disease, but it is not significantly altered in viral hepatitis. Changes in hepatic blood flow are expected to affect the total clearances of drugs with medium and high extraction ratios. Blood flow probably plays a role in the decreases in clearances observed with lidocaine and propranolol.

Influence of Age on Drug Kinetics

Most of our knowledge on the effect of age on drug disposition has been acquired in the last few years. Although significant differences in drug kinetics have been found among various age groups, no unifying theory is available. Often, these differences are drug specific, and it is necessary to examine a number of examples in order to obtain a picture of age effects on drug disposition. Fortunately, one book (22) and three reviews on the subject have recently been published (16,23,34).

Newborn, Young Infant, and Child

The plasma protein binding of several drugs is generally reduced in newborns. Such a generalization cannot be extended to infants. Newborns have a lower total plasma protein concentration and high levels of free fatty acids, both of which are compatible with higher free fractions than in adults. For example, phenytoin free fraction in newborn is double the adult value and even larger in hyperbilirubinemia. Interestingly, phenytoin volume of distribution is also approximately twice the adult value. In infants (3–24 months), phenytoin binding approaches adult values. In the case of diazepam, plasma free fraction in newborns is also increased, but the volume of distribution is slightly lower than in adults. This is attributed to the lower body lipid content in neonates. Although phenobarbital is not extensively bound in adults ($f = 0.5$–0.6), its free fraction is slightly increased in the neonate with a corresponding increase in volume of distribution.

Hepatic microsomal activity is reduced in the neonate. Very few clearances have been reported in the literature. However, the half-lives of several drugs including phenobarbital, phenytoin, and valproic acid are longer in the neonate. The pattern of change in drug elimination in the first months of life are drug specific. For phenobarbital, half-life decreases during the first 2 to 4 weeks and remains shorter in infants than in adults. Similarly, diazepam half-life decreases from values of 40 to 400 hr in premature newborns to 8 to 14 hr in infants, whereas adult values range between 20 and 30 hr.

For most antiepileptic drugs, the ratio of steady-state drug level to dose is lower in children than in adults. This reflects the fact that clearance is generally larger in this age group than in adults. In many cases, there appears to be a gradual increase in this ratio from the newborn to the adolescent and the adult.

Drug Disposition in the Aged

Within the last 5 years, a body of data has accumulated indicating that the metabolism of some drugs is impaired with older age (6,27, 32,33). Several possible explanations of these observations have been advanced: decreased intrinsic ability to metabolize drugs; selective mortality (rapid metabolizers die sooner); resistance to environmental enzyme inducers. For example, the recent studies of Vestal and Wood (34) illustrate the effects of increasing age on basic kinetic parameters. These authors examined three model compounds with different extraction ratios: antipyrine (low), indocyanine green (high), and propranolol (medium). For antipyrine, the mean plasma clearance was 39% lower in the older age group (48–68 yr) than in the younger age group (21–37 yr). Volume of distribution was significantly smaller in the older group. As a result, there was no significant difference in half-life between the groups. Also, with respect to antipyrine clearance, there was no age group difference between nonsmokers, whereas younger smokers exhibited a twofold larger clearance than older smokers. For indocyanine green, systemic plasma clearance was 46% larger in the younger group. However, there was no age effect in volume of distribution. Consequently, indocyanine green half-life was longer (40%) in the younger group.

The age effect for propranolol paralleled that observed for indocyanine green. Systemic clearance was significantly larger in the younger than in the older group. There was no difference in volume of distribution, and half-life differences reflected the clearance effect. Calculated intrinsic clearances were different between the two age groups only for smokers. Apparent liver blood flow was 24% lower in the older group. The decrease in intrinsic clearance with age manifests itself also in the form of a reduced first-pass effect when propranolol is given orally.

NONLINEAR PHARMACOKINETICS

This topic is of particular relevance in the clinical pharmacology of antiepileptic drugs since they exhibit both types of nonlinearities observed in pharmacokinetics: dose dependency and time dependency.

Dose-Dependent Kinetics

Dose dependence results from the dependence of rates of transfer or metabolism on concentration. Pharmacokinetically, this results in concentration (or dose) dependence of basic parameters such as free fraction or intrinsic clearance. Thus, plots of area under the curve and steady-state concentration versus dose become nonlinear (Fig. 5), and half-life and the time to reach steady state become dose-dependent. Phenytoin is the classical example of a drug exhibiting a decreasing clearance with increasing dose as the result of saturable metabolism (31). Valproic acid, on the other hand, exhibits increases in clearance and volume of distribution because of increases in free fraction with increasing dose (4).

From a theoretical point of view, it is of interest to review the relationship between linear and nonlinear behavior of clearance in Michaelis–Menten kinetics. The rate of metabolism, V, is assumed to be dependent on plasma concentration according to the relationship

$$V = \frac{V_{max}C}{K_m + C} \qquad [28]$$

where V_{max} and K_m are as previously defined. For phenytoin, V_{max} values range between 100 and 1,000 mg/day, and K_m values between 1 and 15 μg/ml. When concentration is less than 0.1 K_m, V becomes proportional to C in a first-order fashion. The ratio V_{max}/K_m is the clearance and is dose independent. When concentration is much higher than K_m, V becomes equal to V_{max} and is constant and maximum. With concentrations around K_m, V is concentration dependent as described by the above nonlinear relationship.

For a steady state to be achieved, the rate of drug administration, R, has to equal the rate of elimination; i.e.,

$$R = \frac{V_{max}C_{ss}}{K_m + C_{ss}} \qquad [29]$$

From this relationship, it is possible to express C_{ss} as a function of dosing rate

$$C_{ss} = \frac{R \cdot K_m}{V_{max} - R} \qquad [30]$$

When R is smaller than 0.1 V_{max}, C_{ss} is proportional to R, the constant of proportionality being the reciprocal of clearance (kinetics are

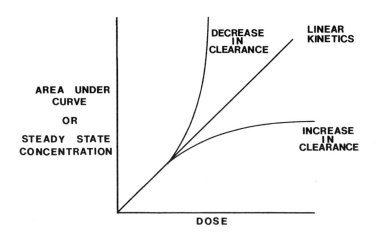

FIG. 5. Relationship between area under the curve or steady-state concentration and dosing rate, illustrating two types of dose dependencies. In linear kinetics, the clearance is constant.

linear). When R is smaller than V_{max} (but larger than 0.1 V_{max}), the increase in steady-state concentration is more than proportional to the increase in R (Fig. 5). As R approaches V_{max}, C_{ss} increases asymptotically. When R is equal to or larger than V_{max}, a steady state is not achieved. Similarly, the time to reach a fraction of steady state increases with R.

In nonlinear kinetics, clearance and half-life have limited utility. The useful parameters are V_{max}, K_m, and volume of distribution. An extensive body of literature describes methods of determination of V_{max} and K_m for phenytoin and their applications to epileptic patients; the reader may wish to consult recent reviews (21,31).

Nonlinearity in plasma protein binding results in increases in total clearance for drugs with low extraction ratios (Fig. 5). Increases in dosing rate result in less than proportional increases in steady-state concentration. However, as shown in equation 26, free concentration should increase in proportion to the dose. In such increases, therapeutic monitoring of free levels proves very useful.

Time-Dependent Kinetics

The time dependencies reported in the literature to date can be classified into two categories: (a) physiologically induced time dependency (chronopharmacokinetics); and (b) chemically induced time dependency (20). Both types of time dependencies are found among antiepileptic drugs.

Chronopharmacokinetics[6]

This type of time dependence is related to the fact that rhythms are a fundamental property of most physiological functions. The word chronopharmacokinetics has been used to describe rhythms in drug absorption, distribution, and elimination. Chronovariability in absorption–elimination parameters (such as peak concentration and peak time) has been observed for

---

[6]References to the examples cited can be found in Levy (20).

many different drugs: phenacetin, acetaminophen, antipyrine, chlorazepate, β-methyldigoxin, indomethacin, theophylline, carbamazepine, valproic acid, and ethanol. Diurnal variations in systemic clearance were reported for ethosuximide, valproic acid, carbamazepine, and clonazepam in rhesus monkeys. Daily variations in enzymatic metabolic activity were also observed with a variety of substrates in rodents. Plasma free fractions of phenytoin and valproic acid were found to vary in a reproducible fashion over a diurnal phase in normal volunteers. Also, several examples have illustrated the fact that the diurnal rhythm in urinary pH influences the excretion of weak acids (salicylic acid, sulfonamides) and bases (amphetamine).

Chemically Induced Time Dependence[6]

Auto- and heteroinduction of drug clearance represent typical examples of this type of time dependence. The time course of change in drug clearance is assessed by following the time course of decreases (addition of inducer) or increases (removal of inducer) in steady-state blood levels. Many examples of such changes have been reported using pharmacokinetic models of induction. Warfarin levels were followed after addition and/or removal of several inducers, dichloral phenazone, antipyrine, amylobarbital, and quinalbarbitone. The time course of autoinduction of carbamazepine was found to be faster in rhesus monkeys (1.5–2 days) than in healthy humans (3 weeks) or epileptic children (3–5 weeks). The decrease in clonazepam levels following the addition of carbamazepine was found to be faster in rhesus monkeys than in humans. The induction of valproic acid and ethosuximide clearances by carbamazepine was also examined in rhesus monkeys and humans.

This second type of time dependence generally has more clinical significance than chronopharmacokinetic phenomena because of the extent of the changes in drug levels. However, chronovariability in pharmacokinetic parameters should be taken into consideration in experimental designs of pharmacokinetic studies.

APPENDIX

The time course of drug concentration following a single oral dose is given by:

$$C = \frac{F D k_a}{V (k_a - K)} (e^{-Kt} - e^{-k_a t}) \quad [A1]$$

All symbols are as defined in the text.

This relationship is analogous to that describing the time course of metabolite concentration following an intravenous dose of parent drug.

$$C_m = \frac{D k_f}{V_{max}(K_m - K)} (e^{-Kt} - e^{-K_m t}) \quad [A2]$$

where $k_f = \dfrac{Cl_f}{V}$, and all other symbols are as defined in the text.

ACKNOWLEDGMENTS

The author acknowledges the assistance of Ms. Ruth Baker, Ms. Raina H. Ballard, and Ms. Colleen D. Timmis in the preparation of this manuscript.

REFERENCES

1. Benet, L. Z. (1976): *The Effect of Disease States on Drug Pharmacokinetics*. American Pharmaceutical Association, Washington.
2. Benet, L. Z., and Galeazzi, R. L. (1979): Noncompartmental determination of the steady-state volume of distribution. *J. Pharm. Sci.*, 68:1071–1074.
3. Blanchard, J., Sawchuk, R. J., and Brodie, B. B. (1979): *Principles and Perspectives in Drug Bioavailability*. S. Karger, Basel.
4. Bowdle, T. A., Patel, I. H., Levy, R. H., and Wilensky, A. J. (1980): Valproic acid dosage and plasma protein binding and clearance. *Clin. Pharmacol. Ther.*, 28:486–492.
5. Branch, R. A., and Shand, D. G. (1976): Hepatic drug clearance in chronic liver disease. In: *The Effect of Disease States on Drug Pharmacokinetics*, edited by L. Z. Benet, pp. 77–86. American Pharmaceutical Association, Washington.
6. Crooks, J., O'Malley, K., and Stevenson, I. H. (1976): Pharmacokinetics in the elderly. *Clin. Pharmacokinet.*, 1:280–296.
7. Dettli, L. (1970): Multiple dose elimination kinetics and drug accumulation in patients with normal and impaired renal function. In: *Advances in the Biosciences, Vol. 5,* edited by G. Raspe, pp. 39–54. Pergamon Press, New York.
8. Dettli, L. C. (1974): Drug dosage in patients with renal disease. *Clin. Pharmacol. Ther.*, 16:274–280.
9. Evans, W. E., Schentag, J. J., and Jusko, W. J. (1980): *Applied Pharmacokinetics: Principles of Therapeutic Drug Monitoring.* Applied Therapeutics, San Francisco.
10. Fingl, E. (1972): Absorption, distribution, and elimination: Practical pharmacokinetics. In: *Antiepileptic Drugs,* edited by D. M. Woodbury, J. K. Penry, and R. P. Schmidt, pp. 7–21. Raven Press, New York.
11. Gibaldi, M., and Perrier, D. (1975): Multicompartment models. In: *Pharmacokinetics,* edited by M. Gibaldi and D. Perrier, pp. 45–96. Marcel Dekker, New York.
12. Gibaldi, M., and Perrier, D. (1975): Multiple dosing. In: *Pharmacokinetics,* edited by M. Gibaldi and D. Perrier, pp. 97–128. Marcel Dekker, New York.
13. Gillette, J. R. (1971): Factors affecting drug metabolism. *Ann. N.Y. Acad. Sci.*, 179:43–66.
14. Gillette, J. R. (1977): The phenomenon of species variations; problems and opportunities. In: *Drug Metabolism—from Microbe to Man,* edited by D. V. Parke and R. L. Smith, pp. 147–168. Taylor and Francis, London.
15. Gugler, R., Shoeman, D. W., Huffman, D. H., Cohlmia, J. B., and Azarnoff, D. L. (1975): Pharmacokinetics of drugs in patients with the nephrotic syndrome. *J. Clin. Invest.*, 55:1182–1189.
16. Hilligoss, D. M. (1980): Neonatal pharmacokinetics. In: *Applied Pharmacokinetics: Principles of Therapeutic Drug Monitoring,* edited by W. E. Evans, J. J. Schentag, and W. J. Jusko, pp. 76–94. Applied Therapeutics, San Francisco.
17. Kunin, C. M. (1967): A guide to the use of antibiotics in patients with renal disease. A table of recommended doses and factors governing serum levels. *Ann. Intern. Med.*, 67:151–158.
18. Lane, E. A., and Levy, R. H. (1980): Prediction of steady state behavior of metabolite from dosing of parent drug. *J. Pharm. Sci.*, 69:610–612.
19. Levy, G. (1976): Clinical implications of interindividual differences in plasma protein binding of drugs and endogenous substances. In: *The Effect of Disease States on Drug Pharmacokinetics,* edited by L. Z. Benet, pp. 137–151. American Pharmaceutical Association, Washington.
20. Levy, R. H. (1981): Time dependent pharmacokinetics. In: *The International Encyclopedia of Pharmacology and Therapeutics, Pharmacokinetics—Theory and Methodology,* edited by M. Rowland and G. Tucker. Pergamon Press, Oxford (*in press*).
21. Ludden, T. M. (1980): Phenytoin. In: *Applied Pharmacokinetics: Principles of Therapeutic Drug Monitoring,* edited by W. E. Evans, J. J. Schentag, and W. J. Jusko, pp. 315–318. Applied Therapeutics, San Francisco.
22. Morselli, P. L. (1977): *Drug Disposition During Development.* Spectrum Publications, New York.
23. Morselli, P. L., Franco-Morselli, R., and Bossi, B. (1980): Clinical pharmacokinetics in newborns and infants: Age-related differences and therapeutic implications. *Clin. Pharmacokinet.*, 5:485–527.

24. Pang, K. S., and Rowland, M. (1977): Hepatic clearance of drugs. I. Theoretical considerations of a 'well-stirred' and a 'parallel tube' model. *J. Pharmacokinet. Biopharm.*, 5:625–653.

25. Pang, K. S., and Rowland, M. (1977): Hepatic clearance of drugs. II. Experimental evidence for acceptance of the 'well-stirred' model over the 'parallel tube' model using lidocaine in the perfused rat liver in situ preparation. *J. Pharmackoinet. Biopharm.*, 5:665–680.

26. Prescott, L. F., and Nimmo, W. S. (1981): *Drug Absorption: Proceedings of the Edinburgh International Conference.* ADIS Press, Sydney, Australia.

27. Richey, D. P., and Bender, D. (1977): Pharmacokinetic consequences of aging. *Annu. Rev. Pharmacol. Toxicol.*, 17:49–65.

28. Rowland, M., Benet, L. Z., and Graham, G. G. (1973): Clearance concepts in pharmacokinetics. *J. Pharmacokinet. Biopharm.*, 1:123–136.

29. Rowland, M., Blaschke, T. F., Meffin, P. J., and Williams, R. L. (1976): Pharmacokinetics in disease states modifying hepatic and metabolic function. In: *The Effect of Disease States on Drug Pharmacokinetics,* edited by L. Z. Benet, pp. 53–75. American Pharmaceutical Association, Washington.

30. Tozer, T. N. (1979): Pharmacokinetic principles relevant to bioavailability studies. In: *Principles and Perspectives in Drug Bioavailability,* edited by J. Blanchard, R. J. Sawchuk, and B. B. Brodie, pp. 120–155. S. Karger, Basel.

31. Tozer, T. N., and Winter, M. E. (1980): Phenytoin. In: *Applied Pharmacokinetics: Principles of Therapeutic Drug Monitoring,* edited by W. E. Evans, J.

J. Schentag, and W. J. Jusko, pp. 275–314. Applied Therapeutics, San Francisco.

32. Triggs, E. J., and Nation, R. L. (1975): Pharmacokinetics in the aged: A review. *J. Pharmacokinet. Biopharm.*, 3:387–418.

33. Vestal, R. E. (1978): Drug use in the elderly: A review of problems and special considerations. *Drugs,* 16:358–382.

34. Vestal, R. E., and Wood, A. J. J. (1980): Influence of age and smoking on drug kinetics in man: Studies using model compounds. *Clin. Pharmacokinet.*, 5:309–319.

35. Wagner, J. G. (1975): Linear compartment models. In: *Fundamentals of Clinical Pharmacokinetics,* edited by J. G. Wagner, pp. 57–126. Drug Intelligence Publications, Illinois.

36. Wilkinson, G. R. (1980): Influence of liver disease on pharmacokinetics. In: *Applied Pharmacokinetics: Principles of Therapeutic Drug Monitoring,* edited by W. E. Evans, J. J. Schentag, and W. J. Jusko, pp. 57–75. Applied Therapeutics, San Francisco.

37. Wilkinson, G. R., and Shand, D. G. (1975): A physiological approach to hepatic drug clearance. *Clin. Pharmacol. Ther.*, 18:377–390.

38. Williams, R. L., Blaschke, T. F., Meffin, P. J., Melmon, K. L., and Rowland, M. (1976): The influence of acute viral hepatitis on the disposition and plasma binding of tolbutamide. *Clin. Pharmacol. Ther.*, 200:290–299.

39. Williams, R. L., and Mamelok, R. D. (1980): Hepatic disease and drug pharmacokinetics. *Clin. Pharmacokinet.*, 5:528–547.

Antiepileptic Drugs, edited by D. M. Woodbury, J. K. Penry, and C. E. Pippenger. Raven Press, New York © 1982.

3

General Principles

Biotransformation

E. Perucca and A. Richens

Many drugs are lipophilic compounds of low molecular weight, so that after being filtered at the renal glomeruli, they are readily reabsorbed by diffusion from the tubular epithelium. In order to be eliminated from the body, these compounds must be transformed into more polar water-soluble metabolites, which are subsequently excreted in urine. In the majority of cases, the biotransformation products are pharmacologically inert, but in other cases, active metabolites may be produced which can be responsible in full or in part for the biological effects of the parent drug. In either situation, changes in the rate of drug metabolism may play a fundamental role in determining the duration and extent of the pharmacological effect.

In this chapter some of the more important concepts relative to the biotransformation of drugs in man are considered, with special attention being focused on those aspects that are most relevant to the disposition of antiepileptic drugs.

PATHWAYS OF DRUG METABOLISM

The biochemical reactions responsible for the biotransformation of drugs in man almost invariably require enzymatic catalysis. The majority of the enzymes involved are located in the smooth endoplasmic reticulum (microsomes) of the hepatic cells, although a lower degree of enzymatic activity can also be detected in the microsomes and the cytosol of other organs such as the kidney, the gut, the lung, and the skin. As a general rule, the biotransformation process involves two phases (215):

$$\text{Parent drug} \xrightarrow[\text{oxidation, reduction}]{\text{Phase I}}$$

$$\text{Phase I metabolite(s)} \xrightarrow[\text{conjugation}]{\text{Phase II}}$$

Final metabolite(s)

In phase I reactions, functional groups such as -OH, -COOH, and $-NH_2$ are introduced into the drug molecule, resulting in the formation of more polar metabolites which may or may not retain pharmacological activity. In phase II reactions, the functional group is coupled with an endogenous substrate such as glucuronic acid, acetic acid, or inorganic sulfate, resulting in the formation of water-soluble conjugated products which are generally inactive and readily eliminated. Sometimes, the metabolic process may be restricted to phase I or phase II reactions only: in the latter case, functional groups suitable for conjugation must obviously be already present in the chemical structure of the parent compound.

Phase I Reactions

Oxidation

The oxidative biotransformation of drugs includes a wide range of biochemical reactions which take place to a large extent in the hepatic microsomes (61). Microsomal oxidative enzymes are often referred to as mixed-function oxidase to indicate the requirement for both molecular oxygen and a reducing agent; the term monooxygenase is also used and indicates that one molecule of oxygen is consumed per molecule of substrate, one atom being incorporated into the substrate and one reduced to H_2O (145). The enzymatic system consists of at least two components, a cytochrome which is termed cytochrome P-450 and a flavoprotein (fp$_1$) which catalyses the reduction of the cytochrome. For hydroxylation, the biochemical characteristics of the interaction among the cytochrome, the substrate, and the cofactors required have been

mostly identified (Fig. 1). The reaction is initiated by the binding of the drug to cytochrome P-450, followed by the interaction of the complex with NADPH-dependent fp$_1$, molecular oxygen, and cytochrome b$_5$ (165). Oxidation finally takes place and is followed by the dissociation of the complex into oxidized drug, oxidized cytochrome P-450, and H_2O.

Apart from drugs and other xenobiotics, numerous lipid-soluble endogenous substances such as free fatty acids, steroid hormones, and vitamins are known to function as substrates for the cytochrome P-450 monooxygenase (49, 63,102,114). Despite the wide variety of biochemical reactions catalyzed, the system is characterized by a high degree of substrate and product specificity, which varies in exacting fashion not only with species, strain, sex, tissue, and subcellular compartment, but also with age, hormonal status, nutritional conditions, disease, and exposure to pharmacological agents (95,114,139,164). Evidence is accumulating that

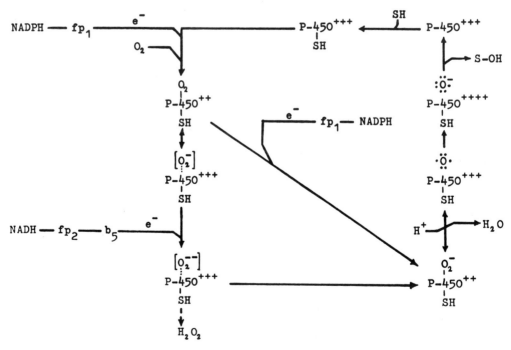

FIG. 1. Schematic representation of cytochrome P-450-dependent drug oxidation in hepatic microsomes and its interaction with cytochrome b$_5$, flavoproteins, NADH, and NADPH. SH, the drug; SOH, the oxidized drug; fp$_1$, NADPH–cytochrome P-450 reductase; fp$_2$, NADH–cytochrome b$_5$ reductase; b$_5$, cytochrome b$_5$. The superscript associated with P-450 indicates the valence state of the heme iron of cytochrome P-450. For details, see Powis and Jansson (165).

this specificity may result from the presence of different forms and different proportions of cytochrome P-450 within the hepatic microsomes (71,76,83,88,201,202,206,208).

The majority of currently used antiepileptic drugs are extensively metabolized by the monooxygenase system. Some important examples of oxidative reactions include the aromatic hydroxylation of phenytoin (66), phenobarbital (210), primidone (58), and carbamazepine (120), the alkyl oxidation of valproic acid (51) and ethosuximide (A.J. Glazko, Chapter 51); the *N*-demethylation of chlordiazepoxide (190) and trimethadione (29); and the S→O substitution in the conversion of thiopental to pentobarbital (215). Some of these reactions occur sequentially at one or multiple sites of the same molecule. Valproic acid, for example, is first ω-hydroxylated to 2-propyl-5-hydroxyvaleric acid and then further oxidized to 2-propylglutaric acid at the extremity of the aliphatic side chain (51,101). Diazepam, on the other hand, is first demethylated in position 1 to nordiazepam and subsequently hydroxylated in position 3 to yield oxazepam, its final phase I metabolite (189).

An important type of oxidative reaction is the formation of epoxides. An epoxide is a three-membered cyclic ether resulting from the enzymatic addition of oxygen across a double bond. A well-known example of epoxide is the 10,11-epoxide of carbamazepine: this active metabolite accumulates in serum during chronic administration of carbamazepine and is likely to be responsible for part of the anticonvulsant effect of the parent drug (14). Unlike carbamazepine-10,11-epoxide, other epoxides are chemically unstable intermediates which can bind covalently to biological macromolecules and thereby produce undesired effects such as mutagenesis (5), carcinogenesis (70), and tissue necrosis (24). Toxic epoxides are possibly formed during the conversion of hydantoin drugs to their dihydrodiol derivatives (59).

Reduction

Several types of reductive reactions of drugs in the body have been described, the most important examples being the reduction of nitro-compounds (e.g., chloramphenicol) and azo-compounds (e.g., Prontosil®) to amines and the reduction of ketones (e.g., cortisone) to secondary alcohols (cortisol). The enzymes catalyzing these reactions are predominantly microsomal; certain azo- and nitro-compounds, however, are reduced by gut bacteria and not by mammalian enzymes (62). The role of reductive reactions in the metabolism of antiepileptic drugs is limited, the best known examples being the reduction of nitrazepam to the corresponding amine (131) and the reduction of chloral hydrate to trichloroethanol (28).

Hydrolysis

Hydrolytic reactions are catalyzed by a variety of enzymatic systems which are located not only in the hepatic cells but also in the kidney, the brain, the serum, and many other tissues. Enzymes such as cholinesterases, carbon anhydrase, and aryl esterases play an important role in phase I metabolism of a number of drugs containing ester groups (107).

Phase II Reactions

Conjugations (phase II reactions) are synthetic reactions and therefore require a source of energy which is generally provided by ATP. With the exception of mercapturic acid formation, these reactions are characterized by the formation of an activated nucleotide as an intermediate and a transferring enzyme which catalyses the final conjugation step (215). The conjugated metabolite is usually more polar, more water soluble, and less extensively bound to plasma proteins; as a result, it is more readily excreted from the body. Most conjugation reactions result in drug inactivation.

Glucuronidation

Conjugation with glucuronic acid, the most common of the synthetic reactions, may occur with compounds containing the hydroxyl, carboxyl, amino, mercapto, or dithiocarboxyl group. The reaction involves the transfer of glucuronic acid from uridine diphosphate (UDP)-

glucuronic acid to the aglycon by UDP-glucuronyltransferase, a microsomal enzyme system independent of but functionally related to the mixed-function oxidase (45). The product of the reaction may be either an ether or an ester glucuronide. Ester glucuronides are unstable in alkaline urine and may be responsible for false positive tests for urinary glucose when the classic cupric ion reduction test is used (64). Apart from drugs, glucuronide-forming enzymes are actively involved in the metabolism of endogenous substrates such as steroids, bilirubin, and catecholamines (45). In humans, hepatic UDP-glucuronyltransferase activity is controlled by genetic and environmental factors and can be

drastically reduced in a number of inherited diseases, e.g., in Gilbert's syndrome, resulting in unconjugated hyperbilirubinemia and abnormal glucuronidation of various drugs (122). Examples of glucuronidation reactions involving antiepileptic drugs are plentiful. The majority of phase I metabolites of phenytoin, phenobarbital, primidone, carbamazepine, ethosuximide, valproic acid, chloral hydrate, and many benzodiazepine drugs are all excreted in urine as glucuronide derivatives. In the case of carbamazepine, the glucuronidation process is not restricted to the oxidized metabolites but may also extend to the amino group of the unmetabolized drug (Fig. 2) (120).

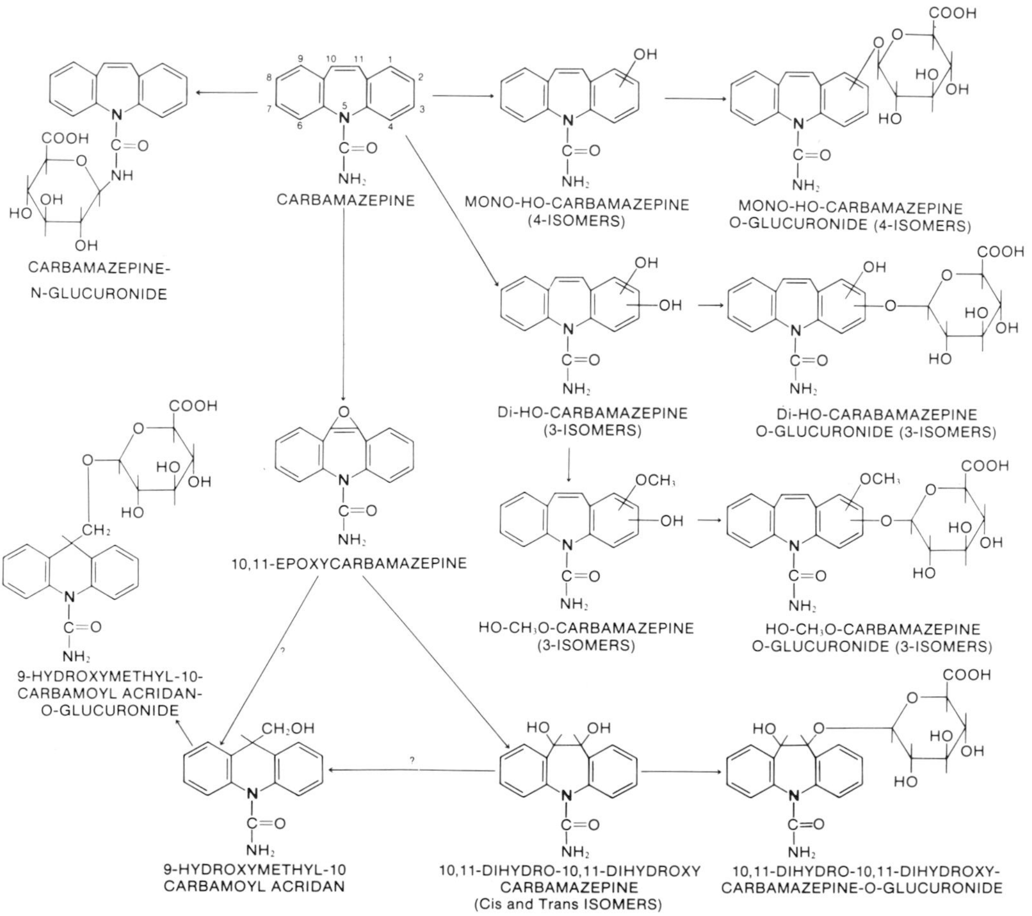

FIG. 2. Scheme of carbamazepine metabolism in man. (From Lynn et al., ref. 120, reproduced with permission. © American Society for Pharmacology and Experimental Therapeutics.)

The benzodiazepine drug lorazepam does not undergo phase I metabolism to any important extent and can be recovered predominantly as the glucuronide in the urine of man (69).

Acetylation

In acetylation reactions, amino groups situated on the drug molecule or its phase I metabolite(s) react with acetyl-CoA to form an amide bond. The reaction is catalyzed by nonmicrosomal enzymes, the activity of which may in some cases exhibit marked genetic polymorphism. Acetylation is the classic metabolic process responsible for the biotransformation of isoniazid, procainamide, hydralazine, phenelzine, dapsone, and various sulfonamide drugs. The 7-amino derivative of nitrazepam is metabolized in this way (93).

Other Conjugation Reactions

Important endogenous substrates that may serve as conjugating agents in humans include sulfate and the amino acids glycine, glutamine, and cysteine. Methylation may also be an important conjugation reaction for certain drugs. These synthetic reactions, which are generally nonmicrosomal, are not frequently involved in antiepileptic drug metabolism, and the reader is referred elsewhere for more detailed information (8,22,64,185,207).

FACTORS INFLUENCING DRUG METABOLISM

The rate at which drugs are metabolized in the body varies considerably, not only among individuals but also within the same individual under the influence of both genetic and environmental factors. The section below deals with some of the most important sources of variation in hepatic drug metabolism in man. It should be understood, however, that the same factors controlling drug metabolism in the liver may also influence the rate of drug metabolism at extrahepatic sites (113). For certain drugs, e.g., estrogens, progestagens, and chlorpromazine, the latter may actually be quantitatively more important than metabolism in the liver itself.

Genetic Factors

The role of genetic factors in controlling the rate of metabolism of drugs is best illustrated by the acetylator phenotype. In a given population, large interindividual differences are observed in the ability to acetylate isoniazid, and subjects can be classified as slow or fast inactivators depending on the rate at which they eliminate the drug. Slow acetylation is inherited as an autosomal recessive trait, and fast acetylation as an autosomal dominant trait (205), the frequency of the latter being approximately 60% in Caucasians. The metabolism of drugs that undergo predominantly oxidative biotransformation is also under genetic control (1,212) and, like the acetylator phenotype, may exhibit typical patterns of genetic polymorphism (84,195). About 9% of whites, for example, show defective oxidative metabolism of drugs such as debrisoquine, phenacetin, guanoxan, metiamide, and *p*-methoxyamphetamine (84,205). The condition is inherited as a recessive trait controlled by gene loci that have recently been shown not to be linked to those responsible for the expression of the slow acetylator phenotype (123).

Another example of a genetically transmitted defect of the mixed-function oxidase in man is provided by the "deficient *para*-hydroxylation" of phenytoin (106). In humans, phenytoin is predominantly metabolized by *para*-hydroxylation of one of the phenyl groups to yield 5-(*p*-hydroxyphenyl)-5-phenylhydantoin (*p*-HPPH), which is subsequently conjugated with glucuronic acid and excreted in urine. Kutt et al. (106) identified a patient who developed unusually high serum phenytoin concentrations and excreted abnormally low amounts of *p*-HPPH in urine while taking a "standard" dose of the drug (300 mg daily). The metabolic handling of phenobarbital and phenylalanine, which are also metabolized by *para*-hydroxylation, was normal in the same patient. Studies of phenytoin metabolism were performed in two generations of the propositus affected. Of the five individuals tested, two (the mother and one sibling) demonstrated a very low capacity of phenytoin elimination, strongly suggesting a genetic mode of inheritance for this condition.

Age

It is well recognized that the human fetus and newborn are more susceptible to adverse drug effects than the adult organism. This can be explained, at least in part, by a reduced ability to metabolize drugs during the early stages of life. Indeed, low or absent hepatic drug-metabolizing enzyme activity during fetal or neonatal life has been detected in numerous animal species including the rat, the mouse, the rabbit, the guinea pig, and the swine (41,53,89,193,194). In the phylogenic series, however, the human being is somewhat atypical in that the presence of a developed smooth endoplasmic reticulum, drug-metabolizing enzyme components, and mixed-function oxidase activity can be demonstrated at significant levels during the first part of gestation (140,168), in some cases as early as 6 weeks (79,147). The metabolizing capacity of the human fetal liver, however, appears to be restricted to only a limited number of substrates, and the relatively well-developed ability to oxidize ethylmorphine, aniline (168), testosterone (218), and other steroid compounds (97) in vitro during the first part of gestation apparently contrasts with the low or absent capacity for 3,4-benzpyrene hydroxylation, aminopyrine N-demethylation (218), glucuronide synthesis (171), and other conjugation reactions (97) in the corresponding stages of intrauterine life.

Although pharmacokinetic studies in the newborn generally demonstrate low drug-metabolizing enzyme activity, as reflected by longer elimination half-lives and/or increased serum drug levels at steady state, it remains to be established whether the impairment of drug metabolism results from incomplete maturation of the relevant enzyme systems, from the presence of endogenous competitive inhibitors, or both. With most drugs, the biotransformation rate increases gradually over a period of several weeks to several years to peak rates in childhood that

are often higher than those observed in adults. A typical example of this phenomenon is provided by the age-dependent differences in the elimination kinetics of diazepam, the apparent serum half-life of the drug varying from 75 ± 35 hr in premature newborns to 31 ± 2 hr in full-term newborns, 10 ± 2 hr in infants, 17 ± 3 hr in children, and 24 ± 12 hr in adults (134). Evidence that the slower elimination in newborns results from impaired metabolism is provided by a decreased rate of formation of both the demethylated and the hydroxylated metabolites of diazepam in this age group. Phenobarbital also shows age-dependent kinetics, its serum half-life ranging from 234 ± 43 hr in premature newborns to 146 ± 23 hr in full-term newborns, 58 ± 7 hr in infants, 38 ± 10 hr in children, and 132 ± 18 hr in adults (data from separate studies) (134).

The metabolic transformation of other antiepileptic drugs in neonates, infants, and children has been less extensively investigated. At least for phenytoin (170) and carbamazepine (169), the elimination rate of transplacentally transferred drug in full-term newborns of epileptic mothers has been reported to be similar to that in adults, suggesting induction of the neonatal metabolizing enzymes during fetal life. In infancy and childhood, the biotransformation of carbamazepine, phenytoin, and ethosuximide appears to be faster than in adult life (134, 167,175), providing an explanation for the observation that younger children (1 to 6 years of age) require larger doses of these drugs for therapeutic serum concentrations to be achieved (134).

At the other extreme of life, in old age, the rate of drug metabolism may be reduced even in the absence of any detectable pathological condition. Because of decreased hepatic elimination, for example, serum chlormethiazole levels after ordinary oral doses may be higher in the elderly than in the young (138). Serum phenytoin levels also tend to be higher in the elderly as compared with younger patients receiving equivalent doses (Fig. 3), suggesting impaired para-hydroxylation capacity with increasing age (82). In elderly patients with hy-

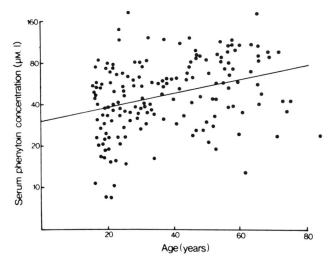

FIG. 3. Relationship between steady-state serum phenytoin concentration and age in 170 patients receiving phenytoin (300 mg daily). Multiple correlation = 0.31, $p < 0.001$. (From Houghton et al., ref. 82, reproduced with permission.)

poalbuminemia, however, the metabolic clearance of phenytoin may paradoxically be accelerated, possibly because the lower degree of plasma protein binding facilitates the uptake of the drug into the hepatic cell (77).

Sex

Very marked sex-linked differences in rate of drug metabolism are seen in laboratory animals, especially in the rat (79,95). In man, these differences are relatively minor and usually unimportant. After correction for height and body weight, serum phenytoin levels are higher in males than in females given an identical dose (82). After administration of the same dose per body weight, serum phenobarbital and primidone levels also tend to be higher in males than in females (204). Whether these findings reflect differences in drug-metabolizing activity or in other pharmacokinetic parameters is not known.

Pregnancy

A number of studies have demonstrated a progressive decline in the serum concentration of phenytoin, phenobarbital, and carbamaze-

pine during pregnancy (see ref. 36 for review). For carbamazepine, the reduction of the serum concentration of the parent drug is associated with a concomitant rise in the ratio of the 10,11-epoxide derivative to the unmetabolized drug in serum. Although changes in absorption and distribution kinetics may also occur, these findings can be explained at least in part by an increased rate of hepatic drug metabolism during pregnancy, possibly secondary to the stimulant effect of progesterone on microsomal enzyme activity (34). Indeed, proliferation of the smooth endoplasmic reticulum has been described in healthy women during the last 3 months of pregnancy (149). In addition, a progressive rise in the urinary excretion of D-glucaric acid, an indirect index of drug-metabolizing enzyme activity, has been shown to occur in normal pregnant women from the 12th week of pregnancy until delivery, with a gradual decline to normal levels by the sixth week post-partum (39).

Enzyme Saturation

The metabolism of most drugs administered in therapeutic doses *in vivo* follows first-order kinetics; i.e., the amount of substrate transformed per unit of time is proportional to the concentration of the same substrate at the biotransformation site. Once distribution in tissues has been completed, the elimination of these drugs from the body is characterized by a monoexponential decline from which the serum half-life can be determined as the time required for the serum concentration to halve. Under these conditions, the serum concentration of the drug at steady state is linearly related to the administered dose.

First-order kinetics do not apply to phenytoin metabolism. The reason for this is that the enzyme system responsible for the conversion of phenytoin to its major metabolite, p-HPPH, easily becomes saturated at serum concentrations commonly encountered in therapeutic practice. The saturable nature of phenytoin metabolism has two important practical implications.

1. The rate of elimination of the drug progressively decreases as dosage and serum concentration are increased (7,81). When the hydroxylating enzyme gradually becomes saturated, the metabolic process approaches zero-order kinetics, i.e., the rate of metabolism proceeds at a constant rate, independent of the amount of drug in the body. Under these conditions, the elimination phase is no longer linear, and the half-life can only be calculated by using particular techniques, e.g., by superimposing radioactive tracer doses on a steady concentration (81).

2. The relationship between the serum concentration and the administered dose is nonlinear, a change in dose producing a disproportionally large change in serum concentration at steady state and, thereby, in pharmacological effect (17,125,179). As illustrated in Fig. 4, the limit at which the dose–concentration relationship steepens shows considerable intersubject variability, making the effect of dose increments on the serum

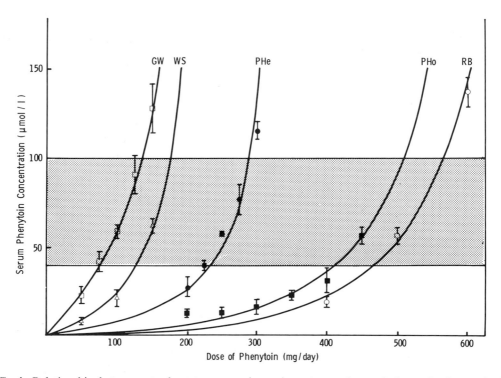

FIG. 4. Relationship between steady-state serum phenytoin concentration and phenytoin dosage in five patients studied at different dose levels. The hatched area represents the therapeutic range. (From Richens and Dunlop, ref. 179, reproduced with permission.)

concentration poorly predictable in the individual patient.

In the presence of saturable metabolism, the metabolic process follows a kinetic pattern intermediate between first-order and zero-order which can at best be described by using the classic equation of enzyme kinetics, the Michaelis–Menten equation. In its original form, the equation states that the velocity of any enzyme-catalyzed reaction (V) is related to the concentration of the substrate (S) by the relationship:

$$V = V_{max}S/(K_m + S) \qquad (1)$$

where V_{max} is the maximum rate of metabolism, and K_m a proportionality constant for that particular enzyme, defined as the concentration of substrate at which the reaction proceeds with a velocity $V = \frac{1}{2}V_{max}$. When the system operates under nonsaturable conditions, $S \ll K_m$, and equation 1 reduces to:

$$V = V_{max} S/K_m \qquad (2)$$

i.e., the velocity of the reaction is linearly related to the concentration of the substrate (first-order kinetics).

In recent years, a rearranged form of the Michaelis–Menten equation has often been used in an attempt to describe the disposition kinetics of phenytoin *in vivo*. The ultimate goal of this exercise is the prediction of the dosage adjustment required to produce a desired serum concentration. Ideally, V_{max} and K_m should be derived for each patient before treatment is begun so that the optimum dose can be calculated, but this is impractical because multiple serum concentration determinations following administration of single doses are necessary (127). Alternatively, individual K_m and V_{max} can be derived from serum drug levels at steady state. By using this approach, Ludden et al. (115,116) suggested that the Michaelis–Menten constants can be satisfactorily estimated by means of a common linear transformation of the Michaelis–Menten equation and only two dose–serum concentration points. A differently rearranged form of the equation, more recently proposed by Mullen (135), also allows calculation of individual Michaelis–Menten parameters *in vivo* when at least two (preferably three) steady-state serum concentration points are known. Once these parameters have been derived, the adjustment in dose necessary to produce a desired change in serum concentration can be easily extrapolated from a direct linear plot.

Obviously, the disadvantage of these methods is the requirement for multiple dose–serum concentration determinations beforehand. A less precise but more practical approach is provided by the use of Richens and Dunlop's nomogram (180) in its recently revised form (166) (Fig. 5). The nomogram, also based on a rearranged form of the Michaelis–Menten equation, has been constructed by using an average K_m value derived from data obtained in a large population of patients. Given a single reliable serum phenytoin concentration value, the nomogram allows prediction of the dosage adjustment necessary to achieve any other concentration. Although, on average, predicted changes in serum phenytoin concentration correlate well with those observed, the authors themselves were careful to point out that the nomogram has several limitations. It is constructed from a mean K_m value, but as K_m varies substantially from subject to subject (and also within the same subject under the influence of such factors as disease or concurrent drug therapy), the nomogram will underestimate the required change in dose in some patients and overestimate it in others.

An alternative nomogram for adjusting phenytoin dosage when a single serum concentration value is known has been proposed by Martin et al (125). In this method, a linearized transformation of the Michaelis–Menten equation is used to construct different dose–serum concentration plots within a given range of individual V_{max} and K_m values. The line providing the best possible fit for the individual data is then selected on the basis of the single serum concentration point. As with Richens and Dunlop's nomogram, predictions based on this method have only limited accuracy and can be grossly misleading if the measurement of the serum concentration is unreliable, if patient's compliance is in doubt, if the bioavailability

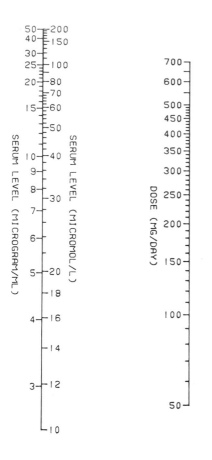

FIG. 5. Nomogram for adjusting phenytoin dosage. Given a single reliable serum concentration on a given daily dose of phenytoin, the dose required to achieve a desired serum concentration can be predicted. A line is drawn connecting the observed serum concentration (*left-hand scale*) with the dose administered (*center scale*) and extended to intersect the *right-hand vertical line*. From this point of intersection, another line is drawn back to the desired serum level (*left-hand scale*). The dose required to produce this level can be read on the *center scale*. Note: this nomogram will give misleading predictions if the serum concentration measurement is inaccurate, if the phenytoin preparation used has incomplete bioavailability, if the patient's compliance is in doubt, or if a change in concurrent treatment has been made since measurement of the serum concentration. (From Rambeck et al., ref. 166, reproduced with permission.)

of the pharmaceutical preparation of phenytoin used is incomplete, or if a change in concurrent drug therapy is made at the same time.

Perhaps the most satisfactory approach to the prediction of the correct dosage adjustment is to combine the nomogram with Mullen's direct linear plot (135) or other similar methods (115,125), using the first when only one serum concentration point is known and then moving to the latter when further data are available (125,166).

Feedback Inhibition by Metabolite Formation

Animal experiments suggest that the dose dependence of phenytoin metabolism may in fact not be caused by enzyme saturation but by feedback inhibition by the main biotransformation product of phenytoin, *p*-HPPH. *In vitro,* the addition of phenytoin at different concentrations to fortified 9,000 × *g* rat liver supernatants does not affect the rate of hydroxylation of the drug, whereas the addition of *p*-HPPH to this system inhibits hydroxylation in a competitive manner (20,65). *In vivo,* administration of salicylamide, which competitively inhibits glucuronide conjugation and thereby produces accumulation of *p*-HPPH in the organism, markedly prolongs the elimination of phenytoin in rats (111). Direct administration of *p*-HPPH to rats (6,48) and to monkeys (67) also has a dramatic inhibitory effect on phenytoin elimination.

In order to examine the possibility that product inhibition may also operate in man, we determined the total body clearance of phenytoin during an intravenous infusion of the metabolite and during a control infusion of the solvent in three healthy volunteers (155). Under these conditions, *p*-HPPH did not produce any consistent change in phenytoin elimination, suggesting that feedback inhibition does not occur in man.

Enzyme Induction

Twenty-two years ago, in the course of investigations designed to assess the mechanism responsible for the development of tolerance to barbiturates, Remmer and Alsleben (174) made the fundamental discovery that phenobarbital treatment stimulates the activity of the hepatic drug-oxidizing enzymes. In male rats, the shortening of the hexobarbital sleeping time produced by phenobarbital pretreatment was associated with a threefold increase in the oxidation rate of hexobarbital and a twofold increase in the N-demethylation rate of pethidine in the liver. It soon became clear that, in addition to phenobarbital, several other pharmacological agents, industrial contaminants, voluntary and dietary substances possess the ability to stimulate microsomal drug metabolism (3,34,40, 91,92). This phenomenon is currently referred to as enzyme induction (173). In recent years, considerable advances have been made in the understanding of enzyme induction at the molecular level. Thus, we now know that during phenobarbital treatment the hepatic microsomal cytochrome P-450 content increases severalfold in a parallel fashion to the increase in drug oxidation rate. Together with cytochrome P-450, a rise in flavoprotein 1 (fp$_1$) content is observed; there is only a slight and delayed rise in cytochrome b$_5$ content and no rise in the second flavoprotein (associated with NADH), fp$_2$ (173). These biochemical modifications are associated with striking morphological changes consisting of marked proliferation of the smooth endoplasmic reticulum and, in certain animal species, hepatic hypertrophy (50,87).

Recent evidence indicates that the mixed-function oxidase response to various enzyme-inducing agents is polymorphic, different substrates stimulating the formation of different types and/or proportions of cytochrome P-450. During treatment with phenobarbital and related compounds, most oxidative reactions catalyzed by cytochrome P-450 are accelerated, including those involving endogenous substrates such as cortisol, testosterone, and vitamin D$_3$. During treatment with carcinogenic hydrocarbons such as benzpyrene and 3-methylcholanthrene, the oxidation of barbiturates and the N-demethylation of ethylmorphine are not accelerated, although the hydroxylation rate of benzpyrene increases severalfold (173). This and additional lines of evidence suggest that polycyclic hydrocarbons induce a different type of cytochrome P-450 which does not take part in the oxidation of barbiturates and related compounds (196).

More recently, up to six different forms of cytochrome P-450 have been identified by chromatographic, immunologic, and electrophoretic techniques in the hepatic microsomes of animals exposed to various enzyme-inducing drugs (76,83,88,201,202,208).

The study of enzyme induction in laboratory animals is relatively easy because samples of hepatic tissue can be readily obtained, and microsomal cytochrome P-450 content and drug metabolizing activity can be directly estimated *in vitro*. This experimental approach, however, is only exceptionally applicable to man, and assessment of induction in this species must almost invariably rely on the measurement of indirect indices of drug-metabolizing activity *in vivo*. These methods can be classified into two categories: (a) those designed to detect changes in rate of metabolic elimination of a marker drug (e.g., antipyrine, warfarin, tolbutamide, hexobarbital, phenylbutazone) and (b) those designed to assess an increased rate of formation of endogenous substances (e.g., serum γ-glutamyltransferase activity, urinary excretion of D-glucaric acid and 6-β-hydroxycortisol). (For a review of the significance, applications, and limitations of these methods, see refs. 23 and 151.) Comparison of these indices in different animal species and in man clearly indicates the occurrence of large interspecies differences in the inductive effects of drugs. Ethosuximide, for example, is a strong enzyme inducer in the rat but appears to be completely devoid of this property in the guinea pig and in man (60). Rifampicin, on the other hand, is a potent inducing agent in man (143) but has little or no effect on microsomal enzyme activity in the rat (10).

In an extensive review published more than a decade ago, Conney (34) quotes at more than 200 the number of substances known to stimulate the hepatic microsomal enzymes in experimental animals. A review of available evidence to date, however, indicates that a definite inducing effect in man has been demonstrated for only a few of these agents (Table 1). Among these, the antiepileptic drugs carbamazepine, phenobarbital, phenytoin, and primidone stand prominently, and not only because of their very

TABLE 1. *Major enzyme-inducing agents in man*

Antipyrine (143)	Pheneturide (109)
Carbamazepine (153)	Phenobarbital and other
Chlorinated insecticides (3)	barbiturates (11,153)
Cigarette smoking (91)	Phenylbutazone (31)
Ethanol (94)	Phenytoin (153)
Glutethimide (85)	Polychlorinated biphenyls
Medroxyprogesterone	(3)
(188)	Polycyclic hydrocarbons
Meprobamate (42)	(3)
Methaqualone–diphen-	Primidone (153)
hydramine (11)	Rifampicin (143)

marked enzyme-inducing potency. Unlike most of the other agents listed in Table 1, antiepileptic drugs are usually prescribed for long periods, often in high dosage, and often in combination. It is hardly surprising, therefore, that patients treated with these drugs show evidence of the highest degree of induction ever described in humans (200), as indicated by a marked increase in hepatic cytochrome P-450 concentration (198), a marked shortening of the serum antipyrine half-life, and a massive increase of the urinary excretion of D-glucaric acid (153,154) (Fig. 6).

The clinical consequences of hepatic microsomal enzyme induction by antiepileptic drugs are considerable (151,177). Self-stimulation of metabolism (autoinduction) is most clearly observed with carbamazepine and is responsible for the progressive decline of the serum concentration at steady state and the shortening of the serum half-life of the drug a few weeks after initiation of treatment (47). Stimulation of metabolism of other concurrently administered drugs also occurs and is responsible for a number of clinically important interactions that are seen in patients treated with phenytoin, barbiturates, carbamazepine, and other enzyme-inducing drugs (152,178). Some of the best-documented examples include: decreased serum warfarin and dicoumarol concentration and reduced anticoagulant response (74,121); enhancement of metabolism, probably in the gastrointestinal tract (12) as well as in the hepatic microsomes (19), of estrogens and progestagens and reduced efficacy of the contraceptive pill (9,18,78); in-

creased rate of quinidine metabolism and decreased antidysrhythmic activity of the latter drug (38); increased elimination of prednisone (26), prednisolone (162), methylprednisolone (27), cortisol (209), dexamethasone (90), and metyrapone (128) and reduced clinical efficacy of these agents when used therapeutically (21,25–27,46,128) or diagnostically (90,129); increased presystemic elimination of alprenolol and consequent reduction of its β-blocking activity (33); increased conversion of pethidine to the more toxic metabolite norpethidine and, possibly, potentiation of the CNS adverse effects of the former drug (199); and increased conversion of paracetamol and isoniazid to toxic nucleophilic metabolites, and possibly enhancement of the hepatotoxicity of the latter drugs (131,159,161,216).

Perhaps even more important are the clinical consequences of stimulation of the metabolism of endogenous substances (see refs. 151,182 for reviews). Increased inactivation of vitamin D, for example, is likely to be implicated in the pathogenesis of anticonvulsant rickets and osteomalacia (13,108,181). Induction of sex hormone metabolism may provide an explanation for the development of certain endocrine abnormalities in epileptic patients, such as acne, hirsutism, and irregularities of the menstrual cycle in females (151) and reduced libido, potency, and fertility in males (32,117). Additional examples of clinical or biochemical abnormalities possibly related to enzyme induction include: modifications of triglyceride, cholesterol, and lipoprotein metabolism (43,44, 118,119,126,130,141), folate deficiency (108), precipitation of attacks of acute intermittent porphyrias (151), increased bile flow (96), increased γ-glutamyltransferase activity in serum (211), and reduced serum bilirubin levels (203). A relatively good correlation ($r = 0.635$, $p < 0.01$) between antipyrine half-life and serum unconjugated bilirubin concentration has recently been described in a large group of subjects that included drug-treated epileptic patients and normal controls (191). The authors went as far as to suggest that a single measurement of unconjugated bilirubin concentration in

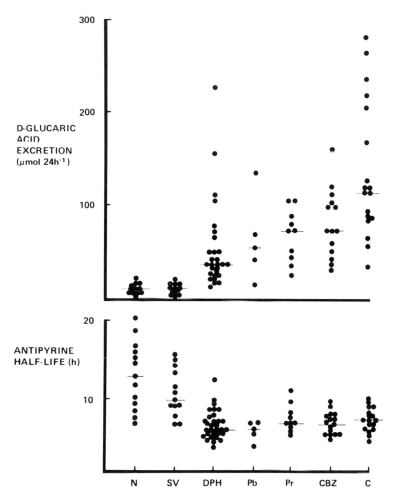

FIG. 6. Serum antipyrine half-life and urinary excretion of D-glucaric acid (as lactone) in normal drug-free control subjects (N) and in patients receiving chronic therapy with antiepileptic drugs, alone or in combination: SV, sodium valproate; DPH, phenytoin; Pb, phenobarbital; Pr, primidone; CBZ, carbamazepine; and C, combination therapy. Note the marked shortening of the antipyrine half-life and the increase in urinary excretion of D-glucaric acid in patients treated with drugs other than sodium valproate.

serum under fasting conditions could be used as an index of enzyme induction.

Enzyme Inhibition

Competitive inhibition among different substrates for the microsomal drug-metabolizing enzymes can be readily demonstrated *in vitro*. *In vivo,* inhibition of metabolism is less common, mainly because the concentrations of drugs achieved in the hepatic microsomes are usually well below those required to saturate the enzyme system, and competition is minimized under these conditions (52). Not surprisingly, many of the best-known examples of interactions resulting in inhibition of metabolism *in vivo* involve those drugs that exhibit saturation kinetics at therapeutic dosages, e.g., dicoumarol (100) and phenytoin (178). The list of drugs known to inhibit phenytoin metabolism in the clinical situation is particularly impressive and includes, besides dicoumarol, phencoupromon,

disulfiram, sulthiame, pheneturide, methsuximide, imipramine, chlorpromazine, methyl-
phenydate, phenyramidol, chlorpheniramine,
propoxyphene, phenylbutazone, chloramphenicol, isoniazid, trimethoprim, and various sulfonamide drugs (152,178). When any of these
agents is administered to patients receiving
chronic therapy with phenytoin, the elimination
of phenytoin may be delayed, and its concentration in serum may rise. Moreover, because
of the saturable nature of phenytoin metabolism, even a moderate degree of enzyme inhibition can result in a disproportionate increase
in the serum concentration at steady state, and
clinical intoxication is particularly likely to occur in these conditions.

From the clinical point of view, enzyme inhibition is potentially more dangerous than enzyme induction because it tends to occur more
rapidly, usually within a few days as opposed
to several days for enzyme induction. In the
case of the inhibition of phenytoin metabolism
by sulthiame, however, a period of 10 to 20
days generally elapses before the interaction may
become manifest after the start of sulthiame
administration, suggesting that a noncompetitive type of inhibition may be operating. Because of this delay, the interaction may not be
readily recognized, and the appropriate adjustments of phenytoin dosage may not be made,
resulting in a disproportionately high incidence
of cases of phenytoin intoxication in patients
receiving sulthiame in combination (80).

Another important interaction occurs between phenytoin and isoniazid (Fig. 7). In the
early 1960s, many physicians used to comment
on the unusual sensitivity of tuberculotic patients to the toxic effects of phenytoin. The possibility of a drug interaction was first considered
when Murray (136) reported the occurrence of
marked drowsiness and unsteadiness of gait in
70 out of 637 institutionalized epileptic patients
who were given isoniazid for prophylaxis against
tuberculosis. It is now known that isoniazid is
one of the most powerful inhibitors of phenytoin metabolism (104). This interaction is of
particular theoretical interest because isoniazid,
unlike phenytoin, is not mainly metabolized by
mixed-function oxidase. *In vivo,* inhibition of

phenytoin metabolism by isoniazid occurs only
in slow acetylators, probably because only these
subjects achieve hepatic concentrations of isoniazid sufficiently high to interfere with phenytoin hydroxylation (104). *In vitro,* and possibly *in vivo,* the inhibition is potentiated by *p*-
aminosalicylic acid (PAS) which is frequently
associated with isoniazid in the treatment of tuberculosis (105).

The metabolism of antiepileptic drugs other
than phenytoin appears to be less susceptible to
being inhibited by other drugs (see refs. 152,
178 for reviews). Methsuximide, sulthiame,
valproic acid, chloramphenicol, dicoumarol, and
methylphenidate have all been shown to elevate
serum phenobarbital concentrations in some patients, presumably by inhibiting the hepatic hydroxylation of the latter drug (152). A particularly important interaction occurs between
carbamazepine and propoxyphene. Drowsiness,
dizziness, headache, and other adverse effects
developed in five out of seven patients with epilepsy or trigeminal neuralgia who were given
propoxyphene hydrochloride, 65 mg t.d.s. for
2 to 7 days (37). The effect was associated in
all patients with a marked rise of the serum
carbamazepine concentration, probably because
of inhibition of carbamazepine metabolism, as
suggested by a concurrent increase of the concentration ratio of carbamazepine to its 10,11-
epoxide in serum. This interpretation is supported by the results of a recent study in which
propoxyphene was shown to inhibit the monooxygenase system *in vitro* in a similar manner
to SKF 525-A, the classic powerful enzyme inhibitor, which it resembles chemically (163). In
the same study, the metabolite norpropoxy-
phene was also shown to be a potent inhibitor
of hepatic oxidative drug metabolism. Like SKF
525-A and many other drugs, propoxyphene is
a potent inhibitor when given acutely and an
inducer when given chronically. The ability of
a given compound to act as an inhibitor and an
inducer at the same time provides an explanation for the apparently inconsistent and contradictory nature of certain drug interactions.
Thus, phenobarbital may either decrease or increase the serum concentration of phenytoin depending on whether stimulation or inhibition of

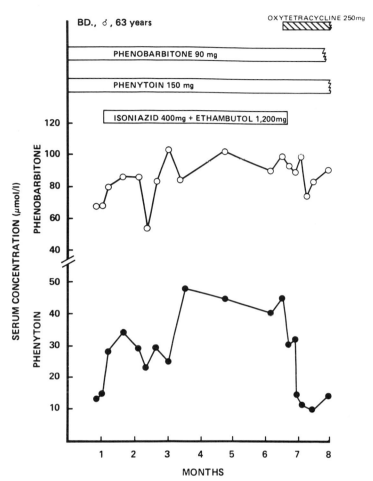

FIG. 7. The effect of subchronic treatment with isoniazid–ethambutol on the serum phenytoin and pheno-barbital concentration in a 63-year-old institutionalized epileptic patient. Note the marked increase in serum phenytoin concentration during antituberculosis therapy. (From Perucca and Richens, ref. 157, reproduced with permission.)

phenytoin metabolism prevails in the individual patient (103). Phenytoin, a potent inducer, may decrease the serum concentration and the phar macological effect of dicoumarol (74) but may also potentiate the anticoagulant action of war-farin, presumably by inhibiting the metabolic elimination of the latter drug (137).

Restrictive Elimination

The majority of the factors considered so far influence the rate of drug metabolism in the body by affecting the activity of the hepatic drug-metabolizing enzymes. The latter effects can usually be readily reproduced or demonstrated *in vitro;* indeed, hepatic microsomal enzymes systems are increasingly used in drug metabolism studies. Obviously, it would be advantageous if data obtained *in vitro* could also be used to predict parameters of drug metabolism and disposition *in vivo*. Unfortunately, this is not simple, nor is it always possible, for at least two reasons:

1. Drug-metabolizing enzymes exist not only in the liver but also in many other organs and tissues.

2. Even for drugs that are metabolized entirely by the liver, the rate of metabolism is dependent not only on the activity of the drug-metabolizing enzymes but also on other factors such as hepatic size, binding of the drug to plasma and red cell constituents, delivery of substrate by blood flow to the organ, and anatomical arrangement of the hepatic vasculature.

The efficiency of any organ in removing a drug from the perfusing blood *in vivo* is best provided by the term "clearance," defined as the volume of blood from which the drug is cleared per unit of time (214). When a drug is eliminated entirely through biotransformation in the liver, the total blood clearance equals the hepatic metabolic clearance (Cl_H) which can be defined as (214):

$$Cl_H = Q \cdot E \qquad (3)$$

where Q is the hepatic blood flow and E is the extraction ratio of the drug across the organ. The hepatic extraction ratio E is a very useful parameter in predicting the relative contribution of enzymic and nonenzymic factors to the rate of metabolism *in vivo*. In the case of highly extracted compounds ($E > 80\%$), the activity of the metabolizing enzymes is so high that almost all of the drug, whether bound or unbound in the blood, is removed. For these drugs (e.g., lidocaine, propranolol), the metabolic clearance is primarily dependent on the rate of hepatic blood flow and is relatively insensitive to changes in activity of the drug-metabolizing enzymes (see below).

The situation is entirely different for drugs characterized by a low extraction ratio ($E < 20\%$). Drugs with a low extraction ratio (e.g., warfarin, phenytoin, valproic acid) are those that the liver has difficulty in clearing, either because they are poor substrates for the enzyme or because their access to the site of metabolism is limited by low diffusibility across biological membranes (146). For these drugs, clearance is largely determined by changes in enzymatic activity as may occur during induc-

tion or inhibition and is virtually independent of the rate of hepatic blood flow. The removal of these drugs from the circulation is always limited to their fraction unbound in blood, which in turn determines drug availability at the metabolic site. Under these conditions, restrictive elimination applies; i.e., the clearance of total drug is positively correlated with the fraction unbound in blood (112,158,192). The latter, in turn, is by no means constant. For many drugs, the fraction unbound in plasma increases as the drug concentration in plasma increases because of partial saturation of plasma protein binding sites. In the presence of restrictive elimination, the metabolic clearance of these drugs will also increase accordingly, the overall effect being a progressive flattening of the total drug concentration–dosage relationship, whereas the relationship between dosage and free drug concentration remains linear throughout. Examples of drugs showing this type of restrictive, dose-dependent elimination include naproxen (186, 187), clofibrate (72), quinidine (55), and valproic acid (68,73). Impairment of plasma protein binding secondary to genetic factors, disease, or concomitant administration of other chemicals that act like competitive displacing agents also results in increased total drug clearance (35,217). The very marked increase of phenytoin clearance in elderly (77) and uremic patients (110,142) with hypoalbuminemia is likely to result at least in part from reduced plasma protein binding of phenytoin in these conditions. Moreover, increased clearance of total phenytoin has recently been demonstrated in normal subjects following displacement of the drug from plasma proteins by salicylic acid (54). Valproic acid has also been shown to displace phenytoin from plasma protein binding sites (133). In a recent study, administration of sodium valproate (1,200 mg daily for 7 days) to seven normal volunteers resulted in an approximate 50% increase of the unbound fraction of phenytoin in plasma; the metabolic clearance of total phenytoin also increased, whereas the clearance of free (unbound) phenytoin was reduced, possibly due to concurrent inhibition of the metabolism of this drug (56,57).

Flow-Dependent Elimination and First-Pass Effect

As discussed above, the metabolic clearance of drugs subject to high hepatic extraction is primarily determined by the rate of delivery of the drug to the organ (hepatic blood flow) and is little influenced by changes in drug-metabolizing activity of the enzymes (146,214). For these drugs, binding to plasma proteins, by increasing the rate of transport of the drug to the liver, may actually enhance rather than restrict the elimination process.

As a result of the high hepatic extraction ratio, these compounds undergo extensive presystemic (first-pass) metabolism in the liver before reaching the systemic circulation after being absorbed from the gastrointestinal tract (184). When administered by the oral route, the whole dose absorbed is presented to the liver; under these circumstances, the amount of the drug metabolized during the first passage through the organ is no longer limited by plasma protein binding or rate of hepatic blood flow, but it directly reflects the activity of the drug-metabolizing enzymes (150,214). When the latter are reduced, such as occurs in the presence of inhibitors, in old age, or in hepatic disease, the fraction of the dose that escapes presystemic elimination may be greatly increased. This mechanism is probably responsible for the 10-fold increase of the oral availability of chlormethiazole in patients with cirrhosis of the liver (148). Conversely, in patients with increased drug-metabolizing capacity, e.g., epileptic patients treated with phenytoin and barbiturates, the oral availability of the same drugs may be reduced. This has indeed been shown to be true in the case of alprenolol (2), lidocaine (160) (Fig. 8), metyrapone (128), and paracetamol (159).

Saturation of first-pass metabolism is frequently observed with drugs that are subject to high hepatic extraction ratios. This can result in disproportionate and potentially hazardous increases in plasma concentrations after relatively small increments in dosage (86).

Disease

Hepatic Disease

The effect of liver disease on the hepatic metabolism of drugs is complex. On one hand, reduction of drug-metabolizing enzyme activity through hepatocellular damage (197) and disruption of hepatic vascular architecture, by reducing drug availability at the site of metabolism (213) tend to decrease the metabolic capacity of the organ. On the other hand, in the case of highly albumin-bound drugs characterized by restrictive elimination (see Chapter 2), the latter effects may be counterbalanced by a concomitant reduction in the degree of plasma protein binding, which increases the amount of free drug available for metabolism in the liver (15). Which of these opposing mechanisms will predominate

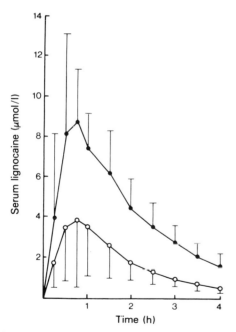

FIG. 8. Serum lignocaine (lidocaine) concentration (mean ± S.D.) after oral administration of lidocaine hydrochloride monohydrate (750 mg) in six normal subjects (*solid circles*) and in six epileptic patients (*open circles*). $P < 0.05$ at all sampling times except 0.25 and 0.5 hr. (1 μmole/liter = 0.23 μg/ml). (From Perucca and Richens, ref. 160, with permission.)

depends on a combination of factors such as the type and the severity of hepatic disease, the degree of hypoalbuminemia, the age of the patient, and the pharmacokinetic properties, dosage, and route of administration of the administered drug (213). With diazepam, available evidence seems to indicate the occurrence of moderate to severe impairment of metabolic elimination in patients with liver disease. In a controlled study in which only age-matched and drug-free subjects were used, the half-life of diazepam was found to be 106 ± 15 hr in patients with cirrhosis compared with 46 ± 14 hr in controls, and 75 ± 28 h in patients with acute viral hepatitis compared with 33 ± 9 hr in controls (98). In patients with hepatic cirrhosis, the metabolic clearance of phenobarbital was also reduced, as suggested by an approximate 50% increase in the elimination half-life and a significantly reduced excretion of its hydroxy-metabolite derivatives in urine (4). In the cases of valproic acid (99) and phenytoin (16), however, the opposing mechanisms, decreased drug-metabolizing capacity and increased unbound drug available for metabolism, appear to balance each other, and no significant change in the metabolic elimination of these drugs was seen in the patients with hepatic disease included in these studies.

A 10-fold increase in the oral availability of chlormethiazole has been reported in patients with hepatic cirrhosis, presumably because of impaired presystemic metabolism of the latter drug (148). Chlormethiazole belongs to the group of drugs that show flow-dependent, nonrestrictive elimination, and no compensatory increase in clearance can occur for these drugs when albumin binding is reduced.

Renal Disease

The metabolic elimination of phenytoin (110) and many other drugs (172) is increased in uremia. At least for phenytoin, the effect cannot be entirely explained by a reduction in the degree of drug plasma protein binding. Odar-Cederlöf and Borgå (142) postulated induction of metabolism in the uremic state.

DRUG METABOLISM: THERAPEUTIC IMPLICATIONS

It is well known that in patients with impaired renal function the dosage of drugs that are excreted unchanged in urine must be individualized on the basis of the glomerular filtration rate. For drugs that are eliminated through biotransformation, the dosage also needs to be individualized to take into account the marked interindividual differences in drug metabolism. As a general rule, patients with reduced drug-metabolizing capacity are more likely to develop signs of toxicity when given "standard" doses of a drug and require doses lower than usual for a satisfactory therapeutic effect to be achieved. Most slow metabolizers of phenytoin, for example, will develop marked ataxia when stabilized on an average (300 mg) dose of the drug, whereas an occasional fast metabolizer will tolerate twice as much without any untoward effect. The clinical usefulness of monitoring the serum phenytoin concentration and the need for careful individualization of dosage are evident under these circumstances.

The situation is more complex when a drug is converted to active metabolites. In this case, the relative contribution of the metabolite to the overall biological effect will depend on a combination of factors such as the relative potency and rate of elimination of the metabolite itself, the duration of treatment, and the route of administration of the parent drug. For primidone, for example, there is considerable evidence that much of the antiepileptic efficacy observed during prolonged treatment is in fact mediated by its conversion into phenobarbital (144). Under these circumstances, an increase in the rate of primidone metabolism, such as may occur during concomitant administration of phenytoin (176), can actually result in enhancement rather than in reduction of the therapeutic effect. Since phenobarbital accumulates slowly in the body, the full pharmacological effect of primidone may not become manifest until 2 or 3 weeks after a change in dosage, even though the serum concentration of the parent compound reaches steady state in less than

3 days. Other antiepileptic drugs, apart from primidone, that are wholly or partly active through metabolite formation include carbamazepine (14), chloral hydrate (75), diazepam (124), methylphenobarbital (30), troxidone (30), and, possibly, sodium valproate (183). In some cases, metabolites may show toxicological properties not apparently shared by the parent compound. Toxic metabolites rather than the parent drug are probably responsible for the development of the acute liver necrosis observed during isoniazid therapy or after paracetamol overdose (132). Experimental and clinical evidence indicates that the hepatotoxic effect of these agents can be potentiated by concomitant treatment with enzyme-inducing drugs (156, 161,216).

CONCLUSION

The examples presented above clearly illustrate the importance of drug metabolism in the modulation of drug response. Yet, it is alarming how little is known about the metabolic fate of many widely used drugs and the pharmacological and toxicological implications of the reactions involved. No doubt, improved understanding of biotransformation processes will result not only in better new drugs for the future but also in safer and more effective ways of using those that we already have.

REFERENCES

1. Alexanderson, B. (1973): Prediction of steady state plasma levels of nortriptyline from single oral dose kinetics: A study in twins. *Eur. J. Clin. Pharmacol.*, 6:44–53.
2. Alvan, G., Piafski, K., Lind, M., and Von Bahr, C. (1977): Effect of pentobarbital on the disposition of alprenolol. *Clin. Pharmacol. Ther.*, 22:316–321.
3. Alvares, A. P. (1978): Interactions between environmental chemicals and drug biotransformation in man. *Clin. Pharmacokinet.*, 3:462–477.
4. Alvin, J., McHorse, T. S., Hoyumpa, A., Bush, M. T., and Schenker, S. (1975): The effect of liver disease in man on the disposition of phenobarbital. *J. Pharmacol. Exp. Ther.*, 192:224–235.
5. Ames, B. N., Sims, P., and Grover, P. L. (1972): Epoxides of carcinogenic polycyclic hydrocarbons are frameshift mutagens. *Science*, 176:47–49.
6. Ashley, J. J., and Levy, G. (1972): Inhibition of diphenylhydantoin elimination by its major metab-

7. olite. *Res. Commun. Chem. Pathol. Pharmacol.*, 4:297–306.
8. Atkinson, A. J., and Shaw, J. W. (1973): Pharmacokinetic study of a patient with diphenylhydantoin toxicity. *Clin. Pharmacol. Ther.*, 14:521–528.
9. Axelrod, J. (1971): Methyltransferase enzymes of physiologically active compounds and drugs. In: *Concepts in Biochemical Pharmacology, Vol. 28*, edited by B. B. Brodie and J. R. Gillette, pp. 609–619. Springer-Verlag, Berlin.
10. Back, D. J., Breckenridge, A. M., Crawford, F., McIver, M., Orme, M. l'E., Park, B. K., Rowe, P. H., and Smith, E. (1979): The effect of rifampicin on norethisterone pharmacokinetics. *Eur. J. Clin. Pharmacol.*, 15:193–197.
11. Back, D. J., Cross, K. J., Hiley, C. R., and Yates, M. S. (1979): The effect of rifampicin on liver blood flow, microsomal enzyme activity and bile flow in the rat. *Biochem. Pharmacol.*, 28:1293–1297.
12. Ballinger, B., Browning, M., O'Malley, K., and Stevenson, I. H. (1972): Drug metabolizing capacity in states of drug dependence and withdrawal. *Br. J. Pharmacol.*, 45:638–643.
13. Barber, H. E., Dawod, S. H., and Hawksworth, G. M. (1979): *Unpublished data.*
14. Bell, R. D., Pak, C. Y. C., Zewekh, J., Barilla, D. E., and Vasko, M. (1979): Effect of phenytoin on bone and vitamin D metabolism. *Ann. Neurol.*, 5:374–378.
15. Bertilsson, L. (1978): Clinical pharmacokinetics of carbamazepine. *Clin. Pharmacokinet.*, 3:128–143.
16. Blaschke, T. F. (1977): Protein binding and kinetic of drugs in liver diseases. *Clin. Pharmacokin.*, 2:32–44.
17. Blaschke, T. F., Meffin, P. J., Melmon, K. L., and Rowland, M. (1975): Influence of acute viral hepatitis on phenytoin kinetics and plasma protein binding. *Clin. Pharmacol. Ther.*, 17:685–691.
18. Bochner, F., Hooper, W. S., Tyrer, J. H., and Eadie, M. J. (1972): Effect of dosage increments on blood phenytoin concentrations. *J. Neurol. Neurosurg. Psychiatry*, 35:873–876.
19. Bolt, H. M., Bolt, M., and Kappus, H. (1977): Interaction of rifampicin treatment with pharmacokinetics and metabolism of ethinyloestradiol in man. *Acta Endocrinol. (Kbh.)*, 85:189–197.
20. Bolt, H. M., Kappus, H., and Bolt, M. (1975): The effect of rifampicin treatment on the metabolism of oestradiol by human liver microsomes. *Eur. J. Clin. Pharmacol.*, 8:301–307.
21. Borondy, P., Chang, T., and Glazko, A. J. (1972): Inhibition of diphenylhydantoin hydroxylation by 5-(p-hydroxyphenyl)-5-phenylhydantoin. *Fed. Proc.*, 31:582.
22. Bouchard, P., Kuttenn, F., Nahoul, K., Mavier, P., Schaison, G., and Mauvais-Jarvis, P. (1979): Déviation du métabolisme du cortisol induite par la rifampicine: Conséquences thérapeutiques au cours de l'insuffisance surrénalienne. *Nouv. Presse Med.*, 8:1651–1654.
23. Boyland, E. (1971): Mercapturic acid conjugation. In: *Concepts in Biochemical Pharmacology, Vol. 28*, edited by B. B. Brodie and J. R. Gillette, pp. 584–608. Springer-Verlag, Berlin.

23. Breckenridge, A. (1975): Clinical implications of enzyme-induction. In: *Enzyme Induction,* edited by D. V. Parke, pp. 273–301. Plenum Press, New York, London.

24. Brodie, B. B., Reid, W. D., Cho, A. K., Sipes, G., Krishna, G., and Gillette, J. R. (1971): Possible mechanism of liver necrosis caused by aromatic organic compounds. *Proc. Natl. Acad. Sci. U.S.A.,* 68:160–164.

25. Brooks, P. S., Buchanan, W. W., Grove, M., and Downie, W. W. (1976): Effects of enzyme induction on metabolism of prednisolone. Clinical and laboratory study. *Ann. Rheum. Dis.,* 35:339–343.

26. Brooks, S. M., Werk, E. E., Ackerman, S. J., Sullivan, I., and Thrasher, K. (1972): Adverse effect of phenobarbital on corticosteroid metabolism in patients with bronchial asthma. *N. Engl. J. Med.,* 286:1123–1128.

27. Buffington, G. A., Dominquez, J. H., Piering, W. F., Hebert, L. A., Kauffman, H. M., and Lennann, J. (1976): Interaction of rifampicin and glucocorticoids: Adverse effect on renal allograft function. *J.A.M.A.,* 236:1958–1960.

28. Butler, T. C. (1948): The metabolic fate of chloral hydrate. *J. Pharmacol. Exp. Ther.,* 92:49–58.

29. Butler, T. C., and Poole, D. T. (1975): Demethylation of trimethadione and metharbital by rat liver microsomal enzymes. *Biochem. Pharmacol.,* 14:937–942.

30. Butler, T. C., and Waddell, W. J. (1958): *N*-Methylated derivates of barbituric acid, hydantoin and oxazolidindione used in the treatment of epilepsy. *Neurology (Minneap.),* 8(Suppl. 1):106–112.

31. Chen, W., Vrindten, P. A., Dayton, P. G., and Burns, J. J. (1962): Accelerated aminopyrine metabolism in human subjects pretreated with phenylbutazone. *Life Sci.,* 1:35–42.

32. Christiansen, C., Deigaard, J., and Lund, M. (1975): Potens, fertilitet og kønshormon-udskillelse hos yngre mandlige epilepsilidende. *Ugeskr. Laeger.,* 137:2402–2405.

33. Collste, P., Seideman, P., Borg, K.-O., Haglund, K., and Von Bahr, C. (1979): Influence of pentobarbital on effect and plasma levels of alprenolol and 4-hydroxy-alprenolol. *Clin. Pharmacol. Ther.,* 25:423–427.

34. Conney, A. H. (1967): Pharmacological implication of microsomal enzyme induction. *Pharmacol. Rev.,* 19:317–366.

35. Crouthamel, W. G., and Cenedella, R. J. (1975): Clofibrate pharmacokinetics: Effect of elevation of plasma free fatty acids. *Pharmacology,* 13:465–473.

36. Dam, M., Christiansen, J., Munck, O., and Mygind, K. I. (1979): Antiepileptic drug metabolism in pregnancy. *Clin. Pharmacokinet.,* 4:53–62.

37. Dam, M., Kristensen, C. B., Hansen, B. S., and Christiansen, J. (1977): Interaction between carbamazepine and propoxyphene in man. *Acta Neurol. Scand.,* 56:633–697.

38. Data, J. L., Wilkinson, G. R., and Nies, A. S. (1976): Interaction of quinidine with anticonvulsant drugs. *N. Engl. J. Med.,* 294:699–702.

39. Davis, M., Simmons, C. J., Dordoni, B., Maxwell, I. D., and Williams, R. (1973): Induction of hepatic enzymes during normal human pregnancy. *Br. J. Obst. Gynaecol.,* 80:690–694.

40. Dollery, C. T., Fraser, H. S., Mucklow, J. C., and Bulpritt, C. J. (1979): Contribution of environmental factors to variability in human drug metabolism. *Drug Metab. Rev.,* 9:221–236.

41. Done, A. K. (1964): Developmental pharmacology. *Clin. Pharmacol. Ther.,* 5:432–479.

42. Douglas, J. F., Ludwig, B. J., and Smith, N. (1963): Studies on the metabolism of meprobamate. *Proc. Soc. Exp. Biol. Med.,* 112:436–438.

43. Durrington, P. N. (1979): Effect of phenobarbitone on plasma lipoprotein B and plasma high-density lipoprotein cholesterol in normal subjects. *Clin. Sci. Mol. Med.,* 56:501–504.

44. Durrington, P. N., Roberts, C. J. C., Jackson, L., Branch, R. A., and Hartog, M. (1976): Effect of phenobarbitone on plasma lipids in normal subjects. *Clin. Sci. Mol. Med.,* 50:349–353.

45. Dutton, G. J. (1971): Glucuronide-forming enzymes. In: *Concepts in Biochemical Pharmacology, Vol. 28,* edited by B. B. Brodie and J. R. Gillette, pp. 378–400. Springer-Verlag, Berlin.

46. Edwards, O. M., Courtenay-Evans, R. J., Galley, J. M., Hunter, J., and Tait, A. D. (1974): Changes in cortisol metabolism following rifampicin therapy. *Lancet,* 2:549–551.

47. Eichelbaum, M., Ekbom, M., Bertilsson, R., Ringberger, V.-A., and Rane, A. (1975): Plasma kinetics of carbamazepine and its epoxide metabolite in man during single and multiple dosing. *Eur. J. Clin. Pharmacol.,* 8:337–341.

48. El Hawari, A. M., and Plaa, G. L. (1978): Role of the enterohepatic circulation in the elimination of phenytoin in the rat. *Drug. Metab. Dispos.,* 6:59–69.

49. Estabrook, R. W., Franklin, M. R., Cohen, B., Shigamatzu, A., and Hildebrandt, A. G. (1971): Influence of hepatic microsomal mixed function oxidation reactions on cellular metabolic control. *Metabolism,* 20:187–199.

50. Feinman, L., Rubin, E., and Lieber, C. S. (1972): Adaptation of the liver to drugs. In: *Liver and Drugs,* edited by F. Orlandi and A.-M. Jezequel, pp. 41–83. Academic Press, London.

51. Ferrandes, B., and Eymard, P. (1977): Metabolism of sodium valproate in rabbit, rat, dog and man. *Epilepsia,* 18:169–182.

52. Fingl, E., and Woodbury, D. M. (1975): General principles. In: *The Pharmacological Basis of Therapeutics,* edited by L. S. Goodman and A. Gilman, pp. 1–46. Macmillan, New York.

53. Fouts, J. R., and Adamson, R. H. (1959): Drug metabolism in the newborn rabbit. *Science,* 129:897–898.

54. Fraser, D. G., Ludden, T., Evens, R. P., and Sutherland, E. W. III. (1979): *In vivo* displacement of phenytoin from plasma proteins with salicylate. *Clin. Pharmacol. Ther.,* 25:226.

55. Fremstad, D., Nilsen, O. G., Storstein, L., Amlie, J., and Jacobsen, S. (1979): Pharmacokinetics of quinidine related to plasma protein binding in man. *Eur. J. Clin. Pharmacol.,* 15:187–192.

56. Frigo, G. M., Gatti, G., Lecchini, S., Hebdige, S.,

Perucca, E., and Crema, A. (1980): Interaction between phenytoin and valproic acid: Plasma protein binding and metabolic effects. *Clin. Pharmacol. Ther.*, 28:779–789.

57. Frigo, G. M., Lecchini, S., Gatti, G., Perucca, E., and Crema, A. (1979): Modification of phenytoin clearance by valproic acid in normal subjects. *Brit. J. Clin. Pharmacol.*, 8:53–56.

58. Gallagher, B. B., Baumel, I. P., and Mattson, R. H. (1972): Metabolic disposition of primidone and its metabolites in epileptic subjects after single and repeated administration. *Neurology (Minneap.)*, 22:1186–1192.

59. Gerber, N., Thompson, R. M., Smith, R. G., and Lynn, R. K. (1979): Evidence for the epoxide–diol pathway in the biotransformation of mephenytoin. *Epilepsia*, 20:287–294.

60. Gilbert, J. C., Scott, A. K., Galloway, D. B., and Petrie, J. C. (1974): Ethosuximide: Liver enzyme induction and D-glucaric acid excretion. *Brit. J. Clin. Pharmacol.*, 1:249–252.

61. Gillette, J. R. (1966): Biochemistry of drug oxidation and reduction by enzymes in hepatic endoplasmic reticulum. *Adv. Pharmacol.*, 4:219–261.

62. Gillette, J. R. (1971): Reductive enzymes. In: *Concepts in Biochemical Pharmacology, Vol. 28*, edited by B. B. Brodie and J. R. Gillette, pp. 349–361. Springer-Verlag, Berlin.

63. Gillette, J. R., Davis, D. C., and Sasame, H. A. (1972): Cytochrome P-450 and its role in drug metabolism. *Ann. Rev. Pharmacol.*, 12:57–84.

64. Glauser, S. C. (1974): Drug metabolism: Conjugation and multiple pathways. *Med. Clin. North Am.*, 58:945–949.

65. Glazko, A. J. (1972): Diphenylhydantoin. *Pharmacology*, 8:163–177.

66. Glazko, A. J. (1973): Diphenylhydantoin metabolism. A prospective review. *Drug. Metab. Dispos.*, 1:711–714.

67. Glazko, A. J., Chang, T., Maschewske, E., Hayes, A., and Dill, W. A. (1976): *Unpublished data.*

68. Gram, L., Flachs, H., Würtz-Jørgensen, A., Parnas, J., and Andersen, B. (1979): Sodium valproate, serum level and clinical effect in epilepsy: A controlled study. *Epilepsia*, 20:303–312.

69. Greenblatt, D. J., Schillings, R. T., Kyriakopoulos, A. A., Shader, R. I., Sisenwine, S. F., Knowles, J. A., and Ruelius, H. W. (1979): Clinical pharmacokinetics of lorazepam. 1. Absorption and disposition of oral ^{14}C-lorazepam. *Clin. Pharmacol. Ther.*, 20:239–247.

70. Grover, P. L., Sims, P., Huberman, E., Marquardt, H., Kuroki, T., and Heidelberger, C. (1971): *In vitro* transformation of rodent cells by K-region derivatives of polycyclic hydrocarbons. *Proc. Natl. Acad. Sci. U.S.A.*, 68:1089–1101.

71. Guengerich, F. P. (1979): Isolation and purification of cytochrome P-450, and the existence of multiple forms. *Pharmacol. Ther.*, 6:99–121.

72. Gugler, R., and Hartlapp, J. (1978): Clofibrate kinetics after single and multiple doses. *Clin. Pharmacol. Ther.*, 24:432–438.

73. Gugler, R., Schell, A., Eichelbaum, M., Fröscher, W., and Schülz, H.-V. (1977): Disposition of valproic acid in man. *Eur. J. Clin. Pharmacol.*, 12:125–132.

74. Hansen, J. M., Siersbaek-Nielsen, K., Kristensen, M., Skovsted, L., and Christensen, L. K. (1971): Effect of diphenylhydantoin on the metabolism of dicoumarol in man. *Acta Med. Scand.*, 189:15–19.

75. Harvey, S. C. (1955): Hypnotics and sedatives. In: *The Pharmacological Basis of Therapeutics,* edited by L. S. Goodman and A. Gilman, pp. 124–136. Macmillan, New York.

76. Haugen, D. A., and Coon, M. J. (1976): Properties of electrophoretically homogeneous phenobarbital-inducible and β-naphthoflavone-inducible forms of liver microsomal cytochrome P-450. *J. Biol. Chem.*, 251:7929–7939.

77. Hayes, M. J., Langman, M. J. S., and Short, A. H. (1975): Changes in drug metabolism with increasing age. Phenytoin clearance and protein binding. *Br. J. Clin. Pharmacol.*, 73–79.

78. Hempel, A., and Klinger, W. (1976): Drug-stimulated biotransformation of hormonal steroid contraceptives: Clinical implications. *Drugs*, 12:442–448.

79. Henderson, P. T. (1978): Development and maturation of drug-metabolizing enzymes. *Eur. J. Drug Metab. Pharmacokinet.*, 1:1–14.

80. Houghton, G. W., and Richens, A. (1974): Phenytoin intoxication induced by sulthiame in epileptic patients. *J. Neurol. Neurosurg. Psychiatry*, 37:275–281.

81. Houghton, G. W., and Richens, A. (1974): Rate of elimination of tracer doses of phenytoin at different steady-state serum concentration in epileptic patients. *Br. J. Clin. Pharmacol.*, 1:155–161.

82. Houghton, G. W., Richens, A., and Leighton, M. (1975): Effect of age, height, weight and sex on serum phenytoin concentration in epileptic patients. *Br. J. Clin. Pharmacol.*, 2:251–256.

83. Huang, M. T., West, S. B., and Lu, A. Y. H. (1976): Separation, purification, and properties of multiple forms of cytochrome P-450 from the liver microsomes of phenobarbital-treated mice. *J. Biol. Chem.*, 251:4659–4665.

84. Idle, J. R., and Smith, R. L. (1979): Polymorphisms of oxidation at carbon centers of drugs and their clinical significance. *Drug. Metab. Rev.*, 9:301–318.

85. Jackson, L., Homeida, M., and Roberts, C. J. C. (1978): The features of hepatic enzyme induction with gluthetimide in man. *Br. J. Clin. Pharmacol.*, 6:525–528.

86. Jacquot, C. (1978): Biodisponibilité et effet de "premier passage" du medicament. *Therapie*, 33:683–697.

87. Jezequel, A.-M., and Orlandi, F. (1972): Fine morphology of the human liver as a tool in clinical pharmacology. In: *Liver and Drugs,* edited F. Orlandi and A.-M. Jezequel, pp. 145–192. Academic Press, London.

88. Johnson, E. F., and Muller-Eberhard, V. (1977): Multiple forms of cytochrome P-450: Resolution and purification of rabbit liver aryl hydrocarbon hydroxylase. *Biochem. Biophys. Res. Commun.*, 76:644–651.

89. Jondorf, W. R., Maickel, R. P., and Brodie, B. B. (1958): Inability of newborn mice and guinea pigs

to metabolize drugs. *Biochem. Pharmacol.*, 1:352–354.

90. Jubiz, W., Meikle, A. W., Levinson, R. A., Mizutani, S., West, C. D., and Tyler, F. H. (1970): Effect of diphenylhydantoin on the metabolism of dexamethasone. *N. Engl. J. Med.*, 283:11–14.

91. Jusko, W. J. (1979): Influence of cigarette smoking on drug metabolism in man. *Drug. Metab. Rev.*, 9:221–236.

92. Kappas, A., Alvares, A. P., Anderson, K. E., Pantuck, E. J., Pantuck, C. B., Chang, R., and Conney, A. H. (1978): Effect of charcoal-broiled beef on antipyrine and theophylline metabolism. *Clin. Pharmacol. Ther.*, 23:445–450.

93. Karim, A.K.M.B., and Evans, D. A. P. (1976): Polymorphic acetylation of nitrazepam. *J. Med. Genet.*, 13:17–19.

94. Kater, R. M. H., Roggin, G., Tobon, F., Zieve, P., and Iber, F. L. (1969): Increased rate of clearance of drugs from the circulation of alcoholics. *Am. J. Med. Sci.*, 258:35–39.

95. Kato, R. (1979): Characteristics and differences in the hepatic mixed function oxidases of different species. *Pharmacol. Ther.*, 6:41–98.

96. Klaassen, C. D. (1969): Biliary flow after microsomal enzyme induction. *J. Pharmacol. Exp. Ther.*, 168:216–223.

97. Klinger, W. (1977): Development of drug metabolizing enzymes. In: *Drug Disposition During Development*, edited by P. L. Morselli, pp. 71–88. Spectrum, New York.

98. Klotz, U., Avant, G. R., Hoyumpa, A., Schenker, S., and Wilkinson, G. R. (1975): The effect of age and liver disease on the disposition and elimination of diazepam in adult man. *J. Clin. Invest.*, 55:347–359.

99. Klotz, U., Rapp, T., and Müller, W. A. (1978): Disposition of valproic acid in patients with liver disease. *Eur. J. Clin. Pharmacol.*, 13:55–60.

100. Koch-Weser, J. (1975): Drug interactions in cardiovascular therapy. *Am. Heart J.*, 90:93–116.

101. Kochen, V. W., Imbeck, H., and Jakobs, C. (1977): Untersuchungen über die Ausscheidung bon Metaboliten der Valproinsäure im Urin der Ratte und des Menschen. *Arzneim. Forsch.*, 27:1090–1099.

102. Kuntzman, R. (1969): Drugs and enzyme induction. *Annu. Rev. Pharmacol.*, 9:21–36.

103. Kutt, H. (1972): Diphenylhydantoin. Interactions with other drugs in man. In: *Antiepileptic Drugs*, edited by D. M. Woodbury, J. K. Penry, and R. P. Schmidt, pp. 169–180. Raven Press, New York.

104. Kutt, H., Brennan, R., Dehejia, H., and Verebely, K. (1970): Diphenylhydantoin intoxication. A complication of isoniazid therapy. *Am. Rev. Respir. Dis.*, 101:377–384.

105. Kutt, H., Verebely, K., and McDowell, F. (1968): Inhibition of diphenylhydantoin metabolism in rats and in rat liver microsomes by antitubercular drugs. *Neurology (Minneap.)*, 18:706–710.

106. Kutt, H., Wolk, M., Scherman, R., and McDowell, F. (1964): Insufficient parahydroxylation as a cause of diphenylhydantoin toxicity. *Neurology (Minneap.)*, 14:542–548.

107. La Du, B. N., and Shady, H. (1971): Esterases of human tissues. In: *Concepts in Biochemical Phar-*

macology, Vol. 28, edited by B. B. Brodie and J. R. Gillette, pp. 477–499. Springer-Verlag, Berlin.

108. Latham, A. N., Millbank, L., Richens, A., and Rowe, D. J. F. (1973): Liver enzyme induction by anticonvulsant drugs, and its relationship to disturbed calcium and folic acid metabolism. *J. Clin. Pharmacol.*, 13:337–342.

109. Latham, A. N., and Richens, A. (1973): Pheneturide, a more potent liver enzyme inducer than phenobarbitone? *Br. J. Pharmacol.*, 47:615P.

110. Letteri, J. M., Melk, H., Louis, S., Kutt, H., Durante, P., and Glazko, A. J. (1971): Diphenylhydantoin metabolism in uraemia. *N. Engl. J. Med.*, 285:648–652.

111. Levy, G., and Ashley, J. J. (1973): Effect of an inhibitor of glucuronide formation on elimination kinetics of diphenylhydantoin in rats. *J. Pharm. Sci.*, 62:161–162.

112. Levy, G., and Yacobi, A. (1974): Effect of plasma protein binding on elimination of warfarin. *J. Pharm. Sci.*, 63:805–806.

113. Litterst, C. L., Mimnaugh, E. G., and Gram, T. E. (1977): Comparative alterations in extra hepatic drug metabolism by factors known to affect hepatic activity. *Biochem. Pharmacol.*, 26:749–755.

114. Lu, A. Y. H., and West, S. B. (1978): Reconstituted mammalian mixed-function oxidases: Requirements, specificites and other properties. *Pharmacol. Ther.* [A], 2:337–358.

115. Ludden, T. M., Allen, J. P., Valutsky, W. A., Vicuna, A. V., Nappi, J. M., Hoffman, S. F., Wallace, J. E., Lalka, D., and McNay, J. L. (1977): Individualisation of phenytoin dosage regimens. *Clin. Pharmacol. Ther.*, 21:287–293.

116. Ludden, T. M., Hawkins, D. W., Allen, J. P., and Hoffman, S. F. (1976): Optimum phenytoin dosage regimens. *Lancet*, 1:307–308.

117. Luhdorf, K., Christiansen, P., Hansen, J. M., and Lund, M. (1977): The influence of phenytoin and carbamazepine on endocrine function: Preliminary results. In: *Epilepsy, Eighth International Symposium,* edited by J. K. Penry, pp. 209–213. Raven Press, New York.

118. Luoma, P. V., Pelkonen, R. O., Myllylä, V., and Sotaniemi, E. A. (1979): Relationship between serum lipid levels and indices of drug metabolism in epileptics. *Clin. Pharmacol. Ther.*, 25:235.

119. Luoma, P. V., Reunanen, M. I., and Sotaniemi, E. A. (1978): Serum lipid levels during long-term therapy with anticonvulsants. *Clin. Pharmacol. Ther.*, 23:119–120.

120. Lynn, R. K., Smith, R. G., Thompson, R. M., Deinzer, M. L., Griffin, D., and Gerber, N. (1978): Characterization of glucuronide metabolites of carbamazepine in human urine by gas-chromatography and mass spectrometry. *Drug Metab. Dispos.*, 6:494–501.

121. MacDonald, M. G., and Robinson, D. S. (1968): Clinical observations of possible barbiturate interference with anticoagulants. *J.A.M.A.*, 204:97–100.

122. Macklon, A. F., Savage, R. L., and Rawlins, M. D. (1979): Gilbert's syndrome and drug metabolism. *Clin. Pharmacokinet.*, 4:223–232.

123. Mahgoub, A., Idle, J. R., and Smith, R. L. (1979): Genetically determined variability in drug metabo-

lism: Dual slow acetylation and drug oxidation traits. *Lancet,* 2:154.

124. Mandelli, M., Tognoni, G., and Garattini, S. (1978): Clinical pharmacokinetics of diazepam. *Clin. Pharmacokinet.,* 3:72–91.

125. Martin, E., Toser, T. N., Sheiner, L. B., and Riegelman, S. (1977): The clinical pharmacokinetics of phenytoin. *J. Pharmacokinet. Biopharm.,* 5:579–596.

126. Martin, P. J., Martin, J. V., and Goldberger, D. M. (1975): γ-Glutamyltranspeptidase, triglycerides and enzyme induction. *Br. Med. J.,* 1:17–18.

127. Mawer, G. E., Mullen, P. W., Rodgers, M., Robins, A. J., and Lucas, S. B. (1974): Phenytoin dose adjustment in epileptic patients. *Br. J. Clin. Pharmacol,* 1:163–168.

128. McLelland, J., and Jack, W. (1978): Phenytoin/dexamethasone interaction: A clinical problem. *Lancet,* 1:1096–1097.

129. Meikle, A. W., Jubiz, W., Matsukura, S., West, C. D., and Tyler, F. (1969): Effect of diphenylhydantoin on the metabolism of metyrapone and release of ACTH in man. *J. Clin. Endocrinol.,* 29:1553–1558.

130. Miller, N. E., and Nestel, P. J. (1973): Altered bile acid metabolism during treatment with phenobarbitone. *Clin. Sci. Mol. Med.,* 45:257–262.

131. Mitchard, M. (1971): Bioreduction of organic nitrogen. *Xenobiotica,* 1:469–481.

132. Mitchell, J. R., and Potter, W. Z. (1975): Drug metabolism in the production of liver injury. *Med. Clin. North Am.,* 59:877–885.

133. Monks, A., Boobis, S., Wadsworth, J., and Richens, A. (1978): Plasma protein binding interaction between phenytoin and valproic acid *in vitro. Br. J. Clin. Pharmacol.,* 6:487–492.

134. Morselli, P. L. (1977): Psychotropic drugs. In: *Drug Disposition During Development,* edited by P. L. Morselli, pp. 431–474. Spectrum, New York.

135. Mullen, P. W. (1978): Optimal phenytoin therapy: A new technique for individualizing dosage. *Clin. Pharmacol. Ther.,* 23:228–232.

136. Murray, F. J. (1962): Outbreak of unexpected reactions among epileptics taking isoniazid. *Am. Rev. Respir. Dis.,* 86:729–732.

137. Nappi, J. M. (1979): Warfarin and phenytoin interactions. *Ann. Intern. Med.,* 90:852.

138. Nation, R. L., Vine, J., Triggs, E. J., and Learoyd, B. (1977): Plasma level of chlormethiazole and two metabolites after oral administration to young and aged human subjects. *Eur. J. Clin. Pharmacol.,* 12:137–145.

139. Nebert, D. W., Robinson, J. R., and Kon, H. (1973): Further studies on genetically mediated differences in monooxygenase activities and spin state of cytochrome P-450 iron from rabbit, rat and mouse liver. *J. Biol. Chem.,* 248:7637–7647.

140. Nemis, A. H., Warner, M., Loughnan, P. N., and Aranda, J. V. (1976): Developmental aspects of the hepatic cytochrome P-450 mono-oxygenase system. *Annu. Rev. Pharmacol.,* 16:427–445.

141. Nikkilä, E. A. Kaste, M., Ehnholm, C., and Viukari, J. (1978): Increase of serum high-density lipoprotein in phenytoin users. *Br. Med. J.,* 2:99.

142. Odar-Cederlöf, I., and Borgå, O. (1974): Kinetics of diphenylhydantoin in uraemic patients: Conse-

quences of decreased plasma protein binding. *Eur. J. Clin. Pharmacol.,* 7:31–37.

143. Ohnhaus, E. E., and Park, B. K. (1970): Measurement of urinary 6-β-hydroxycortisol excretion as an *in vivo* parameter in the clinical assessment of the microsomal enzyme-inducing capacity of antipyrine, phenobarbitone and rifampicin. *Eur. J. Clin. Pharmacol.,* 15:139–145.

144. Olesen, O. V., and Dam, M. (1967): The metabolic conversion of primidone (Mysoline) to phenobarbital in patients under long-term treatment. *Acta Neurol. Scand.,* 43:348–356.

145. Orrenius, S., Von Bahr, C., Jakobsson, S. V., and Ernster, L. (1972): Substrate interaction with microsomal P-450. In: *Structure and Function of Oxidation Reduction Enzymes,* edited by A. Akeson and A. Ehrenberg, pp. 309–320. Pergamon Press, Oxford.

146. Pang, K. S., Rowland, M., and Toser, T. N. (1978): *In vivo* evaluation of Michaelis–Menten constants of hepatic drug eliminating systems. *Drug Metab. Dispos.,* 6:197–200.

147. Pelkonen, O., and Kärki, N. T. (1971): Demonstration of cytochrome P-450 in human fetal liver microsomes in early pregnancy. *Acta Pharmacol. Toxicol. (Kbh.),* 30:158–160.

148. Pentikainen, I., Neuvonen, P. J., Tarpila, S., and Syvalahti, E. (1978): Effect of cirrhosis of the liver on the pharmacokinetics of chlormethiazole. *Br. Med. J.,* 2:861–863.

149. Perez, V., Gorodisch, S., Casavilla, F., and Maruffo, C. (1971): Ultrastructure of human liver at the end of normal pregnancy. *Am. J. Obstet. Gynecol.,* 110:428–431.

150. Perrier, D., and Gibaldi, M. (1974): Clearance and biologic half-life as indices of intrinsic hepatic metabolism. *J. Pharmacol. Exp. Ther.,* 191:17–24.

151. Perucca, E. (1978): Clinical consequences of micro somal enzyme-induction by antiepileptic drugs. *Pharmacol. Ther.,* 2:285–314.

152. Perucca, E. (1981): Antiepileptic drug interactions. In: *A Textbook of Epilepsy,* edited by J. Laidlaw and A. Richens. Churchill-Livingstone, Edinburgh *(in press).*

153. Perucca, E., Hedges, A. M., Makki, K., Hebdige, S., Wadsworth, J., and Richens, A. (1979): The comparative enzyme-inducing properties of antiepileptic drugs. *Br. J. Clin. Pharmacol.,* 7:414–415.

154. Perucca, E., and Richens, A. (1980): Hepatic microsomal enzyme-induction in epileptic patients receiving single and multiple drug therapy. In: *The Place of Sodium Valproate in the Treatment of Epilepsy,* edited by M. Parsonage and A. D. S. Caldwell, pp. 179–183. Academic Press, London.

155. Perucca, E., Makki, K., and Richens, A. (1978): Is phenytoin metabolism dose-dependent by enzyme-saturation or by feedback inhibition? *Clin. Pharmacol. Ther.,* 24:46–51.

156. Perucca, E., and Richens, A. (1981): The pathophysiological basis of drug toxicity. In: *Current Topics in Pathology,* Vol. 69, edited by E. Grundmann, pp. 17–68. Springer-Verlag, Berlin.

157. Perucca, E., and Richens, A. (1981): Anticonvulsant drug interactions in epilepsy. In: *The Treatment of Epilepsy, Current Status of Modern Therapy,* Vol.

5, edited by J. Tyrer, pp. 95–128. M.T.P. Press, Lancaster.

158. Perucca, E., and Richens, A. (1981): Interpretation of serum drug levels: Relevance of protein binding. In: *Drug Concentrations in Neuropsychiatry, Ciba Foundation Symposium 74*, pp. 51–68. Excerpta Medica, Amsterdam.

159. Perucca, E., and Richens, A. (1979): Paracetamol disposition in normal subjects and in patients treated with antiepileptic drugs. *Br. J. Clin. Pharmacol.*, 7:201–206.

160. Perucca, E., and Richens, A. (1979): Reduction of the oral availability of lignocaine by induction of first-pass metabolism in epileptic patients. *Br. J. Clin. Pharmacol.*, 8:21–31.

161. Pessayre, O., Bentata, M., Degott, C., Nouel, O., Miguet Rueff, B., and Benhamou, J. P. (1977): Isoniazid–rifampicin fulminant hepatitis: A possible consequence of the enhancement of isoniazid hepatotoxicity by enzyme induction. *Gastroenterology*, 72:284–289.

162. Petereit, L. B., and Meikle, A. W. (1977): Effectiveness of prednisolone during phenytoin therapy. *Clin. Pharmacol. Ther.*, 22:912–916.

163. Peterson, G. R., Hostetler, R. M., Lehman, T., and Covault, H. P. (1979): Acute inhibition of oxidative drug metabolism by propoxyphene (Darvon). *Biochem. Pharmacol.*, 28:1783–1790.

164. Pohl, L. R., Porter, W. R., Frager, W. F., Fasco, M. J., Baker, F. D., and Fenton, J. W., III (1976): Warfarin—stereochemical aspects of its metabolism by rat liver microsomes. *Biochem. Pharmacol.*, 25:2153–2162.

165. Powis, B., and Jansson, I. (1979): Stoichiometry of the mixed function oxidase. *Pharmacol. Ther.*, 7:297–311.

166. Rambeck, B., Boenigk, H. E., Dunlop, A., Mullen, P. W., Wadsworth, J., and Richens, A. (1979): Predicting phenytoin dose—a revised nomogram. *Ther. Drug Monitor.*, 1:325–334.

167. Rane, A. (1978): Clinical pharmacokinetics of antiepileptic drugs in children. *Pharmacol. Ther.*, 2:251–267.

168. Rane, A., and Ackermann, E. (1972): Metabolism of ethylmorphine and aniline in human fetal liver. *Clin. Pharmacol. Ther.*, 13:663–670.

169. Rane, A., Bertilsson, L., and Palmer, L. (1975): Disposition of placentally transferred carbamazepine (Tegretol®) in the newborn. *Eur. J. Clin. Pharmacol.*, 8:283–284.

170. Rane, A., Borgå, O., Garle, M., and Sjöqvist, F. (1974): Plasma disappearance of transplacentally transferred phenytoin in the newborn studied with mass fragmentography. *Clin. Pharmacol. Ther.*, 15:39–45.

171. Rane, A., Sjöqvist, F., and Orrenius, S. (1973): Drugs and fetal metabolism. *Clin. Pharmacol. Ther.*, 14:666–672.

172. Reidenberg, M. M. (1977): The biotransformation of drugs in renal failure. *Am. J. Med.*, 62:482–485.

173. Remmer, H. (1972): Induction of drug metabolizing enzyme-system in the liver. *Eur. J. Clin. Pharmacol.*, 5:116–136.

174. Remmer, H., and Alsleben, B. (1958): Die Aktivi-

erung der Entgiftung in den Lebermikrosomen wahrend der Gewehnung. *Klin. Wochenschr.*, 36:332–333.

175. Rey, E., D'Athis, P., de Lauture, D., Dulac, O., Aicardi, J., and Olive, G. (1979): Pharmacokinetics of carbamazepine in the neonate and in the child. *Int. J. Clin. Pharmacol. Biopharm.*, 17:90–96.

176. Reynolds, E. H., Fenton, G., Fenwick, P., Johnson, A. L., and Laundy, M. (1975): Interaction of phenytoin and primidone. *Br. Med. J.*, 2:594–595.

177. Richens, A. (1974): The clinical consequences of chronic hepatic enzyme induction by anticonvulsant drugs. *Br. J. Clin. Pharmacol.*, 1:185–187.

178. Richens, A. (1977): Interactions with antiepileptic drugs. *Drugs*, 13:266–275.

179. Richens, A., and Dunlop, A. (1975): Serum phenytoin levels in management of epilepsy. *Lancet*, 2:247–248.

180. Richens, A., and Dunlop, A. (1975): Phenytoin dosage nomogram. *Lancet*, 2:1305–1306.

181. Richens, A., and Rowe, D. J. F. (1970): Interaction between anticonvulsant drugs and vitamin D. *Br. J. Pharmacol.*, 40:593–594.

182. Richens, A., and Woodford, F. P. (1976): *Anticonvulsant Drugs and Enzyme Induction*. Associated Scientific Publishers, Amsterdam.

183. Rowan, A. J., Binnie, C. D., Warfield, C. A., Meinardi, H., and Meijer, J. W. A. (1979): The delayed effect of sodium valproate on the photoconvulsive response in man. *Epilepsia*, 20:61–68.

184. Rowland, M. (1972): Influence of route of administration on drug availability. *J. Pharm. Sci.*, 61:70–74.

185. Roy, A. B. (1971): Sulphate conjugation enzymes. In: *Concepts in Biochemical Pharmacology, Vol. 28*, edited by B. B. Brodie and J. R. Gillette, pp. 536–563. Springer-Verlag, Berlin.

186. Runkel, R., Chaplin, M. D., Sevelius, H., Ortega, E., and Segre, E. (1976): Pharmacokinetics of naproxen overdoses. *Clin. Pharmacol. Ther.*, 20:269–277.

187. Runkel, R., Forchielli, E., Sevelius, H., Chaplin, M., and Segre, E. (1973): Non-linear plasma response to high doses of naproxen. *Clin. Pharmacol. Ther.*, 15:261–266.

188. Saarni, H., Sotaniemi, E. A., and Ahokas, J. (1977): Effect of medroxyprogesterone on the hepatic metabolism. *Acta Pharmacol. Toxicol. (Kbh.)*, 41(Suppl. 4):73.

189. Schwartz, M. A., Koechlin, B. A., Postma, E., Palmer, S., and Krol, G. (1965): Metabolism of diazepam in rat, dog and man. *J. Pharmacol. Exp. Ther.*, 149:423–435.

190. Schwartz, M. A., and Postma, E. (1966): Metabolic N-demethylation of chlordiazepoxide. *J. Pharm. Sci.*, 55:1358–1362.

191. Scott, A. K., Jeffers, T. A., Petrie, J. C., and Gilbert, J. C. (1979): Serum bilirubin and hepatic enzyme-induction. *Br. Med. J.*, 2:310.

192. Shand, D. G., Mitchell, J. R., and Oates, J. A. (1975): Pharmacokinetic drug interactions. In: *Concepts in Biochemical Pharmacology, Vol. 28*, edited by J. R. Gillette and J. R. Mitchell, pp. 272–314. Springer-Verlag, Berlin.

193. Short, C. R., and Davies, L. E. (1970): Perinatal development of drug-metabolizing enzyme activity in swine. *J. Pharmacol. Exp. Ther.*, 174:185–196.
194. Short, C. R., Kinden, D. A., and Stith, R. (1976): Fetal and neonatal development of the monooxygenase system. *Drug Metab. Rev.*, 5:1–42.
195. Sloan, T. P., Mahgoub, A., Lancaster, R., Isle, J. R., and Smith, R. L. (1978): Polymorphism of carbon oxidation of drugs and clinical implications. *Br. Med. J.*, 2:655–657.
196. Snyder, R., and Remmer, H. (1979): Classes of hepatic microsomal mixed function oxidase inducers. *Pharmacol. Ther.*, 7:203–244.
197. Sotaniemi, E. A., Pelkonen, R. O., Ahokas, J. T., Pirttiaho, H. I., and Ahlqvist, J. (1975): Relationship between *in vivo* and *in vitro* drug metabolism in man. *Eur. J. Drug Metab. Pharmacokinet.*, 1:39–45.
198. Sotaniemi, E. A., Pelkonen, R. O., Ahokas, J. T., Pirttiaho, H. I., and Ahlqvist, J. (1978): Drug metabolism in epileptics: *In vivo* and *in vitro* correlations. *Br. J. Clin. Pharmacol.*, 5:71–76.
199. Stambaugh, J. E., Wainer, I. W., Hemphill, D., and Schwartz, I. (1977): A potentially toxic interaction between pethidine (Meperidine) and phenobarbitone. *Lancet*, 1:398–399.
200. Stevenson, I. H., O'Malley, K., and Shepherd, A. M. M. (1976): Relative induction potency of anticonvulsant drugs. In: *Anticonvulsant Drugs and Enzyme Induction*, edited by A. Richens and F. P. Woodford, pp. 37–46. Associated Scientific Publishers, Amsterdam.
201. Thomas, P. E., Lu, A. Y. H., Ryan, D., West, S. D., Kawalek, J., and Levin, W. (1976): Immunochemical evidence for six forms of rat liver cytochrome P-450 obtained using antibodies against purified rat liver cytochromes P-450 and P-448. *Mol. Pharmacol.*, 12:746–758.
202. Thomas, P. E., Lu, A. Y. H., Ryan, D., West, S. B., Kawalek, S., and Levin, W. (1976): Multiple forms of rat liver cytochrome P-450. Immunochemical evidence with antibody against P-448. *J. Biol. Chem.*, 251:1385–1391.
203. Thompson, R. P. H., Eddleston, A. L. W. F., and Williams, R. (1969): Low plasma bilirubin in epileptics on phenobarbitone. *Lancet*, 1:21–22.
204. Travers, R., Reynolds, E. H., and Gallagher, B. (1972): Variation in response to anticonvulsants in a group of epileptic patients. *Arch. Neurol.*, 27:29–33.
205. Vesell, E. S. (1975): Genetically determined variations in drug disposition and response in man. In: *Concepts in Biochemical Pharmacology*, edited by J. R. Gillette and J. R. Mitchell, pp. 169–212. Springer-Verlag, Berlin.
206. Warner, M., Lamarca, M. V., and Neims, A. H. (1978): Chromatographic and electrophoretic heterogeneity of the cytochrome P-450 solubilized from untreated rat liver. *Drug Metab. Dispos.*, 6:353–362.
207. Weber, W. W. (1971): Acetylating, deacetylating and amino acid conjugating enzymes. In: *Concepts in Biochemical Pharmacology, Vol. 28*, edited by B. B. Brodie and J. R. Gillette, pp. 564–583. Springer-Verlag, Berlin.
208. Welton, A. F., O'Neal, O., Chaney, L. C., and Aust, S. D. (1971): Multiplicity of cytochrome P-450 hemoproteins in rat liver microsomes. *J. Biol. Chem.*, 250:5631–5639.
209. Werk, E. E., McGee, J., and Sholiton, L. J. (1964): Effect of diphenylhydantoin on cortisol metabolism in man. *J. Clin. Invest.*, 43:1824–1835.
210. White, M. P., and Dekaban, A. S. (1977): Metabolic fate of phenobarbital. A quantitative study of p-hydroxyphenobarbital elimination in man. *Drug Metab. Dispos.*, 5:63–74.
211. Whitfield, J. B., Moss, D. W., Neale, G., Orme, M. l'E., and Breckenridge, A. (1973): Changes in plasma γ-glutamyltranspeptidase activity associated with alterations on drug metabolism in man. *Br. Med. J.*, 1:316–318.
212. Whittaker, J. B., and Price-Evans, D. A. (1970): Genetic control of phenylbutazone metabolism in man. *Br. Med. J.*, 4:323–328.
213. Wilkinson, G. R., and Schenker, S. (1975): Drug disposition and liver disease. *Drug Metab. Rev.*, 4:139–175.
214. Wilkinson, G. R., and Shand, D. G. (1975): A physiological approach to hepatic drug clearance. *Clin. Pharmacol. Ther.*, 18:377–390.
215. Williams, R. T. (1971): Introduction: Pathways of drug metabolism. In: *Concepts in Biochemical Pharmacology, Vol. 28*, edited by B. B. Brodie and J. R. Gillette, pp. 226–242. Springer-Verlag, Berlin.
216. Wright, N., and Prescott, L. F. (1973): Potentiation by previous drug therapy of hepatotoxicity following paracetamol overdosage. *Scott. Med. J.*, 18:56–58.
217. Yacobi, A., and Levy, G. (1975): Comparative pharmacokinetics of coumarin anticoagulants. XIV. Relationship between protein binding, distribution and elimination kinetics of warfarin in rats. *J. Pharm. Sci.*, 64;1660–1664.
218. Yaffe, S. J., Rane, A., Sjöqvist, F., Boreus, L.-O., and Orrenius, S. (1970): The presence of a monooxygenase system in human fetal liver microsomes. *Life Sci.*, 9:1189–1200.

Antiepileptic Drugs, edited by D. M. Woodbury, J. K. Penry, and C. E. Pippenger. Raven Press, New York © 1982.

4

General Principles

Practical Pharmacokinetics

Pieter J. M. Guelen and Eppo van der Kleijn

In antiepileptic drug therapy the nature and intensity of the seizures, the condition of the patient, and the anticonvulsant spectra, toxicities, and clinical efficacies of the compounds available strongly determine the choice of drugs prescribed. Other factors will dominate their handling in epileptic patients.

It is the aim of chronic (antiepileptic) drug treatment to establish and maintain a constant amount of drug in the body in order to minimize oscillations in clinical effects. This so-called steady-state situation is highly dependent on the dose of the drug administered per unit of time, the fate of that drug in the body, and the processes that control and influence drug transformation. The rates at which these processes occur simultaneously are characteristic for each drug with the restriction of a number of variables and determine the onset, time course, and intensity of beneficial or toxic effect(s) to the body.

The time course of the amounts of drugs and their metabolites in biological fluids, tissues, and excreta in the body can be described according to mathematical models. The study of such models is called pharmacokinetics, a term first introduced by F. W. Dost in 1953 (3). The application of the information obtained from theoretical and experimental pharmacokinetic studies in relation to pharmacological and clinical effects for the treatment of patients is further specified by the term clinical pharmacokinetics (9).

Antiepileptic drug therapy was among the first areas to benefit from clinical pharmacokinetic studies because of the widespread availability of plasma concentration-monitoring methods. Most of these studies have been reviewed in the literature (5,6,8,11,13,17) and are extensively summarized in the various chapters of this book dealing with each specific drug.

Traditionally, dosage schedules in epilepsy have been subjectively based on clinical judgment of the disease state of the patient with successive modifications made of the dose and compounds until a satisfactory condition has been reached. Still, many epileptic patients appear to react inadequately to pharmacotherapy. Antiepileptics as well as other drugs may precipitate clinical symptoms at toxic dosages similar to the symptoms of the original disease. Patients at apparent "normal" dosage regimens may reach toxicity or may fail to reach therapeutic effect because of large variations in individual pharmacokinetics or of factors altering the pharmacokinetic behavior of a drug during long-term treatment (5).

Although the use of plasma level determinations has contributed considerably to an improvement in antiepileptic drug therapy over the past decade, the possibilities of clinical pharmacokinetics in medical practice have not yet been fully utilized. Two important reasons may be cited for this relatively new approach to drug therapy not having attained maximum applicability. One is that one encounters numerous difficulties in defining, observing, and quantifying therapeutic efficacy of drugs in epileptic patients. The other is that the interpretation of plasma concentration data requires a thorough understanding of the contributions of the numerous factors that influence the pharmacokinetics and thus the steady-state levels of drugs in patients to guarantee optimum utilization of these data for dosage regimen adjustment for the benefit of the epileptic patient (16). In general, the average physician may not fully master the pharmacokinetics of antiepileptic drugs, their application for clinical practice, and the various factors that influence the final efficacy of these drugs. The aim is curing the patient and not curing the drug.

In this chapter the basic principles of clinical pharmacokinetics are described, approaching this complicated matter from a practical point of view. The use of inconceivable pharmacokinetic equations and inscrutable mathematical derivations has been avoided as much as possible. The interested reader is referred to various textbooks (14,18–20).

CONCEPTS OF DRUG ACTION

When drugs are administered to the body, a sequence of biochemical and physiological processes is initiated. The active compound must pass several barriers before it can exert a biological effect. In this process, three main phases can be discerned as shown in Fig. 1.

In the pharmaceutic phase the active compound has to be released from its dosage form, e.g., tablet, capsule, solution. The rate and extent of liberation are influenced by crystal structure, particle size, and coating of the drug formulation. In the pharmacokinetic phase, the drug will be distributed all over the body, depending on a number of factors such as absorption, lipophilicity, binding to proteins and tissues, and rates of metabolism and elimination. In practice, it means that only a limited fraction of the active compound administered finally reaches the place where the effects occur, the receptor.

The pharmacokinetic events generally proceed at a rate slower than the very fast formation of drug–receptor complexes in the latter pharmacodynamic phase (18). Therefore, the onset and time course of action of a drug will in many cases depend on the rate-limiting kinetic characteristics of that substance. A single drug evokes as many effects as there are receptors for that drug.

In the scheme presented in Fig. 1, one proceeds on the assumption that there is a direct relationship among the dose administered, the concentration reached in the body (or the plasma concentration), and the ultimate effect. This relationship is the working hypothesis. How difficult it is to describe this relation practically will become apparent.

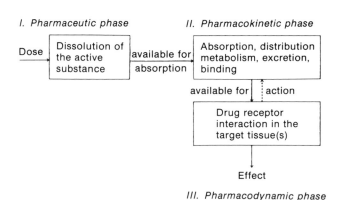

FIG. 1. Three main phases of drug availability.

Dose–Effect Relationship

Depending on the given amount of a drug (the dose), several effects may occur:

$$\text{Dose} \rightarrow \begin{array}{c}\text{Concen-}\\\text{tration}\end{array} \rightarrow \text{Effect} \begin{array}{l}\nearrow \text{Subtherapeutic}\\\rightarrow \text{Therapeutic}\\\searrow \text{Toxic}\end{array}$$

Furthermore, different effects will occur when a given drug is administered to several patients in the same dose as a result of large variations in the plasma concentrations measured because of interindividual variations in pharmacological and pharmacokinetic processes. The range between the minimum effective concentration and the minimum toxic concentration is called the therapeutic (safety) range or therapeutically relevant plasma concentration. The appearance of subtherapeutic and toxic effects in a group of patients will strongly depend on this therapeutic range.

For a theoretical patient population, the therapeutic range is shown in Figs. 2 and 3 for two types of drugs, one with a large therapeutic range and one with a small therapeutic range. In the case of a large therapeutic range (Fig. 2), improvement of the dosage regimen, when subtherapeutic or toxic effects occur, will certainly lead to concentrations of the drug in the body (or plasma concentrations) at which optimum therapeutic efficacy is reached in 95% of the patient population. Different figures will be reached in the case of a small therapeutic range (Fig. 3). Both toxicity and absence of effect are likely to be observed, and optimum therapeutic efficacy within one concentration range will never be found for the majority of the patients.

This very last example often applies to the treatment of epilepsy where symptoms appear to be resistant to drug therapy. Difficulties will increase further for combinations of drugs as are often used in antiepileptic drug therapy and for drugs with pharmacologically active metabolites, e.g., primidone, of which approximately 25% is converted to phenobarbital in addition to other (active) metabolites. To achieve chronic drug therapy in the epileptic patient with the aid of plasma concentration monitoring, plasma concentration values are used that are considered to be therapeutically relevant. These values have been evaluated from careful clinical studies in a number of cases by closely monitoring predefined objective therapeutic effects, adverse effects, or absence of effects. Again, this is done on the assumption that the plasma concentration reflects the total amount of drug in the body and that the relationship between

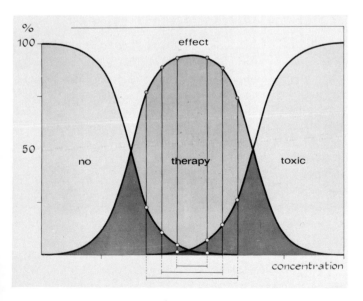

FIG. 2. The therapeutic concentration range of a hypothetical drug in a theoretical infinite patient population. The drug has a rather large therapeutic range. Overly large concentration oscillations may lead to periods of no effect or toxic effect. Improvement of a regimen leading to a concentration coinciding with the optimum of the therapeutic effectivity and a reduction of the oscillations will have a favorable effect on the probability of success.

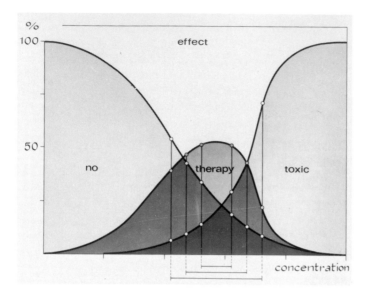

FIG. 3. Similar distribution curve as in Fig. 2 for a hypothetical drug with a small therapeutic range. Both toxicity and absence of effect are likely to be observed within one concentration range, so the probability of optimum therapeutic effect never reaches a value over 50%.

plasma concentration and concentration at the site of the receptor responsible for the effect is linear within the therapeutic working range. However, because of limited standardization in medical terminology and the multitude of experimental variables in epileptic patients, the relative therapeutic plasma concentrations often show large variations, limiting their practical value (12).

Moreover, the relationship between the daily dosage and the measured plasma concentration shows a wide interindividual variation in epileptic patients. These variations are often attributed to unreliable intake of the prescribed drugs by the patients and to interindividual differences in bioavailability. Other factors may also contribute significantly to these dose–concentration variations (5). The optimum plasma concentration for maximum clinical control is strongly dependent on the clinical condition of the individual patient and will vary from patient to patient, so the best therapeutic plasma concentration has to be established for each individual by close monitoring of the clinical effect.

CONCEPTS OF PHARMACOKINETICS

In pharmacokinetics, one tries to establish the rates of absorption, distribution, metabolism,

and excretion by means of mathematical models in order to obtain information on the period of presence of drug in the body. The basic mathematical model including the major pharmacokinetic processes is presented in Fig. 4. In this model, the symbols k_{nm} represent the rate constants at which the indicated processes proceed. For simplification, the body is usually represented as a system of compartments, even though these lack physiological or anatomical reality.

Distribution of Antiepileptic Drugs in the Body

The concepts of pharmacokinetics consider both direct and linear relationships between the concentration of the drug at the site at which it is assayed (usually the plasma concentration) and the concentration in the rest of the body. Variations in general and/or regional distributions of different drugs are reflected in the apparent volume of distribution and in the corresponding elimination rate constant.

In anatomical terms, variations result from differences in flow rate through the different tissues and organs, regional binding to proteins and tissues resulting in a tissue distribution coefficient (TDC) that is different for the various tissues. The TDC is the relationship between the concentration of the drug in the tissue

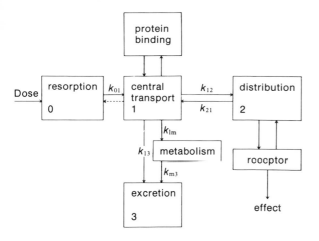

FIG. 4. Basic mathematical model of pharmacokinetic processes.

and the corresponding plasma concentration according to:

$$TDC = C_{tissue}/C_{plasma} \qquad [1]$$

It is generally assumed that only the free (unbound) concentration creates the diffusion gradient in distribution. But since both psychotropic and antiepileptic drugs are usually active in fluids other than plasma, we also have to consider the binding to proteins or other materials in plasma and tissues. As shown earlier (1), the tissue distribution coefficient appears to be very important and largely controls the fraction bound in tissues. Also, the binding capacity (bound fraction) in tissue can vary among different regions in the body. All of these forces create a diffusion gradient and so a final distribution pattern during long-term therapy, the so-called equilibrium or steady state.

Whole-body autoradiographic distribution studies in animals confirm these theoretical suggestions (5). An example of the distribution of ^{14}C-labeled phenytoin in a squirrel monkey is shown in Fig. 5. White areas correspond to the presence of radioactivity as parent compound or as metabolite. The total amount of radioactivity (corresponding to drug concentrations) in various tissues exceeds the concentration of the compound in blood.

Plasma Protein Binding

Antiepileptic drugs bind to a relatively large extent to plasma proteins, mainly the plasma albumin fraction. In general, when plasma concentrations are measured, only the total plasma concentration is determined (bound plus unbound concentration). The binding of drugs to albumin is relatively nonselective and usually reversible. The total plasma concentration is assumed to be in equilibrium with the free plasma concentration:

$$C_{plasma \ (total)} \rightleftharpoons$$
$$C_{bound} + C_{free} \qquad [2]$$

Only the free drug can move across membranes, diffuse all over the body, and finally reach the receptor site. So measurement of the free drug concentration in plasma gives a better correlation with the clinical effect than the total plasma concentration, as proven for phenytoin (1).

In Table 1, the binding fraction of antiepileptic drugs to plasma proteins is shown. Fractional binding usually varies only slightly with drug concentrations in the therapeutic range but varies directly with albumin concentration. Also, other drugs and endogenous compounds may compete with the antiepileptic drugs for the binding sites at proteins (5,15). Although linearity in protein binding seems to appear throughout the therapeutic concentration range for most of the antiepileptic drugs, this does not necessarily mean that linearity appears in all body structures. Nonlinearity most often occurs in case of large tissue distribution coefficients, as is found with phenytoin (2). It should be

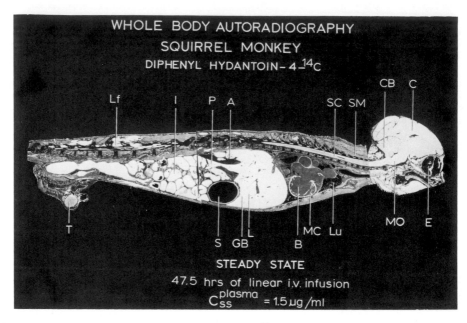

FIG. 5. Whole-body autoradiogram of the distribution of ^{14}C-phenytoin in the squirrel monkey after 47.5 hr of linear i.v. infusion. White areas correspond to the presence of radioactivity. Note the high concentrations in the excretory organs that appear to be mostly metabolites.

noted that most pharmacokinetic parameters are derived from total plasma concentration measurements; therefore, total plasma concentrations are generally meant when plasma concentrations are mentioned.

Some Important Pharmacokinetic Parameters

Many pharmacokinetic processes can be described satisfactorily by a simplification of the complex basic pharmacokinetic model according to a so-called one-compartment model (Fig. 6). In this model, k_0 represents the rate constant of absorption, k_{el} the total elimination rate constant, C_t the concentration of the drug in this compartment at any time after administration (plasma concentration), and V the apparent volume of distribution. The one-compartment model depicts the body as a single homogenous unit in which rates of distribution over the body and elimination from the various organs are of first order and proportional to the drug concentration. The most important pharmacokinetic pa-

rameters defining the fate of drug in the body will be discussed separately.

The Biological Half-Life

The pharmacokinetic parameters, initiated after administration of a drug to a body, result in a plasma concentration–time profile from which the pharmacokinetic parameters can be derived. In Fig. 7, an example of such a plasma concentration–time curve after a single oral administration of 250 mg ethosuximide to a volunteer is shown. After absorption and distribution have been completed, the drug is eliminated from the body at a certain rate. The elimination rate constant (k_{el}) is of first order, which means that the fraction of the drug eliminated from the body in any time period is constant. Therefore, by plotting the concentration data on a logarithmic scale against time, a straight line describing the plasma decay curve is obtained. The biological half-life ($t_{1/2}$) is defined as the time period in which half of the amount present in the body is eliminated.

TABLE 1. *Mean pharmacokinetic parameters of the antiepileptic drugs*

Generic drug name	Therapeutic concentration range (C_{ss}, mg/liter)	Dosage interval (Δt, hr)	Half-life ($t_{1/2}$, hr)	Relative apparent volume (V_d, liter/kg)
Phenobarbital	30–40	8–12	120–150	0.7
Phenytoin	10–15	6–8	20–24	0.7
Primidone	8–12	8	10	1
Ethosuximide	60–80	8	30–40	0.65
2-Propylpentanoate	60–80	6	7–10	0.65
Carbamazepine	5–8	8	35[a]	1.1
Clonazepam	0.03–0.06	8	30	3.3
Diazepam	0.4	8	32	1.8
Nitrazepam	0.08–0.12	8	30	1.8

[a]After chronic medication, the half-life may reduce to 8 to 15 hr because of enzyme stimulation.

The relationship between $t_{1/2}$ and k_{el} can be written as:

$$t_{1/2} = 0.693/k_{el} \qquad [3]$$

The biological half-life of ethosuximide in the volunteer (Fig. 7) appears to be 34 hr, so k_{el} can be calculated. By extrapolation of the elimination part of the curve to time zero (the moment of administration) and assumption of 100% absorption, a theoretical maximum concentration of the elimination phase can be read (C_0). This parameter may be obtained more precisely after i.v. administration of the drug (no absorption problems), but sufficiently reliable parameters may be calculated from oral administration data, assuming complete, rapid absorption.

The biological half-life of a drug varies from individual to individual depending on intraindividual differences in metabolism and elimination. This parameter is very useful to determine optimal dosing intervals during (sub)chronic drug treatment in order to reach adequate steady-state plasma concentrations.

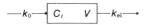

FIG. 6. One-compartment model representing a simplification of the complex basic pharmacokinetic model. k_0, Rate constant of absorption; k_{el}, total elimination rate; C_t, concentration of drug in this compartment at any time after administration (plasma concentration); V, apparent volume of distribution.

The Apparent Volume of Distribution

One defines the magnitude of the various compartments in which all pharmacokinetic processes are indicated in the basic model by the so-called apparent volume of distribution (V_d). It is a proportionality constant in the relationship between the dose administered, or the amount of drug in the body, and the drug concentration in plasma.

The apparent volume of distribution is considered as the volume in which the drug has been dissolved when it is distributed homogeneously over that volume. From distribution studies in animals, it can be learned that this does not necessarily obtain for all of the various organs, depending on regional subdistribution and binding to tissues and protein structures. In fact, in many organs a higher concentration will be reached than in plasma. Still, the drug is considered to be "homogeneously distributed." So the apparent volume of distribution has no direct physiological meaning and, in many cases, might be much larger than the total volume of the body. The apparent volume of distribution is expressed in liters/kg and can be determined in a number of ways: (a) by using the theoretical maximum concentration of the elimination phase (C_0) according to:

$$V_d = D/C_0 \qquad [4]$$

or (b) by using the area under the plasma concentration–time curve (AUC) after a single i.v.

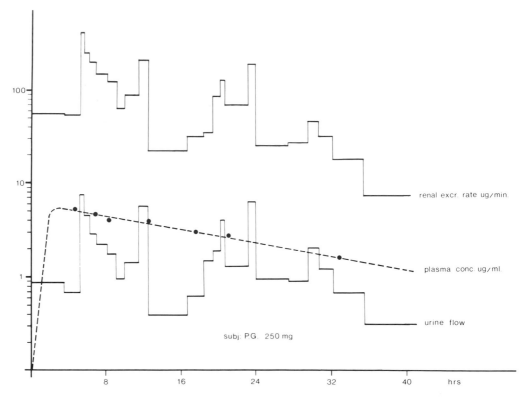

FIG. 7. Plasma concentration–time curve and renal excretion rate of ethosuximide after administration of 250 mg to a volunteer.

administration, or from oral data, assuming rapid and complete absorption, by:

$$V_d = D/\text{AUC} \cdot k_{el} \qquad [5]$$

In both equations, D represents the dose of the drug administered.

Drug Clearance

Deactivation of the drug in the body is done by direct elimination from the body through the kidneys or by metabolism mainly in the liver and elimination of the formed metabolites. Both metabolism and excretion determine the rate at which the active compound will be removed from the body. A measure for the total rate of loss of material from the body is called the total body clearance ($\dot{V}$) and is defined as the part of the apparent volume of distribution (V_d) that is cleared from the drug per unit of time (usu-

ally hours or minutes). It has a dimension of liters/hr or ml/min.

Since it is derived from the sum of all elimination mechanisms, metabolic and renal clearance, the total body clearance of a drug may be written as:

$$\dot{V} = K_m + K_r \qquad [6]$$

in which K_m represents the metabolic and K_r the renal clearance. In the simplified pharmacokinetic model, the product of k_{el} and V_d represents the total body clearance:

$$\dot{V} = k_{el} \cdot V_d \qquad [7]$$

so the total body clearance can be calculated using the AUC by rearranging equation 5 according to:

$$\dot{V} = D/\text{AUC} \qquad [8]$$

Whereas the total body clearance defines the distribution and elimination characteristics of a drug in the body, this parameter may be used for dose regimen calculations (5) provided that the individual clearance value of each particular drug is sufficiently well known. The dose regimen calculation concept for chronic drug treatment will be discussed further on in this chapter.

Bioavailability

When a drug is administered orally, the observed area under the plasma concentration–time curve (AUC) will generally be smaller than the AUC found after i.v. administration of the same dose to the same patient. Because of interindividual differences in absorption kinetics, incomplete absorption, and first-pass metabolism, the actual part of the amount administered orally and thus available for distribution in the body is reduced. These problems do not occur after i.v. administration. The fraction of the drug finally available for distribution (and action) after oral administration is called the bioavailability (F) and may be calculated by measuring AUC after oral and i.v. administration according to:

$$F = \frac{\text{AUC after oral dose}}{\text{AUC after i.v. dose}} \qquad [9]$$

In chronic drug treatment, this parameter is tacitly considered to be constant within a patient or within a group of patients. However, interindividual variations are observed because of variations in absorption kinetics and in the motility of the gastrointestinal tract and may strongly influence the actual amount of drug available for action.

Steady-State Plasma Concentration

In most of the considerations of the concept of pharmacokinetics presented so far, only single-dose kinetics have been discussed. In antiepileptic drug therapy, single doses are seldom used, and the drugs are administered on a long-term basis. During chronic drug treatment with a fixed dose at a fixed time interval (D mg every t hr), the various pharmacokinetic processes, as presented in the basic model, attain an equilibrium. Mathematically, the equilibrium can be derived fairly accurately when the physiological condition of the patient is not changing too much. This is called a steady-state situation. When the biological half-life is large compared with the time interval between two drug administrations (the dosage interval, Δt), long-term drug treatment can be interpreted as a constant supply of the drug in the body, a so-called linear infusion. This is the case with nearly all antiepileptic drugs. In general, it can be assumed that a steady state is reached after administration for a time period of five times the biological half-life of the drug; in steady state, there exists equilibrium between supply and total body clearance of the drug.

During i.v. infusion, the plasma concentration at any time after starting the infusion (C_t) can be calculated by:

$$C_t = \frac{k_0}{k_{el} \cdot V_d}(1 - e^{-k_{el} \cdot t}) \qquad [10]$$

In this equation, k_0 represents the infusion rate constant (mg/hr), k_{el} the total elimination rate constant, and V_d the apparent volume of distribution. When time (t) increases during the infusion, the factor $e^{-k_{el} t}$ approaches zero, so the equation can be simplified:

$$C_t = k_0/k_{el} \cdot V_d \qquad [11]$$

The plasma concentration C_t now represents the steady-state plasma concentration (C_{ss}). In this equation, the product of k_{el} and V_d (liter and hr^{-1}) represents the total body clearance ($\dot{V}$, liter/hr), so equation 11 can be rewritten:

$$C_{ss} = k_0/\dot{V} \qquad [12]$$

The infusion constant k_0 for antiepileptic drugs can be considered as a dosage regimen of D mg per unit of time (mg/hr) or as a dose per dosage interval (Δt, hr) so:

$$k_0 = D/\Delta t \qquad [13]$$

Rearrangement of equations 12 and 13 then yields:

$$C_{ss} = D/\Delta t \cdot \dot{V} \qquad [14]$$

Most often, a linear relationship between clearance and body weight (W) or body surface is assumed, so a new parameter is introduced, the relative clearance ($\dot{V}'$), which is better comparable among individuals. This parameter has a dimension of liter per hour per kg body weight (liter/hr · kg). Equation 14 then reads:

$$C_{ss} = F \cdot D/\Delta t \cdot \dot{V}' \cdot W \qquad [15]$$

in which C_{ss} is the plasma concentration of the drug in steady state, F is the bioavailability factor, D is the dose administered, Δt is the dosage interval, $\dot{V}'$ is the relative clearance of that particular drug, and W is the body weight.

When the plasma concentrations of the antiepileptic drugs are determined at a proper time after administration, the relative clearance values of these drugs can be calculated by using equation 15. For simplification, F is generally assumed to be 1.0. The relative clearance values of the antiepileptic drugs have been calculated and evaluated in a large epidemiological study (5). Although large interindividual variations in the relative clearance values in epileptic patients have been found, a large number of variables could be determined and quantified, allowing dose regimen calculations to be made using the relative clearance value as the starting point.

Different Pharmacokinetic Characteristics

In steady state, the pharmacokinetics of most antiepileptic drugs can be described satisfactorily by the one-compartment model and the plasma concentrations calculated using the equations discussion in the preceding sections. However, some drugs show an altered pharmacokinetic behavior during chronic treatment compared to single-dose administration. These alterations influence the total amount of drug in the body when the dose remains constant, and patients may end up with subtherapeutic or toxic plasma concentrations. Some of these different pharmacokinetic characteristics will be discussed here briefly.

Nonlinear Pharmacokinetics

Some drugs such as phenytoin show an altered pharmacokinetic behavior when the dose of the drug is increased. In man, phenytoin (PHT) is largely metabolized to (*para*-hydroxyphenyl)-phenylhydantoin (HPPH), which is rapidly eliminated, almost exclusively as the glucuronide. The enzyme system responsible for metabolism reaches the point of saturation and metabolizes the increasing amount of drug with an unchanged rate. When this situation occurs, an increase of the dose then causes a disproportionate elevation of the plasma concentration. The characteristics of PHT kinetics mentioned here can be described by a capacity-limited elimination model using the Michaelis–Menten equation derived from enzyme kinetics. For PHT, capacity-limited kinetics are found to occur within the therapeutic concentration range. A measure for capacity-limited or nonlinear kinetics is the so-called Michaelis–Menten constant (K_m). The K_m value represents the concentration of the drug (mg/liter) at which half of the metabolizing enzymes present are occupied. Values of K_m for PHT have been reported varying from 1.5 to 25.2 mg/liter (7,10).

The influence of nonlinear kinetics on the elimination part of the plasma concentration–time curve after administration of different dosages of PHT to the same patient is shown in Fig. 8. At a dose of 250 mg of PHT, the elimination phase of the curve is linear. Increasing the dose to 1,000 mg results in a nonlinear elimination of the drug, with a final half-life equal to the half-life found after a dose of 250 mg.

Under strictly defined conditions, when plasma concentrations of PHT are measured following various dose increments, the proportionality between dose and plasma concentration may be described as:

$$\frac{F \cdot D}{\Delta t} = \frac{V_{max} \cdot C_{ss}}{K_m + C_{ss}} \qquad [16]$$

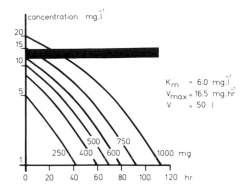

FIG. 8. Nonlinear elimination kinetics of phenytoin after i.v. administration of various dose increments. Nonlinearity begins to appear below the therapeutic concentration range (*shaded area*).

in which the maximum rate of metabolism of the drug for the individual concerned is represented as $V_{\max}$ (mg/hr) and the Michaelis–Menten constant as K_m (mg/liter). This approximation is justified since it may be assumed that the enzymatic mechanism (cytochrome P-450) responsible for the metabolism of PHT will be saturated at higher dosages. In equation 16, the relationship between dose and plasma concentration is now determined by two independent constants (K_m and $V_{\max}$) instead of one clearance value as in linear kinetics. The impact of nonlinear kinetics on dose regimen calculations will be discussed further on in this chapter.

Enzyme Induction

During long-term treatment with antiepileptic drugs, the steady-state plasma concentration of drugs such as phenobarbital and carbamazepine tends to fall gradually. This phenomenon is caused by enzyme induction.

It is known that phenobarbital and carbamazepine, among others, induce an increase in the amount of cytochrome P-450 after administration to laboratory animals and humans. An increasing amount of metabolizing enzyme results in an increased rate of metabolism. The rate at which the amount of enzymes increases in time is relatively high in rats when massive doses of, for example, phenobarbital are given (75 mg/kg). Although these massive doses never

will be prescribed to epileptic patients, the process of enzyme induction will proceed at a lower rate for a longer period of time (some weeks or even months). Changing the daily dose of drugs with enzyme-inducing abilities usually also means an alteration of the level of enzyme induction.

These drugs not only induce their own metabolism (autoinduction) but also the metabolism of other drugs administered simultaneously (heteroinduction). The increased rate of metabolism results in a decreased elimination half-life and thus in an increased total body clearance. Whereas an increased clearance value affects the input–output equilibrium of the drug, the steady-state plasma concentration will gradually decrease until it reaches a new (lower) level of equilibrium.

In Fig. 9, the effects of enzyme induction on the steady-state plasma concentration of carbamazepine are shown. Starting from an initial half-life of 35 hr, maximum steady-state plasma concentrations of 20 mg/liter may be reached when no enzyme induction occurs. The elimination half-life remains 35 hr measured after the last dose. Autoinduction reduces the final elimination half-life to approximately 20 hr, so the maximum concentrations reached will be lower. The addition of other enzyme-inducing agents to the therapy, e.g., phenobarbital, will reduce the final half-life of carbamazepine to 10 hr. Therefore, the total body clearance ($V_d \times k_{el}$) will increase from 1.98 to 6.93 liter/hr. The impact of enzyme-inducing properties of compounds on the drug therapy will be obvious.

Renal Clearance of Antiepileptic Drugs

Antiepileptic drugs are not only cleared by the metabolic route but also directly through the kidneys into the urine. Although the kinetics of renal excretion are generally well understood (18,20), the renal clearance of antiepileptic drugs is often ignored in clinical practice.

Renal clearance of drugs is determined by glomerular filtration rate, tubular reabsorption, urine flow, and urine pH. The last two in particular may vary over the course of a day or differ from day to day. These variations influ-

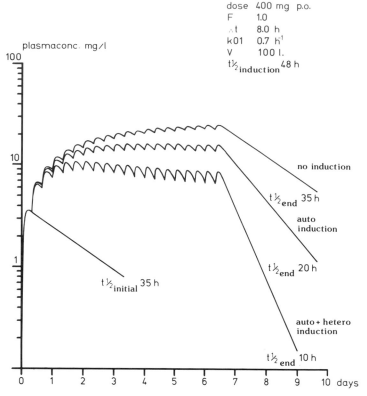

FIG. 9. The effects of enzyme induction (auto- and heteroinduction) on the elimination half-life and steady-state plasma concentrations of carbamazepine during subchronic treatment in a theoretical simulation model.

ence the renal clearance of antiepileptic drugs and thus the total body clearance of these drugs, as shown in equation 6.

In the plasma concentration–time curve of ethosuximide presented in Fig. 7, the renal excretion rate of ethosuximide is also shown. The renal excretion rate is given as the amount of drug excreted per unit of time (μg/min). In this figure, it is obvious that the renal excretion rate fluctuates with the urine flow. From the renal excretion rate and the corresponding plasma concentrations, the renal clearance can be calculated:

$$K_r = \frac{dQ/dt}{C_t} \qquad [17]$$

in which K_r is the renal clearance, dQ/dt is the renal excretion rate, and C_t is the plasma concentration. By plotting the renal clearance ver-

sus the urine flow (Fig. 10), one finds a clear linear relation between these two parameters. The average urine flow over the day is approximately 1.0 ml/min. Small deviations from this average figure increase the renal clearance of ethosuximide. Similar figures are found for other antiepileptic drugs such as primidone, phenobarbital, and carbamazepine. No influence of urine flow rate could be observed for valproic acid (4). Other drugs are currently under investigation.

DOSE CALCULATION CONCEPTS

Whenever decisions are made about choice of drug, route of administration, therapeutic plasma concentration in view of the nature and degree of the disease, and the dosage interval, the amount of drug will be the only variable that has to be established. When the pharma-

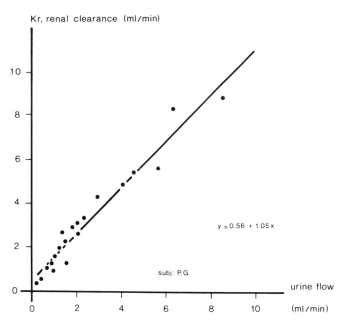

Kr, renal clearance (ml/min)

$y = 0.56 + 1.05 x$

subj: P.G.

urine flow

(ml/min)

FIG. 10. Influence of the urine flow on the renal clearance of ethosuximide in a volunteer. Clearance values are calculated from the plasma concentration and renal excretion rate data as shown in Fig. 7.

cokinetic parameters such as elimination half-life and relative volume of distribution (V_d') of the drug are sufficiently known, they can be used to calculate the maintenance dose, using the rearranged equations 7 and 15:

$$D = k_{el} \times V_d' \times \Delta t \times W \times C_{ss} \quad [18]$$

The mean pharmacokinetic parameters of the antiepileptic drugs for which this calculation can be used are shown in Table 1. If the product of the elimination rate constant and the relative volume of distribution is defined as the relative clearance, a parameter that is less complicated for use in dose regimen calculations, equation 18 may be read as:

$$D = k_{el} \times V' \times \Delta t \times W \times C_{ss} \quad [19]$$

The dose calculated with this equation can be a reliable individual adaptation of the maintenance dose, especially when the individual relative clearance value of the drug in that particular patient is used, whenever this value is sufficiently well known from previous plasma level determinations.

For the calculation of the dose when a new therapy is started, average clearance values obtained from large retrospective studies may be used (5). These clearance values are presented in Table 2. Calculations based on the relative clearance concept are only allowed in cases of linear kinetics and when no major alterations occur in the physiological and clinical condition of the patient. They are based on a linear relationship between the dose administered and the measured plasma concentration as graphically shown in Fig. 11.

From single-point concentration determinations, the dose can be corrected using a simplified equation. When the intended plasma concentration (C_{ther}) and the clinically intended effect have not been reached and the calculated

TABLE 2. *The relative clearance values of the major antiepileptic drugs[a]*

Generic drug name	V' (ml/hr·kg)
Phenobarbital	5.0
Phenytoin	20.0
Primidone	60.0
Carbamazepine	30.0 – 150.0
Ethosuximide	18.0
2-Propylpentanoate	12.0

[a]Data are obtained from a retrospective study in a large group of epileptic patients with a wide variety of co-medication (5).

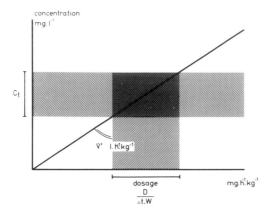

FIG. 11. Graphic presentation of the relationship between the dose administered and the plasma concentration during steady state in linear kinetics used for relative clearance calculations. In this figure, the reciprocal of the slope of the ideal line represents the relative clearance (V', liter/hr/kg) of the drug.

clearance for the individual appears to match the normal clearance value, the dose can proportionally be corrected:

$$\text{New dose} = \frac{\text{previous dose} \times C_{\text{ther}}}{C_{\text{prev}}} \quad [20]$$

Drugs that show enzyme-capacity-limited elimination, including phenytoin, will need a more complicated nonlinear correction for dose calculations. If K_m and $V_{\max}$ values are sufficiently well known in a patient, they may be used to calculate the optimum dose. Rearrangement of equation 16 then leads to:

$$D = \frac{V_{\max}}{K_m + C_{\text{ss}}} \times V_d' \times \Delta t \times W \times C_{\text{ss}}$$

$$[21]$$

When plasma concentrations are measured in a patient under optimum conditions of steady state after two consecutive dosage increments, the K_m value in that patient easily may be calculated from the equation:

$$K_m = \frac{D_2 \times C_1 \times C_2 - D_1 \times C_1 \times C_2}{D_1 \times C_2 - D_2 \times C_1}$$

$$[22]$$

In this equation, D_1 is the initially instituted

dose, D_2 the second dose, and C_1 and C_2 their measured plasma concentrations, respectively. From equation 21 it can be seen that $V_{\max}$ and K_m are related to the total body clearance of a drug according to:

$$V_{\max} = V' \times (K_m + C_{\text{ss}}) \quad [23]$$

So $V_{\max}$ can be calculated when the total body clearance at a single level is sufficiently known. The clearance, however, should be determined in a situation in which nonlinear elimination does not occur, i.e., at low dosages of the drug.

For the dose calculation in nonlinear pharmacokinetics, the $V_{\max}$ value of a drug appears to be of minor importance, and if the K_m can be calculated accurately enough, the following equation may be used to calculate the maintenance dose:

$$\text{New dose } (D) =$$
$$\frac{(K_m + C_{\text{prev}}) \times C_{\text{ther}}}{(K_m + C_{\text{ther}}) \times C_{\text{prev}}} \times \text{previous dose} \quad [24]$$

in which C_{ther} represents the desired plasma concentration, C_{prev} the measured concentration at a previous dose, and K_m the Michaelis–Menten constant of the drug in that particular patient.

Adjustments of dosage regimens of drugs known to have nonlinear pharmacokinetic properties, such as phenytoin, should be done carefully, and the clinical experience of the physician will be as important as pharmacokinetic knowledge to avoid losing sight of the needs of the individual patient.

GENERAL COMMENTS

Unlike infectious diseases for which the discovery of drugs led to an almost complete cure rate, the treatment of epilepsy has not benefited from drugs to the same extent. Although undoubtedly indispensable for the complete or partial control of seizures, the success of drug treatment in epilepsy until now has satisfied neither patients nor physicians.

Even without an understanding of the causes of epileptic seizures, it has become evident that the effectiveness of treatment could gain from individualized adjustments of antiepileptic drug therapy. The concept of taking the individual patient as his own reference standard has changed treatment routines and created possibilities for prospective planning, in-process vigilance, retrospective monitoring, and feedback procedures. Plasma concentration determinations have alerted physicians to the fact that to assume that a prescribed dose always leads to an intended effect is relatively unjustified.

The application of pharmacokinetic logic to the interpretation of plasma concentration data and the use of relative clearance data of drugs now allow the physician to calculate an individual dosage regimen accurately. However, these interpretation and calculation concepts require a thorough understanding of the background of clinical pharmacokinetics and of the pharmacokinetic properties of the compounds involved. For the antiepileptic drugs, the available clinical pharmacokinetic information appears to be rather extensive (5,6,8,11,13,17). However, the interindividual variability in drug handling and response and the difficulties in quantifying therapeutic efficacy in epilepsy strongly reduce the practical application of clinical pharmacokinetics.

REFERENCES

1. Booker, H. E., and Darcey, B. (1973): Serum concentrations of free diphenylhydantoin and their relationship to clinical intoxications. *Clin. Chem.*, 17: 607–611.
2. Dayton, P. G., Israili, Z. H., and Perel, J. M. (1973): Influence of binding on drug metabolism and distribution. *Ann. N.Y. Acad. Sci.*, 226:172–181.
3. Dost, F. H. (1953): *Der Blutspiegel: Kinetic der Konzentrations abläufe in der Kreislaufflüssigkeit*. Georg Thieme, Leipzig.
4. Guelen, P. J. M., Janssen, T. J., and Vree, T. B. (1980): The renal excretion of anti-epileptics. In: *World Conference on Clinical Pharmacology and Therapeutics*, Abstr. 0686. Macmillan, London.
5. Guelen, P. J. M., and van der Kleijn, E. (1978): *Rational Antiepileptic Drug Therapy*. Elsevier/North Holland, Amsterdam.
6. Hvidberg, E. F., and Dam, M. (1976): Clinical pharmacokinetics of anticonvulsants. *Clin. Pharmacokinet.*, 1:161–188.
7. Jusko, W. J., Koup, J. R., and Alvan, G. (1976): Nonlinear assessment of phenytoin bioavailability. *J. Pharmacokinet. Biopharm.*, 4:327–336.
8. Leal, K. W., and Troupin, A. S. (1977): Clinical pharmacology of anti-epileptic drugs, a summary of current information, *Clin. Chem.*, 23:1964–1968.
9. Levy, G. (1974): *Clinical Pharmacokinetics, a Symposium*. American Pharmaceutical Association, Washington.
10. Martin, E., Tozer, T. N., Sheiner, L. B., and Riegelman, S. (1977): The clinical pharmacokinetics of phenytoin. *J. Pharmacokinet. Biopharm.*, 5:579–596.
11. Morselli, P. L., and Franco-Morselli, R. (1980): Clinical pharmacokinetics of anti epileptic drugs in adults. *Pharmacol. Ther.*, 10:65–101.
12. Porter, R. J., and Penry, J. K. (1978): Efficacy and choice of antiepileptic drugs. In: *Advances in Epileptology, 1977*, edited by H. Meinardi and A. J. Rowan, pp. 220–231. Swets & Zeitlinger, Amsterdam.
13. Rane, A. (1978): Clinical pharmacokinetics of anti-epileptic drugs in children, *Pharmacol. Ther.*, 2:251–267.
14. Ritshel, W. A. (1976): *Handbook of Basic Pharmacokinetics*. Drug Intelligence Publications, Hamilton.
15. Rowland, M. (1980): Plasma protein binding and therapeutic drug monitoring. *Ther. Drug Monitor.*, 2: 29–37.
16. Travers, R. D., Reynolds, E. H., and Gallagher, B. B. (1972): Variation in response to anticonvulsants in a group of epileptic patients. *Arch. Neurol.*, 27:29–33.
17. Van der Kleijn, E., Guelen, P. J. M., Baars, A. M., Vree, T. B., and Termond, E. (1976): Clinical pharmacokinetics of anti epileptic drugs. In: *Clinical Pharmacy and Clinical Pharmacology*, edited by W. A. Gouveia, T. Tognaoni, and E. van der Kleijn, pp. 43–66. North-Holland, Amsterdam.
18. Van Rossum, J. M. (1977): *Handbook of Experimental Pharmacology, Vol. 47, Kinetics of Drug Action*. Springer-Verlag, Berlin.
19. Wagner, J. G. (1971): *Biopharmaceutics and Relevant Pharmacokinetics*. Drug Intelligence Publications, Hamilton.
20. Wagner, J. G. (1975): *Fundamentals of Clinical Pharmacokinetics*. Drug Intelligence Publications, Hamilton.

Antiepileptic Drugs, edited by D. M. Woodbury, J. K. Penry, and C. E. Pippenger. Raven Press, New York © 1982.

5

General Principles

Toxicity

Gabriel L. Plaa

The fact that chemicals can induce toxic reactions in biological systems, particularly in man, has been known for a long time. Actually, the mechanisms involved in some of these reactions were discovered before modern pharmacology was established. It is said that Claude Bernard's lectures in 1856 on the toxic effects of noxious gases and curare constituted a course in pharmacology (8). The therapeutic effects of many drugs constitute a response that, if exaggerated, can lead to a toxic reaction. The problem has been to determine the balance necessary so that chemical interactions with the biological system can be more beneficial than harmful.

CLASSIFICATION OF TOXIC REACTIONS

Drug toxicity usually refers to those properties of a drug that are harmful to the organism or are so undesirable that they greatly limit the therapeutic usefulness of the drug in question. Zbinden (25) has classified toxic reactions into three categories of change: functional, biochemical, and structural. By his classification, functional toxicity "is due to the pharmacological effects which are not necessary for the desired action, although they may for another patient and under different circumstances constitute an important therapeutic effect." Table 1 summar-

izes the major categories of "functional side effects" as described by Zbinden. The term "function" is being used here in its broadest sense and actually represents a change in function of an organ system. Each of these major classes can be subdivided into many subcategories. For instance, the following subcategories are ascribed for the central nervous system: ataxia, convulsions, dysarthria, extrapyramidal reaction, headache, hyperreflexia, incoordination, paresthesia, tremor, and vertigo. It is obvious that the more functions attributed to a particular system, the more subclassifications of abnormal effects can be described. These undesirable side effects are usually reversible on discontinuation of the drug.

Included in Zbinden's second classification, "biochemical toxicity," are reactions that do not produce gross evidence of organ damage but cause changes in biochemical reactions associated with the various organs. These biochemical changes by Zbinden's definition are not accompanied by marked anatomical changes. Shifts in hormonal balance and changes in acid–base balance, serum electrolytes, and blood coagulation are examples of this type of drug-related toxic change. Again, these changes are usually reversible on discontinuation of the drug.

The third category, "structural toxicity," involves an actual change in the structure of the

TABLE 1. *Functional side effects associated with drug therapy*

1. Changes of wakefulness, general well-being, emotions, and personality
   Aggressiveness, agitation, anxiety, depression, insomnia, psychosis, sedation, weakness, etc.
2. Central and peripheral nervous system
   Convulsions, ataxia, extrapyramidal reaction, paresthesia, etc.
3. Sensory organs
   Blurred vision, metallic taste, tinnitus, etc.
4. Skin
   Perspiration, pruritus, etc.
5. Musculoskeletal system
   Cramps, fasciculations, etc.
6. Cardiovascular and respiratory system
   Angina, fibrillation, dyspnea, nasal congestion, hypertension, bradycardia, etc.
7. Gastrointestinal system, including salivary glands, pancreas, and liver
   Constipation, dry mouth, emesis, nausea, parotid pain, etc.
8. Urinary system
   Nocturia, voiding difficulty, etc.
9. Genital system, including mammary glands
   Amenorrhea, breast engorgement, decrease of libido, impotence, etc.
10. Local drug effects
    Burning in esophagus, pain on injection, etc.
11. Changes involving the whole body
    Fever, hypothermia, weight gain, etc.

From Zbinden (25), with permission.

organ or the tissue involved. Obviously, these structural changes can also bring about biochemical and functional changes (for example, drug-induced liver injury, granulocytopenia, and cataracts).

In 1963, the results of a retrospective survey were published (25) concerning the frequency of biochemical and structural drug toxicity in humans following the use of drugs. In this survey, all reports involving overdosage or the treatment of very serious diseases were eliminated. More than 20,000 patients were included in this survey, and more than 100 different drugs were involved. Of these patients, 7.3% exhibited structural or biochemical changes related to the drug action. Toxic effects on the hematopoietic system were the most frequent, followed by effects on the liver, skin, sensory organs, pericardium, fetal development, bone and joints, gastrointestinal tract, and kidney.

In the last 10 years, a considerable amount of interest in adverse drug reactions has been generated (4,12,16). Many of the published reports give inadequate information for determination of cause-and-effect relationships. In most reports, there is a notable lack of data concerning appropriate control groups. Therefore, quantitative assessment of incidence and impact of these reactions is difficult. Incidences of 6 to 15%, 1 to 6%, 1 to 28%, and 10 to 20% have been reported (4,12,16); the precise incidence is still unknown.

It is of interest to determine whether these adverse drug reactions represent known properties of the drugs involved or whether they represent aberrant, undetectable types of responses. Such data are also imprecise. Estimates derived from the literature (4,16) indicate that about 80% of the reactions responsible for the patient's hospitalization were considered to be traceable to known pharmacological mechanisms, less than 10% were immunologic (allergic) in character, and less than 5% could be attributed to idiosyncratic and other unknown mechanisms. The data, although imprecise, lead to the conclusion that 70 to 80% of the adverse drug reactions are at least understandable and predictable.

DETECTION OF DRUG TOXICITY

It is now quite apparent that, regardless of the extensive toxicologic testing carried out under the present regulations of government agencies, significant toxic effects can sometimes be discovered only when a drug has been introduced into the market and has been administered to a great number of patients. Several reasons can be invoked to explain why toxic reactions may not be uncovered in preclinical testing.

The toxic reaction may be a rare event. If the occurrence manifests itself only about once in 1,000 cases, or once in 10,000 cases, it is highly unlikely that the toxic reaction will be uncovered in preclinical testing. Only when the substance is used extensively will it be possible to establish a cause-and-effect relationship. An example of this type of toxic event is the aplastic anemia associated with the antibiotic chloramphenicol. It took several years of clinical experience before the association was made between the drug and the toxic reaction. Drug toxicities based on genetic abnormalities are also examples of this type of event.

The toxic reaction may appear only after prolonged drug administration. The possible carcinogenicity of drugs falls into this category.

The toxic effect of a drug may not be reproducible in the particular animal species used for preclinical testing. Reactions that are not readily observable in laboratory animals include headache, nausea, insomnia, and psychotic disturbances. An example of this type of reaction are the episodes that are observed when monoamine oxidase inhibitors are given to individuals who eat foods rich in tyramine. In the area of liver injury, it is common to find drugs associated with cholestatic reactions in man that cannot produce the same effects in laboratory animals. This situation creates problems because it is difficult to determine experimentally whether it is the species that is responding differently or whether the multiple factors involved in the toxic reaction are not reproduced in all species. Toxic reactions involving metabolic transformations (e.g., of the drug) can cause this type of aberrant response in different species.

Loomis (15) has described the various factors that can influence toxicity. These include biological, chemical, and genetic factors, as well as the route of administration. The subcategories for each of these factors are given in Table 2. These have been very well described by Loomis (15), and the interested reader should consult this book.

The mechanisms of harmful effects observed with drugs can also be classified. The classification devised by Loomis (15) and found in Table 3 can be extremely useful for characterizing these effects.

The "idiosyncratic response" does not appear in this classification system, yet one often sees this term applied to some forms of toxic reactions. Unfortunately, the use of the term "idiosyncratic reaction" is confusing. These reactions may be defined by some authors merely

TABLE 2. *Factors affecting toxicity*

A. Biologic factors
   1. Translocation of chemicals
   2. Reserve functional capacity
   3. Storage of chemicals in the organism
   4. Tolerance
B. Chemical factors
   1. Nonspecific chemical action
   2. Selective chemical action
     a. Target organs or receptors
   3. Ionization and lipid solubility on translocation
   4. Biotransformation mechanisms
     a. Inhibition of biotransformation reactions
     b. Induction of biotransformation reactions
C. Genetic factors
   1. Accumulation of chemicals
   2. Prolongation of action of chemicals
   3. Increased sensitivity to chemicals
   4. Species and strain resistance
D. Route of administration

Adapted from Loomis (15), with permission.

in terms of a low incidence regardless of the underlying mechanism. Others may define it as a low-incidence response occurring by an entirely unknown mechanism. Goldstein et al. (8) prefer to restrict the use of the term to describe drug reactions involving a genetically determined abnormal reactivity on the part of the subject. Most toxicologists would agree that mere frequency of reaction should not be the basis of the definition, but some might have reservations to the restriction of the term "drug idiosyncrasy" only to genetically based reactions. Such a restriction necessitates the formulation of an-

TABLE 3. *Classification of mechanisms of harmful effects of drugs*

A. Normal effects associated with
   1. Exposure to normal doses depending on
     a. malfunction of mechanisms for terminating action of the agent
     b. actions on the wrong target system
     c. synergism with other chemicals
   2. Exposure to excessive doses depending on
     a. nonspecific caustic or corrosive action
     b. exaggerated pharmacologic effects
     c. specific toxicologic actions
     d. production of pathologic sequelae
     e. sociologic complications
B. Abnormal effects depending on
   1. Immune mechanisms

Adapted from Loomis (15), with permission.

other category, the "unexplained reaction." The matter is still unresolved, but the reader should be aware that "drug idiosyncrasy" means different things to different authors.

Some mention should be made of the evaluation of drug toxicity in animals and humans. Table 4 summarizes various toxicologic procedures that are more or less routinely employed in the preclinical testing of new potential drugs. Four types of studies are carried out: acute toxicity, subchronic, chronic, and special. In the subchronic and chronic studies, the highest dose level selected is one that is sufficiently high to produce signs of toxicity in that species. In these phases, hematologic and organ function tests are done routinely; also, autopsies and histologic examination of organs are performed.

In acute toxicity studies, one purpose is to determine the toxic signs that occur when the drug is given only once and in high dosages. A second purpose is to obtain some idea of the quantitative relationships involved (toxic dosage versus probable therapeutic dosage). In addition, close observation and physical examination of the animals can yield some insight into the mechanisms involved.

Since most drugs are given to humans for a prolonged period, one must determine the toxicological profile of a new drug under these circumstances. This is the purpose of the subchronic and chronic studies. These are designed to uncover biochemical and morphologic abnor-

TABLE 4. *Routine animal toxicologic tests*

Acute tests with single dose
 1. Median lethal dose (LD_{50}) in rodents
 2. Pyramiding single-dose studies in dogs
 3. Local effects on rabbit skin (for agents to be used topically)
Prolonged tests with daily doses
 1. Subchronic, up to 3 months, using rats and dogs, three dose levels
 2. Chronic, 6 months to 2 years, using rats and dogs, two to three dose levels
Special tests
 1. For effects on fertility and reproduction
 2. For teratogenicity
 3. For carcinogenicity and mutagenicity
 4. For effects on behavior
 5. Interactions with other chemical agents

---

malities that might occur after repetitive exposures. Again, quantitative comparisons of the dosages involved are made to establish the relative safety of the drug.

A battery of special tests are designed to detect toxic manifestations that are not likely to be encountered in routine acute, subchronic, and chronic studies. Such tests include those used for measuring teratogenesis, effects on reproduction, mutagenesis, and carcinogenesis. Quantitative comparisons of the dosages involved are essential for establishing relative safety.

Interest in teratogenicity arose because of the thalidomide tragedy. Since then, suitable methods have been devised for the detection of possible teratogens in laboratory animals. Tests using nonplacental species such as the developing chicken embryo were among the first to be utilized. However, such tests are open to considerable criticism; since many factors influence the results, little confidence can be placed in them. Mice, rats, and rabbits are the test animals most frequently used at the present time. The range of dosages should be such that maternal toxicity itself does not influence the outcome. Live and dead fetuses are counted, the uterus is examined for resorptions, and all fetuses are systematically examined for evidence of malformations.

There are three components to the tests used for assessing reproduction: effects on fertility (both males and females), effects on gestation (fetal development, teratogenicity, mutagenicity, intrauterine mortality), and effects on the progeny (maternal lactation and acceptance of the offspring; growth, development and sexual maturity of the offspring).

Testing for possible carcinogenic properties has become a major preoccupation of toxicologists involved in the safety evaluation process. It is an extremely complex problem and one that has created emotional reactions because of the possible impact on society. Carcinogenicity testing is usually performed in rodents or dogs, and the animals are maintained over their entire life-span. The chemical is given by the intended route of exposure in humans, and at least two dosage levels are used. It is common to describe the chemicals that produce any type of tumor as tumorigenic agents and those that produce malignant tumors are carcinogenic agents. However, a controversy still exists since the ultimate fate of benign tumors in animals has not been resolved. A potentially carcinogenic chemical may produce the following in animals: the occurrence of a type of tumor not seen in normal control animals, an increased incidence of spontaneous tumors of a type seen in normal control animals, and a combination of these two events. Furthermore, qualitative differences between types of carcinogenic agents can be demonstrated. Some agents are strongly carcinogenic (maximally tolerated dosages are not needed to demonstrate the effect, a small number of animals are needed, and the time needed to produce the response is relatively short), whereas others are weak carcinogens (near-toxic dosages have to be employed, a large number of animals are required, and near-lifetime exposures are needed). All of these elements must be considered when making a reasoned judgment on the possible carcinogenic properties of a chemical.

During recent years, there has been considerable interest in the testing of mutagenicity. Both mammalian and nonmammalian (bacteria, yeast, plants, insects) systems have been devised. The latter have one serious disadvantage in that they lack the physiological and biotransformation components known to affect toxicity (Table 2) in mammals. Attempts have been made to overcome the biotransformation aspect by the addition of mammalian metabolizing systems to some of the test systems. Both *in vitro* and *in vivo* assays are utilized, and this field is evolving very rapidly. However, there is considerable controversy concerning the extrapolation of such data to possible toxic manifestations in humans. Among the *in vitro* tests, one finds the Ames *Salmonella* microsomal assay system and variations of this procedure. The suspected mutagen is incubated with a histidine-dependent strain of *Salmonella,* and mutagenesis is indicated when the number of revertant organisms (non-histidine dependent) increases after incubation. For *in vivo* tests, one finds the dominant lethal assay, the host-mediated assay, and various cytogenetic methods. In the dominant lethal assay, male rodents are first treated with the chemical and then mated with females; the latter are sacrificed and examined for abnormal fetal development. In the host-mediated assay, microorganisms are grown in the peritoneal cavity of the rodent host, the test agent is given to the host, and the mutation frequency in the organisms is subsequently measured. The cytogenetic tests make use of various tissues from animals or humans: bone marrow, lymphocytes, skin fibroblasts, gametocytes, and amniotic fluid cells. A battery of mutagenicity tests is employed since no single method is adequate for determining the possible risk to humans. The various tests vary considerably in terms of sensitivity, specificity, and applicability. Furthermore, the distinctively artificial nature of the test systems make interpretations regarding safety rather tenuous; unfortunately, quantitative interpretations needed for safety evaluation are extremely limited.

DOSE–RESPONSE RELATIONSHIPS

The concept of a dose–response relationship is extremely important in toxicologic evaluations. The underlying principle behind this concept is that for all chemicals and all biologic systems, there is a dosage that exerts a maximum response and one that exerts a minimum response. Between these two dosages, a range of responses will be found as the dosage is altered. When lethality is the endpoint being measured, it is obvious that there can only be an all-or-none response. Therefore, if one uses a population of animals given a range of dosages, one calculates the percentage of animals at each dosage that show the lethal response. When this kind of response is established, it is possible to calculate by a number of different statistical procedures (14,17,24) the dosage that kills 50% of the population, the median lethal dosage (LD_{50}). Dose–response relationships can be determined for responses other than lethality. In these cases, the median effective dosage (ED_{50}) is calculated. If quantal (all-or-none) data (e.g., percentage of subjects affected) are desired, the measured responses are merely converted into all-or-none units after establishing the appropriate cutoff value between "no effect" and "effect." Two responses associated with acute liver injury, plasma sulfobromophthalein (BSP) retention and elevated serum transaminase (SGPT) activity, have been utilized (13) to obtain dose–response data for hepatoxicity.

Dose–response curves can be used to compare quantitatively the differences in toxic potencies observed in a series of different drugs. Furthermore, for a single compound one can derive a quantitative estimate of its relative potency for producing several different toxic effects. Dose–response relationships are also used to estimate the "no adverse effect level" in the safety evaluation process of drugs. This is the dosage that results in no detectable injurious effect and is used to establish safety factors.

LOW-INCIDENCE RESPONSES

Some untoward drug reactions in humans are uncovered only after widespread use in large patient populations because the toxic reaction may be a rare event. These have been described as low-incidence toxic reactions. Frequencies of 0.1%, 0.01%, and 0.001% are examples of such reactions. Toxicologists tend to deemphasize abnormal responses in treatment groups if a clear dose–response relationship is not observed, particularly when the abnormal response is observed in a low-dosage group but not at higher dosages. One normally assumes that the laboratory animal sampling selected for test purposes represents a homogeneous population. However, subpopulations can exist within a supposedly homogeneous population; such an occurrence was demonstrated in rats for sodium chloride-induced hypertension (3). Thus, a low-incidence toxic reaction in a test population may be the reflection of the presence of a susceptible subpopulation that is diluted out by a larger subpopulation of nonresponders. One can calculate how many subjects would be required to un-

cover such a situation in a test population (26). If the incidence of the reaction is 1% (1:100), one would have to test 299 subjects in order to have a 95% probability of detecting at least one responder. If the incidence is 0.1% (1:1000), 2,995 subjects would have to be tested to get at least one responder. With incidences of 0.01% (1:10,000) and 0.001% (1:100,000), the required number of test subjects increases to 29,956 and 299,572, respectively, to detect at least one responder. These calculations show why it is virtually impossible to expect to detect low-incidence toxic reactions in animal studies if the dose–response relationship cannot be demonstrated.

DRUG INTERACTIONS

The multiple use of drugs in current medical practice has created the problem of drug interaction and its sequelae of undesirable or even toxic reactions. The clinical implications of such interactions are now reasonably well known, and appropriate references for specific drug interactions mentioned below can be rapidly obtained (1,11). The fact that two or more drugs are administered to a patient does not mean that a drug interaction will necessarily occur. Whether or not an interaction will be seen depends entirely on the particular drugs involved. Also, the fact that an interaction can occur does not mean that it will always occur; patient variability is the most evident feature of drug interactions. If an interaction does occur, it need not always result in a toxic response. Furthermore, among those that do result in toxic effects, fortunately only a few are life threatening. The dangerous drug interactions are those that involve the combination of different drugs that affect the pharmacokinetics of coumarin-type anticoagulants, oral hypoglycemic agents, and cardiotonic drugs. The interaction between the tricyclic antidepressants and guanethidine-type antihypertensive drugs is also dangerous and is due to an interaction at the site of action.

Drug interactions can occur at many levels. However, many of them are due to alterations in pharmacokinetics because of modifications in absorption, distribution, biotransformation, or excretion. Those drugs whose pharmacologic actions are particularly affected by modifications in plasma concentrations are more prone to result in interactions. Furthermore, when the difference between the therapeutic and the toxic plasma concentrations is small, it is more likely that the interaction may result in a toxic effect. However, the interaction can lead to a loss of therapeutic effect if the combined administration of the drugs causes the plasma concentration of the affected agent to drop below its therapeutic level.

Decreased absorption can obviously lower plasma concentrations. Such events have been observed when tetracyclines are coadministered with calcium, aluminum, or ferrous salts. Poorly soluble complexes between the tetracycline and the ions are formed, resulting in poor absorption of these broad-spectrum antibiotics.

Diminished drug binding to plasma proteins can lead to an increase in circulating free drug and an increase in tissue distribution. The problem of sulfonamides and kernicterus in the premature infant (19), due to displacement of bilirubin from plasma protein binding sites is one example. Drugs can also displace each other. Displacement of anticoagulants by phenylbutazone analogs has led to serious bleeding episodes. Methotrexate can be displaced by salicylates and may result in hepatotoxicity.

By far the greatest interest in drug interaction has been at the level of biotransformation. The induction of mixed-function oxidases in the liver by a multitude of drugs increases the possibilities of such drug interactions. The classical example is the inductive effect of phenobarbital on dicoumarol biotransformation in patients on anticoagulant therapy (2). Plaa et al. (22) showed that combined use of phenobarbital and primidone in epileptics could result in toxicity due to the enhanced conversion of primidone to phenobarbital. Adverse effects of phenobarbital on corticosteroids in asthmatics are believed to be due to induction of corticosteroid metabolism. Inhibition of drug metabolism also can

lead to drug interactions. Treatment with disulfiram results in discomforting symptoms when ethanol is ingested (9). This is supposedly due to the accumulation of acetaldehyde caused by an interference of its metabolism by disulfiram. Phenytoin metabolism can be inhibited by several drugs (dicoumarol, chloramphenicol, isoniazid, disulfiram, sulfamethizol) and can result in phenytoin toxicity. Dicoumarol and chloramphenicol can decrease tolbutamide biotransformation.

Interaction at sites of elimination are also known. Both in the kidney and in the liver, transport systems for acidic and basic substances have been demonstrated (23). In the kidney use has been made of this phenomenon to increase blood levels of penicillin by the coadministration of probenecid. The uricosuric effects of sulfinpyrazone are significantly reduced by the concurrent administration of salicylates. It is now believed that it is the nonionic moiety that is involved in back diffusion in the tubules. Therefore, alkalinization has been employed to enhance the excretion of barbiturates and salicylates in drug intoxications. In the liver, much less is known about possible drug interactions. However, it was observed that administration of radiocontrast material can affect the subsequent excretion of BSP, thus resulting in a false abnormal liver function profile. In rats, diazepam and BSP inhibit the biliary excretion of each other (10,21), and diazepam modifies the biliary excretion of phenytoin and certain cardiac glycosides (5,6). Since the importance of the enterohepatic circulation in determining drug action is yet to be determined (20), the clinical implications of possible drug interactions at the level of biliary excretion are unknown. However, it is known that cholestyramine can lower serum levels of digitoxin through binding of the digitoxin in the gut and thereby interrupting the enterohepatic circulation; digitoxin intoxication has been treated successfully by this procedure. Cholestyramine can bind thyroid hormone and warfarin as well.

Another type of interaction has been observed with the monoamine oxidase inhibitors

part 3, edited by O. Eichler, A. Farah, H. Herken, and A. D. Welch, pp. 130–149. Springer-Verlag, New York.

21. Plaa, G. L., Besner, J.-G., and Caillé, G. (1975): Effect of diazepam on sulfobromophthalein excretion. In: *Clinical Pharmacology of Psychoactive Drugs,* edited by E. M. Sellers, pp. 203–218. Addiction Research Foundation, Toronto.

22. Plaa, G. L., Fujimoto, J. M., and Hine, C. H. (1958): Intoxication from primidone due to its biotransformation to phenobarbital. *J.A.M.A.,* 168:1769–1770.

23. Stowe, C. M., and Plaa, G. L. (1968): Extrarenal excretion of drugs and chemicals. *Annu. Rev. Pharmacol.,* 8:337–356.

24. Weil, C. S. (1952): Tables for convenient calculation of median-effective dose (LC_{50} or LD_{50}) and instructions in their use. *Biometrics,* 8:249–263.

25. Zbinden, G. (1963): Experimental and clinical aspects of drug toxicity. In: *Advances in Pharmacology, Vol. 2.* edited by S. Garattini and P. A. Shore, pp. 1–112. Academic Press, New York.

26. Zbinden, G. (1973): *Progress in Toxicology, Vol. 1.* Springer-Verlag, New York.

Antiepileptic Drugs, edited by D. M. Woodbury, J. K. Penry, and C. E. Pippenger. Raven Press, New York © 1982.

6

General Principles

Principles of Drug Action: Structure–Activity Relationships and Mechanisms

Gary L. Jones and Dixon M. Woodbury

HISTORY OF STRUCTURE–ACTIVITY RELATIONSHIPS IN ANTICONVULSANT RESEARCII

At least two million Americans suffer one or more of the many forms of epilepsy, a collection of seizure disorders equally common worldwide (51). However, antiepileptic drug therapy provides some seizure control for only about 70 to 80% and complete control for not more than 50% of the affected population (23). In terms of therapeutic efficacy the most significant progress in seizure control came with the introduction of phenobarbital in 1912 (36) and diphenylhydantoin in 1938 (63). Unfortunately, the decades that followed have witnessed application of the "law of diminishing returns"; that is, expanded programs have produced smaller increments of seizure control in the remaining population. Furthermore, it has become increasingly evident that significant progress toward complete seizure control will continue to elude society as long as the molecular bases of antiepileptic drug action remain unresolved. It is toward this latter goal that many recent investigations of structure–activity relationships (SAR) have been directed. The purpose of this chapter is fourfold: (a) to document the progress of an-

ticonvulsant SAR research in terms of qualitative and quantitative developments; (b) to discuss the probable causes of failure in such research; (c) to consider certain aspects of experimental design; and (d) to provide a recent example of the application of quantitative SAR in anticonvulsant research.

QUALITATIVE SAR

Selective antiepileptic drug therapy with organic compounds became a reality in 1912 when Hauptmann (36) reported the clinical effectiveness of phenobarbital. Prior to this the only effective drug therapy for epilepsy involved the use of the highly toxic bromide ion, introduced clinically in 1857 (56). Not only did the bromide ion have a very low therapeutic index, but it was also devoid of the structural content necessary for the design of superior antiepileptic agents. The discovery of the action of phenobarbital against generalized tonic–clonic seizures was significant because it afforded a relatively low-risk modality of antiepileptic therapy, and it also provided the first structural information to which an enormous SAR data base would eventually be added. However, almost a quarter century elapsed before deliberate and systematic efforts were undertaken in the search for alternative agents.

The epochal studies of Merritt and Putnam (63) in 1938 provided the first unquestionable breakthrough since the introduction of phenobarbital. Their documentation of the clinical efficacy of diphenylhydantoin (phenytoin) marked the beginning of an era which continues to this day; phenytoin and phenobarbital remain the two most useful drugs employed in the treatment of epileptic patients. The introduction of phenytoin was also significant for a variety of reasons unrelated to its immediate therapeutic application. It provided the first evidence of the selective nature of antiepileptic therapy. Phenytoin proved somewhat effective in the treatment of complex partial seizures (psychomotor epilepsy) as well as generalized tonic–clonic seizures (grand mal), whereas phenobarbital was notably ineffective against the former. Because it is not a sedative, phenytoin was also responsible for the recognition that sedation is not a requisite for anticonvulsant efficacy.

Evidence for the selective nature of antiepileptic therapy was further strengthened by the discovery of the anticonvulsant properties of trimethadione (50). Unlike phenobarbital and phenytoin, trimethadione was ineffective against generalized tonic–clonic seizures, but it proved to be the first effective drug for the treatment of absence (petit mal) seizures. Neither phenobarbital nor phenytoin is effective against absence seizures. Aside from its almost immediate acceptance into therapeutics, trimethadione was significant because it reaffirmed the value of laboratory screening in the search for new anticonvulsants and it emphasized the necessity of a battery of screening tests to avoid the exclusion of potentially useful drugs. For example, the most thoroughly documented experimental model of generalized tonic–clonic seizures, the maximal electroshock (MES) test (101), will detect drugs potentially useful against this type of seizure. However, trimethadione and other drugs not effective against generalized tonic–clonic seizures fail in nontoxic doses to modify the seizure pattern elicited in this test.

Such drugs require an alternative experimental model, one germane to the particular type of seizure under investigation. The most thoroughly documented and successful model of absence seizures is the pentylenetetrazol (Metrazol)-induced threshold seizure. Drugs effective in the prevention of the clonic threshold seizure induced by pentylenetetrazol (MET) in mice almost always have antiabsence activity in humans (101). Thus, the usual practice in the gross screening of potential antiepileptic drugs is to employ both the MES and the threshold MET models of generalized tonic–clonic and absence seizures, respectively.

The intense synthetic and screening activity that followed the introduction of phenytoin and trimethadione has produced thousands of compounds, hundreds with some degree of anticonvulsant activity, but relatively few with a useful place in therapeutics. A partial list of those that have at one time or another been found to be clinically useful includes a variety of substituted barbiturates, hydantoins, oxazolidinediones, succinimides, acetylureas, benzodiazepines, tricyclic carboxamides, and sulfonamides (Fig. 1A,B). For an extensive documentation of the many thousands of compounds synthesized and subjected to various screening tests, the reader may refer to a monograph by Close and Spielman (22) or to a more recent book edited by Vida (97). The former covers the literature through 1958; the latter from 1959 to 1976.

Although the purpose of this chapter is not to review the myriad of structures known to be associated with anticonvulsant activity, certain qualitative indices of the structure–activity relationship have long been recognized. For example, at least one phenyl or similar aromatic group is required at R_1 or R_2 (Fig. 1A) for optimal activity against most partial and generalized seizures. An exception is that alkyl substitution at R_1 (R_2) seems to be necessary (in most cases) for antiabsence action. Alkyl substitution elsewhere on the molecule can attenuate to some degree the selective influence of aromatic or alkyl groups at R_1 (R_2), providing that anticonvulsant activity is judged on the basis of certain

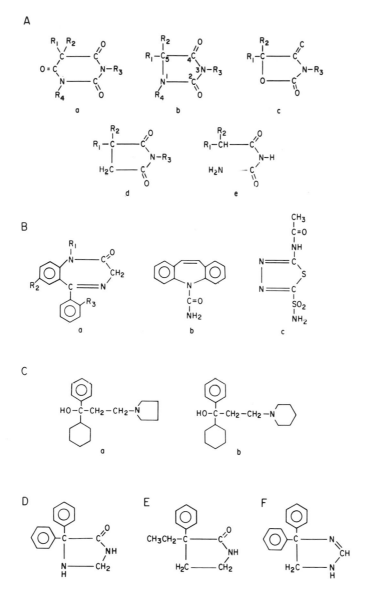

FIG. 1. A variety of substituted anticonvulsant compounds found to be clinically useful includes those depicted in **A** and **B**. Included in **A** are barbituric acid derivatives (**a**) such as phenobarbital (R_1 = phenyl, R_2 = ethyl, R_3 = R_4 = hydrogen), hydantoins (**b**) such as phenytoin (R_1 = R_2 = phenyl, R_3 = R_4 = hydrogen), oxazolidinediones (**c**) such as trimethadione (R_1 = R_2 = R_3 = methyl), succinimides (**d**) such as ethosuximide (R_1 = ethyl, R_2 = methyl, R_3 = hydrogen), and acetylureas (**e**) such as phenacemide (R_1 = phenyl, R_2 = hydrogen). Included in **B** are benzodiazepines (**a**) such as diazepam (R_1 = methyl, R_2 = chlorine, R_3 = hydrogen), tricyclic carboxamides such as carbamazepine (**b**), and sulfonamides such as acetazolamide (**c**). The structures in **B** bear a less obvious structural similarity among themselves than do those in **A**, and substituent effects on selectivity are different. The compounds in **C–F** have not been found clinically useful but are active in various experimental models of epilepsy. Procyclidine (**Ca**) and trihexyphenidyl (**Cb**) lack obvious structural similarities to the compounds in **A** (and **B**). The structures in **D–F** possess greater structural similarity to those in **A**, but the composition of the heterocyclic ring differs. See text for discussion.

experimental models; but if activity is judged on the basis of clinical experience, the nature of substituents R_1 and R_2 uniquely determine a drug's efficacy either for absences or for a variety of other seizure types.

However, the structural common denominator of anticonvulsant activity continues to elude investigators. Among the many factors hampering progress is the chemical diversity of structures known to possess such activity. Included are the hydantoins, succinimides, barbiturates, and oxazolidinediones, which are chemically different yet structurally quite similar; and the acetylureas, benzodiazepines, sulfonamides, tricyclic carboxamides (e.g., carbamazepine), and pyrrolidino- and piperidinopropanols (e.g., procyclidine and trihexyphenidyl, respectively) (Fig. 1A–C). To the latter compounds, which are not only chemically dissimilar but also lack obvious stereochemical similarities, can be added scores of additional cyclic and acyclic structures.

It was not until 1970, when Camerman and Camerman (8) demonstrated a not-so-obvious conformational similarity between phenytoin and diazepam, that a more comprehensive appreciation of the structural basis of anticonvulsant action began to unfold. The Camermans' X-ray crystallography studies revealed conformational and other similarities among phenytoin (9), diazepam (10), procyclidine (14), trihexyphenidyl (15), phenacemide (12), and ethylphenacemide (12). They found that all of these drugs possess hydrophobic regions and electron-donor groups with similar stereochemical features. For example, the two phenyl rings of phenytoin share a similar mutual orientation in space with the phenyl and clorophenyl rings in diazepam and with the phenylcyclohexyl moiety in procyclidine and trihexyphenidyl. When these hydrophobic groups were approximately superimposed, it was found that two electron-donor functions (either oxygen or nitrogen) also occupy similar positions and orientations in space. This was true even for the open-chained acetylureas (phenacemide and ethylphenacemide) because the acetylurea moiety

folds back on itself to form a six-atom "ring" stabilized by hydrogen bonding.

These observations led the Camermans to propose that stereochemical properties form the basis of selective anticonvulsant action and that anticonvulsant potential in new compounds might be predictable from this knowledge (13). A quantitative measure of the stereochemical similarities among these drugs was provided as the interatomic distance between electron-donor atoms and the distance between these atoms and the hydrophobic groups. For example, the two electronegative atoms in phenytoin thought to best approximate the optimal configuration for anticonvulsant action are the two carbonyl oxygens. The distance between these atoms is 4.56 Å. The respective atoms in diazepam (those that best approximate the carbonyl oxygens in phenytoin when the phenyl groups of the two molecules are superimposed) are the carbonyl oxygen and the trigonal nitrogen at the 4-position of the azepine ring (see Fig. 1B). Their interatomic distance is 3.35 Å. Based on a comparison of these distances with the respective interatomic distances for a variety of benzodiazepine (13) and sulfonamide (11) compounds, the Camermans proposed that a critical lower limit (approximately 2.4 Å) must be exceeded before a particular compound will possess significant anticonvulsant activity (13).

However, a quantitative relationship between interatomic distance and anticonvulsant activity should not be inferred. As a practical necessity one must define what kind of anticonvulsant activity is being measured; i.e., the experimental model. As already noted, the MES model of generalized tonic–clonic seizures frequently detects a different pharmacological group of drugs than does the threshold MET model of absence seizures. Therefore, the demonstration of a quantitative relationship must be consistent with a particular model.

A comparison of interatomic distances with anti-MET and anti-MES potencies is depicted for seven drugs in Table 1. The interatomic distance is between the two electron-donor atoms thought to most closely approximate the car-

TABLE 1. *Comparison of interatomic distance with potency in the MES and scMET tests*

Drug	Interatomic distance (Å)[a]	MES ED$_{50}$[b]	scMET ED$_{50}$[b]
Phenytoin	4.56	9.5	N.A.
Diazepam	3.35	19.1	0.17
Phenobarbital	4.51	21.8	13.2
Procyclidine	3.55	33.6	N.A.
Trihexyphenidyl	2.76	75.7	N.A.
Pheneturide	4.12	77.4	41.5
Phenacemide	4.13	87.3	116.0

[a]The interatomic distances were taken from Camerman and Camerman (13) and represent the distance (in angstroms) between the two electron-donor atoms thought to be involved in anticonvulsant activity.

[b]MES and scMET refer to the maximal electroshock and subcutaneous pentylenetetrazol threshold tests, respectively. The ED$_{50}$s represent the intraperitoneal dosage (mg/kg) necessary to protect 50% of the test population (mice) against the experimentally induced seizures. These data were taken from Krall et al. (47). N.A., not active.

bonyl oxygens of phenytoin when the hydrophobic groups of the molecules are maximally superimposed. It is clear that drugs totally ineffective against MET-induced seizures have interatomic distances that include the extremes (i.e., trihexyphenidyl, 2.76 Å; procyclidine, 3.55 A; phenytoin, 4.56 Å). Furthermore, an 8.8-fold difference in anti-MET potency (comparing phenacemide and phenobarbital) can be compared with only a very modest difference in interatomic distance. Unfortunately, the comparison of anti-MES potencies with interatomic distances also fails to demonstrate a simple correlation.

These findings are not remarkable considering the diversity of potent anticonvulsants that clearly do not conform to the structural prescription discussed above. Doxenitoin, for example, is a phenytoin-like structure, the only difference being reduction of the carbonyl at the 2-position to a methylene group (Fig. 1D). Yet, this drug retains significant anticonvulsant potency when evaluated by the MES test (31). It is possible that the nitrogen in the 1-position suffices as the second electron donor in the absence of the carbonyl oxygen; the distance between *N*-1 and the remaining carbonyl oxygen is 3.5 Å (an estimate taken from Drieding ster-

eomodels) compared with 4.56 Å between the two oxygens in phenytoin. The distance between the *N*-3 nitrogen and the single oxygen in doxenitoin (approximately 2.3 Å, estimated) would not satisfy the critical distance defined in the above formulation. However, a reasonably potent 2-pyrrolidinone has been described which is in essence a hydantoin with the *N*-1 nitrogen and *C*-2 carbonyl replaced by methylene groups (61) (Fig. 1E). This compound, 3-ethyl-3-phenyl-2-pyrrolidinone, has two relatively electronegative atoms, but their separation is estimated to be only about 2.3 Å. Furthermore, an imidazole derivative, 4,4-diphenylimidazolidine, is an effective anticonvulsant even though it is totally without oxygen (30) (Fig. 1F). Thus, the possibility exists that two nitrogens (approximately 2.2 Å apart) suffice as the requisite electron donors even though they are separated by less than the critical distance already discussed.

These observations support a less rigorous hypothesis of activity against generalized tonic clonic (GTC) seizures: simply, two electron donors are required in some proximity to a bulky hydrophobic moiety. Although it is possible to cite exceptions even to the "two-electron-donor" requirement (6), it is not clear that these exceptions represent drugs with "selective" anticonvulsant action (as opposed to general CNS depression).

On the basis of the existing knowledge that a phenyl or similar aromatic group is necessary for anti-GTC activity, each of the compounds employed in the Camermans' studies could be expected to possess such activity; and, indeed, they do. Therefore, the stereochemical dependence defined in the above studies seems to apply only to the group of anticonvulsants with activity against GTC seizures. It is clear, for example, that trimethadione (3,5,5-trimethyl-2,4-oxazolidinedione) and similar alkyl-substituted compounds having selective action against absence seizures do not conform to the structural prescription defined for the anti-GTC drugs. Although many drugs that are effective in the MES test are also variably effective in the MET model, these are structures that (with few exceptions) possess a combination of aromatic and alkyl substitution, usually on a tetrahedral carbon. Thus, phenacemide, pheneturide, and phenobarbital (among many others) have some degree of anti-MET activity in addition to their anti-MES efficacy. (Because of special problems such as a paradoxical exacerbation of absence seizures or an unwarranted risk of serious toxicity, these drugs are normally used to treat partial seizures and generalized seizures exclusive of absences.)

Drugs with exclusive alkyl or aromatic substitution are almost always effective only in the MET or MES models, respectively. However, diazepam and similar 1,4-benzodiazepines represent exceptions to this general rule. These structures have two bulky hydrophobic groups with the prescribed stereochemistry for purely anti-GTC action, but they are actually considerably more potent when tested in the threshold MET model than in the MES model. This incongruity probably implies a unique mechanism of action for these compounds. Although conformational similarities between phenytoin and diazepam led the Camermans to propose a common mechanism, evidence accruing from quantitative SAR studies supports the concept of a fundamentally different mechanism (see below), even for the anti-GTC component of diazepam's action.

Quantitative SAR

Whereas the independent variables in qualitative SAR studies are most often drawn from physicochemical intuition, the variables employed in quantitative SAR investigations are necessarily defined in numerical terms. It should be apparent from the foregoing discussion that the types and positional status of atomic nuclei provide only very limited information, and this information is frequently not well suited for quantitative correlation. After all, it is the electrons in the vicinity of nuclei that are involved in the variety of forces presumed responsible for the drug–receptor interaction. Indices that provide a measure of the electronic properties of a molecule should therefore be of considerable

value in the resolution of SAR problems. Experimental techniques that might provide such information include X-ray crystallography, X-ray photoelectron shifts, ^{13}C NMR shifts, and measurements of dipole moments. These methods provide information only for the equilibrium (least-energy) conformation. However, it is perfectly reasonable to expect that nonequilibrium conformations play a vital role in certain types of drug action. For example, a drug might have to pass through an unstable conformation in order to gain access to the receptor, or it might have to assume an unstable conformation to permit binding to the receptor (77). Theoretical calculations presently offer the only access to electron distribution information in nonequilibrium as well as equilibrium states.

Molecular orbital theory has been employed with increasing success during the past two decades to assist in the definition of electronic correlates of drug action (4,16,42,45). Simple and modified Huckel π-electron approximations (39,99) have been employed by early workers in medicinal chemistry, but interpretation was complicated because only "half" the story was told; that is, σ-bond electrons and saturated systems were not considered. Although there has been occasional success using these theories, it has been achieved in studies confined to a closely related series of homologous planar molecules. The most debilitating handicap in these methods is the neglect of electron repulsion terms, which leads to poor estimates of energy level transitions, but in rigorously controlled studies charge-transfer mechanisms and mechanisms related to covalent bond formation have been elucidated (28,87). A self-consistent field π-electron approximation has been described in which there is an attempt to account for the electron repulsion terms, but there is still neglect of the overlap integral as in the Huckel theories (71). Although it should be superior to the simpler theories in predicting excited states and charge densities, it has not been used to nearly the same extent.

There are several all-valence-electron methods presently available that provide energy values as a function of geometry. Thus, these should be superior in the estimation of molecular conformation. The earliest, known as the extended Huckel theory (EHT), again neglected the electron and nuclear repulsion terms, but overlap integrals were retained, and the resonance integrals were considered between bonded and nonbonded atoms (37). As with the other methods that ignore repulsion terms, EHT is not a good estimator of bond lengths and charge densities (except when dealing with molecules whose atoms are very close on the electronegativity scale). But EHT has been very useful in predicting preferred conformations, even though the barriers to internal rotation are usually exaggerated (43,44).

An all-valence-electron theory that neglects the overlap integral but treats the repulsion terms has been described by Pople et al. (72). In this method, there is complete neglect of differential overlap (CNDO), and the theory expectedly provides poor estimates of preferred conformation. However, it possibly provides the most accurate semiempirical estimate of charge densities and dipole moments. A "compromise" between the CNDO and EHT theories has been described in the iterative extended Huckel method (IEHT). Here, the overlap and resonance integrals are retained as with EHT, but an attempt to account for the repulsion terms has also been incorporated (104,105). Thus, IEHT has been useful in the prediction of preferred conformation, and charge densities are more realistic than those calculated with EHT (57,58,75,76).

Additional semiempirical methods and the more accurate *ab initio* Hartree–Fock methods have been described (1,49). However, most SAR investigations require data for a relatively large number of molecules, and it is often necessary to study each in a variety of tautomeric and conformational forms. This, of course, will limit the sophistication with which individual calculations can be performed. Thus, for a reasonably homologous series of molecules, sacrifice of the "pure" methods for economy is frequently justified and can, in fact, lead to useful data that are accurate in a relative, if not absolute, sense.

Although molecular orbital theory has been widely employed in the study of structures having pharmacological importance, very few such studies have involved the anticonvulsant drugs. Andrews (2) performed EHT and CNDO calculations on a series of anticonvulsants and related compounds in order to assess the role that atomic charge might play in their action. Two hypotheses were tested. (a) Because the imide group is so commonplace in anticonvulsant drugs, hydrogen bonding involving this group is related to activity. (b) The electron density on the substituent-bearing tetrahedral carbon is related to anticonvulsant action. The second hypothesis was derived from Perkow's (69) postulate that the actions of many drugs result from low electron density at a "biologically active center," the tetrahedral carbon in this series of drugs. When the calculated charge densities were employed as a predictor of hydrogen-bonding strength, an overt correlation was not found to occur with anti-MES potency or with anti-MET potency. Nor did the electron density at the heterocyclic tetrahedral carbon seem to correlate with biological activity. These results led Andrews to conclude that neither hydrogen bonding nor the charge at Perkow's "biologically active center" was involved in determining anticonvulsant selectivity or potency. Despite Andrews' negative results, additional efforts to test this hypothesis should be encouraged. For example, there is some question regarding the choice of ground state charge densities to predict hydrogen bond strength. The suggestion has been made that a change in charge density occurs on hydrogen bonding that parallels bond strength (38) and might therefore be a more relevant index to correlate with activity. A model comprising the anticonvulsant and a standard hydrogen bond donor–acceptor might be useful for such correlation analysis (46). Furthermore, Andrews' study did not employ multivariate analysis. It remains distinctly possible that hydrogen bonding is involved in the "drug–receptor" interaction but that other structural or electronic properties modify the association to varying degrees. The use of multivariate analysis is discussed below.

More recently, a molecular orbital study of

the anticonvulsant 1,3-dihydro-5-phenyl-1,4-benzodiazepine-2-ones was reported. Lucek et al. (59) employed the CNDO/2 method in an attempt to characterize the electronic correlates of anti-MET activity. They failed to show significant correlations between anticonvulsant activity and lipophilicity (estimated from hydrophobic constants, π), total electronic charge at any atom, or the energies of the highest occupied or lowest empty molecular orbitals (HOMO or LEMO, respectively).[1]

The lack of correlation with hydrophobicity is not surprising in view of the finding by Lien et al. (54) that only 24% of the variability ($r = 0.489$) of 1,4-benzodiazepines as anti-MET agents could be accounted for by π alone. However, a significant correlation was observed with the electron density in the p_y orbital at the aromatic carbon adjacent to the amide (N-1) nitrogen. This directional dependence of the electron density might explain the loss of activity when the A ring (Fig. 1) is substituted at positions 6, 8, or 9 (90). Because Lien et al. (54) were able to improve their correlation by addition of the Hammet σ constant (32), it would be interesting to include in their multivariate analysis the p_y orbital charge densities calculated by Lucek et al (59). A high degree of colinearity (between σ and the p_y charge densities) or an effective substitution of either parameter might imply that the two indices are estimates of the same phenomenon. Furthermore, it should be of special interest to apply multiple regression analysis to the data of Lucek et al. (59). Although a dependence on

lipophilicity was apparently not significant from simple regression analysis, its contribution might become apparent when evaluated as a partially independent variable. Precedent has already been established for such an effect (see below). A conceptual explanation might be that lipophilicity governs access of a drug to its site of action (because of its effect on the penetration of membranes), whereas the electronic properties relate to its interaction with a receptor.

A special discussion is warranted concerning the anti-MET models employed in the above studies. Andrews (2) used data reported by others (18–21,25) for the subcutaneous MET threshold test. This test, a fairly reliable predictor of antiabsence activity (92), measures the ability of a drug to prevent the clonic seizure in mice produced by the subcutaneous administration of $\sim$ 85 mg/kg of pentylenetetrazol. Drugs such as phenytoin and carbamazepine have no activity in this test. However, the benzodiazepine data employed by Lien et al. (54) and Lucek et al. (59) were obtained by a maximal pentylenetetrazol (mMET) seizure test (91). This test measures the ability of a drug to prevent the tonic seizure produced by a large subcutaneous dose (e.g., 125 mg/kg) or a smaller intravenous dose (e.g., 38 mg/kg) of pentylenetetrazol. The mMET tests often are effective discriminators of anti-GTC drugs; drugs such as ethosuximide and trimethadione do not prevent the tonic component of seizures induced in this test except in very high dosage. Many of the benzodiazepine compounds are effective antagonists of both maximal and threshold seizures, but they are usually most potent when evaluated by the threshold model (47). However, because none of the quantitative SAR studies of the benzodiazepine class has been based on the latter model, the benzodiazepine data used by Lien et al. (54) and Lucek et al. (59) should be interpreted in the context of anti-GTC activity, whereas the anti-MET data in Andrews' (2) study of miscellaneous compounds should be interpreted in the context of antiabsence activity.

Although the benzodiazepines can be potent antagonists of both maximal and threshold sei-

---

[1]Although the orbital energies were not found to contribute to activity, they have been implicated in the action of antimalarial (85), hallucinogenic (87), carcinogenic (17), and other drugs and have been investigated for a different class of anticonvulsant drugs, as described below. The HOMO refers to the energy of the two most energetic electrons in a molecule, or the minimum amount of energy necessary to remove an electron from that orbital. The LEMO refers to the energy of the unoccupied orbital that would be the first to receive additional electrons should they be provided or, more accurately, the amount of energy given off if electrons are added. It is commonly assumed that the HOMO and LEMO might relate to the propensity of a molecule to engage in a charge-transfer interaction with a particular receptor molecule provided certain conditions are met (46).

zures, they can also be extensively metabolized in the time frame normally required (as much as 30 min) for the subcutaneous test. For example, there is very little parent compound in mouse brain 30 min after a single intraperitoneal dose of diazepam; the metabolites nordiazepam and oxazepam predominate (74). Thus, it is not reasonable to expect accurate correlations with physicochemical and theoretical indices when activity is not known to result from those structures for which the indices were determined. Because Lien et al. (54) employed the subcutaneous anti-mMET potencies reported by Sternbach et al. (91), it is possible that their correlation analysis is complicated by metabolism. However, the benzodiazepine data employed by Lucek et al. (59) were obtained with the "1-min intravenous" anti-mMET test. The protocol involved the intravenous administration of a 70 mg/kg dose of pentylenetetrazol just 1 min after an intravenous dose of benzodiazepine (W. Dairman, *personal communication*). Thus, the problem of metabolism may have been largely overcome in Lucek's study. However, it is possible that the rates of penetrance of the blood–brain barrier by benzodiazepine derivatives are not very uniform; hence, the intravenous dose might not represent a uniform estimate of drug concentrations in the brain at the time of testing.

Several other molecular orbital studies of benzodiazepine derivatives have been reported recently. A CNDO study was reported by Blair and Webb (5). Their results, like those of Lucek's group (59), failed to demonstrate a significant contribution of lipophilicity to anticonvulsant activity [the anticonvulsant data, taken from Sternbach et al. (91), was for the subcutaneous mMET test], and their demonstration of a negative dependence of potency on the total molecular dipole moment was consistent with reported studies (to be discussed below) of miscellaneous compounds (53–55). However, a unique observation was the reasonably strong correlation between anticonvulsant activity and charge density on the carbonyl oxygen. Although the regression was not as strong ($r = 0.73$) as that for the dipole moment

($r = 0.82$) in simple regression analysis, both regressions were highly significant ($p < 0.001$). The improvement in regression on either parameter after inclusion of the other generally was not significant because of the familiar interdependence (covariance) among calculated electronic indices (see below).

Again, caution is warranted in the interpretation of these data because of the significant metabolism that has possibly occurred during the time frame of the subcutaneous mMET test. [Although seizures will normally occur within a few minutes after the subcutaneous administration of 125 mg/kg pentylenetetrazol in mice, the data reported by Sternbach et al. (91) are for benzodiazepines administered by the oral route; thus, a significant amount of time might have been required to achieve effective brain concentrations before the MET test was conducted.] Furthermore, the results cannot be directly compared with those of Lucek's group (59) because of the difference in the anti-mMET tests performed (subcutaneous versus intravenous).

Information about the participation of HOMO in the activity of the benzodiazepines was provided by Lukovits and Otvos (60) using simple Huckel theory. In this study, both binding to human serum albumin (HSA) and pharmacological activity were dependent on HOMO: higher energies resulted in more favorable binding to HSA but lower pharmacological activity. The pharmacological activity was protection against the subcutaneous mMET seizure, taken from Sternbach et al. (91). The conclusion was that the derivatives with higher HOMOs are less potent because of a charge-transfer association with "nonspecific acceptor" sites which reduces the concentration in equilibrium with the receptor.

Another study of the involvement of HOMO in the anticonvulsant activity of benzodiazepines was reported by Sarrazin et al. (82). They attempted to correlate the minimal electroshock data of Sternbach et al. (91) not only with HOMO but with LEMO as well. Because only relatively weak correlations were obtained ($r = 0.47$ and 0.67 for HOMO and LEMO, respectively) in single variate analysis, they concluded that charge transfer probably does not contribute to the drug–receptor interaction for this class of compounds. However, we have performed simple linear regression analyses on these data and find that the correlation is fairly significant ($p < 0.013$) for LEMO, even though the correlation is small. The equation we derived is $\log 1/C_{min} = 21.1\ \text{LEMO} - 3.46$, which indicates a positive dependence of potency on LEMO (C is equivalent to ED_{50}, the dose that is required to produce a specified response in 50% of the test population; thus, potency increases with $\log 1/C$.) This leads us to suspect that a charge-transfer interaction may, in fact, be involved as a partial contributor in the determination of relative benzodiazepine potencies.

Because an increase in LEMO should have the effect of diminishing a charge-transfer interaction (recall that LEMO represents the energy given off when electrons are added), these data support the suggestion made by Lukovits and Otvos (60) that "nonspecific acceptor" sites are involved in an association that reduces the drug concentration at the receptor. Thus, higher LEMOs should be associated with less charge-transfer binding to nonspecific sites and higher concentrations of free drug at the site of action. However, according to the data of Sarrazin et al. (82), the electron is presumably transferred from the macromolecule to the benzodiazepine; hence, the term "nonspecific donor" sites might be more appropriate. The other equation we derived ($\log 1/C_{min} = 18.4\ \text{HOMO} + 5.62$) indicates that higher HOMOs are also related to greater potency. (The latter equation is significant only at the 89% level.) The prediction that increasing values of HOMO should enhance potency is not in agreement with the data of Lukovits and Otvos (60) or with their interpretation that association with nonspecific sites occurs by virtue of an electron transfer from the drug to the macromolecule. Although the equation correlating HOMO with potency is less significant than that for LEMO, the sign indicated that if HOMO is involved it might be relevant to a specific drug–receptor interaction. The dis-

crepancy between the two studies might have resulted from the use of the mMET test data by Lukovits and Otvos (60) and of minimal electroshock data by Sarrazin et al. (82).

Sarrazin et al. (82) also suggested that potency in the minimal and maximal electroshock tests depends on the electronic charge on the azepine N_4 atom, and the respective equations were written as

$$\log \frac{1}{C_{min}} = -29{,}700\ Q^2_{N_4}$$
$$-9{,}670\ Q_{N_4} - 970 \quad [1]$$

$$\log \frac{1}{C_{max}} = -64{,}500\ Q^2_{N_4}$$
$$-2.09\ Q_{N_4} - 1{,}690 \quad [2]$$

where Q_{N_4} is the calculated electronic charge on the N_4 atom. The charge Q_{N_4} was corrected for the various derivatives to account for the influence of the dihedral angle N_4–C_5–$C_1{}'$–$C_2{}'$ on electron distribution. The reported correlation coefficients were 0.97 and 0.89, respectively. However, it is not apparent from their data that these equations provide accurate estimates of the dependent variable ($\log 1/C$). Evaluation of the above polynomials using their corrected atomic charges (Q_{N_4}) resulted in very poor estimates of potency. The application of their data in a least-squares multiple-regression analysis performed by the present authors produced the more accurate equations given below:

$$\log \frac{1}{C_{min}} = -30547\ Q^2_{N_4}$$
$$-9954\ Q_{N_4} - 812.6 \quad [3]$$

$$\log \frac{1}{C_{max}} = -65983\ Q^2_{N_4}$$
$$-21360\ Q_{N_4} - 1729.3 \quad [4]$$

The multiple correlation coefficients are 0.98 and 0.90, respectively. Evaluation of these quadratics with respect to the corrected charges produced estimates of potency very close to the experimental values of Sternbach et al. (91).

Thus, it is apparent that the conclusion of Sarrazin et al. (82) that a relationship exists between anticonvulsant potency and charge on the azepine N_4 nitrogen is a valid one, even though the accuracy of the reported equations is in doubt. However, their suggestion that the drug–receptor interaction likely involves hydrogen bonding between the N_4 nitrogen of the azepine ring and a hydrogen atom on the receptor must remain somewhat tenuous. This is because the relationship between potency and N_4 charge is parabolic: an increase in charge will initially increase potency, but further increases will eventually diminish potency. Because a conceptual understanding of this phenomenon is not as easy as the parabolic dependence of potency on lipid solubility (discussed below), we must assume for the present that hydrogen bonding is not the only interaction mechanism influenced by the electronic charge on the N_4 nitrogen.

In the study by Lien et al. (54), the pharmacological activities of 16 anticonvulsant compounds (including only two benzodiazepine derivatives) were compared with a variety of independent variables. The pharmacological endpoints included anti-MES and anti-MET potencies, and the median toxic dose (TD_{50}) was based on the rotorod measurement of ataxia. The anti-MET activities were for the subcutaneous threshold model. All of the pharmacological data were taken from Krall et al. (47). With all 16 compounds included, the best correlation (eq. 1 of Table 2) for the anti-MES test was obtained with log P (log partition coefficient). Although the correlation improved very slightly on addition of the parabolic $[(\log P)^2]$ term and/or the dipole moment, the standard deviations also increased. When diazepam, clonazepam, and carbamazepine were deleted from the regression analysis, the best correlation (eq. 2 of Table 2) was obtained with log MW (molecular weight), although the correlation with log P was as good as (or better than) before the deletion. The rationale for deleting the two benzodiazepines was based on a recent study suggesting that these drugs occupy specific receptors (65). However, the rationale for deleting carbamazepine was not as clear, except that it was a drug structurally "quite different" from the remaining compounds.

On the basis of molecular models, it is apparent that carbamazepine has structural properties quite similar to phenytoin: when the two phenyl rings in each molecule are brought into approximate coincidence, the C_4 carbonyl and the N_3 imide group of phenytoin approximate similar positions with the carbonyl and amide groups, respectively, in carbamazepine. Because this and other data are consistent with a greater similarity of carbamazepine to phenytoin than to the benzodiazepines, it is not clear that carbamazepine should have been deleted. The authors have performed calculations using the data given by Lien et al. (54) but have deleted only the benzodiazepine compounds.

We found that the best equation for the MES data is one that includes the dipole moment (μ)

TABLE 2. *Survey of quantitative structure–activity relationships of anticonvulsants*

Equation	Reference	n	r	s	Model
1. $\log 1/C = 0.627 \log P + 2.588$	54	16	0.874	0.342	MES
2. $\log 1/C = 7.776 \log MW - 14.438$	54	13	0.941	0.241	MES
3. $\log 1/C = -0.301 (\log P)^2 + 0.852 \log P$ $- 0.629 \mu + 4.139$	54	12	0.915	0.227	MET (threshold)
4. $\log 1/C = 15.939 \log MW - 0.972 \log P$ $+ 0.549 \mu - 33.187$	54	16	0.933	0.388	TD_{50} (rotorod)
5. $\log 1/C = -0.222 (\log P)^2 + 1.153 \log P$ $- 0.368 \mu + 2.994$	55	18	0.92	0.24	MES
6. $\log 1/C = 0.720 \log P - 0.396 \mu + 3.144$	53	11	0.967	0.189	MES
7. $\log 1/C = -0.226 (\log P)^2 + 0.800 \log P$ $- 0.361 \mu + 0.175$	55	10	0.99	0.11	LD_{50} (acute)

as well as the log MW term. The regression, described by the equation log $1/C = 8.4$ log MW $+ 0.3\mu - 16.3$, is slightly stronger ($r = 0.954$) and has a smaller standard error (0.230) than that described for the log MW term alone (with carbamazepine deleted). Both equations are highly significant ($p < 0.00001$). However, the sign on the dipole moment is positive, an observation that is not in harmony with other multivariate regressions involving this parameter (see below).

The best correlation (eq. 3 of Table 2) for the anti-MET test was also achieved only after the two benzodiazepines were deleted. Phenytoin and carbamazepine were not included because they are inactive in this test. Two properties of this correlation deserve mention. First, the equation is parabolic in the log P term; that is, potency increases with an increase in log P until an optimal value is attained, further increases diminishing activity. A quantitative description of this phenomenon has been expressed for a variety of drugs according to the following equation (35):

$$\log \frac{1}{C} = -k(\log P)^2 + k' \log P + k'' \quad [5]$$

A conceptual explanation of this phenomenon is that most drugs must have a minimal degree of lipid solubility to permit their penetration of membranes and eventual access to receptors. However, as the lipid solubility increases beyond an optimal value, the drug becomes sequestered within the lipid matrix of the membrane, with a reduction in the probability that it will ever find a receptor.

Perceptive discussions of this parabolic relationship between potency and hydrophobicity have been presented by Penniston et al. (68) and McFarland (62). The second interesting property is the negative dependence of potency on the dipole moment, a finding in agreement with previous observations (53,55). The physical meaning of a negative correlation of dipole moment with activity is not easily ascertained, especially if the assumption is made that the dipole moment is causally related to activity.

Given the present knowledge, it seems more likely that the dipole moment relates to a binding process that decreases drug concentrations at the receptor. The fact that the benzodiazepines are potent anticonvulsants (especially with respect to the MET threshold test) yet have relatively large dipole moments, together with the finding that better correlations were obtained in both experimental models when they were deleted, supports earlier suggestions (65) that they act by a different mechanism.

The most successful correlation (eq. 4 of Table 2) for the rotorod ataxia test was obtained when all 16 compounds were included in the analysis. Notable in these results was the positive dependence of toxicity on the dipole moment and its negative dependence on the log P term. The reciprocal relationship of the dipole moment in the comparison of anticonvulsant and neurotoxic properties is consistent with the idea that neurotoxicity results from a separate drug–receptor interaction and is not an extension of the anticonvulsant action. As already suggested, a large dipole moment might result in a relative distribution of drug away from its site of anticonvulsant action, possibly to sites involved in conferring toxicity, hence, the positive dependence of toxicity on dipole moment. The negative dependence of toxicity on the log P term also supports this contention; it is possible that toxicity results from an interaction with relatively hydrophilic (and polar) sites, whereas anticonvulsant activity depends on interaction at relatively hydrophobic sites (where dipolar interactions are not so prominent). The dependence of anti-MES potency and neurotoxicity on log MW (eqs. 2 and 4 of Table 2) is evidence that van der Waals interactions might play an important role in anticonvulsant actions and effects. However, because of the expected colinearity between the log MW and log P terms, it is difficult to ascribe a physical interpretation to either term. In fact, it is possible that van der Waals forces are the major ingredient of hydrophobic bonding (81).

In an earlier study by Lien et al. (55), the correlates of anti-MES activity were reported for a more diverse group of chemical structures than employed in the later study (54). Included were cyclohexanone and other derivatives unrelated to the traditional anticonvulsants. There was no simple dependence on log P or log MW such as was reported for the more limited group of compounds. Instead, the correlates in this larger, miscellaneous series bore a greater resemblance to those reportedly involved in anti-MET activity (compare eqs. 3 and 5 of Table 2); in both cases there was a parabolic relationship with log P and a negative dependence on the dipole moment.

There might be several explanations for this apparent difference between the two studies. The earlier study involved 18 compounds having a much greater range of log P values than the 13 drugs employed in the more recent study. Also, many of the dipole moments used in the two studies were estimated from experimental moments of similar structures. With accurate dipole moments (experimental or theoretical) a stronger correlation with anti-MES activity might have been demonstrated in the later investigation. Some results presented below indicate that the estimates of dipole moments used in the previous studies have not been exceptionally accurate. Thus, the more accurate relationship with anti-MES activity is probably that expressed in equation 5 of Table 2 rather than equations 1 or 2 of that table. However, in yet another study by Lien (53), the analysis of a smaller group of drugs yielded an equation (eq. 6 of Table 2) with a higher correlation coefficient and a lower standard error than any of those already discussed. This equation also demonstrates a negative dependence of anti-MES potency on the dipole moment, but the dependence on log P is not parabolic in this case. It should thus be clear that much further study is necessary before a definitive quantitative SAR can be described for the anticonvulsant drugs.

It is interesting to note that the equation that characterizes the dependence of acute lethal toxicity (eq. 7 of Table 2) includes a negative dipole moment and is qualitatively very similar to the equations (eqs. 3 and 5 of Table 2) that were written for the subcutaneous MET and MES tests. Because this negative dependence contrasts with the positive dependence of neurotoxicity (eq. 4 of Table 2) on dipole moment, it is tempting to speculate that the mechanisms involved in lethality are not simple extensions of those that confer neurotoxicity (as measured in the rotorod test). This thought is strengthened by the fact that both equations (eqs. 4 and 7 of Table 2) were derived from data for similar, if not identical, compounds (including barbiturates, hydantoins, and other imides). A useful exercise might be the separate analyses of sedative and nonsedative anticonvulsants (e.g., barbiturates versus hydantoins) in terms of their $TD_{50}s$ and $LD_{50}s$ to determine if the dipole moment likewise exerts an opposing influence in each category.

All of the equations depicted in Table 2 were derived from studies in which the anticonvulsant data were obtained from mice. Furthermore, the electroshock parameters in the MES equations were, as far as we know, identical. It should go without saying that great mischief can result from attempts to compare structure–activity data obtained in studies conducted with different animal species and experimental models.

PROBABLE CAUSES OF FAILURE IN ANTICONVULSANT SAR RESEARCH

Several major factors can be cited that have impeded progress in anticonvulsant SAR research: (a) the chemical diversity of molecules known to possess anticonvulsant activity; (b) the anatomic, physiological, and biochemical complexity of the central nervous system; and (c) the lack of entirely suitable models of epilepsy. The confusional role of chemical diversity has been documented above. An even greater handicap is that imposed by the approximately 10 billion neurons and an even greater number of neuroglia that comprise the central nervous system. The anatomic organization of neurons into structures such as the cerebrum, cerebellum, medulla, and spinal cord provides an obvious (albeit gross) basis for selective drug action, and the neuroglia should not be excluded as possible participants in anticonvulsant drug action (102). Furthermore, the neuronal subdivision into nuclei and tracts, and the functions thus subserved, provide an even greater foundation for selectivity.

From a biochemical aspect, the numerous enzymes that regulate permeability and transport phenomena, energy and neurotransmitter metabolism, and even macromolecular metabolism are all potential targets for an anticonvulsant mechanism. For example, within a particular anatomic or functional subdivision of the central nervous system, there may be a diversity of proven or putative neurotransmitters, some mediating excitatory processes while others mediate inhibitory phenomena.

Because in the normal state brain function is at equilibrium with excitatory and inhibitory processes, excessive neuronal activity (e.g., seizures) can result from an increase in excitatory transmission or, alternatively, from a decrease in inhibitory transmission. Thus, changes in the concentrations of either excitatory or inhibitory neurotransmitters represent potential mechanisms of anticonvulsant action. Finally, considering the extensive interaction that occurs among the various anatomic, biochemical, and functional levels and the bewildering technical problems encountered in the isolation for study of any particular subdivision, and the difficulty in reintegrating the results for meaningful interpretation, it is truly remarkable that our current state of knowledge is where it is. The problem is not simply to resolve from the anatomic and functional complexity a subdivision to which one can attribute an effect, but it is also to recognize that multiple actions and effects at multiple levels will occur, there being a requirement to identify which effect might be causally related to anticonvulsant action.

The premature identification of a physiological or biochemical effect as one causally related to anticonvulsant action is an all-too-common scenario, when, in fact, the measured effect is simply a correlate of drug action resulting from parallel or divergent effector systems. A schematic representation of such possibilities is depicted below.

$$D + R \longrightarrow A \longrightarrow B \longrightarrow C \longrightarrow etc. \qquad [6]$$
$$D + R' \longrightarrow A' \longrightarrow B' \longrightarrow C' \longrightarrow etc.$$
$$\qquad\qquad\qquad\qquad\qquad\qquad [7]$$
$$D + R \begin{cases} \longrightarrow A \longrightarrow B \longrightarrow C \longrightarrow etc. \\ \longrightarrow A' \longrightarrow B' \longrightarrow C' \longrightarrow etc. \end{cases}$$

The symbols D and R (R') represent drug and receptor, respectively, and A (A'), B (B'), C (C'), etc., represent effects consequent to the drug–receptor interaction. The symbols A (A') through C (C'), etc. collectively constitute an effector system. It is entirely conceivable that for both models the structure–activity relationships along one effector system might exist in others as well. In the example of a parallel effector system (eq. 6), the anticonvulsant effect might be the terminal effect along one effector system, although the effect to which one is ascribing mechanistic significance actually arises from a different drug–receptor interaction. In the model of a divergent effector system (eq. 7), the common receptor might eventually be identified, but useful information pertinent to the effector system might be overlooked.

One need consider only a relatively few of the "modern" anticonvulsant drugs in order to demonstrate how the complexity of the central nervous system interacts to impede resolution of their mechanisms. Phenytoin is thought to limit the propagation of seizure discharge by its very pronounced ability to inhibit posttetanic potentiation (PTP) (26). This phenomenon, the facilitation of synaptic transmission following rapid, repetitive presynaptic stimulation, is thought to be involved in the initiation of seizure spread from a local area to the entire brain. However, other anticonvulsants appear to have relatively little effect on this phenomenon. Phenobarbital has no clear-cut effect on PTP (48). Carbamazepine seems to inhibit PTP, but only in the early periods after administration (20 min); later, PTP is elevated (24). Another report has indicated that therapeutic concentrations of carbamazepine have no effect on PTP (40). Trimethadione, a prototype antiabsence agent, has no effect on PTP (27); nor does clonazepam (93), even though the benzodiazepine compounds are known to limit seizure spread (95).

A more consistent finding among the anticonvulsant compounds is their ability to interfere in some capacity with γ-aminobutyric acid (GABA) metabolism. For example, phenytoin (96), phenobarbital (80), ethosuximide (83), diazepam (67), and others have been shown to produce increased brain concentrations of this inhibitory neurotransmitter. Data are not yet available for carbamazepine. However, the apparent mechanism for this increase is not uniform. Because therapeutic concentrations of phenytoin do not inhibit GABA transaminase or succinate semialdehyde dehydrogenase (the two enzymes responsible for GABA degradation), the increase in GABA concentration is thought to result from increased synthesis (83). Similarily, phenobarbital inhibits GABA transaminase only at very high (supratherapeutic) concentrations (83). On the other hand, ethosuximide (83) and diazepam (67) in therapeutic concentrations do inhibit this enzyme. Nonuniform data have also been reported regarding GABA utilization. Phenytoin and phenobarbital (98) both stimulate the uptake of GABA into rat brain synaptosomes, whereas diazepam inhibits GABA uptake into mouse brain synaptosomes (66). Numerous other biochemical effects, the most interesting being alterations in cation transport (70,88,103), have been demonstrated. However, all have likewise failed to provide a uniform model that correlates with the clinical or *in vivo* efficacy of these agents.

Does the apparently unique inhibition of PTP by phenytoin relate causally to its anticonvulsant action, or is the inhibition of PTP simply a physiological correlate of phenytoin action in an effector system not shared by other drugs? Similar questions might be asked of GABA's role in anticonvulsant action. Certainly, the complexity of the central nervous system provides an adequate basis for the expectation that multiple anticonvulsant mechanisms might exist. Indeed, the diverse patterns of clinical epilepsy are clearly expressions of such complexity (29). It is only logical to expect that a drug

selective for GTC seizures will act by a different mechanism than one selective for absence seizures.

However, the common structural information contained in the numerous anticonvulsant molecules suggests that at the most fundamental level there is a common physicochemical mechanism. For example, electronic indices that govern the ability to participate in hydrogen-bonding, dipole–dipole, charge-transfer, or other bonding mechanisms might also uniformly govern the activity of all anticonvulsant molecules. Thus, it is conceivable that selectivity arises not as a result of a fundamentally different physical interaction at the site of action but rather as a result of variations in the nature of the particular effector systems where the drug, because of its physicochemical properties, might happen to be localized. A challenge in quantitative structure–activity investigation is to characterize drug action not only in terms of the electronic indices that govern the physical interaction with the receptor but also in terms of other physicochemical properties as they might relate to differences in the molecular localization of such drugs.

The third major factor that has hampered progress in anticonvulsant SAR investigation has been the dearth of entirely suitable experimental models. The currently available models have several limitations, but the most serious problem relates to the fact that there are no adequately documented *in vitro* models of epilepsy. Most of the quantitative SAR studies of anticonvulsants reported thus far have employed as the dependent variable estimates of potency based on the amount of drug administered systemically. Such studies are usually inaccurate and result in failure because the variables of absorption, distribution, biotransformation, and excretion preclude a reliable expression of the drug's concentration in equilibrium with its receptor. An *in vitro* model, on the other hand, would insure to a reasonable approximation that the drug–receptor interaction will be uncomplicated by membrane penetration and metabolism. To the extent that *in vivo* models are useful for qualitative analysis,

bamazepine, and cyheptamide) were obtained from commercial sources. The remaining compounds, α,α-diphenylsuccinimide (64), diphenylacetylurea (89), and 5,5-diphenylbarbituric acid (3), were synthesized according to their respective published methods. The drug concentrations in blood and brain tissue were analyzed by gas–liquid chromatography using either published or novel assays. The details of the analyses will be published in a separate communication.

The log P values (Table 3) were calculated in each case by using the measured log P of a suitable parent compound and adding the appropriate hydrophobic substituent constants (π) (34). Although experimental log P values are available for phenytoin and phenobarbital (34), the above procedure was maintained for consistency. The pertinent calculations will be presented in a separate publication.

The electronic indices depicted in Table 3 were derived (to a noniterative approximation) using an EHT molecular orbital program obtained through the Quantum Chemistry Program Exchange (QCPE) of Indiana University.[2] Input for the EHT program includes the cartesian coordinates of each atom in the molecule. These coordinates were obtained with the aid of a separate program, QCPE 94, which computes the geometry of the molecule given bond angles, bond lengths, and information defining conformation.

As stated above, HOMO (Table 3) is an expression of the minimum amount of energy necessary to remove an electron from the molecule. Higher-lying (less negative) HOMOs are associated with a relatively greater ability to transfer the electrons they contain to a particular electron acceptor, possibly a receptor having an especially low-lying (less positive) LEMO.

Hence, a strong correlation of drug activity with HOMO is frequently interpreted in terms of a charge-transfer interaction between the drug and its receptor.

The dipole moment term, μ (Table 3), is an expression of the asymmetric distribution of bonding electrons in a molecule as a result of differences in the electronegativities of the composite atoms. The displacement is toward the more electronegative atom. Most drug molecules are a composite of atoms with different electronegativities and will therefore have permanent dipole moments. The interaction of two dipoles is thought by many to constitute a major stabilizing force in the association of numerous drugs with their receptors. For example, the polar carbonyl group might interact in a dipolar configuration with a variety of polar groups in proteins or other macromolecules. Although these forces are relatively weak, they might be the determinant factor where a weak secondary binding site must be present to impart stereoselective activity. Actually, there are three different bonding mechanisms that might involve dipolar forces. The strongest is the ion–dipole interaction, which ranks just below the ionic bond in terms of stability. The dipole–dipole interaction is relatively weaker, and the dipole–induced dipole interaction the weakest. The latter occurs when a molecule having a permanent dipole approaches a nonpolar molecule, inducing an asymmetric distribution of electrons which results in a temporary dipole moment. Although the weakest of the dipolar interactions, it is stronger than van der Waals bonds.

One of the deficiencies of the EHT method results from its neglect of electron repulsion terms; as a result, the calculated dipole moments are exaggerated. This is evident from a comparison of the calculated and experimental moments of phenobarbital; the calculated moment is about four times the measured value. (Experimental values are not available for most of the compounds in this study.) However, the relationships among experimental values among reasonably homologous structures should be maintained in the calculated values despite the exaggeration of absolute values. This has been

[2]This program is available in either of two versions; QCPE 358 is IBM compatible, whereas QCPE 380 is adapted for CDC computers with the CDC extended FORTRAN compiler. The programs can handle atoms in the first five rows of the periodic table and can accommodate up to 150 orbitals (including s, p, and d), 23 main atoms and 21 hydrogen atoms. The latter dimensions can be readily altered by changing the variable dimension statements. Calculations can be executed in an iterative or noniterative format.

verified by the authors for a number of compounds with known experimental dipole moments.

The final two variables include the electrostatic interaction energy (E) calculated according to Schuster (84) and the molecular weight (MW). The variable E can be thought of as a measure of the attraction of the valence electrons by their nucleus; the more negative the value, the stronger the attraction. Hence, more positive values would be consistent with a greater potential for electrostatic interaction. The MW term was included because previous studies (54,55) have demonstrated its possible involvement in anticonvulsant action or toxicity (although the log MW term was used). The interpretation was that van der Waals forces were possibly involved in a drug–receptor interaction or an interaction with nonspecific macromolecules.

The dependence of anticonvulsant activity on log P and the calculated electronic indices were analyzed by a least-squares multiple-regression method. The dependent variable in each calculation was the ED_{50}, expressed in one of the three formats given in Table 3 (intraperitoneal dosage, brain concentration, or blood concentration). The independent variables included not only the indices listed in Table 3 but the transformation log P^2 and a variety of additional electronic parameters (e.g., atomic charges). However, Table 3 contains only the independent variables that were found to contribute significantly to a strong overall regression equation. The effect of the independent variables on the overall regression was individually determined by a stepwise deletion method. The best-fit equations for anticonvulsant potency are presented in Table 4. It is perhaps noteworthy that the best equation in each case was obtained when potency was expressed directly as the ED_{50} rather than as the log of the reciprocal ED_{50} as is commonly done. Of some surprise was the reasonably good equation derived for potency based on parenteral dosage (eq. 1 of Table 4). The correlation is very strong ($r = 0.993$), and the overall regression is reasonably significant ($p = 0.027$). The most significant partial regression coefficient is E, the electrostatic interaction energy, but the log P term and dipole moment μ are also significant at an acceptable level. Although the significance of HOMO might be questionable, deletion of this term resulted in a large increase in the standard error (s) and a decrease in the correlation coefficient (r).

The equation based on measured brain concentrations (eq. 2 of Table 4) contained the same independent variables as eq. 1 (Table 4), and the partial coefficients were not substantially different (except, perhaps, for HOMO). How-

TABLE 4. *Selected equations correlating anti-MES activity with physicochemical and theoretical indices*

		r	s	Significance level (p), overall regression	Significance level (p), partial coefficients
1. ED_{50} (i.p.)[a]	= 94.6 log P + 29.5 HOMO − 26.9 E + 4.8 μ − 102.9	0.993	12.97	0.027	0.009 0.090 0.006 0.050
2. ED_{50} (Brain)[a]	= 83.7 log P − 29.8 E + 19.7 HOMO + 2.1 μ − 179.7	0.997	7.29	0.010	0.003 0.0008 0.066 0.081
3. ED_{50} (Blood)[a]	= 56.3 log P − 22.3 E − 0.8 MW − 82.6	0.992	6.49	0.004	0.001 0.0001 0.011

[a]Potency is expressed in the same units used in Table 3.

ever, the significance of the overall regression was greater ($p = 0.010$), the standard error less ($s = 7.29$), and the multiple correlation coefficient slightly higher ($r = 0.997$) than for eq. 1. The contribution of E was again most significant ($p = 0.0008$), and the significance of the log P term likewise increased ($p = 0.003$). Although HOMO was more significant ($p = 0.066$) in this equation, the significance of the dipole moment was less ($p = 0.081$).

The best equation for predicting potency based on blood concentrations involved a somewhat different set of indices. Again, the log P and E terms were very significant ($p = 0.001$ and 0.0001, respectively), and their signs were the same, but the MW term was also significant ($p = 0.011$). On the other hand, HOMO and μ did not improve the regression.

It is interesting that none of the best-fit regression equations included the parabolic log P^2 term. Furthermore, the sign of the log P term is positive. Therefore, an increase in log P will result in a decreased potency (i.e., larger ED_{50}). Although at first this might appear suspicious considering our knowledge that lipid solubility is a requirement for membrane penetration, further inspection reveals that the equation is in fact consistent with the parabolic dependence of potency on log P. This is because the regression was analyzed for a relatively few compounds, all of which had very substantial lipid solubilities (log $P = 1.61$ to 3.02). As described above, lipid solubilities of this magnitude should exert a negative influence on potency because of the drug's tendency to remain dissolved within the lipid matrix of the membrane. (This argument presupposes that the site of action will not be found within the lamella of the first membrane encountered, which, of course, is a safe assumption.) Had the analysis been conducted with a larger data set including compounds having a wider range of log P values, the equations may have been parabolic (i.e., $ED_{50} = a + b \log P^2 - c \log P \ldots + nN$).

The same interpretation of the involvement of HOMO in anticonvulsant action might be applied here as was done for the benzodiazepine compounds by Lukovits and Otvos (60). Because HOMO is a negative number, a more energetic HOMO (i.e., more positive) will have the effect of lowering potency (i.e., increasing the ED_{50}). This is not consistent with a drug–receptor interaction involving a charge-transfer mechanism. Thus, the positive dependence of ED_{50} on HOMO possibly relates to the involvement of HOMO in a charge-transfer interaction between the drug and nonselective binding sites. More energetic HOMOs might thereby decrease drug concentration in equilibrium with the receptor.

The most significant partial regression coefficient in each equation (Table 4) was for the electrostatic interaction energy (E). Because the sign of the regression coefficient was in each case negative, and the value of E is itself negative, a greater potency (lower ED_{50}) is associated with higher (more positive) values of E. Thus, the lower the attraction of an electron for its core the more likely it is that the molecule will be a potent anticonvulsant. In other words, anticonvulsant potency seems to be directly related to the ability of a molecule to participate in an electrostatic interaction with an acceptor molecule.

The positive dependence of ED_{50} on dipole moment in equations 1 and 2 of Table 4 is consistent with earlier findings for the benzodiazepines (5) and miscellaneous compounds (53–55), which is gratifying in view of the modest level of significance for this term. The interpretation of this positive dependence might be the same as that already suggested above. [Note, however, that in reference to the work of Lien et al. (54) the dependence was described as negative. This is because potency in their work is described as the log of the inverse ED_{50} as opposed to the ED_{50} directly.] That is, the larger the dipole moment the lower the potency (larger ED_{50}), presumably because of a dipole–dipole interaction between the drug and a nonreceptor binding site, resulting in a decrease in drug concentration in equilibrium with the receptor. This is the same principle as was discussed for HOMO's involvement.

However, another interpretation is quite possible. Dipolar interactions are highly dependent on orientation of the participant dipoles. For the dipole–dipole interaction, the most stable configuration is a head-to-tail orientation described by the following equation

$$E = 2\mu_a\mu_b/d^3D \qquad [8]$$

where μ is the dipole moment for each dipole (a and b), d is the distance between the centers of the two moments, and D is the dielectric constant of the separating medium. Deviations from the head-to-tail orientation decrease the stability of the complex, and an antiparallel orientation of the two dipoles would, in fact, destabilize the drug–receptor complex. Thus, steric factors might exist that restrict the interacting (drug–receptor) dipoles to an antiparallel configuration. Larger dipole moments would thereby lower the association constant for the two species and not necessarily lower the drug concentration in equilibrium with the receptor.

The involvement of the molecular weight (MW) term in anticonvulsant SAR analysis has been documented previously (Table 2, eqs. 2 and 4), and the interpretation was that van der Waals interactions might play an important role in the drug–receptor interaction (54). (Note that the log MW term had been applied in previous studies.) However, because of the familiar covariance of the lipid/water partition coefficient and molecular weight, it has not yet been possible to ascertain in greater detail the physical meaning of this term (54). It is even more difficult at this time to provide a physical explanation for the unique occurrence of the MW term in equation 3 of Table 4. If the MW term did, in fact, express the involvement of van der Waals forces (or any bonding mechanism for that matter) in a drug–receptor complex, one would certainly expect to find that term in the regression based on brain concentration as well. Hence, this is a matter that requires further study.

The relative success of the equations depicted in Table 4 can be judged by the accuracy of their predictions (Table 5). Even though equation 1 of Table 4 described a very strong and reasonably significant regression, the predicted ED_{50}s are of only marginal value, as their comparison with the actual values demonstrates. The more potent drugs were predicted with less accuracy. The difference between the predicted and actual value was only 2.8% of the actual value for diphenylacetylurea but 350% of the actual value for phenytoin, the most potent drug when expressed in terms of the intraperitoneal dosage. The accuracy improved markedly when equation 2 of Table 4 was used to predict potency on the basis of brain concentrations. The full range of potencies were predicted exceptionally well, as illustrated in Table 5. The largest difference between predicted and actual values was only 26.1% of the actual value for carbamazepine, and the smallest difference (except for phenobarbital which was predicted exactly) was only 1.3% of the actual value (diphenylacetylurea). The accuracy of equation 3 of Table 4 was generally intermediate between

TABLE 5. *Comparison of actual potencies with potencies predicted using equations in table 4.*[a]

Drug	Actual			Predicted			Difference		
	I.p.	Brain	Blood	I.p.	Brain	Blood	I.p.	Brain	Blood
Phenytoin	2.8	21.0	8.7	−7.0	18.4	9.8	9.8	2.6	1.1
Phenobarbital	8.2	64.6	74.1	13.1	64.6	72.5	−4.9	0.0	1.6
α,α-Diphenylsuccinimide	10.5	33.4	19.9	18.6	37.6	22.9	−8.1	−4.2	−3.0
Carbamazepine	4.1	20.7	10.2	9.9	26.1	15.6	−5.8	−5.4	−5.4
Cyheptamide	34.3	37.7	23.3	28.7	31.3	15.1	5.6	6.4	8.2
Diphenylacetylurea	159.7	157.3	90.4	164.2	159.4	93.5	−4.5	−2.1	−3.1
5,5-Diphenylbarbituric acid	123.1	144.8	77.8	115.0	142.1	75.0	8.1	2.7	2.8

[a]Potencies are listed as ED_{50}s and are expressed in the same units as used in Table 3.

mazepine: Mechanism of action. *Ad. Neurol.,* 11:263–276.

41. Kannan, K. K., Vaara, I., Nostrand, B., Lovgren, S., Borell, A., Fridborg, K., and Petef, M. (1977): Structure and function of carbonic anhydrase: Comparative studies of sulphonamide binding to human erythrocyte carbonic anhydrases B and C. In: *Drug Action at the Molecular Level,* edited by G. C. K. Roberts, pp. 73–91. University Park Press, Baltimore.

42. Kaufman, J. J., and Kerman, E. (1974): Quantum chemical and other theoretical techniques for the understanding of the psychoactive action of the phenothiazines. *Biochem. Psychopharmacol.,* 9:55–75.

43. Kier, L. B. (1967): Molecular orbital calculation of preferred conformations of acetylcholine, muscarine and muscarone. *Mol. Pharmacol.,* 3:487–494.

44. Kier, L. B. (1968): Molecular orbital calculations of the preferred conformations of histamine and a theory on its dual activity. *J. Med. Chem.,* 11:441–445.

45. Kier, L. B. (1970): *Molecular Orbital Studies in Chemical Pharmacology.* Springer-Verlag, New York.

46. Kier, L. B. (1971): *Medicinal Chemistry, Vol. 10, Molecular Orbital Theory in Drug Research.* Academic Press, New York.

47. Krall, R. L., Penry, J. K., White, B. G., Kupferberg, H. J., and Swinyard, E. A. (1978): Antiepileptic drug development: II. Anticonvulsant drug screening. *Epilepsia,* 19:409–428.

48. Kutt, H. (1974): Mechanism of action of antiepileptic drugs. *Handbook of Clinical Neurology, Vol. 15,* edited by P. J. Vinken and G. W. Bruyn, pp. 621–663. North-Holland, Amsterdam.

49. Lathan, W. A., Curtiss, L. A., Hehre, W. J., Lisle, J. B., and Pople, J. A. (1974): Molecular orbital structures for small organic molecules and cations. *Prog. Phys. Org. Chem.,* 11:175–261.

50. Lennox, W. G. (1945): The petit mal epilepsies: Their treatment with Tridione. *J.A.M.A.,* 129:1069–1073.

51. Lennox, W. G., and Lennox, M. A. (1960): *Epilepsy and Related Disorders, Vol. I.* Little, Brown, Boston.

52. Li, J. C. R. (1964): *Statistical Inference, Vol. II.* Edwards Brothers, Ann Arbor.

53. Lien, E. J. (1970): Structure–activity correlations for anticonvulsant drugs. *J. Med. Chem.,* 13:1189–1191.

54. Lien, E. J., Liao, R. C. H., and Shinouda, H. G. (1979): Quantitative structure–activity relationships and dipole moments of anticonvulsants and CNS depressants. *J. Pharm. Sci.,* 68:463–465.

55. Lien, E. J., Tong, G. L., Chou, J. T., and Lien, L. L. (1973): Structural requirements for centrally acting drugs I. *J. Pharm. Sci.,* 62:246–250.

56. Locock, C. (1857): Contribution to discussion on paper by E. H. Sieveking. *Lancet,* 1:528.

57. Loew, G., Motulsky, H., Trudell, J., Cohen, E., and Hjelmeland, L. (1974): Quantum chemical studies of the metabolism of the inhalation anesthetics methoxyflurane, enflurane, and isoflurane. *Mol. Pharmacol.,* 10:406–418.

58. Loew, G., Trudell, J., and Motulsky, H. (1973): Quantum chemical studies of the metabolism of a series of chlorinated ethane anesthetics. *Mol. Pharmacol.,* 9:152–162.

59. Lucek, R. W., Garland, W. A., and Dairman, W. (1979): CNDO/2 molecular orbital study of selected 1,3-dihydro-5-phenyl-1,4-benzodiazepin-2-ones. *Fed. Proc.,* 38:541.

60. Lukovits, I., and Otvos, L. (1978): Correlation between the protein binding, biological activity and energy of the highest occupied molecular orbital of benzodiazepine derivatives. *Stud. Biophys.,* 69:187–191.

61. Marshall, F. J. (1958): Some 3,3-disubstituted-2-pyrrolidinones. *J. Org. Chem.,* 23:503–505.

62. McFarland, J. W. (1970): On the parabolic relationship between drug potency and hydrophobicity. *J. Med. Chem.,* 13:1192–1196.

63. Merritt, H. H., and Putnam, T. J. (1938): Sodium diphenyl hydantoinate in treatment of convulsive disorders. *J.A.M.A.,* 111:1068–1073.

64. Miller, C. A., and Long, L. M. (1951): Anticonvulsants. I. An investigation of N-R-α-R_1-α-phenylsuccinimides. *J. Am. Chem. Soc.,* 73:4895–4898.

65. Mohler, H., and Okuda, T. (1977): Benzodiazepine receptor: Demonstration in the central nervous system. *Science,* 198:849–851.

66. Olsen, R. W., Lamar, E. E., and Bayless, J. D. (1977): Calcium-induced release of γ-aminobutyric acid from synaptosomes: Effects of tranquilliser drugs. *J. Neurochem.,* 28:299–305.

67. Ostravskaya, R. U., Molodavkin, G. M., Porfireva, R. P., and Zubovskaya, A. M. (1975): Mechanism of the anticonvulsant action of diazepam. *Bull. Exp. Biol. Med.,* 79:270–273.

68. Penniston, J. T., Beckett, L., Bentley, D. L., and Hansch, C. (1969): Passive permeation of organic compounds through biological tissue: A non-steady-state theory. *Mol. Pharmacol.,* 5:333–341.

69. Perkow, W. (1966): Constitution and action of biologically active compounds. XVII. Common structural principles in drugs. *Arzneim. Forsch.,* 16:1287–1297.

70. Pincus, J. H., Grove, I., Marino, B. B., and Glaser, G. H. (1970): Studies on the mechanisms of action of diphenylhydantoin. *Arch. Neurol.,* 22:566–577.

71. Pople, J. A. (1953): Electron interaction in unsaturated hydrocarbons. *Trans. Faraday Soc.,* 49:1375–1385.

72. Pople, J. A., Santry, D. P., and Segal, G. A. (1965): Approximate self-consistent molecular orbital theory. I. Invariant procedures. *J. Chem. Phys.,* 43:S129–S135.

73. Purpura, D. P., Penry, J. K., Tower, D. B., Woodbury, D. M., and Walters, R. D. (1972): *Experimental Models of Epilepsy—A Manual for the Laboratory Worker.* Raven Press, New York.

74. Randall, L. O., Schallek, W., Sternbach, L. H., and Ning, R. Y. (1974): Chemistry and pharmacology of the 1,4-benzodiazepines. In: *Psychopharmacological Agents,* edited by M. Gordon, pp. 175–281. Academic Press, New York.

75. Rein, R., Fukuda, N., Clarke, G. A., and Harris, F. E. (1968): Iterative extended Huckel study of nucleic acid bases. *J. Theor. Biol.,* 21:88–96.

76. Rein, R., Fukuda, N., Win, H., Clarke, G. A., and Harris, F. W. (1966): Iterative extended Huckel theory. *Chem. Phys.*, 45:4743–4744.

77. Richards, W. G. (1977): Calculation of essential drug conformations and electron distributions. In: *Drug Action at the Molecular Level*, edited by G. C. K. Roberts, pp. 41–54. University Park Press, Baltimore.

78. Roberts, G. C. K. (1977): Substrate and inhibitor binding to dihydrofolate reductase. In: *Drug Action at the Molecular Level*, edited by G. C. K. Roberts, pp. 127–150. University Park Press, Baltimore.

79. Rogers, K. S., and Cammarata, A. (1969): Superdelocalizability and charge density. A correlation with partition coefficients. *J. Med. Chem.*, 12:692–693.

80. Saad, S. F., El Masry, A. M., and Scott, P. M. (1972): Influence of certain anticonvulsants on the concentration of γ aminobutyric acid in the cerebral hemispheres of mice. *Eur. J. Pharmacol.*, 17:386–392.

81. Salem, L. (1964): Intermolecular forces in biological systems. In: *Electronic Aspects of Biochemistry: Proceedings*, edited by B. Pullman, pp. 293–299. Academic Press, New York.

82. Sarrazin, M., Bourdeaux, M., and Briand, C. (1976): Etude de quelques relations structure–activite des benzodiazepines. *Ann. Phys. Biol. Med.*, 9:211–220.

83. Sawaya, M. C. B., Horton, R. W., and Meldrum, B. S. (1975): Effects of anticonvulsant drugs on the cerebral enzymes metabolizing GABA. *Epilepsia*, 16:649–655.

84. Schuster, P. (1969): Coulomb Energiekorrekturen in der erweiterten Huckelmethode. *Monatsschr. Chem.*, 100:1033–1040.

85. Singer, J. A., and Purcell, W. P. (1967): Hueckel molecular orbital calculations for some anti-malarial drugs and related molecules. *J. Med. Chem.*, 10:754–762.

86. Snedecor, G. W., and Cochran, W. G. (1980): *Statistical Methods*, Seventh Edition. The Iowa State University Press, Ames.

87. Snyder, S. H., and Merril, C. R. (1965): A relation between the hallucinogenic activity of drugs and their electronic configuration. *Proc. Natl. Acad. Sci. U.S.A.*, 54:258–266.

88. Sohn, R. S., and Ferrendelli, J. A. (1976): Anticonvulsant drug mechanisms. Phenytoin, phenobarbital, and ethosuximide and calcium flux in isolated presynaptic endings. *Arch. Neurol.*, 33:626–629.

89. Spielman, M. A., Geisler, A. O., and Close, W. J. (1948): Anticonvulsant drugs. II. Some acylureas. *J. Am. Chem. Soc.*, 70:4189–4191.

90. Sternbach, L. H. (1973): Chemistry of 1,4-benzodiazepines and some aspects of the structure-activity relationship. In: *The Benzodiazepines*, edited by S. Garratini, E. Mussini, and L. O. Randall, pp. 1–26. Raven Press, New York.

91. Sternbach, L. H., Randall, L. O., Banziger, R., and Lehr, H. (1968): Structure-activity relationship in the 1,4-benzodiazepine series. *Drugs Affecting the Central Nervous System, Vol. 2*, edited by A. Burger, pp. 237–264. Marcel Dekker, New York.

92. Swinyard, E. A. (1969): Laboratory evaluation of antiepileptic drugs. Review of laboratory methods. *Epilepsia*, 10:107–119.

93. Swinyard, E. A., and Castellion, A. W. (1966): Anticonvulsant properties of some benzodiazepines. *J. Pharmacol. Exp. Ther.*, 151:369–375.

94. Toman, J. E. P., Swinyard, E. A., and Goodman, L. S. (1946): Properties of maximal seizures and their alteration by anticonvulsant drugs and other agents. *J. Neurophysiol.*, 9:231–240.

95. Tsuchiya, T., Fukushima, H., and Kitagawa, S. (1976): Effect of benzodiazepines on penicillin induced epileptic discharges. *Folia Pharmacol. Jpn.*, 72:861–877.

96. Vernadakis, A., and Woodbury, D. M. (1960): Effect of diphenylhydantoin and adrenocortical steroids on free glutamic acid, glutamine and gamma-aminobutyric acid concentrations of rat cerebral cortex. In: *Inhibition in the Nervous System and Gamma-Aminobutyric Acid*, edited by E. Roberts, C. F. Barden, A. van Harreveld, C. A. G. Wiersma, W. R. Adey, and K. F. Killam, pp. 242–248. Pergamon Press, New York.

97. Vida, J. A. (1977): *Anticonvulsants*. Academic Press, New York.

98. Weinberger, J., Nicklas, W. J., and Berl, S. (1976): Mechanism of action of anticonvulsants. Role of the differential effects on the active uptake of putative neurotransmitters. *Neurology Minneapol.*, 26:162–166.

99. Wheland, G. W., and Pauling, L. (1935): A quantum-mechanical discussion of orientation of substituents in aromatic molecules. *J. Am. Chem. Soc.*, 57:2086–2095.

100. Wohl, A. J. (1970): Electronic molecular pharmacology: The benzothiadiazine antihypertensive agents. II. Multiple regression analyses relating biological potency and electronic structure. *Mol. Pharmacol.*, 6:195–205.

101. Woodbury, D. M. (1972): Applications to drug evaluations. In: *Experimental Models of Epilepsy—A Manual for the Laboratory Worker*, edited by D. P. Purpura, J. K. Penry, D. B. Tower, D. M. Woodbury, and R. D. Walters, pp. 557–601. Raven Press, New York.

102. Woodbury, D. M. (1980): Phenytoin: Introduction and history. In: *Antiepileptic Drugs: Mechanisms of Action*, edited by G. H. Glaser, J. K. Penry, and D. M. Woodbury, pp. 305–313. Raven Press, New York.

103. Woodbury, D. M. (1980): Phenytoin: Proposed mechanisms of anticonvulsant action. In: *Antiepileptic Drugs: Mechanisms of Action*, edited by G. H. Glaser, J. K. Penry and D. M. Woodbury, pp. 447–471. Raven Press, New York.

104. Zerner, M., and Gouterman, M. (1966): Porphyrins. IV. Extended Hueckel calculations on transition metal complexes. *Theor. Chim. Acta.*, 4:44–63.

105. Zerner, M., Gouterman, M., and Kobayashi, H. (1966): Porphyrins. VIII. Extended Hueckel calculations on iron complexes. *Theor. Chim. Acta*, 6:363–400.

Antiepileptic Drugs, edited by D. M. Woodbury,
J. K. Penry, and C. E. Pippenger. Raven Press,
New York © 1982.

7

General Principles

Experimental Detection, Quantification, and Evaluation of Anticonvulsants

Ewart A. Swinyard and Jose H. Woodhead

More than four decades have passed since Putnam and Merritt (8) first demonstrated that drugs effective in epilepsy can be distinguished from other organic chemicals by testing their ability to suppress experimentally induced convulsions in normal laboratory animals. During this time, virtually all species of laboratory animals have been subjected to a wide variety of electrical, chemical, and sensory seizure-evoking techniques in anticipation of finding a model that would be representative of the clinical disorder. Ideally, such models should duplicate the human clinical condition. Unfortunately, knowledge of the underlying causes of various types of convulsive disorders is still incomplete, and the development of laboratory models based on etiology is not yet possible. Consequently, most experimental models of epilepsy are designed to simulate in laboratory animals various chemical, electrical, or overt manifestations of the disorder (7).

Anticonvulsant drug activity can also be determined at various biological levels, such as axons; intact single cells; groups of cells, including pre- and postsynaptic events; suborgan cellular connections, including spinal cord pathways; organ systems, including the whole brain; and modified intact animals in which the

brain has been surgically or chemically altered (7). Many of these sophisticated procedures are extremely valuable, especially as penultimate tests prior to clinical drug trials and as models for the study of seizure mechanisms. Unfortunately, many of them are also tedious, time consuming, and costly. Consequently, they do not lend themselves to the routine screening of the large numbers of chemicals one must test in the search for new agents with antiepileptic potential. For these and other reasons, intact normal rodents are preferred for this purpose (4).

At present, no single laboratory test will in itself establish the presence or absence of anticonvulsant activity in a chemical substance. Therefore, a battery of tests should be employed for identifying and evaluating substances with anticonvulsant potential. These tests should be selected for their ability to detect substances with anticonvulsant activity, to show whether such activity results from the prevention of seizure spread or from the elevation of seizure threshold, and to provide some insight as to their mechanisms of action. Since antiepileptic drugs must be taken chronically and, in many instances, throughout the life of the patient, it is equally important to include a battery of toxicity tests in the procedure. The toxicity tests should not only enable the investigator to determine accurately the minimal median neurotoxic dose and the 24-hr median lethal dose but should also provide a profile of the overt toxic manifestations between these two dose levels. A procedure specifically designed to accomplish these objectives will be described in this chapter. The authors have used this procedure for approximately 7 years in an anticonvulsant drug development program (4). During this time, over 5,500 chemical substances have been screened for anticonvulsant activity and neurotoxicity. In addition, more than 900 chemicals shown to have activity by the anticonvulsant identification procedure have been subjected to various levels of anticonvulsant quantification and evaluation. Thus, these procedures have been shown to be reliable and reproducible.

It is hoped that this chapter will afford interested readers some insight into the principles and procedures involved in the detection, quantification, and evaluation of anticonvulsant drugs.

MATERIALS AND METHODS

Experimental Animals

Adult male CF No. 1 albino mice (18 to 25 g in weight) and adult male Sprague–Dawley albino rats (100 to 150 g in weight) are used as experimental animals. The animals are maintained on an adequate diet (S/L Custom Lab Diet-7) and allowed free access to food and water except during the short time they are removed from their cages for testing. Animals newly received in the laboratory are allowed 3 or 4 days to correct for the food and water restriction incurred during transit before being employed in these procedures. All animals are housed, fed, and handled in a manner consistent with the recommendations in HEW publication (NIH) No. 7423, *Guide for the Care and Use of Laboratory Animals*. As animals are set up for each experimental procedure, they are carefully identified in order to record drug doses administered and responses observed during the course

of the entire experiment. Animals should be used only once and then disposed of in a humane manner. In the event animals are in short supply, however, they may be used a second time provided at least 1 week is allowed for the animal to eliminate the test drug.

Electroshock Apparatus and Chemicals

For the test based on maximal electroshock convulsions (MES test), corneal electrodes are used, and 60-Hz alternating current is delivered for 0.2 sec by means of an apparatus similar to that originally designed by Woodbury and Davenport (16); the current delivered by this instrument is independent of the external resistance. Maximal seizures are elicited with a current intensity five to seven times that necessary to evoke minimal electroshock threshold seizures, i.e., 50 mA in mice and 150 mA in rats.

For tests based on chemically induced convulsions, the convulsant chemical is made up in a concentration that will induce convulsions in more than 97% of animals (CD_{97}) when injected in mice in a volume of 0.01 ml/g body weight or in rats in a volume of 0.02 ml/10 g body weight. Pentylenetetrazol (Metrazol®) (CD_{97}, 85 mg/kg in mice; 70 mg/kg in rats) is administered to mice as a 0.85% solution in 0.9% sodium chloride or to rats as a 3.5% solution in 0.9% sodium chloride. Bicuculline (CD_{97}, 2.70 mg/kg in mice) is administered as a 0.027% solution prepared as follows: the requisite amount of bicuculline is dissolved in 1.0 ml of warmed 0.1 N HCl with the aid of a micromixer, and sufficient 0.9% sodium chloride solution is added to make a 0.027% solution. This solution must be made up fresh and used immediately. Picrotoxin (CD_{97}, 3.15 mg/kg) is administered as a 0.032% solution in 0.9% sodium chloride. Strychnine (CD_{97}, 1.20 mg/kg) is administered as a 0.012% solution in 0.9% sodium chloride. All chemical convulsants are administered subcutaneously into a loose fold of skin in the midline of the neck. Shoulder and pelvic areas are avoided in order to eliminate sequelae of the injection which might erroneously be interpreted as neuromuscular deficit. Since the doses employed in the above tests induce convulsions in over 97% of mice, it is unnecessary to run control groups simultaneously with the test groups.

Preparation and Injection of Test Drugs

Test drugs soluble in water are administered in 0.9% sodium chloride solution; those insoluble in water are administered in 30% polyethylene glycol 400 (PEG). The test substance is given in a concentration that permits optimal accuracy of dosage without the volume contributing excessively to total body fluid. Thus, the volume employed in mice is 0.01 ml/g body weight; the volume employed in rats is 0.04 ml/10 g body weight. Test drugs are administered either intraperitoneally (i.p.) or orally (p.o.) as indicated in Table 1. The subcutaneous (s.c.) route is reserved for the administration of the chemical convulsants. No other drugs or chemicals should be injected at the same subcutaneous site.

Anticonvulsant Tests

Five tests are used in the identification, quantification, and evaluation of anticonvulsant activity. The methods employed in these tests have been reported previously (4,9–11,14). The important details are summarized below.

Maximal Electroshock Seizure Test

At the previously determined time of peak effect (TPE) of the test substance, a drop of electrolyte solution (0.9% sodium chloride solution) is applied to the eyes of each animal, the corneal electrodes are applied to the eyes, and the electrical stimulus (50 mA in mice; 150 mA in rats; 60 Hz) is delivered for 0.2 sec. The animals are restrained only by hand and are released at the moment of stimulation in order to permit observation of the seizure throughout its entire course. Abolition of the hindleg tonic extensor component after drug treatment is taken as the endpoint for this test. The tonic component is considered abolished if the hindleg tonic extension does not exceed a 90° angle with the

TABLE 1. *Flow chart for anticonvulsant drug screening[a]*

Phase I.	Anticonvulsant identification Mice, i.p. administration Dose range: 30, 100, 300, and 600 mg/kg Tests: MES, sc Met, rotorod, and observation of general behavior Time of test: ½ and 4 hr
Phase II.	Anticonvulsant quantification in mice i.p. TPE: MES, sc Met, rotorod ED_{50}: MES, sc Met, rotorod
Phase III.	Toxicity profile in mice i.p. Observation of general behavior induced by 1 TD_{50}, 2 TD_{50}s and 4 TD_{50}s Determination of HD_{50} and LD_{50}
Phase IV.	Anticonvulsant quantification in mice p.o. TPE: MES, sc Met, rotorod ED_{50}: MES, sc Met, rotorod
Phase V.	Antiepileptic drug differentiation in mice i.p. ED_{50}s sc pentylenetetrazol [stimulates neuronal membranes directly, induces minimal-threshold (cl) seizures]; sc bicuculline [blocks GABA receptors and, thus, interferes with GABA-inhibitory function, induces both clonic and tonic extensor (cl, TE) seizures]; sc picrotoxin [blocks presynaptic inhibition mediated by GABA, induces minimal-threshold (cl) seizures]; sc strychnine [blocks postsynaptic inhibition mediated by glycine, induces maximal (TE) seizures]; and other chemical convulsants considered essential. Compare with the profile of clinically effective antiepileptic drugs.
Phase VI.	Anticonvulsant quantification in rats p.o. TPE: MES, sc Met, minimal neurotoxicity ED_{50}: MES, sc Met, minimal neurotoxicity

[a]The various neurotoxicity and anticonvulsant tests described in the text have been integrated into an anticonvulsant screening procedure designed to identify, quantify, and evaluate the anticonvulsant potential of candidate chemical substances.

plane of the body and indicates that the test substance has the ability to prevent seizure spread.

Subcutaneous Pentylenetetrazol Seizure Threshold Test

The CD_{97} of pentylenetetrazol (85 mg/kg, mice; 70 mg/kg, rats) is injected subcutaneously in a volume of 0.01 ml/g body weight into each of the requisite number of mice (0.02 ml/

10 g body weight in rats) at the previously determined TPE for the test substance. The animals are placed in isolation cages and observed for the next 30 min for the presence or absence of a seizure. A threshold convulsion is defined as one episode of clonic spasms that persists for at least a 5-sec period. Absence of a threshold convulsion during the 30-min period of observation is taken as the endpoint and indicates that the test substance has the ability to elevate the pentylenetetrazol seizure threshold.

Subcutaneous Bicuculline Seizure Threshold Test

The CD_{97} of bicuculline (2.70 mg/kg) is injected subcutaneously in a volume of 0.01 ml/g body weight into each of the requisite number of mice at the previously determined TPE for the test substance. The mice are placed in isolation cages and observed for the next 30 min for the presence or absence of a threshold seizure as described under the subcutaneous pentylenetetrazol (sc Met) test. Absence of a threshold seizure indicates that the test substance has the ability to elevate the bicuculline seizure threshold.

Subcutaneous Picrotoxin Seizure Threshold Test

The CD_{97} of picrotoxin (3.15 mg/kg) is injected subcutaneously in a volume of 0.01 ml/g body weight into each of the requisite number of mice at the previously determined TPE for the test substance. The mice are placed in isolation cages and observed for the next 45 min for the presence or absence of a threshold convulsion. Absence of a threshold convulsion is taken as the endpoint and indicates that the test substance has the ability to elevate the picrotoxin seizure threshold.

Subcutaneous Strychnine Seizure Pattern Test

The CD_{97} of strychnine (1.20 mg/kg) is injected subcutaneously in a volume of 0.01 ml/g body weight into each of the requisite number

of mice at the previously determined TPE of the test substance. The mice are placed in isolation cages and observed for 30 min for the presence or absence of the hindleg tonic extensor component of the seizure. Abolition of the hindleg tonic extensor component is taken as the endpoint for this test and indicates that the test substance has the ability to prevent seizure spread.

Determination of Acute Toxicity

Acute toxicity induced by candidate anticonvulsant drugs in laboratory animals is usually characterized by some type of neurological abnormality. In mice, these abnormalities can easily be detected by the rotorod test (2). The rotorod test is somewhat less useful in rats and must usually be supplemented by the positional sense test and gait and stance test. For quick reference, the muscle tone test and the righting test are also described. The names assigned to these tests are those employed in our laboratory and do not necessarily refer to the specific neurological reflexes involved (9,10).

Rotorod Test

This test is used exclusively in mice to assess neurotoxicity. When a normal mouse is placed on a rod that rotates at a speed of 6 rpm, the mouse can maintain its equilibrium for long periods of time. Neurological deficit is indicated by inability of the animal to maintain its equilibrium for 1 min on this rotating rod in each of three trials.

Positional Sense Test

If the hindleg of a normal mouse or rat is gently lowered over the edge of a table, the animal will quickly lift its leg back to a normal position. The animal's inability to rapidly correct such an abnormal position of the limb indicates neurological deficit.

Gait and Stance Test

Neurological deficit is indicated by a circular or zig-zag gait, ataxia, abnormal spread of the legs, abnormal body posture, tremor, hyperactivity, lack of exploratory behavior, somnolence, stupor, or catalepsy, among other signs.

Muscle Tone Test

Normal animals have a certain amount of skeletal muscle tone which is apparent to the experienced handler. A loss of skeletal muscle tone characterized by hypotonia or flaccidity indicates neurological deficit.

Righting Test

If a mouse or rat is placed on its back, the animal will quickly right itself and assume a normal posture. The animal's inability to rapidly correct for the abnormal body posture is evidence of neurological deficit.

Abnormal neurological status disclosed by the rotorod test is commonly taken as the endpoint for the toxicity determination in mice. Abnormal neurological status disclosed by the rotorod test, positional sense test, or the gait and stance test is taken as the endpoint for the toxicity determination in rats. Inability of a rat to perform normally on at least two of the above three tests indicates that the animal has some neurological deficit.

Acute Toxicity Profile

The overt signs and symptoms of acute toxicity induced by each test substance may be determined in intact animals by a modification of the procedure described by Irwin (3). Six mice are randomly divided into three groups of two mice each, and each group is administered a dose equivalent to either 1 TD_{50}, 2 TD_{50}s, or 4 TD_{50}s of the test substance. A comprehensive assessment of the symptoms of toxicity is made 10, 20, and 30 min and 1, 2, 4, 6, 8, and 24 hr after administration of the test substance. The data obtained provide valuable insight not only as to the symptoms and kind of toxicity induced but also as to the approximate level of the median effective hypnotic (HD_{50}) and median lethal (LD_{50}) doses of the test substance.

Time of Peak Effect

Quantitative anticonvulsant tests and the determination of the median neurotoxic dose of the candidate substance should be conducted at the time of peak effect (TPE) as determined by the specific test procedure (e.g., rotorod test, MES test, sc Met test). Examination of the phase I results (see Table 2) will usually reveal the approximate range between no anticonvulsant activity or no neurotoxicity and some anticonvulsant activity or some neurotoxicity. An approximate ED_{50} or TD_{50} is then estimated by giving four groups of animals (two animals in each group) a range of four doses between no activity or no toxicity and some activity or some toxicity; these animals are then subjected to the appropriate anticonvulsant or neurotoxicity test(s) at ½, 1, 2, and 4 hr. The approximate ED_{50} is then administered to four groups of animals (four animals in each group) and tested at ½, 1, 2, and 4 hr, respectively. The data obtained are plotted against time on linear graph paper; the TPE is then determined by visual inspection of the graph. In the determination of the TPE for toxicity, an approximate TD_{50} is administered to a single group of eight animals, all of which are then subjected to the appropriate toxicity test(s) for mice or rats at the time intervals indicated above or until peak toxicity has obviously passed. Similarly, the results are plotted on graph paper, and the TPE determined by visual inspection of the graph.

TABLE 2. *Phase I: anticonvulsant identification*

Test	Time (hr)	Dose (mg/kg)			
		30	100	300	600
MES	½	1/1[a]	1/1	1/1	1/1
sc Met	½	0/1	1/1	1/1	1/1
Toxicity	½	0/4	4/4	4/4	4/4
MES	4	0/1	1/1	1/1	1/1
sc Met	4	0/1	0/1	1/1	1/1
Toxicity	4	0/2	0/2	2/2	2/2

[a]No. protected or toxic/No. tested

Determination of the Median Effective or Toxic Dose

In general, the procedure employed to determine the median effective or toxic dose is the same as for TPE, except that animals subjected to anticonvulsant tests can only be used once. In the determination of the median effective dose (ED_{50}) by an anticonvulsant procedure, eight animals are injected with the dose used in the determination of the TPE and subjected to the anticonvulsant test at the TPE. The percent of animals protected is plotted against the dose on log-probit paper, and another dose level is selected. This procedure is repeated until at least four points have been established between the dose level that protects 0% of the animals and the dose level that protects 100% of the animals. These data are then subjected to statistical analysis (see below), and the ED_{50}, 95% confidence interval, and slope of the regression line are recorded in the experimental protocol.

In the determination of the median toxic dose (TD_{50}), it should be remembered that one point was previously established in the TPE experiments. The percent toxic response is plotted against the dose on log-probit paper, and another dose is selected. This dose is administered to eight animals. The animals are then subjected to the respective toxicity test for mice or rats at ½, 1, 2, and 4 hr. This procedure is repeated until four points have been established between the dose level that induces no signs of toxicity in any of the animals and the dose that is toxic to all of the animals. These data are then subjected to statistical analysis (see below), and the calculated results are recorded in the experimental protocol book.

The procedures for the determination of the median hypnotic dose (HD_{50}) and the 24-hr median lethal dose (LD_{50}) are the same as those described for the median toxic dose. Information on the approximate dose level can usually be obtained for both the hypnotic dose and the lethal dose from the toxicity profile studies. The endpoints employed are the loss of righting reflex for the HD_{50} and the occurrence of death within 24 hr for the LD_{50}. The data obtained are subjected to statistical analysis as described below.

Statistical Analysis

The various median effective doses (MES, sc Met, bicuculline, picrotoxin, and strychnine) and median toxic doses (TD_{50}, HD_{50}, and LD_{50}) are calculated by a FORTRAN probit analysis program. This program also provides the 95% confidence intervals and the slopes of the regression lines along with the standard error of the slopes. Reasonable estimates of these values may be determined by the log-probit method of Litchfield and Wilcoxon (5). This kind of statistical treatment provides the kind of data essential to a critical evaluation of either anticonvulsant activity and toxicity or structure-activity relations.

SPECIAL PRECAUTIONS

Davenport and Davenport (1) have shown that starvation increases the severity of maximal electroshock seizures, i.e., shortens tonic flexion and prolongs tonic extension. Therefore, all animals used in anticonvulsant tests should be allowed free access to food and water except during the actual test. Male CF No. 1 mice and Sprague–Dawley rats are preferred for anticonvulsant studies because these strains are more docile. Moreover, maximal electroshock seizures, particularly if a drop of electrolyte solution (local anesthetic solution or 0.9% sodium chloride solution) is applied to the eyes before the application of the corneal electrodes, are rarely lethal in CF No. 1 mice (15). Also, these tests are more reproducible if animals of the same sex, age, and weight are employed (18). Except for phenytoin, the ED_{50} of which is the same in both young and old rats or mice, aging in rats is associated with decreased ED_{50} values for selected anticonvulsant drugs and in mice with increased ED_{50} values (6). Also, approximately 10% of rats fail to give a full maximal seizure; the incidence of this is higher in older rats and in animals that struggle during electrode placement. Animals that struggle excessively should be discarded.

Rats that are to be used for evaluating drug toxicity should be examined by the battery of toxicity tests before the test drug is administered. Individual animals may have peculiarities in gait, equilibrium, muscle tone, or placing response that might otherwise erroneously be attributed to the test substance.

In general, chemical convulsants such as pentylenetetrazol should be administered subcutaneously in a dose that will induce minimal convulsions in 97% of the animals. Such dose levels reveal the ability of the candidate substance to alter (increase or decrease) seizure threshold. Higher doses, such as those sufficient to evoke maximal tonic–clonic seizures, usually provide information on the ability of the test substance to alter seizure spread but very little enlightenment relative to effects on seizure threshold. It should also be emphasized that when the chemical convulsant is given subcutaneously, the test substance should be given either intraperitoneally or orally. If it becomes necessary to give the test substance subcutaneously, the substance should be injected in an area removed from the site in which the convulsant agent is to be injected. This procedure will avoid false positives induced by vasoconstrictor substances retarding the absorption of the convulsant agents (A. K. Shenoy and E. A. Swinyard, *unpublished observations*).

It is well known that aggregation alters the susceptibility of mice to various chemical substances, including amphetamine and pentylenetetrazol (12). For this reason, animals injected with a convulsant drug are immediately placed in individual cages and remain in this environment during the time they are under observation.

A frequently ignored precaution concerns the quality control of laboratory utensils and glassware. Disposable test tubes, hypodermic syringes, needles, etc. should be employed whenever possible. If very insoluble, highly potent materials must be triturated with an organic solvent in a mortar and pestle (either porcelain or glass), meticulous washing procedures must be followed to avoid contamination of the next substance triturated in this same mortar and pestle. For example, Swinyard and Woodhead (13) have shown that as much as 20 times the sc Met ED$_{99}$ (66.25 μg) of clonazepam can remain in an insufficiently washed mortar and pestle. They suggest that an internal control test should be designed in order to determine when implements that must be reused are "clean." Observations of this kind indicate that investigators must be constantly alert for procedures that may compromise experimental results.

DETECTION AND QUANTIFICATION OF ANTICONVULSANT ACTIVITY

Detection of Anticonvulsant Activity

The profiles of experimental anticonvulsant activity of all clinically useful antiepileptic drugs are characterized by their ability to prevent seizure spread and/or to increase minimal seizure threshold. Drugs useful in generalized tonic–clonic (grand mal) and complex partial (temporal lobe) seizures, *e.g.,* phenytoin, are characterized by the ability to prevent seizure spread and may or may not increase minimal seizure threshold. Drugs useful in absence seizures, *e.g.,* ethosuximide, are characterized by the ability to elevate seizure threshold and have only limited, if any, ability to prevent seizure spread. Some investigators have suggested that the timed i.v. infusion of pentylenetetrazol should be used as a screening procedure so that agents that modify either one or both of these endpoints can be identified in a single animal. The timed i.v. infusion of pentylenetetrazol is one of the most sensitive measures of seizure threshold; however, the time to the onset of tonic extension is so variable (SD of the mean 6 to 10 times that for minimal threshold) that it cannot be relied on to detect seizure spread. For these reasons, the procedures to be described utilize two tests for the detection of anticonvulsant activity in candidate substances: the maximal electroshock seizure (MES) pattern test to detect agents that prevent seizure spread and the subcutaneous pentylenetetrazol (sc Met) threshold test to detect agents that elevate minimal seizure threshold.

The intraperitoneal route of administration is employed in phases I, II, III, and V of this screening procedure (Table 1) in order to avoid false negative data that may result from vagaries in the oral absorption of the test substance. The oral route of administration is used in phases IV and VI. Since the cost of mice is only approximately one-fourth that of rats, mice are used in phases I through V and rats in phase VI. However, rats are occasionally given an intraperitoneal dose of the test substance in order to establish the extent of oral absorption in this species.

Phase I, anticonvulsant identification, is used to identify active and relatively nontoxic substances. Sixteen mice are randomly divided into four groups of four mice each; each group is then given either 30, 100, 300, or 600 mg/kg of the test substance intraperitoneally. Thirty minutes after administration of the test substance, all four animals in each group are subjected to the rotorod test, and immediately thereafter one animal in each group is subjected to the MES test, and one animal in each group to the sc Met test. Four hours after drug administration, the remaining two mice in each group are subjected to the rotorod test, and immediately thereafter, one animal is subjected to the MES test and the other animal to the sc Met test. Thus, it requires only 16 mice to cover the dose range of 30, 100, 300, and 600 mg/kg and the time periods of ½ and 4 hr.

The results obtained from the phase I procedure enable the investigator to identify active and relatively nontoxic substances as well as to identify inactive and/or toxic substances, to determine the approximate effective dose level and the approximate minimal toxic dose level of active substances, to obtain an early insight as to time of onset and duration of action of the test substance, to estimate the approximate protective indices, and to decide if further work is justified.

Typical results obtained from the phase I screening procedure are shown in Table 2 which shows that the test substance is effective in nontoxic doses against the MES test but effective only at or near the toxic dose level (100 mg/kg) by the sc Met test. Thus, the protective indices appear to be approximately 3 and 1 by the MES and sc Met tests, respectively. The test substance also appears to have a relatively rapid onset and short duration of action, since both the anticonvulsant effects and neurotoxic effects are significantly greater at 30 min than at 4 hr. These data indicate that further experimental work is justified, since the favorable anticonvulsant profile suggests possible clinical usefulness in generalized tonic–clonic and complex partial seizures.

Krall et al. (4) have shown that the phase I procedure has a high level of reproducibility. As shown in Table 3, five randomly selected compounds were subjected to five repeated, blind phase I evaluations. Only two of the 25 evaluations differed from the initial screen. In one case, the repeated trial showed rotorod toxicity at 300 mg/kg instead of 100 mg/kg in the initial trial. In the other case, one repeat sc Met test

TABLE 3. *Comparison of initial and 25 repeated phase I evaluations[a]*

Repeated results	All tests			MES			sc Met			Rotorod		
>300	0	0	33	0	0	12	0	0	14	0	0	7
300	1	21	1	0	9	0	0	4	1	1	8	0
100 30	19	0	0	4	0	0	6	0	0	9	0	0
Dose (mg/kg)	30 100	300	>300	30 100	300	>300	30 100	300	>300	30 100	300	>300

[a]Data from Krall et al. (4).

showed activity at 300 mg/kg, whereas the initial trial failed to demonstrate activity at any of the dose levels tested. Thus, this test system is simple, rapid, and reliable; the endpoints are clear and easily determined; the procedure lends itself to the screening of large numbers of chemicals; the tests give very few false positives or false negatives; and all clinically useful antiepileptic drugs and agents active in other test systems are active by one or another of these test procedures.

Quantification of Anticonvulsant Activity

Phase II, anticonvulsant quantification, serves to quantitate in mice the anticonvulsant activity and minimal neurotoxicity of the substances identified in phase I. This is accomplished by first resolving the TPE (see above) for anticonvulsant activity (MES and sc Met tests) and toxicity (rotorod test). The median effective dose by the MES and sc Met tests and the median toxic dose by the rotorod test are then determined at the previously determined TPE after drug administration as already discussed. Thus, phase II reveals the TPE, the ED_{50}s by the MES and sc Met tests, the TD_{50} by the rotorod test, the 95% confidence intervals, slopes of the regression lines, and protective indices. The TPE data provide further insight into the time of onset and the duration of anticonvulsant and toxic activity. The ED_{50}s and TD_{50} lend themselves to structure–activity studies. Also, the median effective dose information and protective indices reveal for the first time reliable information as to possible clinical usefulness. Quantitative data of this kind are essential for making a judgment as to whether a more complete evaluation of the anticonvulsant potential of the test substance is justified.

Phase III, toxicity profile, and the median hypnotic dose (HD_{50}) and median lethal dose (LD_{50}) after intraperitoneal administration in mice reveal the dose–time relationship and the profile of overt toxic manifestations as well as two additional quantitative measures of toxicity (HD_{50} and 24-hr LD_{50}). Since all of this information is obtained in mice after the intraperitoneal administration of the test substance, data obtained in phases II and III provide a good profile of the acute dose–effect relationship from minimal anticonvulsant activity through maximal anticonvulsant activity and from minimal neurotoxicity through overt signs of toxicity including the median hypnotic dose to the dose lethal to 50% of mice within 24 hr. From these kinds of data one can determine if the test substance has a profile of action that warrants testing the drug after oral administration in mice.

Phase IV, anticonvulsant quantification in mice, provides the same kind of information as phase II except that the test substance is given by the oral route of administration. These data, the TPE, ED_{50} MES test, ED_{50} sc Met test, and TD_{50}, are important for several reasons. They reveal whether the substance is active when given orally; the TPE indicates how rapidly it is absorbed; and a comparison of the ED_{50}s and TD_{50} with similar data obtained after intraperitoneal administration (phase II) discloses how adequately the test substance is absorbed after oral administration. All of these factors are important because clinically useful antiepileptic drugs are usually given by the oral route of administration. Consequently, test substances that reach this point and still exhibit a satisfactory anticonvulsant activity, margin of safety, and adequate absorption after oral administration usually proceed to phase V, particularly if they also have a unique chemical structure.

Phase V, antiepileptic drug differentiation in mice, is designed to delineate more precisely the antiepileptic potential of the candidate substance. Four chemical convulsants are used for this purpose: pentylenetetrazol, bicuculline, picrotoxin, and strychnine. Since each of these convulsants acts through a somewhat different neurotransmitter system, the ED_{50}s obtained by these procedures reflect the profile of antiepileptic activity of the test substance. This profile can then be compared with the antiepileptic profiles of the prototype agents. Thus, the antiepileptic activity of the test substance can be more carefully differentiated and some insight obtained as to its possible mechanism of action.

Test substances that reach this point in the

TABLE 4. *Profile of anticonvulsant activity of intraperitoneally administered prototype antiepileptic drugs in mice (phases II and V)[a]*

Drug	Time of test (hr)	Rotorod TD$_{50}$ (mg/kg)	ED$_{50}$s (mg/kg)				
			MES	sc Met	Bicuculline	Picrotoxin	Strychnine
Phenytoin	2	65.46 (52.49–72.11) [15.23]	9.50 (8.13–10.44) [13.66] PI = 6.89[b]	No protection	No protection	No protection	Max. protection 50% at 55–100 mg/kg
Carbamazepine	¼, ¼	71.56 (45.91–134.79) [4.77]	8.81 (5.45–14.09) [3.62] PI = 8.12	Potentiates	Max. protection 62.5% at 50–130 mg/kg	37.20 (25.32–59.69) [3.86] PI = 1.92	78.83 (39.39–132.03) [2.85] PI = 0.91
Phenobarbital	½, 1, 1	69.01 (62.84–72.89) [24.67]	21.78 (14.99–25.52) [14.98] PI = 3.17	13.17 (5.87–15.93) [5.93] PI = 5.24	37.72 (26.49–47.39) [4.07] PI = 1.83	27.51 (20.88–34.82) [4.79] PI = 2.51	95.30 (91.31–99.52) [18.51] PI = 0.72
Valproate	¼	425.84 (368.91–450.40) [20.84]	271.66 (246.97–337.89) [12.83] PI = 1.57	148.59 (122.64–177.02) [11.84] PI = 2.87	359.95 (294.07–438.54) [7.51] PI = 1.18	387.21 (341.37–444.38) [8.35] PI = 1.10	292.96 (261.12–323.43) [11.80] PI = 1.45
Ethosuximide	½	440.83 (383.09–485.34) [18.37]	>1000 PI < 0.44	130.35 (110.99–150.46) [10.06] PI = 3.38	459.01 (349.92–633.13) [10.06] PI = 0.96	242.69 (227.84–255.22) [26.43] PI = 1.82	Max. protection 62.5% at 360 mg/kg
Clonazepam	½	0.184 (0.163–0.227) [14.44]	92.65 (44.86–189.34) [1.90] PI = 0.002	0.009 (0.0046–0.0165) [13.90] PI = 20.44	0.0086 (0.004–0.021) [1.35] PI = 21.40	0.043 (0.027–0.059) [3.51] PI = 4.28	No protection

[a]The 95% confidence interval is given in parentheses; the slope of the regression line is in brackets.
[b]Protective index (PI) = TD$_{50}$/ED$_{50}$.

screening program are likely candidates for pharmacokinetic and chronic toxicity studies prior to cautious clinical trial. Phase VI, anticonvulsant quantification in rats after oral administration, is intended to verify the experimental anticonvulsant activity and neurotoxicity in another rodent species and to develop the dose information prerequisite to chronic toxicity studies in this species. More importantly, the phase VI studies in rats provide information that must be carefully reviewed before one can determine if the accumulated experimental data are sufficiently promising to warrant moving the candidate substance into costly pharmacokinetic and chronic toxicity studies.

Six commonly used antiepileptic drugs have been subjected to the procedures described above. The drugs were selected for two reasons: (a) they are representative of the chemical structures of commonly employed antiepileptic agents: hydantoin (phenytoin), iminostilbene (carbamazepine), barbiturate (phenobarbital), succinimide (ethosuximide), carboxylic acid (valproate), and benzodiazepine (clonazepam); and (b) they are the drugs of choice or alternates for generalized tonic–clonic (grand mal) and complex partial (psychomotor) seizures or absence (petit mal) seizures. Table 4 summarizes the results obtained from phases II and V after intraperitoneal administration of the drugs to mice; Table 5 the results from phase III, also after intraperitoneal administration of the drugs to mice; and Table 6 the results from phases IV and VI after oral administration of the drugs to mice and rats, respectively. Such data correlate well with the clinical use of these agents and provide a basis for the evaluation of the antiepileptic potential of candidate substances.

TABLE 5. *Toxicity profile of some intraperitoneally administered prototype antiepileptic drugs in mice (phase III)*

Drug	Dose 50 (mg/kg)		
	Lethality[a]	Righting reflex[b]	Rotorod[c]
Phenytoin	229.61 (216.44–259.10)[d] [15.89][e]	178.34 (152.93–195.45) [14.03]	65.46 (52.49–72.11) [15.23]
Carbamazepine	628.70 (555.77–707.67) [10.11]	172.24 (134.12–197.79) [5.92]	71.56 (45 91–134.79) [4.77]
Phenobarbital	264.70 (241.55–285.52) [15.95]	135.45 (114.90–177.42) [8.41]	69.01 (62.89–72.89) [24.67]
Valproate	1104.62 (1021.54–1253.66) [11.41]	885.53 (820.86–957.04) [12.46]	425.84 (368.91–450.40) [20.84]
Ethosuximide	1813.55 (614.04–1918.93) [21.63]	850.61 (751.19–917.93) [16.43]	440.83 (383.09–485.34) [18.37]
Clonazepam	>6000	>6000	0.184 (0.163–0.227) [14.40]

[a]Measured as 24-hr LD_{50}.
[b]Measured as HD_{50}.
[c]Measured as TD_{50}.
[d]95% confidence interval in parentheses.
[e]Slope of regression line in brackets.

TABLE 6. *Profile of anticonvulsant activity of orally administered prototype antiepileptic drugs in mice and rats (phases IV and VI)*

Drug	Time of test (hr)		Rotorod TD_{50} (mg/kg)		MES ED_{50} (mg/kg)		sc Met ED_{50} (mg/kg)	
	Mice	Rats	Mice	Rats[a]	Mice	Rats	Mice	Rats
Phenytoin	2,2	½,4	86.71 (80.39–96.09)[b] [13.01][c]	>3000	9.04 (7.39–10.62) [6.28] PI = 9.59[d]	29.82 (21.92–38.91) [2.82] PI > 100	No protection	No protection
Carbamazepine	½,½,½	2,1	217.21 (131.49–270.11) [3.47]	813.06 (488.76–1233.87) [6.07]	15.44 (12.44–17.31) [9.07] PI = 14.06	8.50 (3.39–10.53) [4.50] PI = 95.65	48.07 (40.75–57.35) [5.50] PI = 4.52	No protection
Phenobarbital	2,2,2	½,5,5	96.78 (79.88–115.00) [8.51]	61.09 (43.72–95.85) [3.00]	20.09 (14.78–31.58) [5.20] PI = 4.82	9.14 (7.58–11.86) [4.12] PI = 6.68	12.59 (7.99–19.07) [3.84] PI = 7.62	11.55 (7.74–15.00) [4.08] PI = 5.29
Valproate	2,1,1	1,½,½	1264.39 (800.0–2250.0) [4.80]	280.26 (191.32–352.76) [4.63]	664.80 (605.33–718.00) [18.17] PI = 1.90	489.54 (351.14–728.37) [2.90] PI = 0.57	388.31 (348.87–438.61) [8.12] PI = 3.26	179.62 (146.73–210.35) [8.62] PI = 1.56
Ethosuximide	1,½,½	2,2,2	879.21 (839.89–933.51) [30.50]	1012.31 (901.66–1109.31) [15.33]	>1000 PI < 0.88	>1200 PI < 0.84	192.71 (158.59–218.44) [7.39] PI = 4.36	53.97 (45.57–60.85) [9.05] PI = 18.76
Clonazepam	½,½,1	½,1,1	3.39 (1.30–4.51) [2.49]	71.64 (35.70–101.21) [3.66]	78.35 (55.80–110.01) [2.30] PI = 0.04	186.04 (70.0–500.0) [1.17] PI = 0.39	0.06 (0.01–0.12) [2.85] PI = 56.50	0.062 (0.016–0.131) [1.167] PI = 1,155.5

[a] Minimal neurotoxicity based on ataxia.
[b] 95% confidence interval in parentheses.
[c] Slope of regression line.
[d] Protective index (PI) = TD_{50}/ED_{50}.

EVALUATION OF ANTIEPILEPTIC POTENTIAL

The anticonvulsant potential of a candidate substance is usually assessed by comparing the results obtained from well-standardized test procedures such as those described herein with similar results obtained with prototype agents (see Tables 4–6). Such an assessment usually starts with a comparison of the minimal neurotoxic dose (TD_{50}), anticonvulsant efficacy as indicated by the various tests ($ED_{50}s$), and protective indices (PIs). Although the $TD_{50}s$ and $ED_{50}s$ do provide important information, they reveal little when viewed alone. For example, Table 4 shows that the $TD_{50}s$ of the six prototype agents range from 0.184 to 440.83 mg/kg, whereas the $ED_{50}s$ by the MES test range from 8.81 to 271.66 mg/kg, and those for the sc Met test from 0.009 to 148.59 mg/kg. Considerably more can be learned from a comparison of protective indices (PI = TD_{50}/ED_{50}), since this ratio reflects the spread between the median effective dose and the median minimal neurotoxic dose.

Protective indices may also provide some insight into possible clinical use. A summary evaluation of the PIs listed in Tables 4–6 is shown in Table 7. It may be seen from this table that the three drugs clinically useful in generalized tonic–clonic and complex partial (temporal lobe) seizures (phenytoin, carbamazepine, and phenobarbital) are characterized in the laboratory by marked ability to prevent seizure spread (anti-MES activity) and may (phenobarbital and carbamazepine) or may not (phenytoin and carbamazepine) increase pentylenetetrazol seizure threshold. On the other hand, the three drugs effective in absence seizures (ethosuximide, valproate, and clonazepam) are characterized by a marked ability to increase pentylenetetrazol seizure threshold and may (valproate) or may not (ethosuximide and clonazepam) have any significant effect on seizure spread (anti-MES activity). The other three tests, sc bicuculline, sc picrotoxin, and sc strychnine, not only provide some enlightenment on the mechanism of action of these drugs, but the profile obtained correlates well with their spectrum of clinical use. Thus, valproate is the only one of the six substances that is effective by all five tests in nontoxic doses. The broad

TABLE 7. *Anticonvulsant activity of prototype drugs based on protective index*[a]

Antiepileptic drug	Route of administration	Seizure spread		Seizure threshold		
		MES	sc Strych	sc Met	sc Bic	sc Pic
Phenytoin	i.p.	+ + +	–	–	–	–
	oral[b]	+ + + +		–		
Carbamazepine	i.p.	+ + +	–	–	–	+
	oral	+ + + +		+ + +[c]		
Phenobarbital	i.p.	+ +	–	+ + +	+	+ +
	oral	+ + +		+ + +		
Ethosuximide	i.p.	–	–	+ +	–	+
	oral	–		+ + + +		
Valproate	i.p.	+	+	+ +	+	+
	oral	+[c]		+[c], + +		
Clonazepam	i.p.	–	–	+ + + +	+ + + +	+ + +
	oral	–		+ + + +		

[a]TD_{50}/ED_{50} = protective index (PI).
[b]Mice and rats.
[c]Mice only.

$$- = \text{PI} < 1$$
$$+ = 1 < \text{PI} < 2$$
$$+ + = 2 < \text{PI} < 4$$
$$+ + + = 4 < \text{PI} < 10$$
$$+ + + + = \text{PI} > 10$$

anticonvulsant profile of valproate correlates well with its wide spectrum of clinical use.

Since PIs are based on the assumption that the slope of the two regression lines (toxicity and activity) are parallel, these values are only valid when the slopes of the dose–activity regression lines are not significantly different. If the regression lines are parallel, the calculated PI will be the same at any particular point on the regression lines. If the regression lines are not parallel, the PI is only valid at the D_{50} level. Above or below this median level, the PI may be either higher or lower. Therefore, in terms of drug safety, the calculated PI may be misleading.

Ideally, an anticonvulsant drug should be capable of suppressing experimental seizures in all animals at dose levels devoid of even minimal toxic effects. Thus, it is informative to calculate a "safety ratio" (TD_3/ED_{97}) for the candidate substance and to compare this with similar ratios for prototype drugs. Table 8 shows a comparison of valproate and phenobarbital on the basis of the "safety ratio." Valproate can completely suppress pentylenetetrazol seizures in 97% of animals at dose levels devoid of even minimal neurotoxicity, and phenobarbital can afford a similar level of protection against both maximal electroshock and pentylenetetrazol seizures. This more limited profile of anticonvulsant efficacy is in keeping with the fact that valproate is most widely employed in absence and myoclonic seizures, and phenobarbital in generalized tonic–clonic and complex partial (temporal lobe) seizures.

Since antiepileptic drugs are generally administered orally, it is important to determine how well the candidate drug is absorbed from the gastrointestinal tract. Some answers to this question can be obtained by comparing the data obtained after oral and intraperitoneal administration of the candidate substance. For example, Table 6 shows that the oral TD_{50} and ED_{50}s for MES and sc Met in mice for phenobarbital are 96.87, 20.09, and 12.59 mg/kg, respectively, whereas Table 4 indicates the intraperitoneal TD_{50} and ED_{50}s for MES and sc Met are 69.01, 21.78, and 13.17 mg/kg, respectively. Thus, the ratios (oral dose/intraperitoneal dose) are 1.40, 0.92, and 0.96 for the TD_{50} and ED_{50}s for MES and sc Met, respectively. This indicates that phenobarbital is completely absorbed after oral administration.

Another example involving a species pharmacokinetic problem may be cited. Table 6 shows that the oral TD_{50} and ED_{50} by the MES test for phenytoin in rats are >3,000 and 29.82 mg/kg, respectively, whereas other data from this laboratory indicate that the intraperitoneal TD_{50} and ED_{50} by the MES test are 111.47 and 15.55 mg/kg, respectively. Thus, the ratios for the TD_{50}s and ED_{50}s are 26.91 and 1.92, respectively. It is generally agreed that for a candidate antiepileptic agent to be worthy of further study, this ratio should be ≤4; ideally, the ratio should be < 2. When evaluated by these criteria, the ratio of the TD_{50}s for phenytoin (26.91) suggests that phenytoin is not absorbed adequately after oral administration in rats. However, the ratio of the oral ED_{50}s (1.92) sug-

TABLE 8. *Safety ratios (TD_3/ED_{97}) for intraperitoneally administered valproate and phenobarbital in mice*

Drug	Parameter	Test and effective dose (mg/kg)				
		MES	sc Strych	sc Met	sc Bic	sc Pic
Valproate	TD_3	345	345	345	345	345
	ED_{97}	382	420	210	640	660
	Safety ratio[a]	0.90	0.82	1.64	0.54	0.52
Phenobarbital	TD_3	49	49	49	49	49
	ED_{97}	29	122	28	112	68
	Safety ratio[a]	1.69	0.40	1.75	0.44	0.72

[a]Ratios >1 indicate that maximum anticonvulsant protection is achieved in nontoxic doses.

gests that the drug is adequately absorbed. Such ambiguities must be resolved before a final judgment can be made with respect to absorption after oral administration. Previous studies (17) indicate that the maximal level of absorption of phenytoin from the gastrointestinal tract in rats is 66 mg/kg. Since this is unique to this particular drug in this particular species, one must conclude that phenytoin is absorbed adequately after oral administration.

It should be mentioned that for a candidate antiepileptic agent to be useful in humans, the "margin of safety" in rats (ratio between the 5-day oral LD_{50} and the oral ED_{50} for the desired activity) should be ≥ 10. For this reason, one should determine the 5-day oral LD_{50} of promising substances in rats prior to subjecting them to further pharmacological or subacute toxicity studies. This not only provides additional evidence relative to the agent's potential clinical usefulness but also makes available data helpful in planning subsequent subacute toxicity studies. Finally, it should be remembered that the ultimate value of an anticonvulsant drug must be determined in clinical practice. Laboratory methods of assay are valid only to the extent that their results correlate with clinical experience. The results obtained by methods described herein correlate well with the clinical usefulness of all currently available antiepileptic drugs.

SUMMARY

The technical procedures and statistical analyses employed in the anticonvulsant drug screening program of the National Institute of Neurological and Communicative Disorders and Stroke, officially known as the "Early Pharmacological Evaluation of Anticonvulsant Drugs," have been described. In addition, special attention has been directed to factors that may compromise the results. A six-phase anticonvulsant drug-screening flow chart has been presented (Table 1), and the use of these phases in the detection and quantification of anticonvulsant activity has been explained. Data obtained by subjecting six prototype antiepileptic

drugs (phenytoin, carbamazepine, phenobarbital, valproate, ethosuximide, and clonazepam) to this procedure are provided as a basis of comparison with data from candidate substances. Also, the anticonvulsant profiles of these prototype drugs have been correlated with their clinical use in epilepsy. Particular attention has been given to the use of anticonvulsant efficacy, acute toxicity, protective indices (TD_{50}/ED_{50}), safety ratio (TD_3/ED_{97}), extent of oral absorption (oral ED_{50}/i.p. ED_{50}), and margin of safety (5-day oral LD_{50}/oral ED_{50}) in evaluating antiepileptic potential. Examples are given as to how these identification, quantification, and evaluation procedures are applied in order to assist the inexperienced investigator in the evaluation of candidate substances.

ACKNOWLEDGMENT

Supported by a contract (NO1-NS-5-2302) from the National Institute of Neurological and Communicative Disorders and Stroke.

REFERENCES

1. Davenport, V. D., and Davenport, H. W. (1948): The relation between starvation, metabolic acidosis and convulsive seizures in rats. *J. Nutr.*, 36:139–152.
2. Dunham, N. W., and Miya, T. A. (1957): A note on a simple apparatus for detecting neurological deficit in rats and mice. *J. Am. Pharm. Assoc. Sci. Ed.*, 46:208–209.
3. Irwin, S. (1968): Comprehensive observational assessment: Ia. A systematic, quantitative procedure for assessing the behavioral and physiologic state of the mouse. *Psychopharmacologia*, 13:222–257.
4. Krall, R. L., Penry, J. K., White, B. G., Kupferberg, H. J., and Swinyard, E. A. (1978): Antiepileptic drug development: II. Anticonvulsant drug screening. *Epilepsia*, 19:409–428.
5. Litchfield, J. R., Jr., and Wilcoxon, R. (1949): A simplified method of evaluating dose–effect experiments. *J. Pharmacol.*, 96:99–113.
6. Petty, W. C., and Karler, R. (1965): The influence of aging on the activity of anticonvulsant drugs. *J. Pharmacol. Exp. Ther.*, 150:443–448.
7. Purpura, D. P., Penry, J. K., Tower, D., Woodbury, D. M., and Walter, R. (1972): *Experimental Models of Epilepsy—A Manual for the Laboratory Worker.* Raven Press, New York.
8. Putnam, T. J., and Merritt, H. H. (1937): Experimental determination of the anticonvulsant properties of some phenyl derivatives. *Science*, 85:525–526.

9. Swinyard, E. A. (1949): Laboratory assay of clinically effective antiepileptic drugs. *J. Am. Pharm. Assoc.,* 38:201–204.

10. Swinyard, E. A. (1969): Laboratory evaluation of antiepileptic drugs. Review of laboratory methods. *Epilepsia,* 10:107–119.

11. Swinyard, E. A., Brown, W. C., and Goodman, L. S. (1952): Comparative assays of antiepileptic drugs in mice and rats. *J. Pharmacol. Exp. Ther.,* 106:319–330.

12. Swinyard, E. A., Clark, L. D., Miyahara, J. T., and Wolf, H. H. (1961): Studies on the mechanism of amphetamine toxicity in aggregated mice. *J. Pharmacol. Exp. Ther.,* 132:97–102.

13. Swinyard, E. A., and Woodhead, J. H. (1978): Drug contamination of mortars and pestles. *J. Pharm. Sci.,* 67:1758–1759.

14. Toman, J. E. P., Swinyard, E. A., and Goodman, L. S. (1946): Properties of maximal seizures and their alteration by anticonvulsant drugs and other agents. *J. Neurophysiol.,* 9:231–240.

15. Torchiana, M. L., and Stone, C. A. (1959): Postseizure mortality following electroshock convulsions in certain strains of mice. *Proc. Soc. Exp. Biol. Med.,* 100:290–293.

16. Woodbury, L. A., and Davenport, V. D. (1952): Design and use of a new electroshock seizure apparatus, and analysis of factors altering seizure threshold and pattern. *Arch. Int. Pharmacodyn. Ther.,* 92:97–104.

17. Woodbury, D. M., and Swinyard, E. A. (1972): Diphenylhydantoin: Absorption, distribution, and excretion. In: *Antiepileptic Drugs,* edited by D. M. Woodbury, J. K. Penry, and R. P. Schmidt, pp. 113–123. Raven Press, New York.

18. Woolley, D. E., Timiras, P. S., Rosenzweig, M. R., Krech, D., and Bennett, E. L. (1961): Sex and strain differences in electroshock convulsions of the rat. *Nature,* 190:515–516.

Antiepileptic Drugs, edited by D. M. Woodbury,
J. K. Penry, and C. E. Pippenger. Raven Press,
New York © 1982.

8

General Principles

Experimental Quantification and Evaluation of Anticonvulsant Drugs in a Primate Model

Joan S. Lockard and René H. Levy

Our primate model is a model of alumina gel-induced chronic partial epilepsy as developed by Kopeloff et al. (11). It has spontaneous motor and secondarily generalized tonic–clonic seizures and no other seizure types. Its seizures and associated clinical manifestations can be continuously and automatically recorded for months at a time (20). This monkey model can provide a research window between acute animal models and difficult clinical trials. Its utility is multifaceted, serviceable both in the study of epileptic phenomena and in a wide range of pharmacological problems. Our primate model permits evaluation of drug efficacy and toxicity, of drug interaction in polytherapy, of drug tolerance and withdrawal problems, and studies of single- and multiple-dose pharmacokinetics. The model is also equipped to evaluate other variables in epilepsy, such as learning impairment (48), psychosocial influences (19), emotional factors (36), endogenous effects (28), and non-drug therapies exemplified by cerebellar stimulation (34) and attentional tasks (37). Finally, its methods for frequent sampling of epileptiform activity and CSF and plasma drug concentrations convert these normally diagnostic and therapeutic indicators of epilepsy to quantitative tools for assessing brain function and fundamental drug disposition processes.

This primate model differs specifically from rodent drug screens (12,13) in several important ways. The screens use drug-challenge methodology that provide dose–response rather than plasma level–response data on the test compounds. Clinical trials of the last decade have confirmed Brodie and Reid's classical hypothesis (2) that plasma concentrations of lipid-soluble drugs are a more reliable meter of pharmacological effect than is dose when the efficacious and toxic ranges are studied across species. Moreover, the question of acute versus chronic testing is not addressed in the rodent drug screens by their very nature. In comparison, this primate model is not a monkey screen but provides the equivalent of prehuman clinical trials.

Chronic investigations have been conducted for 11 years in our primate model encompassing approximately 12,000 recording hours of monkey EEG (interictal spikes, background rhythms, and sleep stages) and a comparably large number of plasma drug level determinations. Obviously, space does not allow an in-depth review of all the applications of this model. The objective of this chapter is to familiarize the reader with the methods involved, the research possibilities they allow, and some of the model's therapeutic contributions to date.

METHODS

Pharmacokinetic Studies

Preclinical Studies

Analytical methods.

Studies in the preclinical phase (Fig. 1, top) are initiated at least 3 to 6 months prior to the scheduled implementation of an efficacy study (Fig. 1, bottom). Initially, these studies involve the development of an analytical method for the parent drug (and less often, metabolites). Gas and liquid chromatography (GLC and HPLC) have been useful because they afford the rapid turnover required in efficacy studies. Occasionally, however, as was the case for carbamazepine and its 10,11-epoxide (29), parent drug and metabolite were assayed by chemical ionization mass spectrometry with isotopically labeled internal standards (46).

Solubility studies.

These include determination of saturation solubility in water at room temperature. Initially, this information facilitates drug administration in kinetic studies, and later, it is useful in the selection of dosing regimen.

Phase I Studies

Pilot kinetic studies.

Pilot kinetic studies are necessary since, generally, no knowledge is available on the pharmacokinetic behavior of new drugs in macaques. The selection of a dose for the first preliminary study is based on the results of the NINCDS Anticonvulsant Screening Project (12,13) or similar data available from the parent pharmaceutical company. The NINCDS Screen 2 yields a maximal electroshock seizure test (MES) ED_{50} and a subcutaneous pentylenetetrazol (ScMet) seizure threshold test ED_{50} (median effective dose) as well as a rotorod test TD_{50} (minimal neurological deficit). Screen 3 provides additional measures of activity and, in particular, a delineation between the rotorod TD_{50} and the LD_{50} (median lethal dose). The initial pilot study is performed with the MES ED_{50} administered as a single intravenous dose to three monkeys. It yields two pieces of information: an assessment of the toxicity of this dose in the monkey and an initial conversion factor between dose and plasma level. If the MES ED_{50} yields no observable toxicity, the rotorod TD_{50} is used in the same monkeys. If the TD_{50} produces no toxicity, a dose higher than the TD_{50} but lower than the LD_{50} is used in the same monkeys. The objective of this approach is to obtain an estimate of toxic doses and corresponding blood levels. Once these "ceiling" doses are known, the range of doses to be used in the random design of single-dose studies can be easily determined (the lowest doses are often limited by assay sensitivity).

Single and multiple dose studies.

These studies (Phase IA, Fig. 1) are performed at several random levels, using the doses and sampling schedules derived from the pilot studies to obtain the following pharmacokinetic parameters of the parent drug and subsequently, if appropriate, of metabolite(s): (a) clearances

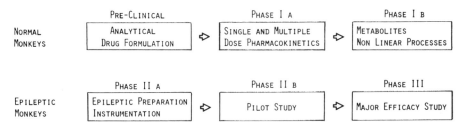

FIG. 1. The phases of drug evaluation in primate model. **Top row,** sequence of kinetic studies in normal monkeys; **bottom row,** the steps involved in prehuman clinical trials.

(systemic and intrinsic; metabolic and renal); (b) volume(s) of distribution; (c) resulting half-life; (d) extent of plasma protein binding and blood binding (free fraction in plasma and blood/plasma partition ratio); (e) bioavailability (role of first-pass effect); (f) fraction of dose metabolized to a particular metabolite; (g) more importantly, such designs allow an assessment of the presence of dose dependency in any of the basic parameters.

Subchronic studies.

Semichronic studies are then conducted (again in normal monkeys) to provide a means of testing the mode of administration of the drug. These studies reveal whether the clearances remain constant over time (autoinduction or autoinhibition). Typically, the drug is administered for 7 to 14 days by constant-rate intravenous infusion or multiple oral doses, and the pharmacokinetic parameters obtained are compared with the single-dose values. If nonlinearity is present, it is pursued later (Phase IB, Fig. 1) in an attempt to quantify it. Several such examples have been encountered, e.g., carbamazepine autoinduction (40) and diurnal oscillations in clearance of valproic acid (17) and ethosuximide (39).

While these studies are ongoing, the data on toxicity and kinetic parameters in normal monkeys are utilized to plan the pilot and main efficacy studies with epileptic monkeys (Phases II and III, Fig. 1, bottom).

Development of a dosing regimen.

The key parameters considered are drug clearance, aqueous solubility, and half-life. A knowledge of the parent drug systemic clearance (Cl_s) permits an estimation of the required rate of administration (R) to achieve any target level (C^*): $R = C^* \times Cl_s$. The maximum rate of intravenous administration is the product of the drug water solubility and the infusion flow rate (0.5–2 ml/hr).

In the simpler cases, the new drug has a low extraction ratio, i.e., a low systemic (or intrinsic) clearance combined with adequate water solubility. The required rate of administration is smaller than the maximum rate. Examples are

valproic acid and ethosuximide. In such cases, administration by constant-rate intravenous infusion (through a femoral catheter) in saline is preferred, independent of the drug half-life. This mode of administration has two advantages: it enables maximum control of the rate of administration and thus opens the possibility of "titration" and individualization of regimen by changing the concentration of the infusion solution or by modifying the flow rate. Constant-rate infusion also permits minimization of the extent of fluctuation in levels. The only oscillations that are seen are those resulting from diurnal effects on drug clearance.

In the more complicated cases, the required rate of administration exceeds the maximum rate. This occurs when the new drug has a medium or high extraction ratio and/or a low water solubility. This situation leaves only the option of multiple dosing. Drugs with relatively long half-lives (longer than 6–8 hr) are administered by gastric intubation. Drugs with short half-lives (0.5–5 hr) are administered through a chronic intraperitoneal catheter. This approach requires the preparation of an aqueous suspension of the new drug and documentation of the reproducibility of the absorption kinetics of that formulation.

Efficacy Studies

Phase II and III Methods

Epileptic preparation.

For any given efficacy study in this primate model, some 6 to 12 rhesus (*Macaca mulatta;* e.g., ref. 25) or crab-eating monkeys (*Macaca fascicularis;* 23) are made experimentally epileptic (Phase IIA, Fig. 1, bottom). Approximately 0.2 cc of aluminum hydroxide is injected subpially in the left (or right) pre- and postcentral gyrus, sensory–motor, hand and face areas as confirmed by electrical cortical stimulation during sterile craniotomy. The animals start to exhibit both EEG epileptiform activity and focal seizures at about the same time, between 6 and 10 weeks post-injection. Subsequently, in a Jacksonian-like sequence of greater body involvement (9), the monkeys gradually manifest secondarily generalized tonic–clonic seizures, reaching a relatively stable baseline of both partial and generalized seizure frequency by 4 to 6 months post-injection (21). The baseline frequency for each animal usually remains the same for years unless treatment intervention or changes in health occur. The disease process is reversible by surgical excision of the epileptogenic focus even after several years of seizures (7).

EEG methods.

Several months prior to the commencement of a drug study, each monkey is implanted with an EEG head plug, which comprises a nine-skull-screw, eight-channel electrode montage (20) for sleep staging (0–4, REM) and for detection and quantification of interictal EEG epileptiform activity. At a standard EEG polygraph speed of 30 mm/sec, the number of spikes/10 sec page or the number of spikes/min for lengthy records is obtained. Interictal spikes are defined as unilateral phase-reversed fast activity, less than 80 msec in duration, more than 100 mV in amplitude, with a velocity of the rising phase of 2 mV/msec or greater. At least two half-hour day EEG recordings per animal per week are used to ascertain diurnal spike frequency. One all-night recording is conducted every 2 to 3 weeks for each monkey for the duration of a study to quantify nocturnal interictal spikes and to correlate them with the sleep stages in which they occur.

Drug administration and sampling.

Several months prior to the commencement of a drug study, each animal is trained to accept a nasogastric tube for oral dosing or is equipped, depending on the alternative mode of drug administration, with two or three of six chronically tested indwelling catheters (18): (a) a jugular catheter for blood sampling to ascertain plasma drug concentrations, (b) a jejunum cannula for gastric administration of drug in suspension, (c) an i.p. catheter to allow periodic bolusing of drug into the intraperitoneal cavity, (d) a femoral catheter for constant-rate intravenous drug infusion, (e) an intrathecal catheter in

the fourth ventricle for periodic sampling of CSF drug concentrations, and (f) another intrathecal catheter in cisternum magna for drug transport studies.

Each monkey has its own drug delivery pump and shares a saline pump with one other monkey to sustain the integrity of the blood-sampling catheter. Individualized drug administration is essential to compensate for animal differences in total body clearance. To prevent disturbances to the monkeys once a study is in progress, access to the cannulation tubing is accomplished in an adjacent room. Flushing of the sampling tubing at night is done with water-bath-maintained saline so as not to awaken an animal by venous temperature change.

During a drug study, either two blood and/or two CSF samples (steady-state samples) are taken on different days of the week at the same time of day for each animal to ascertain steady-state concentrations of the compound(s) under investigation. In addition, three different series of five to seven blood and/or CSF samples are obtained: (a) one at the commencement of drug administration (drug distribution phase) prior to the achievement of steady state, (b) a second every 2 weeks which involves diurnal and nocturnal sampling (one sample every 2–3 hr for 24 hr), and (c) a third period of samples at the time of drug withdrawal, during the drug elimination phase. For purposes of health and exercise the monkeys are caged before and after a study; their cannulation tubing is closed off in a heparin lock and sterilely tucked under the skin for the duration of the caging. The cages are equipped for seizure recording during the interim (if necessary), and the catheters are usually viable for up to 3 months of dormancy.

Seizure monitoring.

During a study, the animals are housed in one of two facilities, restrained or free-moving. In the restrained research environment (capacity $N = 12$), each monkey is maintained in a primate chair with an accelerometer for continuous polygraph readout of all gross motor activity. Groups of three adjacent monkeys are monitored continuously by a closed-circuit TV system with infrared vidicon and video recorder (for a total of four systems). Infrared lights at night (1800–0600 hr), video time/date generators, and constant-speed polygraph recordings allow 24-hr coverage of clinical seizures. Just beneath the motor activity channel for each monkey, a single channel of slow-speed EEG (¼ mm/sec; ref. 20) is also read out. A minicomputer programmed to detect seizure envelopes on the polygraphs automatically activates the respective videotape recorder to visually record the clinical seizures. The criteria for detection of the seizure envelopes are contiguous pen excursions simultaneously on any pair of motor and slow-speed EEG channels that are of a particular minimal duration and amplitude.

The video tapes are reviewed daily for clinical verification of seizures. The motor activity envelopes of the verified seizures become the permanent data from which frequency, duration, severity (i.e., mean amplitude of the envelope), and time of occurrence are automatically saved by the computer. This methodology for the restraint experimental situation provides nearly 100% accuracy in seizure detection and quantification (18).

In the free-moving primate facility, which houses a socially interacting group of monkeys (maximum capacity, $N = 9$), seizure detection is accomplished by telemetry of a single channel of EEG per animal emanating from miniature, battery-equipped EEG headplugs (19). The batteries are externalized and easily replaced monthly. Again, the EEG polygraph readout is slow speed (¼ mm/sec), and the computer uses only this single channel of output (at a slight cost in accuracy of detection) to activate video cassette recorders (two 12-hr cassettes cover a 24-hr period) in a closed-circuit TV system. A camera with a fish-eye lens and infrared vidicon provides 24-hr monitoring of the entire facility housing the monkeys. The group behaviors preceding and following each time-ticked detected seizure and the clinical description of the seizures are tabulated from the cassettes played back the following day. In this way, the psychosocial influence on seizures during drug therapy and baseline periods may be quantified.

Behavioral and health measures.

For the monkeys in the free-moving research situation, 100 two-digit codes of solitary and social behaviors have been delineated so as to frequently monitor and quantify the interactions and general activity of the animals (19). Normal, feral macaques have a rich repertoire of dominant, submissive, play, and affiliative behaviors. The associative and agonistic behaviors of stable groups of normal rhesus monkeys in our facility have provided a standard for evaluating the behavior of epileptic monkeys. Specific problems of possible side effects (e.g., ataxia) and psychotropic consequences of certain therapies (e.g., carbamazepine) may also be described in detail since the monkeys are free moving.

In our research studies necessitating restraint of the animals, operant conditioning techniques have been utilized to assess behavior. During a study, the monkeys are automatically fed, with each animal having a food pellet dispenser on its primate chair, a lever for activating the dispenser, and a panel of stimulus lights to indicate the particular operant schedule of reinforcement required to achieve the pellets. Seven different combinations of time and number of lever responses (i.e., rate) are computer programmed, the particular schedule for any given study being determined to optimize the behavioral assessment of the treatment under evaluation. For instance, in a study of clonazepam efficacy for partial seizures (30), drug tolerance and drug withdrawal were reflected in operant performance, permitting quantification of these effects.

Daily charts of water, food pellet, and fruit consumption and urine and feces elimination are maintained as additional indicators of the health of the monkeys. Laboratory tests including red and white blood cell counts, hematocrits, platelet counts, urine analyses, and kidney and liver function, BUN, albumin, and fibrinogen tests are done routinely (usually one every 1–3 weeks). Also, daily collations of seizure and EEG data are made for immediate feedback regarding the state of health of the animals under study. For example, we were able to follow closely the increase in seizures and EEG spikes when, in the study of clonazepam, the drug was withdrawn and to intervene on behalf of the monkeys had it become necessary.

Pilot Studies

Preliminary studies (Phase IIB, Fig. 1) are conducted in this primate model to determine which variables (seizures, EEG spikes, operant behavior, social behavior, and laboratory tests) should be monitored, and the length of time and at what levels they are to be monitored in the major efficacy studies. This phase also tests the drug vehicle(s) (solvent systems) to be utilized, the dosing regimens to be followed, the range of drug concentrations in plasma and CSF to be achieved in evaluating the parent drug(s) and/ or their metabolite(s), the number of dose steps needed to cover the efficacy range, and the criteria to be utilized in assessing drug efficacy and toxicity. Pilot studies eliminate many of the undesirable surprises in major testing efforts of experimental anticonvulsants in particular and help to dictate optimal research design and assessment guidelines in more extensive studies.

The starting point in testing new anticonvulsants involves ascertaining the plasma drug concentration range of effect in monkey and the drug formulation and mode of administration that will achieve steady-state levels within that range. The approach utilized is to work backward from the plasma drug levels that realized toxicity in normal monkeys (Preclinical Phase, Fig. 1). Therefore, several different dose equivalents (in terms of mg/kg of body weight) of plasma drug levels up to the toxic threshold of the multiple-dose studies (Phase IA, Fig. 1) are selected as likely to reveal a range of pharmacological effect in the pilot study. The outcome of the range tested in the preliminary study is then used to determine the doses to be administered in the main study.

Preliminary studies also allow possible problems to surface that may be specific to chronic evaluation of new drugs, such as drug tolerance, enzyme induction, dose dependency, diurnal oscillations in drug level, or, in polytherapy, drug interactions. Awareness of one or more of these factors facilitates the planning of the main study so as to either more adequately quantify or control for their effects.

Major Studies

The objective of major efficacy studies is to test chronically the efficacy and toxicity of new antiepileptic drugs in comparison to those of standard anticonvulsants. These studies not only are serviceable in decisions as to the possible clinical utility of new compounds but they provide additional data not readily obtained from patients. Information may be gathered on clinically elusive or difficult drug management problems such as the consequences of drug withdrawal or the role of active metabolites in therapeutic outcome. Quantification of the effects of exogenous and endogenous factors, such as the test drug's influence on endocrine levels (e.g., growth hormone) and/or on sleep and ultimately on seizures, is also possible during these studies. Moreover, these chronic evaluations allow the acquisition of data on time-dependent processes such as prophylaxis or nonreversibility of pharmacological effects.

In the sections to follow, a spectrum of findings from efficacy studies in this primate model are provided to illustrate its research contributions and future potential. No attempt at a comprehensive review has been made, but rather, the findings represent a somewhat biased selection of studies to show the variety of data possible.

OVERVIEW OF FINDINGS

Seizures and EEG Spikes

Our primate model by design has many more spontaneous seizures per unit of time than would be allowed for patients in order to maximize the data that can be gathered in a given study. Moreover, quantification of EEG interictal spikes in the model has been used to assess therapeutic efficacy, providing even more data per epoch of research time. In patients, however, EEG interictal spikes have been used almost exclusively as a diagnostic tool or to facilitate the localization of epileptic foci. Interictal spikes are not usually quantified, nor is their frequency systematically employed as an indicator of the degree of severity of the disease, as is seizure frequency. Although the patient studies that have correlated EEG interictal fast activity with frequency of seizures have not generally found a strong relationship, serial EEG recordings in the same patients with singular seizure types under well-controlled conditions and monotherapy have not usually been achieved. In contrast, standardized serial recordings of long duration are the rule in this monkey model, and correlations between number of interictal spikes and overt seizures have been generally high. For instance, in a study of the comparative efficacy of phenytoin, phenobarbital, and primidone (35), the frequency and severity of seizures correlated significantly with number of interictal spikes in the majority of animals ($r = 0.42$ to 0.87; $p < 0.05$). Similar relationships have been found in most of our drug-testing research, and in some studies (e.g., 29) the correlation coefficient has been even higher ($r = 0.98$, $p < 0.01$).

Antiepileptic Drug Evaluation

In the last decade some 40 quantitative studies on anticonvulsants in monkey have been conducted in our laboratories (see ref. 18 for review). With respect to efficacy in the crab-eating macaque, several studies (23) of monotherapy and polytherapy with phenytoin, phenobarbital, primidone, and valproate have been carried out. However, the vast majority of chronic drug testing has been conducted in rhesus monkeys: two hydantoins, albutoin and phenytoin; prophylactic polytherapy with phenytoin and phenobarbital on seizure development; the assessment of two compounds pertinent to absence seizures, ethosuximide and valproate; newer drugs more specific to partial seizures, carbamazepine and the experimental compound cinromide; more recently, the drug interactions of valproate and phenytoin; and a study just completed in the model on the comparative efficacy of phenytoin, phenobarbital,

diazepam, valproate, and carbamazepine in a new paradigm for status epilepticus. The pharmacokinetics of most of these anticonvulsants has also been investigated in single-dose and multiple-dose studies in rhesus monkeys.

Efficacious Plasma Drug Levels

In all these studies, the efficacious plasma drug concentrations in monkey overlapped reasonably well with the effective ranges in epileptic patients. For instance, the therapeutic plasma level range in the primate model is 5 to 12 μg/ml for phenytoin (35), 20 to 40 μg/ml for phenobarbital (35), 50 to 150 μg/ml for valproate (25), and 60 to 100 ng/ml for clonazepam (30). The optimal range for carbamazepine, 4 to 10 μg/ml, has not been achieved chronically because of the drug's insolubility and short half-life in the monkey (29,33). The effective levels of cinromide are best indicated by its major active metabolite whose effective range is 7 to 14 μg/ml (26,27). In general, the above plasma level ranges in the primate model decreased (with few exceptions) the frequency of EEG interictal spikes as well as the numbers of both partial and secondarily generalized clinical seizures.

Testing New Anticonvulsants

The value of this primate model is most evident in the testing of new antiepileptic drugs. For example, as was the case in evaluating valproate in the model, several unsuspected but important findings became evident: (a) valproate is a broad-spectrum anticonvulsant, effective against gross motor seizures (28); (b) its plasma concentrations fluctuate in a diurnal cycle (16,28); and (c) it has three time effects (Fig. 2), a temporary one lasting 2 days only, a later more permanent decrease in seizure frequency after several weeks of drug administration, and a carryover effect of seizure reduction for several weeks post-drug when, in fact, no valproate is detectable in plasma after the initial postdrug day (24).

Similarly, in the evaluation of the experi-

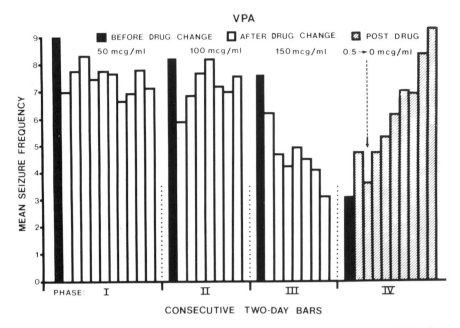

FIG. 2. Mean seizure frequency in primate model ($N = 12$) as a function of valproate (VPA) plasma levels. Drug administration was by constant-rate intravenous infusion. Note (a) the temporary effect of VPA in the first 2 days of phases I and II, (b) the permanent effect of VPA in phase III, and, (c) in phase IV, the nonreversibility of pharmacological effect for 2 weeks when the plasma drug concentrations were essentially zero after day 2.

mental drug cinromide in the primate model (26,27) several findings were germane to its subsequent evaluation in clinical trials: (a) the pharmacological effectiveness of cinromide was found to be individual specific, efficacious against partial seizures only in some monkeys; (b) cinromide usually decreased seizure duration whether or not it attenuated seizure frequency; and (c) its major metabolite at plasma levels of 7 to 14 μg/ml was primarily responsible for its efficacy, whereas the activity of the parent compound and its secondary metabolite did affect the therapeutic outcome because of their short half-life and the first-pass effect of the parent compound. Obviously, as was found in our monkey model, cinromide's success as an antiepileptic drug will depend, in part, on whether a delicate balance of plasma concentrations among the three active agents involved can be maintained in some patients (15).

Drug Interactions

The CSF/plasma drug concentration ratios that have been determined in rhesus monkeys to date have corresponded relatively closely with those in humans. Phenytoin and valproate are highly protein bound (greater than 80% and 98%, respectively), whereas phenobarbital is less so (approximately 60%). These findings suggest that there may be different pharmacological effects from a combined regimen of any two of these drugs as compared to either alone. For example, toxicity has been found to increase in patients when valproate is added to a phenobarbital regimen since plasma phenobarbital levels rise (3,6,45) as a consequence of the inhibition of phenobarbital metabolism by valproate (10).

A similar situation occurred in the combined regimen of valproate and phenytoin in monkey

(31). When valproate (VPA) was added to phenytoin (PHT), seizure frequency decreased ($p < 0.01$). However, when PHT was added to VPA, seizure frequency did not decrease beyond the effect of VPA alone, although seizure duration and severity decreased initially ($p < 0.05$). These different outcomes as a function of drug order were paralleled by an increase ($p < 0.002$) in the free fraction of PHT (after the addition of VPA) and an increase ($p < 0.07$) in the clearance of VPA (after the addition of PHT). In the former case, VPA inhibited the metabolism of PHT, and in the latter, PHT facilitated the metabolism of VPA by enzyme induction.

Seizure Development
and Pharmacologic Prophylaxis

Our monkey model also allows studies of drug effects on the development of epilepsy. A 12-month prophylaxis study using polytherapy of phenytoin and phenobarbital (21) documented the development of the epileptogenic focus in monkey and the influence of these drugs on that process. After a year of treatment which began within 48 hr of the alumina gel injections, only partial seizures were manifested in the drug group, whereas secondarily generalized tonic–clonic seizure were exhibited by the placebo group. However, in the 4-month no-drug follow-up study (22), only those drug-treated animals that had received higher concentrations of phenytoin in weeks 6 through 12 of treatment fared better than the placebo-treated animals when the treatment period was over.

What transpired during the treatment period was that the drug-treated monkeys had lower plasma concentrations of phenytoin than expected, since not only did phenytoin self-induce its own metabolic enzymes but phenobarbital also facilitated the induction. The polytherapy reduced both plasma levels and half-life of phenytoin to approximately two-thirds of what they would have been during monotherapy with phenytoin alone. Therefore, to compensate for this reduction, the phenytoin dose for half of

the drug group was increased during weeks 6 through 12. The elevation in plasma phenytoin levels from 3 to 9 μg/ml to 6 to 13 μg/ml (a) temporarily decreased tonic–clonic seizures while simultaneously increasing the frequency of focal seizures (paradoxical seizures during phenytoin therapy have also been documented in patients; 47) and (b) permanently decreased the seizure frequency that the animals would have had during the follow-up period.

Subsequently, with regard to these same monkeys, the following questions were asked: was their epilepsy reversible by resection of the epileptic focus (7), and were the levels of the membrane enzyme Na^+,K^+-ATPase in epileptic cortex different from those in normal cortex (42)? Excision of only the alumina-induced granuloma (first resection) still left some seizures, but with the removal of the cortex immediately around the granuloma (second resection), the animals were seizure-free and had no independent focus (in terms of EEG spikes) on the contralateral homotopic hemisphere.

When Na^+,K^+-ATPase was measured in serially excised specimens of cerebral cortex in normal as well as the epileptic monkeys, the epileptic cortex showed significantly lower values than did the normals as is the case in human epilepsy (41). There were no differences between the levels of the placebo- versus the drug-treated epileptic monkeys. Moreover, the levels of the contralateral homotopic tissue (third resection) of the epileptic monkeys were no different from those of normal monkeys.

FUTURE APPLICATIONS OF THE MODEL

Drug Distribution Processes

The capability of chronically sampling CSF drug concentrations in our monkey model is beginning to provide a better understanding of drug processes and their effects on epilepsy. For example, the sampling of CSF concentrations of valproate during treatment has revealed that (a) the drug is in CSF immediately with its appearance in blood; (b) it is not in CSF when it is not in blood; (c) when plasma levels of the drug endogenously cycle during chronic administration by constant-rate intravenous infusion, so too do the CSF levels; and (d) the concentration of the drug in CSF is reliably less than the free concentration in blood (Fig. 3). These data are starting to form a cogent picture. They suggest that the nonreversibility of pharmacological effects of valproate (Fig. 2; 24) cannot be explained by lagging levels of the drug in CSF and that, in fact, valproate may be actively transported out of CSF (14). Therefore, other hypotheses are being explored such as the possibility of a secondary process involving changing levels of neurotransmitters such as GABA. A recent preliminary study in the model suggests that this may be the case (1). Also, with an intrathecal catheter for administration of valproate into CSF, active transport processes and

mechanisms of drug action may be studied more directly. As Sackellares et al. (43) indicated for patients, "If further instances of unexplained stupor occur with valproic acid, studies of free drug concentrations are warranted."

Status Epilepticus Paradigm

A review of clinical status epilepticus (8) has indicated that fatality results in up to 20% of affected patients and that the likelihood of a fatal outcome covaries with the frequency of severe seizures and the duration of the status. A variety of anticonvulsants have been prescribed for the treatment of status epilepticus, but there still exist considerable discrepancies regarding their efficacy (4). Moreover, status epilepticus is not a singular concept; there are many different seizure categories of status epi-

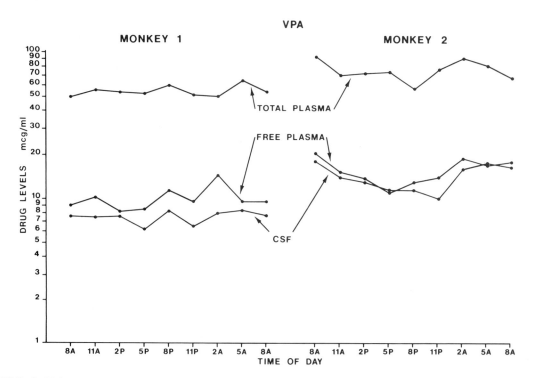

FIG. 3. Valproate levels in two rhesus monkeys as a function of time of day. From **top** to **bottom,** total plasma, unbound in plasma, and CSF drug concentrations. Drug administration was by constant-rate intravenous infusion. Note (a) the diurnal oscillations in both plasma and CSF concentrations and (b) that the CSF levels are generally lower than the free levels in plasma.

lepticus (5). Even the diagnosis of status epilepticus is variable, with different interpretations of its definition depending upon the particular circumstances.

Status epilepticus has been evinced spontaneously and during withdrawal of certain anticonvulsants in our primate model. It manifests itself in this model as frequent discrete seizures, with an animal-specific, relatively fixed interseizure interval. In some monkeys the interval may be as short as 4 to 5 min, and in others, as long as an hour. In any event, if pharmacological intervention does not transpire, death usually ensues within 24 hr.

Obviously, what is needed to combat status epilepticus is an experimental paradigm of frequent seizures that can be easily reversed so as to determine, without risk of life, highly effective therapies for this disease process. Therefore, 4-deoxypyridoxine hydrochloride (4-DP; 38) is being used in the monkey model to reliably precipitate discrete, recurrent seizures that can be stopped immediately by administration of the antagonist, pyridoxine hydrochloride (vitamin B_6) if the need should arise. A 100 to 150 mg/kg intravenous dose of 4-DP elicits (usually within ½ hr) paroxysms in the model at the site of the alumina gel epileptogenic focus (left sensory–motor cortex) that culminate in a series of secondarily generalized tonic–clonic seizures with a largely invariant (≤20%) interseizure interval.

A very recent study of the comparative efficacy of five anticonvulsants (phenytoin, phenobarbital, diazepam, carbamazepine, and valproate) in the 4-DP status epilepticus paradigm has been conducted (32). After the 4-DP injection and the occurrence of the first serial seizure, each animal ($N = 5$) was treated with a loading dose (infused intravenously over a 10-min period) followed by a 1-hr constant-rate infusion calculated to maintain normally efficacious plasma levels of the given antiepileptic agent (treatment period) or an equivalent volume of solvent (control solution). If seizures were prevented during the treatment period, the anticonvulsant was regarded as therapeutic. If 3 to 5 seizures occurred during the treatment period (unchecked by the test or control solution), then additional seizures were prevented by an injection intravenously of vitamin B_6. The results indicate that (a) when certain plasma and CSF levels of phenytoin and carbamazepine were attained, seizures stopped, (b) valproate only delayed seizure onset, (c) the effectiveness of phenobarbital or diazepam was animal specific, and (d) if seizures were not stopped, the drugs differentially influenced seizure severity, interseizure interval, and/or frequency of EEG spike activity. These data have validated the paradigm and will provide the comparative standard for testing new anticonvulsants in the future so as to increase the arsenal of effective drugs for status epilepticus.

Social Model Paradigm

Another important area of concern that interacts with epilepsy is the influence of social phenomena on seizures. Sorting out those psychosocial variables from among the many that may have a significant impact on the success of the patients' adjustment and therapy is clinically a most difficult task. Our primate model in the free-moving research situation (i.e., social model) could be instrumental in narrowing the field of possibilities. Also, the data gathered would have utility in clarifying the interplay of these parameters with drug therapy.

For instance, in a study currently ongoing in the social model, the problem of neonatal psychophysical development after fetal exposure to anticonvulsants is being conducted. Control data are already available from this laboratory on the social and physical maturation of infants born to epileptic rhesus monkeys who did not receive drugs during pregnancy (19). During this first drug study, the three adult females that are presently pregnant (in a group of six animals) have been receiving phenytoin orally since their introduction to the three males in the group. The births of the monkey infants are imminent, and periodic data collection on their health and subsequent growth rates, activity levels and mother–offspring interactions will commence shortly. Documentation of a drop in plasma drug levels of the females during pregnancy, as has been found in patients (44), will also be attempted. Systematic observations on the social associations and behaviors of the entire group have been ongoing and will continue for the first 3 months of neonatal life. Subsequent studies will follow in which primidone and ethosuximide will be administered, respectively, to new groups of monkeys. These data will then be compared to information from our facility and from field and other captive-animal studies on normal rhesus monkeys. Such comparisons may allow a partitioning of the effects of seizure, anticonvulsant, and social interactions on the development of infants and on social behaviors more generally.

SUMMARY

In conclusion, this chronic primate model of partial seizures provides a clinical research opportunity simulating gross motor epilepsy in patients. It allows an evaluation of difficult clinical problems of drug therapy such as tolerance, toxicity, and drug interactions. It also permits the chronic testing of new anticonvulsants so as to increase the antiepileptic armament available to patients both in situations when the disease process is stable or in precipitous situations such as during drug withdrawal or status epilepticus. Moreover, this monkey model may be used to assess the influence on seizures of emotional, psychosocial, and developmental factors. Finally, the model is serviceable in the pursuit of therapeutic mechanisms of action and in the study of drug distribution processes.

ACKNOWLEDGMENTS

The authors are Affiliates of the Child Development and Mental Retardation Center, Seattle. This research was supported by NINCDS Contract Nos. NO1-NS-2282 and NO1-NS-1-2349 and Grant No. NS 04053. The authors wish to thank Laurie L. Peterson for her efforts in the final preparation of this manuscript.

REFERENCES

1. Bakay, R. A., Harris, A. B., Lockard, J. S., and Levy, R. H. (1982): The effects of acute and chronic administration of VPA on CSF neurotransmitters. (*In preparation.*)
2. Brodie, B. B., and Reid, W. D. (1969): Is man a unique animal in response to drugs? *Am. J. Pharm.,* 141:21–27.
3. Bruni, J., and Wilder, B. J. (1979): Valproic acid: Review of a new antiepileptic drug. *Arch. Neurol.,* 36:393–398.
4. Froscher, W. (1979): *Treatment of Status Epilepticus.* University Park Press, Baltimore.
5. Gastaut, H. (1982): Classification of status epilepticus. In: *Status Epilepticus: Mechanisms of Brain Damage and Treatment,* edited by A. V. Delgado-Escueta, C. G. Wasterlain, D. M. Treiman, and R. J. Porter. Raven Press, New York (*in press*).
6. Gram, L., Wulff, K., Rasmussen, K. E., Flachs, H., Wurtz-Jorgensen, A., Sommerbeck, K. W., and Lohren, V. (1977): Valproate sodium: A controlled clinical trial including monitoring of drug levels. *Epilepsia,* 18:141–148.
7. Harris, A. B., and Lockard, J. S. (1981): Absence of seizures or mirror foci in experimental epilepsy after excision of alumina and astrogliotic scar. *Epilepsia,* 22:107–122.
8. Heintel, H. (1972): *Der Status Epilepticus, Seine Atiologie, Klinik und Letalitat.* Fischer, Stuttgart.
9. Jackson, J. H. (1870): A study of convulsions. *Transactions St. Andrews Medical Graduates' Association,* Vol. iii. Reprinted in: *Selected Writings of John Hughlings Jackson,* Vol. 1, *On Epilepsy and Epileptiform Convulsions,* edited by J. Taylor, pp. 8–36, 1958. Basic Books, New York.
10. Kapatanovic, I., Kupferberg, H. J., Porter, R. J., and Penry, J. K. (1980): Valproic acid–phenobarbital interaction: A systematic study using stable isotopically labeled phenobarbital in an epileptic patient. In: *Antiepileptic Therapy: Advances in Drug Monitoring,* edited by S. I. Johannessen, P. L. Morselli, C. E. Pippenger, A. Richens, D. Schmidt, and H. Meinardi, pp. 373–379. Raven Press, New York.
11. Kopeloff, L. M., Barrera, S. E., and Kopeloff, N. (1942): Recurrent convulsive seizures in animals produced by immunological and chemical means. *Am. J. Psychiatry,* 98:881–902.
12. Krall, R. L., Penry, J. K., Kupferberg, H. J., and Swinyard, E. A. (1978): Antiepileptic drug development: I. History and a program for progress. *Epilepsia,* 19:393–408.
13. Krall, R. L., Penry, J. K., White, B. G., Kupferberg, H. J., and Swinyard, E. A. (1978): Antiepileptic drug development: II. Anticonvulsant drug screening. *Epilepsia,* 19:409–428.
14. Levy, R. H. (1980): CSF and plasma pharmacokinetics: Relationship to mechanisms of action as exemplified by valproic acid in monkey. In: *Epilepsy: A Window to Brain Mechanisms,* edited by J. S. Lockard and A. A. Ward, Jr., pp. 191–200. Raven Press, New York.

15. Levy, R. H., Lockard, J. S., Lane, E. A., and Wilensky, A. L. (1981): Preclinical evaluation of cinromide in the primate model: Relevance to the design of phase II clinical trials. In: *Advances in Epileptology: XIIth Epilepsy International Symposium,* edited by M. Dam, L. Gram, and J. K. Penry, pp. 35–44. Raven Press, New York.

16. Levy, R. H., Lockard, J. S., Patel, I. H., and Congdon, W. C. (1977): Time-dependent kinetics III: Diurnal oscillations in steady-state plasma valproic acid levels in rhesus monkeys. *J. Pharm. Sci.,* 66:1154–1156.

17. Levy, R. H., Lockard, J. S., Patel, I. H., and Lai, A. A. (1977): Efficacy testing of valproic acid compared to ethosuximide in monkey model: I. Dosage regimen design in the presence of diurnal oscillations. *Epilepsia,* 18:191–203.

18. Lockard, J. S. (1980): A primate model of clinical epilepsy: Mechanisms of action through quantification of therapeutic effects. In: *Epilepsy: A Window to Brain Mechanisms,* edited by J. S. Lockard and A. A. Ward, Jr., pp. 11–49. Raven Press, New York.

19. Lockard, J. S. (1980): Social primate model of epilepsy. In: *Epilepsy: A Window to Brain Mechanisms,* edited by J. S. Lockard and A. A. Ward, Jr., pp. 165–190. Raven Press, New York.

20. Lockard, J. S., Congdon, W. C., DuCharme, L. L., and Finch, C. A. (1980): Slow-speed EEG for chronic monitoring of clinical seizures in monkey model. *Epilepsia,* 21:325–334.

21. Lockard, J. S., Congdon, W. C., DuCharme, L. L., and Huntsman, B. J. (1976): Prophylaxis with diphenylhydantoin and phenobarbital in alumina-gel monkey model: I. Twelve months of treatment: Seizure, EEG, blood and behavioral data. *Epilepsia,* 17:37–47.

22. Lockard, J. S., DuCharme, L. L., Congdon, W. C., and Franklin, S. C. (1976): Prophylaxis with diphenylhydantoin and phenobarbital in alumina-gel monkey model: II. Four month period of post-treatment: Seizure, EEG, blood, and behavioral data. *Epilepsia,* 17:49–57.

23. Lockard, J. S., and Harris, A. B. (1979): Crab-eating macaque (*Macaca fascicularis*): A substitute for the rhesus (*Macaca mulatta*) epileptic monkey model. *Epilepsia,* 20:425–430.

24. Lockard, J. S., and Levy, R. H. (1976): Valproic acid: Reversibly acting drug? *Epilepsia,* 17:477–479.

25. Lockard, J. S., Levy, R. H., Congdon, W. C., DuCharme, L. L., and Patel, I. H. (1977): Efficacy testing of valproic acid compared to ethosuximide in monkey model: II. Seizure, EEG, and diurnal variation. *Epilepsia,* 18:205–224.

26. Lockard, J. S., Levy, R. H., DuCharme, L. L., and Congdon, W. C. (1979): Experimental anticonvulsant cinromide in monkey model: Preliminary efficacy. *Epilepsia,* 20:339–350.

27. Lockard, J. S., Levy, R. H., DuCharme, L. L., and Congdon, W. C. (1980): Cinromide's metabolite in monkey model: Gastric administration and seizure control. *Epilepsia,* 21:177–182.

28. Lockard, J. S., Levy, R. H., DuCharme, L. L.,

Congdon, W. C., and Patel, I. H. (1977): Diurnal variation of valproic acid plasma levels and day–night reversal in monkey. *Epilepsia,* 18:183–189.

29. Lockard, J. S., Levy, R. H., DuCharme, L. L., Congdon, W. C., and Patel, I. H. (1979): Carbamazepine revisited in a monkey model. *Epilepsia,* 20:169–173.

30. Lockard, J. S., Levy, R. H., DuCharme, L. L., and Salonen, L. D. (1979): Clonazepam in focal-motor monkey model: Efficacy, tolerance, toxicity, withdrawal and management. *Epilepsia,* 20:683–695.

31. Lockard, J. S., Levy, R. H., Kirkevold, B. C., and Ludwick, T. (1982): A monkey model for drug interaction: Exemplified by valproate and phenytoin. In: *Advances in Epileptology: The XIIIth Epilepsy International Symposium,* edited by H. Akimoto, H. Kazamatsuri, and M. Seino. Raven Press, New York (*in press*).

32. Lockard, J. S., Levy, R. H., Koch, K. M., Maris, D. O., and Friel, P. N. (1982): A monkey model for status epilepticus: Carbamazepine and valproate compared to three standard anticonvulsants. In: *Status Epilepticus: Mechanisms of Brain Damage and Treatment,* edited by A. V. Delgado-Escueta, C. G. Wasterlain, D. M. Treiman, and R. J. Porter. Raven Press, New York (*in press*).

33. Lockard, J. S., Levy, R. H., Uhlir, V., and Farquhar, J. A. (1974): Pharmacokinetic evaluation of anticonvulsants prior to efficacy testing exemplified by carbamazepine in epileptic monkey model. *Epilepsia,* 15:351–359.

34. Lockard, J. S., Ojemann, G. A., Congdon, W. C., and DuCharme, L. L. (1979): Cerebellar stimulation in alumina-gel monkey model: Inverse relationship between clinical seizures and EEG interictal bursts. *Epilepsia,* 20:223–234.

35. Lockard, J. S., Uhlir, V., DuCharme, L. L., Farquhar, J. A., and Huntsman, B. J. (1975): Efficacy of standard anticonvulsants in monkey model with spontaneous motor seizures. *Epilepsia,* 16:301–317.

36. Lockard, J. S., Wilson, W. L., and Uhlir, V. (1979): Spontaneous seizure frequency and avoidance conditioning in monkeys. *Epilepsia,* 13:437–444.

37. Lockard, J. S., and Wyler, A. R. (1979): The influence of attending on seizure activity in a monkey model. *Epilepsia,* 20:157–168.

38. Meldrum, B. S., and Horton, R. W. (1971): Convulsive effects of 4-deoxypyridoxine and bicuculline in photosensitive baboons (*Papio papio*) and in rhesus monkeys (*Macaca mulatta*). *Brain Res.,* 35:419–436.

39. Patel, I. H., Levy, R. H., and Lockard, J. S. (1977): Time-dependent kinetics II: Diurnal oscillations in steady state plasma ethosuximide levels in rhesus monkeys. *J. Pharm. Sci.,* 66:650–653.

40. Pitlick, W. H., and Levy, R. H. (1977): Time-dependent kinetics I: Exponential autoinduction of carbamazepine in monkeys. *J. Pharm. Sci.,* 66:647–649.

41. Rapport, R. L., Harris, A. B., Friel, P. N., and Ojemann, G. A. (1975): Human epileptic brain Na,K-ATPase activity and phenytoin concentrations. *Arch. Neurol.,* 32:549–554.

42. Rapport, R. L., Harris, A. B., Lockard, J. S., and Clark, A. F. (1981): Na$^+$ + K$^+$-ATPase in serially excised segments of epileptic monkey cortex. *Epilepsia,* 22:123–127.

43. Sackellares, J. C., Lee, S. I., and Dreifuss, F. E. (1979): Stupor following administration of valproic acid to patients receiving other antiepileptic drugs. *Epilepsia,* 20:697–703.

44. Sherwin, A. L., Loynd, J. S., Bock, G. W., and Sokolowski, C. D. (1974): Effects of age, sex, obesity and pregnancy on diphenylhydantoin levels. *Epilepsia,* 15:507–521.

45. Simon, D., and Penry, J. K. (1975): Sodium di-*N*-propylacetate (DPA) in the treatment of epilepsy. *Epilepsia,* 16:549–574.

46. Trager, W. F., Levy, R. H., Patel, I. H., and Heal, J. M. (1978): Simultaneous analysis of carbamazepine and carbamazepine-10,11-epoxide by GC/CI/MX stable isotope methodology. *Anal. Lett.,* B11:119–133.

47. Troupin, A. L., and Ojemann, L. M. (1976): Paradoxical intoxication—A complication of anticonvulsant administration. *Epilepsia,* 16:753–758.

48. Wyler, A. R., and Lockard, J. S. (1977): Seizure severity and the acquisition and performance of operant tasks in monkey model. *Epilepsia,* 18:109–116.

Antiepileptic Drugs, edited by D. M. Woodbury,
J. K. Penry, and C. E. Pippenger. Raven Press,
New York © 1982.

9

General Principles

Testing of Antiepileptic Drugs in Humans: Clinical Considerations

James J. Cereghino and J. Kiffin Penry

HISTORY AND REGULATION OF ANTIEPILEPTIC DRUG TESTING IN HUMANS

The pharmacological therapy of epilepsy parallels the development of science. At first, it had no scientific rationale. Then the keen observation of clinicians led to the discovery of the antiepileptic effectiveness of bromide and phenobarbital—drugs being used in humans for other purposes. Phenytoin was introduced into clinical use after a deliberate, rational laboratory search for new antiepileptic drugs. Because of important species differences in drug metabolism and drug action, the ultimate value of any new drug must be proven clinically. Increased scientific knowledge and a greater consciousness of human rights and human dignity now mandate that the clinical efficacy of new antiepileptic drugs be determined as rapidly as possible so that efficacious and safe drugs may be made available to individuals whose seizures are not controlled by the available antiepileptic drugs or to those who have adverse reactions to these drugs. At the same time, ineffective or potentially hazardous drugs must be identified quickly to minimize the number of individuals exposed. Although the mechanisms of antiepileptic drug action have been well explored (45), the ulti-

mate physiological and biochemical actions are not known; this tremendously increases the challenge in the clinical evaluation of new antiepileptic drugs.

The history and regulation of antiepileptic drug testing in humans were reviewed in an earlier edition of this book (5). The development and evaluation of new drugs in the United States are controlled by Federal regulations of the Food and Drug Administration (FDA) of the Department of Health and Human Services (DHHS), formerly the Department of Health, Education, and Welfare (DHEW) (24–26). Similar regulatory bodies exist throughout the world (66), but criteria for approval for marketing vary. In the United States, the safety, efficacy, and bioavailability of new drugs must be demonstrated, whereas in other countries only the safety of new drugs need be demonstrated.

All new drugs in the United States must be studied under a "Notice of Claimed Investigational Exemption for a New Drug" (IND), a procedure first introduced in the Drug Amendments Act of 1962 (commonly referred to as the Kefauver–Harris Amendment) (24). The IND requires sponsors of new drugs to supply complete chemical and manufacturing information and results of preclinical investigations, including animal studies; to assure that there will not be unreasonable hazard to humans; to provide a description of the proposed investigation, credentials of the investigators, and copies of informational material supplied each investigator; to agree to notify the FDA promptly of adverse effects; to obtain informed consent from patients; and to submit annual progress reports. The sponsor of an IND is usually a pharmaceutical firm, which then appoints investigators.

The FDA regulations further require that the investigation be conducted in three phases. Phase I determines the safety of the drug in humans, usually in normal volunteers. Phase II determines if the drug treats or prevents the disease for which it is intended and gives estimates of its safety and efficacy. Phase III evaluates the long-term efficacy and safety of the drug by means of extensive clinical trials. Two adequate and well-controlled clinical trials performed by independent investigators or a multiclinic study in which the data of at least three investigators can be evaluated independently are considered minimal to establish the efficacy of a new drug (39). Although not a published regulation, it is generally implied that at least one of these trials must be performed in the United States.

In 1977, with the development of the science of biopharmaceutics and pharmacokinetics, the FDA noted that it is possible to characterize a drug product more fully by determining its biological availability, and thus the agency promulgated regulations for demonstration of bioequivalence requirements for certain drug products (35). After completion of these pharmacological, clinical, and bioequivalence studies in humans, a manufacturer's "New Drug Application" (NDA) with supporting data and proposed labeling may be reviewed by the FDA. If the FDA approves the NDA, the new drug may then be marketed (27). One of the major delays in approval of new antiepileptic drugs can be attributed to deficiencies in clinical protocols, particularly when efficacy is not clearly defined (28,38).

Definitions of "safe" and "effective" are not easily formulated, because no drug is completely safe or completely effective for everyone. Furthermore, the terms may be defined by scientific, medical, and regulatory criteria. Wardell (65) has summarized the situation thus:

The more stringently an agency defines "efficacy" and "safety," the more it will inhibit innovation. The dilemma is that on the one hand patients may be harmed by unsafe or ineffective drugs if regulatory standards are inadequate; on the other hand they may be equally—or more—harmed by their diseases if the regulatory criteria for drug approval are so high that they deny effective existing drugs to patients who need them, or suppress research aimed at developing new therapies.

The introduction of phenytoin in 1938 (53,54) initiated a new era in the pharmacotherapy of epilepsy. Thirteen additional antiepileptic drugs were marketed from 1946 to 1960. From 1938 to 1962, the FDA reviewed only the safety of new drugs marketed in the United States (26). Their efficacy was usually determined in clinical practice. A quotation from Lord Bertrand Russell could well be used to summarize the evaluation of efficacy during that time period: "The opinions that are held with passion are always those for which no good ground exists" (61). Coatsworth (8), in a 1971 report, analyzed published clinical evaluations of antiepileptic drugs and was unable to establish the true efficacy of many of these drugs. The Drug Amendments Act of 1962 (24) required the demonstration of both safety and efficacy of new drugs. As a result, drugs marketed between 1938 and 1962 on the basis of safety alone were reviewed for efficacy. The National Academy of Sciences/National Research Council (NAS/NRC) was asked to evaluate the efficacy claims for each indication of approximately 4,000 drug formulations (30,31). The FDA has published periodic compilations of drugs included in the efficacy review as part of the Drug Efficacy Study Implementation Project (DESI) (42). The following brands of antiepileptic drugs have been evaluated to date: Dilantin® (phenytoin), oral (29,36); Dilantin®, powder for injection, parenteral (20); Zarontin® (ethosuximide), Mysoline® (primidone), Milontin® (phensuximide), Celontin® (methsuximide), Peganone® (ethotoin), Tridione® (trimethadione), Paradione® (paramethadione), Mesantoin® (mephenytoin),

Gemonil® (metharbital), and Phenurone® (phenacemide), all oral (29).

Recommended guidelines for testing of antiepileptic drugs in the United States have been published in the first edition of this book (5) and have also been published by the FDA (32–34,40). Recognizing the need to facilitate the international exchange of data supporting the investigation of new antiepileptic agents, the Commission on Antiepileptic Drugs of the International League Against Epilepsy developed and published principles for clinical testing of antiepileptic drugs (56). Reviewing the unsatisfactory aspects of the drug treatment of epilepsy, the Commission concluded that "Even in the best of hands, existing drugs are not sufficient for the task, and hence an urgent need exists for the development of new drugs" (59). Further, this group acknowledged "that the general standard of evaluation of antiepileptic drugs had been, and still was, poor" (60). The poor quality of clinical trials most often resulted from correctable factors, such as investigator naivety in clinical trials, poor compliance with the protocol, inadequate monitoring, or incorrect use of statistical techniques. The Commission has instituted the Ciba–Geigy Award for the best controlled clinical trial of an antiepileptic drug published in each calendar year (60). In reviewing trials, the Commission has observed that all are still deficient in one or more respects but, nevertheless, embody elements of a good controlled trial. The first award was given retrospectively for the best controlled clinical trial published prior to January 1, 1976; the recipients were Cereghino et al. (4). The award went to Simonsen et al. (63) in 1976 and to Troupin et al. (64) in 1977.

DRUG DEVELOPMENT

The development of a new antiepileptic drug follows an orderly sequence: from synthesis to anticonvulsant screening to preclinical development to clinical development to marketing (Fig. 1). Table 1 indicates the time involved in the development of the three antiepileptic drugs most recently marketed in the United States.

The three phases of antiepileptic drug development overlap to some extent, but Phase I studies in humans usually do not begin before completion of animal studies. A primate model is being developed which may provide useful information for this phase of evaluation (52). Information from an earlier phase will be relevant in designing and executing later phases.

There are three major sources of potential new antiepileptic drugs (49,50): (a) agents developed specifically for epilepsy, (b) compounds serendipitously discovered to have an anticonvulsant effect, and (c) drugs initially developed for another condition. Before a new drug is tested in humans, its structure–activity relationships, relevant physical properties, purity, and stability are determined (Fig. 1). Results of the laboratory screening for anticonvulsant properties are reviewed. Information on the drug's mechanisms of action, absorption, distribution, biotransformation, and excretion is obtained in several species. Acute and chronic toxicity studies are performed. The dosage required in humans is estimated. If questions arise after the drug has been administered to humans, further animal studies should be done.

Drug development has become an increasingly costly and time-consuming proposition. It is recognized that for every new product, thousands of compounds have been prepared, isolated, or extracted, pharmacologically screened and tested, and then rejected. As scientific findings have developed, more extensive tests of efficacy and safety are now required. For example, in order to reduce risks of adverse effects, more extensive tests of carcinogenicity, mutagenicity, and teratogenicity are now required. In addition, advancements in clinical techniques and instrumentation become the standards by which ensuing developments are evaluated. Although the intent is to speed the availability and increase the safety of needed medications, the actual result appears to have been to increase development time.

The problems involved in the development and evaluation of new antiepileptic drugs in the United States were reviewed by the Commission for the Control of Epilepsy and Its Conse-

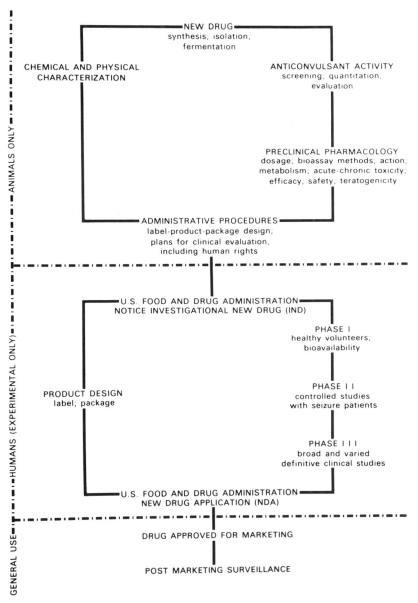

FIG. 1. Major steps in the development of an antiepileptic drug. Decision to return to a previous step or to terminate development may occur at any stage.

quences (9,10). This group made a number of specific recommendations to increase the development, evaluation, and marketing of new antiepileptic drugs (11).

Antiepileptic drugs frequently fall into categories designated as "therapeutic orphan drugs" and "drugs of little commercial value." "Ther-

apeutic orphan drugs" are those that have not received FDA approval for use in a certain group of individuals (usually children) because their efficacy or safety has not yet been demonstrated in that group. The drug is marketed and usually contains a warning for that group of individuals. "Drugs of little commercial value" are

TABLE 1. *Development time for the three antiepileptic drugs most recently marketed in the United States*

Drug	Year synthesized	Year anticonvulsant activity identified	First clinical reports in epilepsy	Year first marketed	Epilepsy indication filed with U.S. FDA	Approved for epilepsy use by U.S. FDA
Carbamazepine	Early 1950s	Early 1950s	1962	1969	1969	1974
Clonazepam	1961	1961	1969	1973	1973	1975
Valproate	1881	1963	1964	1967	1974	1978

either drugs whose efficacy and potential sales are limited to a small group of persons or drugs that are not patentable. It is unlikely that a pharmaceutical firm would recover its research and development costs from a small market or from a drug it could not patent.

CLINICAL STUDIES WITH HEALTHY VOLUNTEERS (PHASE I)

Phase I studies should provide data on the safety, pharmacological effects, pharmacokinetics, and side effects of the drug. Healthy (''normal'') adult volunteers usually participate in Phase I testing. Since abnormalities of disease need not be considered, subjects are more readily available, and interpretation of findings is easier, but the results may not have direct application to those patients for whom the drug is being developed. Particularly with antiepileptic drugs, healthy volunteers may differ from patients in their ability to tolerate the side effects of large doses of the drug. Informed consent (see below) is obtained, and close observation and expert supervision are mandatory. The investigators must be experienced in clinical pharmacology and medicine and must be willing to perform the tedious, frequent, and thorough examination of subjects.

The predicted effective dosage is calculated from animal studies based on knowledge of the metabolism, distribution, and excretion of the drug and body weight of the subject. Because of physiological differences between humans and animals, a small initial dosage is usually used and is then gradually increased to the predicted effective dosage.

Phase I studies usually consist of a rising sin-gle-dose safety study, single-dose pharmacokinetic studies, multiple-dose safety studies, and multiple-dose pharmacokinetic studies (12). The studies to evaluate drug effect usually use a random-assignment, single- or double-blind design, since antiepileptic drugs may have a central nervous system effect that may produce signs and symptoms difficult to evaluate objectively. In addition, all subjects will necessarily be informed of potential signs and symptoms of toxicity, and some individuals will be subject to suggestibility. Evaluation includes physical examination, vital signs, psychological examination, physiological measurements, subjective impressions, and a battery of laboratory studies, with a minimum of hematological, renal, and cardiac measurements (67).

The use of subjects with known convulsive disorders is generally contraindicated in early Phase I testing. Women of childbearing potential are excluded. Abstinence from all drugs, both prescribed and nonprescribed, and from alcohol for at least 1 week and preferably longer before the trial period are desirable, and no other drugs or alcohol may be given during the test period. It may be necessary to test a very promising drug with significant potential for adverse effects in highly refractory patients who have frequent seizures and a poor prognosis. In some instances, children may need to be included, for example, those with infantile spasms.

Few Phase I studies of antiepileptic drugs have been published. Most often, these studies are performed by pharmaceutical firms and are used in designing subsequent studies, but they are not reported in the literature. Phase I testing of cinromide, a potential new antiepileptic drug, has recently been reported (7). Study documentation must include subject identification, demographic data, medical history, vital statistics, pre- and posttreatment physical examination, medication administration and dosage records, drug batch number, observed or reported physical or behavioral effects, laboratory data, including normal ranges, and adverse reactions. Information on adverse reactions should include the date and time of the reactions, time of onset in relation to last dose, a description of the reaction, including its severity and duration, the investigator's judgment as to whether the reaction was drug related, and the control measures used, with the response of the reaction to those measures. It is ideal, but not always practical, to determine the serum concentration of the drug at the time of the reaction.

Information on bioavailability of the drug at the administered dosages is of extreme importance during this phase. The drug's rate of absorption, steady-state blood level at various dosages, and metabolic half-life are determined in Phase I. Excretion studies and identification of major metabolites (which may later be shown to have anticonvulsant activity) are highly recommended during this phase, although they have seldom been performed.

EARLY CLINICAL STUDIES WITH EPILEPTIC PATIENTS (LATE PHASE I AND PHASE II)

Phase II demonstrates the efficacy of the drug in epileptic patients. At the same time, the therapeutic dose range is determined, and individual variability within this range is observed.

Adult patients experiencing incomplete seizure control are suitable subjects for Phase II testing. Patients whose seizures are well controlled on current therapy are not suitable subjects for Phase II studies unless their current medication is causing excessive side effects. Seizures must be classified according to the International Classification of Epileptic Seizures (11a,44). Adult subjects are preferable in Phase II testing unless the seizure type is restricted to the young age period, for example, absence attacks, infantile spasms, and atonic

seizures. Children with other forms of epilepsy must be selected on the basis of extreme refractoriness to current medication. The FDA has issued recommendations for study setting, patient characteristics, exclusion criteria, study designs, and monitoring (32–34,40). Informed consent (see below) must be obtained.

In initial Phase II studies, the investigational drug is generally added to existing therapy in an open manner. Later, after some evidence of efficacy of the new drug in humans has been obtained, existing therapy may be withdrawn if satisfactory seizure control is achieved through addition of the new agent. Study documentation is similar to Phase I testing.

Patients who participate in early clinical studies of a drug are generally excluded from participating in later definitive clinical studies. One reason for this exclusion is that patients who have already participated in a trial may bring with them preconceived ideas of the effectiveness of the drug, which would bias later studies.

DEFINITIVE CLINICAL STUDIES WITH EPILEPTIC PATIENTS (LATE PHASE II AND PHASE III)

Phase III testing begins after the decision has been made that a drug has sufficient therapeutic potential in relation to its safety to warrant a formal therapeutic trial. Phase III permits more variability in the experimental design.

Objectives of a Clinical Trial

In designing a clinical trial of an antiepileptic drug, the investigator must clearly define the questions that will be asked during the trial. This has been a serious deficiency in many clinical trials. The major objective is to determine the degree of efficacy of the treatment and to provide some comparisons between the effectiveness of the new drug and that of other currently available drugs.

A clinical trial can also assess the potential side effects of the drug and the practical problems that may interfere with the ability of patients to adhere to the treatment regimen even if the drug effectively controls seizures. Other potentially burdensome problems to the patient, such as frequency of drug administration or the need for repeated hematological studies, can be evaluated.

Response to an antiepileptic drug can be widely defined (see below). There may be remote and not easily defined or quantified changes, such as an improvement in mood or behavior. It is easy to postulate so many of these factors that sight of the initial study objectives may be lost.

Because a clinical trial is expensive and anxiety provoking to the subjects and their families, the objectives must be clearly formulated so that it is not done for limited or trivial purposes. Neither should the number of objectives be so unwieldy that the trial is doomed to failure.

Experimental Design

Clinical observations of a drug treatment are useful, but controlled clinical trials are required in Phases II and III before a new drug can be marketed (24,38). Such trials must be designed so that meaningful conclusions can be drawn and extended to other populations. The trial design must allow for the systematic collection of data so that appropriate statistical analyses can be carried out. Experimental designs of clinical trials and various methods used for the control of bias are further discussed in Chapter 10.

The statistical design of a clinical trial is not the work of a biostatistician alone. The subtleties of seizures and clinical observations require close interaction between clinicians with experience in neurology and controlled clinical trials and statisticians with experience in the design of clinical trials and knowledge of neurological disease. The physician must carefully define the patient population and recognize limitations that may be imposed on the study by problems of patient availability. The effect on the patient's life of participating in such a study must be considered. Can a young individual be hospitalized for the duration of a study during the school year? Can a patient leave an institution over a holiday period without jeopardizing

compliance, evaluation methodology, or safety? Such factors may impose very practical limitations on study design.

Relevant findings from previous clinical trials must be carefully documented and considered because of their relevance to planning for sample size, hypotheses, experimental design, and general application of the findings.

Subject Selection

Animal studies and early Phase II studies are used to delineate the seizure type or types most responsive to a new antiepileptic drug. Controlled clinical trials will thus usually be restricted to these types of seizures. The accurate specification of the seizure type is crucial—but often overlooked—to the success of the trial. The International Classification of Epileptic Seizures (11a,44) is most frequently used. Because of the multiple terminologies used to describe seizures, any clinical trial must clearly define the seizure type specified in order to make the trial comprehensible to other workers in the field. Seizures are usually classified by the description given by the patient or other observer, and rarely can an adequate and detailed description of the seizures be obtained in this way. It is possible for several different types of seizures to be considered the same type by the patient. Accurate diagnosis of seizure type by video monitoring must be considered for drug trials.

Clinical trials are further complicated by the fact that many potential participants have multiple seizure types. A new drug effective for one type of seizure may have no effect on another type. Other medications may be required when multiple seizure types coexist. However, most of the currently available antiepileptic drugs are enzyme inducers and may have an effect on the metabolism of the test drug.

Several difficulties may be encountered in selecting a seizure type for a study. First, clinical studies are usually initiated with the hope of marketing a drug. It would be desirable to have the drug marketed for all types of seizures for which it is effective, but the cost of mounting controlled studies for several seizure types is considerable. In practice, an NDA is usually sought for a specific seizure type, and additional indications are requested later. Second, a particular seizure type often varies. For example, should complex partial seizures only, complex partial seizures secondarily generalized, and elementary partial seizures progressing to complex partial seizures be considered as a single entity in a drug trial? If too much "splitting" is done, an extremely large pool of patients will be required for the trial; if too much "lumping" is done, the efficacy of a drug limited to a particular seizure type may be missed.

Moral and ethical considerations limit the testing of new drugs for some seizure types to individuals who are continuing to have seizures despite optimal therapy with existing drugs or to those who are experiencing adverse reactions to these drugs. In reality, these individuals usually have associated mental and motor handicaps from an underlying cerebral disease state that also produces the seizures. Whether these individuals are representative of the spectrum of individuals with seizures is certainly questionable.

It becomes apparent, then, that statistical evidence of the efficacy of a new antiepileptic drug may be difficult to demonstrate. The selection of subjects for a clinical trial forces the burden of proof of efficacy onto the trial design. The clinician bears the responsibility for careful and correct subject selection and must make certain that the methods of collecting data are clinically feasible and that the data are objective and worthwhile. No study should be started without an estimation of sample size based on power considerations.

Patients with treatable causes of seizures should be excluded from drug studies. The list of exclusion criteria has expanded as clinical trials have become more sophisticated. Some newly diagnosed seizure patients may not be suitable candidates. Because of the long time required for some antiepileptic drugs to reach a steady-state blood level, and because the currently available appropriate drugs should be tried, it has been suggested that epileptic patients should not be considered for drug studies for at least 6 to 9 months following initial diagnosis. However, this is not intended to exclude previously untreated patients with certain seizure types (e.g., absence seizures) from clinical trials. Other excludable categories include patients whose seizures are associated with tumors or progressive brain lesions, progressive degenerative or demyelinating neurological disorders, metabolic diseases, or active CNS infections, as well as those whose seizures are believed to be of psychogenic origin. Patients with chronic medical disorders of clinical significance are excluded, as are abusers of drugs or alcohol. Patients with conditions that may interfere with absorption (such as partial gastrectomy or iliectomy), distribution, metabolism, or excretion of drugs are excluded. Patients with recent status epilepticus or psychotic episodes are frequently excluded. Nonambulatory patients are excluded since this may affect the metabolic rate. Also frequently excluded are patients with low IQs (below 50) or those who have a history of noncompliance or inability to cooperate.

The number of individuals suitable for a well-controlled study will, in reality, be quite limited. This phenomenon has been described by Lasagna (51):

It can be represented graphically by a square wave, the periodicity of which is determined by the duration of the clinical trial. As soon as the trial begins, the supply of suitable patients becomes one-tenth of what it was said to be before the trial began. I have assumed that it returns to the pre-trial level as soon as the trial ends.

Human Rights—Informed Consent

Enlisting the cooperation of subjects in a clinical trial is mandatory. Some subjects are reluctant to have anything to do with new treatment procedures, whereas others are eager to participate in new treatment modalities. In most countries, informed consent must be obtained in writing before an individual can participate in a clinical trial. In the United States, "informed consent" means the knowing consent of an individual or his legally authorized representative, so situated as to be able to exercise free power of choice without undue inducement or any element of force, fraud, deceit, duress, or other form of constraint or coercion. Both the FDA and the HHS have proposed regulations for informed consent (13,21,57). The basic elements of information necessary to such consent include:

1. A statement that the clinical investigation involves research and that an institutional review board has approved the solicitation of subjects to participate in research; see HHS policy regulations (21) for definitions.
2. An explanation of the scope, aims, and purposes of the research, the procedures to be followed, and their purposes and duration, including the identification of any experimental procedures.
3. A description of reasonably foreseeable discomforts and risks.
4. A description of any benefits reasonably to be expected.
5. The disclosure of any appropriate alternative procedures or courses of treatment that might be advantageous for the subject.
6. An offer to answer any inquiries concerning the procedures, the subject's rights, or related procedures.
7. A statement that participation is voluntary and instruction that the person is free to withdraw consent and to discontinue participation in the project or activity at any time without penalty or loss of benefits (including continued treatment) to which the subject is otherwise entitled.
8. A statement of the nature of financial compensation, if any, to the subject.
9. An explanation as to the availability or unavailability of medical treatment or compensation for injury incurred as the result of participating in research, what it consists of, and where further information may be obtained.
10. A statement that new information developed during the course of the research that may relate to the subject's willingness to continue participation will be provided.
11. A statement describing the maintenance of confidentiality of records identifying the subject and that the records may be made available to the FDA.
12 Instructions as to whom the subject should contact if there are questions or problems or if harm occurs.

An unresolved moral and ethical question, particularly pertinent in seizure disorders, is the fact that children and institutionalized adults with no known relatives are usually excluded from clinical trials. At question is the right of the individual to participate with dignity in a clinical trial in order potentially to share in the benefits of advances in medical knowledge. Society must yet decide whether this right outweighs the individual's inability to appreciate fully the risk involved in a clinical trial. Does the right to treatment include the right to unproven treatment when conducted under carefully monitored conditions?

Specific regulations for prisoners (14–16, 21,37,41), persons institutionalized as mentally disabled (18,20,21), and children (17,19,21) have been developed in the United States.

Pilot Studies

The term "pilot study" has different meanings to different individuals. For example, Phase II pharmacokinetic studies may be termed pilot studies. Later, in planning for a controlled clinical trial, it may be necessary to do additional pharmacokinetic studies for the specific population. A "pilot study" may also be done in an open manner to determine how rapidly the drug may be initiated, how frequent dosing must be, or how the drug is tolerated. Another type of "pilot study" may actually be a small version of the proposed study to determine procedural problems in advance. There may need to be several "pilot studies" before a controlled clinical trial is begun.

There is a very real danger of commencing a controlled clinical trial prematurely. As many problems as possible must be anticipated before the trial begins. Failure to do so may invalidate all data collected up to the point of the problem. Each study will have unique problems because of the drug or the population under study. Table 2 lists some, but by no means all, of the topics that must be addressed in the pretrial period.

One of the major objectives to be determined from the pilot study process is the appropriate dosage for the population under consideration and the rate at which the dosage can be initiated. The occurrence of side effects during initiation of dosage must be minimized. Such reactions need not break the blind nature of a study, however, since clinically identical "side effects" may occur with placebo treatment.

From the experimental methodology, a protocol is devised to instruct the involved personnel on procedures to be followed during the study. Pilot studies allow the personnel to become familiar with patient management and the recording system. The pilot study may also allow for a trial of response measurements.

The availability of a method for determining the amount of drug in the blood is crucial not only to defining the pharmacokinetics of the drug for establishment of a dosage regimen, but also to evaluating compliance and results. For example, we were involved in a study of a potential antiepileptic drug in which serum drug levels were not measured during early clinical testing. When a methodology was later developed, it became apparent that the drug was not being entirely absorbed and that increasing the dosage in an attempt to produce higher serum concentrations caused adverse reactions (2,3).

TABLE 2. *Pretrial considerations in a controlled clinical trial*

Patient selection
  Seizure type(s) and accuracy of classification
  Prestudy seizure frequency
  Presumed cause of seizures
  Associated physical and mental problems
  Duration of seizures
  History of another seizure type now quiescent (e.g., absence seizures)
  Other drugs (e.g., antiepileptic, tranquilizers, vitamins, laxatives)
  Prior therapy and prior serum drug concentrations (i.e., are seizures refractory?)
  Consent form
  Age
  Race
  Sex
  Potential for pregnancy
  Competency
Trial design
  Control for investigator and patient bias and identification of placebo effect
  Method of subject assignment
  Drug packaging, unit dose
  Buildup of drug(s), final dose
  Duration of medication
  Minimum number of subjects
  Treatment setting
  Dosage schedule
  Prehuman pharmacology
Clinical trial
  Control of administration schedule
  Evaluators
  Observational methodology and frequency
  Data collection for side effects
  Criteria and protocol for removal from study
  Protocol for continued seizures
  Protocol for intercurrent illness or injury
  Protocol for side effects
  Arrangements for sample collection
Statistical analysis
  Statement of null hypothesis
  Basis for judgment
  Did study answer objective?
  Data management
  Data analyses

The Clinical Trial

A reasonable time schedule for a clinical trial must be established. The short-term and long-term efficacy of a drug need to be evaluated and may require different designs. Availability of subjects will also affect the study design. It is unusual to have enough patients in one place at one time to start studying all of them simultaneously. Subjects may need to be entered into a trial as they become available, and provisions must be made in the design to allow for randomization of such variables as age, weight, sex, race, and seizure frequency.

Multicenter or collaborative studies may be needed to ensure the collection of sufficient data in a reasonable length of time. Adherence to identical protocols at each center is crucial to permit pooling of data for analysis. Statistical justification must be presented for combining results from different centers.

Planned interim examinations of the data may be necessary, but the methods and rules for doing so must be specified in advance. The effect that this examination will have on the ultimate outcome of the study must be considered. Patients or their ombudsmen may need to be informed about information developed during the course of the study that may alter their willingness to continue to participate in the trial. In some cases, it may be necessary for ethical reasons to examine the data during the study.

All data should be analyzed as rapidly as possible. Errors in original data entries are more easily reconstructable if little time has passed.

The problem of sample attrition must be considered in advance in consultation with the biostatistician. In some cases, new patients may be added during the study when criteria for doing so are specified in advance. In other studies, sample size may be large enough to absorb some patient attrition.

A means of monitoring the drug administration schedule needs to be devised and may include pill counting and determination of serum drug levels. Unit packaging of each dose may increase compliance, and marking each dose with the day and time will assist the person in knowing if a dose has been missed. Instructions must also be given for forgotten doses. Protocols must be devised in advance to deal with adverse reactions to the drug, continued seizures, and intercurrent illness or injury. Criteria and a protocol for removing a subject from the study must be designated in advance, and all personnel must be carefully trained in the application of these procedures. The criteria for terminating the study before the planned completion must be specified. Criteria for breaking the blind on an individual subject or for the whole study must also be specified. The procedure to be followed if a patient dies while participating in a study must be specified in advance. Decisions to terminate a study prematurely must be based on rational scientific facts, not on an emotional response to an acute crisis.

Selection of dosage may present considerable difficulty. A fixed dosage for all individuals greatly simplifies packaging and maintenance

of the blind. On a fixed dosage, however, some individuals may have seizures because of inadequate dosage, and others may experience side effects because the dosage is too high. An alternative is to adjust the dosage during the study based on serum drug concentration, even though maintenance of the blind becomes more difficult, as does packaging of the medication. Another problem occurs if the FDA sets a limit on dosage, and it develops during the study, on the basis of data from other sources, that the study dosage is too low. Such a problem occurred with the study of valproate.

The investigators must be experienced in drug testing and in epilepsy. The study design must appropriately control both investigator and patient bias and identify placebo forces in shaping responses. Anxiety about the use of blind studies prevents some investigators from performing such studies. Since most antiepileptic drugs have side effects during the initiation of therapy, the physician directly responsible for the subject's care must be sensitive to patient safety without withdrawing the drug prematurely.

In the United States, the investigator is required to maintain adequate records of the disposition of all receipts of the drug, including dates, quantity, and use by subjects. If the clinical trial is suspended or terminated, the investigator must return to the sponsor any unused supply of the drug. The investigator is also required to maintain case histories designed to record all observations and other data pertinent to the clinical trial. Each page of material submitted to the FDA must be personally signed by the investigator, a task that can be particularly onerous. The drug disposition records and the case histories must be kept for 2 years after the date of approval of the New Drug Application. If no application is filed, records must be kept for 2 years after the FDA is notified of discontinuation of the IND trials.

Methods for Objective Measurement of Efficacy

Objective assessment of response during a clinical trial is of paramount importance and raises a host of issues that need to be clarified before a trial begins. Methodologies for determining the safety and efficacy of a drug tend to be expensive and technically difficult. A distinction must be made between the demonstration of efficacy of a drug for marketing purposes and for an individual patient. The demonstration of efficacy in an individual patient consists of a trial of a drug selected from among those marketed, followed by a joint decision between the patient and physician concerning the desired results. The proof of efficacy required for marketing approval is defined by regulatory bodies and varies among countries and among classes of drugs. This section on evaluation methodology will primarily address marketing efficacy.

Seizure Frequency

At first glance, the objective measurement of a new antiepileptic drug seems deceptively easy. Seizures either occur or they do not. But even for generalized tonic–clonic seizures—those most easily observed and counted—the situation becomes complicated. Although patients may report that the seizure frequency has not changed, they may note a change in the character ("they are not as hard") or the time frame ("they all occur at one time of day") of the seizures. Usually these changes occur during the trial, are not anticipated from pilot studies, are not consistent from patient to patient, and, despite attempts at quantitation, do not produce analyzable results.

The simplest record of seizures is a calendar, either a listing of their occurrence by date and time on a blank sheet of paper or a more formal scorecard type of record (6). These are maintained by the patient or a relative or companion and are most suitable for generalized tonic–clonic seizures. For an individual constantly with someone, this method should be fairly accurate. Problems arise in forgetting to record seizures and in omission of seizures that occur during sleep and other periods of nonobservation. In the New Castle efficacy studies (2–4,6) performed in an institution, three types of seizure

records were kept: (a) a form devised for the study, (b) a running log of activities in a unit, and (c) a form for monthly summary of seizures, kept in the patient's institutional chart. One individual was assigned to make certain that all three records matched. A formal comparison of the accuracy of the three forms was not made, but circumstances did arise when seizures were not recorded on at least one of the forms. Seizures were most apt to be recorded erroneously when the patient was about to leave the unit, such as going to a meal, was away from the unit, such as in school or vocational workshop, or sustained minor injury during the seizure.

In absence seizures, the problem of measuring seizure frequency is even more complicated. Clinical estimates of absence seizure frequency are significantly related to the duration of spike-wave bursts recorded on the EEG. Bursts lasting less than 3 sec are generally unidentified by intensive clinical observation unless the patient is engaged in speaking, writing, or fine movements of the upper extremities. Bursts lasting less than 1 sec generally do not produce clinically observable behavioral alterations (1,55). Browne et al. (1) found that the 12-hr telemetered EEG was the most reliable method of estimating the number of absence seizures, both before and after treatment in a drug trial, and assessment by a trained observer was the next best method. Estimates of mothers and routine observation by hospital staff were usually much lower.

A sophisticated system for monitoring infantile spasms has been developed (43,48). A 24-hr recording system graphically displays concurrent, time-synchronized data on a wide range of physiological functions.

Equipment for monitoring the EEG by use of portable, wearable recorders is being developed by several firms. Sato et al. (62) have described an eight-channel EEG digital cassette recorder useful for home monitoring. Technical problems, such as signal dropout, still need to be corrected, and existing models tend to be heavy and bulky for prolonged wear.

With combined video and electroencephalographic recording of seizures (58), it is possible to document objectively the effect of a specific drug on some specific seizure types, but the evaluation methodology is expensive. The question may rightfully be asked, "Is it worth the expense, or can new drugs be evaluated by more traditional, less costly techniques?" The new methodologies do permit rapid short-term evaluation of a new drug while exposing the least number of patients to ineffective or potentially hazardous drugs. Humanistic aspects may thus outweigh cost considerations.

Once an accurate and objective measure of seizure frequency is assured, other measures of a drug's efficacy, such as seizure-free interval, can be considered. Without an accurate, objective count of seizures, other measures are useless.

Serum Drug Concentrations

The measurement of serum drug concentrations is an objective means of determining patient compliance, determining toxic drug levels, identifying pharmacokinetic problems, and defining effective drug levels. Drug interaction can be defined in patients receiving multiple drugs. The measurement of serum drug concentrations during a trial allows the possible identification of other causes of what appears to be ineffectiveness of the drug.

Neuropsychological Tests

The role of neuropsychological testing in clinical evaluation of drugs is currently limited. A review of the literature reveals a gradual progression toward improved research design in psychological evaluation. Sophisticated test batteries are being developed and standardized specifically for patients with epilepsy to provide objective measures of intelligence, cognitive function, emotional status, and psychological correlates of cerebral damage (22). Objective measures of psychological and social function are also being developed (23). It is not now possible to identify firmly the mechanism involved in producing changes in ability, but it

may be possible to measure objectively the direction of changes in function. Incidentally, a drug trial must be long enough to allow such changes to occur.

The collection of "neuropsychological" data in clinical trials has been based on clinical impressions—sometimes recorded in a uniform way (4), but more often not. The inclusion of new methodologies increases trial cost and time, and the value of including these tests must be assessed in relation to the overall study objectives.

Laboratory Monitoring

As a minimum, laboratory tests of hematopoietic, hepatic, renal, and cardiovascular function must be done before a clinical trial begins. Additional laboratory tests are based on the chemical structure of the drug and acute and chronic animal toxicity studies. Once the drug has been administered to humans, the occurrence of side effects and subjective observations by the subjects determine the need for additional tests. For multiple reasons, the current trend is to do more and more laboratory monitoring. Before each test is added, however, the objectives of that particular measurement should be clearly stated, and it should be determined, with statistical consultation, the number of patients to be monitored before the test is considered no longer necessary (presuming no abnormalities are found). The procedure to be followed if the test result deviates from normal must be specified in advance.

Preference Ratings

It has been suggested, particularly for double-blind studies, that both physicians and patients should, subjectively or objectively (using a standardized scale), rate the drug being compared. Such ratings give an indication of subjective factors that might influence future use of the drug. When preference ratings are used, meaningful criteria should be established to insure consistent results.

Side Effects

The protocol should be designed to anticipate side effects of the drug and should indicate the procedure to be followed when they occur. The central nervous sytem effects of antiepileptic drugs may be subtle and should be measured objectively when possible. Examples of such measures are steadiness on standing (47), the rotary pursuit meter (46,55), and a variety of reaction time tests (47).

The adverse effects of the drug should be carefully documented, with a description of the presumed effect, time of onset, duration, serum drug concentration, time of onset in relation to last dose, and confounding variables. Any adverse effect that may reasonably be regarded as caused by, or is probably caused by, the new drug must be reported to the sponsor promptly; if the adverse effect is alarming, it must be reported immediately.

SUMMARY

The ultimate value of any new antiepileptic agent must be proved in the clinic as rapidly as possible so that the new drug may be made accessible to those individuals whose seizures are not controlled by available medications or to those who have adverse reactions to the available drugs. At the same time, as few individuals as possible should be exposed to an ineffective drug. In most countries throughout the world, regulatory bodies require proof of a new drug's safety and, in some countries, of its efficacy and bioavailability before permitting it to be marketed. Unfortunately, the poor quality of many clinical trials of antiepileptic drugs has often delayed their availability. International attention has now been focused on the problem, and guidelines or principles for testing of antiepileptic drugs have been promulgated. Clinical trials must have a clear statement of objectives, and human rights must be carefully safeguarded.

Clinical testing of a new antiepileptic drug follows an orderly progression. Safety is first determined in humans, usually normal volunteers. Testing then determines if the drug treats or prevents the disease for which it is intended and is followed by short-term and long-term efficacy and safety evaluation.

Particular problems confront the investigator of new antiepileptic drugs because of unique features of the disease. The intensity and characteristics of epilepsy vary among individuals. The occurrence of seizures may modify an individual's behavior, which may in turn modify the manifestations of the disease. Rate of absorption, genetic differences in bioabsorption, modification of liver enzyme systems by previous therapy, and central nervous system variations may all modify the effects of drugs in humans. Variations in the drug itself, such as formulation, may also affect its bioavailability. The selection of an epileptic population for study and the choice of a study design thus become extremely complex.

The clinician bears the responsibility for careful and correct subject selection and must make certain that the data to be collected are worthwhile and clinically obtainable by objective methods. A clinical trial must be carefully designed to collect data systematically for appropriate statistical hypotheses and analyses. A study should not be started without an estimation of sample size based on power considerations.

Recent years have witnessed the development of clinical techniques and instrumentation that improve the objective evaluation of drug efficacy. Their use is becoming standard practice in drug evaluation. Although expensive, these techniques can lead to a vast increase in our knowledge of epilepsy and the mechanisms of action of antiepileptic drugs.

REFERENCES

1. Browne, T. R., Penry, J. K., Porter, R. J., and Dreifuss, F. E. (1974): A comparison of clinical estimates of absence seizure frequency with estimates based on prolonged telemetered EEGs. *Neurology (Minneap.)*, 24:381–382.
2. Cereghino, J. J., Brock, J. T., and Penry, J. K. (1972): Other hydantoins: Albutoin. In: *Antiepileptic Drugs*, edited by D. M. Woodbury, J. K. Penry, and R. P. Schmidt, pp. 283–291. Raven Press, New York.

3. Cereghino, J. J., Brock, J. T., Van Meter, J. C., Penry, J. K., Smith, L. D., Fisher, P., and Ellenberg, J. (1974): Evaluation of albutoin as an antiepileptic drug. *Clin. Pharmacol. Ther.*, 15:406–416.

4. Cereghino, J. J., Brock, J. T., Van Meter, J. C., Penry, J. K., Smith, L. D., and White, B. G. (1974): Carbamazepine for epilepsy: A controlled prospective evaluation. *Neurology (Minneap.)*, 24:401–410.

5. Cereghino, J. J., and Penry, J. K. (1972): General principles: Testing of anticonvulsants in man. In: *Antiepileptic Drugs*, edited by D. M. Woodbury, J. K. Penry, and R. P. Schmidt, pp. 63–73. Raven Press, New York.

6. Cereghino, J. J., Van Meter, J. C., Brock, J. T., Penry, J. K., Smith, L. D., and White, B. G. (1973): Preliminary observations of serum carbamazepine concentration in epileptic patients. *Neurology (Minneap.)*, 23:357–366.

7. Cloutier, G., Gabriel, M., Geiger, E., Cook, L., Rogers, J., Cummings, W., and Cato, A. (1980): Cinromide: Phase I testing of a potential antiepileptic. In: *Advances in Epileptology. The Xth Epilepsy International Symposium*, edited by J. A. Wada, and J. K. Penry, p. 351. Raven Press, New York.

8. Coatsworth, J. J. (1971): *Studies on the Clinical Efficacy of Marketed Antiepileptic Drugs*, NINDS Monograph No. 12. U.S. Government Printing Office, Washington.

9. Commission for the Control of Epilepsy and Its Consequences (1977): *Workshop on Antiepileptic Drug Development. April 15, 1977. Arlington, Virginia. Edited Transcript.* HEW Publication No. (NIH)77–185.

10. Commission for the Control of Epilepsy and Its Consequences (1977): *Workshop on Antiepileptic Drug Development. April 15, 1977. Arlington, Virginia. Summary, Tables, and Appendices.* HEW Publication No. (NIH)77–186.

11. Commission for the Control of Epilepsy and Its Consequences (1977): *Plan for Nationwide Action on Epilepsy, Vol. I*, pp. 45–60. HEW Publication No. (NIH)78–276.

11a. Commission on Classification and Terminology of the International League Against Epilepsy (1981): Proposal for revised clinical and electroencephalographic classification of epileptic seizures. *Epilepsia*, 22:489–501.

12. Czerwinski, A. W. (1974): The Phase I drug study. In: *Drug Induced Clinical Toxicity*, edited by F. G. McMahon, pp. 37–44. Futura Publishing, Mount Kisco, New York.

13. DHEW, Food and Drug Administration, Office of the Secretary (1979): [45 CFR, Part 46] Proposed regulations amending basic HEW policy for protection of human research subjects. *Fed. Register*, 44:47688–47729.

14. DHEW, General Administration (1978): [45 CFR Part 46] Protection of human subjects. Additional protections pertaining to biomedical and behavioral research involving prisoners as subjects. *Fed. Register*, 43:53652–53656.

15. DHEW, Office of the Secretary (1977): [45 CFR, Part 46] Protection of human subjects. Research involving prisoners and notice of report and recommendations

of the National Commission of the Protection of Human Subjects of Biomedical and Behavioral Research. *Fed. Register*, 42:3076–3091.

16. DHEW, Office of the Secretary (1978): [45 CFR, Part 46] Protection of human subjects. Proposed regulations on research involving prisoners. *Fed. Register*, 43:1050–1053.

17. DHEW, Office of the Secretary (1978): Research involving children. Report and recommendations of the National Commission for the Protection of Human Subjects of Biomedical and Behavioral Research. *Fed. Register*, 43:2084–2114.

18. DHEW, Office of the Secretary (1978): Protection of human subjects. Research involving those institutionalized as mentally infirm. Report and recommendations of the National Commission for the Protection of Human Subjects of Biomedical and Behavioral Research. *Fed. Register*, 43:11328–11358.

19. DHEW, Office of the Secretary (1978): [45 CFR, Part 46] Protection of human subjects. Proposed regulations on research involving children. *Fed. Register*, 43:31786–31794.

20. DHEW, Office of the Secretary (1978): [45 CFR, Part 46] Protection of human subjects. Proposed regulations on research involving those institutionalized as mentally disabled. *Fed. Register*, 43:53950–53956.

21. DHHS, Office of the Secretary (1981): Final regulations amending basic HHS policy for protection of human research subjects. *Fed. Register*, 46:8366–8392.

22. Dodrill, C. B. (1978): A neuropsychological battery for epilepsy. *Epilepsia*, 19:611–623.

23. Dodrill, C. B., Batzel, L. W., Queisser, H. R., and Temkin, N. R. (1980): An objective method for the assessments of psychological and social problems among epileptics. *Epilepsia*, 21:123–135.

24. Drug Amendments Act of 1962. Public Law 87–781, 21 USC 355.

25. Federal Food and Drug Act of 1906. Public Law 384, 59th Congress.

26. Federal Food, Drug, and Cosmetic Act of 1938. Public Law 717, 75th Congress.

27. FDA (1967): Clinical testing: Synopsis of new drug regulations. *FDA Papers*, 1 21–25.

28. FDA (1970): Chapter 1—Food and Drug Administration, Department of Health, Education, and Welfare. Subchapter C—Drugs. Part 130—New drugs. Part 146—Antibiotic drugs; procedural and interpretive regulations. Hearing regulations and regulations describing scientific content of adequate and well-controlled clinical investigations. *Fed. Register*, 35:7250–7253.

29. FDA (1970): [Docket No. FDC-D-187; NDA 5–856, etc.] Certain anticonvulsant drugs. Drugs for human use; Drug Efficacy Study Implementation. *Fed. Register*, 35:13594–13596.

30. FDA (1972): [21 CFR, Part 130 1] Drug Efficacy Study Implementation notices. Applicability of DESI notices to identical, related, and similar drug products. *Fed. Register*, 37:2969–2970.

31. FDA (1972): Chapter I, Food and Drug Administration, Department of Health, Education, and Welfare, Subchapter C—Drugs. Part 130—New Drugs. Subpart A—Procedural and interpretive regulations.

Applicability of DESI notices and notices of opportunity for hearing to identical, related, and similar drug products. *Fed. Register,* 37:23185–23187.

32. FDA (1977): *General Considerations for the Clinical Evaluation of Drugs.* HEW Publication No. (FDA)77–3040.

33. FDA (1977): *General Considerations for the Clinical Evaluation of Drugs in Infants and Children.* HEW Publication No. (FDA)77–3041.

34. FDA (1977): *Guidelines for the Clinical Evaluation of Anticonvulsant Drugs (Adults and Children).* HEW Publication No. (FDA)77–3045.

35. FDA (1977): Chapter I, Food and Drug Administration, Department of Health, Education, and Welfare. Subchapter D—Drugs for human use. Part 314—New Drug Applications. Part 320—Bioavailability and bioequivalence requirements. Procedures for establishing a bioequivalence requirement. *Fed. Register,* 42:1624–1653.

36. FDA (1977): [Docket No. 76N–0245; DESI 5856] Phenytoin and phenytoin sodium. Drug for human use; efficacy study implementation; followup notice. *Fed. Register,* 42:39721–39724.

37. FDA (1978): (21 CFR Part 50) [Docket No. 78N–0049] Protection of human subjects. Proposed establishment of regulations. *Fed. Register,* 43:19417–19422.

38. FDA (1978): [Docket No. 77N–0278] Obligations of clinical investigators of regulated articles. *Fed. Register,* 43:35210–35236.

39. FDA (1979): Isocarboxazid; drugs for human use; Drug Efficacy Study Implementation; permission for drugs to remain on the market; amendment. *Fed. Register,* 44:50409–50410.

40. FDA (1980): *Guidelines for the Clinical Evaluation of Antiepileptic Drugs (Adults and Children).* HHS Publication No. (FDA)81–3110.

41. FDA (1980): 21 CFR, Part 50 [Docket No. 78N–0049] Protection of human subjects; prisoners used as subjects in research. *Fed. Register,* 45:36386–36392.

42. FDA, Bureau of Drugs, DESI Project (1979): *FDA Interim Index to Evaluations Published in the Federal Register for NAS/NRC Reviewed Prescription Drugs. Volume IX Cumulative up to December 1, 1979.* Food and Drug Administration, Rockville, Maryland.

43. Frost, J. D., Jr., Hrachovy, R. A., Kellaway, P., and Zion, T. (1978): Quantitative analysis and characterization of infantile spasms. *Epilepsia,* 19:273–282.

44. Gastaut, H. (1970): Clinical and electroencephalographical classification of epileptic seizures. *Epilepsia,* 11:102–113.

45. Glaser, G. H., Penry, J. K., and Woodbury, D. M., editors (1980): *Antiepileptic Drugs: Mechanisms of Action.* Raven Press, New York.

46. Goode, D. J., Penry, J. K., and Dreifuss, F. E. (1970): Effects of paroxysmal spike-wave on continuous visual–motor performance. *Epilepsia,* 11:241–254.

47. Ideström, C.M. (1960): Experimental psychologic methods applied in psychopharmacology. *Acta Psychiatr. Neurol. Scand.,* 35:302–313.

48. Kellaway, P., Hrachovy, R. A., Frost, J. D., Jr., and Zion, T. (1979): Precise characterization and quantification of infantile spasms. *Ann. Neurol.,* 6:214–218.

49. Krall, R. L., Penry, J. K., Kupferberg, H. J., and Swinyard, E. A. (1978): Antiepileptic drug development: I. History and a program for progress. *Epilepsia,* 19:393–408.

50. Krall, R. L., Penry, J. K., White, B. G., Kupferberg, H. J., and Swinyard, E. A. (1978): Antiepileptic drug development: II. Anticonvulsant drug screening. *Epilepsia,* 19:409–428.

51. Lasagna, L. (1976): On the other hand. *Med. World News,* 17(25):112.

52. Lockard, J. S. (1980): A primate model of clinical epilepsy: Mechanisms of action through quantification of therapeutic effects. In *Epilepsy: A Window to Brain Mechanisms,* edited by J. S. Lockard and A. A. Ward, Jr., pp. 11–49. Raven Press, New York.

53. Merritt, H. H., and Putnam, T. J. (1938): Sodium diphenylhydantoinate in treatment of convulsive disorders. *J.A.M.A.* 111:1068–1073.

54. Merritt, H. H., and Putnam, T. J. (1945): Experimental determination of anticonvulsant activity of chemical compounds. *Epilepsia (Second Series),* 3:51–75.

55. Penry, J. K. (1973): Behavioral correlates of generalized spike-wave discharges in the electroencephalogram. In: *Epilepsy: Its Phenomena in Man,* edited by M. A. B. Brazier, pp. 171–188. Academic Press, New York.

56. Penry, J. K. (1973): Principles for clinical testing of antiepileptic drugs. *Epilepsia,* 14:451–458.

57. Petricciani, J. C. (1979): *Comparison of the HEW and FDA Proposed Regulations for IRBs and Informed Consent.* DHEW, PHS, FDA, Bureau of Biologics, Rockville, Maryland.

58. Porter, R. J., Penry, J. K., and Wolf, A. A., Jr. (1976): Simultaneous documentation of clinical and electroencephalographic manifestations of epileptic seizures. In: *Quantitative Analytic Studies in Epilepsy,* edited by P. Kellaway and I. Petersén, pp. 253–268. Raven Press, New York.

59. Reynolds, E. H. (1976): Editorial: Unsatisfactory aspects of the drug treatment of epilepsy. *Epilepsia,* 17:xiii–xv.

60. Reynolds, E. H. (1978): Report of the Commission on Antiepileptic Drugs of the International League Against Epilepsy, 1974–1977. *Epilepsia,* 19:115–117.

61. Russell, B. (1961): *Basic Writings of Bertrand Russell,* edited by L. E. Denonn and R. E. Egner, p. 28. Simon & Schuster, New York.

62. Sato, S., Penry, J. K., and Burch, J. D. (1978): Eight-channel EEG digital cassette recorder for monitoring partial and generalized seizures. In: *Proceedings of the Second International Symposium on Ambulatory Monitoring,* edited by F. D. Stott, E. B. Raftery, P. Sleight, and L. Goulding, pp. 93–103. Academic Press, London.

63. Simonsen, N., Zander Olsen, P., Kühl, V., Lund, M., and Wendelboe, J. (1976): A comparative controlled study between carbamazepine and diphenylhydantoin in psychomotor epilepsy. *Epilepsia,* 17:169–176.

64. Troupin, A., Moretti Ojemann, L., Halpern, L., Dodrill, C., Wilkus, R., Friel, P., and Feigl, P. (1977): Carbamazepine—a double blind comparison with phenytoin. *Neurology (Minneap.),* 27:511–519.

65. Wardell, W. M. (1978): Human data requirements for acceptance of new drugs: Are these requirements enough or too much? In: *The Scientific Basis of Official Regulation of Drug Research and Development,* edited by A. F. De Schaepdryver, F. H. Gross, L. Lasagna, and D. R. Laurence, pp. 66–81. Heymans Foundation, Ghent.

66. Wardell, W. M. (1978): *Controlling the Use of Therapeutic Drugs. An International Comparison.* American Enterprise Institute for Public Policy Research, Washington, D.C.

67. Zarafonetis, C. J. D., Riley, P. A., Jr., Willis, P. W. III, Power, L. H., Werbelow, J. D., Farhat, L., Beckwith, W., and Marks, B. H. (1978): Clinically significant adverse effects in a Phase I testing program. *Clin. Pharmacol. Ther.,* 24:127–131.

Antiepileptic Drugs, edited by D. M. Woodbury,
J. K. Penry, and C. E. Pippenger. Raven Press,
New York © 1982.

10

General Principles

Testing of Antiepileptic Drugs in Humans: Statistical Considerations

B. G. White

In 1946, the British Medical Research Council set up the first large-scale randomized clinical trial to evaluate streptomycin in the therapy of pulmonary tuberculosis (18). Since then, controlled clinical experimentation has become established as the principal means of collecting scientific data on the relative merits of medical treatments. However, with the increased awareness of patients' rights (28) and the rise to prominence of human experimentation review committees in the United States, several ethical issues have been raised concerning the conduct of clinical trials. The basic issues are: (a) a fear that the trial, by withholding a favorable new therapy, demands an unneeded sacrifice from some patients; and (b) a concern that an untested new therapy exposes some patients to unneeded additional risk.

Responses to such issues are currently developed on an *ad hoc* basis. Most people recognize that the primary objective of medical science is to cure the diseases of individual patients, but they also recognize that the necessary knowledge has to be accumulated slowly. The specter of "unneeded sacrifice" or "additional risk" is real, but a balance must be struck among the conflicting requirements of medicine, law, economics, and ethics (4,9).

Tukey (33) has expressed the consensus among researchers: "Many of us are concerned, by what seems to me to be very strong evidence, that the only source of reliable evidence about the usefulness of almost any sort of therapy or surgical intervention is that obtained from well planned and carefully conducted randomized, and, when possible, double-blind clinical trials." The United States Food and Drug Administration (FDA) has issued guidelines for currently acceptable approaches to the study of investigational drugs in man (13). These guidelines state that "the objective of clinical investigations is to assess whether a drug is of value in the treatment or prophylaxis of a disease. Investigations of this nature must be conducted in such a way that the participating subjects, or patients, are exposed to the least possible risk consistent with the anticipated benefit." The FDA has also released guidelines for the evaluation of several specific classes of compounds, including anticonvulsants (14).

CONTROLLED CLINICAL TRIALS

Definition

Clinical trials are defined as prospective experiments of new therapies or diagnostic procedures carried out with human beings (36).

Certain general criteria are needed to insure that a clinical trial is an "adequate and well controlled clinical investigation." These criteria are:

1. Clearly stated study objectives.
2. A well-specified population subgroup (i.e., target population) with adequate selection criteria.
3. Allocation of patients to treatments so that valid statistical analysis is possible.
4. Inclusion, if possible, of a concurrent control or comparison group.
5. Single-blind or double-blind study design.
6. Plan of study so structured that measurements of effectiveness are well defined.
7. Maintenance of strict protocol adherence.
8. Detailed documentation of study dropouts or withdrawals.

Several other criteria depend on the class of drugs being tested. For instance, in the testing of antiepileptic therapies, a trial would not be considered "adequate and well controlled" if the measurement of serum antiepileptic drug levels was omitted.

Classification

Clinical trials (especially as carried out in the United States) can be divided into two broad classifications: randomized and nonrandomized trials.

Randomized trials employ a chance mechanism to allocate patients to the therapies. These trials, by their nature, are comparative and may be (a) single-blind—only the patient is unaware of the treatment administered; (b) double-blind—both patient and physician are unaware of the treatment administered; or (c) open—both patient and physician are aware of the treatment assigned. Randomized trials may also include such design features as placebo lead-in periods to establish the magnitude of the placebo effect; blocking, which involves the random assignment of patients within groups expected to respond similarly to therapy; or crossover to an alternate therapy, which allows intraindividual comparisons.

Nonrandomized trials typically consist of prospective data collections on a single new therapy. Evaluation is then based on a retrospective comparison of the new data with historical data not collected specifically for the comparison. The relative merits of these two broad classes of clinical trial designs are still being debated (1,17,23).

Controlled clinical trials may also be classified by the manner in which the sample size is selected—fixed in advance or determined sequentially. Fixing the sample size allows calculation of the probability of showing a statistically significant result for clinically relevant differences in treatments. In sequential randomized designs, the trial size is determined by the accumulating response data. Most sequential clinical trials involve adaptive treatment assignment, which utilizes accumulating information on the relative merits of treatments to assign the best treatment to the most patients. Weinstein (34) and Hoel et al. (20) have given numerous examples of designs based on adaptive treatment assignment. These sequential designs are used infrequently in clinical investigations, mainly because:

1. Double-blind trials are often impossible to conduct; in "play-the-winner" assignment the physician may know the treatment assignment before the next patient enters the trial.
2. These trials are difficult to understand.
3. Although fewer patients may be assigned to the poorer treatment in an adaptive trial, the total number of patients needed for the trial may be greater than in a trial of fixed sample size (31,32).

Randomized clinical trials of fixed sample size may be further classified by the number of treatments given each patient—single-period trials and multiple-period trials. Single-period trials consist of only one treatment period. The sample is randomly divided into mutually exclusive and exhaustive subgroups, and each subgroup receives one of the trial treatments for the entire study period. In multiple-period trials, the sample is also divided into mutually exclusive and exhaustive subgroups, but each subgroup receives more than one treatment. The treatments are administered serially, and effects are observed for a specified period. Multiple-period designs typically include a suitable lag or "washout" period between treatments. Multiple-period designs are of many types, including cross-over designs (26), cyclical designs (11), switchback designs (27), two-stage adaptive designs (8), and Latin square and lattice designs (7).

New Approaches

In designing a clinical trial, one must weigh carefully the sometimes opposing considerations of ethics, medicine, biostatistics, law, and economics. Clinical trials should be designed according to the fundamentally sound and efficient experimental principles developed by Fisher (12). They must also be subject to current ethical and informed consent guidelines applicable to human experimentation (28). These considerations may require that optimal statistical designs be replaced by designs that conform to both moral and legal constraints. The heightened awareness of patients' rights with a concomitantly intense focusing on the informed consent procedure has led to the development of several new single-period and multiple-period clinical trial designs.

Single-Period Designs

Zelen (36) has proposed a class of single-period designs called "patient consent" designs (Fig. 1). Both designs incorporate a decision by the patient only on the experimental treatment. In Design I, eligible patients are randomized into one of two groups: N_1, the investigator does not seek informed consent; N_2, the investigator seeks informed consent. Patients assigned to N_1 are given the best available standard treatment, T_1. Patients assigned to N_2 are asked to accept the new therapy, T_2. Patients who refuse the new therapy receive the standard therapy, T_1. Design II incorporates a slight modification of the previous design: patients in the N_2 group are

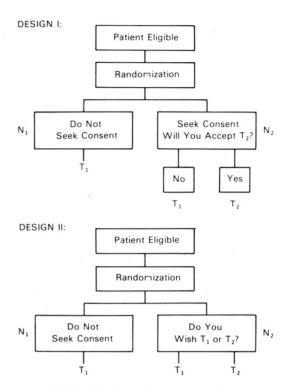

FIG. 1. Zelen's patient consent designs.

given the option of receiving the standard therapy, T_1, or the new therapy, T_2.

Although they increase the possibility of recruitment rates, these "patient consent" designs have several disadvantages. For one thing, they cannot be used when a double-blind experiment is needed. Also, the practical and ethical appropriateness of excluding a portion of the eligible patients without their knowledge is questionable (10,15,29). Statistical analysis of these designs is still unreported.

Lindley (21) has proposed a "less than efficient" single-period design. This "ethical" design assumes a dichotomous (binary) response variable—positive response or not—and assigns patients to treatment on the basis of an assessment of their potential response to the standard treatment, T_1. According to Lindley, "it is possible to make sound judgments about, for example, the comparative effects of two or more treatments, when the design incorporates an assignment to treatment."

Two-Period Designs

The most common multiple-period design is the two-period crossover design (Fig. 2). This design randomly assigns each patient to receive both treatments, either in sequence T_1, T_2 or sequence T_2, T_1. In an attempt to balance the number of patients completing each sequence, the randomization process is restricted. After a specified number of patients (a block) have been accessioned, each treatment sequence can be expected to have an identical number of patients. This restriction in the randomization process is called "randomized permuted blocks."

The use of this design, however, has been criticized on two fronts (2,3,25). In one area, the criticisms focus on the ethical dilemma of withdrawing an effective treatment in order to administer the alternative treatment. For example, in a clinical trial involving patients who have a high frequency of absence seizures, a complete crossover design would require that treatment be withdrawn from all patients, even those it had benefited in period I. A "wash-out" period would be followed by the alternative treatment, which might or might not be effective. In this situation, the alternative treatment, whether it is the standard or the new treatment, could at best maintain the patient's current state of seizure control and at worst result in severe complications. Because of such circumstances, the strict application of the classical two-period

crossover design is difficult to justify ethically in certain chronic diseases. The two-period crossover design has also been criticized by the FDA for the implicit assumption that there is no unequal carryover effect of the initial treatment.

A new design has been used which, unlike the single-period design, has the statistical efficiency of a crossover design (35). This design, randomization with incomplete crossover (Fig. 3), is identical to the classical two-period crossover design except that patients who show a positive response to the period I treatment are not switched to the alternative treatment. Only those patients who do not respond to the first treatment are "crossed over." This design has been used in a study of absence seizures (30).

A modification of the incomplete crossover design—profile assessment with incomplete crossover—is shown in Fig. 4. This design incorporates a preentry diagnostic screening and assessment procedure based on existing data, medical judgment, or any other information that would identify patients likely to respond to the standard treatment. Each patient is then assigned to the treatment that promises the highest individual probability of success. In the United States, treatment assignment for controlled clinical trials is usually carried out by a data-coordinating center. Thus, a profile assessment procedure could be incorporated into the study design without sacrificing the advantages of a blinded trial. Applications of this design are

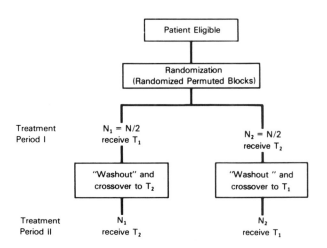

FIG. 2. Classical two-period crossover design.

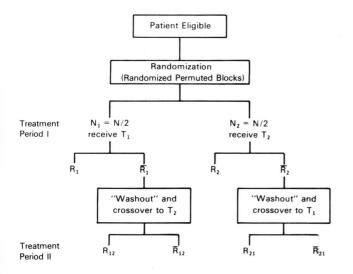

FIG. 3. Two-period incomplete crossover design—patient assignment by randomization.

currently being undertaken for the efficacy evaluation of several types of anticancer therapies.

TESTING OF ANTIEPILEPTIC THERAPIES IN HUMANS: DESIGN OF CHOICE

The types of clinical trial designs used to evaluate the efficacy of antiepileptic therapies were explored by reviewing the published literature for 1970 through 1979. A clinical trial was defined as "any prospective study which utilized some form of experimental design" (6).

The review was not restricted to reports of "controlled" clinical trials, partly because of the relatively recent advent of routine monitoring of serum antiepileptic drug levels. Multiple reports of the same trial were excluded.

A total of 113 reports of clinical trials were found. Twenty-eight were conducted in the United States, and the remainder in other countries (Fig. 5). The various methods used for control of bias in the evaluation of treatment effect are shown in Table 1. Of the 28 United States trials, 16 (57%) reported using either a single- or double-blind technique for the control

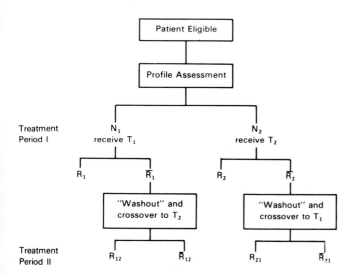

FIG. 4. Two-period incomplete crossover design—patient assignment by profile assessment.

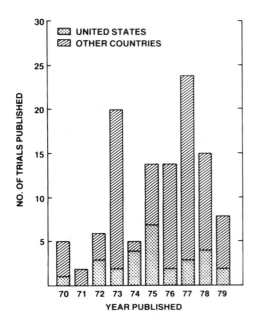

FIG. 5. Clinical efficacy trials of antiepileptic therapies, 1970–1979.

TABLE 2. *Basis for judgment of therapeutic efficacy in clinical efficacy trials of antiepileptic therapies*

	Number of trials	
	United States	Other countries
Clinical judgment	2	43
Frequency summary	5	15
Statistical tests of hypothesis	21	27
Total	28	85

control group, a two-period crossover design was used in 10 (63%) of the 16 United States trials and in 15 (75%) of the 20 trials in other countries. Clearly, the two-period crosover design has been the design of choice for evaluating the clinical efficacy of antiepileptic therapies in the last decade.

Two-Period Crossover Design

The two-period changeover design (27) has gained wide acceptance in many clinical applications. This design has often been used in the efficacy testing of drugs from many classes. In a review of clinical investigations of antianxiety drugs, McNair (22) reported that "two-thirds of the experiments utilized crossover designs." As Grizzle (16) demonstrated for applications in which the response to treatment is measured on a continuous scale, this design is more efficient than a randomized block design if resid-

of bias. Only 23 (27%) of the 85 studies conducted in other countries reported using some form of control for bias.

The most frequent basis for judgment of treatment effect was the statistical tests of the hypothesis (Table 2). No attempt was made to judge the appropriateness of statistical tests or of the resulting inferences. Of the United States studies, 21 (75%) reported using statistical tests as means of assessing efficacy. Statistical tests were used in 27 (32%) of the studies conducted in other countries.

The types of designs used for the 113 trials are shown in Table 3. Of the trials that used a

TABLE 1. *Method of control for bias in clinical efficacy trials of antiepileptic therapies*

	Number of trials	
	United States	Other countries
Single-blind	3	4
Double-blind	13	19
Open or not reported	12	62
Total	28	85

TABLE 3. *Designs of clinical efficacy trials of antiepileptic therapies*

	Number of trials	
Trial design	United States	Other countries
One group	12	61
Parallel groups	3	3
Two-period crossover	10	15
Multiple-period crossover	3	2
Sequential	0	3
Factorial	0	1
Total	28	85

ual treatment effects are equal and if correlation between responses to the two treatments is positive.

The complete two-period crossover design requires each patient to receive both treatments—either T_1 then T_2 or T_2 then T_1 (see Fig. 2). The main statistical concept involved in any crossover design is the ability to capitalize on the correlation between repeated measurements in the same patient compared with independent measurements on two different patients. This is especially relevant to an evaluation of anti-epileptic therapy; since any group of patients differs widely in the frequency of seizures, the intraclass correlation coefficients tend to be well above 50%.

Crossover designs are commonly used in the study of chronic diseases, which are defined as diseases that persist in varying degrees of severity unless treated. In the individual patient, this definition implies that the severity of the untreated disease will not remain constant over time (19).

Crossover designs are best used in short-term studies and are well suited for study of palliative drugs with relatively short half-lives. As Hills and Armitage (19) point out, two assumptions are needed for the analysis of crossover designs. First, "the effect of treating a subject during a specific period is to change the response by a fixed amount, which depends upon the treatment and is the same (apart from a random component) for all subjects." Second, "the fixed amount is the same for both periods." The first assumption is common not only to crossover designs but to parallel single-period studies as well. The second assumption is the important one for crossover trials. This assumption implies that the response to a treatment received during period two should not be influenced by the treatment received during the first treatment period. Clearly, the assumption of no treatment-by-period interaction is not justified under any of the following conditions:

1. If the drug produces a permanent effect or "cure."
2. If the drug is excreted slowly.

3. If the drug produces delayed effects, either beneficial or adverse, beyond the "washout" period.
4. If the natural course of the disease being studied undergoes rapid change or evolution.

Base-line information can be utilized to sharpen estimation of treatment differences. For example, in both complete and incomplete crossover designs, defining the crossover criteria as a reduction from base line essentially negates the carry-over effect. Base line subtraction provides a simple procedure for adjusting the effect of sequence group differences. The only risk in assessing efficacy without the assumption of a sequence effect involves a situation in which a drug shows a carry-over effect without a main effect. In studies of chronic diseases, it is difficult to conceive of a situation in which there is a carry-over effect from a drug that has no main effect (24). Thus, crossover designs should not be employed unless the disease state of each patient is well characterized prior to administration of each treatment. Chassan (5), however, points out that the use of the two-period crossover design should be favored "whenever it is feasible."

The crossover design allows for estimation of parameters not available in a parallel study, that is, the combination of response probabilities to each drug. In phase II clinical testing, where sample size is small and no attempt is made to carry out a definitive study, the estimation of these individual response probabilities is sometimes more important than the estimation of the overall response rates. This is especially true in the treatment of neurological disorders, where both the standard drug and the investigational drug are sometimes generally ineffective, yet the investigational drug could possibly increase response by 30% more than if only the standard treatment were available.

REFERENCES

1. Atkins, H. (1966): Conduct of a controlled clinical trial. *Br. Med. J.,* 2:377–379.
2. Brown, B. W., Jr. (1978) *Statistical Controversies*

in *The Design of Clinical Trials. Technical Report No. 37.* Stanford University Press, Stanford, California.

3. Brown, B. W., Jr. (1979): *The Crossover Experiment for Clinical Trials. Technical Report No. 43.* Stanford University Press, Stanford, California.

4. Byar, D. P., Simon, R. M., Friedewald, W. T., Schlesselman, J. J., DeMets, D. L., Ellenberg, J. H., Gail, M. H., and Ware, J. H. (1976): Randomized clinical trials. Perspectives on some recent ideas. *N. Engl. J. Med.,* 295:74–80.

5. Chassan, J. B. (1970): Letter to the editor: A note on relative efficiency in clinical trials. *J. Clin. Pharmacol.,* 10:359–360.

6. Coatsworth, J. J. (1971): *Studies on the Clinical Efficacy of Marketed Antiepileptic Drugs.* DHEW Publication No. 73–51. National Institutes of Health, Bethesda, Maryland.

7. Cochran, W. G., and Cox, G. M. (1957): *Experimental Designs,* Second edition. John Wiley & Sons, New York.

8. Colton, T. (1963): A model for selecting one of two medical treatments. *J. Am. Stat. Assoc.,* 58:388–400.

9. Cournand, A. (1977): The code of the scientist and its relationship to ethics. *Science,* 198:699–705.

10. Curran, W. J. (1979): Reasonableness and randomization in clinical trials: Fundamental law and governmental regulation. *N. Engl. J. Med.,* 300:1273–1275.

11. Davis, A. W., and Hall, W. B. (1969): Cyclic changeover designs. *Biometrika,* 56:283–293.

12. Fisher, R. A. (1970): *Statistical Methods for Research Workers,* 14th edition. Hafner Press, New York.

13. Food and Drug Administration (1977): *General Considerations for the Clinical Evaluation of Drugs.* HEW (FDA) 77–3040. United States Government Printing Office, Washington, D.C.

14. Food and Drug Administration (1977): *Guidelines for the Clinical Evaluation of Anticonvulsant Drugs (Adults and Children).* HEW (FDA) 77-3045. United States Government Printing Office, Washington, D.C.

15. Fost, N. (1979): Consent as a barrier to research. *N. Engl. J. Med.,* 300:1272–1273.

16. Grizzle, J. E. (1965): The two-period change-over design and its use in clinical trials. *Biometrics,* 21:467–480.

17. Herbert, V. (1977): Acquiring new information while retaining old ethics. *Science,* 198:690–693.

18. Hill, A. B. (1948): Streptomycin treatment of pulmonary tuberculosis. A Medical Research Council investigation. *Br. Med. J.,* 2:769–782.

19. Hills, M., and Armitage, P. (1979): The two-period cross-over clinical trial. *Br. J. Clin. Pharmacol.,* 8:7–20.

20. Hoel, D. G., Sobel, M., and Weiss G. H. (1975): A survey of adaptive sampling for clinical trials. In: *Perspectives in Biometry,* edited by R. Elashof, pp. 29–60. Academic Press, New York.

21. Lindley, D. V. (1975): The effect of ethical design considerations on statistical analysis. *Appl. Stat.,* 24:281–228.

22. McNair, D. M. (1973): Antianxiety drugs and human performance. *Arch. Gen. Psychiatry,* 29:611–617.

23. Mike, V., and Good, R. A. (1977): Old problems, new challenges. *Science,* 198:677–678.

24. O'Neill R. (1977): Current status of crossover designs. Pharmaceutical Manufacturers Association Statisticians Meeting General Session, October 27, 1977, Arlington, Virginia.

25. O'Neill, R. T., and Cornfield, J. (1976): *Minutes of the Meeting of the Biometric and Epidemiological Methodology Advisory Committee, June 23, 1976.* Bureau of Drugs, United States Food and Drug Administration, Rockville, Maryland.

26. Patterson, H. D. (1951): Change-over trials. *J. R. Stat. Soc. [B.],* 13:256.

27. Patterson, H. D., and Lucas, H. L. (1962): *Change-over designs. Technical Bulletin No. 147.* NC Agricultural Experiment Station and U.S. Dept. of Agriculture, Washington, D.C.

28. Privacy Protection Study Commission (1977): *Personal Privacy in an Information Society.* United States Government Printing Office, Washington, D.C.

29. Relman, A. S. (1979): The ethics of randomized clinical trials: Two perspectives. *N. Engl. J. Med.,* 300:1272.

30. Sato, S., Penry, J. K., White, B. G., Dreifuss, F. E., and Sackellares, J. C. (1979): Double-blind crossover study of sodium valproate and ethosuximide in the treatment of absence seizures. *Neurology (Minneap.),* 29:603.

31. Simon, R. (1977): Adaptive treatment assignment methods and clinical trials. *Biometrics,* 33:743–749.

32. Simon, R., Weiss, G. H., and Hoel, D. G. (1975): Sequential analysis of binomial clinical trials. *Biometrika,* 62:195–200.

33. Tukey, J. (1977): Some thoughts on clinical trials, especially problems of multiplicity. *Science,* 198:679–684.

34. Weinstein, M. C. (1974): Allocation of subjects in medical experiments. *N. Engl. J. Med.,* 291:1278–1285.

35. White, B. G. (1979): *A Class of Ethical Designs for Controlled Clinical Trials.* Doctoral Dissertation, The Johns Hopkins University, Baltimore.

36. Zelen, M. (1979): A new design for randomized clinical trials. *N. Engl. J. Med.,* 300:1242–1245.

Antiepileptic Drugs, edited by D. M. Woodbury,
J. K. Penry, and C. E. Pippenger. Raven Press,
New York © 1982.

11

General Principles

Clinical Efficacy and Use of Antiepileptic Drugs

Roger J. Porter

This chapter discusses the clinical efficacy of antiepileptic drugs as determined from a review of 120 clinical trials published mostly between 1970 and 1980, using criteria set forth by Coatsworth (2) but including few of the studies from his review. It also discusses the selection of appropriate drug therapy based on the various seizure types.

CLINICAL EFFICACY

The first step in evaluating the efficacy of antiepileptic drugs is to determine what criteria will be used in deciding whether a drug actually works. Coatsworth (2) found that the deficiencies of many studies are primarily twofold: (a) failure to control data collection to insure that measurements are valid, reliable, and unbiased, and (b) failure to specify the types of attacks to be studied and to use the most objective methods of determining seizure frequency. He evaluated 110 clinical trials of antiepileptic drugs and found that only 12 to 15 of these trials were controlled; nearly 90% of the studies were only an open comparison of therapy added to previous standard medication.

Some of the clinical trials not included in Coatsworth's monograph were reviewed in 1977 (9), at which time it was recognized that the three most important additions to the antiepilep-

tic armamentarium had received the greatest attention from clinical investigators. These three drugs, carbamazepine, clonazepam, and valproate, continue to be the most prominent drugs in clinical studies.

Review of Clinical Trials

In the 120 clinical trials reviewed here, "excellent control" is defined as 50 to 100% reduction in seizures in at least 51% of the patients, "moderate control" indicates a 1 to 49% reduction in at least 51% of the patients, and "unchanged or worse" includes patients who derived no benefit from the trial or even became worse (2,9).

The operational definition of a clinical trial required that each study must be prospective, with an experimental design or plan (2). The majority of the 120 trials were uncontrolled. Only three, all studies of carbamazepine, occurred before 1970. It is of interest to note the different kinds of drugs or treatments, aside from clonazepam, valproate, and carbamazepine, that were studied (Table 1). There was considerable interest in the newer derivatives of successful antiepileptic drugs with sedative properties such as barbiturates and benzodiazepines and only minor interest in other compounds. There were no studies on the hydantoins or the diones.

TABLE 1. *Distribution of drugs or treatments in 32 clinical trials*

Drug or treatment[a]	Number of trials
Benzodiazepines	11
Barbiturates	5
Folate	3
Corticotropin (ACTH)	2
Ethosuximide	2
Taurine	2
Steroids	2
Albutoin	1
Cerebral phospholipids	1
Dantrolene	1
Depamide	1
Furosemide	1
γ-Amino-β-hydroxybutyric acid (GABOB)	1
Imipramine	1
Ketogenic diet	1
Lithium carbonate	1
Sulthiame	1

[a]Except clonazepam, valproate, and carbamazepine.

The study of barbiturates and benzodiazepines is an intriguing effort. Clinically, these potent antiepileptic drugs rarely manifest life-threatening toxicity, but even at usual doses, their sedative effects may be prominent in children and are too often ignored in adults (10,16). Clearly, the search continues for a less sedative but equally effective barbiturate or benzodiazepine. It is not known whether the mechanism of action of either of these classes of drugs is inextricably related to their sedative action, in which case this search is futile.

The most widely studied drug was clonazepam. It is the most potent antiepileptic drug marketed, and 39 trials were carried out on various seizure types (Table 2). Enthusiasm was strongest for its use in absence seizures, with some suggestion of effectiveness for partial and generalized tonic–clonic seizures. Objectionable features of this benzodiazepine are the primarily dose-related side effects of sedation, hyperactivity, and behavioral changes, which are especially notable in children (15). Another problem is the development of tolerance to its beneficial effects.

The second most studied drug was valproate or valproic acid; 30 trials were carried out. Again,

the drug resembles clonazepam in that its most impressive efficacy is for absence seizures. Although valproate is anecdotally reported to be effective for myoclonic seizures, this indication cannot be ascertained from this analysis of clinical trials, in which it appears to be no more effective than clonazepam. Valproate does appear to be effective against generalized tonic–clonic seizures, at least in some cases. Its effectiveness against partial seizures is less impressive.

There were 19 studies of carbamazepine. Presumably because of the established notion that this drug is most effective in partial and generalized tonic–clonic seizures, virtually all studies were in these seizure types, and all were enthusiastic about its efficacy.

Although it is difficult to obtain from the clinical trial data any clear indication of which drug is best for each seizure type, there are definitely preferred drugs in each case (Table 3).

CLINICAL USE

The proper use of antiepileptic drugs depends not only on a thorough understanding of their pharmacological characteristics, which are well described throughout this volume, but also on the knowledge of how these drugs are applied to the patient with epilepsy. Although efforts to relate drug efficacy to fundamental etiological processes are continuing, the most useful clinical criteria for deciding which drug is best for the patient comes from a knowledge of the patient's seizure type.

Seizure Classification

The application of appropriate drug therapy to the epilepsies requires knowledge of the seizure types and their classification. Continuous efforts have been undertaken to improve our ability to classify seizures empirically. Following the most notable advance in seizure classification (5), a series of three videotape workshops were conducted in the late 1970s under the auspices of the International League Against Epilepsy. Emerging from this effort is the most

TABLE 2. *Results of 88 clinical trials of clonazepam, valproate, and carbamazepine*

Drug	Number of trials	No. of trials by seizure type[a]							
		Simple partial	Complex partial	Generalized tonic–clonic	Absence	Myoclonic	Atonic	Infantile spasms	"Mixed" or undesignated
Excellent control									
Clonazepam	39	1	9	7	15	3	6	1	2
Valproate	30	1	4	5	17	3	3	1	1
Carbamazepine	19	2	12	13	1	0	0	0	1
Moderate control									
Clonazepam	39	4	8	6	4	2	0	3	5
Valproate	30	2	9	8	3	2	5	0	0
Carbamazepine	19	0	0	1	0	0	0	0	0
Unchanged or worse									
Clonazepam	39	2	5	5	1	0	1	3	0
Valproate	30	0	3	0	0	2	2	1	0
Carbamazepine	19	0	0	0	0	0	0	0	0

[a]Many trials included more than one seizure type.

TABLE 3. *Recommended drugs for various seizure types*

Decreasing likelihood of effectiveness	Partial seizures				Generalized seizures			
	Simple partial seizures	Complex partial seizures	Generalized tonic–clonic seizures	Absence seizures	Myoclonic seizures	Atonic seizures	Infantile spasms
1	Phenytoin	Carbamazepine	Phenytoin	Ethosuximide	Valproate	Valproate	ACTH
2	Carbamazepine	Phenytoin	Carbamazepine	Valproate	Ethosuximide		Steroids
3	Primidone	Primidone	Phenobarbital	Clonazepam	Clonazepam		Nitrazepam
4	Phenobarbital	Phenobarbital	Valproate	Methsuximide			Clonazepam

recent classification, generated from an analysis of the clinical and electroencephalographic characteristics of the recorded seizures. This classification is summarized below, but those who treat epilepsy will undoubtedly wish to refer to the original source (3).

Virtually all epileptic seizures can be divided into partial seizures and generalized seizures. Partial seizures are distinguished from generalized seizures by local onset, either clinically or electroencephalographically. Rarely, some seizures may not be classifiable in either of these categories.

Partial Seizures

Partial seizures are divided into three subgroups: simple, complex, and secondarily generalized. Simple partial seizures are characterized by preservation of normal consciousness. The attack is usually highly localized, such as jerking of one arm, and is limited in most cases to one hemisphere. The patient can describe the attack, either during or after its occurrence. Complex partial seizures are characterized by alteration of consciousness. They may be preceded by a simple partial seizure ("aura"), which warns the patient of possible progression to altered consciousness. Typically, complex partial attacks are accompanied by automatisms for which the patient has no memory. The patient usually recovers gradually and may be confused or lethargic for several minutes. Finally, any type of partial seizure may progress to a generalized tonic–clonic seizure or, in other words, become "secondarily generalized."

Generalized Seizures

Generalized seizures are a more heterogeneous group than the partial seizures. The most prominent is the generalized tonic–clonic (grand mal) seizure in which generalized muscle rigidity with opisthotonus gradually yields to increasing duration of the relaxation phases, and tonic rigidity thereby changes to clonic jerking. The jerking gradually wanes and ceases, leaving the patient stuporous or comatose. The attacks are commonly secondary to other seizure types, especially partial seizures, but the characteristics are nonetheless stereotyped.

Generalized tonic–clonic seizures presumably involve a maximum of neuronal systems compared to other types of seizures, but whole neuronal systems may remain uninvolved. Other types of generalized seizures, described below, presumably involve fewer neuronal systems than do generalized tonic–clonic seizures.

Absence seizures begin in childhood or adolescence and are characterized by a brief (usually less than 10–15 sec) interruption of consciousness. The attack is often accompanied by mild clonic jerking, usually of the eyelids, by increased or decreased postural tone, and by automatic behavior. The seizure almost always ceases abruptly, a useful criterion for separating absence seizures from complex partial seizures; such distinction is critical for appropriate drug therapy.

Atonic seizures are associated with a sudden loss of postural tone, and some patients wear helmets for head and face protection from resultant falls.

Clonic seizures and the myoclonias are exceedingly heterogeneous, and symptoms of clonic jerking often accompany other seizure types.

Finally, infantile spasms, a heterogeneous syndrome, begin in 90% of affected patients before the age of 1 year. The spasms usually manifest by sudden and often repetitive jerks of the extremities and torso. Most cases are accompanied by mental retardation.

Seizure Diagnosis

The key to the diagnosis and treatment of epilepsy is the patient's history. The history usually gives the information needed to make a "seizure diagnosis," which is generally based on the International Classification of Epileptic Seizures (5). Although not necessarily of etiological significance, the seizure diagnosis is extremely important therapeutically. The failure to establish a proper seizure diagnosis, either by history or special techniques such as intensive monitoring, often leads to poor seizure control and medication toxicity from improper drugs. Furthermore, the physician who is uncertain of the seizure diagnosis may use medications in a nonspecific way, resorting to the prescription of multiple drugs before single drugs have been given an adequate trial. The physician who is unquestionably dealing with absence seizures, for example, will utilize ethosuximide or valproate with confidence and vigor. When the seizure diagnosis is unknown, however, the usual starting medications are phenytoin or phenobarbital or both, often in subtherapeutic doses, and therapeutic efforts frequently end in failure and frustration.

Diagnostic Approach

The first priority, therefore, is to establish the seizure diagnosis. To accomplish this, the physician must obtain a detailed description of the attacks. Many patients are not prepared for this, and some will give a terminology-oriented description, using such terms as "petit mal" or "temporal lobe." The physician must reorient the patient to more fundamental, descriptive terms. If the patient is asked "What is the first thing that happens?" in a typical seizure, more useful information will be obtained. Patients with simple partial seizures, or those with auras only, will be able to describe the entire event by themselves, in logical sequence. Patients with complex partial seizures will need assistance, either from persons who have seen the attacks or from a knowledge of what they have been told. Another good question is, "What do other people see when you have a seizure?" Finally, it is important to learn whether the attack ends abruptly or whether it tapers into a postictal state. A positive response to the question "Do you feel 'bad' or 'tired' after an attack?" strongly suggests the presence of an abnormal postictal state, which would generally rule out, for example, absence seizures. Except when hysteria is suspected, it is not usually necessary to obtain a detailed description of generalized tonic–clonic seizures. They are generally stereotyped and often accompany a wide variety of more fundamental seizure types.

When the seizure diagnosis cannot be made from the history alone, the task becomes more difficult. Routine EEGs will be of some assistance, and activation procedures such as hyperventilation, photic stimulation, and sleep deprivation should always be included. Naturally, the physical and neurological examinations should be performed, but they are infrequently useful in making a seizure diagnosis. Computer-assisted tomography is also not particularly useful in this regard but may be helpful in finding unsuspected lesions; this is especially true in patients with chronic epilepsy who are not often restudied.

Intensive Monitoring of Intractable Seizures

Many patients with epilepsy are subject to seizures that are apparently resistant even to vigorous therapeutic efforts. Every seizure type is represented among these patients, but especially prevalent are infantile spasms and atonic/myoclonic attacks in children and partial seizures in both children and adults. A growing number of centers are beginning to recognize the value of the seizure diagnosis for these difficult patients and to utilize advanced techniques to obtain this information, especially when the historical data are inadequate and confirmation by more objective means is desired. Because a maximum degree of observation and control must be exercised for the period of evaluation, these techniques have been grouped under the heading "intensive monitoring" (12). Intensive monitoring consists of prolonged EEG recording, videotape recording of clinical seizures, and frequent determination of plasma antiepileptic drug concentrations.

Long-term EEG recording is useful when an ictal recording of a seizure is needed to assist in determining the seizure type. It also gives objective information about the severity of the disorder, as in absence seizures, where the number of spike–wave bursts may be counted; these have a high correlation with decreased mental function (1,11). Quantitation of these abnormal paroxysmal discharges also allows evaluation of the efficacy of therapy in absence seizures (6).

Long-term EEG recording is accomplished either by direct connection to the EEG machine or by telemetry; the latter allows freedom of movement for the patient and encourages a more normal environment. The various systems have been reviewed (14).

Videotape recording of seizures is the most effective way of establishing the seizure diagnosis. When the history is inadequate or even, surprisingly, when it appears to be rather good, a recorded attack can be revealing. Video analysis has been utilized to define the characteristics of absence seizures (7) and complex partial seizures (4,17), but much work remains for other types of attacks. Several methods of combining the televised view of the patient with the simultaneously recorded EEG have been developed (13).

Finally, frequent determination of antiepileptic drug concentrations is critical to intensive monitoring. These measurements should be performed daily and more often when indicated. The blood should be drawn prior to the morning dose of medication; the drug concentrations obtained at that time are more easily compared, as they are least affected by peaks of drug absorption. The following key elements are important in the proper utilization of antiepileptic drug determinations:

1. Antiepileptic drug monitoring is used only as a guide to changes in therapy; it is not a substitute for clinical judgment.
2. The determinations help achieve maximal effects of each medication.
3. Expected therapeutic concentrations are average values; each patient will have an individually optimal concentration.
4. The determinations are invaluable in the presence of toxic effects, especially in patients taking multiple drugs.
5. Noncompliance, malabsorption, and altered metabolism can be identified, but only the first is a common problem.
6. A reliable laboratory is critical to proper interpretation of the results (8).

Intensive monitoring helps to obtain, first, a correct diagnosis, and, second, maximal drug efficacy without toxicity. With the patient in the hospital, long-term videotape and EEG recordings are best obtained at the same time that medications are gradually discontinued. This discontinuation serves two purposes: it eliminates drugs that are thought to be inappropriate or unnecessarily toxic, and it causes a gradually increasing seizure frequency. The latter increases the yield of videotape and EEG recordings, permitting a seizure diagnosis as early as possible. Some medications, such as anti-absence drugs, can be stopped abruptly. Primidone and carbamazepine should be discontinued more slowly, and phenytoin, often the last drug to be removed, is removed cautiously to avoid excessive generalized tonic–clonic attacks.

Appropriate Drug Therapy

The selection of an appropriate antiepileptic drug depends on whether the patient has generalized or partial seizures (see Table 3). In some seizure types, such as certain myoclonic or atonic attacks in the Lennox–Gastaut syndrome, all drug therapy is of such dubious value that it is difficult to name any drugs that would have a high likelihood of success.

Partial Seizures

Partial seizures respond to the same drugs used for generalized tonic–clonic seizures, a coincidence that may reflect the secondary origin of most generalized tonic–clonic attacks. Phenytoin and carbamazepine are effective for partial seizures, and neither has a prominent sedative effect. In intractable cases, the two drugs can be used together; the use of barbiturates should be reserved for cases not responsive to this combination.

Generalized Seizures

Generalized tonic–clonic seizures are usually the easiest to treat. They respond to phenytoin or carbamazepine. In resistant cases, both drugs should be used together. If control is not possible with these drugs, it may be necessary to resort to a barbiturate or desoxybarbiturate.

In patients with absence attacks, three drugs, ethosuximide, valproate, and clonazepam, are all effective in a large percentage of cases. It is intriguing to note that the structures of these compounds are surprisingly different, suggesting that these drugs have different mechanisms of action. Of the other medications, phensuximide is too rapidly metabolized, methsuximide is more toxic than ethosuximide and probably is no more efficacious, and trimethadione, the first drug marketed as an antiabsence medication, has a relatively high toxicity potential. Of the three preferred drugs, clonazepam frequently causes sedation, irritability, and behavioral changes, and valproate, although nonsedative, has rare, but sometimes fatal idiosyncratic hepatotoxicity. Ethosuximide is therefore the drug of first choice, with valproate the second choice. Both of these drugs can cause nausea and vomiting, which is the most common complaint in treated children. Neither drug has significant sedative potential at usual doses, and the use of the two medications together may significantly reduce seizure frequency in the more refractory cases. In the 40 to 50% of patients with absence attacks who also have generalized tonic–clonic seizures, there may be some value in choosing valproate because of its wider spectrum of efficacy. The anectodal reports of worsening of generalized tonic–clonic seizures by ethosuximide are not generally substantiated, but neither does this compound have any efficacy for these major attacks.

Infantile spasms are an especially difficult syndrome. The prognosis is dismal, not so much for the attacks, which often respond at least temporarily, but for the associated mental retardation. ACTH or corticosteroids are moderately successful in controlling the frequency of the seizures. The benzodiazepines, notably clonazepam and nitrazepam (the latter is unavailable in the United States), also have some usefulness. Some European investigators who have experience with both nitrazepam and clonazepam find the former to be more efficacious.

Other agents used to treat this syndrome include valproate, mephobarbital, and phenobarbital.

Atonic seizures are also extremely resistant to therapy. The drugs most commonly used to treat this seizure type are valproate, clonazepam, and nitrazepam. None is very successful, but valproate may be the most effective.

CONCLUSION

The appropriate drug therapy for patients with epilepsy can only be indirectly inferred from clinical trials. Most important is the establishment of the seizure diagnosis. Antiepileptic drug therapy is most efficacious when the seizure type is correctly diagnosed so that the appropriate drug can be prescribed.

REFERENCES

1. Browne, T. R., Penry, J. K., Porter, R. J., and Dreifuss, F. E. (1974): Responsiveness before, during, and after spike–wave paroxysms. *Neurology (Minneap.),* 24:659–665.
2. Coatsworth, J. J. (1971): *Studies on the Clinical Efficacy of Marketed Antiepileptic Drugs, NINDS Monograph No. 12.* U.S. Government Printing Office, Washington.
3. Commission on Classification and Terminology of the International League Against Epilepsy (1981): Proposal for revised clinical and electroencephalographic classification of epileptic seizures. *Epilepsia,* 22:489–501.
4. Escueta, A. V., Kunze, U., Waddell, G., Boxley, J., and Nadel, A. (1977): Lapse of consciousness and automatisms in temporal lobe epilepsy: A videotape analysis. *Neurology (Minneap.),* 27:144–155.
5. Gastaut, H. (1970): Clinical and electroencephalographical classification of epileptic seizures. *Epilepsia,* 11:102–113.
6. Penry, J. K., Porter, R. J., and Dreifuss, F. E. (1972): Ethosuximide. Relation of plasma levels to clinical control. In: *Antiepileptic Drugs,* edited by D. M. Woodbury, J. K. Penry, and R. P. Schmidt, pp. 431–441. Raven Press, New York.
7. Penry, J. K., Porter, R. J., and Dreifuss, F. E. (1975): Simultaneous recording of absence seizures with video tape and electroencephalography. A study of 374 seizures in 48 patients. *Brain,* 98:427–440.
8. Pippenger, C. E., Paris-Kutt, H., Penry, J. K., and Daly, D. (1977): Proficiency testing in determinations of antiepileptic drugs. *J. Anal. Toxicol.,* 1:118–122.
9. Porter, R. J., and Penry, J. K. (1978): Efficacy and choice of antiepileptic drugs. In: *Advances in Epileptology, 1977: Psychology, Pharmacotherapy, and New Diagnostic Approaches,* edited by H. Meinardi and

A. J. Rowan, pp. 220–231. Swets & Zeitlinger, Amsterdam.

10. Porter, R. J., and Penry, J. K. (1980): Antiepileptic drugs. Phenobarbital: Biopharmacology. *Adv. Neurol.*, 27:493–500.

11. Porter, R. J., Penry, J. K., and Dreifuss, F. E. (1973): Responsiveness at the onset of spike–wave bursts. *Electroencephalogr. Clin. Neurophysiol.*, 34:239–245.

12. Porter, R. J., Penry, J. K., and Lacy, J. R. (1977): Diagnostic and therapeutic reevaluation of patients with intractable epilepsy. *Neurology (Minneap.)*, 27:1006–1011.

13. Porter, R. J., Penry, J. K., and Wolf, A. A., Jr. (1976): Simultaneous documentation of clinical and electroencephalographic manifestations of epileptic seizures. In: *Quantitative Analytic Studies in Epilepsy*, edited by P. Kellaway and I. Petersén, pp. 253–268. Raven Press, New York.

14. Porter, R. J., Wolf, A. A., Jr., and Penry, J. K. (1971): Human electroencephalographic telemetry. A review of systems and their applications and a new receiving system. *Am. J. EEG Technol.*, 11:145–159.

15. Sato, S., Penry, J. K., Dreifuss, F. E., and Dyken, P. R. (1977): Clonazepam in the treatment of absence seizures: A double-blind clinical trial. *Neurology (Minneap.)*, 27:371.

16. Theodore, W. H., and Porter, R. J. (1980): The removal of sedative antiepileptic drugs from the regimens of patients with intractable epilepsy (abstr). *Ann. Neurol.*, 8:93.

17. Theodore, W. H., Porter, R. J., and Penry, J. K. (1981): Complex partial seizures: A videotape analysis of 108 seizures in 25 patients (abstr). *Neurology (NY)* 31:108.

Antiepileptic Drugs. edited by D. M. Woodbury,
J. K. Penry, and C. E. Pippenger. Raven Press,
New York © 1982.

12

Phenytoin

Chemistry and Methods of Determination

Anthony J. Glazko

Phenytoin is the generic name for 5,5-diphenylhydantoin[1] (acid form), commonly known in this country as Dilantin® or diphenylhydantoin. It has the chemical structure shown in Fig. 1.

The free acid has a molecular weight of 252.26; the sodium salt has a molecular weight of 274.25, equivalent to acid content of 91.98%.

The acid form is used in formulations of aqueous suspensions (Pediatric Dilantin-30 Suspension® and Dilantin-125 Suspension®) containing 30 mg or 125 mg of phenytoin acid per 5 ml. The free acid is also used in formulating chewable tablets (Dilantin Infatabs®) containing 50 mg phenytoin acid per tablet. However, other products are formulated with the sodium salt of phenytoin (phenytoin sodium; acid equivalents = 91.98%). With these preparations, the drug content is expressed in terms of the sodium salt rather than the free acid. Thus, the gelatine capsules (Dilantin Sodium Kapseals®) are formulated to contain either 30 mg or 100 mg of phenytoin sodium (= 27.6 mg or 92.0 mg of phenytoin acid equivalents) per capsule. This 8% difference in drug content should be taken into account when changing from one product to another. The sodium salt is also used in combination with phenobarbital (Dilantin Sodium with Phenobarbital, Kapseals®) and in parenteral formulations (Parenteral Dilantin® = phenytoin sodium injection). The drug content is given in terms of the sodium salt.

To eliminate any confusion in terminology, phenytoin assays are expressed in terms of free acid equivalents. Concentrations are usually reported as micrograms of phenytoin per milliliter of biological fluid (μg/ml = mg/liter), but there has been a trend toward expressing concentrations on a molar basis (e.g., micromoles of phenytoin per liter). See formula for conversion, page 185.

Phenytoin is a weak organic acid that is poorly soluble in water. The apparent dissociation constant (pK_a'), representing the pH at which half the drug is ionized, was found to be in the range of 8.3 to 9.2 by nonaqueous titration in earlier

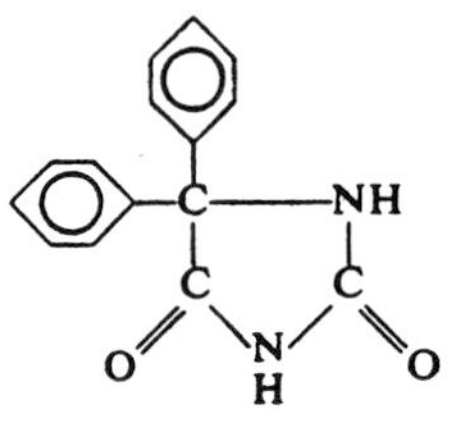

FIG. 1. Structure of phenytoin.

---

[1] *Chemical Abstracts* name is 5,5-diphenyl-2,4-imidazolidinedione.

work (3,39). Recent experiments by Schwartz et al. (78) based on solubility measurements indicated a true pK_a' of 8.06 in water. The acid was essentially nonionized at pH 5.4 (solubility about 19.4 μg/g at 25.4°C), whereas the data at pH 7.4 (about 80% nonionized) indicated a water solubility of 20.5 μg/g (25.2°C). Higher concentrations of phenytoin required strongly alkaline solutions, with solubility measurements of 165 μg/ml at pH 9.1 (borate buffer), and 1,520 μg/ml at pH 10 (sodium hydroxide) (38). Parenteral phenytoin sodium is made up in an aqueous vehicle containing propylene glycol, ethanol, and sodium hydroxide. It contains 50 mg phenytoin sodium per ml (= 46 mg phenytoin acid per ml). The solubility of phenytoin in blood plasma is about 75 μg/ml (37°C), at least in part because of binding of the drug on the plasma proteins (38).

Phenytoin sodium is not recommended as an analytical standard because of its variable water content and partial conversion to the free acid on exposure to carbon dioxide (38). Ishiguro et al. (49) measured the vapor pressure of hydrated forms of the sodium salt at different temperatures and concluded that the mono-, tetra-, hepta-, octa-, and hendecahydrates were present. The tetra- and heptahydrates appeared to be most stable under conditions of high humidity, with a moisture content of 20.8% and 31.5%, respectively. This group also reported that the absorption of CO_2 by phenytoin sodium increased with the degree of hydration, forming sodium bicarbonate and phenytoin acid (48).

ASSAY OF PHENYTOIN

The high degree of clinical interest in accurate phenytoin assays is reflected in the large number of papers on this subject that have appeared since our last review (38). This period has been marked by rapid expansion in high-performance liquid chromatography (HPLC), enzyme immunoassay (EMIT), and radioimmunoassay (RIA) techniques. At the same time, many improvements have been made in spectrophotometric techniques based on oxidation procedures and in gas–liquid chromatography (GLC) techniques. The latter have become especially valuable for the rapid detection and measurement of many different anticonvulsant drugs in single plasma specimens.

Spectrophotometric Methods

The colorimetric procedure for phenytoin originally described by Dill et al. (27) has been compared with GLC assays by Berlin et al. (9) using a modification of the procedure described by MacGee (59). Samples included those of patients taking phenobarbital and other drugs as well as those from patients taking phenytoin alone. The two procedures gave essentially the same results, but the standard deviation for single estimates was 0.2 μg/ml for the GLC procedure and 0.6 μg/ml for the colorimetric procedure. At low concentrations of phenytoin, the GLC procedure could be used down to 0.2 μg/ml with 200 μl of plasma, whereas the corresponding limit for the colorimetric procedure was 2 μg/ml with 3-ml plasma samples.

Similar comparisons have been made by Janz and Schmidt (50), between the GLC method of Kupferberg (56) and the UV absorbance procedure of Svensmark and Kristensen (87). Samples were taken from patients receiving only phenytoin. Assays on the same plasma samples were significantly higher by spectrophotometric assay (mean $\pm$ SD = 17.4 $\pm$ 11.3 μg/ml) than by GLC assay (11.7 $\pm$ 9.2 μg/ml).

Oxidation Procedures

A major step forward in spectrophotometric methods came with the introduction of oxidative procedures by Wallace et al. (95) in which phenytoin was converted to benzophenone. Bromine was first used to effect this conversion, later being replaced by alkaline permanganate (94). The beauty of this procedure is that phenobarbital and most other drugs do not interfere with the assay. However, the original Wallace procedure required large volumes of plasma (5–10 ml), involved extraction with chloroform, which interfered with the assay, and required specialized glassware for refluxing and distillation steps. As a result, numerous modifications of the Wallace procedure were introduced to make the procedure suitable for clinical use. Lee and Bass (85) used micro-Kjeldahl equipment to reduce the plasma volume to 1 ml. Morselli (65) eliminated the distillation step by extracting the benzophenone with benzene. Vessman et al. (93) used gas–liquid chromatography to measure the benzophenone. Dill et al. (25) eliminated the use of chloroform from the procedure and used powdered potassium permanganate to insure an excess of this reagent. They also eliminated the need for specialized reflux and distillation equipment by using glass-stoppered test tubes. A similar technique was described several years later by Fellenberg et al. (35).

Bock and Sherwin (10), Thurkow et al. (89), Meulenhoff et al. (62), and Saitoh et al. (75) further modified the Wallace procedure, reducing the volume of plasma to 0.1 ml. Wallace and Hamilton (96) also recognized the need for scaling down the assay procedure but retained their use of specialized reflux equipment. A major breakthrough in 1972 by Dill and Glazko (26) involved the development of a simple fluorometric assay procedure for benzophenone, resulting in greater sensitivity of the assay. Several years later, Morrison and O'Donnell (64) reported a phosphorescence procedure for benzophenone, requiring liquid nitrogen temperatures. In a more recent modification of the fluorometric procedure, Dill et al. (28) ran the permanganate oxidation directly on 0.2 ml of plasma, eliminating the need for preliminary extraction with organic solvents. Ordinary test tubes were used for the oxidation step, the benzophenone was extracted by vortexing with heptane, and fluorescence was developed by vortexing the heptane extract with concentrated sulfuric acid. There were no significant differences in plasma levels of phenytoin in 154 clinical specimens assayed by on-column methylation techniques (GLC) and by the fluorometric assay procedure. One operator can handle 40 to 60 samples per day, and the unit cost per sample is remarkably low.

Gas–Liquid Chromatography

By far the largest number of publications on assay methods for phenytoin deal with gas–liquid chromatography (GLC) procedures. The early phases of development in this area have been covered thoroughly in the first edition of *Antiepileptic Drugs* (38). MacGee's on-column methylation procedure with tetramethylammonium hydroxide (TMAH) (59) and Kupferberg's procedure with trimethylanilinium hydroxide (TMPAH) (56) are still widely used today, as is 5-(4-methylphenyl)-5-phenylhydantoin (MPPH), the internal standard originally introduced by Chang and Glazko (16,17). Dudley (32) discussed the desirable features of this internal standard, recommending it for use in GLC assays of multiple antiepileptic drugs. However, problems may arise because of differences in the chemical reactivity or thermal stability of certain drugs, making the use of multiple internal standards desirable.

Current trends are toward multidrug determinations, with equal emphasis on derivative and nonderivative techniques. Derivative formation is to be preferred because of more symmetrical peaks and better separation, better thermal stability, and shorter retention times. Also, the added time factor for on-column methylation techniques is negligible. Solow and co-workers (83,84) used a temperature-programmed version of MacGee's on-column methylation procedure (59) to quantitate numerous hydantoins, succinimides, and barbiturates. A typical run is shown in Fig. 2. Perchalski et al. (67,68) combined the best features of the MacGee (59) and Kupferberg (56) procedures and ran simultaneous assays for phenytoin, phenobarbital, and primidone. Cremers and Verheesen (23) extended the range of assays, using flash methylation for some components, with GLC being run on one column at three different temperatures. More recent multidrug assay procedures with on-column methylation in-

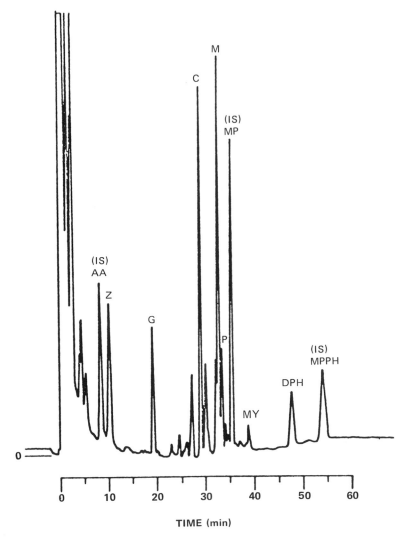

FIG. 2. Chromatograms showing peaks from antiepileptic drug analyses. On-column methylation procedure with tetramethylammonium hydroxide and 5% OV-17 on Gas Chrom Q (100/120 mesh) at 230°C. Z = Zarontin® (ethosuximide); G = Gemonil® (metharbital); C = desmethyl Celontin® (desmethylmethsuximide); M = Milontin® (phensuximide); P = phenobarbital; MY = Mysoline® (primidone); DPH = diphenylhydantoin; AA = α,dimethyl-β-methylsuccinimide; MP = 5-ethyl-5-tolylbarbituric acid; MPPH = 5-(*p*-methylphenyl)-5-phenylhydantoin. From Solow et al. (84), with permission of authors and Preston Publications, Inc.

clude those of Dorrity and Linnoila (29), Abraham and Joslin (1), and Hill and Latham (44). Different methylation conditions have been examined by Estes and Dumont (33) and by Serfontein and de Villiers (80). Other alkylating agents have also been employed, including flash ethylation with triethylammonium hydroxide (36)

and hexylation with tetrahexylammonium hydroxide (37). These may be of value in distinguishing *N*-demethylated metabolites from the parent compounds but offer no real advantages in the assay of phenytoin.

The GLC assay of phenytoin and other anticonvulsant drugs without derivatization has also been explored in depth, with numerous papers appearing in the past 11 years (57,60, 61,70,72–74,76,88,92). Pippenger and Gillen (70) used 1% HIEFF-8BP columns for the separation of a series of drugs without forming derivatives, but a plot of peak heights versus amount of drug did not produce a straight line passing through the origin (56). Sampson et al. (76) used a clean-up step to remove lipids as a possible source of interference. The precipitation of cholesterol as the digitonide was used by Driessen and Emonds (30) to reduce plasma blanks. Ritz and Warren (72) reported that a relatively polar liquid phase (3% OV-225) produced chromatograms comparable to those obtained with derivatization techniques. Brien and Inaba (12) used SE-30 columns with good results. Thoma et al. (88) acidified 0.25 to 0.5 ml plasma with 0.5 ml 1.5 M ammonium sulfate plus 3 drops 3 N HCl and extracted by shaking with 5 ml methylene chloride, resulting in a remarkably clean extract; GLC assays were carried out for underivatized phenobarbital, carbamazepine, primidone, phenytoin, and appropriate internal standards, using a newly developed column (2% SP 2110 + 1% SP2510-DA; Supelco, Inc., Bellefonte, PA). Toseland et al. (91) reported the use of nitrogen-selective detectors (Hewlett-Packard Model 1516A Nitrogen Detector) with nonderivatized anticonvulsant drugs. Because of the simplicity of these procedures and their applicability to the detection and measurement of many different anticonvulsant drugs, they may find a useful place in the clinical laboratory. However, to the analytical chemist, and for reasons already discussed, it seems likely that on-column methylation techniques will continue to find favor for most clinical applications.

Mass Spectrometry

Although the mass spectrometer is too highly specialized an instrument to be considered for general use, it can be used as a rather expensive detector for GLC analyses, extending the range of sensitivity five- to tenfold or more. It plays a more appropriate role as a tool for the structural identification of various derivatives and metabolites of drug products. MacGee (59) showed that the product of on-column methylation of phenytoin was the N,N-dimethyl derivative. This was confirmed by Estas and Dumont (33) who also identified the methylated derivative of the major metabolite of phenytoin (p-HPPH) as 1,3-dimethyl-5-(p-methoxyphenyl)-5-phenylhydantoin. Earlier work by Grimmer et al. (40) indicated that the methylation of phenytoin with diazomethane gave the N-3 monomethyl substituent, whereas similar treatment of p-HPPH produced the N-3 methyl, p-methoxyphenyl (dimethylated) derivative.

Rane et al. (71) used mass fragmentography and multiple ion detection to achieve a sensitivity of 0.01 µg phenytoin per ml. They were able to follow the transplacental passage of drug from mother to fetus using 100 µl of plasma for analysis. Hoppel et al. (45) also described the mass fragmentography of phenytoin and p-HPPH after extractive alkylation, using 10 to 100 µl of plasma. Baty and Robinson (8) used single and multiple ion detection to study the metabolic profile of subjects who had reached steady-state levels of phenytoin. Horning et al. (46) used chemical ionization techniques and selective ion detection to correlate blood plasma levels and breast milk levels after single 100-mg doses of phenytoin. Diazomethane was used as the alkylating agent prior to the introduction of the sample into the mass spectrometer. Lehrer and Karmen (58) also used chemical ionization techniques for the detection and rapid assay of a variety of drugs in serum, including phenytoin (with MPPH internal standard), barbiturates, carbamazepine, nicotine, and caffeine. Assay time in the mass spectrometer was 2 min per sample with direct probe insertion of samples.

High-Performance Liquid Chromatography

The use of HPLC has expanded rapidly in the past few years, with simplified instrumentation and more versatile detection systems readily available. Procedures are rapid, and derivative formation is not usually required. Solvent extraction steps can be eliminated by resorting to protein precipitation with acetonitrile, with assays being run directly on the supernatant. The HPLC technique is amenable to quantitation of multiple drugs in a single run, and it could readily displace GLC from its present favored position.

Anders and Latorre (5) reported the separation of phenytoin and p-HPPH by HPLC on an ion-exchange column, using only standard samples of drug. Evans (34) achieved better separation on silica gel columns and applied the technique to phenytoin and phenobarbital assays on 100-μl serum samples. This was preceded by ether extraction, and the time requirements were about the same as in the usual GLC procedures. Atwell et al. (7) used a silicic acid column but developed a better extraction procedure with methylene dichloride and used an internal standard. Inaba and Brien (47) worked with silica gel columns, but their methodology was directed primarily toward the assay of p-HPPH. Similarly, Albert et al. (4) assayed HPPH but reverted to the use of ion-exchange columns. Adams and Vandemark (2) separated a number of anticonvulsant drugs from serum by absorption on charcoal and elution with acetonitrile : water (17 : 83), the same solvent system used later for chromatography on a reverse-phase column. Phenacetin was used as the internal standard, and the phenytoin assay sensitivity was 0.1 μg/ml with 0.5-ml serum samples.

Kabra et al. (51) used MPPH as a more appropriate internal standard for phenytoin assays. Initial separation procedures included solvent extraction of drugs followed by HPLC on silicic acid columns. Later (53), the conditions were altered by eliminating the extraction step, using 2.5 volumes of acetonitrile to precipitate the proteins from 200-μl samples of plasma or serum. The supernatant was then injected onto a reverse-phase μBondapak®-C_{18} column (Waters Associates, Inc., Milford, MA) and developed with a mobile phase consisting of acetonitrile : pH 4.4 phosphate buffer (19 : 81). Soldin and Hill (82) employed a similar technique with acetonitrile and reverse-phase column chromatography, using a more alkaline

solvent. Slonek et al. (81) used essentially the same technique with a more acidic solvent system. Pesh-Imam et al. (69) also used a reverse-phase column with 5-μm Spherisorb-ODS particles (Altex, Inc., Berkeley, CA) and a mobile phase consisting of acetonitrile, water, and 1.75 M phosphoric acid (27 : 72.8 : 0.2). The method compared favorably with EMIT assays for phenobarbital, primidone, phenytoin, and carbamazepine.

Chamberlain et al. (15) compared their HPLC procedure [extraction with dichloromethane and chromatography on a Partisil®-10 column (Whatman, Clifton, NJ) using MPPH as an internal standard] with the on-column methylation procedure of MacGee (59) and found no statistically significant differences. The HPLC procedure had the lowest day-to-day variation (CV = 4.0%), cost factors were considerably lower than with the GLC procedure, and assay times were about the same. Helmsing et al. (42) and Schweizer (79) used Extrelut® columns (E. Merck, Darmstadt) for preliminary separation of drugs from plasma and other biological fluids, subsequently concentrating the ether eluate with good recovery of drug prior to HPLC or GLC.

Immunoassay Procedures

Two major advances have been made in this area: (a) application of radioimmunoassay procedures (RIA) to drug analysis (21,90) and (b) development of an enzyme-mediated immunoassay technique (EMIT) by the Syva Corp., Palo Alto, CA (77). Radioimmunoassay procedures are based on the binding of a radioisotope-labeled drug to a specific antibody and subsequent measurable displacement of the labeled drug by the addition of a sample containing an unknown amount of unlabeled drug. Assays for radioactivity can be run either on the residual protein-bound drug or on the displaced drug in the supernatant fluid.

Tigelaar et al. (90) prepared an antigen by coupling p-HPPH with chicken γ-globulin and produced an antiserum in rabbits. The RIA with ^{14}C-labeled phenytoin (4.65 mCi/mole) had adequate sensitivity to detect 0.03 μg phenytoin in 0.1 ml of sample, but there was strong cross reactivity with the metabolite p-HPPH. Similar products are marketed by Wien Laboratories, Inc., Succasunna, NJ, and by Clinical Assays, Inc., Cambridge, MA. Cook et al. (22) attached phenytoin to bovine serum albumin through a 5-carbon side chain in the N-3 position of the hydantoin ring and produced an antiserum with high specific activity for phenytoin and virtually no cross reactivity with p-HPPH. Orme et al. (66) compared the RIA procedure of Cook et al. (22) with the GLC procedure of Berlin et al. (9), and found excellent correlation.

The EMIT system eliminated the use of radioactivity as a measure of substrate release from the antibody. The drug is conjugated with a bacterial enzyme (glucose-6-phosphate dehydrogenase) that has no activity when bound to a drug-specific antibody. Thus, an antibody containing a fixed number of binding sites will equilibrate with free drug to reduce the number of available binding sites. Addition of the drug–enzyme complex will result in less binding to the antibody. This is illustrated schematically in Fig. 3. The decrease in enzyme activity provides a measure of drug concentration present in the EMIT system. The enzyme activity is measured by the rate of reaction with glucose-6-phosphate in the presence of the coenzyme factor NAD (nicotinamide adenine dinucleotide). This in turn is reduced to NADH and

measured by its absorbance at 340 nm. This method offers convenience and great rapidity of assay, but reagent costs are high.

Wong et al. (98) recently published a substrate-labeled fluorescent immunoassay (SLFIA) procedure using a single fluorometric reading rather than measurement of enzyme reaction rates. Galactosyl umbelliferone is coupled to a derivative of phenytoin and then bound to a specific antibody. In this form, the substrate is nonfluorescent in the presence of bacterial β-galactosidase. When phenytoin is added to this system, the drug–substrate conjugate is displaced in proportion to the concentration of phenytoin, and enzymatic hydrolysis takes place with the appearance of a fluorescent product. The assay procedure is highly sensitive, with assays possible on 2 μl of undiluted serum or 100 μl of 50-fold diluted serum. There is a 20-min equilibration period, and up to 40 assays can be set up in this time. No interference was encountered from other commonly used drugs. The metabolite p-HPPH at concentrations of 10- to 100-fold greater than normally encountered showed slight interference (10% error at concentrations greater than 35 μg/ml). A side-by-side comparison of clinical serum assays with the SLFIA procedure, the EMIT system, and a GLC assay showed good correlation for all three methods.

Booker and Darcey (11) compared EMIT with

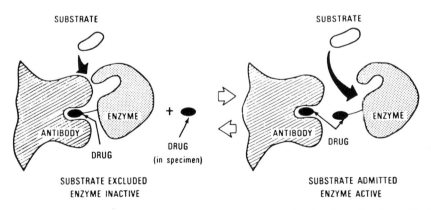

SUBSTRATE EXCLUDED
ENZYME INACTIVE

SUBSTRATE ADMITTED
ENZYME ACTIVE

FIG. 3. Homogeneous enzyme immunoassay. *Left:* enzyme labeled with drug bound to the antibody (enzyme inactive). *Right:* drug in patient's serum bound to the antibody, thus preventing binding of the drug-labeled enzyme (enzyme active). From Schottelius (77), with permission of author and publisher.

their own GLC procedure (chloroform extraction, residue dissolved in carbon disulfide, and GLC on 3% OV-17 with MPPH internal standard) and found good correlation. Spiehler et al. (86) compared phenytoin assays obtained with a commercially available RIA procedure (Wein Lab., Inc.), the EMIT system (Syva Corp.), and the GLC procedure of Perchalski et al. (67). A phenytoin level of 10 μg/ml by GLC corresponded with an average value of 12.7 ± 2.2 μg/ml (RIA), or 11.5 ± 1.0 μg/ml (EMIT). Castro et al. (14) also compared different assay procedures, including RIA (Wein) and EMIT (Syva), and concluded that the EMIT and HLPC procedures (2) were promising alternatives to the GLC and spectrophotometric methods. The same group (60) automated the EMIT system and found generally good correlation with other methods. Kampa et al. (54) compared the EMIT system with the RIA procedures of Wien Laboratories and Clinical Assays, Inc., and found good correlation among all three procedures.

Differential Pulse Polarography

Brooks et al. (13) applied the principle of controlled nitration to the assay of phenytoin and phenobarbital by differential pulse polarography, with a sensitivity of 1 to 2 μg/ml of blood. Practical difficulties in sample preparation and in the separation of phenobarbital from phenytoin prohibit its application to routine assays, but the technique is of interest from a research standpoint.

METABOLITES OF PHENYTOIN

The major metabolite of phenytoin in human subjects is 5-(4-hydroxyphenyl)-5-phenylhydantoin,[2] commonly known as p-HPPH. It has the chemical structure shown in Fig. 4. Its molecular weight is 268.26, and phenytoin acid equivalents are 94.04%.

This metabolite is excreted in the urine as a

---

[2]*Chemical Abstracts* name is 5-(4-hydroxyphenyl)-5-phenyl-2,4-imidazolidinedione.

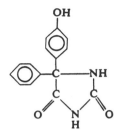

FIG. 4. Structure of 5-(4-hydroxyphenyl)-5-phenyl-hydantoin (p-HPPH).

conjugate of the phenolic group with glucuronic acid, yielding a highly water-soluble product. In order to extract the p-HPPH with an organic solvent, the conjugate must first be hydrolyzed by heating with hydrochloric acid or by treatment with an enzyme preparation containing β-glucuronidase, such as Glusulase® (Endo Laboratories, Inc., Garden City, NY). Dog urine contains large amounts of *meta*-hydroxylated phenytoin (m-HPPH) as well as p-HPPH, but only traces of m-HPPH are found in human urine. Most of the analytical methods that have been reported for phenytoin metabolites are directed toward p-HPPH because of clinical interest in this product. There are no well-established assay procedures for the dihydrodiol metabolite at the present time or for a number of minor catechol derivatives (see Chapter 14), although all have been characterized by GLC procedures (18–20).

Early reports indicated that derivatives of phenytoin and p-HPPH could be separated by GLC procedures and assayed. Chang and Glazko (16,17) used TMS derivatives and two internal standards (S_1 = MPPH; S_2 = m-HPPH). We provided MacGee with both internal standards for his work with dog urine. S_2 turned out to have the same retention time as an unknown peak in acid-hydrolyzed dog urine, later identified by Atkinson et al. (6) as m-HPPH. Consequently, we abandoned the use of S_2 as an internal standard for p-HPPH assays, replacing it with S_1. About the same time, Grimmer et al. (40) published a GLC assay procedure for p-HPPH using diazomethane for methylation and benz(a)anthracene as an internal standard.

Hammer et al. (41) used flash methylation with trimethylanilinium hydroxide to assay p-HPPH. During this period (1968–1971), Dill et al. (24) developed a solvent extraction procedure that effected nearly complete separation of phenytoin and p-HPPH, so that separate colorimetric assays could be run on these compounds. The benzophenone procedure does not work with p-HPPH, and colorimetric methods lack the sensitivity for good plasma level work with p-HPPH. With single 250-mg i.v. doses of phenytoin in adult subjects, the total p-HPPH levels in blood plasma after β-glucuronidase hydrolysis were all below 1 μg/ml. In more recent work, Glazko et al. (39), using a GLC assay procedure, reported total p-HPPH plasma levels after 300-mg doses of phenytoin once daily for 15 days to range from 1 to 3 μg/ml for subjects with short phenytoin half-lives and < 1 μg/ml for subjects with long phenytoin half-lives.

Other work on GLC procedures includes the use of flash methylation by Estas and Dumont (33) with MPPH as the internal standard and a 3% OV-17 column. Karlen et al. (55) also used flash methylation techniques. Urine was preextracted with isoamyl alcohol to remove the dihydrodiol metabolite which could interfere with the assay (20). Midah et al. (63) used enzymatic hydrolysis with β-glucuronidase, ether extraction, and flash methylation. Witkin et al. (97) used on-column methylation for GLC determination of p-HPPH, using a newly developed internal standard, 5-(p-hydroxyphenyl)-5-(p-methylphenyl)hydantoin. Acid-treated urine gave p-HPPH assays that were not significantly different from those obtained with β-glucuronidase-treated urine.

Driessen and Emonds (31) used short semi-capillary columns packed with a mixture of 2.6% OV-17 and 0.4% OV-225 at 260°C to run extracts of underivatized p-HPPH after enzymatic hydrolysis. The chemical identity of the p-HPPH peak was confirmed by mass spectroscopy. Hoppel et al. (45) used an extractive alkylation procedure with methyl iodide and mass fragmentography for the determination of unconjugated and total p-HPPH in 50 μl of plasma. Baty and Robinson (8) used a trimethylsilyl (TMS) derivative for mass fragmentography of p-HPPH. Deuterated internal standards were used in both of the mass spectrometry methods.

High-precision liquid chromatography assay methods for p-HPPH were introduced by Anders and Latorre (5) using an ion-exchange column, but they did not apply this to biological specimens. Inaba and Brien (47) used small-particle silica gel columns following acid hydrolysis of urine and extraction with ethyl acetate. Albert et al. (4) injected plasma samples directly into DEAE–cellulose anion-exchange columns before and after enzymatic hydrolysis. More recent work has gone in the direction of reversed-phase columns. Kabra and Marton (52) used μBondapak®-C$_{18}$ columns with acetonitrile : water (37 : 63) as the mobile phase and MPPH as the internal standard. Urine samples were acid hydrolyzed and extracted with ethyl acetate : dichloroethane (1 : 2). Hermansson and Karlen (43) were able to determine conjugated p-HPPH in urine by preliminary extraction with isoamyl alcohol to remove interfering substances, acid hydrolysis of the aqueous residue at 100° for 150 min, subsequent extraction at pH 7.5 with diethyl ether, and return to 0.1 M sodium hydroxide. The HPLC was carried out without derivatization on μBondapak®-C$_{18}$ with 27% ethanol in pH 3.2 acetate buffer (0.1 M). Slonek et al. (81) also used μBondapak®-C$_{18}$ columns with a mobile phase consisting of acetonitrile : water (30 : 70), acidified with phosphoric acid to pH 2.65 to 2.69. Deproteinization of spiked plasma specimens with acetonitrile resulted in the recovery of 100% phenytoin and 96% p-HPPH.

CONVERSION

Conversion factor:

$$CF = \frac{1000}{mol.\ wt.} = \frac{1000}{252.3} = 3.96$$

Conversion:

$$(\mu g/ml) \times 3.96 = (\mu moles/liter)$$

$$(\mu moles/liter) \div 3.96 = (\mu g/ml)$$

REFERENCES

1. Abraham, C. V., and Joslin, H. D. (1976): Simultaneous gas-chromatographic analysis for phenobarbital, diphenylhydantoin, carbamazepine, and primidone in serum. *Clin. Chem.*, 22:769–771.
2. Adams. R. F., and Vandemark, F. L. (1976): Simultaneous high-pressure liquid-chromatographic determination of some anticonvulsants in serum. *Clin. Chem.*, 22:25–31.
3. Agarwal, S. P., and Blake, M. I. (1968): Determination of the pK_a' value for 5,5-diphenylhydantoin. *J. Pharm. Sci.* 57:1434–1435.
4. Albert, K. S., Hallmark, M. R., Carroll, M. E., and Wagner, J. G. (1973): Quantitative separation of diphenylhydantoin and its parahydroxylated metabolites by high-performance liquid chromatography. *Res. Commun. Chem. Pathol. Pharmacol.*, 6:845–854.
5. Anders, M. W., and Latorre, J. P. (1970): High-speed ion exchange chromatography of barbiturates, diphenylhydantoin, and their hydroxylated metabolites. *Anal. Chem.*, 42:1430–1432.
6. Atkinson, A. J., MacGee, J., Strong, J., Garteiz, D., and Gaffney, T. E. (1970): Identification of 5-*meta*-hydroxyphenyl-5-phenylhydantoin as a metabolite of diphenylhydantoin. *Biochem. Pharmacol.*, 19: 2483–2491.
7. Atwell, S. H., Green, V. A., and Haney, W. G. (1975): Development and evaluation of method for simultaneous determination of phenobarbital and diphenylhydantoin in plasma by high-pressure liquid chromatography. *J. Pharm. Sci.*, 64:806–809.
8. Baty, J. D., and Robinson, P. R. (1977): Single and multiple ion recording techniques for the analysis of diphenylhydantoin and its major metabolite in plasma. *Biomed. Mass Spectrom.*, 4:36–41.
9. Berlin, A., Agurell, S., Borga, O., Lund, L., and Sjoqvist, F. (1972): Micromethod for the determination of diphenylhydantoin in plasma and cerebrospinal fluid—A comparison between a gas chromatographic and a spectrophotometric method. *Scand. J. Clin. Lab. Invest.*, 29:281–287.
10. Bock, G. W., and Sherwin, A. L. (1971): The rapid quantitative determination of diphenylhydantoin in plasma, serum, and whole blood of patients with epilepsy. *Clin. Chim. Acta*, 34:97–103.
11. Booker, H. E., and Darcey, B. A. (1975): Enzymatic immunoassay vs. gas/liquid chromatography for determination of phenobarbital and diphenylhydantoin in serum. *Clin. Chem.*, 21:1766–1768.
12. Brien, J. F., and Inaba, T. (1974): Determination of low levels of 5,5-diphenylhydantoin in serum by gas–liquid chromatography. *J. Chromatogr.*, 88: 265–270.
13. Brooks, M. A., de Silva, J. A. F, and Hackman, M. R. (1973): The determination of phenobarbital and diphenylhydantoin in blood by differential pulse polarography. *Anal. Chim. Acta*, 64:165–175.
14. Castro, A., Ibanez, J., DiCesare, J. L., Adams, R. F., and Malkus, H. (1978): Comparative determination of phenytoin by spectrophotometry, gas chromatography, liquid chromatography, enzyme immunoassay, and radioimmunoassay. *Clin. Chem.*, 24:710–713.

15. Chamberlain, R. T., Stafford, D. T., Maijub, A. G., and McNatt, B. C. (1977): High-pressure liquid chromatography and enzyme immunoassay compared with gas chromatography for determining phenytoin. *Clin. Chem.*, 23:1764–1766.
16. Chang, T., and Glazko, A. J. (1968): Quantitative assay of 5,5-diphenylhydantoin (DPH) and 5-(*p*-hydroxyphenyl)-5-phenylhydantoin (HPPH) in plasma and urine of human subjects. *Clin. Res.*, 16:339.
17. Chang, T., and Glazko, A. J. (1970): Quantitative assay of 5,5-diphenylhydantoin (Dilantin®) and 5-(*p*-hydroxyphenyl)-5-phenylhydantoin by gas–liquid chromatography. *J. Lab. Clin. Med.*, 75:145–155.
18. Chang, T., Okerholm, R. A., and Glazko, A. J. (1972): A 3-0-methylated metabolite of diphenylhydantoin (Dilantin®) in rat urine. *Res. Commun. Chem. Pathol. Pharmacol.*, 4:13–23.
19. Chang, T., Okerholm, R. A., and Glazko, A. J. (1972): Identification of 5-(3,4-dihydroxyphenyl)-5-phenylhydantoin: A metabolite of 5,5-diphenylhydantoin (Dilantin®) in rat urine. *Anal. Lett.*, 5:195–202.
20. Chang, T., Savory, A., and Glazko, A. J. (1970): A new metabolite of 5,5-diphenylhydantoin (Dilantin®). *Biochem. Biophys. Res. Commun.*, 38:444–449.
21. Cook, C. E. (1978): Radioimmunoassay. In: *Antiepileptic Drugs: Quantitative Analysis and Interpretation*, edited by C. E. Pippinger, J. K. Penry, and H. Kutt, pp. 163–173. Raven Press, New York.
22. Cook, C. E., Kepler, J. A., and Christensen, H. D. (1973): Antiserum to diphenylhydantoin: Preparation and characterization. *Res. Commun. Chem. Pathol. Pharmacol.*, 5:767–774.
23. Cremers, H. M. H. G., and Verheesen, P. E. (1973): A rapid method for the estimation of antiepileptic drugs in blood serum by gas–liquid chromatography. *Clin. Chim. Acta*, 48:413–420.
24. Dill, W. A., Baukema, J., Chang, T., and Glazko, A. J. (1971): Colorimetric assay of 5,5-diphenylhydantoin (Dilantin®) and 5-(*p*-hydroxyphenyl)-5-phenylhydantoin. *Proc. Soc. Exp. Biol. Med.*, 137:674–679.
25. Dill, W. A., Chucot, L., Chang, T., and Glazko, A. J. (1971): Simplified benzophenone procedure for determination of diphenylhydantoin in plasma. *Clin. Chem.*, 17:1200–1201.
26. Dill, W. A., and Glazko, A. J. (1972): Fluorometric assay of diphenylhydantoin in plasma or whole blood. *Clin. Chem.*, 18:675–676.
27. Dill, W. A., Kazenko, A., Wolf, L. M., and Glazko, A. J. (1956): Studies on 5,5-diphenylhydantoin (Dilantin®) in animals and man. *J. Pharmacol. Exp. Ther.*, 118:270–279.
28. Dill, W. A., Leung, A., Kinkel, A., and Glazko, A. J. (1976): Simplified fluorometric assay for diphenylhydantoin in plasma. *Clin. Chem.* 22:908–911.
29. Dorrity, F., Jr., and Linnoila, M. (1976): Rapid gas-chromatographic measurement of anticonvulsant drugs in serum. *Clin. Chem.*, 22:860–862.
30. Driessen, O., and Emonds, A. (1974): Simultaneous determination of anti-epileptic drugs in small samples of blood plasma by gas chromatography, column technology and extraction procedure. *Proc. Kon. Med. Acad. von Wetenschr.*, C77:171–181.
31. Driessen, O., and Emonds, A. (1975): Routine anal-

ysis of 5-(p-hydroxyphenyl)-5-phenylhydantoin in plasma. Proc. Kon. Med. Acad. von Wetenschr., C78:449–460.

32. Dudley, K. H. (1978): Internal standards in gas–liquid chromatographic determination of antiepileptic drugs. In: Antiepileptic Drugs: Quantitative Analysis and Interpretation, edited by C. E. Pippenger, J. K. Penry, and H. Kutt, pp. 19–34. Raven Press, New York.

33. Estas, A., and Dumont, P. A. (1973): Simultaneous determination of 5,5-diphenylhydantoin and 5-(p-hydroxyphenyl)-5-phenylhydantoin in serum, urine and tissues by gas–liquid chromatography after flash-heater methylation. J. Chromatogr., 82:307–314.

34. Evans, J. E. (1973): Simultaneous measurement of diphenylhydantoin and phenobarbital in serum by high performance liquid chromatography. Anal. Chem., 45:2428–2429.

35. Fellenberg, A. J., Magarey, A., and Pollard, A. C. (1975): An improved benzophenone procedure for the micro-determination of 5,5-diphenylhydantoin in blood. Clin. Chim. Acta, 59:155–160.

36. Friel, P., and Troupin, A. S. (1975): Flash-heater ethylation of some antiepileptic drugs. Clin. Chem., 21:751–754.

37. Giovanniello, T. J., and Pecci, J. (1976): Simultaneous isothermal determination of diphenylhydantoin and phenobarbital serum levels by gas–liquid chromatography following flash-heater hexylation. Clin. Chim. Acta, 67:7–13.

38. Glazko, A. J. (1972): Diphenylhydantoin: Chemistry and methods of determinaton. In: Antiepileptic Drugs, edited by D. M. Woodbury, J. K. Penry, and R. P. Schmidt, pp. 103–112. Raven Press, New York.

39. Glazko, A. J., Peterson, F. E., Smith, T. C., Dill, W. A., and Chang, T. (1980): Phenytoin metabolism in human subjects with short and long plasma half-lives. Fed. Proc., 39:1099.

40. Grimmer, G., Jacob, J., and Schäfer, H. (1969): Die gaschromatographische Bestimmung von 5,5-diphenylhydantoin und 5-(p-Hydroxyphenyl)-5-phenylhydantoin im Blut. Arzneim. Forsch., 19:1287–1290.

41. Hammer, R. H., Wilder, B. J., Streiff, R. R., and Mayersdorf, A. (1971): Flash methylation and GLC of diphenylhydantoin and 5-(p-hydroxyphenyl)-5-phenylhydantoin. J. Pharm. Sci., 60:327–329.

42. Helmsing, P. J., Van Der Woude, J., and Van Eupen, O. M. (1978): A micromethod for simultaneous estimation of blood levels of some commonly used antiepileptic drugs. Clin. Chim. Acta, 89:301–309.

43. Hermansson, J., and Karlen, B. (1977): Assay of the major (4-hydroxylated) metabolite of diphenylhydantoin in human urine by reversed-phase high-performance liquid chromatography. J. Chromatogr., 130:422–425.

44. Hill, R. E., and Latham, A. N. (1977): Simultaneous determination of anticonvulsant drugs by gas–liquid chromatography. J. Chromatogr., 131:341–346.

45. Hoppel, C., Garle, M., and Elander, M. (1976): Mass fragmentographic determination of diphenylhydantoin and its main metabolite, 5-(4-hydroxyphenyl)-5-phenylhydantoin, in human plasma. J. Chromatogr., 116:53–61.

46. Horning, M. G., Lertratanangkoon, K., Nowlin, J.,

Stillwell, W. G., Stillwell, R. N., Zion, T. E., Kellaway, P., and Hill, R. M. (1974): Anticonvulsant drug monitoring by GC-MS-COM techniques. J. Chromatogr. Sci., 12:630–635.

47. Inaba, T., and Brien, J. F. (1973): Determination of the major urinary metabolite of diphenylhydantoin by high-performance liquid chromatography. J. Chromctogr., 80:161–165.

48. Ishiguro, T., Kozatani, J., and Otsuka, A. (1955): Absorption of carbon dioxide on diphenylhydantoin sodium hydrates. J. Pharm. Soc. Jpn., 75:1556–1559.

49. Ishiguro, T., Kozatani, J., and Shibata, K. (1958): Physico–chemical studies of sodium salts of diphenylhydantoin hydrates. VI. Hygroscopic behavior and dissociation pressure of diphenylhydantoin sodium hydrates. J. Pharm. Soc. Jpn., 78:391–394.

50. Janz, D., and Schmidt, D. (1974): Comparison of spectrophotometric and gas–liquid chromatographic measurements of serum diphenylhydantoin concentrations in epileptic out-patients. J. Neurol., 207:109–116.

51. Kabra, P. M., Gotelli, G., Stanfill, R., and Marton, L. J. (1976): Simultaneous measurement of phenobarbital, diphenylhydantoin, and primidone in blood by high-pressure liquid chromatography. Clin. Chem., 22:824–827.

52. Kabra, P. M., and Marton, L. J. (1976): High-pressure liquid-chromatographic determination of 5-(4-hydroxyphenyl)-5-phenylhydantoin in human urine. Clin. Chem. 22:1672–1674.

53. Kabra, P. M., Stafford, B. E., and Marton, L. J. (1977): Simultaneous measurement of phenobarbital, phenytoin, primidone, ethosuximide and carbamazepine in serum by high-pressure liquid chromatography. Clin. Chem., 23:1284–1288.

54. Kampa, I. S., Jarzabek, J., and Hundertmark, J. M. (1978): A comparison of the "EMIT" assay with two iodinated radioimmunoassays for diphenylhydantoin. Clin. Biochem., 11:167–168.

55. Karlen, B., Garle, M., Rane, A., Gutova, M., and Lindborg, B. (1975): Assay of the major (4-hydroxylated) metabolites of diphenylhydantoin in human urine. Eur. J. Clin. Pharmacol., 8:359–363.

56. Kupferberg, H. J. (1970): Quantitative estimation of diphenylhydantoin, primidone and phenobarbital in plasma by gas–liquid chromatography. Clin. Chim. Acta, 29:283–288.

57. Latham, A. N., and Varlow, G. (1976): Simultaneous quantitative gas-chromatographic analysis of ethosuximide, phenobarbitone, primidone and diphenylhydantoin. Br. J. Clin. Pharmacol., 3:145–150.

58. Lehrer, M., and Karmen, A. (1976): Chemical ionization mass spectrometry for rapid assay of drugs in serum. J. Chromatogr., 126:615–623.

59. MacGee, J. (1970): Rapid determination of diphenylhydantoin in blood plasma by gas–liquid chromatography. Anal. Chem., 42:421–422.

60. Malkus, H., DiCesare, J. L., Meola, J. M., Pippenger, C. E., Ibanez, J., and Castro, A. (1978): Evaluation of EMIT methods for the determination of the five major antiepileptic drugs on an automated kinetic analyzer. Clin. Biochem., 11:139–142.

61. Meijer, J. W. A. (1971): Simultaneous quantitative

determination of anti-epileptic drugs, including carbamazepine, in body fluids. *Epilepsia,* 12:341–352.

62. Meulenhoff, J. S., and Lojenga, J. C. K. (1972): Details of the Wallace method for the determination of phenytoin in blood, plasma and serum. *Pharm. Weekbl.,* 107:737–744.

63. Midah, K. K., McGilveray, I. J., and Wilson, D. L. (1976): Sensitive GLC procedure for simultaneous determination of phenytoin and its major metabolite from plasma following single doses of phenytoin. *J. Pharm. Sci.,* 65:1240–1243.

64. Morrison, L. D., and O'Donnell (1974): Determination of diphenylhydantoin by phosphorescence spectrometry. *Anal. Chem.,* 46:1119–1120.

65. Morselli, P. L. (1970): An improved technique for routine determinations of diphenylhydantoin in plasma and tissues. Clin. Chim. Acta, 28:37–40.

66. Orme, M. l'E., Borga, O., Cooke, C. E., and Sjoqvist, F. (1976): Measurement of diphenylhydantoin in 0.1-ml plasma samples: Gas chromatography and radioimmunoassay compared. *Clin. Chem.,* 22:246–249.

67. Perchalski, R. J., Scott, K. N., Wilder, R. J., and Hammer, R. H. (1973): Rapid, simultaneous GLC determination of phenobarbital, primidone and diphenylhydantoin. *J. Pharm. Sci.,* 62:1735–1736.

68. Perchalski, R. J., and Wilder, B. J. (1974): GLC microdetermination of plasma anticonvulsant levels. *J. Pharm. Sci.,* 63:806–807.

69. Pesh-Imam, M., Fretthold, D. W., Sunshine, I., Kumar, S., Terrentine, S., and Willis, C. E. (1979): High-pressure liquid chromatography for simultaneous analysis of anticonvulsants: Comparison with EMIT® system. *Ther. Drug Monit.,* 1:289–299.

70. Pippenger, C. E., and Gillen, H. W. (1969): Gas chromatographic analysis for anticonvulsant drugs in biological fluids. *Clin. Chem.,* 15:582–590.

71. Rane, A., Garle, M., Borga, O., and Sjoqvist, F. (1974): Plasma disappearance of transplacentally transferred diphenylhydantoin in the newborn studied by mass fragmentography. *Clin. Pharmacol. Ther.,* 15:39–45.

72. Ritz, D. P., and Warren, C. G. (1975): Single extraction GLC analysis of six commonly prescribed antiepileptic drugs. *Clin. Toxicol.,* 8:311–324.

73. Rutherford, D. M., and Flanagan, R. J. (1978): Rapid micro-method for the measurement of phenobarbitone, primidone and phenytoin in blood plasma or serum by gas–liquid chromatography. *J. Chromatogr.,* 157:311–320.

74. Sabih, K., and Sabih, K. (1969): Gas chromatographic method for determination of diphenylhydantoin blood level. *Anal. Chem.,* 41:1452–1454.

75. Saitoh, Y., Nishihara, K., Nakagawa, F., and Suzuki, T. (1973): Improved microdetermination for diphenylhydantoin in blood by UV spectrophotometry. *J. Pharm. Sci.,* 62:206–210.

76. Sampson, D., Harasymiv, I., and Hensley, W. J. (1971): Gas chromatographic assay of underivatized 5,5-diphenylhydantoin (Dilantin) in plasma extracts. *Clin. Chem.,* 17:382–385.

77. Schottelius, D. D. (1978): Homogeneous immunoassay system (EMIT) for quantitation of antiepileptic

drugs in biological fluids. In: *Antiepileptic Drugs: Quantitative Analysis and Interpretation,* edited by C. E. Pippenger, J. K. Penry, and H. Kutt, pp. 95–108. Raven Press, New York.

78. Schwartz, P. A., Rhodes, C. T., and Cooper, J. W., Jr. (1977): Solubility and ionization characteristics of phenytoin. *J. Pharm. Sci.,* 66:994–997.

79. Schweizer, K., Wick, H., and Brechbühler, T. (1978): An improved method for preparation of samples for the simultaneous assay of some antiepileptic drugs by gas–liquid chromatography. *Clin. Chim. Acta,* 90:203–208.

80. Serfontein, W. J., and de Villiers, L. S. (1977): Quantitative gas chromatographic analysis of barbiturates and hydantoins with quarternary ammonium hydroxides. *J. Chromatogr.,* 130:342–345.

81. Slonek, J. E., Peng, G. W., and Chiou, W. L. (1978): Rapid and micro high-pressure liquid chromatographic determination of plasma phenytoin levels. *J. Pharm. Sci.,* 67:1462–1464.

82. Soldin, S. J., and Hill, J. G. (1976): Rapid micromethod for measuring anticonvulsant drugs in serum by high-performance liquid chromatography. *Clin. Chem.,* 22:856–859.

83. Solow, E. B., and Green, J. B. (1972): The simultaneous determination of multiple anticonvulsant drug levels by gas–liquid chromatography. *Neurology, (Minneap.),* 22:540–550.

84. Solow, E. B., Metaxas, J. M., and Summers, T. R. (1974): Antiepileptic drugs: A current assessment of simultaneous determination of multiple drug therapy by gas liquid chromatography on-column methylation. *J. Chromatogr. Sci.,* 12:256–260.

85. Soo Ik Lee, and Bass, N. H. (1970): Microassay of diphenylhydantoin. Blood and regional brain concentrations in rats during acute intoxication. *Neurology (Minneap.),* 20:115–124.

86. Spiehler, V., Sun, L., Miyada, D. S., Sarandis, S. G., Walwick, E. R., Klein, M. W., Jordan, D. B., and Jessen, B. (1976): Radioimmunoassay, enzyme immunoassay, spectrophotometry, and gas–liquid chromatography compared for determination of phenobarbital and diphenylhydantoin. *Clin. Chem.,* 22:749–753.

87. Svensmark, O., and Kristensen, P. (1963): Determination of diphenylhydantoin and phenobarbital in small amounts of serum. *J. Lab. Clin. Med.,* 61:501–507.

88. Thoma, J. J., Ewald, T., and McCoy, M. (1978): Simultaneous analysis of underivatized phenobarbital, carbamazepine, primidone, and phenytoin by isothermal gas–liquid chromatography. *J. Anal. Toxicol.,* 2:219–225.

89. Thürkow, I., Wesseling, H., and Meijer, D. K. F. (1972): Estimation of phenytoin in body fluids in the presence of sulfonyl urea compounds. *Clin. Chim. Acta,* 37:509–513.

90. Tigelaar, R. E., Rapport, R. L., Inman, J. K., and Kupferberg, H. J. (1973): A radioimmunoassay for diphenylhydantoin. *Clin. Chim. Acta,* 43:231–241.

91. Toseland, P. A., Albani, M., and Gauchel, F. D. (1975): Organic nitrogen-selective detector used in gas-chromatographic determination of some anticon-

vulsant and barbiturate drugs in plasma and tissues. *Clin. Chem.,* 21:98–103.

92. Van Meter, J. C., Buckmaster, H. S., and Shelley, L. L. (1970): Concurrent assay of phenobarbital and diphenylhydantoin in plasma by vapor-phase chromatography. *Clin. Chem.,* 16:135–138.

93. Vessman, J., Hartvig, P., and Strömberg, S. (1970): Gas chromatography and electron capture detection of benzophenone formed by chromic acid oxidation. Part 3. Applications in the determination of *gem*-diphenyl-substituted compounds. *Acta Pharm. Suec.,* 7:373–388.

94. Wallace, J. E. (1966): Spectrophotometric determination of diphenylhydantoin. *J. Forensic Sci.,* 11:552–559.

95. Wallace, J., Biggs, J., and Dahl, E. V. (1965): De-termination of diphenylhydantoin by ultraviolet spectrophotometry. *Anal. Chem.,* 37:410–413.

96. Wallace, J. E., and Hamilton, H. E. (1974): Diphenylhydantoin microdetermination in serum and plasma by UV spectrophotometry. *J. Pharm. Sci.,* 63:1795–1798.

97. Watkin, K. M., Bius, D. L., Teague, B. L., Wiese, L. S., Boyles, L. W, and Dudley, K. H. (1979): Determination of 5-(*p*-hydroxyphenyl)-5-phenylhydantoin and studies relating to the disposition of phenytoin in man. *Ther. Drug. Monitor,* 1:11–34.

98. Wong, R. C., Burd, J. F., Carrico, R. J., Buckler, R. T., Thoma, J., and Boguslaski, R. C. (1979): Substrate-labeled fluorescent immunoassay for phenytoin in human serum. *Clin. Chem.,* 25:686–691.

Antiepileptic Drugs, edited by D. M. Woodbury, J. K. Penry, and C. E. Pippenger. Raven Press, New York © 1982.

13

Phenytoin

Absorption, Distribution, and Excretion

Dixon M. Woodbury

The many sites at which phenytoin (PHT) acts, its receptors, must be reached before its action can take place. This involves movement of PHT from the site of entrance into the body into the blood stream (absorption), distribution in blood and extracellular fluids to the cell boundaries, and passage across the cell membranes into cells and across subcellular membranes into subcellular organelles. The amount of PHT that reaches the receptor and its duration of stay there depend on its rate of biotransformation and excretion from the body. It is the purpose of this chapter to describe the absorption, distribution, and excretion of PHT in the body and to discuss the factors that affect these processes. This is of obvious clinical importance, for therapy with the drug is useless if sufficient drug does not reach its site of action. A knowledge and proper use of this information will often change a therapeutic failure into a triumphant success.

ABSORPTION

The absorption of PHT from its site of entrance into the body (e.g., oral, intramuscular) as is the case with other drugs, depends on the following factors: its pK_a and lipid solubility, the pH of the medium in which PHT is dis-

solved, its solubility in the medium, and its concentration.

These factors are frequently altered by the presence of certain foods or drugs in the intestinal tract and by the formulations employed. The latter is of particular importance, since aqueous liquids of the pure chemical are commonly employed in the laboratory, whereas more complex formulations of liquids, capsules, and tablets are employed clinically. As is now well known, the chemical form employed, the particle size, the filler and masking agents used in the clinical formulation, and the tablet hardness, all of which can affect dissolution rate, may have a marked effect on the absorption of PHT from the gastrointestinal tract.

In the stomach, little absorption of PHT occurs because it is extremely insoluble at the pH of gastric juice (about 2.0). Thus, despite the fact that at the reported pK_a value of 8.31 (16, see also 45) PHT exists predominantly in the un-ionized form and should be absorbed readily by passive diffusion, it achieves only a very low concentration in the gastric juice and consequently is only poorly and slowly absorbed (16). The simultaneous administration of PHT and an antacid decreases the absorption of PHT and thereby decreases the plasma level below the value it would normally attain.

On passage into the duodenum where the pH is approximately 7 to 7.5, more of the drug exists in the ionized form and hence is considerably more soluble in the intestinal fluid. The bile salts also increase the solubility of the drug. In addition, the surface area for absorption is much larger in the duodenum. Thus, absorption can take place rapidly, and it is at this site that the maximum absorption of PHT occurs. Absorption from the jejunum and ileum is slower than from the duodenum and is poor from the colon (53,71). Rectal absorption does not occur (53). The distal portion of the duodenum is also the site of maximum reabsorption of PHT after its intravenous injection (57). As shown in Table 1, 4 hr after 100 mg of PHT was injected into the isolated stomach, Dill et al. (16) demonstrated that the plasma contained 0.6 μg/ml of PHT, whereas with the drug in the upper and lower small intestine, the plasma levels were 3.8 and 1.5 μg/ml, respectively. Lesser amounts, 0.9 and 0.7 μg/ml, appeared in the plasma when the same dose was placed in the caecum and large intestine, respectively. These observations support the fact that PHT is relatively insoluble at the pH of the gastric juice and that significant absorption does not take place until the drug reaches the upper part of the small intestine. However, PHT can rapidly cross the intestinal wall in both directions in all portions of the intestinal tract (57).

Even at the higher pH of the intestinal fluid, PHT is relatively insoluble, and its rate of absorption depends mainly on the rate at which it can enter the blood stream, as discussed below. At pH 7.8 and 37°C, PHT is soluble in intestinal fluid to the extent of about 100 μg/ml. In man, the usual single oral dose is 100 mg, and this is distributed only in a maximum of 1,000 ml of intestinal fluid even if complete mixing occurs. Since it is soluble to the extent of only 100 μg/ml, and the amount of fluid in which it is actually dissolved is much less than 1,000 ml, some is left undissolved. This remaining portion can be solubilized only after that already in solution is absorbed, a process that is limited by the fact the solubility of PHT in plasma is only 75 μg/ml at 37°C. Thus, absorption can occur only at the rate at which PHT is removed from the blood stream by storage in fat, binding to plasma and tissue constituents, biotransformation by liver, and excretion into bile or urine. Since most of the PHT in solution is in the unionized form and is relatively lipid soluble (log octanol/water partition coefficient, 2.23), it is readily absorbed across the lipid membranes of the mucosal cells of the intestinal tract; hence, passage across these cells is not a limiting factor. Thus, dissolution in the gastrointestinal fluids is the rate-limiting process in the absorption of PHT.

The results of experiments in rats and mice (94) show that there is a linear relationship between the percent of PHT absorbed and the dose of drug placed in isolated intestinal loops. Absorption was virtually 100% complete within 90 min in both species when the concentration of PHT was 100 μg/ml. With solutions of 500 μg/ml and above, there was a linear relationship between the log dose placed in the loops and the percent absorbed. Thus, it would appear that the rate of absorption in the two species is the same.

After oral doses of 5 to 250 mg/kg of PHT were given to rats and mice, the plasma levels in the rats were always considerably lower than those of the mice. A dose–effect relationship between plasma levels of PHT and oral dosage was noted for mice but not for rats, where the levels reached a plateau with dosages above 66 mg/kg. It is likely that this plateau represents a dose range at which PHT is saturating the intestinal fluids and has reached the limit of solu-

TABLE 1. *Absorption of PHT[a] from isolated segments of rat gastrointestinal tract*

Segment injected	Plasma PHT level (μg/ml)
Stomach	0.6
Upper small intestine	3.8
Lower small intestine	1.5
Caecum	0.9
Large intestine	0.7

[a]100 mg placed in each section; plasma PHT levels determined 4 hr after dosage.

After Dill et al. (16), with permission.

bility. Thus, the plateau represents an equilibration between the stabilizing of the PHT in the gastrointestinal tract and absorption into the plasma at a rate determined by the factors mentioned above, of which metabolism by the liver and protein binding are probably most important, since the former is faster and the latter larger in the rat than in the mouse. These differences between rats and mice can explain the greater LD_{50} and TD_{50} in rats than in mice.

Thus, any factor that interferes with the dissolution of PHT or its solubility in intestinal fluids will delay its absorption. For example, the formulation of PHT preparations for oral use is important, as documented by Glazko and Chang (26). They compared in dogs the absorption of different size particles of PHT. The dissolution rate of the large particles was slower than that of the small ones; hence, the plasma levels were correspondingly different. That these factors are important in humans has been demonstrated by reports from Australia (19, 66,83) that show that a large number of patients showed toxicity with usual doses of PHT given to epileptics because the formulation of the PHT in the capsules given the patients had been changed. The usual capsules contained PHT with an excipient of calcium sulfate, whereas the capsules that produced toxicity in the same dose had lactose as an excipient. Changing back to the usual preparation restored normal plasma drug levels, and the toxic manifestations disappeared. Obviously, the excipient blocked the absorption of the drug by an as yet unknown mechanism. However, in another study (64) in which different brands of PHT were compared in epileptic patients, no significant differences in serum levels were found. Thus, bioavailability of the drug is variable, and it is advisable when using this drug that the physician not change preparations once the dose and steady-state plasma level have been established. It is evident, therefore, that in humans the rate of absorption (rate constant, k_a) of PHT is somewhat irregular, not first order, and prolonged (37).

Studies on the bioavailability of PHT have shown that the drug is absorbed nonlinearly and,

therefore, that bioavailability must be measured by methods that employ nonlinear pharmacokinetics as described by Martis and Levy (51) and applied to PHT by Jusko (37).

Utilizing the data of Lund et al. (48) from patients in whom serum concentrations of PHT were compared on intravenous and oral administration of 4.6 mg/kg of this drug, Jusko (37) showed that absorption of PHT was not uniform and that the data could be fitted by nonlinear kinetics. Thus, on oral administration there was an initial absorption peak at 4 to 7 hr and a secondary peak of 8 to 15 hr after injection of PHT. Thereafter, the absorption continued for a prolonged period of about 2 days. The decline was much flatter with the orally administered drug than with the intravenous. In intoxicated patients, gastrointestinal absorption of PHT continued for as long as 60 hr after ingestion (87). The secondary absorption peak was assumed to result from dissolution of an appreciable fraction of the residual dosage form when food was ingested. Estimation of the bioavailability of PHT by linear (comparative areas under the plasma concentration-versus-time curves after intravenous and oral administration) and nonlinear calculations showed that the linear method yielded a mean bioavailability estimate of 0.87, whereas the nonlinear method generated a mean value of 0.98 (37). Thus, the direct use of area ratios underestimates the essentially complete absorption of PHT from oral capsules. This is explained by the fact that the intravenous route produces an initially higher serum concentration because of the saturation kinetics of these drugs, and this causes a more prolonged retention of phenytoin in the body and produces a slightly larger area value for the intravenous dose.

Therefore, linear (area values) kinetics for bioavailability studies with PHT preparations can be applied only when the study is carried out at relatively low dosages where such kinetics are present. This value for PHT in normal subjects represents an absorption half-life of about 8 hr, but studies are difficult to carry out because the K_m of PHT is small and highly variable ($\sim$3.4 mg/kg), as discussed below.

Kutt et al. (40) reported one case of a defect

in gastrointestinal absorption of PHT. In this patient, plasma levels of PHT remained below 1 μg/ml on daily administration of 300 mg given orally; the urinary excretion of the major metabolite of PHT, 5-(p-hydroxyphenyl)-5-phenylhydantoin (HPPH), was also low (14% of ingested dose). Intravenous injection produced a rise in the plasma level after 5 days to 42 μg/ml, and excretion of HPPH increased to over 60% of the injected dose. During oral administration, large amounts of PHT were recovered from feces. Absorption of other drugs such as salicylates, sulfonamides, and tetracyclines was not impaired, and there was no evidence of malabsorption of fat and carbohydrate. The mechanism of this defect has not been elucidated.

In humans, after oral administration of a single dose, peak blood levels are generally reached between 4 and 8 hr after administration, although the peak may be reached as early as 3 hr and as late as 12 hr after ingestion of the drug (16,60). The time of peak effect appears to be independent of the dose. The levels may remain at the peak values for 24 hr.

In newborns and in younger infants (up to 3 months of age), PHT appears to be absorbed very slowly and incompletely after both oral and intramuscular administration (36). In older infants and children, in contrast, the drug is absorbed very efficiently by the oral route, with peak plasma levels usually attained 2 to 6 hr after dosing (8,85).

The absorption of PHT from the gut can be delayed and reduced by concurrent administration of phenobarbital (55,81). Phenytoin is absorbed more slowly when injected intramuscularly than when it is given orally (14,88,89). This is because of its poor water solubility which makes it act as a repository preparation because of deposition of PHT crystals in the muscle. This causes hemorrhagic areas around the crystals (89). It is absorbed only as the free drug is cleared from the plasma by binding to plasma proteins, distribution and binding in tissues, storage in fat, biotransformation in liver, and excretion. If PHT must be given parenterally, it should be administered intravenously rather than intramuscularly. However, brief periods of intramuscular administration after the steady-state has been reached can be used without alterations in serum levels (10,88) because over a 5-day period, complete absorption of the precipitated drug in the muscle does take place (39). The plasma concentration attained after intramuscular administration fits a pharmacokinetic model derived from precipitation and redissolution of PHT at the intramuscular injection site (see 37 for discussion).

DISTRIBUTION

Plasma Binding and Half-Life

Binding

On entering the circulatory system, PHT is rapidly and reversibly bound to proteins. The percent bound to protein for different species is shown in Table 2. In man, the average is about 90% (69 to 96%) at 37°C (33,49). The percent bound varies little with plasma concentration, but in the clinically occurring plasma concentration range (5 to 50 μg/ml), there is a small increase in the unbound fraction of PHT with increasing total concentration (15,49). Newborn infants exhibit significantly lower protein binding of PHT than do adults (69), as do newborn kittens (21). The percent unbound increases (percent bound decreases) with age in normal individuals (90.1% at 17 years and 87.3% bound at 53 years) (33). Binding in males (89.4%) does not differ from that in females (89%). Binding is directly correlated with plasma albumin and total bilirubin (33). There is probably competition between PHT and endogenous bilirubin for binding sites on the albumin molecule. A Scatchard plot of PHT binding indicates that PHT is bound to several sites on the plasma proteins. At therapeutic concentrations of PHT (<20 μg/ml), one or several sites seem to be involved (49).

Previous studies in neonatal animals had suggested a reciprocal relationship between the unbound fraction of PHT and the albumin level in plasma (69) and indicated that PHT was bound to serum albumin. However, proof of this was not forthcoming until the studies of Lightfoot and Christian (46). They identified by radioimmunoelectrophoresis of human serum that PHT is bound to albumin and two α-globulin proteins which are identical with those to which thyroxine is bound. However, unlike thyroxine, PHT is not bound to prealbumin. The observed affinity of both PHT and thyroxine for albumin and the two α-globulins is direct confirmation of previous studies (20,47,61–63,78,90) reporting competition among thyroxine, triiodothyronine, and PHT for binding proteins. The failure of PHT to bind to prealbumin probably accounts for the ability of this drug to displace thyroxine from the thyroxine-binding globulin onto prealbumin (62,78,90); it also displaces thyroxine onto albumin. Fichsel and Knöpfle (20) showed that long-term therapy with PHT in epileptic children produced considerable alterations in the thyroidal hormonal state. These consisted of dose-dependent decreases in protein-bound iodine, thyroxine, free thyroxine, triiodothyronine, and also a slight decrease in plasma thyrotropin (TSH). These were a result of displacement of thyroxine and triiodothyronine from their plasma protein binding sites as well as a more rapid conversion and metabolism of thyroxine and triiodothyronine induced by PHT. The decreased TSH was also partly a result of PHT-induced inhibition of TRH release from the hypothalamus. Carbon dioxide decreases the binding power of the α-globulins and presumably therefore decreases the ability of both thyroxine and PHT to bind to them (63).

In addition to thyroxine and triiodothyronine, other drugs bind to these same proteins and compete for the binding sites. Thus, salicylic acid, phenylbutazone, sulfafurazol, and acetazolamide, in concentrations that may be obtained clinically, compete with PHT for these sites and displace it from them (49). Also, endogenous compounds such as fatty acids displace PHT from plasma proteins and are a potential source of drug interactions (30). When these substances (e.g., salicylates) are given, the level of free PHT in the blood increases and, conversely, when PHT is given, the plasma levels of free salicylate and thyroxine, increase. The unbound fraction of PHT has been reported to increase between 16 and 200% in the presence of salicylate (49), an effect that takes place only with high doses of salicylate and is not clinically important (44). The increased free level increases the anticonvulsant effect of the drug which depends on the unbound drug concentration and not the total plasma concentration (75); it also allows more of the PHT to reach the liver per unit time, and increased biotransformation results, with a consequent more rapid decline in the level of the drug in the plasma. However, this is true only if the enzyme system in the liver that metabolizes PHT is not saturated. If the enzyme is saturated, as is often the case, the plasma half-life increases in the presence of these other drugs. Phenytoin binding is decreased in uremia (e.g., 84.2%) and in hepatic disease (e.g., 84.1%) (5,33,34,74) mainly because of the decrease in plasma proteins. It is not altered by pregnancy and oral contraceptives (33). A review of PHT binding has been provided by Porter and Layzer (65).

Half-Life

The plasma half-life of PHT in the body is defined as the time it takes for the concentration of the drug in plasma, at the time of its peak level after a single dose or the steady-state level after multiple doses, to decline by 50%. This value is a measure of the rate of metabolism and excretion of the drug and varies quantitatively from species to species as shown in Table 2. In humans, the half-life after oral administration of doses that result in therapeutic levels averages about 22 hr with a range of 7.0 to 42.0 hr (2,16); the half-life after intravenous administration is shorter and ranges from 10 to 15 hr (27,79). This difference undoubtedly results from the slow rate of absorption of PHT from the gut, as discussed previously, which maintains the plasma concentration at a high level for a longer period of time.

However, since the half-life increases with dose and exhibits large individual variations, an average value is meaningless. For example,

TABLE 2. *Plasma and brain binding, CSF/plasma, brain/plasma, and brain/CSF ratios, apparent volume of distribution (V_D), plasma half-life, K_m and V_{max} values of PHT in various species*

Species	Protein binding		Ratios			$T_{\frac{1}{2}}$ (hr)	V_D (liter/kg)	K_m (mg/liter)	V_{max} (mg/kg per day)	References
	Plasma (%)	Brain (%)	CSF to plasma	Brain to plasma	Brain to CSF					
Humans (4.4→6.5→13.6 mg/kg orally)	86 (73–93)		0.17				0.59			22,93,94
Normal adults						22 → 40 → 59	0.36–0.43			See 94
								5.46	6.13	37
								6.77	6.07	25
								4.20	4.76	23
							0.775			3
	88					15.4[a]	0.724	14.40	16.3	29
90.3(86.9–91.9)			0.12	0.63	5.29			11.54	10.3	50
Nonseizure adults (autopsy)										
Gyrus from temporal lobe				1.35						
Gyrus from parietal lobe				1.40						
Gyrus from frontal lobe (gray)				1.20						
Gyrus from frontal lobe (white)				2.25						
Cerebellar hemisphere				1.37						
Midbrain				1.85						73
Thoracic spinal cord				1.7						
Sciatic nerve				1.0						
Median nerve				0.95						
Epileptic adults (16.0 mg/kg i.v.)	88		0.12	0.75 (temporal lobe)	6.25	51	0.78			11
										84
	88		0.12	1.13 gray 1.33 white	9.4 11.1					76
								3.34	9.93	37
							0.829	14.5	10.9	3

									Reference
Frontal lobe (gray)				1.0					
(white)				0.83					76
Parietal lobe (gray)				0.90					
(white)				1.51					
Temporal lobe (gray)				1.39					
(white)				1.73					
Gyrus from temporal lobe				1.55					73
Gyrus from frontal lobe (gray)				1.73					
Gyrus from frontal lobe (white)				2.73					
Normal child				1.72		$6–8^a$	0.783	3.06, 6.37	23 / See 94
Monkey, fetal				1.78					26
Dog ($20 \rightarrow 50$ mg/kg i.v.)		64, 65	0.36, 0.27, 0.30	1.89, 3.50	7.09, 11.70	$2.2 \rightarrow 6.4$	1.04		15 / 56 / 67
Cat Adult (15 mg/kg i.v.)	90.3	76.1	0.25	2.17	8.76	~72	1.49		21
Newborn (15 mg/kg i.v.)	84.3	69.3	0.32	1.82	5.78	>96	1.32		
Rat (33 mg/kg i.p.)	86	80		1.35, 1.50, 0.95		3.4	1.30	13	16 / 58 / 52 / 25 / 38
Mouse			0.16	1.42					52

^{a}Calculated from formula $T_{\frac{1}{2}}(\text{min}) = \dfrac{0.693 K_m}{V_{max}}$.

Cranford et al. (11) showed that after intravenous infusion of 15 to 18 mg/kg of PHT, the half-lives varied from 10 to 160 hr, with most values ranging from 20 to 70 hr. The distribution was bimodal, and the long half-lives probably occurred in patients with insufficient parahydroxylation, as originally described by Kutt et al. (42). Drugs that interfere with the metabolism of PHT by the liver (e.g., sulthiame, bishydroxycoumarin, sulfaphenazole, disulfiram, and phenyramidol, and simultaneous administration of *p*-aminosalicylate and isoniazid) increase its plasma half-life (31,32,41, 59,77). Conversely, drugs that accelerate its metabolism by enzyme induction, e.g., phenobarbital (12), shorten its half-life under certain conditions, as discussed elsewhere (H. Kutt and H. Paris-Kutt, Chapter 24). For example, sulthiame increased the half-life of a patient on PHT from 12 to 32 hr (31). Genetic factors such as inability of the liver to *p*-hydroxylate PHT also lengthen its half-life and increase blood levels (42). Although an earlier report (8) presents some evidence that children may metabolize PHT at a slower rate than do adults and that the half-life is longer, subsequent reports (see 55, also 13,17,18,23) clearly indicate that PHT is disposed at a faster rate in infants and children than in adults. The $T_{\frac{1}{2}}$ in infants and children is 1.2 to 16.1 hr at low doses but 11.6 to 31.5 hr at higher doses when plasma levels are between 10 and 20 μg/ml (18). Thus, saturation kinetics are present in infants and children as well as adults. Younger children (<5–6 years of age), therefore, require larger doses per kilogram than do adults to reach therapeutic levels. Therefore, there is a lower plasma concentration–dose ratio than in adults (7,68).

It is evident, therefore, that an important determinant of PHT plasma half-life is the dose of the drug. In man (2), dog (31), and mouse (24), increasing the dose of PHT increases the plasma half-life (see Table 2). The dose dependency is best explained by saturation of a rate-limiting enzyme reaction in the metabolism of the drug. Saturation of the biotransformation enzymes can also explain the observed fact (2) that the PHT plasma fall-off curves at high doses are not first-order processes (linear on semilogarithmic paper), whereas they are at low doses, before saturation occurs. At saturating doses, the curves are characteristic of a zero-order process (linear with time on rectangular paper). Arnold and Gerber (2) have shown that there is a wide variation in the rate of plasma decline of PHT in the population. This variation is probably caused by differences in liver drug-metabolizing activity, variation in the degree of dose dependency among individuals, differences in the plasma concentration of PHT at which enzyme induction may occur, or differences in the level at which rate-limiting, drug-metabolizing enzyme reactions become saturated. Since the variability in the half-life of PHT is much less in identical twins than in fraternal twins, the individual variability has been attributed to genetic factors (1). The marked variation in plasma half-life of PHT in individual patients emphasizes the importance of tailoring the dose of the drug to each patient and of monitoring the patient by measurement of plasma PHT levels.

The dose-dependent kinetics of PHT have been expressed in quantitative terms by using a nonlinear pharmacokinetic model (3,23,25, 37,50). Such a model is able to predict plasma levels of the drug based on the dose given and the K_m, $V_{\max}$, and V_D as obtained from experimental subjects. The equation used is based on Michaelis–Menten kinetics and is as follows:

$$[\text{PHT}] = \frac{K_m R}{(V_{\max} - R)}$$

where R is the dosing rate in mg/kg per day, $V_{\max}$ is the maximum rate of metabolism of PHT in mg/kg per day, and K_m is the Michaelis–Menten constant equal to the plasma concentration in mg/liter at which the metabolic rate is one-half maximum. Values of K_m range around 6 to 12 mg/liter. Above these values, zero-order kinetics are more pronounced, and below them, first-order kinetics become more pronounced. The K_m values are usually lower and $V_{\max}$ values higher in children than in adults. It is evident from these pharmacokinetic data that a very small dosage increment of only 50 to 100 mg can produce an increase in steady-state plasma concentrations over a two- to threefold range. Prediction of the adjustments needed to obtain proper therapeutic blood levels can be made from these equations. Nomograms to aid in calculation of dosage changes have been developed by Richens and Dunlop (72) and Martin et al. (50).

As already mentioned, induction of PHT drug-metabolizing enzyme activity by other drugs or by self-induction appears to occur and results in a decreased plasma half-life. However, this generally takes place only after long-term administration of doses large enough to exceed the saturation concentration of the enzymes; at low doses, PHT does not cause self-induction (9).

On intravenous administration of PHT to humans (or animals), two components are observed in the plasma decay curve (79). The first component is very rapid and has a half-life of about 6 min and a volume of distribution (based on the free level of PHT in plasma) of 0.79 liters/kg (79%). This probably represents rapid distribution of PHT into extracellular space, cell water, and slight binding to subcellular constituents, particularly the nuclei, as described below. The second component is slow and has a half-life of 9 hr. Its volume of distribution is 1.75 liters/kg (175%) and undoubtedly represents further binding to the endoplasmic reticulum in cells, since the binding to tissue fractions is greater than that to plasma proteins or than metabolism of the drug by the liver and its subsequent excretion. Distribution into the gastrointestinal tract via biliary excretion of the metabolites from the liver probably also accounts in part for the large volume of distribution of this component.

Volume of Distribution

Following absorption, PHT distributes freely in the body because at the pH of plasma (7.4) it exists predominantly in the un-ionized form, which allows rapid movement across cell membranes by the process of nonionic diffusion. Much of the drug that enters cells binds to subcellular fractions (see below). Within 15 min, the drug has reached its maximum volume of distribution. Values for V_D based on the total level in the plasma are shown in Table 2 and average about 0.78 liter/kg in humans. Since the free level is 10% of the total, the V_D based on the free level is 10 times higher. Thus, the drug is present in higher concentration in cells than in the extracellular fluid. This is due to avid binding in cells, storage in fat, and binding to plasma proteins. It can be seen in Table 2 that the binding of PHT to brain constituents of adult cats is 90% and to plasma proteins 76%. From the data presented in Fig. 1, it is evident that in rats PHT is present in brain, liver, muscle, and fat at a higher concentration than in plasma. This is also the case for the same tissues of mice and cats and probably for those of humans. The accumulation of PHT in tissues occurs mainly by binding, since the concentration of free PHT in all tissues of the body is the same as that in plasma, as shown for the CSF in Table 2. In cats and dogs, chronic administration of PHT (100 mg/kg for 14 to 16 months) results in very high concentrations of the drug in the pituitary and adrenal glands (56).

Phenytoin also distributes into all transcellular fluids as the free form. These fluids include CSF (Table 2), saliva, semen, milk, gastrointestinal fluids, and bile (16,57,58,80,82). Phenytoin also freely crosses the human placental barrier and reaches equilibrium between mother and fetus (4,54). The levels of the drug were found to be the same in mother's plasma, cord blood, and in the infant's serum at the time of delivery. The plasma half-life of PHT in the serum of the newborn infant was 19 hr in one study (4) (which is the same order of magnitude as that of adults), but in another study (54), it was 50 to 60 hr (a value considerably greater than that of adults). However, in the latter study the methods were not described, and therefore, it is difficult to evaluate the results. A longer half-life would be expected in fetal and newborn animals than in adults, because the drug-metabolizing systems in the liver endoplasmic

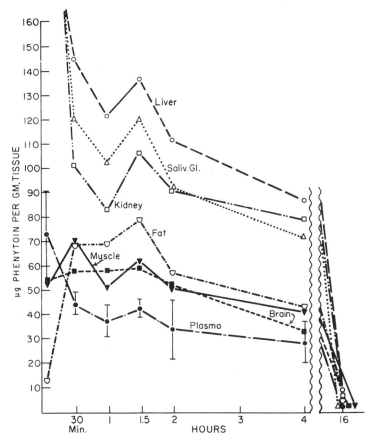

FIG. 1. Distribution of radioactive PHT in various tissues after intravenous administration of 22 mg of PHT labeled with 2-^{14}C-PHT. The ordinate is µg/g tissue, and the abscissa is time (hr) after administration. (From Noach et al., ref. 58, with permission.)

reticulum are poorly developed in immature animals. Phenytoin also crosses the placenta in monkeys and in rats (86).

Bile contains mainly the metabolites of PHT which are formed in the liver and excreted in the bile. Most of the injected dose is excreted in the bile as metabolites, then enters the intestinal fluid and is subsequently reabsorbed into the blood and excreted in the urine (58). G. Ringham and D. M. Woodbury (*unpublished data*) demonstrated that in normal rats 60% of an injected dose of ^{14}C-PHT was excreted from the body in a 48-hr period; of this total, 46% was excreted in urine, and 14% excreted in feces. However, when the bile duct of the rat was cannulated and the bile collected over a 48-hr period, the total excretion was 66 to 72%; the bile contained 43% of the injected radioactivity, whereas urine contained only 28%, and feces only 0.6%. Thus, the bile constitutes a major route of initial excretion of the drug and its metabolites, although ultimately it is mainly excreted from the body in the urine by reabsorption from the intestinal tract.

The amount of PHT that appears in the bile, mainly as HPPH, is influenced by the levels of other drugs. For example, in rats, phenobarbital given acutely appears to compete with the hepatic enzyme that hydroxylates PHT and thereby reduces the rate at which HPPH enters the bile (91). There is indirect evidence that this also occurs in humans.

Brain and CSF Distribution

The phenomenon of redistribution of PHT occurs after a single dose of the drug. This is analogous to the redistribution of thiopental to muscle and fat following a single dose. On intravenous injection in humans or intraperitoneal administration in rats (see Fig. 2), PHT, because of its high lipid solubility, rapidly enters the brain of either species and reaches a peak level in less than 15 min. However, the concentration immediately falls thereafter as the plasma level declines as a result of redistribution of the drug to binding, storage, or depot sites in other tissues (muscle, liver, fat, or lung). Consequently, the neurophysiological effects of the drug rapidly disappear. This redistribution phenomenon is important to recognize in the treatment of status epilepticus with intravenous PHT, as the seizures may recur unless further drug is given after the initial dose. On continued administration of the drug, these sites are saturated, and the brain concentration again increases, paralleling the increase in the plasma level; within 4 to 5 days, it reaches a steady-state level. This is why it takes several days for a therapeutic plasma level of PHT to be reached when therapy is first initiated. However, the steady-state level can be reached rapidly by initial administration of loading doses.

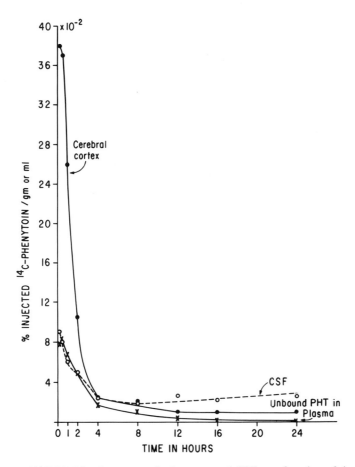

FIG. 2. Distribution of ^{14}C-PHT in plasma, cerebral cortex, and CSF as a function of time in rats. Ordinate is percent of injected dose of ^{14}C-PHT/g wet brain tissue or ml of plasma and CSF, and abscissa is time (hr). The values for plasma represent the free levels of the drug and not the total amount. (From Woodbury and Swinyard, ref. 94, with permission.)

The concentration of PHT in brain is about one to three times the concentration of total drug in the plasma and about six to 10 times the concentration of the free drug in plasma (16,21,38,56,58,86). This is a result of binding to various subcellular fractions of brain cells (38, see 92 for review of this aspect).

Preferential accumulation of PHT in the superior and inferior colliculus, amygdala, and hippocampus, compared with 16 other areas of the brain, was observed in dogs and cats receiving PHT at an oral dose of 10 mg/kg for 14 to 16 months (56). The functional significance of this differential distribution in brain is not yet clear. The simultaneous uptake of PHT into the CSF and brain of dogs has been evaluated (67). Two components of uptake into the brain are present. The first has a half-life of 2.1 min and a V_D of 1.9; it represents uptake into the extracellular fluid and cells. The second component has a half-life of 13 min and a V_D of 1.6; it represents penetration into and binding by subcellular fractions of the brain; uptake into the brain is faster than into the CSF ($T_{\frac{1}{2}}$, 7 min) across the choroid plexus (see 93 for discussion).

The levels of PHT in the brain of humans have been tested in patients who have died from overdosage of the drug and in epileptic patients undergoing brain surgery (43,73,84). In these cases, the concentration in brain is about one to two times the plasma levels, as is the case for experimental animals. Hence, at least at the levels attainable in humans, the binding to brain substituents is not altered by the dose level in the plasma. This is also the case in mice. In man (73,76,84), rats (52,73), and mice (52), there is a significant correlation between brain and plasma PHT concentrations. In humans, the brain/plasma ratio for PHT averages about 1.52, but white matter (2.73) contains approximately twice as much PHT as gray matter (1.73). In brain tissues obtained from an autopsy of an individual patient (73), PHT concentrations in cortical gyri containing mostly gray matter averaged 1.3 times the plasma concentration, values close to those observed in tissues obtained from patients in surgery. White matter tissues averaged twice the values in plasma. Cerebellum had the same levels as the cerebrum. Peripheral nerves (sciatic and median) had values equal to those in the plasma. In rats (16,52,58), the brain/plasma ratio ranges from 0.95 to 1.5, and in mice is 1.42 (52) (see Table 2).

In another study, Vajda et al. (84) found that the brain/plasma ratio of PHT was 0.75 in epileptic patients undergoing temporal lobectomy, and the CSF/plasma ratio was 0.12. Thus, the brain/CSF ratio (equivalent to brain/free plasma concentration ratio) is 6.25. There was a significant correlation between brain and plasma levels. Sironi et al. (76) also found that brain, CSF, and plasma levels were correlated. In addition, they found that PHT was slightly higher in white matter than in gray matter in different areas of brain removed surgically from epileptic patients and in normal and scar tissue. The brain/plasma ratio was 1.13 in gray matter and 1.33 in white matter. Phenytoin concentration in the temporal lobes was twice as high as in the frontal lobes, and that in the parietal lobe was also higher than that in the frontal area. These patients were medically resistant and had therapeutic or higher molar levels of PHT in the brain. Thus, despite adequate levels, the drugs were pharmacologically ineffective. The mechanism of this is not known, but the observations of Rapport et al. (70) that PHT concentration in the areas of maximum epileptogenic activity and astrogliosis in patients with epilepsy was much lower than its concentration in normal brain of four controls suggest that the lack of activity may result from failure to bind the drug in the area of the focus. Evidence suggests that binding may be involved in the action of this drug (see 28, 92 for review).

The higher levels of PHT in white matter are in part undoubtedly a result of the high lipid content of this tissue which is 2.5 times greater than in gray matter of cerebral cortex. This can be explained by the observations of Goldberg and colleagues (28,29) and others (see 28,92 for review) that PHT accumulates in brain by avidly binding to brain proteins and phospholipids. The binding to phospholipids depends on the partition coefficient (PC) which is high for PHT (log PC = 2.23) and is altered by the Ca^{2+} concentration (28). They showed that brain levels in humans were four to 10 times higher than the free PHT as measured in the CSF.

The binding in the brain may, however, be influenced by pH, since CO_2 administration increases the level of PHT in brain and lowers the plasma level (91). It is likely that this effect is not related to the pH change increasing the amount of nonionized drug in the plasma. The percentage change in un-ionized drug is much too small to account for the change, and it is more likely that binding to plasma or brain proteins is altered by the pH shift induced by CO_2. In this connection, it is of interest that CO_2 does decrease α-globulin binding sites in plasma, as described above.

Since the level of free PHT in plasma is the same as in CSF, it distributes passively between these two fluids (see 93 for review), and the CSF concentration can be used to determine the free level in the plasma and the percentage bound to plasma proteins.

EXCRETION

Phenytoin is excreted in urine and feces mainly as its metabolites. Less than 5% of the total drug is excreted as the un-metabolized form in the urine in experimental animals and humans; only a very small amount is excreted in this form in the feces. In rats, about 70% of PHT is ultimately secreted as HPPH, mainly as HPPH glucuronide (only 1% of unconjugated HPPH is excreted in urine), and about 25% as other metabolites (58). In humans, the amount excreted as HPPH is dose dependent. On oral administration, at a dose of 100 mg, only 50% is excreted as HPPH. However, in clinical doses, the excretion of HPPH varies little with dose; about 63% is excreted as this compound. Values as high as 80 to 90% have been reported, but these are probably high. In the first 24 hr after single oral administration of 100 to 150 mg to humans, less than 1% is excreted as PHT, and 27 to 34% as HPPH; after intravenous injection of 50 to 250 mg, 50 to 61% is excreted as HPPH. The dihydrodiol, as well as the

catechol and 3-*O*-methyl catechol derivatives of PHT are formed by rat liver and excreted in urine. However, they have been detected only in small quantities in human urine and are not major excretory products.

Phenytoin must be in the ionized form to be adequately excreted, a process efficiently carried out by the liver to produce HPPH, the dihydroxylated derivative, and the dihydrodiol. The ionized metabolites are excreted by active tubular secretion, as are most organic anions and cations. Thus, Bochner et al. (6) demonstrated that the clearance of PHT (3 to 23 ml/min, depending on urine flow rate) was considerably less than expected for inulin; therefore, it undergoes net resorption in its passage through the kidney. The HPPH glucuronide clearance (76 to 420 ml/min, depending on urine flow rate) exceeded expected inulin clearance if urine flow rates were sufficiently high; thus, this metabolite exhibits net secretion by the renal tubules. However, Hoppel et al. (35) suggest that both HPPH and its glucuronide are mainly filtered in the glomeruli in proportion to creatinine clearance. This is probably true at low urine flow rates, but at high rates, net secretion appears to occur. Alkalinization of the urine enhances the excretion of PHT because the higher pH allows more of the drug to exist in the ionized form; consequently, more leaves by way of tubular secretion, and less is reabsorbed, because this occurs by passive diffusion of the un-ionized, lipid-soluble form. The rate of excretion depends on the extent of binding in the plasma, and, since this is high for PHT (80 to 90%), excretion is slow. In rats about 48 to 60 hr is required for complete excretion of an orally or intravenously administered dose; in humans, excretion requires 72 to 120 hr after oral ingestion and about the same time after intravenous administration (27,79).

The excretion of phenytoin in milk, semen, and saliva has implications for its effects on sperm, on nursing infants, and on teeth and gums, especially if toxic doses are attained. Some evidence suggests that viability of sperm may be affected (80). The effects of long-term PHT in milk on the child have not been evaluated, and there is evidence that the level of PHT in saliva is unrelated to the degree of gum hyperplasia produced. The levels in these fluids are about the same as the free levels in the plasma.

SUMMARY

Phenytoin is rapidly and passively absorbed across the intestinal mucosa in the un-ionized form, but absorption is limited by its extremely low solubility in gastrointestinal fluids. Absorption is a nonliner saturation process that occurs only as the drug is cleared from the plasma and as it goes into solution in the intestinal fluids. After entering the blood, PHT is bound avidly to plasma proteins, but the free form rapidly enters all tissues where it is bound (at least in liver, brain, and muscle) to proteins and phospholipids. Thus, total concentrations in these tissues are higher than in extracellular fluid, but the free levels are the same. Storage in fat also occurs. Concentrations of PHT in transcellular fluids such as CSF, gastrointestinal fluids, bile, saliva, semen, milk, and plasma are the same as the free levels in the blood.

Binding to plasma proteins can be inhibited by drugs such as salicylates, thyroxine, phenylbutazone, and others that compete for the binding sites of the protein. The plasma half-life of the drug in humans is about 22 hr but is dose dependent and obeys saturation (Michaelis–Menten) kinetics. This can be altered by drugs that compete for binding or inhibit or accelerate biotransformation of the drug in the liver. Large doses of the drug that saturate the enzyme that biotransforms PHT in the liver also increase the plasma half-life.

Phenytoin is handled in the urine by glomerular filtration and tubular resorption, whereas its chief metabolite, HPPH, which represents about 70% of the total excretion of PHT in the urine is excreted by glomerular filtration and tubular secretion and obeys saturation kinetics in its elimination.

Most of the drug is excreted in the bile as metabolites which are then reabsorbed from the intestinal tract and excreted in the urine; very little drug is lost in the feces.

Saturation of body binding and storage sites is essential before stable plasma and brain levels can be attained.

ACKNOWLEDGMENTS

Unpublished data presented in this chapter were supported by a Program-Project Grant 5-PO 1-NS-15767 from the National Institute of Neurological and Communicative Disorders and Stroke, N.I.H.

The author is a Research Career Awardee (5-K06-NS13838) of the National Institute of Neurological and Communicative Disorders and Stroke, N.I.H.

REFERENCES

1. Andreasen, P. B., Frøland, A., Skovsted, L., Andersen, S. A., and Hauge, M. (1972): Diphenylhydantoin half-life in man and its inhibition by phenylbutazone: The role of genetic factors. *Acta. Med. Scand.,* 193:561–564.
2. Arnold, K., and Gerber, N. (1970): The rate of decline of diphenylhydantoin in human plasma. *Clin. Pharmacol. Ther.,* 11:121–134.
3. Atkinson, A. J., and Shaw, J. M. (1973): Pharmacokinetic study of a patient with diphenylhydantoin toxicity. *Clin. Pharmacol. Ther.,* 14:521–528.
4. Baughman, F. A., Jr., and Randinitis, E. J. (1970): Passage of diphenylhydantoin across the placenta. *J.A.M.A.,* 213:466.
5. Blum, M. R., Riegelman, S., and Becker, C. E. (1972): Altered protein binding of diphenylhydantoin in uremic plasma. *N. Engl. J. Med.,* 286:109.
6. Bochner, F., Hooper, W. O., Sutherland, J. M., Eadie, J. J., and Tyrer, J. H. (1973): The renal handling of diphenylhydantoin and 5-(*p*-hydroxyphenyl)-5-phenylhydantoin. *Clin. Pharmacol. Therap.,* 14:791–796.
7. Borofsky, L. G., Louis, S., Kutt, H., and Roginsky, M. (1972): Diphenylhydantoin: Efficacy, toxicity and dose–serum level relationships in children. *J. Pediatr.,* 81:995–1002.
8. Buchanan, R. A., Heffelfinger, J. C., and Weiss, C. F. (1969): The effect of phenobarbital on diphenylhydantoin metabolism in children. *Pediatrics,* 43:114–116.
9. Buchanan, R. A., Kinkel, A. W., Goulet, J. R., and Smith, T. C. (1972): The metabolism of diphenylhydantoin (Dilantin®) following once daily administration. *Neurology (Minneap.),* 22:325–336.
10. Cantu, R. C., Schwab, R. S., and Timberlake, W. H. (1968): Comparison of blood levels with oral and intramuscular diphenylhydantoin. *Neurology (Minneap.),* 18:782–784.
11. Cranford, R. E., Leppik, I. E., Patrick, B., Anderson, C. B., and Kostick, B. (1978): Intravenous

phenytoin: Clinical and pharmacokinetic aspects. *Neurology (Minneap.)*, 28:874–880.

12. Cucinelli, A. A., Koster, R., Conney, A. H., and Burns, J. J. (1963): Stimulatory effect of phenobarbital on the metabolism of diphenylhydantoin. *J. Pharmacol. Exp. Ther.*, 141:157–160.

13. Curless, R. G., and Watson, P. D. (1975): Rapid diphenylhydantoin metabolism in infants. *Pediatr. Res.*, 9:282.

14. Dam, M., and Olesen, V. (1966): Intramuscular administration of phenytoin. *Neurology (Minneap.)*, 16:288–292.

15. Dayton, P. G., Cucinell, S. A., Weiss, M., and Perel, J. M. (1967): Dose-dependence of drug plasma level decline in dogs. *J. Pharmacol. Exp. Ther.*, 158:305–316.

16. Dill, W. A., Kazenko, A., Wolff, L. M., and Glazko, A. J. (1956): Studies on 5,5-diphenylhydantoin (Dilantin®) in animals and man. *J. Pharmacol. Exp. Ther.*, 118:270–279.

17. Dodson, W. E. (1980): Phenytoin kinetics in children. *Clin. Pharmacol. Ther.*, 27:704–707.

18. Dodson, W. E. (1980): Phenytoin elimination in childhood: Effect of concentration dependent kinetics. *Neurology (Minneap.)*, 30:196–199.

19. Eadie, M. J., Sutherland, J. M., and Tyrer, D. H. (1968): Dilantin overdosage. *Med. J. Aust.*, 2:515.

20. Fichsel, H. and Knöpfle, G. (1978): Effects of anticonvulsant drugs on thyroid hormones in epileptic children. *Epilepsia*, 19:323–336.

21. Firemark, H., Barlow, C. F., and Roth, L. J. (1963): The entry, accumulation and binding of diphenylhydantoin-2-C^{14} in brain. Studies on adult, immature and hypercapnic cats. *Int. J. Neuropharmacol.*, 2:25–38.

22. Ganshorn, A., and Kurz, H. (1968): Unterschiede zwischen der Protein bindung Neugeborener und Erwachsener und ihre Bedeutung für die pharmakologische Wirkung. *Naunyn Schmiedebergs Arch. Pharmacol.*, 260:117–118.

23. Garrettson, L. K., and Jusko, W. J. (1975): Diphenylhydantoin elimination kinetics in overdosed children. *Clin. Pharmacol. Ther.*, 17:481–491.

24. Gerber, N., and Arnold, K. (1969): Studies on the metabolism of diphenylhydantoin (DPH) in mice. *J. Pharmacol. Exp. Ther.*, 167:77–90.

25. Gerber N., and Wagner, J. G. (1972): Explanation of dose-dependent decline of diphenylhydantoin plasma levels by fitting to the integrated form of the Michaelis–Menten equation. *Res. Commun. Chem. Pathol. Pharmacol.*, 3:455–466.

26. Glazko, A. J., and Chang, T. (1972): 12-Diphenylhydantoin: Absorption, distribution, and excretion (continued). In: *Antiepileptic Drugs*, edited by D. M. Woodbury, J. Kiffin Penry, and R. P. Schmidt, pp. 127–136. Raven Press, New York.

27. Glazko, A. J., Chang, T., Baukema, J., Bill, W. A., Goulet, J. R., and Buchanan, R. A. (1969): Metabolic disposition of diphenylhydantoin in normal human subjects following intravenous administration. *Clin. Pharmacol. Ther.*, 10:498–504.

28. Goldberg, M. A. (1980): Phenytoin: Binding. *Adv. Neurol.* 27:323–337.

29. Goldberg, M. A., and Crandall, P. H. (1978): Human

binding of phenytoin. *Neurology (Minneap.)*, 28:881–885.

30. Gugler, R., Shoeman, D. W., and Azarnoff, D. L. (1974): Effect of *in vivo* elevation of free fatty acids on protein binding of drugs. *Pharmacology*, 12:160–165.

31. Hansen, J. M., Kristensen, M., and Skovsted, L. (1966): Sulthiame (Ospolot®) as inhibitor of diphenylhydantoin metabolism. *Epilepsia*, 9:17–22.

32. Hansen, J. M., Kristensen, M., Skovsted, L., and Christensen, L. K. (1966): Dicoumarol induced diphenylhydantoin intoxication. *Lancet*, 2:265–266.

33. Hooper, W. D., Bochner, F., Eadie, M. J., Tyrer, J. H. (1973): Plasma protein binding of diphenylhydantoin. Effects of sex hormones, renal and hepatic disease. *Clin. Pharmacol. Ther.*, 15:276–282.

34. Hooper, W. D., Sutherland, J. M. Bochner, F., Tyrer, J. H., and Eadie, M. J. (1973): The effect of certain drugs on the plasma protein binding of phenytoin. *Aust. N.Z. J. Med.*, 3:377–381.

35. Hoppel, C., Garle, M., Rane, A., and Sjöquist, F. (1977): Plasma concentrations of 5-(4-hydroxyphenyl)-5-phenylhydantoin in phenytoin-treated patients. *Clin. Pharmacol. Ther.*, 21:294–300.

36. Jalling, B., Boreus, L. O., Rane, A., and Sjöquist, F. (1970): Plasma concentrations of diphenylhydantoin in young infants. *Pharmacol. Clin. (Berl.)*, 2:200–202.

37. Jusko, W. J. (1976): Bioavailability and disposition kinetics of phenytoin in man. In: *Quantitative Analytic Studies in Epilepsy*, edited by P. Kellaway and I. Petersen, pp. 115–136. Raven Press, New York.

38. Kemp, J. W., and Woodbury, D. M. (1971): Subcellular distribution of 4-^{14}C-diphenylhydantoin in rat brain. *J. Pharmacol. Exp. Ther.*, 177:342–349.

39. Kostenbauder, H. B., Rapp, R. P., McGoveen, J. P., Foster, T. S., Perrier, D. G., Blacker, H. M., Hulon, W. C., and Kinkel, A. W. (1975): Bioavailability and single dose pharmacokinetics of intramuscular diphenylhydantoin. *Clin. Pharmacol. Ther.*, 18:449–456.

40. Kutt, H., Haynes, J., and McDowell, F. (1966): Some causes of ineffectiveness of diphenylhydantoin. *Arch. Neurol.*, 14:489–492.

41. Kutt, H., Winters, W., and McDowell, F. (1966): Depression of parahydroxylation of diphenylhydantoin by antituberculosis chemotherapy. *Neurology (Minneap.)*, 16:594–602.

42. Kutt, H., Wolk, M., Scherman, R., and McDowell, F. (1964): Insufficient parahydroxylation as a cause of diphenylhydantoin toxicity. *Neurology (Minneap.)*, 14:542–548.

43. Laubscher, F. (1966): Fatal diphenylhydantoin poisoning. *J.A.M.A.*, 198:1120–1121.

44. Leonard, R. F., Knott, P. J., Rankin, G. O., Robinson, D. S., and Melnick, D. E. (1981): Phenytoin-salicylate interaction. *Clin. Pharmacol. Ther.*, 29:56–60.

45. Levy, R. H. (1980): Phenytoin: Biopharmacology. *Adv. Neurol.* 27:315–321.

46. Lightfoot, R. W., Jr., and Christian, C. L. (1966): Serum protein binding of thyroxine and diphenylhydantoin. *J. Clin. Endocrinol. Metab.*, 16:305–308.

47. Loeser, E. H., Jr. (1961): Studies on the metabolism

of diphenylhydantoin (Dilantin®). *Neurology (Minneap.),* 11:424–429.

48. Lund, L., Alvan, G., Berlin, A., and Alexanderson, B. (1974): Pharmacokinetics of single and multiple oral doses of phenytoin in man. *Eur. J. Clin. Pharmacol.,* 7:81–86.

49. Lunde, P. K. M ., Anders, R., Yaffe, S. J., Lund, L., and Sjöqvist, F. (1970): Plasma protein binding of diphenylhydantoin in man. Interaction with other drugs and the effect of temperature and plasma dilution. *Clin. Pharmacol. Ther.,* 11:846–855.

50. Martin, E., Tozer, T. N., Scheiner, L. B., and Riegelman, S. (1977): The clinical pharmacokinetics of phenytoin. *J. Pharmacokinet. Biopharm.,* 5:579–596.

51. Martis, L., and Levy, R. H. (1973): Bioavailability calculations for drugs showing simultaneous first order and capacity-limited elimination kinetics. *J. Pharmacokinet. Biopharm.,* 1:283–294.

52. Masuda, Y., Utsui, Y., Shiraishi, Y., Karasawa, T., Yoshida, K., and Shimizu, M. (1979): Relationships between plasma concentrations of diphenylhydantoin, phenobarbital, carbamazepine, and 3-sulfamoylmethyl-1,2-benzisoxazole (AD-810), a new anticonvulsant agent and their anticonvulsant or neurotoxic effects in experimental animals. *Epilepsia,* 20:623–633.

53. Meinardi, H., Kleijn, E. van der, Meijer, J. W. A., and Rees, H. van (1975): Absorption and distribution of antiepileptic drugs. *Epilepsia,* 16:353–365.

54. Mirkin, B. L. (1971): Placental transfer and neonatal elimination of diphenylhydantoin. *Am. J. Obstet. Gynecol.,* 109:930–933.

55. Morselli, P. L. (1977): Pharmacokinetics of antiepileptic drugs during development. In: *Antiepileptic Drug Monitoring,* edited by C. Gardner-Thorpe, D. Janz, H. Meinardi, and C. E. Pippinger, pp. 57–72. Pitman Medical, Kent.

56. Nakamura, K., Masuda, Y., Nakatsuji, K., and Kiroka, T. (1966): Comparative studies on the distribution and metabolic fate of diphenylhydantoin and 3-ethylcarbonyldiphenylhydantoin (P-6127) after chronic administration to dogs and cats. *Naunyn Schmiedebergs Arch. Pharmacol.,* 254:406–417.

57. Noach, E. L., and van Rees, H. (1964): Intestinal distribution of intravenously administered diphenylhydantoin in the rat. *Arch. Int. Pharmacodyn. Ther.,* 150:52–61.

58. Noach, E. L., Woodbury, D. M., and Goodman, L. S. (1958): Studies on absorption, distribution, fate and excretion of 4-C^{14} labeled diphenylhydantoin. *J. Pharmacol. Exp. Ther.,* 122:301–314.

59. Olesen, O. V. (1966): Disulfiramum (Antabuse®) as inhibitor of phenytoin metabolism. *Acta Pharmacol. Toxicol. (Kbh.),* 24:317–322.

60. O'Malley, W. E., Denckla, M. A., and O., Doherty, D. S. (1969): Oral absorption of diphenyl-hydantoin as measured by gas liquid chromatography *Trans. Am. Neurol. Assoc.,* 94:318–319.

61. Oppenheimer, J. H., Fisher, L. V., Nelson, K. M., and Jailer, J. W. (1961): Depression of the serum protein-bound iodine level by diphenylhydantoin. *J. Clin. Endocrinol.,* 21:252–262.

62. Oppenheimer, J. H., and Tavernetti, R. R. (1962): Studies on the thyroxine–diphenylhydantoin interaction: Effect of 5,5'-diphenylhydantoin on the displacement of L-thyroxine from thyroxine-binding globulin (TBG). *Endocrinology,* 71:496–504.

63. Osorio, C., Jackson, D. J., Gartside, J. M., and Goolden, A. W. G. (1962): Effect of carbon dioxide and diphenyldantoin on the partition of triiodothyronine labelled with iodine-131 between the red cells and the plasma proteins. *Nature,* 196:275–276.

64. Partington, M. W., Reilly, D. M., Stewart, J. H., and Vickery, S. K. (1973): Serum diphenylhydantoin levels following a change in drug brand. *Can. J. Pharm. Sci.,* 9:31–32.

65. Porter, R. J., and Layzer, R. B. (1975): Plasma albumin concentration and diphenylhydantoin in man. *Arch. Neurol.,* 32:298–303.

66. Rail, L. (1968): Dilantin overdosage. *Med. J. Aust.,* 2:339.

67. Ramsay, R. E., Hammond, E. J., Perchalski, R. J., and Wilder, B. J. (1979): Brain uptake of phenytoin, phenobarbital, and diazepam. *Arch. Neurol.,* 36:535–539.

68. Rane, A., Lunde, P. K. M., Jalling, B., Yaffee, S. J., and Sjöqvist, F. (1971): Plasma protein binding of diphenylhydantoin in normal and hyperbilirubinemic infants. *Pediatr. Pharmacol. Ther.,* 78:877–882.

69. Rane, A., and Wilson, J. T. (1976): Clinical pharmacokinetics in infants and children. *Clin. Pharmacokinet.,* 1:2–24.

70. Rapport, R. L. II, Harris. A. B., Friel, P. N., and Ojemann, G. A. (1975): Human epileptic brain. Na, K, ATPase activity and phenytoin concentrations. *Arch. Neurol.,* 32:549–554.

71. Rees, H. van, and Noach, E. L. (1973): The intestinal absorption of diphenylhydantoin from a suspension in rats. *Arch. Int. Pharmacodyn. Ther.,* 206:76–83.

72. Richens, A., and Dunlop. A. (1975): Serum phenytoin levels in management of epilepsy. *Lancet,* 2:247–248.

73. Sherwin, A. L., Eisen, A. A., and Sokolowski, C. D. (1973): Anticonvulsant drugs in human epileptogenic brain. Correlation of phenobarbital and diphenylhydantoin levels with plasma. *Arch. Neurol.,* 29:73–77.

74. Shoeman, D. W., and Azarnoff, D. L. (1972): The alteration of plasma proteins in uremia as reflected in their ability to bind digitoxin and diphenylhydantoin. *Pharmacology,* 7:169–177.

75. Shoeman, E. W., and Azarnoff, D. L. (1975): Diphenylhydantoin potency and plasma protein binding. *J. Pharmacol. Exp. Ther.,* 195:83–86.

76. Sironi, V. A., Cabrini, G., Porro, M. G., Ravagnati, L., and Marossero, F. (1980): Antiepileptic drug distribution in cerebral cortex, Ammon's horn, and amygdala in man. *J. Neurosurg.,* 52:686–692.

77. Solomon, H. M., and Schrogie, J. J. (1967): The effect of phenyramidol on the metabolism of diphenylhydantoin. *Clin. Pharmacol. Ther.,* 8:554–556.

78. Squef, R., Martinez, M., and Oppenheimer, J. H. (1963): Use of thyroxine displacing drugs in identifying serum thyroxine-binding proteins separated by starch gel electrophoresis. *Proc. Soc. Exp. Biol. Med.,* 113:837–840.

79. Suzuki, T., Saitoh, Y., and Nishihara, K. (1970): Kinetics of and diphenylhydantoin disposition in man. *Chem. Pharm. Bull. (Tokyo)*, 18:405–411.

80. Swanson, B. N., Leger, R. M., Gordon, W. P., Lynn, R. K., and Gerber, N. (1978): Excretion of phenytoin into semen of rabbits and man. Comparison with plasma levels. *Drug Metab. Dispos.*, 6:70–74.

81. Tramposch, A. (1977): The effect of simultaneous administration of phenytoin and phenobarbital on their individual absorption from rat ileum *in situ*. M.S. Thesis, St. John's University, New York.

82. Troupin, A. S., and Friel, P. (1975): Anticonvulsant level in saliva, serum, and cerebrospinal fluid. *Epilepsia*, 16: 223–227.

83. Tyrer, J. H., Eadie, M. J., Sutherland, J. M., and Hooper, W. D. (1970): Outbreak of anticonvulsant intoxication in an Australian city. *Br. Med. J.*, 4:271–273.

84. Vajda, F., Williams, F. M., Davidson, S., Falconer, M. A., and Breckenridge, A. (1974): Human brain, cerebrospinal fluid, and plasma concentration of diphenylhydantoin and phenobarbital. *Clin. Pharmacol. Ther.*, 15:597–603.

85. Weiss, C. F., Heffelfinger, J. C., and Buchanan, R. A. (1969): Serial Dilantin® levels in mentally retarded children. *Am. J. Ment. Defic.*, 73:826–830.

86. Westmoreland, B., and Bass, N. H. (1971): Diphenylhydantoin intoxication during pregnancy. A chemical study of drug distribution in the albino rat. *Arch. Neurol.*, 24:158–164.

87. Wider, B. J., Buchanan, R. A., and Serrono, E. E. (1973): Correlation of acute diphenylhydantoin intoxication with plasma levels and metabolite excretion. *Neurology (Minneap.)*, 23:1329–1332.

88. Wilder, B. J., and Ramsay, R. E. (1976): Oral and intramuscular phenytoin. *Clin. Pharmacol. Ther.*, 19:360–364.

89. Wilensky, A. J., and Lowden, J. A. (1973): Inadequate serum levels after intramuscular administration of diphenylhydantoin. *Neurology (Minneap.)* 23:318–324.

90. Wolff, J., Standaert, M. E., and Rall, J. E. (1961): Thyroxine displacement from serum proteins and depression of serum protein-bound iodine by certain drugs, *J. Clin. Invest.*, 40:1373–1379.

91. Woodbury, D. M. (1969): Role of pharmacological factors in the evaluation of anticonvulsant drugs. *Epilepsia*, 10:121–124.

92. Woodbury, D. M., (1980): Phenytoin: Proposed mechanisms of anticonvulsant action. *Adv. Neurol.*, 27:447–471.

93. Woodbury, D. M. (1981): Pharmacology of anticonvulsant drugs in CSF. In: *Neurobiology of Cerebrospinal Fluid 2*, edited by J. H. Woods. Plenum Press, New York *(in press)*.

94. Woodbury, D. M., and Swinyard, E. A. (1972): Diphenylhydantoin: Absorption, distribution, and excretion. In: *Antiepileptic Drugs*, edited by D. M. Woodbury, J. K. Penry, and R. P. Schmidt, pp. 113–123. Raven Press, New York.

Antiepileptic Drugs, edited by D. M. Woodbury,
J. K. Penry, and C. E. Pippenger. Raven Press,
New York © 1982

14

Phenytoin

Biotransformation

Tsun Chang and Anthony J. Glazko

Phenytoin (5,5-diphenylhydantoin[1]; Dilantin®) is eliminated almost entirely by metabolic transformation prior to excretion in the form of metabolites. Less than 5% of the administered dose is excreted unchanged in the urine (32,46,67,80,82). Up until a decade ago, only a few metabolites of phenytoin were known (19,67). With rapid advances in analytical techniques, a number of new metabolites were identified in animals and in man. This chapter updates our current knowledge regarding the chemical and pharmacological aspects of phenytoin biotransformation.

METABOLIC PATHWAYS

On the basis of known metabolites established to date, the most likely pathways involved in the biotransformation of phenytoin are shown in Fig. 1. Since each of these products is a distinct entity in the overall scheme, the individual metabolites are discussed separately in the following sections.

Diphenylhydantoic Acid and Diphenylglycine (α-Aminodiphenylacetic Acid)

In an initial attempt to define the metabolic fate of phenytoin, Kozelka and Hine (67) reported the identification of diphenylhydantoic acid (DPHA) and diphenylglycine (DPG) in dog and in man, presumably formed via hydrolytic cleavage of the hydantoin ring (Fig. 2).

Using an iodometric titration technique, they found that 1 to 4% of the dose was excreted in dog and human urine as unchanged phenytoin, 1 to 5% as DPHA, and 10 to 27% as DPG. Only 30 to 35% of the dose was accounted for, and the authors concluded that the remainder of the dose could be completely destroyed by further degradation of DPG. This was found later to be a relatively minor pathway. Using ^{15}N-labeled phenytoin, Maynert (80) could detect only traces of DPHA and DPG in dog urine, with small amounts of ^{15}N present as urinary ammonia. Subsequent studies by Chang and Glazko (22) and by Butler et al. (20) showed that DPHA was a relatively minor metabolic product in most species of laboratory animals; however, greater amounts of DPHA were consistently found in the cat (22). These observations eliminated the hypothesis that rupture of the hydantoin ring was

[1]*Chemical Abstracts* nomenclature: 5,5-diphenyl-2,4-imidazolidinedione.

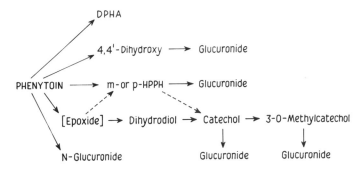

FIG. 1. Proposed pathways of phenytoin metabolism.

a significant factor in the metabolism of phenytoin. In agreement with these *in vivo* observations, Dudley et al. (33) reported that phenytoin was not a substrate for the enzyme dihydropyrimidinase *in vitro*.

Following extensive chromatographic studies of the metabolites in the urine of dogs and Rhesus monkeys receiving [^{14}C]phenytoin and in a few samples of human urine, we were unable to obtain any clear-cut evidence for the presence of DPG as a metabolite of phenytoin (22). In the absence of solid evidence to the contrary, DPG cannot be regarded as a normal metabolite of phenytoin.

Para-HPPH and Meta-HPPH

In 1956, Dill et al. (32) introduced the first quantitative analytical procedure for the assay of phenytoin in biological specimens. They also studied phenytoin metabolism in animals and in man and identified unchanged drug in rat and dog liver as well as in human plasma. They reported the excretion of small amounts of unchanged drug in rat urine and detected at least three metabolites by paper chromatography. A year later, Butler (19) isolated and identified 5-(4-hydroxyphenyl)-5-phenylhydantoin[2] (*p*-HPPH) as the principal urinary metabolite in man and dog. Fifty to 60% of the administered dose was recovered in the urine as an acid-labile conjugate of *p*-HPPH, but only traces of free *p*-

HPPH were detected. Using [^{14}C]phenytoin, Noach et al. (82) demonstrated that 95% of the dose appeared as metabolites in rat urine and that *p*-HPPH accounted for 60 to 70% of the total metabolites present. Maynert (80) clearly established that the conjugate was a glucuronide from which *p*-HPPH could be released by incubation with β-glucuronidase. Direct evidence for the structure of *p*-HPPH glucuronide was provided by Thompson et al. (100), using a permethylation and gas chromatography–mass spectrometry (GC–MS) technique. The *p*-HPPH preparations isolated by Butler (19) from the urine of man and dog appeared to be identical in their physical and chemical properties, but there were marked differences in their optical rotation. The *p*-HPPH isolated from human urine was levorotatory, whereas the *p*-HPPH from dog urine was dextrorotatory. Butler (19) concluded that only one phenyl ring could be hydroxylated in man, whereas either ring could be hydroxylated in the dog. A great deal of new information on the stereoselective hydroxylation of phenytoin in man and in the dog has appeared in the last few years. This will be discussed later in this chapter.

The possible existence of a sulfate conjugate of *p*-HPPH was considered by Maynert (80) and rejected when treatment with phenol sulfatase failed to liberate *p*-HPPH from its conjugate. The absence of a sulfate conjugate was later confirmed by Chang and Glazko (22) by comparing the rate of release of *p*-HPPH from a conjugate isolated from rat urine and from a synthetic *p*-HPPH ethereal sulfate in the pres-

[2]*Chemical Abstracts* nomenclature: 5-(4-hydroxyphenyl)-5-phenyl-2,4-imidazolidinedione.

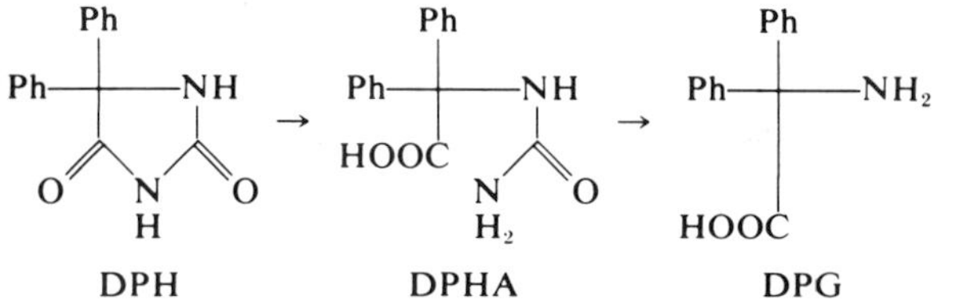

FIG. 2. Structures of phenytoin (DPH), diphenylhydantoic acid (DPHA), and diphenylglycine (DPG).

ence of aryl sulfatase. The synthetic conjugate was completely hydrolyzed in 1 hr, whereas no p-HPPH was released from the urinary conjugate.

Para-hydroxylation has generally been regarded as the major pathway for phenytoin metabolism in man (19,46,80) and in laboratory animals (19,22,80,82). However, in 1970, using the GC–MS technique, Atkinson et al. (4) reported that the major metabolite in dog was m-HPPH, with lesser, variable amounts of p-HPPH also present. The relative proportions of these two metabolites in acid-hydrolyzed dog and human urine are shown in Table 1 (4). Initially, we were unable to confirm the presence of m-HPPH in human urine following enzymatic hydrolysis (22), and the m-HPPH detected by Atkinson et al. (4) was thought to be formed entirely by degradation of the dihydrodiol metabolite (25) during acid hydrolysis of the glucuronides. However, recent work in our laboratory (49) as well as published reports (20) showed that traces of m-HPPH could be found in human urine after treatment with β-glucuron-

idase. According to Butler et al. (20), the ratio of total m-HPPH to p-HPPH in two patients was approximately 1 to 400, considerably less than that reported by Atkinson et al. (4) in acid-hydrolyzed human urine. We had no difficulty in confirming Atkinson's observation in dogs when enzymic hydrolysis was used in place of the acid treatment. Further examination of urine from the cat, mouse, rat, rabbit, and rhesus monkey by gas–liquid chromatographic (GLC) procedures after enzymatic hydrolysis revealed no significant amounts of m-HPPH present.

The identification of both m-HPPH and p-HPPH in dog urine raised questions regarding the homogeneity of the p-HPPH isolated in earlier studies (4,25). Butler et al. (20) then reexamined an authentic sample of p-HPPH isolated in 1957 with modern gas chromatography techniques, and found that the material was indeed pure p-HPPH. Butler et al. (20) recognized the shortcomings of the countercurrent extraction system used in the 1957 study and suggested that the two metabolites were effectively separated by the crystallization steps that followed.

TABLE 1. *Comparison of meta-hydroxylation and para-hydroxylation in man and in dog*

Subject	m-HPPH		p-HPPH	
	μg/ml	%	μg/ml	%[a]
Dog				
1	180.0	74.0	64.0	26.0
2	52.0	82.0	12.0	18.0
3	76.0	78.0	21.0	22.0
4	250.0	65.0	135.0	35.0
Patient				
J.G.	9.0	7.0	116.0	93.0
E.C.	3.0	6.0	51.0	94.0
H.W.	3.0	5.0	56.0	95.0
G.P.	6.0	13.0	39.0	87.0
R.M.	21.0	6.0	359.0	94.0

[a]Results are expressed as percent of total m-HPPH plus p-HPPH.
From Atkinson et al. (4) with permission of the publisher.

As a result, pure p-HPPH was obtained in crystalline form, whereas m-HPPH was lost in the mother liquors.

The *meta*-hydroxylation pathway in dogs appears to be limited to the metabolism of phenytoin. When racemic p-HPPH or m-HPPH was administered to dogs, the compounds were excreted in the urine as glucuronide conjugates with no change in optical rotation (19,20,22). Similarly, the administration of racemic p-HPPH to man or of p-HPPH isolated from rat urine to other rats failed to produce any evidence of further metabolism (19,22). However, in a later study by Gerber and Thompson (39), traces of dihydroxyphenyl metabolites were detected in rat bile following administration of either m-HPPH or p-HPPH.

Dihydrodiol Metabolite

Earlier studies carried out by Noach et al. (82) and Woodbury (103) suggested the presence of hydroxylated metabolites other than p-HPPH. In a preliminary report, Woodbury (103) postulated that two other metabolites might be present in rat urine: (a) one with both phenyl rings hydroxylated in the *para* position, and (b) the other with the *meta* and *para* positions of one ring hydroxylated to form a catechol. No evidence was present to support the proposed chemical structures at that time. Interestingly, both of these products were identified several years later by other investigators (23,99).

Meanwhile, Chang et al. (25) isolated a dihydrodiol metabolite from rat and monkey urine and identified the structure as 5-(3,4-dihydroxy-1,5-cyclohexadien-1-yl)-5-phenylhydantoin.[3] This involved conversion of a phenyl ring to the cyclohexadiene diol with loss of aromaticity. The dihydrodiol metabolite did not have any of the physical and chemical characteristics of the dihydroxyphenyl derivative suggested by Woodbury (103). When an acidic solution of the dihydrodiol or the dry powder was heated, equal amounts of m-HPPH and p-HPPH were

formed (25). Preliminary evidence suggested that the two hydroxyl groups of the dihydrodiol were oriented in the trans configuration (22). The structure of the dihydrodiol was confirmed by Horning et al. (58) using the GC–MS technique. The metabolite was detected in the urine of newborn human infants and subsequently, by others, in the urine of rats (41), mice (98), and men (37,55).

Although dihydrodiols have been identified as metabolites of halobenzenes (91), polycyclic aromatic hydrocarbons (10,11,15,16), and some nonaromatic hydrocarbons (18,73), the dihydrodiol of phenytoin represented the first example of such a metabolite for therapeutic agents. Since then similar metabolites have been identified for a number of drugs (56,59), indicating that this pathway may occur frequently.

Dihydrodiols are known to be formed from arene oxides (14,15,29,51,63–65,83), suggesting that an arene oxide (epoxide) might be an intermediate in phenytoin metabolism. The evidence in support of this hypothesis is largely indirect (22). Incubation of [^{14}C]phenytoin with rat liver $9,000 \times g$ supernatant and reduced glutathione resulted in formation of a product that, when heated with acid, produced p-HPPH (22). However, the chemical nature of the complex has not been established. Other possible metabolites that could arise from arene oxides are permercapturic and mercapturic acids (63,64), but no such metabolites of phenytoin have been identified. In addition, arene oxides are known to undergo nonenzymatic isomerization to phenolic products (29). The role of arene oxide in the possible formation of monohydroxylated metabolites of phenytoin is not clear. Recent evidence seems to favor the arene oxide pathway in some species (20,77,77a,101). On the other hand, a separate hydroxylation mechanism has been postulated for the formation of certain phenols (101).

Arene oxides have attracted considerable attention because of their reactivity and possible role in toxicity mechanisms (17,28,42,83). The teratogenic effect of phenytoin (53,79) suggests that such an intermediate may be in-

---

[3]*Chemical Abstracts* nomenclature: 5-(3,4-dihydroxy-1,5-cyclohexadien-1-yl)-5-phenyl-2,4-imidazolidinedione.

volved. This possibility was investigated by Martz et al. (78). When Swiss mice (day 11 of gestation) were given teratogenic doses of phenytoin (50, 75, and 100 mg/kg) together with 1,2-epoxy-3,3,3-trichloropropane (TCPO, 100 mg/kg), an epoxide hydratase inhibitor, the incidence of cleft lip and palate increased significantly over the phenytoin control group, and the embryo lethality doubled. Covalent binding of ^{14}C radioactivity in the fetus and placenta 4 hr after administration of [^{14}C]phenytoin plus TCPO was twofold greater than with [^{14}C]phenytoin alone. The TCPO had no marked effect on maternal plasma phenytoin levels or on fetal or placental uptake of phenytoin. The authors concluded that the teratogenesis was caused by arene oxide formation and covalent binding to constituents of the gestational tissue.

Catechol and 3-0-Methyl Catechol Metabolites

Using radioisotopes and GC–MS, Chang et al. (23) identified a 3,4-catechol metabolite, 5-(3,4-dihydroxyphenyl)-5-phenylhydantoin, in rat urine following administration of phenytoin in the diet over a period of 2 weeks. In the meantime, Borga et al. (12) detected the same metabolite in rat urine and human urine. Further work by Chang et al. (24) resulted in the identification of a 3-0-methylcatechol metabolite in rat urine as 5-(4-hydroxy-3-methoxyphenyl)-5-phenylhydantoin. The thin-layer chromatographic (TLC) characteristics of the two metabolites in rat urine are shown in Fig. 3. The catechol and the 3-0-methylcatechol represented approximately 2% and 10%, respectively, of the total phenytoin metabolites in rat urine. The use of trimethylsilyl derivatives (23,24) was the key step in identification of these metabolites by making it possible to distinguish between the catechol and 3-0-methylcatechol. Borga et al. (12), using an on-column methylation technique, were unable to distinguish between the two metabolites because they formed the same end product, 1,3-dimethyl-5-(3,4-dimethoxy-phenyl)-5-phenylhydantoin. Later, Midha et al. (81) reported positive identification of the

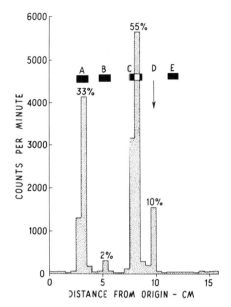

FIG. 3. TLC of phenytoin metabolites in rat urine. Band A, dihydrodiol; B, catechol; C, *p*-HPPH; D, 3-*O*-methylcatechol. Figures express percent of ^{14}C in each fraction. (From Chang et al., ref. 24, with permission of PJD Publications, Ltd., Westbury, N.Y. 11590, USA)

catechol and 3-0-methylcatechol in human, monkey, and dog urine. The same metabolites were also identified as glucuronides in the bile from isolated perfused rat liver (38).

The mechanism by which the catechol is formed has not been clearly established. It could be formed via dehydrogenation of the dihydrodiol metabolite by a mechanism similar to those described by Ayengar et al. (7). In a preliminary experiment, the ^{14}C-labeled dihydrodiol metabolite isolated from rat urine was administered perorally to rats. It did not result in the appearance of the catechol metabolite in the urine (23). However, it should be noted that the catechol was isolated from rat urine following repeated doses of phenytoin administered over extended periods of time. In earlier single-dose studies, no significant amounts of the catechol metabolite could be detected in the urine (25). Horning and Lertratanangkoon (57) reported that the urinary excretion of catechol metabolites increased approximately 10-fold following chronic administration of phenytoin in rats. Possibly, the catechol metabolite could be formed by further hydroxylation of *m*-HPPH or *p*-HPPH. Gerber and Thompson (39) identified small amounts of the catechol and 3-*O*-methylcatechol in rat bile by GC–MS techniques following administration of *m*-HPPH or *p*-HPPH to rats or by addition of these compounds to an isolated perfused rat liver preparation. However, other studies (20,22) in which *p*-HPPH or *m*-HPPH was administered to rats or dogs failed to produce any new metabolic products other than the glucuronic acid conjugates.

In rat urine, the concentration of the 3-*O*-methylcatechol metabolite was approximately fivefold greater than that of the catechol, indicating extensive *O*-methylation in this species (24). Evidence obtained in our laboratory indicates that the 3-*O*-methylcatechol metabolite of phenytoin is formed from the catechol. Administration of the synthetic 3,4-dihydroxycatechol to rats resulted in the prompt appearance of 3-*O*-methylcatechol in the urine (24). It is reasonable to assume that the enzyme catechol-*O*-methyltransferase is involved in the formation of this metabolite, since it is known to methylate other catechols including catecholamines (6). This is of interest in terms of mechanism of action, since the phenytoin catechol metabolite could compete with other catechols or catecholamines for 3-*O*-methylation pathways. Hadfield (52) reported that the administration of phenytoin influenced the uptake and binding of catecholamines in rat brain.

4,4′-Dihydroxy Metabolite and *N*-Glucuronide of Phenytoin

Two minor metabolites of phenytoin, the 5,5-*bis*(4-hydroxyphenyl) hydantoin (99) and an *N*-glucuronide of phenytoin (92), were recently identified in rat and in man. The 4,4′-dihydroxy metabolite was excreted as a glucuronide and accounted for about 1% of the total hydroxylated metabolites. The pathway that leads to the formation of this metabolite is not known. When *p*-HPPH was added to the perfusate of an isolated rat liver preparation, there was no evidence for the formation of the 4,4′-dihydroxy metabolite (99). However, addition of the synthetic 4,4′-dihydroxy compound to the same *in vitro* preparation (99) resulted in the formation of a monoglucuronide, a trihydroxyphenytoin glucuronide, and a dihydroxymethoxyphenytoin glucuronide, indicating further hydroxylation of the dihydroxy metabolite. Whether the trihydroxylated product represents normal phenytoin metabolites in intact animals is not known at the present time.

The glucuronide of phenytoin was isolated from an epileptic patient receiving phenytoin and characterized as the N-3 glucuronide by GC–MS. The same metabolite was also present in the bile of an isolated perfused rat liver preparation. The structure assignment was based on the mass spectra of various permethylated derivatives and a comparison of the reaction of the metabolite and 5,5-diphenyl-3-methylhydantoin with diazomethane (92).

STEREOSELECTIVE HYDROXYLATION OF PHENYTOIN

Because of the steric configuration of the hydantoin ring, the two identical phenyl groups of phenytoin attached to carbon 5 are spatially distinguishable and are not necessarily equally susceptible to enzymatic hydroxylation. Introduction of a hydroxyl group in one of the phenyl rings leads to the creation of a chiral center and results in the formation of optically active phenolic metabolites.

Early work by Butler (19) showed that the *p*-HPPH isolated from human urine was levorotatory ($[\alpha]_D^{28} = -16°$) and had the properties of an optically pure enantiomer. The *p*-HPPH specimens isolated from the urine of two different dogs were slightly dextrorotatory and contained slightly different proportions of dextro- and levorotatory isomers (63 : 37 and 56 : 44). Butler (19) concluded that only one phenyl ring was hydroxylated in man, whereas either ring could be hydroxylated in the dog. A levorotatory *p*-HPPH ($[\alpha]_D^{28} = -13.5°$) from rabbit urine has been reported by Gorvin and Brownlee (50).

In 1970, Atkinson et al. (4) identified *m*-HPPH as a major metabolite in dog urine, but the optical rotation was not measured. Chang and Glazko (22) separated *m*-HPPH and *p*-HPPH from enzyme-hydrolyzed dog urine by column chromatography and TLC. The *m*-HPPH had an optical rotation of $[\alpha]_D^{25} = +3.2°$ and the *p*-HPPH showed an opposite rotation of $-2.5°$. In addition, *p*-HPPH was also isolated from rat and monkey urine. Some major differences were noted in the optical rotation of *p*-HPPH isolated from the urine of dog ($-2.5°$), rat ($-18.2°$), and monkey ($-7.0°$) (25). The dihydrodiol metabolite from rat urine showed an optical rotation of $-163°$ (25).

Butler et al. (20) reinvestigated the stereochemistry of phenytoin hydroxylation in man and in the dog. The metabolites (*m*-HPPH or *p*-HPPH) were purified from β-glucuronidase-treated urine using solvent partitioning without crystallization. The results of their study revealed a profound difference in stereoselectivity of phenytoin hydroxylation in the two species. The *m*-HPPH from dog urine was dextrorotatory ($[\alpha]_D^{28} = +8.3°$ and $+8.0°$ for two dogs) and was entirely in the form of a pure optical isomer. The *p*-HPPH from dog and human urine consisted of a 2 : 1 and 10 : 1 mixture, respectively, of levo- and dextrorotatory isomers. The amount of *m*-HPPH in human urine was too low to permit isolation and measurement of optical rotation. The absolute configuration of the optical isomers of *p*-HPPH and *m*-HPPH were established by Poupaert et al. (87) and Maguire et al. (77). The predominant metabolite in human urine, ($-$)-*p*-HPPH, was shown to have the *S* configuration (87), whereas the ($+$)-*m*-HPPH from dog urine had the *R* configuration (77).

The steric configurations of phenytoin and its phenolic metabolites, as summarized by Butler et al. (20), are shown in Fig. 4. To explain the differences in phenytoin hydroxylation for the two species, Butler et al. (20) suggested that at least two functional types of hydroxylating enzymes were present with different stereospecificities and mechanisms of action. The predominant enzyme in man attacks the pro-*S* phenyl ring (A) in the *para* position, resulting in the formation of (*S*)-($-$)-*p*-HPPH. The small amounts of dextrorotatory *p*-HPPH [(*R*)-($+$)-*p*-HPPH] found in man could be produced by the same enzyme or, alternatively, by a second highly stereospecific enzyme. The ratio of (*S*)-($-$)-*p*-HPPH/(*R*)-($+$)-*p*-HPPH in human urine is about 10 : 1. In contrast, the principal enzyme in the dog attacks the pro-*R* ring (B) in the *meta* position with complete stereospecificity, producing the optical isomer (*R*)-($+$)-*m*-HPPH. In addition, the dog has a *para*-hydroxylating enzyme similar to the one in man, and the predominant product is (*S*)-($-$)-*p*-HPPH,

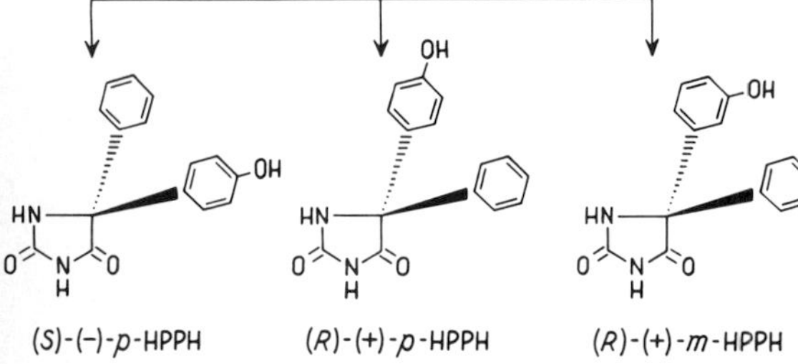

FIG. 4. Steric configurations of the major urinary metabolites of phenytoin in men and in the dog. (From Butler et al., ref. 20, with permission of the publisher.)

with lesser amounts of (R)-(+)-p-HPPH present. The ratio of (S)-(−)-p-HPPH/(R)-(+)-p-HPPH/(R)-(+)-m-HPPH in the dog is approximately 2 : 1 : 18.

The oxidative pathways for the formation of phenytoin metabolites have not been clearly established. The metabolites may be formed by direct hydroxylation of the phenyl rings and/or via intermediate arene oxide metabolites (20,77,101). Maguire et al. (77a) have shown that the dihydrodiol metabolite has an S-configuration in rat and man, whereas the dog produces a 2:1 ratio of the R- and S-diastereoisomers. Although this suggests that the R- and S-arene oxides could be intermediates in the formation of the dihydrodiol and phenolic metabolites, direct hydroxylation has not been ruled out.

SPECIES DIFFERENCES IN METABOLISM

Using [^{14}C]phenytoin, we have chromatographed urine specimens from different species of laboratory animals with the results shown in Table 2 (22). With the exception of the dog,

the major product in all species was a glucuronic acid conjugate of p-HPPH. Significant amounts of free p-HPPH were observed in the urine of mouse, rat, and cat. The dihydrodiol metabolite was found to be present in higher concentrations in the urine of rat and monkey than in the mouse or dog. Small amounts of DPHA were present in the urine of all species examined, but consistently greater amounts were found in the cat. The catechol and 3-0-methylcatechol metabolites were detected in rat urine after repeated administration of phenytoin in the diet and accounted for 2% and 10%, respectively, of the total metabolites present (24). In dog urine, the major metabolite was a glucuronic acid conjugate of m-HPPH. When synthetic p-HPPH was administered to a dog, the compound was excreted unchanged (except for conjugation), and no dihydroxy metabolites were found, indicating that p-HPPH does not undergo further hydroxylation to form a catechol in this species (19,20,22).

Preliminary GLC examination of a number of urine specimens from normal adult subjects and uremic patients receiving phenytoin, as well as from young children, indicated that only

TABLE 2. *Distribution of phenytoin metabolites in animal urine*

Species	TLC solvent systems[a]	Phenytoin metabolites (% of total radioactivity on TLC plates)			
		Conjugated HPPH	DPHA	Diol	Free HPPH
Mouse	A	62	5	14	19
	B	60	5	17	18
Rat	A	58	—	28	14
	B	45	6	29	20
Rabbit	A	95	—	5	—
	B	89	2	9	—
Cat	A	66	13	—	21
	B	67	11	7	15
Dog[b]	A	85	—	15	—
	B	80	6	14	—
Monkey	A	68	—	32	—
	B	66	2	30	2

[a]System A: Silica gel GF with chloroform : methanol : glacial acetic acid (90 : 20 : 1). System B: Silica gel GF with chloroform : methanol (70 : 30).

[b]GLC indicated that m-HPPH was the major metabolite in dog urine.

From Chang et al. (22) with permission of the publisher.

traces of *m*-HPPH and the dihydrodiol metabolite were present. A subsequent crossover study (26) was carried out with six adult male volunteers (three short and three long phenytoin half-life subjects) receiving [^{13}C,^{14}C]-double-labeled phenytoin administered (a) as single 250-mg intravenous doses, (b) as single 250-mg peroral doses, and (c) as single 250-mg intravenous doses following peroral administration of unlabeled phenytoin (100 mg t.i.d.) for 14 days. The urine specimens were examined for ^{14}C activity by TLC following β-glucuronidase treatment. The metabolite distribution patterns were similar in all three treatment groups (% of urinary radioactivity): 68 to 81% *p*-HPPH, 7 to 11% dihydrodiol, 3 to 6% unknown (at the origin), 2.5% 3-0-methylcatechol, 1 to 2% unchanged phenytoin, and about 1% dihydroxycatechol. The subjects with short phenytoin half-lives (<15 hr) generally excreted more *p*-HPPH and less dihydrodiol metabolite, although these differences were not statistically significant. Typical metabolite profiles following peroral doses are shown in Table 3. Metabolites in feces (% of fecal radioactivity) were identified as *p*-HPPH (50–80%), dihydrodiol (15–35%), and the dihydroxycatechol (5–10%).

The routes of excretion of phenytoin metabolites also showed species differences. The dog consistently excreted large amounts of metabolites in the bile (33% of a given dose), whereas the rhesus monkey excreted only 10% in the bile. The nature of the metabolites in monkey and dog bile is of interest because of these differences. Direct TLC of bile from dogs receiving [^{14}C]phenytoin indicated that most of the radioactivity remained at the origin because of polar conjugates. Following enzymatic hydrolysis with β-glucuronidase (Glusulase®), GLC of the bile extract revealed a mixture of *m*-HPPH and *p*-HPPH. Monkey bile contained mainly conjugated *p*-HPPH together with a small amount of unchanged phenytoin.

Species differences in the formation of glucuronic acid conjugates of *m*-HPPH or *p*-HPPH in rat or dog liver supernatant were reported by Gabler (35). Conjugation of *m*-HPPH was greater than that of *p*-HPPH in the dog liver, whereas the opposite effect was found with rat liver supernatant, reflecting, perhaps, a basic species difference in metabolism.

Sex differences in the metabolism of phenytoin should also be mentioned. Conard (27) reported that male rats had a plasma phenytoin half-life of about 0.5 hr and female rats showed a half-life of 2 hr. When the females were pretreated with SKF 525-A (50 mg/kg i.p.) 40 min before dosing with phenytoin, the normal 2-hr half-life was extended to 17 hr. This was accompanied by a reduction in plasma *p*-HPPH levels, indicating that SKF 525-A interfered with the hydroxylation process.

IN VITRO HYDROXYLATION OF PHENYTOIN AND ITS INHIBITION BY HYDROXYLATED METABOLITES

Phenytoin is hydroxylated primarily in the liver by the mixed-function oxidases associated

TABLE 3. *Relative concentrations^a of metabolites in the urine of subjects receiving single 250-mg i.v. doses of labeled phenytoin*

	Subject no.	Phenytoin	*p*-HPPH	3,4-DiOH	3-0-Me	Diol	Origin
Short half-life	4	1.3	88.4	<1	1.6	6.8	2.2
	8	1.7	82.4	<1	1.8	8.8	5.3
	23	1.6	85.1	<1	1.4	6.3	5.5
	Mean	1.5	85.3	<1	1.6	7.3	4.2
Long half-life	14	1.6	80.2	<1	2.4	12.0	3.3
	27	1.1	89.5	<1	0.4	3.7	5.0
	30	1.4	76.7	<1	3.4	15.5	3.1
	Mean	1.4	82.1	<1	2.1	10.4	3.8

^{a}Percent of total ^{14}C on TLC plate.

with the smooth endoplasmic reticulum of the hepatocytes. The rate of hydroxylation appears to be slow, as reflected by the relatively long plasma phenytoin half-lives. It is influenced in part by genetic factors (72), dose-dependent kinetics (1,30,36,41,46,88,89), enzyme induction (36), and by the presence of other drugs (8,60,68,71). The greatly delayed appearance of p-HPPH in the plasma and urine following administration of phenytoin may provide a clue to the mechanism responsible for the extended half-life of this drug. With 0.5-g oral doses of phenytoin administered in gelatin capsules to normal human subjects, peak plasma levels were observed 4 to 12 hr after dosing, whereas the peak urinary excretion of p-HPPH occurred mainly in the 12- to 24-hr period after dosing. Some subjects showed maximum p-HPPH excretion rates as long as 24 to 48 hr after dosing (48). With 250-mg intravenous doses of phenytoin, maximum p-HPPH excretion occurred 6 to 8 hr after dosing (46), showing good correspondence with peak plasma p-HPPH levels (31). These observations suggest that the hydroxylation of phenytoin and the release of p-HPPH into the circulation may be rate-limiting factors in the disposition of this drug. Several in vitro preparations, including isolated perfused liver, isolated hepatocytes, 9,000 × g supernatant, and isolated liver microsomes, have been used to characterize the enzyme system responsible for the hydroxylation of phenytoin.

A dose-dependent metabolism of phenytoin was demonstrated in isolated perfused rat liver preparation (41,61) and in isolated rat hepatocytes (62). The results of these studies also indicated a rapid initial hepatic uptake of phenytoin and extensive binding of the drug in the liver. The principal end product was p-HPPH which was conjugated with glucuronic acid and excreted. The conversion of phenytoin to p-HPPH appeared to be the rate-limiting step in the elimination of phenytoin (41,61).

The microsomal phenytoin hydroxylation system was characterized using rat liver 9,000 × g supernatant or washed liver microsomes (69,70). The cofactor requirements included NADP, NAD, ATP, and oxygen, with an optimal pH of 7.4 and temperature of 37°C. The in vitro hydroxylation of phenytoin in this system exhibited typical saturable enzyme kinetics, with an apparent K_m value of 3.73×10^{-5} M (range 3 to 5×10^{-5} M) (70). The addition of isoniazid (71), SKF 525-A, phenobarbital (70), d-propoxyphene (102), ethosuximide (84), valproate (84), sulthiame (84), or a number of commonly used drugs (70) to the reaction mixture inhibited the reaction. SKF 525-A inhibition was noncompetitive, whereas phenobarbital inhibition was competitive (70). Pretreatment of rats with phenobarbital, chlordane, or DDT prior to sacrifice resulted in a moderate increase in the activity of the microsomal enzymes (69). Pretreatment of rats with phenytoin for 7 days had no apparent effect on the microsomal enzymes, although enzyme induction by phenytoin has been suggested by others (34,36). On the basis of their in vitro kinetic studies, Kutt and Fouts (69), concluded that phenytoin is bound weakly to the microsomal enzymes, accounting for existing clinical observations on the effects of other drugs as inhibitors of phenytoin metabolism and for the relatively low effect of microsomal enzyme inducers on phenytoin metabolism.

Butler et al. (21) succeeded in generating trace amounts of m-HPPH and p-HPPH in vitro using dog liver 9,000 × g supernatant or isolated microsomes. The hydroxylation efficiency of the system was rather poor when compared with similar preparations from rat liver. The quantity of m-HPPH was too low to permit accurate quantitative measurements. Trace amounts of p-HPPH were also detected. The optimal conditions for maximum enzyme activity have not been established. It is possible that the cofactor requirements for stability of the dog hepatic microsomal enzyme system may be entirely different from those of the rat.

In an effort to determine the effect of p-HPPH on the hydroxylation of phenytoin and the effect of phenytoin on the conjugation of p-HPPH with glucuronic acid, a series of in vitro studies were initiated in our laboratory. The addition of synthetic p-HPPH and p-HPPH isolated from rat urine to fortified 9,000 × g rat liver supernatant inhibited phenytoin hydroxylation in a competitive manner ($K_I = 6.4 \times 10^{-5}$ M) (13,43). The inhibitory effect of *p*-HPPH isolated from rat urine is shown in Fig. 5. The addition of phenytoin (2 to 4×10^{-4} M), however, had no marked effect on the rate of formation of *p*-HPPH (43) or on the kinetics of *p*-HPPH conjugation *in vitro* (13). This led to our proposal (43) that the inhibition of DPH hydroxylation could be the result of a feedback mechanism in which the hydroxylated metabolite competes with phenytoin for binding sites on the enzyme complex. In subsequent studies, the catechol and 3-*0*-methylcatechol metabolites of phenytoin were also found to inhibit the *in vitro* hydroxylation of phenytoin (44,45). We also observed that *p*-HPPH inhibited the *in vitro* hydroxylation of phenylbutazone and ripazepam; conversely, oxyphenylbutazone inhibited the hydroxylation of phenytoin (44,45). Stavchansky and associates (76,94–96) reported that *p*-HPPH inhibited the *in vitro* metabolism

of hexobarbital, ethylmorphine, zoxazolamine, and aniline in rat liver $9,000 \times g$ supernatant. The inhibition of ethylmorphine demethylation appeared to be competitive ($K_I = 1.2 \times 10^{-4}$ M), and the inhibition of aniline metabolism was noncompetitive. The inhibition of nicotine metabolism by *p*-HPPH was also reported (75). Spectral changes (95) in microsomal suspensions produced by *p*-HPPH alone or in combination with type I (hexobarbital) or type II (aniline) substrates strongly suggested that *p*-HPPH interacted with cytochrome P-450, resulting in possible interference with the binding and metabolism of drug substrates.

ROLE OF HYDROXYLATED METABOLITES OF PHENYTOIN IN DOSE DEPENDENCY

The dose-dependent phenytoin elimination kinetics observed in laboratory animals (30,

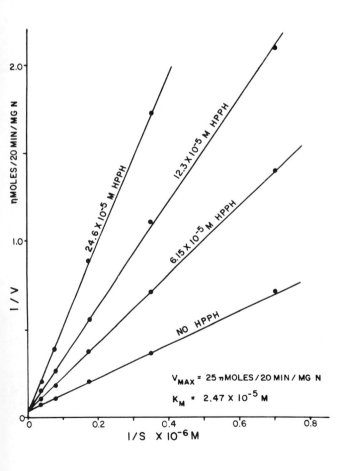

FIG. 5. Inhibition of phenytoin hydroxylation by *p*-HPPH isolated from rat urine (Lineweaver–Burke plot).

36,41) and in man (1,46) are generally attributed to capacity-limited metabolism, adequately described by the Michaelis–Menten equation (5,40). However, this does not necessarily indicate what mechanisms are involved. Clinical manifestations include a curvilinear decline of plasma phenytoin levels (1,30,36,41,43,46), dependence of plasma phenytoin half-life on dosage (30,36), abrupt nonlinear increase in plasma phenytoin levels with minor increases of dosage (9,88,89), and a difference in the area under curve for oral and intravenous routes of administration (66). Data obtained in our laboratory also showed a greatly delayed appearance of *p*-HPPH in the plasma and urine following phenytoin administration (46) as well as dose-dependent excretion of *p*-HPPH.

In searching for an alternative explanation other than capacity-limited metabolism, we first observed that *p*-HPPH inhibited the *in vitro* hydroxylation of phenytoin in a competitive manner (13). In addition, the catechol and 3-*0*-methylcatechol metabolites of phenytoin were also found to inhibit phenytoin hydroxylation *in vitro* (44). This formed the basis of our proposal (43) that product inhibition might be involved in the nonlinear elimination kinetics of phenytoin.

Following completion of our initial *in vitro* studies (13), Ashley and Levy (2) reported that *p*-HPPH given intravenously (25 mg/kg) every 30 min to male rats resulted in a considerable prolongation of plasma phenytoin half-life, 27.5 hr for phenytoin alone versus 126 hr for phenytoin plus *p*-HPPH. The authors concluded that their observation was consistent with product inhibition of phenytoin metabolism. Additional support for the suggested role of product inhibition came from a follow-up study by Levy and Ashley (74) in which they showed that coadministration of phenytoin and salicylamide, a potent inhibitor of glucuronide formation, greatly decreased the rate of phenytoin metabolism. The inhibitory effect presumably resulted from endogeneous *p*-HPPH accumulating at the site of biotransformation. There are indications that *p*-HPPH must be conjugated with glucu-

ronic acid at or close to the site of hydroxylation before it can be released. More information is needed on the sequential steps involved in the metabolism of phenytoin before the mechanism of *p*-HPPH inhibition can be fully understood.

Ashley and Levy (3) reported that the elimination kinetics of phenytoin in rats following 10-mg/kg and 40-mg/kg intravenous doses of phenytoin could not be described by simple Michaelis–Menten kinetics but were qualitatively consistent with product inhibition of phenytoin metabolism. Computer simulation (85) indicated that the dose-dependent change in plasma half-life of some drugs could be explained by product inhibition rather than Michaelis–Menten kinetics. In related developments, Stavchansky et al. (94,96) demonstrated that *p*-HPPH produced a fivefold increase in the hexobarbital sleeping time in mice and produced a twofold increase in the zoxazolamine paralysis time in rats (76). Soda and Levy (93) reported the inhibition of phenytoin metabolism by oxyphenylbutazone in rats. However, the elimination kinetics of sulfanilamide (93), a drug that is not metabolized by oxidative pathways, was not affected by oxyphenylbutazone or 4-hydroxyantipyrine. These observations are compatible with the suggestion (95) that product inhibition or cross-product inhibition may be caused by interaction of the hydroxylated metabolites with cytochrome P-450.

Later, the dose-dependent elimination of phenytoin and the inhibition of phenytoin metabolism by *p*-HPPH were studied in rhesus monkeys (47). Two rhesus monkeys were dosed with [^{14}C]phenytoin intravenously at 10 mg/kg and 50 mg/kg, respectively. At the 10-mg/kg dose level, the plasma phenytoin level was 10 μg/ml 1 hr after dosing and fell with a half-life of 9 hr. The total (free plus conjugated) *p*-HPPH levels rose to a maximum of 2.5 μg/ml in 2 to 4 hr and then declined with a half-life of 16 hr. In the monkey receiving a 50-mg/kg dose, the peak phenytoin levels were about 55 μg/ml, falling slowly over the first 24-hr period with a half-life of 22 hr and then more rapidly as the plasma phenytoin levels continued to fall with a half-life of about 9 hr. The total plasma *p*-

HPPH levels reached a peak of 9 μg/ml about 4 to 8 hr after dosing, nearly double the time required at the lower dose. The p-HPPH half-life in this animal was about 18 hr. Approximately two-thirds of the p-HPPH was conjugated in the monkey plasma regardless of dose, indicating that the glucuronidation of p-HPPH was not affected by high concentrations of phenytoin.

The effects of p-HPPH on plasma phenytoin levels and half-lives were examined in the same animal that had received the single 10-mg/kg [14C]phenytoin dose. This time, a 50-mg/kg intravenous dose of synthetic p-HPPH was administered 2 hr before a 10-mg/kg intravenous dose of [14C]phenytoin. This was followed 2 hr later by a second 50-mg/kg intravenous dose of p-HPPH. The results are graphically illustrated in Fig. 6. Without added p-HPPH, the plasma phenytoin half-life was about 9 hr. The [14C]-p-HPPH levels rose to an early peak 2 to 4 hr after dosing and then declined with a half-life of 16 hr. In the presence of exogenous p-HPPH, the plasma phenytoin levels fell more slowly with a half-life of about 21 hr over the first 24-

hr period and then more rapidly with a half-life of 12 hr in the 24- to 48-hr period after dosing. The plasma [14C]-p-HPPH levels rose more slowly in the presence of exogenous p-HPPH, reached peak value in the 8- to 24-hr period, and then fell more slowly with an estimated half-life of 25 hr. The extent of p-HPPH conjugation remained unchanged despite the high p-HPPH dose. In addition, the peak 14C urinary excretion rate without the loading dose of p-HPPH occurred in the 2- to 4-hr period, whereas the peak excretion rate with the loading dose occurred in the 8- to 24-hr period. The overall urinary recovery of 14C was the same in both cases, representing about 80% of the dose. The data clearly indicate that the normal rate of hydroxylation of phenytoin is significantly reduced in the presence of excess p-HPPH, resulting in a marked increase in the plasma half-life of phenytoin.

The clinical significance of p-HPPH inhibition of phenytoin metabolism in man has not been established. Perucca et al. (86) investigated this possibility in three normal human subjects receiving 100-mg doses of phenytoin, with and without intravenously infused p-HPPH. Their observations indicated that p-HPPH did not produce any significant change in the rate of elimination of phenytoin, apparent volume of distribution, or plasma clearance. The disparity between the animal and human data could have resulted from a number of factors, e.g., species differences in phenytoin metabolism or differences in dosage of p-HPPH used. The 100-mg phenytoin doses used in the study by Perucca et al. (86) were about five-fold lower on an mg/kg basis than those used in the animal experiments (2,47) and actually were not in a range where "saturation" of enzyme capacity would be expected.

The genetic make-up of individual subjects is another factor that may contribute to the large intersubject variation in the rate of phenytoin metabolism. Phenytoin intoxication has been reported in one family with a genetically determined limited capacity to hydroxylate phenytoin (72). This has been confirmed by Vasko et al. (101a), who found four slow phenytoin me-

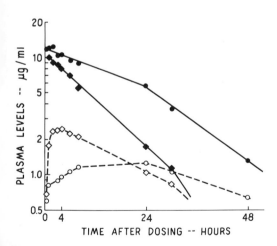

FIG. 6. Effect of loading doses of non-labeled p-HPPH on plasma levels and half-lives of 14C-labeled phenytoin and p-HPPH in a rhesus monkey following a single 10-mg/kg intravenous dose of [14C]phenytoin. *Squares*, no p-HPPH was administered; *circles*, 50-mg/kg intravenous doses of p-HPPH given 2 hr before and 2 hr after the [14C]phenytoin. (From Glazko et al., ref. 47, with permission of the publisher.)

tabolizers out of seven family members examined, representing three generations. Using inbred strains of genetically responsive and nonresponsive aryl hydrocarbon-treated mice as well as hybrids from certain genetic crosses, Robinson and Nebert (90) showed that phenytoin hydroxylation might involve a different cytochrome P-450 species regulated by an "aromatic hydrocarbon-responsive" genetic locus other than the Ah locus. More recently, Atlas et al. (5a) identified "fast metabolizers" and "slow metabolizers" among twelve inbred strains of mice. Heterozygotes showed intermediate values expressed as an additive trait. The data showed good correlation with *in vitro* hepatic P-450 mediated metabolism of phenytoin. Sloan et al. (90a) studied phenytoin hydroxylation in eleven subjects who had previously been characterized as fast and slow metabolizers of debrisoquine. They concluded that the oxidation of these two drugs was controlled by the same gene locus.

Recently, we have examined the metabolic disposition of phenytoin in normal adult volunteers with short and long plasma phenytoin half-lives following repeated oral doses of the drug (49). Five subjects with short half-lives (mean, 14 hr) and four subjects with long half-lives (mean, 30 hr) were selected from a group of 20 subjects following a single 500-mg oral dose of phenytoin. Both groups were given 300 mg of phenytoin (Dilantin® sodium) once daily for 15 days. For the short-half-life group, the mean steady-state phenytoin level ($\overline{C}_{ss}$) was 3.6 μg/ml. In the long-half-life group, the $\overline{C}_{ss}$ was 13.4 μg/ml, almost fourfold greater than in the short-half-life group. Plasma half-lives selected on the basis of the single-dose study were not always predictive of the half-lives following repeated dose administration. In the long-half-life group, two subjects showed a reduction of phenytoin half-life, one was unchanged, and one showed a twofold increase in half-life. Most of the short-half-life group showed a sharp reduction in half-life after termination of dosage. Peak plasma phenytoin levels and area under curve at steady state showed excellent correlation with the plasma half-life of phenytoin. Plasma half-lives for total *p*-HPPH (free plus conjugated)

averaged about 30% greater than phenytoin half-lives in the short-half-life group, and 50% or more in the long-half-life group. The $\overline{C}_{ss}$ plasma levels for total *p*-HPPH were 1.9 μg/ml for the short-half-life group and 0.7 μg/ml for the long-half-life group. Urinary excretion of total *p*-HPPH accounted for 65 to 94% of the dose in the short half-life group, and 52 to 72% of dose in the long half-life group. These differences in the rate of hydroxylation of phenytoin may well be caused by genetically determined differences among the individual subjects, representing fast and slow hydroxylators.

REFERENCES

1. Arnold, K., and Gerber, N. (1970): The rate of decline of diphenylhydantoin in human plasma. *Clin. Pharmacol. Ther.*, 11:121–134.
2. Ashley, J. J., and Levy, G. (1972): Inhibition of diphenylhydantoin elimination by its major metabolite. *Res. Commun. Chem. Pathol. Pharmacol.*, 4:297–306.
3. Ashley, J. J., and Levy, G. (1973). Kinetics of diphenylhydantoin elimination in rats. *J. Pharmacokinet. Biopharm.*, 1:99–102.
4. Atkinson, A. J., Jr., MacGee, J., Strong, J., Garteiz, D., and Gaffney, T. E. (1970): Identification of 5-metahydroxyphenyl-5-phenyl-hydantoin as a metabolite of diphenylhydantoin. *Biochem. Pharmacol.*, 19:2483–2491.
5. Atkinson, A. J., and Shaw, J. M. (1973): Pharmacokinetic study of a patient with diphenylhydantoin toxicity. *Clin. Pharmacol. Ther.*, 14:521–528.
5a. Atlas, S. A., Zweier, J. L., and Nebert, D. W. (1980): Genetic differences in phenytoin pharmacokinetics. *In vivo* clearance and *in vitro* metabolism among inbred strains of mice. *Dev. Pharmacol. Ther.*, 1:281–304.
6. Axelrod, J., and Tomchick, R. (1958): Enzymatic *O*-methylation of epinephrine and other catechols. *J. Biol. Chem.*, 233:702–705.
7. Ayengar, P. K., Hayaishi, O., Nakajima, M., and Tomida, I. (1959): Enzymatic aromatization of 3,5-cyclohexadiene-1,2-diol. *Biochim. Biophys. Acta.*, 33:111–119.
8. Ballek, R. E., Reidenberg, M. M., and Orr, L. (1973): Inhibition of diphenylhydantoin metabolism by chloramphenicol. *Lancet*, 1:150.
9. Bochner, F., Hooper, W. D., Tyrer, J. H., and Eadie, M. J. (1972). Effect of dosage increment on blood phenytoin concentrations. *J. Neurol. Neurosurg. Psychiatry*, 35:873–876.
10. Booth, J., and Boyland, E. (1949): Metabolism of polycyclic compounds. 5. Formation of 1:2-dihydroxy-1,2-dihydronaphthalenes. *Biochem. J.*, 44:361–365.
11. Booth, J., and Boyland, E. (1958): Metabolism of

polycyclic compounds. 13. Enzymic hydroxylation of naphthalene by rat liver microsomes. *Biochem. J., 70*:681–688.

12. Borga, O., Garle, M., and Gutova, M. (1972): Identification of 5-(3,4-dihydroxyphenyl)-5-phenylhydantoin as a metabolite of 5,5-diphenylhydantoin (phenytoin) in rats and man. *Pharmacology, 7*:129–137.

13. Borondy, P., Chang, T., and Glazko, A. J. (1972): Inhibition of diphenylhydantoin hydroxylation by 5-(*p*-hydroxyphenyl)-5-phenylhydantoin. *Fed. Proc., 31*:582.

14. Boyland, E. (1950): The biological significance of metabolism of polycyclic compounds. *Biochem. Soc. Symp., 5*:44–54.

15. Boyland, E., and Sims, P. (1960): Metabolism of polycyclic compounds. 16. The metabolism of 1:2-dihydronaphthalene and 1:2-epoxy-1:2:3:4-tetrahydronaphthalene. *Biochem. J., 77*:175–181.

16. Boyland, E., and Sims, P. (1962): Metabolism of polycyclic compounds. 21. The metabolism of phenanthrene in rabbit and rats: Dihydrodihydroxy compounds and related glucosiduronic acids. *Biochem. J., 84*:571–582.

17. Brodie, B. B., Reid, W. D., Cho, A. K., Sipes, G., Krishna, G., and Gillette, J. R. (1971): Possible mechanism of liver necrosis caused by aromatic organic compounds. *Proc. Natl. Acad. Sci. U.S.A., 68*:160–164.

18. Brooks, C. J. W., and Young, L. (1956): Biochemical studies of toxic agents. 9. The metabolic conversion of indene into *cis*- and *trans*-indane-1:2-diol. *Biochem. J., 63*:264–269.

19. Butler, T. C. (1957): The metabolic conversion of 5,5-diphenylhydantoin to 5-(*p*-hydroxyphenyl)-5-phenylhydantoin. *J. Pharmacol. Exp. Ther., 119*:1–11.

20. Butler, T. C., Dudley, K. H., Johnson, D., and Roberts, S. B. (1976): Studies of the metabolism of 5,5-diphenylhydantoin relating principally to the stereoselectivity of the hydroxylation reactions in man and the dog. *J. Pharmacol. Exp. Ther., 199*:82–92.

21. Butler, T. C., Dudley, K. H., Mitchell, G. N., and Johnson, D. (1977): Hydroxylation of 5,5-diphenylhydantoin (phenytoin) by dog liver microsomes. *Arch. Int. Pharmacodyn., 228*:4–9.

22. Chang, T., and Glazko, A. J. (1972): Diphenylhydantoin: Biotransformation. In: *Antiepileptic Drugs,* edited by D. M. Woodbury, J. K. Penry, and R. P. Schmidt, pp. 149–162. Raven Press, New York.

23. Chang, T., Okerholm, R. A., and Glazko, A. J. (1972): Identification of 5-(3,4-dihydroxyphenyl)-5-phenylhydantoin: A metabolite of 5,5-diphenylhydantoin (Dilantin) in rat urine. *Anal. Lett., 5*:195–202.

24. Chang, T., Okerholm, R. A., and Glazko, A. J. (1972). A 3-*O*-methylated catechol metabolite of diphenylhydantoin (Dilantin) in rat urine. *Res. Commun. Chem. Pathol. Pharmacol., 4*:13–23.

25. Chang, T., Savory, A., and Glazko, A. J. (1970): A new metabolite of 5,5-diphenylhydantoin (Dilantin). *Biochem. Biophys. Res. Commun. 38*:444–449.

26. Chang, T., Young, R., Maschewske, E., Croskey,

L., Smith, T. C., Buchanan, R. A., and Glazko, A. J. (1977): Metabolite studies with $^{13}C-^{14}C$ doubly labeled phenytoin in human subjects. *Epilepsia,* 18:191.

27. Conard, G. J. (1970): *Pharmacological Aspects of Diphenylhydantoin Disposition,* Ph.D. Thesis. University of Wisconsin, Madison.

28. Daly, J. W., Jerina, D. M., and Witkop, B. (1972): Oxides and the NIH shift: The metabolism, toxicity, and carcinogenicity of aromatic compounds. *Experientia, 28*:1129–1264.

29. Daly, J., Jerina, D., Witkop, B., Zaltzman-Nirenberg, D., and Udenfriend, S. (1969): Identification of 1,2-naphthalene oxide as an intermediate in the enzymatic conversion of naphthalene to 2-naphthol and naphthalene-1,2-dihydrodiol. *Fed. Proc., 28*:546.

30. Dayton, P. G., Cucinell, S. A., Weiss, M., and Perel, J. M. (1967): Dose-dependence of drug plasma level decline in dogs. *J. Pharmacol. Exp. Ther., 158*:305–316.

31. Dill, W. A., Baukema, J., Chang, T., and Glazko, A. J. (1971). Colorimetric assay of 5,5-diphenylhydantoin (Dilantin) and 5-(*p*-hydroxyphenyl)-5-phenylhydantoin. *Proc. Soc. Exp. Biol. Mea., 137*:674–679.

32. Dill, W. A., Kazenko, A., Wolf, L. M., and Glazko, A. J. (1956): Studies on 5,5-diphenylhydantoin (Dilantin) in animals and man. *J. Pharmacol. Exp. Ther., 118*:270–279.

33. Dudley, K. H., Butler, T. C., and Bius, D. L. (1974): The role of dihydropyrimidinase in the metabolism of some hydantoin and succinimide drugs. *Drug Metab. Dispos., 2*:103–112.

34. Eling, T. E., Harbison, R. D., Becker, B. B., and Fouts, J. R. (1970): Diphenylhydantoin effect on neonatal and adult rat hepatic drug metabolism. *J. Pharmacol. Exp. Ther., 171*:127–134.

35. Gabler, W. L. (1974): A method for assaying conjugation of diphenylhydantoin metabolites. *Fed. Proc., 33*:525.

36. Gerber, N., and Arnold, K. (1969): Studies on the metabolism of diphenylhydantoin in mice. *J. Pharmacol. Exp. Ther., 167*:77–90.

37. Gerber, N., Lynn, R., and Oates, J. (1972): Acute intoxication with 5,5-diphenylhydantoin (Dilantin) associated with impairment of biotransformation: Plasma levels and urinary metabolites; and studies in healthy volunteers. *Ann. Intern. Med., 77*:765–771.

38. Gerber, N., Seibert, R. A., and Thompson, R. M. (1973): Identification of a catechol glucuronide metabolite of 5,5-diphenylhydantoin (DPH) in rat bile by gas chromatography (GC) and mass spectrometry (MS). *Res. Commun. Chem. Pathol. Pharmacol., 6*:499–511.

39. Gerber, N., and Thompson, R. M. (1974): Identification of catechol glucuronide metabolites of hydroxydiphenylhydantoins (*m*-HPPH, *p*-HPPH) in rat bile. *Fed. Proc. 33*:525.

40. Gerber, N., and Wagner, J. (1972): Explanation of dose-dependent decline of diphenylhydantoin plasma levels by fitting to the integrated form of the Michaelis–Menten equation. *Res. Commun. Chem. Pathol. Pharmacol., 3*:455–466.

41. Gerber, N., Weller, W. L., Lynn, R., Rangno, R. E., Sweetman, B. J., and Bush, M. T. (1971): Study of dose dependent metabolism of 5,5-diphenylhydantoin in the rat using new methodology for isolation and quantitation of metabolites *in vivo* and *in vitro*. *J. Pharmacol. Exp. Ther.*, 178:567–579.

42. Gillette, J. R. (1974): A perspective on the role of chemically reactive metabolites of foreign compounds in toxicity. I. Correlation of changes in covalent binding of reactive metabolites with changes in the incidence and severity of toxicity. *Biochem. Pharmacol.*, 23:2785–2794.

43. Glazko, A. J. (1972): Diphenylhydantoin. NAS/NRC/USP Conference on Bioavailability of Drugs, Washington, D.C., November 22–23, 1971. *Pharmacology*, 8:163–177.

44. Glazko, A. J. (1973): Diphenylhydantoin metabolism. A prospective review. *Drug Metab. Dispos.*, 1:711–714.

45. Glazko, A. J. (1975): Antiepileptic drugs: Biotransformation, metabolism, and serum half-life. *Epilepsia*, 16:367–391.

46. Glazko, A. J., Chang, T., Baukema, J., Dill, W. A., Goulet, J. R., and Buchanan, R. A. (1969): Metabolic disposition of diphenylhydantoin in normal human subjects following intravenous administration. *Clin. Pharmacol. Ther.*, 10:498–504.

47. Glazko, A. J., Chang, T., Maschewski, E., Hayes, A., and Dill, W. A. (1977): Role of hydroxylated metabolites of phenytoin in dose-dependency. In: *Microsomes and Drug Oxidations,* edited by V. Ullrich, A. Hildebrandt, I. Roots, R. W. Estabrook, and A. H. Conney, pp. 508–515. Pergamon Press, New York.

48. Glazko, A. J., Dill, W. A., Drach, J. C., and Chang, T. (1968): Biological availability of drugs; evaluation from blood level and urinary excretion data. In: *Fifth National Symposium of the APhA Academy of Pharmaceutical Sciences,* pp. 326–343. American Pharmaceutical Association, Academy of Pharmaceutical Sciences, Washington.

49. Glazko, A. J., Peterson, F. E., Smith, T. C., Dill, W. A., and Chang, T. (1980): Phenytoin metabolism in human subjects with short and long plasma half-lives. *Fed. Proc.*, 39:1099.

50. Gorvin, J. H., and Brownlee, G. (1957): Metabolism of 5,5-diphenylhydantoin in the rabbit. *Nature*, 179:1248.

51. Grover, P. L., Hewer, A., and Sims, P. (1971): Epoxides as microsomal metabolites of polycyclic hydrocarbons. *FEBS Lett.*, 18:76–80.

52. Hadfield, M. G. (1972): Uptake and binding of catecholamines. Effect of diphenylhydantoin and a new mechanism of action. *Arch. Neurol.*, 26:78–84.

53. Harbison, R. D., and Becker B. A. (1969): Relation of dosage and time of administration of diphenylhydantoin to its teratogenic effect in mice. *Teratology*, 2:305–312.

54. Harvey, D. J., Glazener, L., Stratton, C., Nowlin, J., Hill, R. M., and Horning, M. G. (1972): Detection of a 5-(3,4-dihydroxy-1,5-cyclohexadien-1-yl)-metabolite of phenobarbital and mephobarbital in rat, guinea pig, and human. *Res. Commun. Chem. Pathol. Pharmacol.*, 3:557–565.

55. Holcomb, R., Lynn, R., Harvey, B., Sweetman, B. J., and Gerber, N. (1972): Intoxication with 5,5-diphenylhydantoin (Dilantin): Clinical features, blood levels, urinary metabolites and metabolic changes in a child. *J. Pediatr.*, 80:627–632.

56. Horning, M. G., Butler, C., Harvey, D. J., Hill, R. M., and Zion, T. E. (1973): Metabolism of *N*,2-dimethyl-2-phenylsuccinimide (methsuximide) by the epoxide–diol pathway in rat, guinea pig, and human. *Res. Commun. Chem. Pathol. Pharmacol.*, 6:565–578.

57. Horning, M. G., and Lertratanangkoon, K. (1977): Effect of chronic administration on urinary profiles of phenytoin metabolites. *Fed. Proc.*, 36:966.

58. Horning, M. G., Stratton, C., Wilson, A., Horning, E. C., and Hill, R. M. (1971): Detection of 5-(3,4-dihydroxy-1,5-cyclohexadien-1-yl)-5-phenylhydantoin as a major metabolite of 5,5-diphenylhydantoin (Dilantin) in the newborn human. *Anal. Lett.*, 4:537–545.

59. Horning, M. G., Zion, T. E., and Butler, C. M. (1977): Metabolism of *N*-methyl-2-phenylsuccinimide (phensuximide) by the epoxide–diol pathway. *Fed. Proc.*, 33:525.

60. Houghton, G. W., and Richens, A. (1974): Inhibition of phenytoin metabolism by sulthiame in epileptic patients. *Br. J. Clin. Pharmacol.*, 1:59–66.

61. Inaba, T., Umeda, T., Endrenyi, L., Mahon, W. A., and Kalow, W. (1978): Uptake and metabolism of diphenylhydantoin in the isolated perfused rat livers. *Biochem. Pharmacol.*, 27:1151–1158.

62. Inaba, T., Umeda, T., Mahon, W. A., Ho, J., and Jeejeebhoy, K. N. (1975): Isolated rat hepatocytes as a model to study drug metabolism: Dose-dependent metabolism of diphenylhydantoin. *Life Sci.*, 16:1227–1232.

63. Jerina, D. M., and Daly, J. W. (1974): Arene oxides: A new aspect of drug metabolism. *Science*, 185:573–582.

64. Jerina, D., Daly, J., Witkop, B., Zaltzman-Nirenberg, P., and Udenfriend, S. (1968): Role of the oxide–oxepin system in the metabolism of aromatic substrates. 1. *In vitro* conversion of benzene oxide to a permercapturic acid and dihydrodiol. *Arch. Biochem. Biophys.*, 128:176–183.

65. Jerina, D. M., Daly, J. W., Witkop, B., Zaltzman-Nirenburg, P., and Udenfriend, S. (1970): 1,2-Naphthalene oxide as an intermediate in the microsomal hydroxylation of naphthalene. *Biochemistry*, 9:147–155.

66. Jusko, W. J. Koup, J. R., and Alvan, G. (1976): Nonlinear assessment of phenytoin bioavailability. *J. Pharmacokinet. Biopharm.*, 4:327–336.

67. Kozelka, F. L., and Hine, C. H. (1943): Degradation products of Dilantin. *J. Pharmacol. Exp. Ther.*, 77:175–179.

68. Kutt, H., (1972): Diphenylhydantoin. Interactions with other drugs in man. In: *Antiepileptic Drugs,* edited by D. M. Woodbury, J. K. Perry, and R. P. Schmidt, pp. 169–180. Raven Press, New York.

69. Kutt, H., and Fouts, J. R. (1971): Diphenylhydantoin metabolism by rat liver microsomes and some of the effects of drugs or chemical pretreatment on diphenylhydantoin metabolism by rat liver micro-

somal preparations. *J. Pharmacol. Exp. Ther.*, 176:11–26.

70. Kutt, H., and Verebely, K. (1970): Metabolism of diphenylhydantoin by rat liver microsomes; characteristics of the reaction. *Biochem. Pharmacol.*, 19:675–686.

71. Kutt, H., Verebely, K., and McDowell, F. (1968): Inhibition of diphenylhydantoin metabolism in rats and in rat liver microsomes by anti-tubercular drugs. *Neurology (Minneap.)*, 20:706–710.

72. Kutt, H., Wolk, M., Scherman, R., and McDonald, F. (1964): Insufficient parahydroxylation as a cause of diphenylhydantoin toxicity. *Neurology (Minneap.)*, 14:542–548.

73. Leibman, K. C., and Ortiz, E. (1969): Oxidation of styrene in liver microsomes. *Biochem. Pharmacol.*, 18:552–554.

74. Levy, G., and Ashley, J. J. (1973): Effect of an inhibitor of glucuronide formation on elimination kinetics of diphenylhydantoin in rats. *J. Pharm. Sci.*, 62:161–162.

75. Lubawy, W. C., Kostenbander, H. B., and Mc-Govern, J. P. (1978): *In vivo* and *in vitro* alteration of nicotine metabolism by the major metabolite of phenytoin. *Res. Commun. Chem. Pathol. Pharmacol.*, 19:257–269.

76. Lubawy, W. C., Kostenbander, H. B., and Stavchansky, S. A. (1974): Cross-inhibition of drug metabolism by drug metabolites. Increase of zoxazolamine paralysis time by the major metabolite of diphenylhydantoin. *Res. Commun. Chem. Pathol. Pharmacol.*, 8:75–82.

77. Maguire, J. H., Butler, T. C., and Dudley, K. H. (1978): Absolute configuration of (+)-5-(3-hydroxyphenyl)-5-phenylhydantoin, the major metabolite of 5,5-diphenylhydantoin in the dog. *J. Med. Chem.*, 21:1294–1297.

77a. Maguire, J. H., Butler, T. C., and Dudley, K. H. (1980): Absolute configurations of the dihydrodiol metabolites of 5,5-diphenylhydantoin (phenytoin) from rat, dog and human urine. *Drug Metab. Dispos.*, 8:325–331.

78. Martz, F., Failinger, C. III, and Blake, D. (1977): Phenytoin teratogenesis: Correlation between embryopathic effect and covalent binding of putative arene oxide metabolite in gestational tissue. *J. Pharmacol. Exp. Ther.*, 203:231–239.

79. Massey, K. M. (1966): Teratogenic effect of diphenylhydantoin sodium. *J. Oral Ther. Pharmacol.*, 2:380–385.

80. Maynert, E. W. (1960): The metabolic fate of diphenylhydantoin in the dog, rat and man. *J. Pharmacol. Exp. Ther.*, 130:275–284.

81. Midha, K. K., Hindmarsh, K. W., McGilvray, I. J., and Cooper, J. K. (1977): Identification of urinary catechol and methylated catechol metabolites of phenytoin in human, monkeys, and dogs by GLC and GLC–mass spectrometry. *J. Pharm. Sci.*, 66:1596–1602.

82. Noach, E. L., Woodbury, D. M., and Goodman, L. S. (1958): Studies on the absorption, distribution, fate and excretion of 4-^{14}C-labeled diphenylhydantoin. *J. Pharmacol. Exp. Ther.*, 122:301–314.

83. Oesch, F., Kaubisch, N., Jerina, D. M., and

Daly, J. W. (1971): Hepatic epoxide hydrase. Structure–activity relationships for substrates and inhibitors. *Biochemistry*, 10:4858–4866.

84. Patsalos, P. N., and Lascelles, P. T. (1977): *In vitro* hydroxylation of diphenylhydantoin and its inhibition by other commonly used anticonvulsant drugs. *Biochem. Pharmacol.*, 26:1929–1933.

85. Ferrier, D., Ashley, J. J., and Levy, G. (1973): Effect of product inhibition on kinetics of drug elimination. *J. Pharmacokinet. Biopharm.*, 1:231–242.

86. Ferucca, E., Makki, K., and Richens, A. (1978): Is phenytoin metabolism dose-dependent by enzyme saturation or by feedback inhibition? *J. Clin. Pharmacol. Ther.*, 24:46–51.

87. Poupaert, J. H., Cavalier, R., Claesen, M. H., and Dumont, P. A. (1975): Absolute configuration of the major metabolite of 5,5-diphenylhydantoin, 5-(4'-hydroxyphenyl)-5-phenylhydantoin. *J. Med. Chem.*, 13:1268–1271.

88. Remmer, H., Hirschmann, J., and Greiner, I. (1969): Die Bedeutung von Kumulation und Elimination für die Dosierung von phenytoin (Diphenylhydantoin). *Deutsch. Med. Wochenschr.*, 94:1265–1272.

89. Richens, A., and Dunlop, A. (1975): Serum phenytoin levels in the management of epilepsy. *Lancet*, 2:247–248.

90. Robinson, J. R., and Nebert, D. W. (1974): Genetic expression of aryl hydrocarbon hydroxylase induction. Presence or absence of association with zoxazolamine, diphenylhydantoin, and hexabarbital metabolism. *Mol. Pharmacol.*, 10:484–493.

90a. Sloan, T. P., Idle, J. R., and Smith, R. L. (1981): Influence of D^H/D^L alleles regulating debrisoquine oxidation on phenytoin hydroxylation. *Clin. Pharmacol. Ther.*, 29:493–497.

91. Smith, J. N., Spencer, B., and Williams, T. T. (1950): Studies in detoxication. 34. The metabolism of chlorobenzene in the rabbit. Isolation of dihydrodihydroxychlorobenzene, p-chlorophenyl glucuronide, 4-chlorocatechol glucuronide and p-chlorophenoxy mercapturic acid. *Biochem. J.*, 47:284–293.

92. Smith, R. G., Daves, G. D., Jr., Lynn, R. K., and Gerber, N. (1977): Hydantoin ring glucuronidation: Characterization of a new metabolite of 5,5-diphenylhydantoin in man and the rat. *Biomed. Mass Spectrom.*, 4:275–279.

93. Soda, D. M., and Levy, G. (1975): Inhibition of drug metabolism by hydroxylated metabolites: Cross-inhibition and specificity. *J. Pharm. Sci.*, 64:1928–1931.

94. Stavchansky, S. A. (1974): *Cross-Inhibition of Drug Metabolism by Drug Metabolites.* Ph.D. Thesis, University of Kentucky, Lexington.

95. Stavchansky, S. A., Kostenbauder, H. B., and Lubawy, W. C. (1975): Kinetic and spectral studies of type I and type II compounds with rat hepatic microsomes in the presence of the major metabolite of diphenylhydantoin. *Drug Metab. Dispos.*, 3:557–564.

96. Stavchansky, S. A., Lubawy, W. E., and Kostenbauder, H. B. (1974): Increase of hexobarbital sleeping time and inhibition of drug metabolism by the major metabolite of diphenylhydantoin. *Life Sci.*, 14 1535–1539.

97. Stillwell, W. G., Stafford, M., and Horning, M. G.

(1973): Metabolism of glutethimide (Doriden) by the epoxide diol pathway in the rat and guinea pig. *Res. Commun. Chem. Pathol. Pharmacol.,* 6:579–590.

98. Sweetman, B. J., Lynn, R., Weller, W. L., Gerber, N., and Bush, M. T. (1977): The urinary metabolite pattern of 5,5-diphenylhydantoin (DPH) in control mice and mice pretreated with DPH. *Pharmacologist,* 13:220.

99. Thompson, R. M., Beghin, J., Fife, W. K., and Gerber, N. (1976): 5,5-Bis(4-hydroxyphenyl)hydantoin, a minor metabolite of diphenylhydantoin (Dilantin) in the rat and human. *Drug Metab. Dispos.,* 4:349–356.

100. Thompson, R. M., Gerber, N., Seibert, R. A., and Desiderio, D. M. (1973): A rapid method for the mass spectrometric identification of glucuronides and other polar drug metabolites in permethylated rat bile. *Drug Metab. Dispos.,* 1:489–505.

101. Tomaszewski, J. E., Jerina, D. M., and Daly, J. W. (1975): Deuterium isotope effects during formation of phenols by hepatic monoxygenases. Evidence for an alternative to the arene oxide pathway. *Biochemistry,* 14:2024–2031.

101a. Vasko, M. R., Bell, R. D., Daly, D. D., and Pippenger, C. E. (1979): Inheritance of phenytoin hypometabolism: a kinetic study of one family. *Clin. Pharmacol. Ther.,* 27:96–103.

102. Verebey, K. (1978): Interaction of *d*-propoxyphene and diphenylhydantoin in rat liver microsomal preparation. *Res. Commun. Chem. Pathol. Pharmacol.,* 20:21–29.

103. Woodbury, D. M. (1969): Role of pharmacological factors in the evaluation of anticonvulsant drugs. *Epilepsia,* 10:121–144.

Antiepileptic Drugs, edited by D. M. Woodbury, J. K. Penry, and C. E. Pippenger. Raven Press, New York © 1982.

15

Phenytoin

Interactions with Other Drugs

Henn Kutt

Numerous interactions between phenytoin and other drugs have been observed. These have been reviewed recently by Kutt (49), Richens (78), and Eadie and Tyrer (22). The vast majority of these interactions manifest in some changes of the pharmacokinetic parameters of phenytoin or the other drug. Interactions involving pharmacodynamic parameters have been assumed to take place with some drug combinations, but clearcut documentation of those remains a task for future efforts.

Pharmacokinetic interactions often become evident by the appearance of signs of intoxication in patients receiving common doses of phenytoin in combination with another drug. Less often, the indication of an interaction is lack of effectiveness. As determinations of plasma drug concentrations became available, the pharmacokinetic nature of these interactions was confirmed and further studied. The common sequence of events in an interaction is that after addition of another drug, the plasma concentration of the first drug will rise or fall, depending on the mechanism by which the pharmacokinetic interaction comes about.

It is important to realize that the same drug in combination with phenytoin may not have the same effect in all patients; in fact, opposite effects in different patients are not uncommon. Clearly predictable unidirectional effects in the majority of patients occur only with relatively few drugs when these are given in combination with phenytoin. The reasons for the variability among individuals in the magnitude or direction of the interaction are only partially understood. Genetic factors play a role; a patient who is a slow metabolizer of the interacting drug is more likely to have a severe interaction. The extent of inducibility of hepatic drug-metabolizing enzymes appears also to be genetically controlled. Environmental factors such as previous drug exposure can influence the extent and direction of an interaction, as does the dual effect of some drugs that cause induction of drug-metabolizing enzyme production but inhibit its action. Variable individual susceptibility may be a useful phrase to use in this context.

Whether or not an interaction is to be considered clinically significant depends on the definition of clinical significance. This author believes that the most important criteria in this respect are whether or not an interaction leads to a need to change the drug dosages and whether or not the interaction with a given drug combination is likely to occur in the majority of patients. But with these criteria, one also needs further considerations regarding the end result in an individual patient. A modest or marked elevation of a low phenytoin level through an interaction may merely improve seizure control;

a small elevation of a nearly toxic level may cause intoxication; a marked elevation in a susceptible individual with a combination that has little, if any, effect in the vast majority of patients is obviously significant in that patient.

Also relevant to the clinical significance of phenytoin interactions with other drugs is the manner of use of the other drug. If the latter is taken sporadically, there is less chance for significant changes to develop than with a drug that is taken chronically.

The early reports about interactions sometimes warned not to use the "reported" drug in combination with phenytoin. Empirically, it has become clear now that, particularly with monitoring of plasma drug levels and adjustment of dosages, no drug combination with phenytoin is totally incompatible. It appears that many of the reported interactions, although fascinating biochemical phenomena, are generally of small concern in clinical management of the majority of patients.

MECHANISMS INVOLVED IN PHARMACOKINETIC INTERACTIONS

Absorption

Only a few interactions based on interference with the absorption of phenytoin have been reported.

Calcium sulfate reduces phenytoin bioavailability. This was demonstrated in Australia during a period when calcium sulfate dihydrate was used as the filler in a commercial phenytoin preparation (5). When the filler was changed to lactose, many patients who had been stabilized with the calcium sulfate-containing phenytoin preparation became clinically intoxicated on the same dose of phenytoin. Laboratory studies revealed that an increased amount of phenytoin was present in the feces of patients taking the calcium sulfate-containing drug. The *in vitro* solubility in organic solvents of phenytoin containing calcium sulfate was reduced, indicating chelation.

Antacids have been implicated as agents that can reduce phenytoin absorption (28,49), par-

ticularly if taken at the same time or near the time of phenytoin ingestion. Lack of such effect has also been reported (11). Nevertheless, it may be practical to stagger the ingestion times of phenytoin and antacids in patients whose plasma levels of phenytoin are on the low side.

There is little evidence that phenytoin would interfere with the absorption of other drugs. In one report, phenytoin reduced the plasma metyrapone level when the latter was given orally but not when metyrapone was given intravenously (58).

Protein Binding

About 90% of the total phenytoin in the plasma is protein bound; less binding occurs in the very young and in subjects with renal or hepatic disease. Other strongly binding drugs, such as tolbutamide (95), salicylates (27), valproate (18), and phenylbutazone (84) among others, can displace phenytoin from the binding sites. This effects an increase in the unbound fraction of phenytoin which often leads to increased clearance as the free drug reaches the liver. The result is some lowering of the total plasma concentration of phenytoin; yet, loss of effectiveness may not occur, since at the new lower steady state, the percent of free phenytoin is greater than it was before the displacing drug was added. If the displacing drug, however, also happens to be an inhibitor of the phenytoin-metabolizing system and/or this system was nearly saturated already, the displacing drug may lead to elevation of the total plasma phenytoin level.

Biotransformation

Induction

Phenytoin is metabolized by the hepatic microsomal mixed-function oxidase system, hydroxylation followed by glucuronidation being the major pathway. The production of these enzymes is induced by inducer drugs (such as phenobarbital) or chemicals (such as insecticides), as demonstrated in experimental animals (48). Induction of hepatic drug-metabolizing enzymes in general and phenytoin metabolism in particular also appears to take place in man (17). As evidence of induction of phenytoin metabolism, plasma phenytoin half-life studies with fixed test doses have been carried out before and after or during the administration of the inducing drug. Shortening of the half-life seems to indicate the trend but does not always correlate with the extent of induction during chronic drug administration. This is because of the complexity of phenytoin half-life which is concentration dependent. Other indirect parameters of induction, such as urinary output of D-glucaric acid or plasma γ-glutamyltransferase, have been investigated and found to indicate the trend for induction but not to correlate well with all parameters of induction.

On the other hand, phenytoin can also act as an inducer of the metabolism of various other drugs in animals (24) and in humans, notably that of carbamazepine (23) and anticoagulants (32). Thus, induction is one of the mechanisms involved in the interactions between phenytoin and other drugs. (For more information on induction, see Chapter 24).

Inhibition

Inhibition of metabolism is the other major mechanism by which interactions between phenytoin and other drugs occur, and interactions based on inhibition actually outnumber those caused by induction. The binding of phenytoin (a Type I substrate) with the enzyme is somewhat unstable, as the magnitude of the phenytoin-induced difference spectra in microsomal preparations is easily reduced by a variety of drugs and chemicals (48). It has been shown that some drugs, such as phenobarbital (48,69) and sulthiame (69) are competitive, and others, such as disulfiram (51) and isoniazid (48), are noncompetitive inhibitors of phenytoin metabolism. This distinction has some theoretical relevance: a noncompetitive inhibitor may cause marked accumulation of phenytoin, whereas a competitive inhibitor would only raise the level to a higher plateau at which phenytoin is again able to compete successfully if the entire system

is not yet saturated. To demonstrate the occurrence of inhibition in humans, plasma phenytoin half-life studies have been used, as have measurements of urinary output of the major metabolite, *p*-HPPH. Again, the half-life studies indicate the trend for inhibition but often are not an accurate measure of the extent of inhibition during chronic drug administration. Similarly, the measurements of *p*-HPPH have not contributed much to determining the extent of inhibition, partly because the change of *p*-HPPH output may be only transitory and relatively small in magnitude.

The extent of inhibition of phenytoin metabolism *in vitro* is related to the inhibitor's concentration. *In vivo,* increasing accumulation of phenytoin has been observed after an increase of sulthiame dose. With drugs given in conventional fixed doses, such as isoniazid, the plasma concentration depends on the genetically determined acetylator phenotype: slow acetylators have a higher plasma concentration of isoniazid than fast acetylators, and they also develop higher phenytoin accumulations.

Induction–Inhibition

The induction and inhibition of phenytoin metabolism can take place at the same time if a drug induces the enzyme production but inhibits its action, as is the case with phenobarbital and probably with pheneturide and ethanol. The net result is no change if both effects are equal, or a rise or fall of plasma phenytoin level if one dominates. The alterations of phenytoin level in this context may also change with time. If the inducer–inhibitor was just started, the inhibition may dominate first, leading to an early rise of the phenytoin level. Induction takes some time to develop but may then become dominant and cause a fall of phenytoin level later. Other factors that influence the net result of these opposing effects are the state of induction from previous drug contacts and probably the genetic make-up. The extent of inducibility has been shown to be genetically determined (94); a "good" inducer is likely to have a fall, whereas a "poor" inducer would show no change or a rise of phenytoin level following inducing–inhibiting drug addition.

CLINICAL INTERACTIONS IN WHICH PHENYTOIN KINETICS ARE ALTERED BY OTHER DRUGS

Disulfiram–Phenytoin

Disulfiram, an enzyme inhibitor, appears to inhibit phenytoin metabolism, as it has been reported to cause accumulation of phenytoin and intoxication in the majority of patients taking it together with phenytoin (53,67). After disulfiram is discontinued, the plasma phenytoin level slowly declines (67), probably reflecting the slow elimination of disulfiram. A study by Svendsen et al. (90) with normal volunteers demonstrated that disulfiram reduced phenytoin clearance from approximately 50 ml/min to 34 ml/min. Dosage adjustment of phenytoin is necessary if these two drugs are administered together.

Sulthiame–Phenytoin

Sulthiame has caused elevations of plasma phenytoin levels ranging from modest to considerable and becoming obvious within days (68) or weeks after addition of sulthiame to phenytoin (30,37,38). Comparison of patients taking phenytoin and sulthiame with patients taking phenytoin without sulthiame indicated that plasma phenytoin levels were higher in patients taking both drugs, as was the incidence of clinical phenytoin intoxication (37,38). It is of importance to note that the phenytoin dose was nearly the same in all these patients. In another comparison study (55), little, if any, effect of sulthiame on plasma phenytoin level was observed. Thus, again, not all patients are alike, and reduction of the phenytoin dose may become necessary if its plasma concentration reaches the toxic range and continuation of sulthiame seems to be indicated.

Measurements of plasma phenytoin half-life and the urinary output of p-HPPH have been carried out in some patients before and after the addition of sulthiame (37,68). The results of these studies have failed to provide clear-cut evidence that inhibition of phenytoin metabolism had taken place because of complexities in interpreting the phenytoin half-life and p-HPPH output data. Yet, the sulthiame-induced inhibition of phenytoin metabolism *in vitro* (69) and the general course of events in this interaction suggest that inhibition is the most likely mechanism involved.

Isoniazid–Phenytoin

Isoniazid is an inhibitor of phenytoin metabolism as is demonstrable *in vitro* with microsomal preparations (48) (see Fig. 1). The inhibition is noncompetitive, and the mechanism by which it comes about has not yet been clarified. Noticeable *in vitro* inhibition of phenytoin metabolism occurs with isoniazid concentrations (5 μg/ml) (51) that have been measured in the plasma of patients taking isoniazid, particularly in those individuals who are slow acetylators of isoniazid (48).

In patients taking phenytoin and isoniazid together, the clinical consequences vary and depend on the patient's acetylator phenotype (8,48). The conventional division into fast and slow acetylator phenotype has recently been modified to include an intermediate group (10). This is based on the consideration that the polymorphism in acetylation is controlled by two autosomal alleles on a single gene locus: R and r. This allows three combinations, RR, Rr, and rr, and agrees with the fact that three modes can be distinguished clinically. The fast acetylators generally do not maintain high enough isoniazid concentration to inhibit phenytoin metabolism noticeably. In the intermediate group, a modest elevation of phenytoin level may take place, whereas in the very slow acetylators in whom isoniazid levels are high enough, a considerable phenytoin accumulation may take place (48) as seen in Fig. 2. In groups of patients taking phenytoin and isoniazid together, significant phenytoin accumulation and intoxication has been reported to occur in 10 to 15% of the subjects (8,60,64) who, in some studies, were identified as very slow acetylators (8).

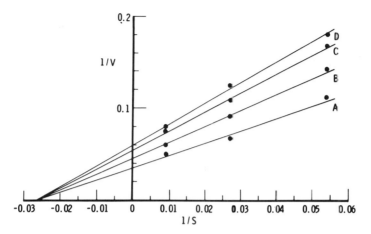

FIG. 1. Noncompetitive inhibition of phenytoin metabolism by isoniazid in rat liver microsomal (9000 × g supernatant) fraction. *Curve* A, control; *curves* B, C, and D, isoniazid added in concentrations of 3.6 × 10^{-5} M; 1.1 × 10^{-4} M; and 5.4 × 10^{-4} M, respectively. (From Kutt, ref. 48, with permission.)

Clinical management of this interaction in patients whose acetylator phenotype is not known is handled best by frequent monitoring of plasma phenytoin levels after the onset of combined therapy with conventional doses. If the plasma phenytoin level continues to rise, as is likely in a slow acetylator, phenytoin dose is reduced, and a new maintenance dose is calculated based on the plasma drug level (48). The isoniazid–phenytoin interaction is thus an example of a situation in which the genetic phenotype with regard to one drug determines the extent of its interaction with another and defines one reason for the "individual susceptibility."

Chloramphenicol–Phenytoin

Chloramphenicol has caused modest elevation of plasma phenytoin levels in some and marked elevations in a few patients (14,38, 46,80). How often this interaction would lead to a need to reduce the phenytoin dose is unclear. It is likely that such need might be infrequent in patients receiving chloramphenicol for 10-day or 2-week courses, whereas this possibility might increase when courses of several weeks are needed, such as in typhoid fever treatment.

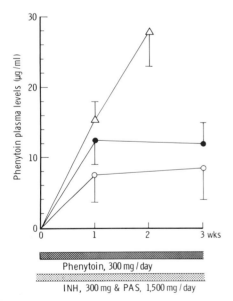

FIG. 2. Plasma levels of phenytoin of patients taking phenytoin and isoniazid together. *Open circles,* fast acetylators; *closed circles,* intermediate slow acetylators; *open triangles,* very slow acetylators. Based on data of Brennan et al. (8).

Propoxyphene–Phenytoin

A small increase of plasma phenytoin level in five patients was observed by Dam et al. (19) after giving the patients 65 mg of propoxyphene three times daily for 6 days. In another patient who took large amounts (10 or more times 65 mg) of propoxyphene for several days (49), phenytoin accumulation to the toxic range did occur. In laboratory studies using rat liver microsomal preparations, propoxyphene has been shown to inhibit phenytoin metabolism (51). In clinical practice, however, with the conventional use of propoxyphene, there is little concern, and significant elevations of plasma phenytoin levels are not expected.

Phenobarbital–Phenytoin

Phenobarbital effectively induces the production of the enzyme(s) involved in phenytoin biotransformation (48). Phenobarbital, however, also competes as a substrate with phenytoin for that enzyme, as competitive inhibition of phenytoin metabolism by phenobarbital is demonstrable *in vitro* (see Fig. 3) (48,69). This dual effect leads to variable results in patients taking phenytoin and phenobarbital together. The opposing effects may cancel each other or lead to a rise or a fall of plasma phenytoin level if one dominates. What to expect in an individual patient is unpredictable and may depend on the state of induction by previous drug intake, the doses of phenytoin and phenobarbital, and probably on the genetic background of the pa-

tient. Genetic control over the extent of phenobarbital induction of metabolism of other drugs has been demonstrated (94) (see genetic influences on induction in Chapter 24).

Comparison of groups of patients taking phenytoin alone and phenytoin together with phenobarbital reveals, in general, that inductions predominate to some extent, as the phenytoin levels in the combined-therapy groups are usually somewhat lower than in monotherapy groups (1,50,63,67,89). In individual patients taking phenytoin, the addition of phenobarbital may cause no change (6,50,55) or may lead to a decline (6,17,50,63) or an elevation (6,50) of plasma phenytoin level. The changes are rarely of large magnitude (1,50,55) and seldom lead to a need for dosage adjustments.

Pheneturide (Phenylethylacetylurea)–Phenytoin

In groups of patients taking phenytoin with or without pheneturide, the plasma phenytoin levels were somewhat higher in the combined therapy group (36,39). When pheneturide was added to the medication of patients stabilized on phenytoin, elevations of plasma phenytoin levels occurred. These elevations were higher in the early phase of combined therapy and de-

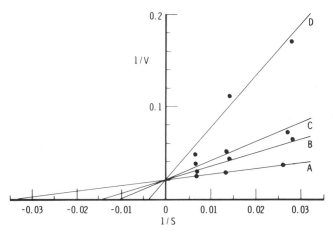

FIG. 3. Competitive inhibition of phenytoin metabolism by phenobarbital in rat liver microsomal (9,000 × g supernatant) fraction. *Curve* A, control; *curves* B, C, and D, phenobarbital added in concentrations 5.9 × 10^{-4} M; 1.1 × 10^{-3} M and 2.3 × 10^{-3} M, respectively. (From Kutt, ref. 48, with permission.)

clined in later weeks (36). This sequence of events appears to indicate that both inhibition and induction are involved in this interaction. Inhibition can start almost immediately, whereas induction takes time to develop. In the long run, inhibition would dominate slightly. The changes were generally not of great magnitude with this drug combination (36,78).

Ethanol–Phenytoin

Chronic use of ethanol has been reported to reduce the plasma phenytoin level (45), perhaps through induction. Elevation of plasma phenytoin level, on the other hand, has been observed during occasional moderate or heavy intake of ethanol (49). Thus, a dual action is likely: chronic intake may have an inducing effect and acute intake an inhibiting effect. The need for dosage adjustments based on this interaction should not be frequent.

Valproate–Phenytoin

The effect of valproate on plasma phenytoin level varies among patients and may vary in the same patient during the course of therapy. Thus, a transient fall (2,9,62) or rise (96) within days after addition of valproate occurs in some patients, with a return to previous values after days or weeks. In other patients, the recovery may take longer and may not quite reach the starting value (9). In general, marked changes are less frequent than smaller changes, and in many patients no significant change in plasma phenytoin level takes place after addition of valproate. A lowering effect is probably more frequent than an elevation (2,9,93). Clinically, the need to adjust phenytoin dose is not frequent.

The mechanism for this interaction is not yet fully clarified, but changes in binding to plasma proteins probably play a role (18,62). Both drugs are bound to a high degree to plasma proteins and compete for binding sites. There is evidence that valproate in higher concentrations (near 100 μg/ml) reduces phenytoin binding from the usual near 90% to 85%. The increase in the free fraction of phenytoin in a patient with unsaturated clearing capacity would result then in a somewhat lower total steady-state phenytoin level (62). Since, however, the valproate level fluctuates considerably during the 24-hr cycle, the effective displacement periods are not long, and the increased clearing of phenytoin is not extensive. Elevation of the plasma phenytoin level might occur in patients whose phenytoin-clearing system is almost saturated, particularly in view of the fact that valproate has been shown to inhibit phenytoin metabolism *in vitro* (69).

Carbamazepine–Phenytoin

The effect of carbamazepine on plasma phenytoin level varies among patients and is generally not of great magnitude. Several authors have reported a lowering effect (33,96), whereas others have found no significant changes, and still others have found that, if anything, there is a slight upward trend (55). What to expect in an individual patient is largely unpredictable.

Benzodiazepines–Phenytoin

The effect of diazepam on plasma phenytoin level varies among patients. In some studies, elevations of phenytoin levels in some patients have been reported (92), whereas in other studies and other patients the opposite has occurred (36,78). In the majority of patients, the commonly used diazepam doses do not seem to cause significant changes of plasma phenytoin levels.

Clonazepam has been found to lower plasma phenytoin level in some patients concomitant with an increase of conjugated *p*-HPPH (22). In other studies, clonazepam has been observed to cause a rise of phenytoin level (96), but more often than not, no significant changes were found (44,65). This suggests that in the majority of patients, alterations of plasma phenytoin levels by clonazepam are not of great clinical concern.

Chlordiazepoxide also has caused phenytoin accumulation in some patients (49,92), but this occurs as a rare exception rather than a rule.

Phenothiazines–Phenytoin

In some instances, chlorpromazine (38,49), prochlorperazine (49), and thioridazine have caused phenytoin accumulation and intoxication. These instances represent exceptionally susceptible individuals, and it is not known what makes them susceptible. In general, phenothiazine drugs do not cause significant alterations of plasma phenytoin levels in the majority of patients taking them together with phenytoin (74,83).

Anticoagulant–Phenytoin

Bishydroxycoumarin (31,85) and to a lesser extent phenprocoumon (85) have been reported to cause elevation of plasma phenytoin levels in some patients. Warfarin (85) and phenindione (85) have caused no change of plasma phenytoin levels. The general experience has been that patients taking phenytoin and anticoagulants together tolerate common doses of phenytoin well.

Methylphenidate–Phenytoin

The effect of methylphenidate on plasma phenytoin level has varied among patients. A rise has been observed in a few patients (29,49), but no change occurred in others (47), possibly the majority.

Tolbutamide–Phenytoin

Tolbutamide was found to alter plasma phenytoin levels in patients (95). Adding 1,000 mg of tolbutamide daily to the medication regimen of patients stabilized on phenytoin caused a small decline (10%) of the total plasma phenytoin level in the majority of the 17 patients studied. The unbound fraction of phenytoin increased considerably at first and then declined but remained elevated above its percent concentration prior to tolbutamide administration. *In vitro* studies indicated some displacement of phenytoin from its binding sites in human plasma by tolbutamide (95). The clinical

effects of this interaction in the majority of patients are likely to be negligible, since the slight fall of total phenytoin concentration is compensated for by the slight increase of the unbound fraction. Problems may occur in patients whose starting phenytoin level was high and whose phenytoin elimination system was nearly saturated; in these, the increase of free phenytoin would not lead to more efficient clearance.

Salicylate–Phenytoin

Salicylates have been shown to displace phenytoin from the plasma protein binding sites *in vitro* and *in vivo*. In clinical studies, an increase of the unbound fraction of phenytoin from the usual 10% to near 16% and an increase of phenytoin clearance by acetylsalicylic acid were demonstrated (27). These changes were to some degree proportional to the acetylsalicylic acid dose, which ranged from 900 mg to 3,600 mg per day. In epileptic patients, high repeated doses of acetylsalicylic acid are expected to cause a small decline of total plasma phenytoin level but a slight increase in the relative percent of free phenytoin (70). Thus, in terms of effectiveness of phenytoin, no change is expected under these circumstances, and a need for dosage adjustment is unlikely to occur.

Additional drugs reported to alter phenytoin kinetics are listed in Table 1.

CLINICAL INTERACTIONS IN WHICH THE KINETICS OF OTHER DRUGS ARE ALTERED BY PHENYTOIN

Phenytoin–Carbamazepine

Phenytoin appears to be a potent inducer of carbamazepine biotransformation. In numerous studies, the plasma concentration of carbamazepine was found to be higher in those patients taking carbamazepine alone than in those taking phenytoin as well (13,23,43,55,81). In individual patients taking carbamazepine, addition of phenytoin often causes the carbamazepine level to fall as much as one-half of the original value (see Fig. 4). Lander et al. (55) calculated that

TABLE 1. *Additional drugs altering phenytoin kinetics*

Reference	Drug	Effect on plasma phenytoin level
Perucca and Richens (71)	Imipramine	Elevation
Olesen (67)	Calcium carbimide	Elevation
Pugh et al. (75)	Chlorpheniramine	Elevation
Eadie and Tyrer (22)	Furosemide	Elevation
Skovsted et al. (84)	Clofibrate	Elevation
Skovsted et al. (84)	Phenylbutazone	Elevation
Solomon and Schrogie (88)	Phenyramidol	Elevation
Eadie and Tyrer (22)	Propranolol	Elevation
Roe et al. (79)	Diazoxide	Lowering
Hansson and Sillanpää (34)	Pyridoxine	Lowering
Baylis et al. (4)	Folate	Lowering
Lander et al. (55)	Ethosuximide	Elevation
Mølholm Hansen et al. (61)	Sulfaphenazole	Elevation
Mølholm Hansen et al. (61)	Sulfamethizole	Elevation
Mølholm Hansen et al. (61)	Sulfadiazine	Elevation
Rambeck (76)	Methsuximide	Elevation
Houghton and Richens (38)	Nortriptylene	Elevation
Windorfer and Sauer (96)	Primidone	Lowering

in their patients, daily phenytoin doses of 1 mg/ kg caused a fall of about 0.5 µg/ml in the carbamazepine plasma level. The plasma concentration of 10,11-carbamazepine epoxide, which usually equals one-third that of the parent compound in patients on monotherapy, may remain unchanged after addition of phenytoin or may undergo a small rise or fall. In most cases, the ratio of the parent compound to metabolite is lowered by phenytoin; its extent is subject to individual variations (23,81). Since the plasma carbamazepine level tends to decline through autoinduction in the early phase of carbamazepine therapy, it may be difficult to discern the effect of phenytoin if the latter is added soon. Whether the mechanism of this interaction is an increased conversion to the 10,11-epoxide metabolite (23,81) or acceleration of some other biotransformation step (22) has not yet been fully clarified. Clinically, increases in the carbamazepine dose may become necessary if maintenance of a desired plasma carbamazepine concentration seems to be indicated.

Phenytoin–Primidone

Phenytoin appears to influence primidone biotransformation. The ratio of primidone-derived phenobarbital to primidone in the plasma of patients taking primidone alone usually ranges from 1.5 to 2.5; if phenytoin is added to the medication, this ratio may increase to 4 or higher (25). The extent of increase of this ratio varies

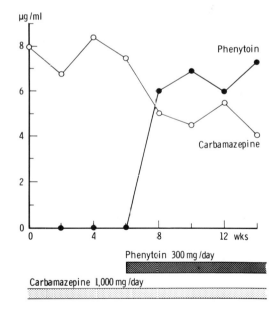

FIG. 4. Decline of plasma carbamazepine level following addition of phenytoin. (From author's unpublished patient data.)

among individual patients, and it may occur either on account of a decrease of primidone or because of an increase of derived phenobarbital concentration or both. As an explanation for this interaction, acceleration of primidone metabolism by phenytoin is usually mentioned (25,82). Theoretically, inhibition of phenobarbital elimination may also play a role, at least in some patients (see phenytoin–phenobarbital). This phenomenon is not of great clinical concern, since it rarely leads to a need for dosage adjustments.

Phenytoin–Phenobarbital

Phenytoin has been reported to cause an elevation of plasma phenobarbital levels in some patients (54,63,96). Also, in some patients stabilized on combination therapy, a fall of plasma phenobarbital level was noted after phenytoin was discontinued (63). In the majority of patients, however, phenytoin has not caused significant changes of plasma phenobarbital levels, and the need to adjust dosages because of this interaction is expected to be quite infrequent (21). The mechanism is likely to be competitive inhibition.

Phenytoin–Contraceptives

Contraceptive failure has been reported in some epileptic patients taking antiepileptic drugs, including phenytoin (35,42). This has led to the hypothesis that the metabolism of synthetic steroids may be induced by phenytoin (16,35). If so, then the extent of this phenomenon apparently varies considerably among individuals and is generally small, since numerous epileptic patients have remained protected by oral contraceptives.

PHENYTOIN EFFECT ON ENDOGENOUS SUBSTANCES AND VITAMINS

Phenytoin is known to accelerate cortisol metabolism, but this usually does not lead to clinical consequences, as a homeostatic mechanism compensates with increased synthesis of cortisol (12). Vitamin K-dependent coagulation factors may become reduced by phenytoin, occasionally leading to bleeding in neonates born to mothers taking phenytoin (86). Osteomalacia in some patients taking phenytoin is thought to be related in part to acceleration of the cholecalciferol biotransformation pathway (40). Plasma folate levels have been found to be reduced in patients taking phenytoin (20), sometimes leading to macrocytic anemia.

Additional drugs whose kinetics have been reported to be altered by phenytoin are listed in Table 2.

PHARMACODYNAMIC INTERACTIONS BETWEEN PHENYTOIN AND OTHER DRUGS

Since most interactions between phenytoin and other drugs involve some pharmacokinetic changes, it is extremely difficult to rule in or out the simultaneous presence of alterations of pharmacodynamic parameters. Is the improved seizure control after adding a second drug to phenytoin simply additive or is there potentiation? Measurements of brain phenytoin and phenobarbital concentrations and comparison of the antiepileptic effect in animals by Leppik and Sherwin (56) indicated that the effect was additive under their experimental conditions. Tunnicliff et al. (91) have found that phenytoin competes with diazepam for binding sites at rat cortex synaptosomal membranes. What does that mean in terms of effectiveness? Refinement of techniques and application of new approaches may help to gain a better understanding in this matter.

Cohan et al. (15) have postulated that suppression of afferent discharges from muscle spindles by phenytoin would potentiate the effectiveness of chlorpromazine in diminishing the extensor tone of decerebrate rigidity in cats. Mendez et al. (59) have found that phenytoin blocked levodopa effects in patients with parkinsonism and postulated that phenytoin may inhibit the uptake or utilization of dopamine by basal ganglia. Ahmad (3) has suggested that

TABLE 2. *Additional drugs whose kinetics are altered by phenytoin*

Reference	Drug	Phenytoin effect on plasma drug level
Kwalick (52)	DDT	Lowering
Solomon et al. (87)	Digitoxin	Lowering
Hvidberg and Sjo (41)	Clonazepam	Lowering
Petruch et al. (73)	Antipyrine	Lowering
Neuvonen et al. (66)	Doxycycline	Lowering
Braithwaite et al. (7)	Nortriptyline	Lowering
Reinken (77)	Pyridoxine	Lowering
McLelland and Jack (57)	Dexamethazone	Lowering
Petereit and Meikle (72)	Prednisolone	Lowering
Meikle et al. (58)	Metyrapone	Lowering
Forsman and Öhman (26)	Haloperidol	Lowering
Hansen et al. (32)	Bishydroxycoumadin	Lowering

renal sensitivity to furosemide is reduced by antiepileptic drugs including phenytoin. These are a few examples of pharmacodynamic interactions, and it is obvious that more work in this field is needed.

CONCLUSION

Numerous interactions between phenytoin and other drugs have been reported. The majority of these are pharmacokinetic in nature and involve induction or inhibition of biotransformation or alteration of plasma protein binding. The result is a rise or decline in the plasma level of phenytoin or that of the other drug.

With many of the reported drug combinations with phenytoin, small changes of plasma levels are not infrequent, but marked changes occur only rarely in apparently unusually susceptible individuals.

The plasma level changes may be in opposite directions in different individuals with the same drug combination, particularly if the interacting drug induces enzyme production but inhibits its action.

Interactions with a predictable potential to necessitate adjustment of dosages occur only with a few drugs in combination with phenytoin. Disulfiram, sulthiame, and isoniazid (in very slow acetylators) cause elevations of plasma phenytoin levels in the majority of patients. Conversely, phenytoin often causes a decline of plasma carbamazepine level. A need to adjust

dosages depends on the magnitude of these changes.

REFERENCES

1. Abarbanel, J., Herishanu, Y., Rosenberg, P., and Eylath, U. (1978): *In vivo* interaction of anticonvulsant drugs. The mathematical correlation of plasma levels of anticonvulsant drugs in epileptic patients. *Isr. J. Neurol.*, 218:137–144.
2. Adams, D. J., Luders, H., and Pippenger, C. (1978): Sodium valproate in the treatment of intractable seizure disorders: A clinical and electroencephalographic study. *Neurology (Minneap.)*, 28:152–157.
3. Ahmad, S. (1974): Renal insensitivity to furosemide caused by chronic anticonvulsant therapy. *Br. Med. J.*, 3:657–659.
4. Bayles, E. M., Crowley, J. M., Preece, J. M., Sylvester, P. E., and Marks, V. (1971): Influence of folic acid on blood phenytoin levels. *Br. Med. J.*, 1:62–64.
5. Bochner, F., Hooper, W. D., Tyrer, J. H., and Eadie, M. J. (1972): Factors involved in an outbreak of phenytoin intoxication. *J. Neurol. Sci.*, 16:481–487.
6. Booker, H. E., Tormey, A. and Toussaint, J. (1971): Concurrent administration of phenobarbital and diphenylhydantoin: Lack of an interference effect. *Neurology, (Minneap.)*, 21:383–385.
7. Braithwaite, R. A., Flanagan, R. A., and Richens, A. (1975): Steady state plasma nortriptyline concentrations in epileptic patients. *Br. J. Clin. Pharmacol.*, 2:469–471.
8. Brennan, R. W., Dehejia, H., Kutt, H., Verebely, K., and McDowell, F. (1970): Diphenylhydantoin intoxication attendant to slow inactivation of isoniazid. *Neurology (Minneap.)*, 20:687–693.
9. Bruni, J., Wilder, B. J., Willmore, L. J., and Barbour, B. (1979): Valproic acid and plasma levels of phenytoin. *Neurology (Minneap.)*, 29:904–905.
10. Chapron, D. J., Blum, M. R., and Kramer, P. A. (1978): Evidence of a trimodal pattern of acetylation

of isoniazid in uremic subjects. *J. Pharm. Sci.,* 67:1018–1019.

11. Chapron, D. J., Kramer, P. A., Mariano, S. L., and Hohnadel, D. C. (1979): Effect of calcium and antacids on phenytoin bioavailability. *Arch. Neurol.,* 36:436–438.

12. Choi, Y., Thrasher, K., Werk, E., Sholiton, L. J., and Olinger, C. (1971): Effect of diphenylhydantoin on cortisol kinetics in humans. *J. Pharmacol. Exp. Ther.,* 176:27–34.

13. Christiansen, J., and Dam, M. (1973): Influence of phenobarbital and diphenylhydantoin on plasma carbamazepine levels in patients with epilepsy. *Acta Neurol. Scand.,* 49:543–546.

14. Christensen, L. K., and Skovsted, L. (1969): Inhibition of drug metabolism by chloramphenicol. *Lancet,* 2:1397–1399.

15. Cohan, S. L., Anderson, R. J., and Raines, A. (1976): Diphenylhydantoin and chlorpromazine in the treatment of spasticity. *Neurology (Minneap.),* 26:367.

16. Coulam, C. B., and Annegers, J. F. (1979): Do anticonvulsants reduce the efficacy of oral contraceptives. *Epilepsia,* 20:519–525.

17. Cucinell, S. A., Conney, A. H., Sansur, M. S., and Burns, J. J. (1965): Drug interactions in man. I. Lowering effect of phenobarbital on plasma levels of bishydroxycoumarin (Dicumarol®) and diphenylhydantoin (Dilantin®). *Clin. Pharmacol. Ther.,* 6:420–429.

18. Dahlqvist, R., Borga, O., Rane, A., and Sjöqvist, F. (1979): Decreased plasma protein binding of phenytoin in patients on valproic acid. *Br. J. Clin. Pharamacol.,* 8:547–552.

19. Dam, M., Christensen, J. M., Brandt, J., Hansen, B. S., Hvidberg, E. F., Angelo, H., and Lous, P. (1980): Antiepileptic drugs: Interaction with dextropropoxyphene. In: *Antiepileptic Therapy: Advances in Drug Monitoring,* edited by S. I. Johannessen, P. L. Morselli, C. E. Pippenger, A. Richens, D. Schmidt, and H. Meinardi, pp. 299–304. Raven Press, New York.

20. Davis, R. E., and Woodliff, H. J. (1971): Folic acid deficiency in patients receiving anticonvulsant drugs. *Med. J. Aust.,* 2:1070–1072.

21. Eadie, M. J., Lander, C. M., Hooper, W. D., and Tyrer, J. H. (1977): Factors influencing plasma phenobarbitone levels in epileptic patients. *Br. J. Clin. Pharmacol.,* 4:541–547.

22. Eadie, M. J., and Tyrer, J. H. (1980): *Anticonvulsant Therapy. Pharmacological Basis and Practice.* Churchill Livingstone, Edinburgh, London, New York.

23. Eichelbaum, M., Kothe, K. W., Hoffmann, F., and von Unruh, G. E. (1979): Kinetics and metabolism of carbamazepine during combined antiepileptic therapy. *Clin. Pharmacol. Ther.,* 26:366–371.

24. Eling, T. E., Harbison, R. D., Becker, B. A., and Fouts, J. R. (1970): Diphenylhydantoin effect on neonatal and adult rat drug metabolism. *J. Pharmacol. Exp. Ther.,* 171:127–134.

25. Fincham, R. W., Schottelius, D. D., and Sahs, A. L. (1974): The influence of diphenylhydantoin on primidone metabolism. *Arch. Neurol.,* 30:259–262.

26. Forsman, A., and Öhman, R. (1977): Applied pharmacokinetics of haloperidol in man. *Curr. Ther. Res.,* 21:396–411.

27. Fraser, D. G., Ludden, T. M., Evens, R. P., and

Sutherland, E. W. (1980): Displacement of phenytoin from plasma binding sites by salicylate. *Clin. Pharmacol. Ther.,* 27:165–169.

28. Garnett, W. R., Carter, B. L., and Pellock, J. M. (1979): Bioavailability of phenytoin administered with antacids. *Ther. Drug Monit.,* 1:435–436.

29. Garrettson, L. K., Perel, J. M., and Dayton, P. G. (1969): Methylphenidate interactions with both anticonvulsant and biscoumacetate. *J.A.M.A.,* 207: 2053–2056.

30. Hansen, J. M., Kristensen, M., and Skovsted, L. (1968): Sulthiame (Ospolot) as inhibitor of diphenylhydantoin metabolism. *Epilepsia,* 9:17–22.

31. Hansen, J. M., Kristensen, M., Skovsted, D. L., and Christensen, L. K. (1966): Dicoumarol-induced diphenylhydantoin intoxication. *Lancet,* 2:265–266.

32. Hansen, J. M., Siersbaek-Nielsen, K., Kristensen, M., Skovsted, L., and Christensen, L. K. (1971): Effect of diphenylhydantoin on the metabolism of dicoumarol in man. *Acta Med. Scand.,* 189:15–19.

33. Hansen, J. M., Siersbaek-Nielsen, K., and Skovsted, L. (1971): Carbamazepine-induced acceleration of diphenylhydantoin and warfarin metabolism in man. *Clin. Pharmacol. Ther.,* 12:539–543.

34. Hansson, O., and Sillanpää, M. (1976): Pyridoxine and serum concentrations of phenytoin and phenobarbitone. *Lancet,* 1:256.

35. Hempel, E., and Klinger, W. (1976): Drug stimulated biotransformation of hormonal steroid contraceptives: Clinical implications. *Drugs,* 12:442–448.

36. Houghton, G. W., and Richens, A. (1974): The effect of benzodiazepines and pheneturide on phenytoin metabolism in man. *Br. J. Clin. Pharmacol.,* 1:344–345.

37. Houghton, G. W., and Richens, A. (1974): Inhibition of phenytoin metabolism by sulthiame in epileptic patients. *Br. J. Clin. Pharmacol.,* 1:59–66.

38. Houghton, G. W., and Richens, A. (1975): Inhibition of phenytoin metabolism by other drugs used in epilepsy. *Int. J. Clin. Pharmacol. Biopharm.,* 12:210–216.

39. Huisman, J. W., Van Heycop Ten Ham, M. W., and Van Zijl, C. W. H. (1970): Influence of ethylphenacetamide on serum levels of other antiepileptic drugs. *Epilepsia,* 11:207–215.

40. Hunter, J. (1976): Effects of enzyme induction on vitamin D_3 metabolism in man. In: *Anticonvulsant Drugs and Enzyme Induction,* edited by A. Richens and F. P. Woodford, pp. 77–84. Elsevier Excerpta Medica North Holland, Amsterdam.

41. Hvidberg, E. F. and Sjo, O. (1975): Clinical pharmacokinetic experience with clonazepam. In: *Clinical Pharmacology of Antiepileptic Drugs,* edited by H. Schneider, D. Janz, C. Gardner-Thorpe, H. Meinardi, and A. Sherwin, pp. 242–246. Springer Verlag, Berlin.

42. Janz, D., and Schmidt, D. (1974): Antiepileptic drugs and failure of oral contraceptives. *Lancet,* 1:1113.

43. Johannessen, S. I., and Strandjord, R. E. (1975): The influence of phenobarbitone and phenytoin on carbamazepine serum levels. In: *Clinical Pharmacology of Antiepileptic Drugs,* edited by H. Schneider, D. Janz, C. Gardner-Thorpe, H. Meinardi, and A. Sherwin, pp. 201–205. Springer Verlag, Berlin.

44. Johannessen, S. I., Strandjord R. E., and Munthe-

kaas, A. W. (1977): Lack of effect of clonazepam on serum levels of diphenylhydantoin, phenobarbital and carbamazepine. *Acta Neurol. Scand.*, 55:506–512.

45. Kater, R. M . H., Roggin, G., Tobon, F., Zieve, P., and Iber, F. L. (1969): Increased rate of clearance of drugs from circulation of alcoholics. *Am. J. Med. Sci.*, 258:35–39.

46. Koup, J. R. (1978): Interaction of chloramphenicol with phenytoin and phenobarbital. A case report. *Clin. Pharmacol. Ther.*, 24:571–575.

47. Kupferberg, H. J., Jeffrey, W., and Hunninghake, D. B. (1972): Effect of methylphenidate on plasma anticonvulsant level. *Clin. Pharmacol. Ther.*, 13: 201–204.

48. Kutt, H. (1974): Interactions with antiepileptic drugs involving multiple mechanisms. In: *Drug Interactions*, edited by P. L. Morselli, S. Garattini, and S. N. Cohen, pp. 211–222. Raven Press, New York.

49. Kutt, H. (1975): Interactions of antiepileptic drugs. *Epilepsia*, 16:393–402.

50. Kutt, H., Haynes, J., Verebely, K., and McDowell, F. (1969): The effect of phenobarbital on plasma diphenylhydantoin level and metabolism in man and in rat liver microsomes. *Neurology (Minneap.)*, 19:611–616.

51. Kutt, H., and Verebely, K. (1970): Metabolism of diphenylhydantoin by rat liver microsomes. I. Characteristics of the reaction. *Biochem. Pharmacol.*, 19:675–686.

52. Kwalick, D. S. (1971): Anticonvulsants and DDT residues. *J.A.M.A.*, 215:120–121.

53. Labram, C. (1975): Dangerous combinations: Phenytoin and disulfiram. *Concours Med.*, 97:6490–6493.

54. Lambie, D. G., Nanda, R. M., Johnson, R. H., Shakir, R. A. (1976): Therapeutic and pharmacokinetic effects of increasing phenytoin in chronic epileptics on multiple drug therapy. *Lancet*, 2:386–389.

55. Lander, C. M., Eadie, M. J., and Tyrer, J. H. (1975): Interactions between anticonvulsants. *Proc. Aust. Assoc. Neurol.*, 12:111–116.

56. Leppik, I. E., and Sherwin, A. (1977): Anticonvulsant activity of phenobarbital and phenytoin in combination. *J. Pharmacol. Exp. Ther.*, 200:570–575.

57. McLelland, J., and Jack, W. (1978): Phenytoin dexamethasone interaction: A clinical problem. *Lancet*, 1:1096–1097.

58. Meikle, A. W., Jubiz, W., Matsakura, S., West, C. D., and Tyler, F. H. (1969): Effect of diphenylhydantoin on the metabolism of metyrapone and release of ACTH in man. *J. Clin. Endocrinol.*, 29:1553–1558.

59. Mendez, J. S., Cotzias, G. C., Mena, I., and Papavasiliou, P. S. (1975): Diphenylhydantoin. Blocking of levodopa effects. *Arch. Neurol.*, 32:44–46.

60. Miller, R. R., Porter, J., and Greenblatt, D. J. (1979): Clinical importance of the interaction of phenytoin and isoniazid. *Chest*, 75:356–358.

61. Mølholm Hansen, J., Kampmann, J. P., Siersbaek-Nielsen, K., Lumholtz, I. B., Arrøe, M., Abilgaard, U., and Skovsted, L. (1979): The effect of different sulfonamides on phenytoin metabolism in man. *Acta Med. Scand. [Suppl.]*, 624:106–110.

62. Monks, A., and Richens, A. (1980): Effects of single doses of sodium valproate on serum phenytoin levels and protein binding in epileptic patients. *Clin. Pharmacol. Ther.*, 27:89–95.

63. Morselli, P. L., Rizzo, M., and Garattini, S. (1971): Interaction between phenobarbital and diphenylhydantoin in animals and in epileptic patients. *Ann. N.Y. Acad. Sci.*, 179:88–107.

64. Murray, F. J. (1962): Outbreak of unexpected reactions among epileptics taking isoniazid. *Am. Rev. Respir. Dis.*, 86:729–731.

65. Nanda, R. N., Johnson, R. H., Keogh, H. J., Lambie, D. G., and Melville, I. D. (1977): Treatment of epilepsy with clonazepam and its effect on other anticonvulsants. *J. Neurol. Neurosurg. Psychiatry*, 40:538–543.

66. Neuvonen, P. J., Penttila, O., Lehtovaara, R., and Aho, K. (1975): Effects of antiepileptic drugs on the elimination of various tetracycline derivatives. *Eur. J. Clin. Pharmacol.*, 9:147–154.

67. Olesen, O. V. (1967): The influence of disulfiram and calcium carbimide on the serum diphenylhydantoin. *Arch. Neurol.*, 16:642–644.

68. Olesen, O. V., and Jensen, O. N. (1969): Drug-interaction between sulthiame (Ospolot) and phenytoin in the treatment of epilepsy. *Dan. Med. Bull.*, 16:154–158.

69. Patsalos, P. M., and Lascelles, P. T. (1977): *In vitro* hydroxylation of diphenylhydantoin and its inhibition by other commonly used anticonvulsant drugs. *Biochem. Pharamcol.*, 26:1929–1933.

70. Paxton, J. W. (1980): Effects of aspirin on serum phenytoin kinetics in healthy subjects. *Clin. Pharmacol. Ther.*, 27:170–178.

71. Perucca, E., and Richens, A. (1977): Interaction between phenytoin and imipramine. *Br. J. Clin. Pharmacol.*, 4:485–486.

72. Petereit, L. B., and Meikle, A. W. (1977): Effectiveness of prednisolone during phenytoin therapy. *Clin. Pharmacol. Ther.*, 22:912–916.

73. Petruch, F., Schueppel, R. V. A., and Steinhilber, G. (1974): Effect of diphenylhydantoin on hepatic drug hydroxylation. *Eur. J. Clin. Pharmacol.*, 7:281–285.

74. Pippenger, C. E., Siris, J. H., Werner, W. L., and Masland, R. L. (1975): The effect of psychotropic drugs on serum antiepileptic levels in psychiatric patients with seizure disorders. In: *Clinical Pharmacology of Antiepileptic Drugs*, edited by H. Schneider, D. Janz, C. Gardner-Thorpe, H. Meinardi, and A. L. Sherwin, pp. 135–142. Springer Verlag, Berlin.

75. Pugh, R. N. H., Geddes, A. M., and Yeoman, W. B. (1975): Interaction of phenytoin and chlorpheniramine. *Br. J. Clin. Pharmacol.*, 2:173–174.

76. Rambeck, B. (1979): Pharmacological interactions of mesuximide with phenobarbital and phenytoin in hospitalized epileptic patients. *Epilepsia*, 20:147–156.

77. Reinken, L. (1973): Die Wirkung von Hydantoin und Succinimid auf den Vitamin B_6 Stoffwechsel. *Clin. Chim. Acta*, 48:435–436.

78. Richens, A. (1977): Interactions with antiepileptic drugs. *Drugs*, 13:266–275.

79. Roe, T. F., Podosin, R. L., and Blaskovics, M. E. (1975): Drug interaction: Diazoxide and diphenylhydantoin. *J. Pediatr.*, 87:480–484.

80. Rose, J. Q., Choi, H. K., and Shentag, J. J. (1977):

Intoxication caused by interaction of chloramphenicol and phenytoin. *J.A.M.A.*, 237:2630–2631.

81. Schneider, H. (1975): Carbamazepine: The influence of other antiepileptic drugs on its serum level. In: *Clinical Pharmacology of Antiepileptic Drugs,* edited by H. Schneider, D. Janz, C. Gardner-Thorpe, H. Meinardi, and A. L. Sherwin, pp. 189–195. Springer Verlag, Berlin.

82. Schottelius, D. D., and Fincham, R. W. (1977): Clinical application of serum primidone levels. In: *Antiepileptic Drugs: Quantitative Analysis and Interpretation,* edited by C. E. Pippenger, J. K. Penry, and H. Kutt, pp. 273–282. Raven Press, New York.

83. Shader, R. I., Weinberger, D. R., and Greenblatt, D. J. (1978): Problems with drug interactions in treating brain disorders. *Psychiatr. Clin. North Am.,* 1:51–69.

84. Skovsted, L., Hansen, J. M., Kristensen, M., and Christensen, L. K. (1974): Inhibition of drug metabolism in man. In: *Drug Interactions,* edited by P. L. Morselli, S. Garattini, and S. N. Cohen, pp. 81–90. Raven Press, New York.

85. Skovsted, L., Kristensen, M., Mølholm Hansen, J., and Siersbaek-Nielsen, K. (1976): The effect of different oral anticoagulants on diphenylhydantoin (DPH) and tolbutamide metabolism. *Acta Med. Scand.,* 199:513–515.

86. Solomon, G. E., Hilgartner, M. W., and Kutt, H. (1972): Coagulation defects caused by diphenylhydantoin. *Neurology (Minneap.,)* 22:1165–1171.

87. Solomon, H. M., Reich, S., Spirt, N., and Abrams, W. B. (1971): Interaction between digitoxin and other drugs *in vitro* and *in vivo*. *Ann. N.Y. Acad. Sci.,* 79:362–369.

88. Solomon, H. M., and Shrogie, J. J. (1967): The effect of phenyramidol on the metabolism of diphenylhydantoin. *Clin. Pharmacol. Ther.,* 8:554–556.

89. Sotaniemi, E., Arvela, P., Hakkarainen, H., and Huhti, E. (1970): The clinical significance of microsomal enzyme induction in the therapy of epileptic patients. *Ann. Clin. Res.,* 2:223–227.

90. Svendsen, T. L., Kristensen, M., Hansen, J. M., and Skovsted, L. (1976): The influence of disulfiram on the half-life and metabolic clearance rate of diphenylhydantoin and tolbutamide in man. *Eur. J. Clin. Pharmacol.,* 9:439–441.

91. Tunnicliff, G., Smith, J. A., and Ngo, T. T. (1979): Competition for diazepam receptor binding by diphenylhydantoin and its enhancement by γ-aminobutyric acid. *Biochem. Biophys. Res. Commun.,* 91:1018–1024.

92. Vaijda, F. J. E., Prineas, R. J., and Lowell, R. R. H. (1971): Interaction between phenytoin and the benzodiazepines. *Br. Med. J.,* 1:346.

93. Vakil, S. D., Critchley, E. M. R., Philips, J. C., Fahim, Y., Haycock, C., Cocks, A., and Dyer, T. (1976): The effect of sodium valproate (Epilim) on phenytoin and phenobarbitone blood levels. In: *Clinical and Pharmacological Aspects of Sodium Valproate (Epilim) in the Treatment of Epilepsy,* edited by N. J. Legg, pp. 75–77. M.C.S. Consultants, Tunbridge Wells, England.

94. Vesell, E. S., and Page, J. G. (1969): Genetic control of the phenobarbital-induced shortening of plasma antipyrine half-lives in man. *J. Clin. Invest.,* 48:2202–2209.

95. Wesseling, H., and Molsthurkow, I. (1975): Interaction of diphenylhydantoin (DPH) and tolbutamide in man. *Eur. J. Clin. Pharmacol.,* 8:75–78.

96. Windorfer, A., Jr., and Sauer, W. (1977): Drug interactions during anticonvulsant therapy in childhood: Diphenylhydantoin, primidone, phenobarbitone, clonazepam, nitrazepam, carbamazepine and dipropylacetate. *Neuropaediatrie,* 8:29–41.

Antiepileptic Drugs, edited by D. M. Woodbury,
J. K. Penry, and C. E. Pippenger. Raven Press,
New York © 1982.

16

Phenytoin

Relation of Plasma Concentration
to Seizure Control

Henn Kutt

Attempts to evaluate the correlation between plasma phenytoin levels and seizure control have produced different opinions. These range from finding no obvious correlation (17,45,46) to finding a reasonably good correlation (6–8,23,32,41). In analyzing the reasons for the differences of opinion, it becomes obvious that the study designs and methods of analysis have varied, as has the basic philosophy of the observers. By and large, if the purpose of the analysis was to find retrospectively a clear-cut relationship between a certain numerical value of plasma phenytoin level and the degree of seizure control in a large group of patients of all ages, i.e., a universally applicable "therapeutic" level, the results have been disappointing. If the purpose of the study was to evaluate prospectively the relationship between the plasma phenytoin level and the degree of seizure control in an individual patient or a group of patients, the results have been quite encouraging in that the seizure frequency usually declined as the plasma phenytoin level increased (4,5, 9,11,32,41). The numerical values of levels above which cessation of or a significant decline in the number of seizures occurred, however, varied considerably among individual patients (4,5,8,16,17,19,20,25,36,43). It ap-

pears, therefore, that, strictly speaking, there are as many "therapeutic" plasma levels of phenytoin as there are individual patients.

THERAPEUTIC RANGE OF PLASMA PHENYTOIN CONCENTRATIONS

The often quoted therapeutic range of 10 to 20 µg/ml or mg/liter probably evolved from the basic desire of humans to have quotable numbers. Many factors have contributed to the genesis of these numbers. Long before the "blood level era," empirical wisdom had already developed that a phenytoin dose of 300 to 400 mg daily was effective in many patients, and this dose was, therefore, commonly used. In the majority of patients with an average phenytoin elimination rate (i.e., excluding fast and slow metabolizers), these doses usually produce plasma levels near or slightly above 10 µg/ml. From measurements of plasma phenytoin levels in a large number of patients, it became obvious that the value of 10 µg/ml (or 8 or 12 µg/ml) was desirable since many patients were well controlled or considerably improved at that level (5,8,22,23,33). It may well be, however, that some of these patients needed lower phenytoin levels, since in most surveys patients have been observed who did well with plasma phenytoin levels below 10 μg/ml. A few patients are known to have been seizure-free for a long time with phenytoin levels around 2 or 3 μg/ml. When the drug was discontinued under the assumption that it was no longer needed, the seizures soon recurred but were abolished again when the previous dose producing the levels of 2 to 3 μg/ml was resumed. On the other hand, there are also patients who do best with phenytoin levels around 25 μg/ml (8,23,43). Finally, there are some patients in whom seizure frequency increases with high phenytoin concentrations, a paradoxical response (25,27,43).

The upper therapeutic level for phenytoin (20 μg/ml) evolved from observations that mild signs of intoxication started to develop in the majority of patients when the level exceeded 20 μg/ml and increased in severity as the level continued to rise. Again, individual variations were observed, a few patients showing signs of intoxication with lower values (3,4,7) but others being symptom-free with values well above 20 μg/ml. The symptom-free stage with high phenytoin levels more often than not develops following an initial period of some symptoms. Most observers agree that phenytoin levels over 30 μg/ml are likely to cause some intoxication in the majority of patients (5,7,19,22,25,45,47).

Besides the 10 to 20 μg/ml range, other, slightly different, therapeutic ranges have been quoted (Table 1). The lowest "effective" level was 3 μg/ml, the highest 15 μg/ml, with an average of 7.4 μg/ml. The studies recommending lower values usually included children, indicating that particularly in children phenytoin levels below 10 μg/ml are often effective. Toxicity might be expected at values ranging from 15 μg/ml to 25 μg/ml, with an average of 20.5 μg/ml (Table 1). Allowing for the composition of the group of patients in which the observations are made, it appears that effectiveness starts with plasma phenytoin levels near 10 μg/ml and potential toxicity with levels near 20 μg/ml in the majority of adult patients. In children, the effectiveness may start with levels near 5 μg/ml (4,36).

The usefulness of having plasma phenytoin levels over 10 μg/ml has been confirmed by several prospective studies. Lund et al. (33) reported that in 32 patients the average seizure frequency was 5.8 per year when the average plasma phenytoin level was 6.1 μg/ml. The seizure frequency dropped to 4.1 when the average level was increased to 11.7 μg/ml and dropped further to 1.6 when the average level was raised to 15.0 μg/ml. Similarly, Reynolds et al. (41) reported achievement of satisfactory seizure control in 90% of patients when phenytoin doses were adjusted to maintain plasma phenytoin levels between 10 and 20 μg/ml.

PROBABLE REASONS FOR VARIATIONS IN THE CLINICALLY EFFECTIVE PLASMA CONCENTRATION OF PHENYTOIN

The reasons for variations in the plasma phenytoin concentrations that achieve control of seizures are not all known. The factors that may play a role include differences in the severity of the seizure process, differences in plasma protein binding of phenytoin, presence of other antiepileptic drugs, nature of the seizure process, erroneous laboratory values, and other factors.

Seizure Severity

The concept of differences in the severity of the seizure process sometimes evoked to explain differences in the effective drug concen-

TABLE 1. *Proposed therapeutic ranges of plasma phenytoin levels*

Reference	Effective (μg/ml)	Toxic (μg/ml)
Borofsky et al. (4)	5	25
Buchthal and Lennox-Buchthal (5)	15	25
Deonna et al. (13)	3	20
van der Kleijn et al. (48)	12	15
Loiseau et al. (29)	7	15
Loiseau et al. (28)	5	18
van Meter et al. (49)	5	15
Norell et al. (37)	12	25
Schobben (44)	5	25
Winek (51)	5	22
Mean	7.4	20.5

tration (22,23,32,43) is still a logical deduction rather than a proven fact. The understanding of biochemical–biophysical (or other) abnormalities involved in the human epilepsies is still incomplete, and there is as yet no instrument that measures the severity of the seizure process directly. In experimental models, however, the effect of increasing the intensity of electrical stimulation (1) is counteracted by increasing the phenytoin concentration and increasing concentrations of intracortically applied penicillin require increasing concentrations of phenytoin to abolish the peripheral seizure manifestations (30,31). Overwhelmingly strong stimuli of the same nature, on the other hand, are influenced only partly or little, if any, by phenytoin (18,31). Furthermore, in patients with ongoing focal seizures, the peripheral seizure manifestations (i.e., clonic limb movements) are gradually decreased in intensity by increasing phenytoin concentrations rather than suddenly stopped by an all-or-none mechanism (22,50). Therefore, there is little doubt that a correlation exists between the severity of the acute seizure process or the intensity of the focus and the concentration of phenytoin.

It may be argued that the mode of action of phenytoin in the acute seizure state may vary from that involved in the prevention of seizures in an epileptic patient. This question cannot be analyzed satisfactorily until further knowledge about the seizure process accumulates. Until then, it seems fair to assume that differences in the severity of the seizure process do exist and reasonable to use that concept as one probable explanation of the variation of effective phenytoin concentrations among epileptic patients (22–24).

Plasma Protein Binding of Phenytoin

An increase of the unbound fraction of phenytoin in the plasma is theoretically expected to increase the brain and plasma total phenytoin concentration ratio (3) and produce increased seizure control. This mechanism may explain why, in patients with chronic uremia and decreased protein binding (21,39) relatively low plasma total phenytoin concentrations are sometimes effective. The same mechanism may be evoked when other drugs competing for binding sites with phenytoin increase the free fraction (10,15,34,38), although the situation becomes complicated if the competing drug also has antiepileptic action (34). Finally, the increased amount of free phenytoin in the plasma may be a factor in the effectiveness of relatively low total phenytoin levels in children (2,14), when the binding of phenytoin may be reduced. Phenytoin binding may also be reduced during pregnancy (12).

Other Antiepileptic Drugs

The presence of other antiepileptic drugs is a factor in seizure control and influences the phenytoin concentrations needed. Equal protection against electrically induced seizures by equimolar concentrations of phenytoin or phenobarbital or the sum total of each in varying ratios was demonstrated by Leppik and Sherwin (26). The measured effective concentrations of phenytoin in patients on combined regimens may therefore be lower than in patients taking phenytoin alone.

The Seizure Process

The nature of the seizure process is expected to influence the concentration of phenytoin needed to control it. Obviously, some seizure types such as absence and some myoclonic seizures are refractory to phenytoin altogether. In others, only a partial beneficial response may occur even with high phenytoin concentrations. How much of this depends on the hypothetical severity of the seizure process and how much on the possible difference in the nature of the seizure process remains to be elucidated.

Laboratory Values

Erroneous laboratory values have not been infrequent, as several surveys have revealed (40,42). This is likely to become less of a problem as the experience of laboratories generally increases. In special situations, however, methodological problems remain. For instance, with immunoassay techniques, the antibody cross reacts with phenytoin metabolites; this becomes a problem in uremic patients as accumulation of metabolites occurs in the plasma of oliguric patients (35).

Other Factors

Differences in the definition of seizure control and in grading the degree of beneficial effects are other factors that may help account for variations in effective phenytoin concentrations.

CONCLUSIONS

A wide range of plasma phenytoin levels has been found in patients who benefited from phenytoin; in the strictest sense, there are as many "therapeutic levels" of phenytoin as there are individual patients. The reasons for this phenomenon include differences in the severity and/or nature of the seizure process, protein binding, and comedication, among others.

The often-quoted "therapeutic range" of 10 to 20 μg/ml is useful in clinical management if it is used with the understanding that it is an empirical range.

The concept of the therapeutic range does a disservice to those physicians who adhere strictly to these numbers, increasing the dose until the concentration reaches 10 μg/ml and promptly decreasing the dose if it exceeds 20 μg/ml, regardless of the clinical condition of the patient.

The therapeutic range may be of great service to those physicians who consider a phenytoin concentration of 10 μg/ml as likely to be effective in adult patients, usually causing no disturbing side effects and possibly providing a margin of safety to some patients. Further adjustments of the dose and level depend on the individual needs of the patient. In patients, particularly children, who are well controlled with levels lower than 10 μg/ml, upward adjustment

may not be necessary. The value of 20 μg/ml is best considered a concentration above which dose-related toxic symptoms may start to occur, usually in a patient who has not yet developed tolerance to the side effects of phenytoin.

REFERENCES

1. Aston, R., and Domino, E. F. (1961): Differential effects of phenobarbital, pentobarbital and diphenylhydantoin on motor cortical and reticular thresholds in the rhesus monkey. *Psychopharmacologia*, 2:304–317.
2. Barth, N., Alvan, G., Borga, O., and Sjoqvist, F. (1976): Two fold interindividual variation in plasma protein binding of phenytoin in patients with epilepsy. *Clin. Pharmacokinet.*, 1:444–452.
3. Booker, H. E., and Darcey, B. (1973): Serum concentrations of free diphenylhydantoin and their relationship to clinical intoxication. *Epilepsia*, 14:177–184.
4. Borofsky, L. G., Louis, S., and Kutt, H. (1973): Diphenylhydantoin in children: Pharmacology and efficacy. *Neurology (Minneap.)*, 23:967–972.
5. Buchthal, F., and Lennox-Buchthal, M. A. (1972): Diphenylhydantoin. Relation of anticonvulsant effect to concentration in serum. In: *Antiepileptic Drugs*, edited by D. M. Woodbury, J. K. Penry, and R. P. Schmidt, pp. 193–209. Raven Press, New York.
6. Buchthal, F., and Svensmark, O. (1959/60): Aspects of the pharmacology of phenytoin (Dilantin®) and phenobarbital relevant to their dosage in the treatment of epilepsy. *Epilepsia*, 1:373–384.
7. Buchthal, F., and Svensmark, O. (1971): Serum concentrations of diphenylhydantoin (phenytoin) and phenobarbital and their relation to therapeutic and toxic effects. *Psychiatr. Neurol. Neurochir.*, 74:117–136.
8. Buchthal, F., Svensmark, O., and Schiller, P. J. (1960): Clinical and electroencephalographic correlations with serum levels of diphenylhydantoin. *Arch. Neurol.*, 2:624–630.
9. Chadwick, D., Vydelingum, L., Galbraith, A., and Reynolds, E. H. (1977): The value of serum phenytoin levels in new referrals with epilepsy. One drug in the treatment of epilepsy. In: *Antiepileptic Drug Monitoring*, edited by C. Gardner-Thorpe, D. Janz, H. Meinardi, and C. E. Pippenger, pp. 187–196. Pitman Medical, Tunbridge Wells, Kent.
10. Dahlqvist, R., Borga, O., Rane, A., and Sjoqvist, F. (1979): Decreased plasma protein binding of phenytoin in patients on valproic acid. *Br. J. Clin. Pharmacol.*, 8:547–552.
11. Dawson, K. P., and Jamieson, A. (1971): Value of blood phenytoin estimation in management of childhood epilepsy. *Arch. Dis. Child.*, 46:386–388.
12. Dean, M., Beresford, S., Patterson, R. J., and Levy, G. (1980): Serum protein binding of drug during and after pregnancy. *Clin. Pharmacol. Ther.*, 28:253–261.
13. Deonna, T., de Crousaz, G., Maquni, G., Bechtel, P., and Schelling, J. L. (1975): Concentration plas-

matique de phenytoine chez les epileptiques-interet pour le clinicien. *Schweiz. Med. Wochenschr.,* 105:936–940.

14. Ehrnebo, M., Agurell, S., Jalling, B., and Boreus, L. O. (1971): Age differences in drug binding by plasma proteins: Studies on human fetuses, neonates and adults. *Eur. J. Clin. Pharmacol.,* 3:189–193.

15. Ehrnebo, M., and Odar-Cederlof, I. (1977): Distribution of pentobarbital and diphenylhydantoin between plasma and cells in blood: Effect of salicylic acid, temperature and total drug concentration. *Eur. J. Clin. Pharmacol.,* 11:37–42.

16. Feldman, R. G., and Pippenger, C. E. (1976): The relation of anticonvulsant drug levels to complete seizure control. *J. Clin. Pharmacol.,* 16:51–59.

17. Gibberd, F. B., Dunne, J. F., Handley, A. J., and Hazleman, B. L. (1970): Supervision of epileptic patients taking phenytoin. *Br. Med. J.,* 1:147–149.

18. Guberman, A., Gloor, P., and Sherwin, A. L. (1975): Response of generalized penicillin epilepsy in the cat to ethosuximide and diphenylhydantoin. *Neurology (Minneap.).,* 25:758–764.

19. Haerer, A. P., and Grace, J. B. (1969): Studies of anticonvulsant levels in epileptics. *Acta Neurol. Scand.,* 45:18–31.

20. Hirschmann, J. (1969): Die Kontrolle der Diphenylhydantoin-Dosierung bei Anfallsleiden durch Bestimmung der Serumspiegel. *Med. Welt,* 5:705–750.

21. Hooper, W. D., Bochner, F., Eadie, M. J., and Tyrer, J. H. (1974): Plasma protein binding of diphenylhydantoin. Effects of sex hormones, renal and liver disease. *Clin. Pharmacol. Ther.,* 15:276–282.

22. Kutt, H. (1972): Diphenylhydantoin. Relation of plasma level to clinical control. In: *Antiepileptic Drugs,* edited by D. M. Woodbury, J. K. Penry, and R. P. Schmidt, pp. 211–217. Raven Press, New York.

23. Kutt, H., and McDowell, F. (1968): Management of epilepsy with diphenylhydantoin. *J.A.M.A.,* 203: 969–972.

24. Kutt, H., and Penry, J. K. (1974): Usefulness of blood levels of antiepileptic drugs. *Arch. Neurol.,* 31:283–288.

25. Lascelles, P. T., Kocen, R. S., and Reynolds, E. H. (1970): The distribution of plasma phenytoin levels in epileptic patients. *J. Neurol. Neurosurg. Psychiatry,* 33:501–505.

26. Leppik, I. E., and Sherwin, A. (1977): Anticonvulsant activity of phenobarbital and phenytoin in combination. *J. Pharmacol. Exp. Ther.,* 200:570–575.

27. Levy, L. L., and Fenichel, G. M. (1965): Diphenylhydantoin activated seizures. *Neurology (Minneap.),* 15:716–722.

28. Loiseau, P., Battellocchi, S., Brachet-Liermain, A., Cenraud, B., Orgogozo, J. M., and Morselli, P. (1980): Evaluation of the role of plasma level monitoring and its consequences in the therapeutic management of epileptics: A longitudinal study with phenobarbitone and phenytoin in 242 patients. In: *Antiepileptic Therapy: Advances in Drug Monitoring,* edited by S. I. Johannessen, P. L. Morselli, C. E. Pippenger, A. Richens, D. Schmidt, and H. Meinardi, pp. 271–276. Raven Press, New York.

29. Loiseau, P., Brachet-Liermain, A., Legroux, M., and Jogeix, M. (1977): Interet du dosage des anticonvul-sivants dans le traitment des epilepsies. *Nouv. Presse Med.,* 6:816–818.

30. Louis, S., Kutt, H., and McDowell, F. (1968): Intravenous diphenylhydantoin in experimental seizures. II. Effect on penicillin-induced seizures in the cat. *Arch. Neurol.,* 18:472–477.

31. Louis, S., Kutt, H., and McDowell, F. (1971): Modification of experimental seizures and anticonvulsant efficacy by peripheral stimulation. *Neurology (Minneap.),* 21:329–336.

32. Lund, L. (1974): Anticonvulsant effect of diphenylhydantoin relative to plasma level. A prospective three year study in ambulant patients with generalized epileptic seizures. *Arch. Neurol.,* 31:289–294.

33. Lund, M., Jorgensen, R. S. and Kühl, V. (1964): Serum diphenylhydantoin (phenytoin) in ambulant patients with epilepsy. *Epilepsia,* 5:51–58.

34. Monks, A., and Richens, A. (1980): The effects of single doses of sodium valproate on serum phenytoin levels and protein binding in man. *Clin. Pharmacol. Ther.,* 27:89–95.

35. Nandedkar, A. K. N., Williamson, R., Kutt, H., and Fairclough, G. F., Jr. (1980): A comparison of plasma phenytoin level determinations by EMIT and gas–liquid chromatography in patients with renal insufficiency. *Ther. Drug Monit.,* 2:427–430.

36. Nolte, R., and Brugmann, G. (1975): Problems in controlled anti-epileptic treatment with phenytoin in children. I. In: *Clinical Pharmacology of Antiepileptic Drugs,* edited by H. Schneider, D. Janz, C. Gardner-Thorpe, H. Meinardi, and A. L. Sherwin, pp. 70–77. Springer, Berlin.

37. Norell, E., Lilienberg, G., and Gamstorp, I. (1975): Systematic determination of the serum phenytoin level as an aid in the management of children with epilepsy. *Eur. Neurol.,* 13:232–244.

38. Paxton, J. W. (1980): Effects of aspirin on serum phenytoin kinetics in healthy subjects. *Clin. Pharmacol. Ther.,* 27:170–178.

39. Perucca, E. (1980): Plasma protein binding of phenytoin in health and disease: Relevance to therapeutic drug monitoring. *Ther. Drug Monit.,* 2:331–344.

40. Pippenger, C. E., Penry, J. K., White, B. G., Daly, D. D., and Buddington, R. (1976): Interlaboratory variability in determination of plasma antiepileptic drug concentrations. *Arch. Neurol.,* 33:351–355.

41. Reynolds, E. H., Chadwick, D., and Galbraith, A. W. (1976): One drug (phenytoin) in the treatment of epilepsy. *Lancet,* 1:923–926.

42. Richens, A. (1975): Quality control of drug estimations. *Acta Neurol. Scand. [Suppl.],* 75:81–84.

43. Schmidt, D., and Janz, D. (1977): Therapeutic plasma concentrations of phenytoin and phenobarbital. In: *Antiepileptic Drug Monitoring,* edited by C. Gardner-Thorpe, D. Janz, H. Meinardi, and C. E. Pippenger, pp. 214–225. Pitman Medical, Tunbridge Wells, Kent.

44. Schobben, A. F. A. M. (1979): *Pharmacokinetics and Therapeutics in Epilepsy,* pp. 67–69. Stichting Studentenpers, Nijmegen, Holland.

45. Travers, R. D., Reynolds, E. H., and Gallagher, B. B. (1972): Variation in response to anticonvulsants in a group of epileptic patients. *Arch. Neurol.,* 27:29–33.

46. Triedman, H. M., Fishman, R. A., and Yahr, M. D.
    (1960): Determination of plasma and cerebrospinal fluid
    levels of Dilantin® in the human. *Trans. Am. Neurol.
    Assoc.,* 85:166–170.
47. Troupin, A. S., and Ojeman, L. M. (1976): Paradox-
    ical intoxication—a complication of anticonvulsant
    administration. *Epilepsia,* 16:753–758.
48. van der Kleijn, E., Guelen, P. J. M., Van Wijk, C.,
    and Baars, I. (1975): Clinical pharmacokinetics in
    monitoring chronic medication with anti-epileptic drugs.
    In: *Clinical Pharmacology of Antiepileptic Drugs,* ed-
    ited by H. Schneider, D. Janz, C. Gardner-Thorpe,
    H. Meinardi, and A. L. Sherwin, pp. 11–13. Sprin-
    ger, Berlin.

49. van Meter, J. C., Buckmaster, H. S., and Shelley, L.
    L. (1970): Concurrent assay of phenobarbital and di-
    phenylhydantoin in plasma by vapour-phase chroma-
    tography. *Clin. Chem.,* 16:135–138.
50. Wallis, W., Kutt, H., and McDowell, F. (1968):
    Intravenous diphenylhydantoin in treatment of acute
    repetitive   seizures.   *Neurology   (Minneap.),*
    18:513–525.
51. Winek, C. L. (1976): Tabulation of therapeutic, toxic,
    and lethal concentrations of drugs and chemicals in
    blood. *Clin. Chem.,* 22:832–836.

Antiepileptic Drugs, edited by D. M. Woodbury,
J. K. Penry, and C. E. Pippenger. Raven Press,
New York © 1982

17

Phenytoin

Toxicity

Mogens Dam

NEUROLOGICAL ASPECTS OF TOXICITY

Encephalopathy

The toxic reactions observed during treatment with phenytoin are usually mild. The reactions usually consist of vertigo, tremor, ataxia, dysarthria, diplopia, nystagmus, and headache. The symptoms disappear when the dose is reduced. Severe side effects are rare at serum phenytoin levels below 30 μg/ml (15). Nystagmus can appear at a serum concentration of about 20 μg/ml, ataxia at 30 μg/ml, and mental changes at 40 μg/ml (54), but great individual differences exist, with toxic symptoms and signs appearing at serum phenytoin levels below what would be expected to be the optimal range and absence of toxic reactions appearing well above this range. The adverse effects on the mental state often lead to a confused state referred to as delirium, psychosis, or encephalopathy. This subacute or chronic reversible impairment of intellectual function, awareness, and mood may be overlooked because of the absence of the usual signs of toxicity. Intellectual deterioration, depression, aggravation of behavioral disorders, impairment of drive and initiative, and

psychomotor slowing are common findings (36,45,72).

Examples of this encephalopathy have been particularly stressed in children, especially in the presence of preexisting brain damage or mental retardation. A deterioration in intellectual function may be overlooked in these patients or regarded as a part of an underlying progressive neurological disease (84). Although blood levels of phenytoin are nearly always in the toxic range, this syndrome may occur with "optimal levels" (40).

In an experimental study of normal students treated with phenytoin, Ideström et al. (46) found a correlation between the serum levels of phenytoin and some measures of concentrational ability and psychomotor performance, although blood phenytoin levels were below optimal range. In a study of 70 adult patients who were given neuropsychological tests while receiving only phenytoin, Dodrill (31) found that blood levels of the drug above optimal range mainly affected tasks involving motor performance. Clinical examination alone seemed to underestimate the degree of central nervous system toxicity and seemed to be inadequate for detecting impaired cognitive function.

The encephalopathy may sometimes be associated with unusual neurological signs, including involuntary movements (4,51,57). Choreoathetosis may be seen in patients with metabolic epilepsy and without neurological deficits when blood levels of phenytoin are above optimal range (19). Otherwise, this symptom is most often seen in connection with brain lesions and may then arise with blood levels in the optimal range (71). Asterixis, which was originally reported in patients with liver disease, is now known to be a common feature of a variety of metabolic and drug-induced encephalopathies including intoxication with phenytoin, primidone, phenobarbital, and carbamazepine. The orofacial dyskinesias, limb chorea, and dystonia caused by intoxication with phenytoin and some other antiepileptic drugs are very similar to the tardive dyskinesias seen in patients on chronic neuroleptic drug therapy. They may be related to the dopamine antagonistic properties of phenytoin (18).

Total external ophthalmoplegia may be observed after administration of large oral or intravenous doses of phenytoin. The return of vestibuloocular responsiveness may lag behind the return of other reflex activity. The mechanism underlying this ophthalmoplegia may be related to the ability of phenytoin to potentiate inhibitory synapses in the vestibulooculomotor pathway and to increase the discharge rate of Purkinje cells which exert an inhibitory influence on the same structures (80).

Spasticity is an uncommon sign of toxicity and is most often caused by excessive blood levels of phenytoin (81). Hyperactive tendon reflexes, clonus, and absent abdominal and cremasteric reflexes may also be present (5). A single case with reversible fasciculations and blood phenytoin levels low in the optimal range has been published. The possibility was suggested that the patient represented an instance of a ''reversible form of motor neuron disease'' as described in connection with lead intoxication and porphyria (30).

Typical of the neurological signs mentioned is that they are all reversible and disappear after reduction in dose or cessation of phenytoin therapy.

Cerebellum

Cerebellar malfunction with ataxia and nystagmus is a well-known manifestation of acute phenytoin toxicity. The symptoms and signs disappear when the dose is lowered or the drug withdrawn. As shown by Kutt and co-workers (54), they are clearly related to the blood levels of phenytoin.

Several cases of poisoning with excessive doses of phenytoin have been reported, but the cerebellar symptoms or signs were not permanent (5,17,33,62,67,69,75). Since the review in 1972 (28), permanent ataxia still has, in some cases, been ascribed to the use of phenytoin by patients with epilepsy (39,70,73,77).

Similarly, a few reports have described experimental cerebellar changes after phenytoin administration to animals (6,49). Karkos (49) described nonspecific, ''degenerative'' changes in rat cerebellum with impairment of the parenchymal and mesenchymal elements after 1 month's administration of phenytoin. However, the same changes were found after treatment with phenobarbital. Further, he observed impairment of the mesenchymal elements before morphological changes in neurocytes and glia after treatment with ethosuximide and primidone. The structure most vulnerable to the effect of all drugs mentioned was found to be the Purkinje cells. He concluded that phenytoin was the most neurotoxic drug, followed by phenobarbital, ethosuximide, and primidone.

Alcala et al. (6) treated three rats with phenytoin over 10-, 20-, and 55-day periods, respectively. The plasma phenytoin level was, in all three animals, well below what was expected to be the optimal range for treatment of epilepsy. Consistent with these blood phenytoin levels, the rats were healthy and showed no neurological signs. Nevertheless, light microscopy findings showed Purkinje cell loss, albeit in only one rat and only minimally. However, they found ultrastructural changes with swollen mitochondria, disrupted cristae, and a whorling arrangement of the rough endoplasmic reticulum in two rats and lipofuscin granules in the third rat. These findings are contrary to earlier ultrastructural studies in which there were no changes in the substructure of the Purkinje cells even though the animals had been treated with toxic but sublethal doses of phenytoin (63).

The light microscopy findings seemed in most studies to be the result of fixation artifacts. Many of the earliest investigations did not use perfusion fixation of the animals. In other studies, the animals were comatose with uncontrolled respiration, which might result in hypoxic changes in the cerebella. Finally, the essential drawback of the light microscopy investigations was the failure to use quantitative methods of Purkinje cell counting. Puro and Woodward (68) were unable to show irreversible cerebellar damage in their phenytoin-treated rats fixated with perfusion. Similarly, we were unable to find any loss of Purkinje cells in monkeys, pigs, and rats intoxicated with phenytoin when we used a quantitative method.

In man, degeneration of Purkinje cells was described in the brains of epileptic patients long before phenytoin was introduced as an anticonvulsant in 1938. There is no convincing pathological evidence of cerebellar changes in man attributable to phenytoin. The significant reduction in the Purkinje cell count of epileptic patients treated with high doses of phenytoin was the result of the epilepsy, as most of these patients were severe epileptics.

It can thus still be concluded that there is no real loss of Purkinje cells in animals and that the cell loss that does occur is caused by the epilepsy rather than by the phenytoin in patients. The current theory tends to emphasize intrinsic metabolic requirements as the basic explanation for the phenomenon of susceptible nerve cells. The abnormal firing creates a complex critical metabolic demand which the compensatory increase in blood flow cannot always meet (76).

Peripheral Neuropathy

Patients receiving long-term phenytoin treatment may develop a predominantly sensory polyneuropathy. The patients seldom complain of symptoms, but a significant correlation is found between areflexia and the development of neuropathy. This development appears to be related to the duration of the phenytoin therapy. Data are not available to indicate the minimum period of treatment after which neuropathy may develop or doses that are able to induce the neuropathy. Patients treated with high doses of phenytoin, e.g., for status epilepticus, may be more apt to develop neuropathy (56,58). The relationship among the number of epileptic seizures, the type of epilepsy, the type of seizures, the duration of the epilepsy, and the neuropathy has not been investigated.

Subnormal serum folate concentrations cannot be demonstrated to be related to the neuropathy, and therapy with folic acid does not result in measurable improvement of the condition (44).

There is no convincing evidence that any of the other commonly used anticonvulsants cause peripheral nerve damage (7).

CHRONIC ASPECTS OF TOXICITY

Hepatic Toxicity

Parker and Shearer (64) reviewed 23 cases of phenytoin-induced liver disease. They found that most patients were adolescents or young adults, equally distributed between the sexes. Black persons outnumbered whites by nearly 2 : 1. Hepatotoxicity developed within 6 weeks of the first phenytoin exposure in the majority, and in most within 1 to 3 weeks, without apparent relation to phenytoin dosage or blood level. A rash was present in all cases, sometimes being mistaken for rubella. More than 90% suffered from fever. Clinical jaundice was observed in 55%, and lymphadenopathy (75%), hepatomegaly (65%), and splenomegaly (35%) were common. In 40%, hemorrhagic tendencies occurred. Two-thirds of the cases had leucocytosis (43). Eosinophilia and atypical lymphocytes were common, which may confuse the syndrome with infectious mononucleosis (10,41,79).

Serum bilirubin, transaminases, and alkaline phosphatases were abnormal in 70%, whereas liver biopsies were always abnormal (16,27, 50,89).

Nothing specific about the liver biopsy points to phenytoin hepatitis, although the histological picture of hepatitis with or without cholestasis with eosinophilia is suggestive (43). There may be fatty and cellular infiltration with variable amounts of mononuclear cells, segmented leucocytes, and eosinophils in the portal and lobular areas and focal or diffuse parenchymal necrosis. Overall, there appears to be mixed hepatocellular damage of cholestasis and necrosis.

In asymptomatic patients on chronic phenytoin therapy, slight biochemical changes with increased serum alkaline phosphatase and alanine aminotransferase activity are found with a few uni- or paucicellular necroses. There are no signs of permanent liver damage (47).

The pathogenesis of phenytoin-induced hepatotoxicity remains unexplained, but the hematologic changes and the skin reactions suggest a hypersensitivity reaction. Circulating antibodies to the drug hapten have been found to be present (50,74). The lack of relationship between dose and blood level of phenytoin excludes a direct toxic effect.

The effectiveness of proposed treatments for phenytoin-induced hepatotoxicity is difficult to evaluate, as some patients may have improved spontaneously (20). Immediate withdrawal of phenytoin is mandatory. Although steroids are thought to suppress the hypersensitivity phenomenon, they may be detrimental, because gastrointestinal hemorrhage and perforation may complicate therapy.

Many drugs with different biochemical and biological properties, including phenytoin, enlarge the liver and cause enzyme induction when used in nontoxic doses for a long time (29,53). The enlargement of the liver seems to be related to the enhancement of drug metabolism in patients treated with phenytoin (66). The inducing effect of phenytoin may explain the raised alkaline phosphatase, serum alanine aminotransferase, and plasma prothrombin time that are often observed in patients treated with phenytoin (14). The dose seems to be important in determining the degree of induction, but a wide variation among patients appears to exist with respect to their responses. The consequence of continued therapy is a state of chronically induced hepatic enzymes. The result may be an altered metabolic activity of a wide spectrum of both endogenous and exogenous substances (11).

Endocrinopathies

Effects on Adrenal Function

Levels of 17-hydroxyketosteroids in plasma are normal during phenytoin therapy. Urinary excretion of 17-hydroxycorticosteroids and 17-ketosteroids may decrease slightly.

The urinary steroid response to the conventional oral metyrapone test is subnormal in persons treated with phenytoin. In subjects treated chronically, administration of the regular oral dose of metyrapone results in plasma metyrapone levels that are lower than those observed in untreated subjects. The lower plasma concentration of metyrapone fails to inhibit 11 β-hydroxylation sufficiently to decrease the plasma cortisol to a concentration low enough to stimulate the release of ACTH. Consequently, plasma 11-deoxycortisol and urinary 17-hydroxycorticosteroid levels are lower than normal. The subnormal plasma levels of unconjugated metyrapone in phenytoin-treated subjects seem to be the result of increased splanchnic metabolism.

In patients on chronic phenytoin therapy, there is no suppression of plasma corticosteroids or urinary 17-hydroxycorticosteroids in the "low-dose" dexamethasone test (2 mg). However, suppression is normal in the "high-dose" test. Phenytoin causes an acceleration of the hepatic conjugation and biliary excretion of dexamethasone. Dexamethasone metabolism involves the formation of polar unconjugated derivatives. Phenytoin enhances hepatic microsomal hydroxylation enzyme activity and stimulates formation of 6-hydroxylated derivatives. Increased conjugation and excretion of dexamethasone lead to lower blood levels of free dexamethasone and less inhibition of ACTH secretion, thereby rendering the "low-dose" dexamethasone test inaccurate (38).

The effect of phenytoin on the clearance of corticoids is proportionately related to the initial plasma half-life of the steroid in the individual. Hydrocortisone, with a relatively short half-life of disappearance from plasma, is less affected than prednisolone and methylprednisolone, which are affected less than dexamethasone, which has the longest half-life. Individual variation in stimulation of hepatic drug-metabolizing enzymes by phenytoin is also a factor (65).

The increased metabolism of corticosteroids may be of clinical importance in epileptic recipients of cadaver renal allografts. A decreased allograft survival has been observed in these patients, possibly caused by an ineffective immunosuppression (87).

Effects on Thyroid Function

A decrease in serum protein-bound iodine (PBI) values in euthyroid patients receiving phenytoin has been widely recognized. This effect has been shown to be extrathyroid. *In vitro*, phenytoin competes with thyroxine (T_4) for binding sites on the thyroxine-binding globulin. A similar competition *in vivo* is thought to explain the low T_4 or PBI value during phenytoin treatment. The effect of phenytoin on serum T_4 or PBI appears after several days of therapy and reaches its maximum at about 2 weeks. The displacement of the thyroid hormones from binding proteins results in reduced serum total hormone, increased free fraction, and resultant increased free hormone concentration (32). These effects are more marked with regard to thyroxine than to triiodothyronine and are reflected in the urinary losses of unconjugated hormones that result from glomerular filtration of serum-free hormones. The uptake of T_4 by the liver is also increased, and there is a greater output of T_4 metabolites. Serum free hormone concentration remains in the euthyroid range, unlike serum total hormone concentrations which may overlap with values in the hypothyroid range.

In vivo, phenytoin therapy consistently produces a gradual decrease of free T_4 concentrations. Despite this, serum thyroid-stimulating hormone (TSH) values remain normal, and the patients remain euthyroid. Phenytoin enhances peripheral conversion of T_4 to T_3, which may explain maintenance of euthyroid status and normal TSH.

The diagnosis of thyrotoxicosis in patients on phenytoin can best be established by means of a radioactive iodine uptake and a suppression study. The laboratory diagnosis of hypothyroidism may be difficult. Serum TSH determination by radioimmunoassay is the most helpful laboratory assessment of thyroid function (38).

Effects on Glucose Metabolism

Phenytoin has been shown to induce hyperglycemia in animals and in man. Marked hyperglycemia, glycosuria, and hyperosmolar nonketotic coma have been recorded in patients receiving phenytoin, orally or intravenously, for epilepsy. Phenytoin seems to inhibit glucose-induced insulin release in the isolated rat pancreas. The decrease in circulating insulin concentration is secondary to a decrease in insulin secretion in response to glucose and not to an enhanced degradation of insulin. This complication may occur with a relatively low dose of phenytoin.

Although the changes in insulin response after administration of therapeutic doses of phenytoin appear to be only moderate in normoglycemic nondiabetic subjects, the implications for the large population with maturity-onset diabetes are apparent. Administration of phenytoin should be especially monitored in patients who have risk factors for diabetes (38).

Effects on Sex Hormones

Phenytoin therapy seems to increase plasma concentration of sex hormone-binding globulin in females (86). A similar rise in sex hormone-binding globulin was found in male patients, associated with an increased plasma concentration of testosterone (8). Others were unable to find any change in testosterone (82). In a group of patients on chronic phenytoin therapy, however, Stewart-Bentley et al. (82) found a decreased concentration of follicle-stimulating hormone (FSH) and a low sperm count with reduced semen volume and motility. Impairment of potency and infertility in patients with epilepsy have been attributed to treatment with antiepileptic drugs. A specific action of these drugs on the germinative tissue has been suggested (24).

There is evidence from animal experiments that estrogens and androgens are metabolized more rapidly when phenytoin is administered chronically (52). Consistent with these findings, it has been suggested that patients on antiepileptic medication may become pregnant despite a regular intake of oral contraceptives (48). Further investigations are needed before firm conclusions can be drawn.

Bone Disorders

Recently, reports of biochemical or radiographic features of rickets have drawn attention to the possible adverse effects of antiepileptic drugs on bone metabolism. Antiepileptic drugs seem to derange bone metabolism, both through induction of liver microsomal mixed-function oxidase enzyme activity, resulting in an increased hepatic catabolism of vitamin D and its biologically active products, and through a direct effect on membrane cation transport systems (42). It has been suggested that the bone disease resulting from phenytoin therapy may be associated with a deficiency of 25-hydroxycholecalciferol and that reduced gastrointestinal absorption of calcium or changes in parathyroid function may not be necessary for the development of the disease (9).

The bone changes found in patients receiving long-term anticonvulsant therapy are similar, in some respects, to those seen in vitamin D deficiency but differ in others. In contrast to vitamin D deficiency, anticonvulsant osteomalacia is characterized by increased bone turnover with, probably, an equal increase in bone formation and bone resorption rates. The bone changes seem to be induced by some alteration in vitamin D metabolism or in the effects of vitamin D metabolites on receptor cells and not by an unspecific effect of anticonvulsant drugs on bone cells (61).

The significant clinical manifestations include rickets, increased risk of pathological fracture, and reduction in serum calcium levels which may predispose to increased seizure frequency (42). Prolonged hypocalcemia with tetany may be seen in infants born at term whose mothers have been treated with phenytoin (37). This may explain the antiepileptic effect of vitamin D_2 reported in a controlled therapeutic trial (24).

Many factors appear to determine the severity of the clinical manifestations, including drug dose, duration of therapy, vitamin D intake, amount of exposure to sunlight, degree of physical activity, and presence of other concurrent diseases (42,60).

The pathological alterations develop in the course of a few months and then remain constant (21). Overt bone disease from phenytoin alone is very uncommon (23). When diagnosed, it requires treatment. The optimal initial dose is 4,000 IU of vitamin D_2 a day for about 4 months. The maintenance dose is 1,000 IU of vitamin D_2 a day (22).

It is controversial whether or not subclinical bone disease should be treated. The presently available data are more in favor of withholding prophylactic treatment than giving it (23). Any prophylactic treatment that leads to the prescribing of relatively large doses of vitamin D needs to be viewed with circumspection and must be firmly based on clinical and not simply biochemical benefit (12).

Hypersensitivity Reactions

Dermatological Reactions

Adverse reactions to phenytoin include hypersensitivity reactions that necessitate drug withdrawal. Severe cases are infrequent, but patients with exfoliative dermatitis and Stevens–Johnson syndrome (41), periarteritis nodosa (85), serum sickness (10), and purpura fulminans with disseminated intravascular coagulation have been reported (83).

A maculopapular erythema has been described as the first manifestation of a syndrome that includes acute renal failure, myositis, fever, lymphadenopathy, exfoliative dermatitis, and hepatitis. Prednisolone sodium phosphate therapy has resulted in the resolution of this hypersensitivity reaction (59). Phenytoin can also cause vasculitis and renal insufficiency by immunologic mechanisms as reported by Watanabe (88) who also found fibrinoid necrosis and cellular infiltration of arteries, venules, and capillaries.

Immunologic Disorders

Serum IgA values were low in 25 of 100 adult epileptic patients treated with phenytoin for at least 6 months (3). The IgA values were normal in untreated patients but fell during treatment with phenytoin. It was suggested that certain constitutional characteristics of epilepsy might predispose to low IgA in the presence of phenytoin (35). The IgA was normal whether or not the patients suffering from epilepsy thought to be secondary to traumatic or infectious events were treated with phenytoin. Others, however, were unable to confirm these findings (1).

Evidence of depressed T-cell function was found in patients with low serum IgA levels treated with phenytoin. No correlation could be demonstrated between the dose and blood level of phenytoin. A correlation was found with HL-A status, as patients with low IgA showed an increased frequency of HL-A2 (78).

Imbalance of the IgG subclasses was often observed, with IgG4 being undetectable in 65% of epileptic patients with constitutional factors for seizures and low IgA (34).

Secretory IgA has a protective function against viral and probably bacterial infections. Patients lacking IgA may therefore manifest an increased susceptibility to gingival inflammation. Gingival inflammation in phenytoin-treated epileptic patients is intimately connected with gingival hyperplasia. A local deficiency of secretory IgA in saliva without a compensatory increase in IgM may cause the development of gingivitis. The connective tissue repair process seems to be altered by phenytoin, which causes fibroblast proliferation with subsequent hyperplasia. It may therefore be suggested that phenytoin in some patients may induce a deficiency of salivary IgA. This deficiency involves an increased susceptibility to gingival inflammation, which, in turn, is considered a predisposing factor for the development of gingival hyperplasia (2). Even if the level of IgA is lowered because of phenytoin treatment, gingival hyperplasia may be limited or prevented by energetic mouth hygiene (13).

It has been suggested that the changed immunologic response in patients treated with phenytoin might be of importance in the development of cancer. Pseudolymphoma has long been known, with the characteristic symptoms of fever, rash, and lymphadenopathy. This syndrome has been judged to lack the sinister prognosis of other lymphomas provided the condition is recognized and the drug withdrawn. The occurrence of true lymphoma has been described in epileptic patients treated with hydantoins for a long time (55). However, in a study of the survival time and occurrence of neoplasms of 9,136 patients treated with anticonvulsants, it was not possible to discover any evidence of an oncogenic effect (26).

REFERENCES

1. Aarli, J. A. (1976): Drug-induced IgA deficiency in epileptic patients. *Arch. Neurol.,* 33:296–299.
2. Aarli, J. A. (1976): Phenytoin-induced depression of salivary IgA and gingival hyperplasia. *Epilepsia,* 17:283–291.
3. Aarli, J. A., and Tönder, O. (1975): Effects of antiepileptic drugs on serum and salivary IgA. *Scand. J. Immunol.,* 4:391–396.
4. Ahmad, S., Laidlaw, J., Houghton, G. W., and Richens, A. (1975): Involuntary movements caused by phenytoin intoxication in epileptic patients. *J. Neurol. Neurosurg. Psychiatry,* 38:225–231.
5. Airing, C. D., and Rosenbaum, M. (1941): Ingestion of large doses of Dilantin sodium. *Arch. Neurol. Psychiatry,* 45:265–270.

6. Alcala, H., Lertratanangkoon, K., Stenbach, W., Kellaway, P., and Horning, M. G. (1978): The Purkinje cell in phenytoin intoxication: Ultrastructural and Golgi studies. *Pharmacologist*, 20:240.

7. Argov, Z., and Mastaglia, F. L. (1979): Drug-induced peripheral neuropathies. *Br. Med. J.*, 1:663–666.

8. Barragry, J. M., Makin, H. L. J., Trafford, D. J. H., and Scott, D. F. (1978): Effect of anticonvulsants on plasma testosterone and sex hormone binding globulin levels. *J. Neurol. Neurosurg. Psychiatry*, 41:913–914.

9. Bell, R. D., Pak, C. Y. C., Zerwekh, J., Barilla, D. E., and Vasko, M. (1979): Effect of phenytoin on bone and vitamin D metabolism. *Ann. Neurol.*, 5:374–378.

10. Braverman, J. M., and Levin, J. (1963): Dilantin-induced serum sickness: Case report and inquiry into its mechanism. *Am. J. Med.*, 35:418–422.

11. Breckenridge, A. M., and Robert, J. B. (1976): Clinical significance of microsomal enzyme induction. *Pharmacol. Res. Comm.*, 8:229–242.

12. *British Medical Journal* (1976): Editorial: Anticonvulsant osteomalacia. *Br. Med. J.*, 2:1340–1341.

13. Bruun Kristensen, C. (1977): One-sided gingival hyperplasia after treatment with diphenylhydantoin. *Acta Neurol. Scand.*, 56:353–356.

14. Buch Andreassen, P., Lyngbye, J., and Trolle, E. (1973): Abnormalities in liver function tests during long-term diphenylhydantoin therapy in epileptic outpatients. *Acta Med. Scand.*, 194:261–264.

15. Buchthal, F., and Svensmark, O. (1960): Clinical and electroencephalographic correlations with serum levels of diphenylhydantoin. *Arch. Neurol.*, 2:624–630.

16. Campbell, C. B., McGuffie, C., and Weedon, A. P. (1977): Cholestatic liver disease associated with diphenylhydantoin therapy: Possible pathogenetic importance of altered bile salt metabolism. *Am. J. Dig. Dis.*, 22:255–262.

17. Cattan, R., Frumusan, P., and Attal, P. (1947): Intoxication aiguë par la diphenylhydantoine. *Bull. Soc. Med.*, 63:346–348.

18. Chadwick, D., Reynolds, E. H., and Marsden, C. D. (1976): Anticonvulsant-induced dyskinesias: A comparison with dyskinesias induced by neuroleptics. *J. Neurol. Neurosurg. Psychiatry*, 39:1210–1218.

19. Chalhub, E. G., and DeVivo, D. C. (1976): Phenytoin-induced choreoathetosis. *J. Pediatr.*, 89:153–154.

20. Chien, L. T., Ceballos, R., and Benton, J. W., Jr. (1970): Diphenylhydantoin fatal hepatic necrosis. *Ala. J. Med. Sci.*, 7:318–322.

21. Christiansen, C. (1976): *Knoglemineralindhold hos Epilepsipatienter i Antikonvulsiv Behandling.* Dansk Undervisningsforlag, Copenhagen.

22. Christiansen, C., and Rødbro, P. (1974): Initial and maintenance doses of vitamin D-2 in the treatment of anticonvulsant osteomalacia. *Acta Neurol. Scand.*, 50:631–641.

23. Christiansen, C., and Rødbro, P. (1977): Anticonvulsant osteomalacia. *Br. Med. J.*, 1:439–440.

24. Christiansen, C., Rødbro, P., and Sjö, O. (1974): ''Anticonvulsant action'' of vitamin D in epileptic patients? A controlled pilot study. *Br. Med. J.*, 2:258–259.

25. Christiansen, P., Deigaard, J., and Lund, M. (1977): Potency, fertility and sexual hormones in young male epileptics. In: *Epileptology*, edited by D. Janz, pp. 190–191. Georg Thieme, Stuttgart.

26. Clemmesen, J., Fuglsang-Frederiksen, V., and Plum, C. M. (1974): Are anticonvulsants oncogenic? *Lancet*, 1:705–707.

27. Crawford, S. E., and Jones, C. K. (1962): Fatal liver necrosis and diphenylhydantoin sensitivity. *Pediatrics*, 30:595–600.

28. Dam, M. (1972): The density and ultrastructure of the purkinje cells following diphenylhydantoin treatment in animals and man. *Acta Neurol. Scand. [Suppl.]*, 48:1–65.

29. Dam, M., Møller, J. E., and Petersen, P. (1969): The effect of diphenylhydantoin and phenobarbital on the liver of the pig. *Epilepsia*, 10:507–519.

30. Direkze, M., and Fernando, P. S. L. (1977): Transient anterior horn cell dysfunction in diphenylhydantoin therapy. *Eur. Neurol.*, 15:131–134.

31. Dodrill, C. B. (1975): Diphenylhydantoin serum levels, toxicity and neuropsychological performance in patients with epilepsy. *Epilepsia*, 16:593–600.

32. Finucane, J. F., and Griffiths, R. S. (1976): Effect of phenytoin therapy on thyroid function. *Br. J. Clin. Pharmacol.*, 3:1041–1044.

33. Floyd, F. W. (1961): The toxic effects of diphenylhydantoin: A report of 23 cases. *Clin. Proc. Child. Hosp.*, 17:195–201.

34. Fontana, A., Joller, H., Skvaril, F., and Grob, P. (1978): Immunological abnormalities and HLA antigen frequencies in IgA deficient patients with epilepsy. *J. Neurol. Neurosurg. Psychiatry*, 41:593–597.

35. Fontana, A., Sauter, R., Grob, P. J., and Joller, H. (1976): IgA deficiency, epilepsy and hydantoin medication. *Lancet*, 2:228–231.

36. Frantzen, E., Hansen, J. M., Hansen, O. E., and Kristensen, M. (1967): Phenytoin (Dilantin) intoxication. *Acta Neurol. Scand.*, 43:440–446.

37. Friis, B., and Sardemann, H. (1977): Neonatal hypocalcaemia after intrauterine exposure to anticonvulsant drugs. *Arch. Dis. Child.*, 52:239–247.

38. Gharib, H., and Munoz, J. M. (1974): Endocrine manifestations of diphenylhydantoin therapy. *Metabolism*, 23:515–524.

39. Ghatak, N. R., Santoso, R. A., and McKinney, W. M. (1976): Cerebellar degeneration following long-term phenytoin therapy. *Neurology (Minneap.)*, 26:818–820.

40. Glaser, G. H. (1972): Diphenylhydantoin toxicity. In: *Antiepileptic Drugs*, edited by D. M. Woodbury, J. K. Penry, and R. P. Schmidt, pp. 219–226. Raven Press, New York.

41. Gropper, A. (1956): Diphenylhydantoin sensitivity: Report of fatal case with hepatitis and exfoliative dermatitis. *N. Engl. J. Med.*, 254:522–523.

42. Hahn, T. J. (1976): Bone complications of anticonvulsants. *Drugs*, 12:201–211.

43. Harinasuta, U., and Zimmerman, H. J. (1968): Diphenylhydantoin sodium hepatitis. *J.A.M.A.*, 203:1015–1018.

44. Horwitz, S. J., Klipstein, F. A., and Lovelace, R. E.

(1967): Folic acid and neuropathy in epilepsy. *Lancet*, 2:1305–1306.

45. Husby, J. (1963): Delayed toxicity and serum concentrations of phenytoin. *Dan. Med. Bull.*, 10:236–239.
46. Ideström, C. M., Schalling, D., Carlquist, U., and Sjöquist, F. (1972): Behavioural and psychophysiological studies: Acute effects of diphenylhydantoin in relation to plasma levels. *Psychol. Med.*, 2:111–120.
47. Jacobsen, N. O., Mosekilde, L., Myhre-Jensen, O., Pedersen, E., and Wildenhoff, K. E. (1976): Liver biopsies in epileptics during anticonvulsant therapy. *Acta Med. Scand.*, 199:345–348.
48. Janz, D., and Schmidt, D. (1973): Anti-epileptic drugs and failure of oral contraceptions. *Lancet*, 1:1113.
49. Karkos, J. (1973): Effect of antiepileptic drugs on the morphological picture of rat cerebellum. *Neuropatol., Pol.*, 11:427–439.
50. Kleckner, H. B., Yakulis, V., and Heller, P. (1975): Severe sensitivity to diphenylhydantoin with circulating antibodies to the drug. *Ann. Intern. Med.*, 83:522–523.
51. Kooiker, J. C., and Sumi, S. M. (1974): Movement disorder as a manifestation of diphenylhydantoin intoxication. *Neurology (Minneap.)*, 24:68–71.
52. Kuntzman, R. (1969): Drugs and enzyme induction. *Annu. Rev. Pharmacol.*, 9:21–36.
53. Kunz, W., Schaude, G., Schmid, W., and Siess, M. (1966): Lebervergrösserung durch Fremdstoffe. *Naunyn Schmiedebergs Arch. Pharmacol.*, 254:470–488.
54. Kutt, H., Winters, W., Kokenge, R., and McDowell, F. (1964): Diphenylhydantoin metabolism, blood levels and toxicity. *Arch. Neurol.*, 11:642–648.
55. *Lancet* (1971): Editorial: Is phenytoin carcinogenic? *Lancet*, 2:1071–1072.
56. Lovelace, R. E., and Horwitz, S. J. (1968): Peripheral neuropathy in long-term diphenylhydantoin therapy. *Arch. Neurol.*, 18:69–77.
57. McLellan, D. L., and Swash, M. (1974): Choreoathetosis and encephalopathy induced by phenytoin. *Br. Med. J.*, 2:204–205.
58. Meienberg, O., and Bajc, O. (1975): Acute polyneuropathy caused by diphenylhydantoin intoxication. *Dtsch. Med. Wochenschr.*, 100:1532–1539.
59. Michael, J. R., and Mitch, W. E. (1976): Reversible renal failure and myositis caused by phenytoin hypersensitivity. *J.A.M.A.*, 236:2773–2775.
60. Mosekilde, L., and Melsen, F. (1976): Anticonvulsant osteomalacia determined by quantitative analysis of bone changes. *Acta Med. Scand.*, 199:349–355.
61. Mosekilde, L., Melsen, F., Christensen, M. S., Lund, B., and Sørensen, O. H. (1977): Effect of long-term vitamin D-2 treatment on bone morphometry and biochemical values in anticonvulsant osteomalacia. *Acta Med. Scand.*, 201:303–307.
62. Nauth-Misir, T. N. (1948): A case of gross overdosage of soluble phenytoin. *Br. Med. J.*, 2:646.
63. Nielsen, M. H., Dam. M., and Klinken, L. (1971): The ultrastructure of Purkinje cells in diphenylhydantoin intoxicated rats. *Exp. Brain Res.*, 12:447–456.
64. Parker, W. A., and Shearer, C. A. (1979): Phenytoin

hepatotoxicity: A case report and review. *Neurology (Minneap.)*, 2:175–178.

65. Petereit, L. B., and Meikle, A. W. (1977): Effectiveness of prednisolone during phenytoin therapy. *Clin. Pharmacol. Ther.*, 22:912–916.
66. Pirttiaho, H. J., Sotaniemi, E. A., Ahokas, J. T., and Pitkänen, U. (1978): Liver size and indices of drug metabolism in epileptics. *Br. J. Clin. Pharmacol.*, 6:273–278.
67. Price, W. C., and Frank. M. E. (1950): Accidental acute Dilantin poisoning. *J. Pediatr.*, 36:652–655.
68. Puro, D. G., and Woodward, D. J. (1973): Effects of diphenylhydantoin on activity of rat cerebellar Purkinje cells. *Neuropharmacology*, 12:433–440.
69. Putnam, T. J., and Rothenberg, S. F. (1953): Results of intensive (narcosis) and standard medical treatment of epilepsy. *J.A.M.A.*, 152:1400–1406.
70. Rapport, R. L., and Shaw, C. M. (1977): Phenytoin-related cerebellar degeneration without seizures. *Ann. Neurol.*, 2:437–439.
71. Rasmussen, S., and Kristensen, M. (1977): Choreoathetosis during phenytoin treatment. *Acta Med. Scand.*, 201:239–241.
72. Reynolds, E. H. (1970): Iatrogenic disorders in epilepsy. In: *Modern Trends in Neurology, No. 5*, edited by D. Williams, pp. 271–286. Butterworths, London.
73. Riley, C. G. (1972): Chronic hydantoin intoxication: Case report. *N.Z. Med. J.*, 76:425–428.
74. Robinson, D. S., MacDonald, M. G., and Hobin, F. P. (1965): Sodium diphenylhydantoin reaction with evidence of circulating antibodies. *J.A.M.A.*, 192:171–172.
75. Robinson, L. J. (1940): Case of acute poisoning from dilantin sodium with recovery. *J.A.M.A.*, 115:289–290.
76. Salcman, M., Defendini, R., Correll, J., and Gilman, S. (1978): Neuropathological changes in cerebellar biopsies of epileptic patients. *Ann. Neurol.*, 3:10–19
77. Selhorst, J. B., Kaufman, B., and Horwitz, S. J. (1972): Diphenylhydantoin-induced cerebellar degeneration. *Arch. Neurol.*, 27:453–456.
78. Shakir, R. A., Behan, P. O., Dick, H., and Lambie, D. G. (1978): Metabolism of immunoglobulin A, lymphocyte function, and histocompatibility antigens in patients on anticonvulsants. *J. Neurol. Neurosurg. Psychiatry*, 41:307–311.
79. Siegal, S., and Berkowitz, J. (1961): Diphenylhydantoin (Dilantin) hypersensitivity with infectious mononucleosislike syndrome and jaundice. *J. Allergy Clin. Immunol.*, 32:447–451.
80. Spector, R. H., Davidoff, R. A., and Schwartzman, R. J. (1976): Phenytoin-induced ophthalmoplegia. *Neurology (Minneap.)*, 26:1031–1034.
81. Stark, R. J. (1979): Spasticity due to phenytoin toxicity. *Med. J. Aust.*, 1:156.
82. Stewart-Bentley, M., Virgi, A., Chang, S., Hiatt, R., and Horton, R. (1976): Effect of dilantin on FSH and spermatogenesis. *Clin. Res.*, 24:101A.
83. Targan, S. R., Chassin, M. R. G., and Grize, L. B. (1975): Dilantin-induced disseminated intravascular coagulation with purpura fulminans. *Ann. Intern. Med.*, 83:227–230.

84. Trimble, M. R., and Reynolds, E. H. (1976): Anti-
    convulsant drugs and mental symptoms: A review.
    Psychol. Med., 6:169–178.
85. Van Wyk, J. J., and Hoffman, C. R. (1948): Periar-
    teritis nodosa: A case of fatal exfoliative dermatitis
    resulting from dilantin sodium sensitization. *Arch. In-
    tern. Med.*, 81:605–611.
86. Victor, A., Lundberg, P. O., and Johansson, E. D.
    B. (1977): Induction of sex hormone binding globulin
    by phenytoin. *Br. Med. J.*, 2:934–935.

87. Wassner, S. J., Pennisi, A. J., Malekzadeh, M. H.
    and Fine, R. N. (1976): The adverse effect of anti-
    convulsant therapy on renal allograft survival. *J. Pe-
    diatr.*, 88:134–137.
88. Watanabe, S. (1964): Angiitis from diphenylhydan-
    toin. *Acta Dermatol.*, 59:121–129.
89. Weedon, A. P. (1975): Diphenylhydantoin sensitiv-
    ity: A syndrome resembling infectious mononucleosis
    with a morbilliform rash and cholestatic hepatitis. *Aust.
    N.Z. J. Med.*, 5:561–563.

Antiepileptic Drugs, edited by D. M. Woodbury, J. K. Penry, and C. E. Pippenger. Raven Press, New York © 1982.

18

Phenytoin

Hematological Toxicity

Anthony V. Pisciotta

For many years, the hydantoin derivatives and the barbiturates have been the mainstays in treatment and control of convulsive disorders. As experience with these drugs accumulated, it became clear that they might be associated with unexpected hematologic reactions. Since these reactions affect a relatively small segment of the population, they are considered "idiosyncratic," that is, expressed only in those patients who have an individual defect that results in unusual susceptibility to the drug's toxic effect. Of the drugs useful in the treatment of epilepsy, the barbiturates have an extremely low incidence of hematologic toxicity. On the other hand, the hydantoin derivatives have been implicated in specific hematologic reactions with sufficient frequency that a relationship has been established.

This chapter deals with the association between phenytoin and specific blood disorders.

The types of hematologic reactions produced by hydantoin derivatives are outlined in Table 1. The designations 0 and 1 + to 4 + are based on data issued by the Registry of Blood Dyscrasias of the American Medical Association (2). The designation 4 + (toxic) means that its incidence of association between a putative drug and a specific blood dyscrasia is greater than double the random occurrence of the blood disorder when the drug is the only one given for 6 months

or more or when it is given together with another drug(s) believed to be innocent of potential hematotoxicity of similar type. The designation 2 + represents an association with stated hematotoxicity although the reaction is rare and occurs simultaneously with administration of another drug known to have similar toxic properties.

By these criteria, phenytoin has been implicated etiologically with megaloblastic anemia, lymphadenopathy (pseudolymphoma), a hypersensitivity syndrome, and, to a lesser degree, aplastic anemia and leukopenia. Mephenytoin is most frequently associated with leukopenia and aplastic anemia, and trimethadione with megaloblastic anemia only.

MEGALOBLASTIC ANEMIA

Megaloblastic anemia is the result of disordered maturation of hematopoietic and other dividing cells that occurs because of deficiency or lack of utilization of vitamin B_{12} or folic acid. It is characterized by a defect in cell division because of perturbation in synthesis of deoxyribonucleic acid (DNA). This results in abnormally large mature and developing cells as well as the characteristic morphologically abnormal nuclear appearance peculiar to this megaloblastic state.

TABLE 1. *Types of hematologic reactions attributed to antiepileptic drugs*

Drug	Megaloblastic anemia	Aplastic anemia	Leukopenia, agranulo-cytosis	Lymphadenopathy (pseudolymphoma)	Generalized hypersensitivity reaction
Phenytoin	+ + + +	+ +	+ +	+ + + +	+ + + +
Mephenytoin	0	+ + + +	+ + + +	0	0
Trimethadione	+ + +	+	0	0	0
Phenobarbital	0	0	0	0	0
Mephobarbital	0	0	0	0	0

Clinical Characteristics

The notion that megaloblastic anemia might be produced by phenytoin was first introduced by Mannheimer and co-workers in 1952 (44) and by Badenoch in 1954 (3). Since then, an ever increasing number of descriptive case reports, reviews, and basic experimental studies have appeared, first in the British literature and later worldwide (59). Although not exhaustive, this review is based on analysis of 60 cases taken from the literature; included were 42 females and 18 males, ranging in age from 10 to 60 years (Fig. 1). In all of these, anemia occurred concomitantly with the administration of phenytoin in doses of 100 to 300 mg given daily for periods ranging from 3 months to 15 years. Diet was probably not important in development of anemia, since an equivalent number of patients were said to have an adequate and a "poor" diet.

Symptomatology in all patients was related to anemia as well as the rapidity with which anemia developed and consisted of weakness, shortness of breath, and easy fatigue. Very few of the patients reported were taking phenytoin alone; other drugs that were given simultaneously included phenobarbital, primidone, trimethadione, and mephobarbital. Megaloblastic anemia rarely appears during treatment with barbiturates alone (27,36). It is more apt to occur when hydantoins are given together with barbiturates or, even more importantly, when hydantoins are used alone (Table 2).

Hematologic Considerations

Megaloblasts are pathologic precursors of erythrocytes that are readily distinguished morphologically from their normal counterparts, the normoblasts (Fig. 2). At each comparable state of maturation, megaloblasts are larger, and their

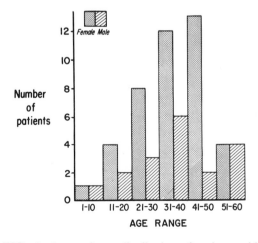

FIG. 1. Age and sex distribution of patients with hydantoin-induced megaloblastic anemia.

TABLE 2. *Megaloblastic anemia in epileptic patients*

Drugs prescribed in combination	Number of cases[a]
Phenytoin	28
Phenobarbital	28
Primidone	13
Ethotoin	1
Mephobarbital	1
Chlorpromazine	1
Trimethadione	2
Alcoholic	1
Phenytoin alone	8
Primidone alone	4
Phenobarbital alone	2

[a]Data from refs. 3,7,11–13,15,16,18,21–27,30,32,35, 36,38–40,44,47,55,59,62,64.

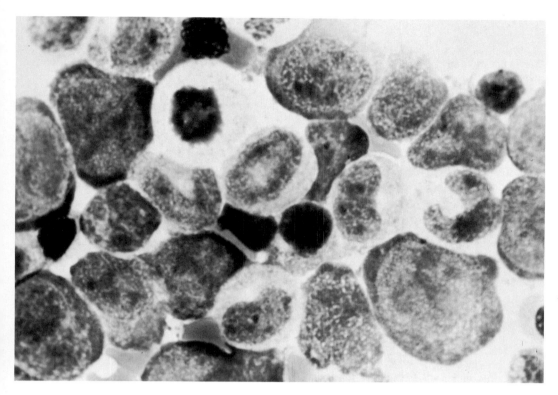

FIG. 2. Representative bone marrow field in megaloblastic anemia secondary to phenytoin (× 850).

cytoplasm stains more deeply basophilic than the corresponding normoblastic stage. In addition, the megaloblastic nucleus reflects a sparse distribution of chromatin, which is carried over to the late stage of development in which the most mature megaloblasts continue to show chromatin deficiency in contrast to the darkly stained pyknotic nucleus that characterizes late normoblasts.

Such changes occur because of deficiency or lack of utilization of vitamin B_{12} or folic acid. Megaloblasts are the products of diminished synthesis of DNA which produces disordered cell division. Such changes result in ineffective erythropoiesis and granulopoiesis which is characterized by intramedullary cell death of hematologic precursors before maturation and release. As a result, the patient develops anemia with a low reticulocyte count as well as leukopenia and thrombocytopenia. Because of the diminished number of mitotic events, the products of disordered maturation are larger in size than normal but are well filled with hemoglobin. Accordingly, the erythrocytes in megaloblastic anemia are large in appearance (macrocytic) and on measurement show an average volume that is greater than normal (mean corpuscular volume) (Fig. 3). These changes in size and nuclear morphology are shared by leuko-

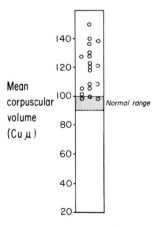

FIG. 3. Elevated mean corpuscular volume in phenytoin-induced megaloblastic anemia.

cytes and platelets as well. The appearance of hypersegmented polymorphonuclear leukocytes together with variations in size and shape of erythrocytes presents a most characteristic picture in the peripheral blood smear. Similarly, the bone marrow picture is characteristic and consists of replacement of normoblastic erythropoiesis by megaloblasts, giant metamyelocytes, and abnormally structured megakaryocytes. Such morphologic changes are characteristic of vitamin B_{12} or folic acid deficiency; morphology alone does not permit a distinction between the two.

Mechanisms of Development

An etiologic relationship between megaloblastic anemia and treatment with phenytoin or primidone indicates that folic acid and not vitamin B_{12} insufficiency represents the basic mechanism (Table 3). Analysis of 61 reported patients showed that 18 treated with vitamin B_{12} alone failed to respond. Instead, 28 of the reported patients, without exception, showed reticulocytosis together with a predictable increment in red cell values within 10 days of inception of folic acid therapy. It is of great interest that 19 patients who responded to folic acid therapy alone continued to receive phenytoin or primidone. Hence, this form of idiosyncratic hematologic reaction is unique, since recovery is expected even though the putative drug is continued as long as folic acid is prescribed.

TABLE 3. *Megaloblastic anemia induced by phenytoin (PHT): results of treatment*[a]

Treatment	Recovered	No response
Folic acid alone	9	0
Folic acid + PHT	19	1
Vitamin B_{12} alone	3	9
Vitamin B_{12} + PHT	4	9
Folic acid + vitamin B_{12}	3	0
Folic acid + vitamin B_{12} + PHT	3	1

[a]Data from refs. 3,7,11–13,15,16,18,21–27,30,32,35, 36,38–40,44,47,55,59,62,64.

Serum vitamin B_{12} levels exceeded 100 pg/ml, except for two patients with levels of 40 and 50 pg/ml each (Fig. 4). Despite this, the patient reported by Kidd and Mollin (36) failed to respond to treatment with vitamin B_{12} but reached normal red cell values when folic acid was given.

Urinary excretion of radioactive vitamin B_{12}, determined by the Schilling procedure, was found to be normal in most patients. However, Lees (38) described eight instances in which, despite a Schilling value on the low normal side, significant increments in vitamin B_{12} excretion occurred after successful treatment.

Following development of appropriate laboratory technology in recent years, serum folic acid levels were all found to be less than 1 ng/ml (Fig. 4). Furthermore, urinary excretion of formiminoglutamic acid during active phases of megaloblastosis exceeded normal limits, indicating further evidence of folate deficiency.

Thus, the concept that folic acid is deficient or not utilized in PHT induced megaloblastosis is incontrovertible. However, the mechanisms of clinical conditions that result in this abnormality are far from understood. In 1958, Chanarin et al. (11) described normal absorption and

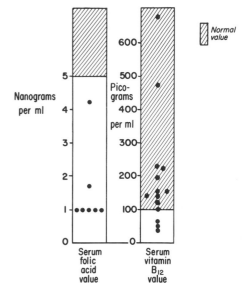

FIG. 4. Serum folic acid and vitamin B_{12} values in phenytoin-induced megaloblastic anemia.

tissue stores of folic acid during treatment with primidone. For this reason, they concluded that the anemia was more likely caused by failure to utilize folic acid rather than its deficiency. Similarly, Girdwood and Lenman (21) found no evidence of malabsorption of folic acid but suggested competitive inhibition of the drugs with folic acid.

Baker et al. (5) noted the structural resemblance of primidone to pyrimidines and to the pteridine portion of folic acid and suggested mutual metabolic competition between these compounds. Interference with proper utilization of pyrimidine groups could result in interference with DNA synthesis and then megaloblastic anemia.

Diet apparently has little to do with production of megaloblastic anemia. Half of the patients were reported to eat a satisfactory diet; in the remainder, the diet was said to be inadequate. In a study of institutionalized patients on a controlled diet, Ibbotson et al. (32) and Weber et al. (65) found consistently low serum and red cell folic acid values in patients treated with phenytoin as compared with control subjects. None of this series of patients had any evidence of megaloblastic anemia at the time of writing. However, 14.6% of Ibbotson's patients had macrocytosis (32). Studies such as this suggest that phenytoin in some way interferes with delivery of folic acid into the peripheral blood or its transport by plasma proteins.

Studies by Hoffbrand and Necheles (28) and by Rosenberg et al. (54) suggest a selective phenytoin-induced malabsorption of folic acid similar to that observed with oral contraceptives (45). The average diet contains a number of folic acid compounds in polyglutamate form which must be broken down to monoglutamates to facilitate absorption. This appears to be accomplished by an enzyme in intestinal epithelial cells (folate conjugase). Using a biopsy capsule to obtain samples of intestinal epithelium, Hoffbrand and Necheles (28) showed that this enzyme was suppressed by addition of phenytoin to intestinal epithelial cells in culture. Furthermore, intestinal epithelium obtained from patients undergoing treatment with phenytoin shows

less folate conjugase activity than those obtained from control subjects. The net effect would be failure to absorb naturally occurring polyglutamic folic acid in foods, an effect that is overcome by offering the patient the more readily absorbable chemically defined monoglutamic folic acid, even while continuing treatment with phenytoin. However, the matter is far from settled, since Baugh and Krumdieck (6) found no evidence of inhibition of conjugase when phenytoin was directly incubated with intestine, liver, or brain. Furthermore, failure to show competitive inhibition of kinetics of enzyme activity casts doubt on this mechanism of phenytoin-induced toxicity.

Moreover, phenytoin has no direct effect on the microbiologic assay of folic acid (17). Taguchi et al. (60) reported that phenytoin, in a concentration of 100 μg/ml, interfered with incorporation of ^{3}H-thymidine into DNA. This concentration exceeds by far any effective therapeutic blood level. Nevertheless, since thymidine incorporated into DNA occurs at a distal point that bypasses folic acid requirements, it was suggested that phenytoin might directly cause cell death and thereby increase folic acid requirements for compensatory renewal of cells.

Whatever the mechanism for megaloblastic anemia may turn out to be, the important point remains that hydantoin-induced megaloblastic anemia is one of those few instances in which the offending drug can continue to be given in a drug-induced blood disorder as long as the patient is treated with folic acid at the same time.

APLASTIC ANEMIA

Aplastic anemia consists of failure of the bone marrow to produce blood cells, resulting in a replacement of recognizable blood cell precursors by fat. It may be total, affecting production of all cells produced in marrow (granulocytes, erythrocytes, and platelets) or selective, affecting any one or two cell types. It is manifested by depletion in numbers of erythrocytes, leukocytes, platelets, and reticulocytes in peripheral blood as well as of their precursors in bone marrow. The reason why aplastic anemia is considered to be the most serious of the various drug-induced blood disorders is related to its protracted if not permanent course, with frequent fatal termination because of uncontrollable hemorrhage or infection. Its prolonged duration is probably related to irreversible damage inflicted on uncommitted hematologic stem cells without which renewal of hematopoiesis is not possible. Less likely, aplastic anemia may occur because of damage directed to the marrow microenvironment whereby growth of marrow stem cells can no longer be supported. However, successful remission induced by engraftment of transplanted compatible marrow cells does not support the latter concept.

Clinical symptomatology is related to anemia, infection associated with leukopenia, and cutaneous or mucosal hemorrhages because of diminished platelet counts. The diagnosis must be confirmed by bone marrow biopsy (Fig. 5) including histologic section of marrow spicules. Generally, marrow spicules are easily aspirated in aplastic anemia; these consist mainly of fat, very few developing bone marrow cells, and a varying number of lymphocytes.

Aplastic anemia sometimes offers a diagnostic dilemma because it has clinical and hematologic features that resemble those produced by other disorders such as miliary tuberculosis, preleukemic or aleukemic leukemia, systemic lupus erythematosus, myelofibrosis, lymphoma, or other malignancies involving the bone marrow. Accordingly, the clinician must carry out diagnostic determinations with care, keeping in mind the abovementioned possibilities as diagnostic alternatives. The bone biopsy is needed to help distinguish among these disorders and facilitates the diagnosis of aplastic anemia.

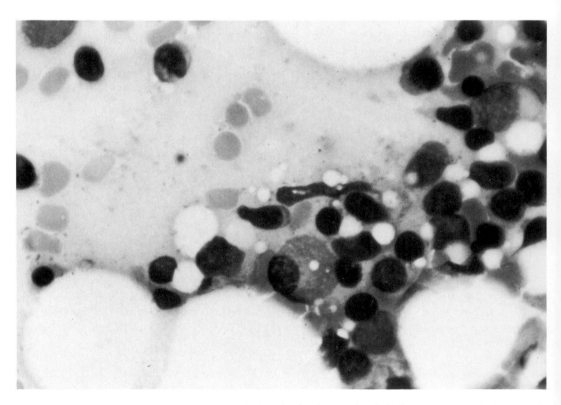

FIG. 5. Bone marrow smear in mephenytoin-induced aplastic anemia. Only lymphocytes and plasma cells persist ($\times$ 850).

The relationship of aplastic anemia to drugs is frequently difficult to establish because the cause-and-effect relationship between them is strictly a matter of circumstantial evidence. Furthermore, the association of aplastic anemia with specific drugs offers a dilemma because it need not occur concomitantly with drug administration, nor does it necessarily become corrected if the drug is discontinued. Moreover, this is such a serious complication of drug therapy that rechallenge of the patient with the drug is never justified.

Fortunately, aplastic anemia is a rare occurrence with antiepileptic drugs. In a review of 48 cases published through 1962 (Table 4), 26 patients were treated with mephenytoin alone, and six with this drug plus other antiepileptic drugs. Twelve patients received trimethadione alone, two were treated with 3-methyl-5-phenylhydantoin (Norantoin®, Nuvarone®), and one each with miscellaneous antiepileptic drugs. No instances of phenytoin-induced aplasia were described, but three patients treated wth phenytoin alone were reported to have pure red blood cell aplasia (10,20,34).

The cases reported in the literature are chiefly of descriptive interest. Few, if any, attempts have been made to describe the mechanism or predictability of the aplastic anemia. The 48 cases reviewed by Robins (51) consisted of 24 females, 23 males, and one patient with sex unidentified, ranging in age between 4 and 68 years. The length of treatment ranged widely, from 14 days to 30 months. Age and sex, therefore, cannot be used as criteria for predicting drug reactivity, nor can duration of treatment. However, where it occurred, aplastic anemia was more likely to have its onset within 1 year of therapy initiation. There was no correlation with the total dose of drug ingested.

That aplastic anemia is a serious complication of drug therapy is attested to by the mortality incidence of 37 out of 48 reported cases. Of this number, all succumbed within 4 months of having developed the disease. Those who survived did so after a prolonged convalescence.

There are presently no identifiable characteristics that would lead to prediction of aplastic anemia in potentially susceptible people. In the absence of these, careful clinical observation is necessary to monitor early phases of aplastic anemia. Even then, no data exist to document the earliest changes that would occur or to suggest whether discontinuing the drug at that point would abort the illness. It is recommended that complete blood cell counts, including platelets and reticulocytes, be done weekly for the first 8 weeks of antiepileptic drug therapy, then monthly for the first year, and then every 3 months thereafter. More frequent monitoring is necessary if the white cell count falls below 2,000/mm^3. It is recommended that treatment be discontinued if leukocytes reach 1,500/mm^3. Sparberg (59) has suggested that aplastic anemia may follow the establishment of megaloblastic anemia, but no evidence of this is available.

Phenytoin has been implicated in pure red cell aplasia. Although only three cases have been reported, one study is remarkable because of a phenytoin-induced biochemical defect produced in a susceptible patient. The patient, a 17-year-old black male, was originally reported by Brittingham et al. (10) and by Yunis et al. (67). He developed pure red cell aplasia during treatment with phenytoin, and he recovered when treatment was stopped. This patient remained normal if not treated with phenytoin or if he received riboflavin together with phenytoin.

Yunis et al. (67) carried out a series of elegant studies describing the incorporation of radioactive substrates into DNA and RNA.

TABLE 4. *Recorded cases of aplastic anemia with use of antiepileptic drugs*

Drug	Number of cases reported[a]
Mephenytoin (MHT) alone	26
Trimethadione alone	12
MHT + other antiepileptic drugs	6
3-methyl-5-phenylhydantoin	2
Methsuximide	1
Phenacemide	1

[a]Data from refs. 8,33,51,59,66.

During periods of normal marrow activity, the yield of radioactive DNA and RNA was suppressed by incubating the marrow with phenytoin. During periods of pure red cell aplasia, when the only cells in bone marrow capable of DNA synthesis were granulocyte precursors, the yield of radioactive DNA and RNA in the presence of phenytoin was similar to that in control preparations, implying that the normoblasts alone were affected by this drug. Autoradiography showed a selective inhibition of incorporation of uridine but not thymidine or deoxyuridine into normoblasts alone. These findings were interpreted to suggest that phenytoin acted specifically to prevent conversion by reduction of ribonucleotides to deoxyribonucleotides.

In our own studies (49) of marrow from patients after recovery from phenytoin-induced aplastic anemia, mephenytoin specifically suppressed incorporation of uridine into marrow cells. This effect was observed in patients recovered from aplastic anemia alone and not in normal controls. Since the tritium label used in our experiments was placed in the carbon-5 position, it would have been lost if the uridine were to be methylated in the same position to produce thymidine in preparation for DNA synthesis. That it did not do so was interpreted as evidence of specific suppression of RNA synthesis.

It is beyond the scope of this chapter to dwell on details of treatment of aplastic anemia. However, it is essential that all drugs suspected of causing aplastic anemia be discontinued when the diagnosis of aplastic anemia is confirmed. Stimulants to resumption of bone marrow activity have only a limited use. The use of riboflavin in preventing pure red cell aplasia has already been mentioned (67). Androgens, either by the oral route (fluoxymesterone, 40 mg/day) or by parenteral administration (e.g., testosterone enanthate, 600 mg/week i.m. or nortestosterone decanoate, 100 mg/week i.m.) should be continued for at least 4 months. The likelihood of recovery remains if an HLA compatible sibling is available; the patient and donor should be referred to a suitable center for a marrow transplant.

LEUKOPENIA AND AGRANULOCYTOSIS

Phenytoin has been implicated as an occasional causative agent in leukopenia and less frequently in agranulocytosis. The distinction between these is a matter of degree of severity. In leukopenia, the total leukocyte count ranges between 2,500 and 4,000/mm^3, and polymorphonuclear leukocytes (PMNs) frequently remain 50 or 60% of that number. Leukopenia is not necessarily accompanied by infection because of the persistence of PMNs and their precursors in peripheral blood and bone marrow. On the other hand, agranulocytosis is characterized by a total leukocyte count well under 2,500/mm^3 and PMNs between 0 and 500/mm^3. In general, agranulocytosis is a selective, sudden depletion of leukocytes induced by drugs. It occurs concomitantly with treatment and generally reverts to normal once the offending drug is discontinued unless uncontrollable infection results in fatality.

The clinical hallmark of agranulocytosis is infection. Patients who develop agranulocytosis during treatment with certain drugs may develop chills, fever, localizing signs such as pharyngitis or proctitis, and collapse by one of several mechanisms. If large numbers of leukocytes are suddenly destroyed in the peripheral blood by antileukocytic antibodies, they may release toxic pyrogenic materials that would produce chills and fever. The prototype drug that is associated with this type of mechanism is aminopyrine. Other drugs produce total bone marrow suppression, which is manifested first by asymptomatic leukopenia. In this case, sooner or later, severe infection would develop and result in a rapidly developing course characterized by chills and fever, leading frequently to fatality because of uncontrolled infection. The drugs most apt to produce agranulocytosis through this mechanism include the phenothiazines.

The hematologic picture of agranulocytosis consists of sudden leukopenia characterized by total absence of polymorphonuclear leukocytes and by normal red cell and platelet values. The bone marrow picture depends on the mechanism of agranulocytosis (48). In immunologically mediated agranulocytosis, granulocyte precursors persist in bone marrow together with aggregates of lymphocytes appearing early, either diffusely or in nodules. This morphologic feature suggests peripheral destruction of leukocytes by drug-induced antibodies. The lymphocytic infiltration is believed to be related to an immune-mediated mechanism.

In agranulocytosis associated with bone marrow suppression (48), the bone marrow morphology is indistinguishable from aplastic anemia. Although this form of agranulocytosis is associated with total suppression of hematopoiesis, it is manifested by a low leukocyte count because of rapid leukocyte turnover compared with that of erythrocytes and platelets. This disorder is too short in duration to result in anemia and thrombocytopenia, which would probably occur if the disease lasted long enough.

In agranulocytosis of this type, the drug's toxic activity is directed to the committed stem cells which are rapidly replaced. In contrast, in aplastic anemia, the drug inflicts damage on uncommitted stem cells and prevents full or rapid recovery because of inability to renew matured marrow cells. The mechanism(s) that underlies agranulocytosis induced by antiepileptic drugs is unknown.

Whether agranulocytosis results from peripheral leukocyte destruction or impaired bone marrow production, the outlook for both types is complete recovery as long as the drug is discontinued and uncontrollable infection or other complications can be avoided or successfully treated.

A common, although nonfatal complication of phenytoin toxicity is mild, nonremitting and nonprogressive leukopenia. In this case, the leukocyte count is modestly diminished (3,000–4,000/mm^3), but with persistence of polymorphonuclear leukocytes in peripheral blood and bone marrow. This is not agranulocytosis because of the persistence of PMNs and their precursors. Furthermore, this type of leukopenia does not usually proceed to complete granulocyte depletion, even though the drug is continued. A normal leukocyte count would be expected if phenytoin were discontinued.

Phenytoin-induced agranulocytosis must be very rare, since only 11 cases (one fatal) have been recorded by the A.M.A. registry (2). The patient who died had cirrhosis and was believed to be incapable of detoxifying phenytoin, allowing a toxic buildup of this drug. Descriptions of bone marrow in three reported cases (37,58,63) shed little light on the basic mechanism of agranulocytosis attributed to phenytoin. All three showed persistence of immature myeloid cells in bone marrow, which suggests peripheral destruction of white blood cells rather than failure of development. Of the nine cases reported in the literature, none offered any data on mechanisms. Two personally studied cases of agranulocytosis failed to disclose any incidence of white blood cell antibodies.

Mild thrombocytopenia has only been recorded in two published reports and in three reports to the A.M.A. registry (2). None of the cases was associated with serious hemorrhage.

PHENYTOIN-INDUCED LYMPHADENOPATHY AND HYPERSENSITIVITY STATES

The effect of phenytoin on the lymphoreticular system is most unique and perplexing. The long-term treatment of a patient with phenytoin may lead to gingival hyperplasia and to lymphadenopathy. The first of these is related to a propensity of phenytoin to stimulate fibroblast development in tissue culture (31). The second is associated with an unexplained effect of phenytoin or its metabolites on lymphocytic proliferation (4,14,19). The subject has been exhaustively explored by Saltzstein and Ackerman (56) who described 32 cases of lymphadenopathy in patients treated variously with phenytoin, mephenytoin, trimethadione, and ethotoin. Treatment with each of these compounds either alone or in combination was carried out for short periods ranging from 2 weeks to 4 months. Each of these patients developed enlargement of cervical, axillary, or inguinal lymph nodes which on biopsy presented a picture suggesting lymphoma or Hodgkin's disease. It is important to note that if hydantoin therapy in such cases is discontinued, the nodes will regress. It is essential to avoid erroneous treatment with irradiation or chemotherapy for conditions that are ordinarily quite benign.

Related to this lymphoproliferative effect of phenytoin is the lupus-like or "hypersensitivity" syndrome it sometimes provokes (1,9, 50,52,53,57,61,68). This disorder is clinically characterized by fever, pruritis, skin rash, sometimes with exfoliation, eosinophilia, and enlargement of liver and spleen as well as lymph nodes. In one instance, vasculitis, disseminated intravascular coagulation, and purpura fulminans, possibly caused by hypersensitivity to phenytoin, was described (61). All of these manifestations rapidly regress if phenytoin is discontinued. Rechallenge with the drug would quickly bring on these manifestations.

Peripheral blood of these patients shows lymphocytosis in addition to eosinophilia. The lymphocytes appear to be reactive, that is, show profuse, deeply basophilic, and vacuolated cytoplasm with irregular cell borders and indented nuclei. These cells resemble those found in infectious mononucleosis, but the heterophil antibody reaction remains negative.

Since laboratory tests shed no light on the diagnostic aspects of this disorder, the most characteristic feature is prompt regression when the drug is discontinued. There would be great confusion if a patient on antiepileptic drugs were also to have a lymphoma. Obviously, such coincidental manifestations of disease would have to be evaluated in individual cases.

Central to explanations of this type of toxicity would be the effect of phenytoin on the lymphocyte population (29,46). In 1965, Holland and Mauer (29) reported studies performed on a woman who had a "hypersensitivity" reaction during treatment with phenytoin. When lymphocytes from this patient were incubated with phenytoin, they enlarged, underwent blast transformation, and engaged in DNA synthesis as manifested by incorporation of ^{3}H-thymidine. If the drug were omitted, or if lymphocytes from normal people were used, such blast transformation failed to develop. This study suggested an important immunologic basis for development of a hypersensitivity reaction to phenytoin.

MacKinney and colleagues (41–43) reported studies on the mechanisms of the proliferative effect of phenytoin in hypersensitivity reactions. They found that it was not even necessary to add phenytoin to lymphocytes from such patients to stimulate DNA synthesis, but spontaneous blastogenesis occurred even in the absence of drugs. In fact, if phenytoin were added to such a culture, incorporation of ^{3}H-thymidine was partially inhibited, which they associated with a colchicine-like effect producing damage to mitotic microtubules. The *in vivo* effect of this drug included suppression in the number of circulating lymphocytes followed by diminished immunoglobulin values. It thus appears that immunosuppression, a lymphoma-like picture, a lupus-like syndrome, and serum sickness may all be interrelated as mechanisms underlying hypersensitivity to phenytoin.

SUMMARY

Phenytoin and its congeners have been implicated in a variety of hematologic reactions. The most common of these, megaloblastic anemia, is responsive to treatment with folic acid and does not require discontinuance of the drug. Aplastic anemia, agranulocytosis, and chronic "benign" leukopenia are less frequently encountered. Lymphadenopathy, sometimes confused clinically and pathologically with lymphoma, is related to a hypersensitivity reaction to phenytoin and regresses when the drug is discontinued.

REFERENCES

1. Aksoy, M., Devrimel, H., and Alpustun, H. (1960): Generalized lymphadenopathy, blood changes, and rash associated with methoin. *Lancet,* 1:605.
2. American Medical Association Study Group on Blood Diseases (1963): *Semi-annual Tabulation of Reports Compiled by the Registry on Blood Dyscrasias of the Study Group on Blood Dyscrasias, Vol. 7.* American Medical Association, Chicago.
3. Badenoch, J. (1954): The use of labelled vitamin B_{12}

and gastric biopsy in the investigation of anaemia. *Proc. R. Soc. Med.*, 47:426–427.

4. Bajoghli, M. (1961): Generalized lymphadenopathy and hepatosplenomegaly induced by diphenylhydantoin. *Pediatrics*, 28:943–945.

5. Baker, H., Frank, O., Hutner, S. H., Aaronson, S., Ziffer, H., and Sobotka, H. (1962): Lesions in folic acid metabolism induced by primidone. *Experientia*, 18:224–226.

6. Baugh, C. M., and Krumdieck, C. L. (1969): Effects of phenytoin on folic-acid conjugases in man. *Lancet*, 2:519–521.

7. Berlyne, N., Levene, M., and McGlashan, A. (1955): Megaloblastic anaemia following anticonvulsants. *Br. Med. J.*, 1:1247–1248.

8. Best, W. R., and Paul, J. T. (1950): Severe hypoplastic anemia following anticonvulsant medication; review of the literature and report of a case. *Am. J. Med.*, 8:124–130.

9. Braverman, I. M., and Levin, J. (1963): Dilantin-induced serum sickness. Case report and inquiry into its mechanisms. *Am. J. Med.*, 35:418–422.

10. Brittingham, T. E., Lutcher, C. L., and Murphy, D. L. (1964): Reversible erythroid aplasia induced by diphenylhydantoin. *Arch. Intern. Med.*, 113:764–768.

11. Chanarin, I., Elmes, P. C., and Mollin, D. L. (1958): Folic-acid studies in megaloblastic anaemia due to primidone. *Br. Med. J.*, 2:80–82.

12. Chanarin, I., Laidlaw, J., Loughridge, L. W., and Mollin, D. L. (1960): Megaloblastic anaemia due to phenobarbitone. The convulsant action of therapeutic doses of folic acid. *Br. Med. J.*, 1:1099–1102.

13. Christenson, W. N., Ultmann, J. E., and Roseman, D. M. (1957): Megaloblastic anemia during primidone (mysoline) therapy. *J.A.M.A.*, 163:940–942.

14. Doyle, A. P., and Hellstrom, H. R. (1963): Mesantoin lymphadenopathy morphologically simulating Hodgkin's disease. *Ann. Intern. Med.*, 59:363–368.

15. Druskin, M. S., Wallen, M. H., and Bonagura, L. (1962): Anticonvulsant-associated megaloblastic anemia. Response to 25 microgm. of folic acid administered by mouth daily. *N. Engl. J. Med.*, 267:483–485.

16. Flexner, J. M., and Hartmann, R. C. (1960): Megaloblastic anemia associated with anticonvulsant drugs. *Am. J. Med.*, 28:386–396.

17. Foster, N., and Campbell, B., Jr. (1976): The effect of diphenylhydantoin on the microbial assay of serum folate. *Clin. Biochem.*, 9:22–23.

18. Fuld, H., and Moorhouse, E. H. (1956): Observations on megaloblastic anaemias after primidone. *Br. Med. J.*, 1:1021–1023.

19. Gams, R. A., Neal, J. A., and Conrad, F. G. (1968): Hydantoin-induced pseudopseudolymphoma. *Ann. Intern. Med.*, 69:557–568.

20. Germano, G., and Scholer, Y. (1968): Erythroblastopenie non megalocytaire et sensible a l'acide folique chez une epileptique. *Acta Haematol. (Basel)*, 39:159–166.

21. Girdwood, R. H., and Lenman, J. A. R. (1956): Megaloblastic anaemia occurring during primidone therapy. *Br. Med. J.*, 1:146–147.

22. Gordin, R. (1958): Megaloblastic anaemia during anticonvulsant therapy. *Acta Med. Scand.*, 162:401–405.

23. Gydell, K. (1957): Megaloblastic anaemia in patients treated with diphenylhydantoin and primidone. *Acta Haematol. (Basel)*, 17:1–15.

24. Hamfelt, A., Killander, A., Malers, E., and de Verdier, C.-H. (1965): Megaloblastic anaemia associated with anticonvulsant drugs. Studies on a case with four relapses. *Acta Med. Scand.*, 177:549–555.

25. Hansen, H. A., Nordqvist, P., and Sourander, P. (1964): Megaloblastic anemia and neurologic disturbances combined with folic acid deficiency. Observations on an epileptic patient treated with anticonvulsants. *Acta Med. Scand.*, 176:243–251.

26. Hawkins, C. F., and Meynell, M. J. (1954): Megaloblastic anaemia due to phenytoin sodium. *Lancet*, 2:737–738.

27. Hobson, Q. J. G., Selwyn, J. G., and Mollin, D. L. (1956): Megaloblastic anaemia due to barbiturates. *Lancet*, 2:1079–1081.

28. Hoffbrand, A. V., and Necheles, T. F. (1968): Mechanism of folate deficiency in patients receiving phenytoin. *Lancet*, 2:528–530.

29. Holland, P., and Mauer, A. M. (1965): Diphenylhydantoin induced hypersensitivity reaction. *J. Pediatr.*, 66:322–332.

30. Horsfield, G. I., and Chalmers, J. N. M. (1963): Megaloblastic anaemia associated with anticonvulsant therapy. *Practitioner*, 191:316–321.

31. Houck, J. C., Cheng, R. F., and Waters, M. D. (1972): The effect of Dilantin upon fibroblast proliferation. *Proc. Soc. Exp. Biol. Med.*, 139:969–971.

32. Ibbotson, R. N., Dilena, B. A., and Horwood, J. M. (1967): Studies on deficiency and absorption of folates in patients on anticonvulsant drugs. *Aust. Ann. Med.*, 16:144–150.

33. Isaacson, S., Gold, J. A., and Ginsberg, V. (1956): Fatal aplastic anemia after therapy with Nuvarone (3-methyl-5-phenylhydantoin). *J. A. M. A.*, 160:1311–1312.

34. Jeong, Y.-G., Jung, Y., and River, G. L. (1974): Pure RBC aplasia and diphenylhydantoin. *J.A.M.A.*, 229:314–315.

35. Kahn, S. B., Lischner, H., Baker, L., and Williams, W. J. (1963): Megaloblastic anemia associated with the ingestion of phenobarbital and primidone. Report of a case in a six-year-old child. *Pediatrics*, 32:376–383.

36. Kidd, P., and Mollin, D. L. (1957): Megaloblastic anaemia and vitamin B_{12} deficiency after anticonvulsant therapy. Report of two cases. *Br. Med. J.*, 2:974–976.

37. Kurtzke, J. F. (1961): Leukopenia with diphenylhydantoin. *J. Nerv. Ment. Dis.*, 132:339–343.

38. Lees, F. (1961): Radioactive vitamin B_{12} absorption in the megaloblastic anaemia caused by anticonvulsant drugs. *Q. J. Med.*, 30:231–248.

39. Long, M. T., Childress, R. H., and Bond, W. H. (1963): Megaloblastic anemia associated with the use of anticonvulsant drugs. *Neurology (Minneap.)*, 13:697–702.

40. Lustberg, A., Goldman, D., and Dreskin, O. H. (1961): Megaloblastic anemia due to Dilantin therapy. *Ann. Intern. Med.*, 54:153–158.

41. MacKinney, A. A., and Booker, H. E. (1972): Diphenylhydantoin effects on human lymphocytes *in vi-*

tro and *in vivo*. An hypothesis to explain some drug reactions. *Arch. Intern. Med.,* 129:988–992.

42. MacKinney, A. A., Jr., Vyas, R., and Powers, K. (1978): Morphologic effect of hydantoin drugs on mitosis and microtubules of cultured human lymphocytes. *J. Pharmacol. Exp. Ther.,* 204:195–202.

43. MacKinney, A. A., Vyas, R. S., and Walker, D. (1978): Hydantoin drugs inhibit polymerization of pure microtubular protein. *J. Pharmacol. Exp. Ther.,* 204:189–194.

44. Mannheimer, E., Pakesch, F., Reimer, E. E., and Vetter, H. (1952): Die hamatologische Komplikationen der Epilepsiebehandlung mit Hydantoinkorpern. *Med. Klin.,* 47:1397–1401.

45. Necheles, T. F., and Snyder, L. M. (1970): Malabsorption of folate polyglutamates associated with oral contraceptive therapy. *N. Engl. J. Med.,* 282:858–859.

46. Neilan, B. A. (1979): Effect of phenytoin on T lymphocyte rosette formation. *Curr. Ther. Res. Clin. Exp.,* 25:557–563.

47. Penny, J. L. (1963): Megaloblastic anemia during anticonvulsant drug therapy. *Arch. Intern. Med.,* 111:744–749.

48. Pisciotta, A. V. (1973): Immune and toxic mechanisms in drug-induced agranulocytosis. *Semin. Hematol.,* 10:279–310.

49. Pisciotta, A. V., Callaghan, J. L., Keller, C., and Kaldahl, J. (1962): The effect of chloramphenicol and methyl-ethyl-phenyl hydantoin (Mesantoin) upon nucleic acid synthesis in marrow cells. *Proc. Cong. Int. Soc. Hematol.,* 9:601–612.

50. Robinow, M. (1963): Diphenylhydantoin hypersensitivity. Treatment with 6-mercaptopurine. *Am. J. Dis. Child.,* 106:553–557.

51. Robins, M. M. (1962): Aplastic anemia secondary to anticonvulsants. *Am. J. Dis. Child.,* 104:614–624.

52. Robinson, D. S., MacDonald, M. G., and Hobin, F. P. (1965): Sodium diphenylhydantoin reaction with evidence of circulating antibodies. *J.A.M.A.,* 192:171–172.

53. Rose, J. Q., Choi, H. K., Schentag, J. J., Kinkel, W. R., and Jusko, W. J. (1977): Intoxication caused by interaction of chloramphenicol and phenytoin. *J.A.M.A.,* 237:2630–2631.

54. Rosenberg, I. H., Godwin, H. A., Streiff, R. R., and Castle, W. B. (1968): Impairment of intestinal deconjugation of dietary folate. A possible explanation of megaloblastic anaemia associated with phenytoin therapy. *Lancet,* 2:530–532.

55. Ryan, G. M. S., and Forshaw, J. W. B. (1955):

Megaloblastic anaemia due to phenytoin sodium. *Br. Med. J.,* 2:242–243.

56. Saltzstein, S. L., and Ackerman, L. V. (1959): Lymphadenopathy induced by anticonvulsant drugs and mimicking clinically and pathologically malignant lymphomas. *Cancer,* 12:164–182.

57. Siegal, S., and Berkowitz, J. (1961): Diphenylhydantoin (Dilantin) hypersensitivity with infectious mononucleosis-like syndrome and jaundice. *J. Allergy,* 32:447–451.

58. Slavin, R. G., and Broun, G. O., Jr. (1961): Agranulocytosis after diphenylhydantoin and chlorothiazide therapy. A case report and discussion of the evidence for the primary role of diphenylhydantoin. *Arch. Intern. Med.,* 108:940–944.

59. Sparberg, M. (1963): Diagnostically confusing complications of diphenylhydantoin therapy. A review. *Ann. Intern. Med.,* 59:914–930.

60. Taguchi, H., Laundy, M., Reid, C., Reynolds, E. H., and Chanarin, I. (1977): The effect of anticonvulsant drugs on thymidine and deoxyribosenucleic acid synthesis by human marrow cells. *Br. J. Haematol.,* 36:181–187.

61. Targan, S. R., Chassin, M. R. G., and Guze, L. B. (1975): Dilantin-induced disseminated intravascular coagulation with purpura fulminans. A case report. *Ann. Intern. Med.,* 83:227–230.

62. Todd, J., and Dewhurst, K. (1964): Macrocytosis and megaloblastic anaemia due to anticonvulsant drugs. *Br. J. Clin. Pract.,* 18:479–480.

63. Turner, P. (1960): Granulocytopenia after treatment with phenytoin sodium. *Br. Med. J.,* 1:1790.

64. Ungar, B., and Cowling, D. C. (1960): Megaloblastic anaemia associated with anticonvulsant drug therapy. *Med. J. Aust.,* 2:461–462.

65. Weber, T. H., Knuutila, S., Tammisto, P., and Tontti, K. (1977): Long-term use of phenytoin: Effects on whole blood and red cell folate and haematological parameters. *Scand. J. Haematol.,* 18:81–85.

66. Witkind, E., and Waid, M. E. (1951): Aplasia of bone marrow during Mesantoin therapy. Report of a fatal case. *J.A.M.A.,* 147:757–759.

67. Yunis, A. A., Arimura, G. K., Lutcher, C. L., Blasquez, J., and Halloran, M. (1967): Biochemical lesion in Dilantin-induced erythroid aplasia. *Blood,* 30:587–600.

68. Zidar, B. L., Mendelow, H., Winkelstein, A., and Shadduck, R. K. (1975): Diphenylhydantoin-induced serum sickness with fibrin-platelet thrombi in lymph node microvasculature. *Am. J. Med.,* 58:704–708.

Antiepileptic Drugs, edited by D. M. Woodbury,
J. K Penry, and C. E. Pippenger. Raven Press,
New York © 1982.

19

Phenytoin

Mechanisms of Action

Dixon M. Woodbury

The preceding chapters have discussed the absorption, distribution, biotransformation, and excretion of phenytoin (PHT) and also the toxicity of this drug. The purposes of this chapter are to discuss the known information about the mechanisms of action of PHT and to present a scheme of its overall mechanism in preventing seizures in experimental animals and man.

Because PHT exerts its effects on many different systems, it is difficult to formulate a single mechanism of action. This chapter will propose several different mechanisms that may explain the diverse effects of this drug. This will involve correlation of data on phylogenetic and ontogenetic effects of PHT, effects on vertebrate and invertebrate membranes, synapses, and receptors, and effects on nonexcitable tissues such as the epithelial cells of toad bladder, gut, choroid plexus, and glia. These effects of PHT will also be correlated with its biochemical effects, and an attempt will be made to identify the mechanisms of its anticonvulsant and, possibly, its toxic actions.

Before discussing the possible mechanisms of action of PHT, it is pertinent to summarize briefly its neurophysiological effects that relate to its anticonvulsant activity. Experimental work on peripheral nerves and neurons has demonstrated that PHT elevates membrane potential, raises threshold, reduces conduction velocity and spike amplitude, and reduces or abolishes repetitive firing. Bursting activity is also suppressed. Posttetanic potentiation in synaptic transmission is strongly inhibited by PHT. It also relaxes smooth muscle *in vitro* and prevents cardiac arrhythmias, particularly those induced by ouabain. In experimental animals, PHT limits the development of maximal seizure activity and, probably related to this, reduces the spread of the seizure process from an active focus. Both of these effects are related to its clinical usefulness in the therapy of generalized tonic–clonic seizures (grand mal). Phenytoin does not elevate the threshold for seizures induced by electric stimulation of the brain or by injection of such convulsant drugs as strychnine, picrotoxin, or pentylenetetrazol. In fact, it potentiates the effects of these convulsants. It does, however, restore excitability to normal when it has been abnormally increased by such procedures as hyponatremia or agents such as cortisone or thyroxine. It also elevates the threshold of cerebral cortex, hippocampus, and amygdala, but not of other subcortical areas (see summaries in 3,16,89,92–95).

From the data available, it appears that the mechanism of PHT can be explained by actions on the basic properties of membranes, synapses, and metabolic processes. Therefore, it appears likely that no single action of the drug

269

can explain all of its manifold effects, although it is possible that one basic action on membranes may explain all its effects. Reviews of the mechanisms of action of PHT can be found in a number of articles (3,13,14,16,18,20,25, 66,89,91,93–95).

The first property to consider is the effects of PHT on membranes. This includes two aspects: effects on ion channels (cation—Na^+, Ca^{2+}; and anion—Cl^-); and effects on active transport processes. In each situation, effects on the plasma membrane and subcellular membranes will be distinguished where possible. A scheme of the mechanisms of action of PHT is shown in Fig. 1.

EFFECTS ON SODIUM INFLUX

The effects of PHT on sodium influx in excitable tissues in both invertebrate and vertebrate nerve fibers have been described by a number of investigators. In peripheral nerve, PHT has, nonspecifically, been considered to be a membrane "stabilizer" because it prevents or interrupts repetitive electrical activity induced by various means (9,36,39,55,82,89). Phenytoin has a marked effect on the nerve membrane to decrease sodium influx by blocking sodium channels in a manner similar to that of tetrodotoxin. It does this by decreasing the early, transient sodium currents in a reversible manner (16,33,46,61–63,65,79,80). Pincus and colleagues (62,63,65), in earlier studies, found the PHT decreased sodium influx in stimulated lobster nerves. Johnston and Ayala (33; also see 3) also observed that PHT decreased sodium influx. They noted that this drug decreased the bursting pacemaker activity in *Aplysia* neurons and found that the results were consistent with its proposed action on the downhill flux of sodium ions, since the regenerative inward sodium current (negative resistance) was abolished by this drug. This action of PHT occurred whether the bursting activity was natural to the cell or induced by a convulsant such as pentylenetetrazol.

Schwartz and Vogel (73) postulated in current- and voltage-clamped myelinated nerves that the excitability-reducing effect of PHT was the result of potential-dependent blockage of the sodium channel by the PHT molecule. The reduction of the sodium current appeared to result from a fast one-to-one reaction of the PHT molecule with a pH-dependent and potential-dependent sodium channel. They postulated that both PHT and procaine bind to sites in the sodium channel that are different from tetrodotoxin and saxitoxin. They also observed that PHT had a stronger effect at pH 7 than at pH 9 and suggested that the molecule is more effective in its neutral, more permeant form. As a result of this action, PHT decreases the action potential amplitude, increases the threshold, and thereby reduces the conduction velocity. There was also an indication that the drug shifted the inactivation (K^+ current) curve in the hyperpolarizing direction, an indication of an increase in potassium permeability.

In squid axons, De Weer (16) and Perry et al. (61) noted that PHT had no effect on sodium efflux but decreased sodium influx by a mechanism similar to that of tetrodotoxin. They concluded that PHT, like tetrodotoxin, blocks both resting and excitable sodium channels as well as those held open by veratridine. They did not find an increase in K^+ permeability. These observations were also confirmed for skeletal muscle by Dwyer (17) who concluded that, since PHT has a chemical structure similar to that of N-ethylmaleimide, it is likely that its effects on the sodium channels, like those of N-ethylmaleimide, are related to its binding to the cell membrane. Phenytoin blocked both open and inactivated channels. An effect of PHT on the cell membrane was also demonstrated by Roses et al. (71) who showed that it normalized the increased fluidity and decreased polarity present in erythrocytes taken from patients with myotonia. This is a change that accounts for stabilization of the membrane by PHT.

Thus, it is evident from these studies that PHT has a marked effect on the membrane to decrease sodium influx by blocking sodium channels in a manner similar to that of local anesthetics or tetrodotoxin. This action of PHT can explain many of its effects on membrane properties and its neurophysiological effects as well as some of its clinical effects.

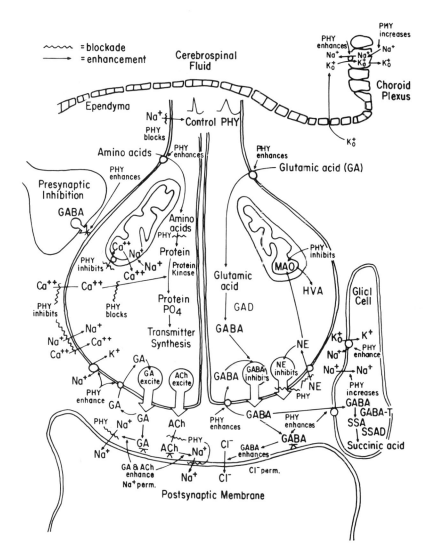

FIG. 1. Proposed mechanisms of action of phenytoin (PHY; note that PHT is used in text) on the central nervous system. Two synapses are shown that represent idealized excitatory (for both glutamic acid and acetylcholine) and inhibitory (for both GABA and norepinephrine) junctions. A presynaptic junction that is GABA mediated is shown with the excitatory synapses. An inhibitory effect of phenytoin is shown by a *wavy line,* and an enhancement by a *straight line*. Active transport systems are shown by a *circle* with an *arrow* pointing toward the direction of transport across the cell membrane. The sequence showing that PHY blocks the Ca^{2+}-dependent phosphorylation of proteins DPH-L and DPH-M that involves protein kinase has been shown by De Lorenzo (see 14) to involve calmodulin and is not shown in this figure. Phenytoin appears to act by preventing the interaction of Ca^{2+} with calmodulin. See text for further discussion.

EFFECTS ON CALCIUM FLUXES

Phenytoin has marked effects on calcium influx across cellular and subcellular membranes. This drug inhibits calcium influx, an action that is either secondary to the decrease in passive sodium influx or due to a direct effect on calcium transport processes (6,7,47). Thus, PHT decreases calcium influx across plasma membranes, particularly in synaptosomes, and also blocks the intracellular uptake of calcium by mitochondria, as discussed below, and microsomes. Sohn and Ferrendelli (74,75) showed that PHT inhibited the uptake of calcium by isolated presynaptic endings prepared from cerebral cortex. This effect has also been noted for lobster walking nerves by Pincus and colleagues (32,64), an effect similar to that of the local anesthetic, procaine.

Thus, PHT blocks sodium channels and limits membrane permeability to calcium. The effect on calcium movements across membranes explains a number of its actions. Thus, PHT inhibits insulin release from pancreatic islet cells, vasopressin and oxytocin release from the neurohypophysis, thyrotropin release from the adenohypophysis, an effect counteracted by strophanthin, adrenocorticotropin release from the adenohypophysis, glucagon release from the isolated perfused pancreas, calcium-, glucagon-, and pentagastrin-stimulated release of calcitonin, catecholamine (norepinephrine) secretion by the adrenal medulla, salivary secretion and release of amylase, and neurotransmitter release (11, 21, 23, 29, 30, 38, 40, 42–44, 51–53, 59, 60, 69, 81,85,90). All these effects are due to a general mechanism of PHT decreasing intracellular calcium by limiting its movement across cell membranes.

In higher doses, PHT is excitatory, an effect presumably due to increased transmitter release as a result of increased intracellular calcium due to inhibition of uptake of calcium by mitochondria, as discussed below. Uptake into microsomes is also inhibited by PHT. The main question with regard to the effects of PHT on calcium influx is whether the decrease is due to a primary action to block calcium channels or is secondary to the decreased passive influx of sodium produced by this drug, as discussed above. The inhibition of passive sodium influx will result in a steepened sodium electrochemical gradient across the cell membrane. Since the sodium gradient is the energy source for cellular uptake of many organic molecules, including transmitters, and is also a major regulator of intracellular calcium levels (6,7,47), most of the effects on calcium produced by PHT can be attributed to inhibition of passive sodium influx. A decrease in sodium influx may limit presyn-

aptic calcium accumulation as a result of limitation of calcium influx through the sodium channel. Since intracellular calcium affects transmitter release, and sodium gradients energize transmitter reuptake, many complex effects of the PHT on transmitter movements should be anticipated, and this has been demonstrated for many systems including the neuromuscular junction as described by Pincus and colleagues (66). However, another possibility is an effect of PHT directly on the cell membrane to block calcium channels. Phenytoin does inhibit the active uptake of calcium by mitochondria, but this only occurs in higher doses and probably accounts for its excitatory effects when toxic levels of the drug are achieved in the plasma. This process is not mediated by an effect on sodium influx. Furthermore, calcium efflux from mitochondria, which is regulated by exchange of cytosolic sodium concentration with intramitochondrial calcium (see 93), is not influenced by PHT. It is obvious that further work in this area to define the effects of calcium at the subcellular molecular levels is highly indicated.

EFFECTS ON ACTIVE SODIUM–POTASSIUM TRANSPORT

A third action of PHT on membranes is exerted mainly on epithelial cells such as those in the choroid plexus, glia, and secretory glands, and also on synaptic membranes, secondary to an influence on calcium binding to the membrane. This is an effect of PHT to increase the permeability of the mucosal cell membrane to sodium and also to stimulate active $Na^+–K^+$ transport. In this case, PHT increases permeability of the mucosal cell membrane to sodium which results in an increase in intracellular sodium, and this leads to an increase in the activity of the sodium pump. This may be due to activation of Na^+, K^+-ATPase or to an increase in its synthesis. The effect has been best demonstrated in frog skin and toad bladder membranes by us (86,87) and others (10,15,68). The increase in sodium permeability is different from that produced by vasopressin and results in an increase in intracellular sodium which is then followed by a decrease in cell sodium through direct stimulation of the sodium–potassium pump. This occurs in the choroid plexus and results in an increase in sodium and a decrease in potassium concentrations in cerebrospinal fluid and an increase in potassium and a decrease in sodium concentrations in glial cells. Both of these effects decrease extracellular potassium and thereby limit its rise induced by excessive neural activity as occurs in seizures. This is particularly prominent with chronic administration of the drug.

To summarize its ionic effects, PHT has three characteristic actions on cell membranes. The first is a well-demonstrated ability to inhibit sodium influx by blocking sodium channels. The second, which may be secondary to the decrease in passive sodium influx or due to a direct effect on calcium transport processes, is a PHT-induced inhibition of calcium influx across cellular and subcellular membranes. The third action, which has been demonstrated mainly on epithelial cells such as glia, choroid plexus, liver cells, gastrointestinal mucosal cells, pancreatic islet cells, salivary gland cells, and probably on other epithelial cells as well, appears to be an effect of PHT to increase permeability of the basal cell membrane to sodium and also to stimulate active sodium–potassium transport across the cell. The latter effect occurs both as a result of the increased intracellular sodium secondary to the increased permeability on the mucosal side membrane to sodium and as a direct action on the sodium pump through either activation of Na^+, K^+-ATPase or an increase in its synthesis. An effect on sodium–potassium transport into synaptosomes, particularly when active Na^+–K^+ transport is compromised, has also been demonstrated (13).

These three basic actions of PHT can explain most of the neurophysiological and toxic effects of this drug when it is used in epileptic patients. The basic effect of PHT thus appears to be directly on the plasma membrane. Limited data available suggest an influence of PHT on the fluidity of the membrane which, in the case of excitable tissues, appears to result in blocking

of sodium channels, possibly by PHT binding to the plasma membrane, or in the case of epithelial tissues, in opening up sodium channels in a manner different from that of vasopressin and thereby allowing increased penetration of sodium into the cell. The mechanisms of these two effects on the cell membrane in the two different types of tissues need further investigation. Also, how PHT stimulates the sodium–potassium pump is unknown at the present time and may be related to an effect on protein synthesis, as will now be discussed.

Under conditions in which PHT stimulates sodium–potassium transport in synaptosomes, it has also been shown to stimulate protein synthesis (13), but when it inhibits sodium transport, it also inhibits protein synthesis (1,13). However, in *in vivo* situations, PHT, even at therapeutic concentrations, inhibits protein synthesis in the brain (35). This inhibition of protein synthesis, demonstrated by others as well, in both adult and immature animals (78,96,98) can explain a number of the effects of PHT on the nervous system. Its most likely effect, however, is on transmitter release from synaptic endings, as postulated by De Lorenzo and colleagues (see 14). They showed that PHT inhibits a calcium-dependent phosphorylation of specific rat and human brain proteins, designated proteins DPH-L and DPH-M. As a result of these studies, they hypothesized that the antagonistic actions of calcium and PHT on the level of phosphorylation of these specific brain proteins may be the underlying basic mechanism mediating the opposing effects of calcium and PHT on the release of neurotransmitter from the presynaptic nerve terminals. Moreover, they demonstrated that calcium and PHT have antagonistic actions on the net level of endogenous phosphorylation of specific rat brain proteins. These specific phosphoproteins were shown to be present in synaptosomal preparations. Evidence was presented for the localization of these phosphoproteins within the vesicles of the presynaptic nerve terminals.

Thus, the data supported their hypothesis that PHT acts by antagonizing the effects of calcium which is essential for phosphorylation of synaptosomal proteins involved in neurotransmitter synthesis. This decreases neurotransmitter production and thereby decreases its release. Thus, the synthesis of those brain proteins that are involved in neurotransmitter synthesis appears to be specifically inhibited by PHT. This group also demonstrated that calmodulin is involved in the regulation of calcium-dependent phosphorylation of these proteins and neurotransmitter release and that PHT may act by preventing this interaction (14).

EFFECTS ON NEUROTRANSMITTERS

The question then arises, what are the effects of PHT on transmitter dynamics and central nervous system synapses? The effects of PHT on neurotransmitters are summarized in Fig. 1 (see 93 for summary). It is evident from this figure that multiple effects on transmitters are present with PHT. For example, PHT decreases norepinephrine uptake and inhibits its secretion, a process that is calcium dependent. Its metabolism by monoamine oxidase may also be inhibited. Thus, the net accumulation of norepinephrine at the receptor depends on a number of factors that include the dose, the time after administration, and the pathological state of the synapses. Decreased secretion is related to inhibition of calcium influx into the presynaptic endings; inhibition of reuptake to decreased sodium influx; and the decreased rate of metabolism to the inhibition of monoamine oxidase by PHT. In addition, since PHT increases the sodium gradient across the cells, this would result in an increase in amino acid uptake which is a sodium-dependent process. Therefore the uptake of any neurotransmitters that are amino acids, such as GABA and glutamic acid, would be increased by PHT. This also appears to be the case as depicted in Fig. 1. In addition, a GABA-like effect of PHT is exerted on the postsynaptic and presynaptic membranes to enhance postsynaptic and presynaptic inhibition. Thus, in invertebrate synapses Ayala et al. (3,5) and Deisz and Lux (12) found that PHT markedly prolonged the GABA-mediated, chloride-dependent IPSP of the crayfish stretch receptor.

Iontophoretic application of GABA produced the same effect as PHT. This drug also prolonged recurrent inhibition, a GABA-mediated process in pyramidal tract cells, as described by Raabe and Ayala (67).

The results of Strejckova and Mares (77) are compatible with an effect of PHT on excitatory as well as inhibitory activity. They noted that in a cortical epileptogenic focus induced in the rat by local application of penicillin, PHT suppressed the excitatory phase of both excitatory and inhibitory units and lengthened the duration of the inhibitory phase and increased the percentage of units in the focus that were inhibitory. These data correlate with the data just discussed that PHT decreases the pacemaker activity of bursting cells in *Aplysia* (2–5,12) and of epileptogenic foci in various animals (54; see 3,16), and that this drug prolongs recurrent inhibition and postsynaptic inhibition. In addition, PHT blocks the effect of acetylcholine to increase sodium permeability of the postsynaptic membrane (Fig. 1). The effects of PHT on neurotransmitter function have been reviewed by Woodbury (89,93).

METABOLIC EFFECTS AND TISSUE BINDING

Another aspect of the mechanisms of action of PHT is its effects on subcellular fractions of cells and on molecular processes. Phenytoin is not a general depressant of the nervous system, and, unlike large doses of phenobarbital and trimethadione, it does not depress the respiration of cerebral tissues. In patients with epilepsy, during the interseizure period, brain respiration is not affected by either PHT or phenobarbital in anticonvulsant doses. Also, *in vitro,* respiration of isolated cerebral tissues in media containing a variety of oxidizable substrates (pyruvate, lactate, or glucose) is unaffected by 10^{-4} M to 10^{-3} M PHT.

These and other data reviewed by Woodbury (89) indicate that PHT does not act by an effect on energy metabolism in the brain. However, in isolated brain mitochondria, PHT (10^{-4} M) inhibits respiration when glutamate–malate is used as a substrate but not when succinate is used. This reduction results in an inhibition of calcium uptake which is coupled to the electron transport respiratory system (M. Lopes-Cardozo, D. M. Woodbury, and R. W. Albers, *unpublished observations*).

Its action, therefore, appears to be restricted to more selective effects on the systems discussed above, namely, movements of ions such as sodium and calcium across the cell membrane. Since PHT is about 90% bound to brain and other tissues (22,24,57), it is pertinent to summarize the role of tissue binding in the possible anticonvulsant action of the drug. As discussed above and by others, it is evident that PHT has a marked membrane-stabilizing effect that is probably related to its anticonvulsant activity. This effect appears to result from a complex interaction between the drug and several membrane components. Protein binding is known to occur and has been shown to be relatively nonspecific in that it is independent of drug concentration, temperature, or tissue origin, and the amount bound is directly proportional to the protein concentration (see 25).

Goldberg and Todoroff (24–27) have demonstrated that PHT, in addition to protein binding, interacts with brain lipids and, particularly, that only phospholipids are capable of this interaction, an effect that involves calcium. The binding of PHT to phospholipids was found to be related to fatty acid composition. Dipalmitoyl and dioleoyl lecithins, the most abundant lecithins in the brain, showed the greatest binding activity (27). In contrast to PHT, phenobarbital showed little interaction with phospholipids. Goldberg (24) also showed that phospholipid binding of $^{45}Ca^{2+}$ could be increased up to five times by the addition of 1×10^{-4} PHT. This calcium phospholipid binding interaction may be an important factor in the stabilizing action of PHT on membranes. These data, together with other observations reviewed by Woodbury (93), indicate that PHT interaction with membrane proteins and phospholipids can result in marked changes in sodium–potassium and calcium transport across membranes. In addition, the calcium–phospho-

lipid–PHT interaction can affect the activity of transport enzymes such as Na^+, K^+-ATPase in the membranes and thereby influence active sodium transport across cell membranes. The nature of this interaction has not yet been elucidated.

Studies of the distribution in subcellular fractions (31,37,56,88,97) of PHT indicate that it binds avidly to the microsomal fraction of brain homogenates. Since the microsomal PHT is bound to the neuronal plasma membrane, it could be responsible for the specific anticonvulsant action of this drug. A review of the subcellular distribution and binding of PHT is found in the article by Woodbury (93). Jones and Woodbury (35) have shown that PHT inhibits protein synthesis. Whether this effect on protein synthesis is mediated through an effect of PHT on amino acid metabolism or on binding to nucleic acids or other fractions has not been settled as yet. *In vitro* experiments generally have tended to show no effect of PHT on protein synthesis or nucleic acid metabolism and binding (8,76). However, in the *in vivo* situation, PHT does inhibit protein synthesis (35,78,96,98). *In vivo*, investigators have found that protein synthesis in both adult and immature rats was inhibited by therapeutic levels of PHT, as measured by incorporation of radioactive leucine into the brain.

Thus, it appears that at least *in vivo*, PHT does inhibit protein synthesis, an effect not related to the uptake of amino acids by the brain. Also, the studies of Jones and Kemp (34) indicate that PHT interacts by strong hydrogen binding with 9-ethyladenine to a higher extent than do other related hydantoins and barbiturates. This suggests that in the cell PHT may well interact with nucleic acids.

Other workers have tested the effects of PHT on nonneural tissues and have shown that it does alter nucleic acid metabolism. For example, MacKinney and Vyas (48,49) demonstrated that PHT inhibits nucleic acid synthesis in cultured human lymphocytes. A relatively high degree of association between adenine and PHT may be responsible for the inhibition of protein synthesis, as already noted above, by interfering with the normal adenine–uracil or adenine–thymine interactions. These data suggest, as reviewed by Woodbury (93), that PHT does have an effect on nucleic acid metabolism and that it does interact with nucleic acids, but much further work is needed to define this interaction and its effect on protein synthesis in the nervous system.

Another effect of PHT on binding in tissues that may partly explain its inhibition of transmitter release and/or secretion of hormones as described above, is its ability to inhibit mitosis of cultured human lymphocytes. MacKinney et al. (50) found that PHT inhibited microtubular polymerization, an indication of a colchicine-like action of the drug. The major metabolite of PHT, HPPH, also inhibited microtubular polymerization, as indicated by metaphase accumulation in these lymphocytes. However HPPH, unlike its parent PHT, enhanced metaphase accumulation without significantly causing inhibition of DNA or protein synthesis. Since colchicine inhibits secretory functions that utilize the microtubular system, such as the release of neurotransmitters, insulin, and other hormones, this colchicine-like effect of PHT may contribute significantly to its inhibitory effects on secretion of norepinephrine and other neurotransmitters and of insulin, calcitonin, salivary amylase, vasopressin, and oxytocin, as described above. However, the relative contribution of this effect, compared with the effects on sodium flux and intracellular calcium, remains to be determined.

Another important aspect of the action of PHT is its effects on cyclic nucleotide regulation in brain, as discussed by Ferrendelli and Kinscherf (19,20; see 18 for summary). It has been established that agents such as veratridine, ouabain, glutamate, and high concentrations of K^+ cause depolarization of excitable cells and markedly elevate levels of adenosine $3':5'$-monophosphate (cyclic AMP) and guanosine $3':5'$-monophosphate (cyclic GMP) in brain tissues *in vitro*. Most of the data indicate that the effects of these depolarizing agents on cyclic AMP and cyclic GMP are a result of the cellular depolarization and not to a direct action on cyclic nucleotide syntheses or degradation. The cellular depolarization enhances Ca^{2+} influx into intracellular fluid, and this increased calcium concentration leads to accumulation of cyclic GMP, probably as a result of activation of guanylate cyclase by Ca^{2+}. Depolarization also increases Ca^{2+}-dependent neurotransmitter release, which in turn activates adenylate cyclases and thereby increases cyclic AMP levels in brain.

Ferrendelli and Kinscherf (20) have demonstrated that PHT, carbamazepine, phenobarbital, primidone, aromatic substituted succinimides, and very high concentrations of clonazepam, agents that block MES seizures and are effective in generalized tonic–clonic seizures, but not ethosuximide, valproic acid, and trimethadione, which block pentylenetetrazol-induced seizures and are effective in absence seizures, inhibit both cyclic AMP and cyclic GMP accumulation produced by veratridine. In addition, PHT selectively inhibits cyclic AMP and cyclic GMP elevations induced by ouabain in a noncompetitive manner. Both veratridine and ouabain cause cellular depolarization by altering Na^+ movements across cell membranes. Veratridine prevents closure of sodium channels, thereby increasing sodium permeability and cell Na^+, and ouabain increases cell Na^+ by inhibiting Na^+, K^+-ATPase and thereby blocks sodium pumping. Cell depolarization can also be induced by glutamate and high concentrations of K^+, but unlike veratridine and ouabain, the depolarization induced by these agents is not blocked by PHT.

Since the cellular depolarization produced by all four of these agents has qualitatively similar effects on Ca^{2+} conductance, neurotransmitter release, cyclic nucleotide regulation, etc., the selective inhibition by PHT of cyclic AMP and cyclic GMP elevations induced by ouabain and veratridine suggests that this anticonvulsant interferes with their depolarizing action. It also appears likely that PHT inhibits veratridine- and ouabain-induced elevation of cyclic AMP and cyclic GMP levels in brain by blocking Na^+ channels. This possibility is supported by the observation that tetrodoxin, which is a known specific blocker of Na^+ channels, has an effect identical to that of PHT on regulation of cyclic nucleotides (19). Whether these effects of PHT on cyclic AMP and/or cyclic GMP regulation are related to its anticonvulsant action awaits further research.

EFFECTS ON EXCITATORY AND INHIBITORY PROCESSES

Unlike phenobarbital and other anticonvulsant drugs that depress the central nervous system, PHT has excitatory effects at high doses. Thus, it has a biphasic effect on the nervous system; that is, it increases excitability and also has an anticonvulsant effect. The question is: how does it exert its effects on both these systems? In neonatal animals, PHT has excitatory effects, and its anticonvulsant effects are exerted in rats only after the 12th day, a time when inhibitory systems in the cerebellum and other parts of the nervous system have developed, and the animal has aquired the ability to have tonic–clonic seizures rather than the purely clonic seizures seen at a younger age (84). Phenytoin also has excitatory effects in high doses, as is evident both from experiments in animals and observations in patients receiving toxic doses of the drug (28,41,45,58, 72,83). In animals, high doses produce irritability, ataxia, and convulsions that are characterized by opisthotonic posturing.

A clinical correlation of the data in animals was reported by Schreiner (72) who described accidental poisoning of a 2-year-old-boy by ingestion of an undetermined number of 100-mg PHT tablets. He developed frequent episodes of opisthotonus and was in a semistuporous state. After hemodialysis, the seizures ceased. Others (45,70,83) also have described PHT-activated seizures. As in the initial report, they were characterized by opisthotonic posturing or generalized tonic–clonic (grand mal) convulsions or both.

Other evidence that PHT stimulates the nervous system is derived from experiments in animals in which chemically induced seizures are produced; PHT enhances seizure activity in animals given pentylenetetrazol, picrotoxin, strychnine, and in animals undergoing CO_2 withdrawal seizures. In such animals, a combination of the chemical convulsant and PHT results in a status epilepticus-like state. The mechanisms involved in these excitatory effects of PHT have been described by Woodbury (93) and need not be detailed here. However, the excitatory effects in animals and the enhancement of the convulsions induced by chemical convulsants indicate that PHT has a general stimulatory effect on both excitatory and inhibitory pathways in the nervous system. In neonatal animals, excitatory pathways appear to predominate because all of the inhibitory ones have not yet developed; thus, the excitatory effects of PHT at this age period appear to be due to an enhanced release of excitatory transmitters such as acetylcholine or glutamic acid. Anticonvulsant effects of PHT then appear at the time when the inhibitory systems have matured and are thus stimulated by PHT. Since inhibition predominates over excitation in this period and later, the stimulatory effect of PHT on the inhibitory systems would result in an anticonvulsant effect. The stimulatory effects on the nervous system may be due to PHT-induced blockade of calcium uptake into mitochondria, a process that increases cytosolic calcium ion concentration and thereby increases transmitter release in both excitatory and inhibitory synapses. The net result is either excitation if excitatory pathways predominate over inhibitory ones or inhibition (anticonvulsant effect) if inhibitory pathways predominate over excitatory pathways.

SUMMARY

The major action of PHT is on the movements of sodium and calcium, by either passive or active transport mechanisms, across cellular or subcellular membranes. In excitable tissues, the major effect appears to be the decrease in sodium influx, which causes a decrease in intracellular sodium and calcium, the net effect of which is blockade of transmitter release. However, in some synapses and at high doses, PHT may block intracellular uptake of calcium by subcellular particles and thereby increase calcium concentration in the cytosol, an effect that could cause an increase in transmitter release and an increase in secretion from endocrine and exocrine glands.

Another effect of PHT that may also be exerted by its influence on phospholipid–calcium interactions in the cell membrane is on the active transport of sodium and potassium across synaptic membranes, particularly when the sodium–potassium transport system is compromised as it is in an epileptogenic focus. In this case, PHT appears to stimulate active sodium–potassium transport, a process that also, like the decrease in sodium influx, increases the sodium gradient across the cell membrane and decreases calcium influx and thereby reduces the release of transmitter from the nerve ending; it also affects the cell membranes and the active reuptake of neurotransmitters.

In nonexcitable tissues, PHT appears to act mainly on active transport of sodium. The main tissues involved are the epithelial cells of the intestinal mucosa, the choroid plexus, possibly glial cells, the salivary glands, and other related epithelial cells. In these cells, PHT increases permeability of the basal membrane to sodium, a process that increases intracellular sodium which then stimulates the sodium–potassium pump in the opposite membrane. In the case of the choroid plexus, for example, this results in a lowering of CSF potassium and constitutes one mechanism whereby the concentration of extracellular potassium in the interstitial fluid of the brain is regulated. Phenytoin may also exert an effect on active sodium–potassium transport in glia, which are epithelial cells, and thereby provide another mechanism by which potassium concentration in the interstitial fluid of the brain is regulated. Thus, these basic effects of PHT on sodium and calcium flux and on active sodium transport across excitable tissue membranes and epithelial cells can explain most of the anticonvulsant, excitatory, and toxic effects of this remarkable agent.

ACKNOWLEDGMENTS

Supported by Program Project Grant Number 1 PO1-NS-15767 from the National Institute of Neurological and Communicative Disorders and Stroke, N.I.H. The author is a recipient of a Research Career Award (5-K6-NB-13,828), NINCDS, National Institutes of Health.

REFERENCES

1. Appel, S. H., Festoff, B. W., Autilio, L., and Escueta, A. V. (1969): Biochemical studies of synapses: III. Ionic activation of protein syntheses. *J. Biol. Chem.*, 244:3166–3172.
2. Ayala, G. F., and Johnston, D. (1977): The influences of phenytoin on the fundamental electrical properties of simple neuronal systems. *Epilepsia*, 18:299–307.
3. Ayala, G. F., and Johnston, D. (1980): Phenytoin: Electrophysiological studies in simple neuronal systems. *Adv. Neurol.*, 27:339–351.
4. Ayala, G. F., Johnston, D., Lin, S., and Dichter, H. N. (1977): The mechanism of action of diphenylhydantoin on invertebrate neurons: II. Effects on synaptic mechanisms. *Brain Res.*, 121:259–270.
5. Ayala, G. F., Lin, S., and Johnston, D. (1977): The mechanism of action of diphenylhydantoin on invertebrate neurons. I. Effects on basic membrane properties, *Brain Res.*, 121:245–258.
6. Baker, P. F., and Blaustein, M. P. (1968): Sodium-dependent uptake of calcium by crab nerve. *Biochim. Biophys. Acta*, 150:167–170.
7. Blaustein, M. P., and Wiesmann, W. P. (1970): The effect of sodium ions on calcium movements in isolated synaptic terminals. *Proc. Natl. Acad. Sci. U.S.A.*, 66:664–671.
8. Boykin, M. E., and Doctor, B. P. (1976): Studies on the binding of 5,5-diphenylhydantoin to nucleic acids *in vitro* and to rat brain subcellular fractions *in vitro* and *in vivo*. *J. Pharmacol. Exp. Ther.*, 196:469–477.
9. Carnay, L., and Grundfest, S. (1974): Excitable membrane stabilization by diphenylhydantoin and calcium. *Neuropharmacology*, 13:1097–1108.
10. Carroll, P. T., and Pratley, J. N. (1970): The effects of diphenylhydantoin on sodium transport in frog skin. *Comp. Gen. Pharmacol.*, 1:365.
11. Cohen, M. S., Bower, R. H., Fidler, S. M., Johnsonbaugh, R. E., and Sode, J. (1973): Inhibition of insulin release by diphenylhydantoin and diazoxide in a patient with benign insulinoma. *Lancet*, 1:40–41.
12. Deisz, R. A., and Lux, H. D. (1977): Diphenylhydantoin prolongs post-synaptic inhibition and iontophoretic GABA action in the crayfish stretch receptor. *Neurosci. Lett.*, 5:199–203.
13. Delgado-Escueta, A. V., and Horan, M. P. (1980): Phenytoin: Biochemical membrane studies. *Adv. Neurol.*, 27:377–398.
14. De Lorenzo, R. J. (1980): Phenytoin: Calcium- and calmodulin-dependent protein phosphorylation and neurotransmitter release. *Adv. Neurol.*, 27:399–414.
15. De Sousa, R. C., and Grosso, A. (1973): Effects of diphenylhydantoin on transport processes in frog skin (*Rana ridibunda*). *Experientia*, 29:1097–1098.
16. De Weer, P. (1980): Phenytoin: Blockage of resting sodium channels. *Adv. Neurol.*, 27:353–361.

17. Dwyer, T. M. (1978): Phenytoin depresses sodium currents in frog skeletal muscle. *Biophys. J.*, 21:41.

18. Ferrendelli, J. A. (1980): Phenytoin: Cyclic nucleotide regulation in the brain. *Adv. Neurol.*, 27:429–433.

19. Ferrendelli, J. A., and Kinscherf, D. A. (1978): Similar effects of phenytoin and tetrodotoxin on cyclic nucleotide regulation in depolarized brain tissue. *J. Pharmacol. Exp. Ther.*, 207:787–793.

20. Ferrendelli, J. A., and Kinscherf, D. A. (1979): Inhibitory effects of anti-convulsant drugs on cyclic nucleotide accumulation in brain. *Ann. Neurol.*, 5:533–538.

21. Fichman, M. P., Kleeman, C. R., and Bethune, J. E. (1970): Inhibition of antidiuretic hormone secretion by diphenylhydantoin. *Arch. Neurol.*, 22:45–53.

22. Firemark, H., Barlow, C. F., and Roth, L. J. (1963): The entry, accumulation, and binding of diphenylhydantoin-2-C^{14} in brain. Studies on adult, immature and hypercapnic cats. *Int. J. Neuropharmacol.*, 2:25–38.

23. Gerich, J. E., Charles, M. A., Levin, S. R., Forsham, P. H., and Grodsky, G. M. (1972): *In vitro* inhibition of pancreatic glucagon secretion by diphenylhydantoin. *J. Clin. Endocrinol. Metab.*, 35:823–824.

24. Goldberg, M. A. (1977): Phenytoin, phospholipids, and calcium. *Neurology (Minneap.)*, 27:827–833.

25. Goldberg, M. A. (1980): Phenytoin: Binding. *Adv. Neurol.*, 27:323–337.

26. Goldberg, M. A., and Todoroff, T. (1973): Binding of diphenylhydantoin to brain protein. *Biochem. Pharmacol.*, 22:2973–2980.

27. Goldberg, M. A., and Todoroff, T. (1976): Diphenylhydantoin binding to brain lipids and phospholipids. *Biochem. Pharmacol.*, 25:2079–2083.

28. Gruber, C. M., Haury, V. G., and Drake, M. E. (1940): The toxic actions of sodium diphenylhydantoinate (Dilantin) when injected intraperitoneally and intravenously in experimental animals. *J. Pharmacol. Exp. Ther.*, 68:433–436.

29. Gutman, Y., and Boonyaviroj, P. (1977): Mechanism of inhibition of catecholamine release from adrenal medulla by diphenylhydantoin and by low concentrations of ouabain (10^{-10} M). *Naunyn Schmiedebergs Arch. Pharmacol.*, 296:293–296.

30. Guzek, J. W., Russell, J. T., and Thorn, N. A. (1974): Inhibition by diphenylhydantoin of vasopressin release from isolated rat neurohypophyses. *Acta Pharmacol. Toxicol. (Kbh.)*, 34:14.

31. Hadfield, M. G., and Bosworth, J. E. (1974): *In vitro* binding of [4-^{14}C] diphenylhydantoin to rat brain microsomes. *Brain Res.*, 71:183–186.

32. Hasbani, M., Pincus, J. H., and Lee, S. H. (1974): Diphenylhydantoin and calcium movement in lobster nerves. *Arch. Neurol.*, 31:250–254.

33. Johnston, D., and Ayala, G. F. (1975): The action of a common anticonvulsant on bursting pacemaker cells in Aplysia. *Science*, 189:1009–1011.

34. Jones, G. L., and Kemp, J. W. (1974): Characteristics of the hydrogen bonding interactions of substituted hydantoins with 9-ethyladenine. *Mol. Pharmacol.*, 10:48–56.

35. Jones, G. L., and Woodbury, D. M. (1976): Effects of diphenylhydantoin and phenobarbital on protein metabolism in the rat cerebral cortex. *Biochem. Pharmacol.* 25:53–61.

36. Julien, R. M., and Halpern, L. M. (1970): Stabilization of excitable membrane by chronic administration of diphenylhydantoin. *J. Pharmacol. Exp. Ther.*, 175:206–212.

37. Kemp, J. W., and Woodbury, D. M. (1971): Subcellular distribution of 4-^{14}C-diphenylhydantoin in rat brain. *J. Pharmacol. Exp. Ther.*, 177:342–349.

38. Kizer, J. S., Cordon, M. V., Brendel, K., and Bressler, R. (1970): The *in vitro* inhibition of insulin secretion by diphenylhydantoin. *J. Clin. Invest.*, 49:1942–1948.

39. Korey, S. R. (1951): Effect of Dilantin and Mesantoin on the giant axon of the squid. *Proc. Soc. Exp. Biol. Med.*, 76:297–299.

40. Krieger, D. T. (1962): Effect of diphenylhydantoin on pituitary–adrenal interrelations. *J. Clin. Endocrinol. Metab.*, 22:490–493.

41. Lascelles, P. T., Kocen, R. S., and Reynolds, E. H. (1970): The distribution of plasma phenytoin levels in epileptic patients. *J. Neurol. Neurosurg. Psychiatry*, 33:501–505.

42. Lee, W. Y., Grumer, H. A., Bronsky, D., and Waldstein, S. S. (1961): Acute water loading as a diagnostic test for the inappropriate ADH syndrome. *J. Lab. Clin. Med.*, 58:937.

43. Levin, S. R., Booker, J. Jr., Smith, D. F., and Grodsky, G. M. (1970): Inhibition of insulin secretion by diphenylhydantoin in the isolated perfused pancreas. *J. Clin. Endocrinol. Metab.*, 30:400–401.

44. Levin, S. R., Charles, M. A., O'Conner, M., and Grodsky, G. M. (1975): Use of diphenylhydantoin and diazoxide upon insulin secretory mechanisms. *Am. J. Physiol.*, 229:49–54.

45. Levy, L. L., and Fenichel, G. M. (1965): Diphenylhydantoin activated seizures. *Neurology (Minneap.)*, 15:716–722.

46. Lipicky, R. J., Gilbert, D. L., and Stillman, I. M. (1972): Diphenylhydantoin inhibition of sodium conductance in the squid giant axon. *Proc. Natl. Acad. Sci. U.S.A.*, 69:1758–1760.

47. Lowe, D. A., Richardson, B. P., Taylor, P., and Donatsch, P. (1976): Increasing intracellular sodium triggers calcium release from bound pools. *Nature*, 260:337–338.

48. MacKinney, A. A. Jr., and Vyas, R. (1972): Diphenylhydantoin-induced inhibition of nucleic acid synthesis in cultured human lymphocytes. *Proc. Soc. Exp. Biol. Med.*, 141:89–92.

49. MacKinney, A. A., and Vyas, R. (1973): The assay of diphenylhydantoin effects on growing human lymphocytes. *J. Pharmacol. Exp. Ther.*, 186:37–43.

50. MacKinney, A. A., Vyas, R., and Lee, S. S. (1975): The effect of parahydroxylation of diphenylhydantoin on metaphase accumulation. *Proc. Soc. Exp. Biol. Med.*, 149:371–375.

51. Malherbe, C., Burrill, K. C., Levin, S. R., Karam, J. H., and Forsham, P. H. (1972): Effect of diphenylhydantoin on insulin secretion in man. *N. Engl. J. Med.*, 286:339–342.

52. Mathews, E. K., and Sakamoto, Y. (1975): Pancreatic islet cells: Electrogenic and electrodiffusional

control of membrane potential. *J. Physiol. (Lond.),* 246:439–457.

53. Mittler, J. C., and Glick, S. M. (1972): Radioimmunoassayable oxytocin release from isolated neural lobes; responses to ions and drugs. In: *IV International Congress of Endocrinology, Washington, 1972. Excerpta Medica Abstracts of Communications,* No. 117, p. 46. Excerpta Medica, Amsterdam.

54. Musgrave, F. S., and Purpura, D. P. (1963): Effects of Dilantin on focal epileptogenic activity of cat neocortex. *Electroencephalogr. Clin. Neurophysiol.,* 15:923.

55. Neumann, R. S., and Frank, G. B. (1977): Effects of diphenylhydantoin and phenobarbital on voltage-clamped myelinated nerve. *Can. J. Physiol. Pharmacol.,* 55:42–47.

56. Nielsen, T., and Cotman, C. (1971): The binding of diphenylhydantoin to brain and subcellular fractions, *Eur. J. Pharmacol.,* 14:344–350.

57. Noach, E. L., Woodbury, D. M., and Goodman, L. S. (1958): Studies on the absorption, distribution, fate and excretion of 4-C^{14}-labeled diphenylhydantoin. *J. Pharmacol. Exp. Ther.,* 122:301–314.

58. Patel, H., and Crichton, J. V. (1968): The neurologic hazards of diphenylhydantoin in childhood. *J. Pediatr.,* 73:676–684.

59. Pento, J. T. (1976): Diphenylhydantoin inhibition of pentagastrin-stimulated calcitonin secretion in the pig. *Horm. Metab. Res.,* 8:399–401.

60. Pento, J. T., Glick, S. M., and Kagan, A. (1973): Diphenylhydantoin inhibition of calcitonin secretion induced by calcium and glucagon. *Endocrinology,* 92:330–333.

61. Perry, J. G., McKinney, L., and De Weer, P. (1978): The cellular mode of action of the antiepileptic drug 5,5-diphenylhydantoin. *Nature,* 272:271–273.

62. Pincus, J. H. (1972): Diphenylhydantoin and ion flux in lobster nerve. *Arch. Neurol.,* 26:4–10.

63. Pincus, J. H., Grove, I., Marino, B. B., and Glaser, G. H. (1970): Studies on the mechanisms of action of diphenylhydantoin. *Arch. Neurol.,* 22:566–577.

64. Pincus, J. H., and Lee, S. H. (1973): Diphenylhydantoin and calcium. Relation to norepinephrine release from brain slices. *Arch. Neurol.,* 29:239–244.

65. Pincus, J. H., and Rawson, M. D. (1969): Diphenylhydantoin and intracellular sodium concentration. *Neurology (Minneap.),* 19:419–422.

66. Pincus, J. H., Yaari, Y., and Argov, Z. (1980): Phenytoin: Electrophysiological effects at the neuromuscular junction. *Adv. Neurol.,* 27:363–376.

67. Raabe, W., and Ayala, G. F. (1976): Diphenylhydantoin increases cortical post-synaptic inhibition. *Brain Res.,* 105:597–601.

68. Riddle, T. G., Mandel, L. H., and Goldner, M. M. (1975): Dilantin–calcium interaction and active Na transport in frog skin. *Eur. J. Pharmacol.,* 33:189–192.

69. Rinne, U. K. (1966): Effect of diphenylhydantoin treatment on the release of corticotropin in epileptic patients. *Confin. Neurol.,* 27:431–440.

70. Roseman, E. (1961): Dilantin toxicity. A clinical and electroencephalographic study. *Neurology (Minneap.),* 11:912–921.

71. Roses, A. D., Butterfield, A., Appel, S. H., and Chestnut, D. R. (1975): Phenytoin and membrane fluidity in myotonic dystrophy. *Arch. Neurol.,* 33:535–538.

72. Schreiner, G. E. (1958): The role of hemodialysis (artificial kidney) in acute poisoning. *Arch. Intern. Med.,* 102:896–913.

73. Schwartz, J. R., and Vogel, W. (1977): Diphenylhydantoin: Excitability reducing action in single myelinated nerve fibers. *Eur. J. Pharmacol.,* 44:241–249.

74. Sohn, R. S., and Ferrendelli, J. A. (1973): Inhibition of Ca^{2+} transport into rat brain synaptosomes by diphenylhydantoin (DPH). *J. Pharmacol. Exp. Ther.,* 185:272–275.

75. Sohn, R. S., and Ferrendelli, J. A. (1976): Anticonvulsant drug mechanisms. Phenytoin, phenobarbital, and ethosuximide and calcium flux in isolated presynaptic endings. *Arch. Neurol.,* 33:626–629.

76. Steinberg, M. S., and Doctor, B. P. (1976): Studies on the effect of 5,5'-diphenylhydantoin on *in vitro* protein synthesis in rat brain. *J. Pharmacol. Exp. Ther.,* 198:648–654.

77. Strejckova, A., and Mares, P. (1981): Effects of diphenylhydantoin on unit activity in a cortical epileptogenic focus in the rat. *Exp. Neurol. (in press).*

78. Swaiman, K. L., and Stright, P. L. (1973): The effects of anticonvulsants on *in vitro* protein synthesis in immature brain. *Brain Res.,* 58:515–518.

79. Swanson, P. D., and Crane, P. O. (1970): Diphenylhydantoin and the cations and phosphates of electrically stimulated brain slices. *Neurology (Minneap.),* 20:1119–1123.

80. Swanson, P. D., and Crane, P. O. (1972): Diphenylhydantoin and movement of radioactive sodium into electrically stimulated cerebral slices. *Biochem. Pharmacol.,* 21:2899–2905.

81. Tokya, K. V., Janka, G. E., Janka, H. U., Forster, C., Butenandt, O., Brugmann, G., and Neiss, A. (1975): Effect of intravenous diphenylhydantoin on glucose tolerance and insulin response in children. *Neuropaediatrie,* 6:176–183.

82. Toman, J. E. P. (1952): Neuropharmacology of peripheral nerve. *Pharmacol. Rev.,* 4:168–218.

83. Troupin, A. S., and Ojemann, L. M. (1975): Paradoxical intoxication—A complication of anticonvulsant administration. *Epilepsia,* 16:753–758.

84. Vernadakis, A., and Woodbury, D. M. (1969): The developing animal as a model. *Epilepsia,* 10:163–178.

85. Watson, E. L., and Siegel, I. A. (1976): Diphenylhydantoin effects on salivary secretion and microsomal calcium accumulation and release. *Eur. J. Pharmacol.,* 37:207–211.

86. Watson, E. L., and Woodbury, D. M. (1972): Effects of diphenylhydantoin on active sodium transport in frog skin. *J. Pharmacol. Exp. Ther.,* 180:767–776.

87. Watson, E. L., and Woodbury, D. M. (1973): Effects of diphenylhydantoin on electrolyte transport in various tissues. In: *Chemical Modulation of Brain Function,* edited by H. C. Sabelli, pp. 187–188. Raven Press, New York.

88. Wilensky, A. J., and Lowden, J. A. (1972): Interaction of diphenylhydantoin-4-^{14}C with subcellular fractions of rat brain. *Can. J. Physiol. Pharmacol.,* 50:346–353.

89. Woodbury, D. M. (1969): Mechanisms of action of anticonvulsants. In: *Basic Mechanisms of the Epilepsies,* edited by H. H. Jasper, A. A. Ward, and A. Pope, pp. 647–681. Little, Brown, Boston.

90. Woodbury, D. M. (1969): Role of pharmacological factors in the evaluation of anticonvulsant drugs. *Epilepsia,* 10:121–143.

91. Woodbury, D. M. (1978): Metabolites and the mechanisms of action of antiepileptic drugs. In: *Advances in Epileptology, 1977: Psychology, Pharmacotherapy, and New Diagnostic Approaches,* edited by H. Meinardi and A. J. Rowan, pp. 134–150. Swets and Zeitlinger, Amsterdam.

92. Woodbury, D. M. (1980): Phenytoin: Introduction and history. *Adv. Neurol.,* 27:305–313.

93. Woodbury, D. M. (1980): Phenytoin: Proposed mechanisms of anticonvulsant action. *Adv. Neurol.,* 27:447–471.

94. Woodbury, D. M., and Esplin, D. W. (1959): Neuropharmacology and neurochemistry of anticonvulsant drugs. *Res. Publ. Assoc. Res. Nerv. Ment. Dis.,* 37:24–56.

95. Woodbury, D. M., and Kemp, J. W. (1971): Pharmacology and mechanisms of action of diphenylhydantoin. *Psychiatr. Neurol. Neurochir.,* 74:91–115.

96. Yanagihara, T., and Hamberger, A. (1971): Effect of diphenylhydantoin on protein metabolism in the central nervous system. Study of subcellular fractions. *Exp. Neurol.,* 31:87–99.

97. Yanagihara, T., and Hamberger, A. (1971): Distribution of diphenylhydantoin in rat organs: Study with neuroglia and subcellular fractions. *J. Pharmacol. Exp. Ther.,* 179:611–618.

98. Yanagihara, T., and Hamberger, A. (1971): Effect of diphenylhydantoin on protein metabolism in neuron and neuroglial fractions of central nervous tissue. *Exp. Neurol.,* 32:152–162.

Antiepileptic Drugs, edited by D. M. Woodbury, J. K. Penry, and C. E. Pippenger. Raven Press, New York © 1982.

20

Other Hydantoins

Mephenytoin and Ethotoin

Harvey J. Kupferberg

MEPHENYTOIN

Mephenytoin (Mesantoin®) has been used successfully for more than 30 years to treat various types of seizures. It is most effective in the treatment of primary and secondary generalized tonic–clonic seizures. Although it is efficacious, mephenytoin often has prominent side effects, the most serious being pancytopenia and irreversible aplastic anemia; the latter is fatal in some patients.

The efficacy and toxicity of mephenytoin may be explained through its metabolic pathways. A primary metabolite, 5-ethyl-5-phenyl-hydantoin (Nirvanol®), has both antiepileptic properties and significant toxicity. It was used clinically in the 1920s for the treatment of chorea in children but caused a high incidence of urticaria and blood dyscrasias. Because 5-ethyl-5-phenylhydantoin appears to contribute to the anticonvulsant activity of mephenytoin, it will also be discussed in detail.

Chemistry and Methods of Determination

Physical and Chemical Properties

Mephenytoin (5-ethyl-3-methyl-5-phenylhydantoin) is a white crystalline compound with a melting point of 137 to 138°C. Its molecular weight is 218.25. Commercially available mephenytoin is a racemic mixture, with both isomers having the same melting point (7). The optical rotations of $R(-)$-mephenytoin are $[\alpha]_D^{25} = -104°$ and $[\alpha]_{365}^{25} = -410°$, and those of $S(+)$-mephenytoin are $[\alpha]_D^{25} = +105°$, $[\alpha]_{365}^{25} = +416°$ (150 mg/10 ml absolute ethanol). The R/S configuration for the enantiomers is correlated on the configuration of $R(-)$, $S(+)$-phenylethylglycine.

Mephenytoin is relatively insoluble in water and lacks a dissociation constant because of the methyl substituent in the 3-position of the hydantoin ring. It is fairly soluble in several organic solvents, and, therefore, partition coefficients between organic solvents and water or aqueous buffer favor extraction into the organic phase (5). The ultraviolet spectrum of mephenytoin does not change between pH 6 and 10.

Nirvanol, like mephenytoin, is supplied for clinical use as the racemic *dl* mixture. It has a melting point of 199 to 200° C. Nirvanol can be resolved into its optically active components by means of brucine, which forms an alcohol-soluble salt that is less soluble in the *d* form than in the *l* form (34). Each isomer has an optical rotation of 115° and a melting point of 237° C. The racemic mixture of Nirvanol is twice as

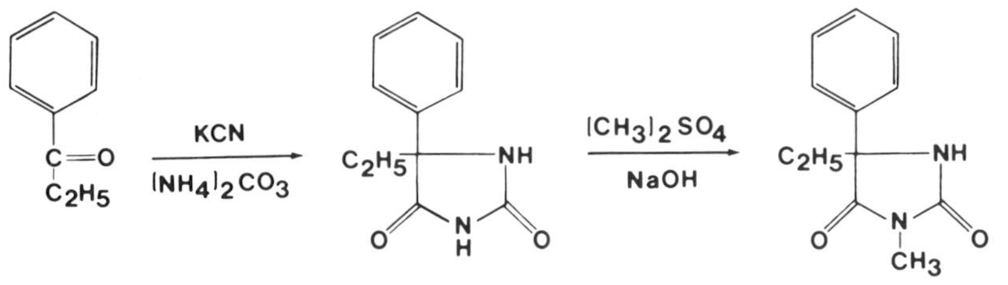

phenylethyl ketone — 5-phenyl-5-ethylhydantoin (Nirvanol) — 5-ethyl-3-methyl-5-phenyl-hydantoin (mephenytoin)

FIG. 1. Synthetic pathway of mephenytoin.

soluble as the *d*-isomer, being 0.66 mg/ml versus 0.33 mg/ml (3). Mephenytoin is highly soluble in benzene, but Nirvanol is not. Nirvanol can be extracted from aqueous solutions (pH 6) with solvents such as ethyl acetate, diethyl ether, ethylene dichloride, or chloroform. Nirvanol is a weak acid with a pK_a of 8.5, and at physiological pH it is predominantly in the un-ionized form.

Synthesis

Mephenytoin is synthesized through the Nirvanol intermediate (Fig. 1). The Bucherer reaction condenses phenylethyl ketone, ammonium carbonate, and potassium cyanide in a mole ratio of 1 : 3 : 2 to produce 5-ethyl-5-phenylhydantoin (Nirvanol). This product is reacted with dimethylsulfate in ethanolic sodium hydroxide to form mephenytoin.

Methods of Determination

Methods for the simultaneous determination of mephenytoin and Nirvanol in body fluids are based on chromatographic techniques. Friel and Troupin (14) described a gas chromatographic method for the determination of several anticonvulsants including mephenytoin and Nirvanol. Derivative formation was accomplished by ''flash-heater'' ethylation, with triethylphenylammonium hydroxide as the ethyl donor. The ethylated derivatives were nearly resolved on a 1.83 m, 3% OV-1 column. The ethylated product of mephobarbital was the only drug found to interfere with the analysis of Nirvanol. In patients on long-term mephenytoin therapy, the levels of mephenytoin were found to be near the method's lower limits of detection (1.5 μg/ml). Kupferberg and Yonekawa (23) assayed mephenytoin and Nirvanol in brain and plasma of mice following the intraperitoneal administration of a 40-mg/kg dose of mephenytoin. Trimethylsilyl derivatives were made of ethylene dichloride tissue extracts prior to gas–liquid chromatography. 3-Methyl-5-cyclopropyl-5-phenylhydantoin was used as the internal standard. The lower limit of sensitivity of this method was approximately 1 μg for each compound.

Küpfer and Bircher (20) formed propyl derivatives of mephenytoin and Nirvanol prior to chromatography. Mephenytoin and Nirvanol were propylated in concentrated base (12 N potassium hydroxide) and propyl iodide combined with plasma extracts dissolved in dimethylsulfoxide. The sensitivity of detection was increased significantly with the use of a nitrogen-selective detector. Blood levels of less than 200 ng/ml of both compounds could be quantitated.

Yonekawa and Kupferberg (38) used a similar alkylation procedure in the determination of plasma levels of mephenytoin and Nirvanol in epileptic patients receiving a single 50-mg dose of mephenytoin. Ethylation of the hydantoin ring was carried out in 2-butanone with ethyl iodide and 10 N potassium hydroxide. The electron-impact mode of the mass spectrometer was used to increase the sensitivity and specificity of the assay. The lower limits of quantitation for mephenytoin and Nirvanol were 10 ng/ml and 50 ng/ml, respectively, and the results were found to be reproducible within 8% on repeated assay.

Absorption, Distribution, and Excretion

Absorption and Distribution

The rate and extent of absorption of mephenytoin have not been studied in detail. Yonekawa and Kupferberg (38) determined the plasma levels of mephenytoin in epileptic patients receiving 50-mg and 400-mg single oral doses of the drug. Mephenytoin was rapidly absorbed from the gastrointestinal tract. Peak plasma mephenytoin levels occurred within 45 min to 2 hr and ranged from 0.4 to 0.6 μg/ml for the 50-mg dose and from 2.3 to 6.7 μg/ml for the 400-mg dose.

The volume of distribution of mephenytoin has not been determined in either humans or experimental animals, and the plasma-to-tissue ratio also has not been reported. Since it is known that methylation enhances the lipid solubility of the barbiturates and thereby leads to an increased volume of distribution (5), methylation of the hydantoins could be expected to have the same effect. Nirvanol is distributed in total body weight (4,5). Kupferberg and Yonekawa (23) found that brain levels of mephenytoin were 1.2 times higher than plasma levels in rats receiving 40 mg/kg of mephenytoin intraperitoneally. Brain levels of Nirvanol were 80% lower than plasma levels in the same rats. At 30 min after administration of mephenytoin, brain levels of mephenytoin and Nirvanol were 19.2 μg/g and 8.1 μg/g, respectively. The brain levels of mephenytoin fell to 5.8 μg/g and those of Nirvanol rose to 18.2 μg/g at 2 hr. The total molar concentration of mephenytoin and Nirvanol, however, did not change more than 10% during the 2-hr period.

Excretion

The amount of mephenytoin excreted in the urine represents a small fraction of the dose ad-

ministered. Initially, it was assumed that this finding represented a complete conversion of mephenytoin to metabolites (3), but later the low excretion was attributed to a low renal clearance (4). The lipid solubility of mephenytoin suggests an increased rate of diffusion back into the renal tubules.

Although mephenytoin is administered as a racemic mixture of equal amounts of $S(+)$ and $R(-)$ isomers, the Nirvanol excreted in the urine is mainly in the l form (90%). The metabolic significance of this finding will be discussed below.

Protein Binding

The plasma protein binding of mephenytoin and Nirvanol in epileptic patients was determined by equilibrium dialysis and measurement of salivary levels (35). The mean free percent of the drugs as determined by equilibrium dialysis was 59.6% and 68.1% for mephenytoin and Nirvanol, respectively. Salivary levels of both drugs were in good agreement with the data obtained by dialysis. These data indicate that changes in binding of these two drugs would not play an important role in either seizure control or toxicity.

Biotransformation

The metabolic pathways of mephenytoin are shown in Fig. 2. Mephenytoin is demethylated to Nirvanol in humans and dogs (3). Butler (4) examined the extent of the demethylation in dogs and found that 88% of an administered dose of mephenytoin is converted to Nirvanol. The rate of conversion is much slower than the elimination rate of Nirvanol, and long-term administration of mephenytoin leads to accumulation of Nirvanol in plasma. Butler (6) then demonstrated that Nirvanol is metabolized to 5-ethyl-5-(p-hydroxyphenyl)hydantoin in humans and dogs. This phenolic product of Nirvanol is formed when either mephenytoin or Nirvanol is administered. The product isolated from human urine contains an equal mixture of both d and l isomers, whereas dog urine contains

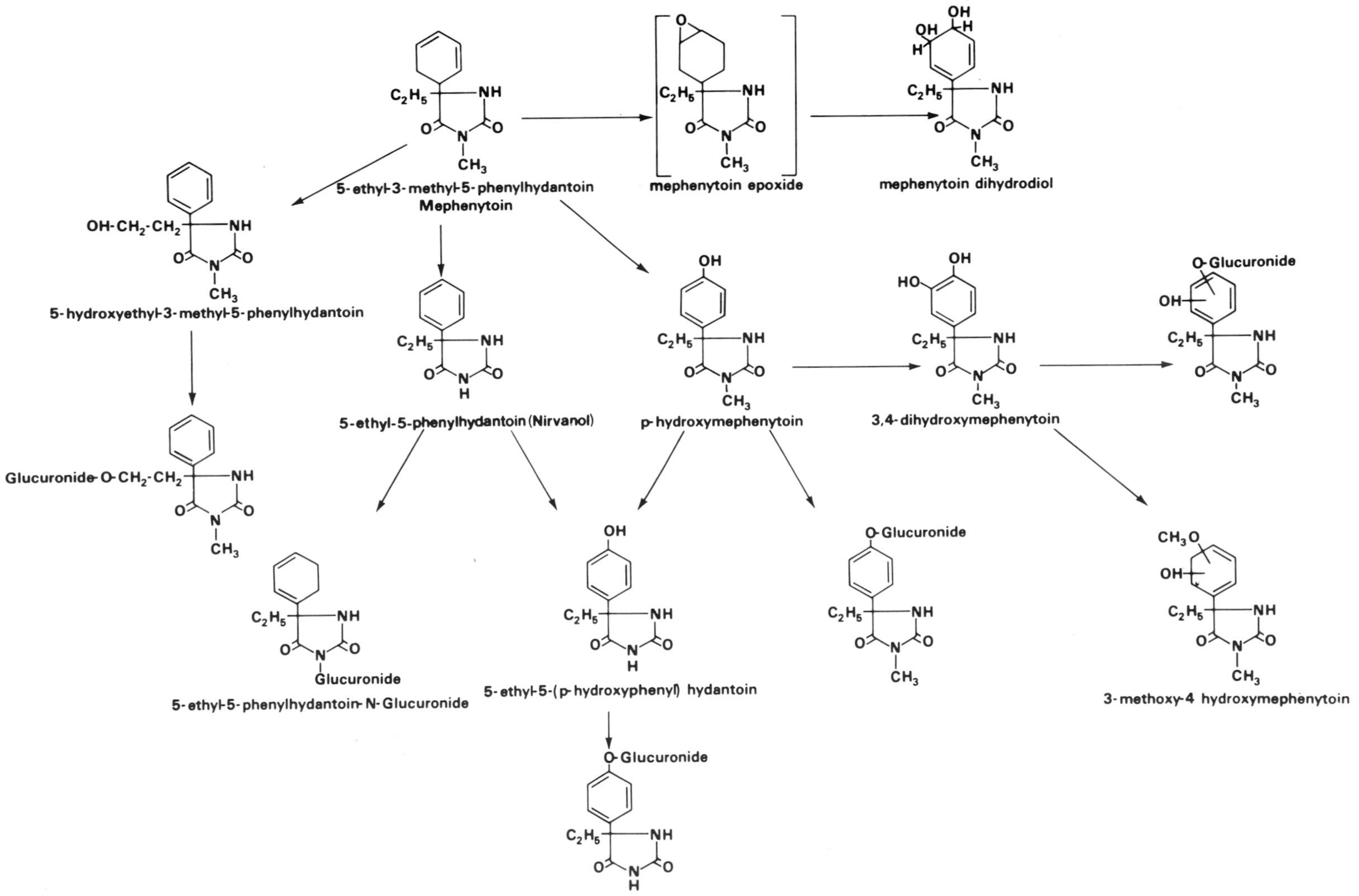

FIG. 2. Metabolic pathways of mephenytoin.

largely the *d* isomer. Most of this phenolic metabolite is conjugated with glucuronic acid.

Recently, several phenolic metabolites of mephenytoin have been identified. Karlaganis et al. (18) identified 5-ethyl-3-methyl-5-(*p*-hydroxyphenyl)hydantoin (*p*-hydroxymephenytoin) and 5-ethyl-3-methyl-5-(*m*-hydroxyphenyl)hydantoin (*m*-hydroxymephenytoin) in the urine of dogs administered 22 mg/kg of mephenytoin orally. *p*-Hydroxymephenytoin can be isolated from rat, guinea pig, and human urine, whereas *m*-hydroxymephenytoin cannot (17). Lynn et al. (25) characterized the glucuronides of 5-hydroxyethyl-3-methyl-5-phenylhydantoin and 5-ethyl-5-(hydroxymethoxyphenyl)-3-methylhydantoin in human urine and tentatively identified the *N*-3 glucuronide of Nirvanol. The dihydrodiol of mephenytoin, as well as 5-ethyl-3-methyl-5-(3,4-dihydroxyphenyl)hydantoin (3,4-dihydroxymephenytoin), has been identified in human (15,17) and guinea pig (17) urine.

Mephenytoin contains an asymmetric carbon atom at the 5-position of the hydantoin ring. Stereoselective metabolism of the enantiomers of mephenytoin have been studied in great detail. Butler and Waddell (7) compared the distribution and elimination of *d* and *l* isomers of Nirvanol in rats. The plasma concentrations of *l*-Nirvanol were considerably higher than those of the *d* isomer when equivalent amounts of each isomer were administered to rats. The volume of distribution and elimination rate constant of the *d* isomer were greater than those of the *l* isomer.

When each isomer of mephenytoin was administered to rats, the rate of production of Nirvanol from *l*-mephenytoin was much greater than that from *d*-mephenytoin (7). Küpfer et al. (21) studied the stereoselective metabolism and pharmacokinetics of Nirvanol in the dog. The volume of distribution and renal clearance of both isomers were identical, whereas the disappearance rate constant and plasma clearance rate were greater for the *l* isomer. The differences in plasma clearance of the two enantiomers could be explained by a stereoselectivity of hepatic hydroxylation. Although the *d* isomer of *p*-hydroxy-

Nirvanol was eliminated in the bile, none of the *l* form could be detected.

These findings confirm those of Butler (3) who found that 90 to 98% of the excreted *p*-hydroxy-Nirvanol was in the *d*-isomer form when either racemic mephenytoin or Nirvanol was administered to dogs.

The stereoselectivity of mephenytoin metabolism in dogs was studied using radiolabeled enantiomers of mephenytoin. The radiolabel, ^{14}C, was located in the 3-methyl position of the molecule. By measuring exhalation of ^{14}C-labeled carbon dioxide and urinary excretion of ^{14}C-hydroxylated mephenytoin metabolites, Küpfer and Bircher (20) confirmed a preferential metabolism of the $R(-)$ enantiomer. Most of the hydroxylated metabolites of mephenytoin were in the $S(+)$ form.

In a preliminary report, Küpfer et al. (22) showed that in humans $R(-)$-mephenytoin undergoes preferential demethylation, whereas $S(+)$-mephenytoin undergoes preferential aromatic hydroxylation.

Smith et al. (33) found that the *l* isomer of mephenytoin, which is of the *R* configuration, is more rapidly demethylated by rat liver microsomes than the *d* isomer.

Experimental Pharmacology

The experimental pharmacology of mephenytoin is described in the following data from the Antiepileptic Drug Development Program (30). Unlike phenytoin, mephenytoin inhibits both electrically and chemically induced seizures. The effective dose (ED_{50}) for maximal electroshock seizures (MES) in mice is 60 mg/kg after intraperitoneal administration and 66 mg/kg after oral administration. The anticonvulsant potency of orally administered mephenytoin in rats is 18 mg/kg. The dose required to cause neurotoxicity, as measured by the rotorod test, was three to six times higher than the ED_{50} in mice and rats. The duration of anticonvulsant activity in mice after intraperitoneal administration is 6 to 10 hr, most likely reflecting the formation of the active metabolite, Nirvanol.

Mephenytoin will also block clonic seizures

induced by pentylenetetrazol, bicuculline, and picrotoxin, the ED_{50} in mice being 30 mg/kg, 124 mg/kg, and 100 mg/kg, respectively. Thus, mephenytoin not only raises the seizure threshold but also prevents the spread of seizures. Mephenytoin is ineffective in preventing strychnine-induced seizures.

Mice receiving intraperitoneally administered doses of mephenytoin exceeding 150 mg/kg exhibit ataxia, decreased motor activity, loss of righting reflex, and decreased respiration. The hypnotic dose (HD_{50}) of mephenytoin administered intraperitoneally to mice is 400 mg/kg, and the lethal dose (LD_{50}) is 570 mg/kg.

Nirvanol has not been studied in great detail, but its anticonvulsant activity is not much different than that of mephenytoin. The MES ED_{50} of intraperitoneally administered Nirvanol in mice is 40 mg/kg.

Clinical Efficacy and Toxicity

Mephenytoin is most effective in the treatment of primary and secondary generalized tonic–clonic seizures (1,19,27). It also satisfactorily controls elementary partial seizures, but its usefulness in treating complex partial seizures has not been fully evaluated. The treatment of absence seizures with mephenytoin has had little or no success.

The serious dose-related toxicity and side effects of mephenytoin, however, have dampened its widespread use. The most serious toxic effects are pancytopenia and irreversible aplastic anemia. Other side effects are skin rash, fever, generalized adenopathy, leukopenia, and ataxia. No fatalities have been reported from overdosage.

The efficacy and toxicity of mephenytoin may be explained by the accumulation of Nirvanol. Introduced in 1916 as a hypnotic, Nirvanol was soon reported to cause toxic manifestations resembling "serum sickness" or hypersensitivity, the so-called Nirvanol disease. Early reports indicated that Nirvanol had more sedative properties than hypnotic effect as compared to phenobarbital (34). This fact prompted its use as the drug of choice in chorea minor and epi-

lepsy. Sobotka et al. (34) were the first to investigate the possibility that the toxicity of Nirvanol was caused by the *l* isomer. Because of its serious side effects, Nirvanol was removed from use as a therapeutic agent.

Steady-state levels of mephenytoin are usually reached within 3 days. The average plasma half-life of mephenytoin is 14 hr. Nirvanol reaches steady-state levels much more slowly than mephenytoin, a reflection of its plasma half-life, an average of 114 hr. The average steady-state plasma Nirvanol level in patients receiving a 400-mg daily dose of mephenytoin was 18 μg/ml, whereas the average steady-state plasma mephenytoin level was 1.5 μg/ml (M. E. Newmark et al., *unpublished data*).

Troupin et al. (36) recently reappraised the clinical use of mephenytoin alone or in combination with other antiepileptic agents. Ninety-three patients were reviewed. Approximately three-fourths of the patients experienced a reduction in seizure frequency or complete seizure control while taking mephenytoin. Many of the objective side effects of cerebellar origin seen with phenytoin were rarely seen with mephenytoin but were qualitatively the same when present. Hirsutism, gingival hypertrophy, and peripheral neuropathies were absent. Performance on psychological tests of cognitive-attentional skills showed a modest improvement during mephenytoin administration.

The fact that both mephenytoin and Nirvanol have been shown to have anticonvulsant activity in experimental animals (23) would argue that seizure control in humans does not result solely from the accumulation of Nirvanol. The relative contribution of each agent to seizure control is difficult to determine. There is no question that seizure control improves as the levels of Nirvanol increase when mephenytoin is administered chronically. Serum Nirvanol–mephenytoin levels of 20 to 30 μg/ml are associated with good seizure control, but plasma levels exceeding 50 μg/ml in patients taking mephenytoin as sole therapy usually lead to toxicity (36).

In most cases mephenytoin is used in combination with other anticonvulsants. Troupin et al. (36) claim that the combined use of me-phenytoin and phenytoin, in somewhat lower doses of each, often leads to improvement in seizure control without side effects. Similar results are observed when mephenytoin and car-bamazepine are used. When mephenytoin is used in combination with a barbiturate, the mephenytoin levels cannot be raised to those attained when mephenytoin is used alone, whereas the barbiturate levels approach the usual therapeutic range. Although mephenytoin lacks many of the side effects of phenytoin, the occurrence of serious toxicity limits its unrestricted use as a primary anticonvulsant.

ETHOTOIN

Ethotoin (Peganone®) was first marketed in the United States in 1957 for the treatment of generalized tonic–clonic seizures. Unfortunately, its usefulness is limited by minimal efficacy despite its relatively minimal side effects as compared with mephenytoin and phenytoin. Therefore, ethotoin is not considered to be a primary antiepileptic agent.

Chemistry and Methods of Determination

Physical and Chemical Properties

Ethotoin (3-ethyl-5-phenylhydantoin) is a white crystalline compound with a melting point of 94° C. Its molecular weight is 204.22. It is insoluble in water and soluble in most organic solvents, e.g., methanol, chloroform, benzene, ethylene dichloride, and methylene chloride. The solubility of ethotoin is essentially unaffected in either dilute acid or base. Strong basic solution will cause its conversion to a dimer through an oxidative process (9).

Synthesis

The synthesis of ethotoin is shown in Fig. 3. The reaction between ethylisocyanate and α-amino-α-phenylacetic acid forms 5-ethyl-2-phenylhydantoic acid; the product is then cyclodehydrated in acid to form ethotoin (10,37).

Methods of Determination

Yonekawa et al. (39) developed a gas chromatographic method specifically for the determination of ethotoin in human plasma. Ethotoin was extracted from plasma (adjusted to a pH of 10) into benzene. (Ethotoin is a neutral compound that is un-ionized at the pH used in the extraction procedure.) The internal standard was 3-methyl-5-cyclopropyl-5-phenylhydantoin. The benzene extract was then washed with 0.5 N HCl. The organic phase was evaporated under water vacuum, and silylated derivatives were formed using *bis*(trimethylsilyl)trifluoroacetamide (BSTFA). The recoveries of ethotoin added to plasma were 85% at concentrations of 2 to 40 μg. The relative standard deviation of five determinations of 10 μg of ethotoin was less than 5%. The method appeared to be relatively free of interference by other agents. Of the

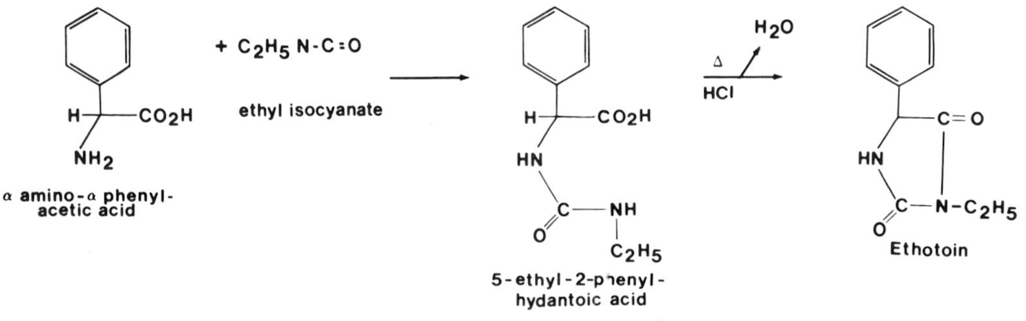

FIG. 3. Synthetic pathway of ethotoin.

antiepileptic drugs, mephobarbital appeared to have a retention time similar to the internal standard.

Naestoft and Larsen (29) developed a mass fragmentographic method for the determination of ethotoin and some of its metabolites in human urine. Ethotoin and the metabolites were extracted from acidified urine with ethyl acetate and silylated before injection into the gas chromatograph. Mephenytoin was used as the internal standard. The mass spectrometer was focused at m/z 261 for ethotoin. Standard curves between 3 and 50 μg were prepared and were linear when the ratio of ethotoin to mephenytoin was plotted against concentration.

Absorption, Distribution, and Excretion

Unlike the case with mephenytoin or phenytoin, many of the pharmacokinetic parameters of ethotoin have not been determined. Peak plasma ethotoin levels following single oral doses of 25 to 30 mg/kg occurred within 2 to 4 hr (35,39). The mean plasma half-life after a single oral dose of ethotoin was 5.1 hr and appeared to be monoexponential with plasma levels of 1 to 30 μg/ml (35,39). Saturation kinetics similar to those of phenytoin did not occur.

Sjö and co-workers (24,32) described nonlinear plasma elimination kinetics for ethotoin after a single oral dose of 30 mg/kg. The elimination of ethotoin became linear below 8 μg/ml. Plasma ethotoin levels more than doubled when the dose was increased from 30 to 60 mg/kg. Plasma clearance of ethotoin decreased by one-third after the dose was doubled. These results were not observed by Troupin et al. (35) or Yonekawa et al. (39) in patients with identical plasma levels.

Naestoft and Larsen (29) found that 14 to 32% of the dose of ethotoin could be accounted for as p-hydroxyethotoin, and 5 to 14% as 5-phenylhydantoin. Although they were not able to identify 5-hydroxy-5-phenylhydantoin, it was estimated that this metabolite accounted for 17 to 34% of the dose. The remaining hydroxylated compounds most likely accounted for less than 5% of the dose. Between 5 and 10% of the dose of ethotoin is excreted unchanged (28).

Protein Binding

The binding of ethotoin to plasma proteins is similar to that of mephenytoin. The percent free drug, based on saliva levels and equilibrium dialysis, is approximately 55%.

Biotransformation

Ethotoin is degraded by two principal routes, one involving metabolic N-deethylation followed by ring cleavage and the other involving phenyl ring hydroxylation (Fig. 4).

Dudley et al. (12) initially studied the metabolism of ethotoin in dogs. They found small amounts of 5-phenylhydantoin and 3-ethyl-5-(4-hydroxyphenyl)hydantoin (p-hydroxyethotoin) and large amounts of 2-phenylhydantoic acid. The hydrolytic ring-opening reaction leading to 2-phenylhydantoic acid was stereospecific and occurred only after a primary N-deethylation reaction of ethotoin.

Bius et al. (2) studied the metabolic fate of ethotoin in humans by use of gas chromatography–mass spectrometry. Eleven metabolites of ethotoin were detected in the urine of a patient receiving 3.0 g of ethotoin daily. Nine of these metabolic products were identified unequivocally by comparing their mass spectra with those of authentic synthetic compounds. Extracts of unhydrolyzed and hydrolyzed (β-glucuronidase) urine were derivatized with BSTFA and subjected to gas chromatography–mass spectrometry in the electron-impact mode. The total ion chromatograms of the extracts are shown in Figs. 5 and 6. The following metabolites were isolated from unhydrolyzed urine: ethotoin, 5-phenylhydantoin, 3-ethyl-5-hydroxy-5-phenylhydantoin (5-hydroxyethotoin), 5-hydroxy-5-phenylhydantoin, 3-ethyl-5-(4-hydroxyphenyl)hydantoin (p-hydroxyethotoin), 3-ethyl-5-hydroxy-5-(4-hydroxyphenyl)hydantoin ("ring-hydroxy"-5-hydroxyethotoin), and ethotoin dihydrodiol. Other metabolites of ethotoin isolated from hydrolyzed urine were: 3-ethyl-5-(2-hydroxyphenyl)hydantoin (o-hydroxyethotoin), 3-ethyl-5-(3-hydroxyphenyl)hydantoin (m-hydroxy-

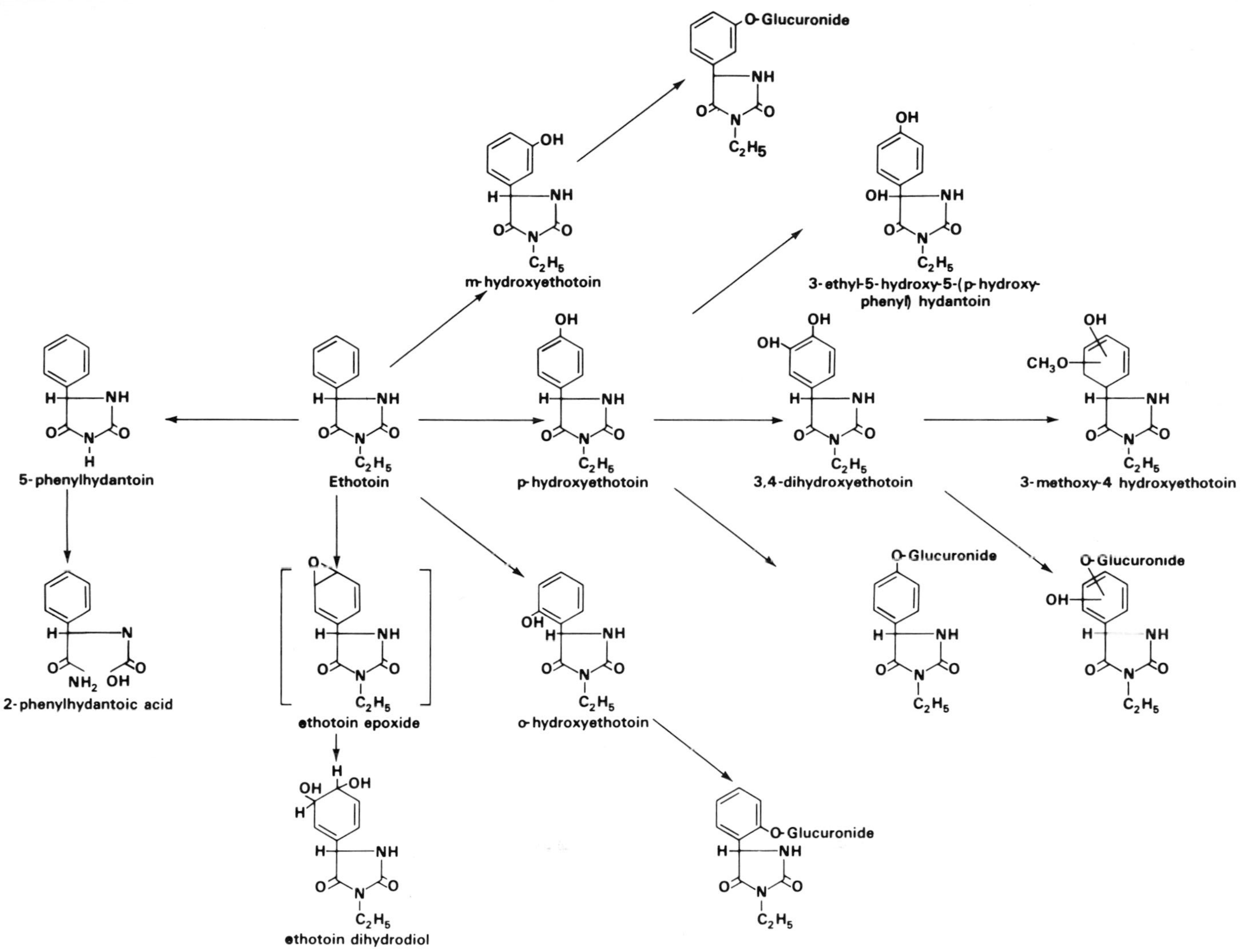

FIG. 4. Metabolic pathways of ethotoin.

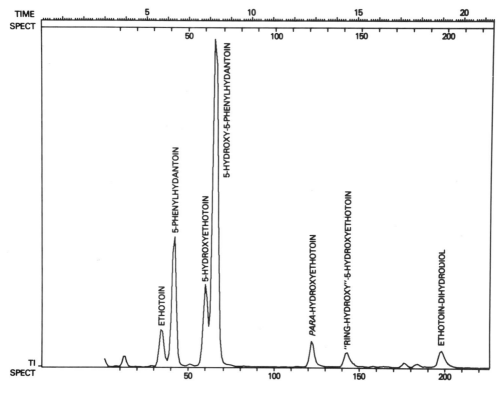

FIG. 5. Total-ion (TI) chromatogram (time in minutes) of a silylated extract of nonhydrolyzed urine of a patient receiving 3.0 g of ethotoin daily. (From Bius et al., ref. 2, with permission. Copyright © 1980 American Society for Pharmacology and Experimental Therapeutics.)

ethotoin), 3-ethyl-5-(3-methoxy-4-hydroxy-phenyl)hydantoin (3-methoxy-4-hydroxyethotoin), 3-ethyl-5-(3,4-dihydroxyphenyl)-hydantoin (3,4-dihydroxyphenylethotoin). Greater quantities of *p*-hydroxyethotoin were recovered from hydrolyzed urine.

The enzyme dihydropyrimidinase (13,26) is responsible for the stereospecific hydrolysis of 5-phenylhydantoin to 2-phenylhydantoic acid. Only the $R(-)$ isomers of the 5-monosubstituted hydantoins, α-phenylsuccinimides, and dihydrouracils are substrates of this enzyme (26). Ethotoin must first undergo *N*-dealkylation to 5-phenylhydantoin before it becomes a substrate. The $R(-)$-2-phenylhydantoic acid excreted in urine counts for approximately 10% of the daily dose. The configuration of 2-phenylhydantoic acid found in the urine of dogs (12) and rats (13) is identical to that of humans. When racemic 5-phenylhydantoin was ad-

ministered to dogs, somewhat more than the theoretical quantity (50 mole % of the dose) of the substances recovered from urine had the $R(-)$ configuration (12). Dudley and Bius (11) demonstrated an *in vitro* interconversion of the optical isomers of 5-phenylhydantoin which could explain the *in vivo* production of $R(-)$-2-phenylhydantoic acid from the S enantiomer of 5-phenylhydantoin.

Experimental Pharmacology

Ethotoin and mephenytoin exhibit similar anticonvulsant profiles in mice (30). The MES ED_{50} in mice is 85 mg/kg following intraperitoneal administration. The dose required to cause neurotoxicity, as measured by the rotorod test, is 171 mg/kg. The duration of anticonvulsant activity in mice following intraperitoneal administration is much shorter than that for me-

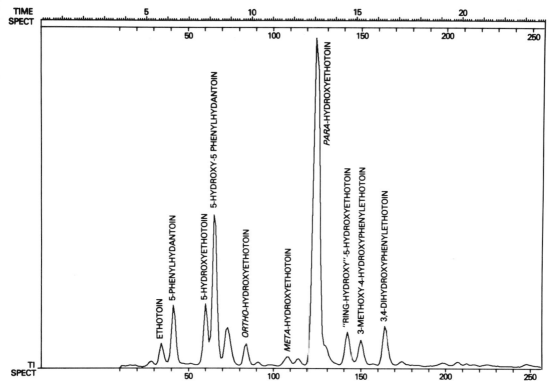

FIG. 6. Total-ion (TI) chromatogram (time in minutes) of a silylated extract of β-glucuronidase-hydrolyzed urine of a patient receiving 3.0 g of ethotoin daily. (From Bius et al., ref. 2, with permission. Copyright © 1980 American Society for Pharmacology and Experimental Therapeutics.)

phenytoin, most likely reflecting the rapid metabolism of ethotoin to inactive metabolites.

Ethotoin also blocks clonic seizures induced by pentylenetetrazol, the ED_{50} being 48 mg/kg following intraperitoneal administration.

Clinical Efficacy and Toxicity

Schwade et al. (31) were the first to evaluate ethotoin clinically; they studied its efficacy in 157 patients with a variety of seizure types. Ethotoin was thought to be less toxic than its analog, 3-methyl-5-phenylhydantoin, which had been evaluated clinically a few years before. Daily dosages in children ranged from 0.5 to 1 g and in adults from 2 to 3 g, given in divided doses. In most cases, ethotoin was added to the existing drug regimen. A combination of ethotoin and phenurone produced serious psychological side effects. Two patients developed mild

rashes. Toxic effects on the hepatic and hematopoietic systems were absent. Carter and Maley (8) found similar results in 38 patients.

Gruber et al. (16) compared the efficacy of seven anticonvulsants and placebo as replacement for regular therapy in a double-blind study in 44 epileptic patients with focal brain damage. Ethotoin in daily doses up to 1,500 mg was the least effective drug in decreasing the seizure frequency.

The side effects of ethotoin are less severe than those of either phenytoin or mephenytoin. Gingival hyperplasia, hirsutism, and urticaria are extremely uncommon. Mild rashes, if they occur, disappear within 3 days after the drug is discontinued. About 5% of the patients complain of gastrointestinal distress.

Teratogenicity may occur with ethotoin as it does with phenytoin. Zablen and Brand (40) reported the occurrence of bilateral cleft lip and cleft palate in a premature infant born to a mother taking ethotoin (500 mg four times a day) and mephobarbital (100 mg four times a day).

The majority of the efficacy studies on ethotoin were carried out at a time when the pharmacokinetic and metabolic parameters of the drug were unknown. The clinical impression is that ethotoin is minimally efficacious and must be given in large doses. Animal studies have shown that ethotoin is one-fourth as potent as phenytoin, and preliminary pharmacokinetic studies indicate that ethotoin must be given at a minimum of four times a day. With an elaboration of these facts and more knowledge of the drug's disposition in epileptic patients, clinicians can then determine the role of ethotoin in the treatment of epilepsy.

CONVERSION

Mephenytoin

Conversion factor:

$$CF = \frac{1000}{mol.\ wt.} = \frac{1000}{218.25} = 4.58$$

Conversion:

$$(\mu g/ml) \times 4.58 = (\mu moles/liter)$$
$$(\mu moles/liter) \div 4.58 = (\mu g/ml)$$

Ethotoin

Conversion factor:

$$CF = \frac{1000}{mol.\ wt.} = \frac{1000}{204.22} = 4.90$$

Conversion:

$$(\mu g/ml) \times 4.90 = (\mu moles/liter)$$
$$(\mu moles/liter) \div 4.90 = (\mu g/ml)$$

REFERENCES

1. Aird, R. B. (1948): The treatment of epilepsy with methylphenylethyl hydantoin (Mesantoin). *Calif. Med.*, 68:141–146.
2. Bius, D. L., Yonekawa, W. D., Kupferberg, H. J.,

Cantor, F., and Dudley, K. H. (1980): Gas chromatographic–mass spectrometric studies on the metabolic fate of ethotoin in man. *Drug Metab. Dispos.*, 8:223–229.
3. Butler, T. C. (1952): Metabolic demethylation of 3-methyl-5-ethyl-5-phenyl hydantoin (Mesantoin). *J. Pharmacol. Exp. Ther.*, 104:299–308.
4. Butler, T. C. (1953): Quantitative studies of the physiological disposition of 3-methyl-5-ethyl-5-phenyl hydantoin (Mesantoin) and 5-ethyl-5-phenyl hydantoin (Nirvanol). *J. Pharmacol. Exp. Ther.*, 109:340–345.
5. Butler, T. C. (1955): The effects of N-methylation in 5,5-disubstituted derivatives of barbituric acid, hydantoin, and 2,4-oxazolidinedione. *J. Am. Pharm. Assoc.*, 44:367–370.
6. Butler, T. C. (1956): The metabolic conversion of 3-methyl-5-ethyl-5-phenyl hydantoin (Mesantoin) and of 5-ethyl-5-phenyl hydantoin (Nirvanol) to 5-ethyl-5-(p-hydroxyphenyl) hydantoin. *J. Pharmacol. Exp. Ther.*, 117:160–165.
7. Butler, T. C., and Waddell, W. J. (1954): A pharmacological comparison of the optical isomers of 5-ethyl-5-phenyl hydantoin (Nirvanol) and of 3-methyl-5-ethyl-5-phenyl hydantoin (Mesantoin). *J. Pharmacol. Exp. Ther.*, 110:120–125.
8. Carter, C. H., and Maley, M. C. (1957): Clinical evaluation of Peganone, a new anticonvulsant. *Am. J. Med.*, 234:74–77.
9. Dudley, K. H., and Bius, D. L. (1969): Diphenylhydantil. *J. Org. Chem.*, 34:1133.
10. Dudley, K. H., and Bius, D. L. (1973): The synthesis of optically active 5-phenylhydantoins. *J. Heterocycl. Chem.*, 10:173–180.
11. Dudley, K. H., and Bius, D. L. (1976): Buffer catalysis of the racemization reaction of some 5-phenylhydantoins and its relation to the *in vivo* metabolism of ethotoin. *Drug Metab. Dispos.*, 4:340–348.
12. Dudley, K. H., Bius, D. L., and Butler, T. C. (1975): Metabolic fates of 3-ethyl-5-phenylhydantoin (ethotoin, Peganone), 3-methyl-5-phenylhydantoin and 5-phenylhydantoin. *J. Pharmacol. Exp. Ther.*, 175:27–37.
13. Dudley, K. H., Butler, T. C., and Bius, D. L. (1974): The role of dihydropyrimidinase in the metabolism of hydantoin and succinimide drugs. *Drug Metab. Dispos.*, 2:103–112.
14. Friel, P., and Troupin, A. S. (1975): Flash-heater ethylation of some antiepileptic drugs. *Clin. Chem.*, 21:751–754.
15. Gerber, N., Thompson, R. M., Smith, R. G., and Lynn, R. K. (1979): Evidence for the epoxide–diol pathway in the biotransformation of mephenytoin. *Epilepsia*, 20:287–294.
16. Gruber, C. M., Jr., Brock, J. T., and Dyken, M. (1962): Comparison of the effectiveness of phenobarbital, mephobarbital, primidone, diphenylhydantoin, ethotoin, metharbital, and methylphenylethylhydantoin in motor seizures. *Clin. Pharmacol. Ther.*, 3:23–28.
17. Horning, M. G., Butler, C. M., Lertratanangkoon, K., Hill, R. M., Zion, T. E., and Kellaway, P. (1976): Gas chromatography–mass spectrometry–computer studies of the metabolism of anticonvulsant drugs. In: *Quantitative Analytic Studies in Epilepsy*, edited by

P. Kellaway and I. Petersen, pp. 95–114. Raven Press, New York.

18. Karlaganis, G., Küpfer, A., Bircher, J., Schlunegger, U. P., Gfeller, H., and Bigler, P. (1980): Identification of mephenytoin metabolites in the dog. *Drug Metab. Dispos.*, 8:173–177.

19. Kozol, H. L. (1950): Mesantoin in treatment of epilepsy. A report on two hundred patients under treatment for periods ranging from two months to four years. *Arch. Neurol.*, 63:235–248.

20. Küpfer, A., and Bircher, J. (1979): Stereoselectivity of differential routes of drug metabolism: The fate of the enantiomers of [^{14}C] mephenytoin in the dog. *J. Pharmacol. Exp. Ther.*, 209:190–195.

21. Küpfer, A., Bircher, J., and Preisig, R. (1977); Stereoselective metabolism, pharmacokinetics and biliary elimination of phenylethylhydantoin (Nirvanol) in the dog. *J. Pharmacol. Exp. Ther.*, 203:493–499.

22. Küpfer, A., Desmond, P., Roberts, R., Schenker, S., and Branch, R. A. (1979): Stereospecific metabolism of the enantiomers of mephenytoin in man. *Fed. Proc.*, 38:742.

23. Kupferberg, H. J., and Yonekawa, W. (1975): The metabolism of 3-methyl-5-ethyl-5-phenylhydantoin (mephenytoin) to 5-ethyl-5-phenylhydantoin (Nirvanol) in mice in relation to anticonvulsant activity. *Drug Metab. Dispos.*, 3:26–29.

24. Lund, M., Sjö, O., and Hvidberg, E. (1975): Plasma concentrations of ethotoin in epileptic patients. In: *Clinical Pharmacology of Anti-Epileptic Drugs*, edited by H. Schneider, D. Janz, C. Gardner-Thorpe, H. Meinardi, and A. L. Sherwin, pp. 111–114. Springer-Verlag, Berlin.

25. Lynn, R. K., Bauer, J. E., Gordon, W. P., Smith, R. G., Griffin, D., Thompson, R. M., Jenkins, R., and Gerber, N. (1979): Characterization of mephenytoin metabolites in human urine by gas chromatography and mass spectrometry. *Drug Metab. Dispos.*, 7:138–144.

26. Maguire, J. H., and Dudley, K. H. (1978): Partial purification and characterization of dihydropyrimidinases from calf and rat liver. *Drug Metab. Dispos.*, 6:601–605.

27. Mallin, A. W., and Gammon, G. D. (1953): A clinical evaluation of Mesantoin in epilepsy. *J. Nerv. Ment. Dis.*, 118:193–203.

28. Naestoft, J., Hvidberg, E. F., and Sjö, O. (1976): Saturable metabolic pathways for ethotoin in man. *Clin. Exp. Pharmacol. Physiol.*, 3:453–459.

29. Naestoft, J., and Larsen, N. E. (1977): Mass fragmentographic quantitation of ethotoin and some of its metabolites in human urine. *J. Chromatogr.*, 143:161–169.

30. National Institute of Neurological and Communicative Disorders and Stroke (1978): *Anticonvulsant Screening Project: Antiepileptic Drug Development Program*. DHEW Publication No. (NIH) 78-1093. National Institutes of Health, Bethesda.

31. Schwade, E. D., Richards, R. K., and Everett, G. M. (1956): Peganone, a new antiepileptic drug. *Dis. Nerv. Syst.*, 17:155–158.

32. Sjö, O., Hvidberg, E. F., Larsen, N.-E., Lund, M., and Naestoft, J. (1975): Dose-dependent kinetics of ethotoin in man. *Clin. Exp. Pharmacol. Physiol.*, 2:185–192.

33. Smith, J. A., Waddell, W. J., and Butler, T. C. (1963): Demethylation of *N*-methyl derivatives of barbituric acid, hydantoin, and 2,4-oxazolidinedione by rat liver microsomes. *Life Sci.*, 7:486–492.

34. Sobotka, H., Peck, S. M., and Kahn, J. (1933): Optically active hydantoins as hypnotics. *J. Pharmacol. Exp. Ther.*, 47:209–215.

35. Troupin, A. S., Friel, P., Lovely, M. P., and Wilensky, A. J. (1979): Clinical pharmacology of mephenytoin and ethotoin. *Ann. Neurol.*, 6:410–414.

36. Troupin, A. S., Ojemann, L. M., and Dodrill, C. B. (1976): Mephenytoin: A reappraisal. *Epilepsia*, 17:403–414.

37. Ware, E. (1950): The chemistry of the hydantoins. *Chem. Rev.*, 46:403–470.

38. Yonekawa, W., and Kupferberg, H. J. (1979): Measurement of mephenytoin (3-methyl-5-ethyl-5-phenylhydantoin) and its demethylated metabolite by selective ion monitoring. *J. Chromatogr.*, 163:161–167.

39. Yonekawa, W., Kupferberg, H. J., and Cantor, F. (1975): A gas chromatographic method for the determination of ethotoin (3-ethyl-5-phenylhydantoin) in human plasma. In: *Clinical Pharmacology of Anti-Epileptic Drugs*, edited by H. Schneider, D. Janz, C. Gardner-Thorpe, H. Meinardi, and A. L. Sherwin, pp. 115–121. Springer-Verlag, Berlin.

40. Zablen, M., and Brand, N. (1977): Cleft lip and palate with the anticonvulsant ethotoin. *N. Engl. J. Med.*, 297:1404.

Antiepileptic Drugs, edited by D. M. Woodbury, J. K. Penry, and C. E. Pippenger. Raven Press, New York © 1982.

21

Phenobarbital

Chemistry and Methods of Determination

Svein I. Johannessen

Phenobarbital was introduced into the treatment of epilepsy in 1912. Following barbital, which was introduced in 1903, phenobarbital was the second derivative of barbituric acid marketed for clinical use, and it was the first effective organic antiepileptic agent. Most other antiepileptic drugs were later developed as structural variations of phenobarbital.

PHYSICAL AND CHEMICAL PROPERTIES

Phenobarbital is a 5,5-substituted barbituric acid, 5-ethyl-5-phenylbarbituric acid. The well-known structural formula is shown in Fig. 1. Other barbiturates are formed by various substitutions in the 1 and 5 positions. Phenobarbital is much more potent as an anticonvulsant than as a sedative and is often capable of being used as an antiepileptic drug in nonsedative doses in contrast to other barbiturates. Slight changes in structure may convert barbituric acid derivatives into convulsants. Thus, convulsant properties may appear as hypnotic activity diminishes, if the alkyl side chains in the C-5 position are too long. A phenyl group at C-5 or N confers selective anticonvulsant activity on a barbiturate.

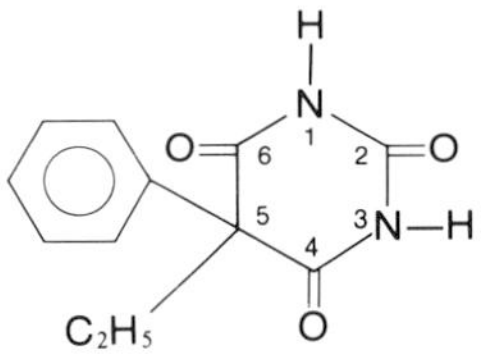

Phenobarbital consists of a white crystalline material with a somewhat bitter taste. The molecular weight is 232.23, and the melting point is 176°C. The free acid is only sparingly soluble in water, whereas the sodium salt is freely soluble. Phenobarbital is soluble in organic solvents such as chloroform, diethyl ether, and ethanol. The partition coefficient between chloroform and water is 4.2 at pH 3.4.

The pK_a is 7.3 (70), and phenobarbital is a considerably stronger acid than other barbiturates. The ionization exponent is lower than that of compounds with only alkyl or alkenyl substituents in the C-5 position. The electron-attracting force of the phenyl group favors the dissociation of a proton from nitrogen. These acidic properties are of importance in relation to the distribution and excretion of the drug. The effects of a change of pH on the distribution of a weak acid across a semipermeable membrane are stronger the lower the pK_a of the acid. The rate of change of the urine/plasma concentration

FIG. 1. Structural formula for phenobarbital (5-ethyl-5-phenylbarbituric acid).

297

ratio with change of urinary pH depends on the pK_a of a weak acid. Thus, the change in the ratio is higher the lower the pK_a of the acid. The pK_a of phenobarbital is such that a change of extracellular pH without a corresponding change of intracellular pH will cause a shift of the drug from one compartment to the other. Metabolic and respiratory alkalosis and acidosis cause important shifts of phenobarbital between the extracellular and intracellular compartments. The clearance of phenobarbital is much higher when urine is alkaline than when it is acidic, since the pK_a of the drug is such that the renal clearance is largely influenced by change of urinary pH. This is of clinical importance in the treatment of phenobarbital intoxication. The rate of renal excretion of unchanged phenobarbital also varies considerably in patients with uncontrolled water intake and diet.

Phenobarbital and other barbiturates are quite stable in aqueous solutions of low pH. Unlike phenytoin, exposure of phenobarbital to strong aqueous alkali and heating will rupture the barbituric acid ring, mostly at the 1,6 or 3,4 bonds.

The physical properties of a compound are of importance for separation methods in drug assays. Differences in ionization in aqueous solutions, partition coefficients between organic solvents and aqueous solutions at various pH values, mobility in chromatographic systems, volatility, stability, and absorbance in ultraviolet light all play important roles in an optimal drug assay.

SYNTHESIS

Various reactions described for the chemical synthesis of barbiturates have been reviewed by Vida and Gerry (69). These reactions may take place in acidic, neutral, or alkaline medium. Some examples are given below.

The barbiturates are commonly synthesized by the condensation of appropriate malonic acid derivatives with urea. Phenobarbital is prepared by ethylating phenylmalonic ester and condensing the product with urea in the presence of sodium alcoholate or, first, preparing phenylbarbituric acid and then ethylating with ethyl

bromide and sodium alcoholate. The condensation of malononitrile with urea in alkaline medium also produces barbiturates in good yield. An appropriate malonic acid can be condensed with urea in the presence of phosphorous oxychloride. It is also possible to synthesize 5,5-disubstituted barbituric acids from alkylation of 5-monosubstituted barbiturates with the powerful phenylating agent diphenyliodonium chloride.

METHODS OF DETERMINATION

A variety of techniques have been used for measuring phenobarbital at biological concentration (34,44,47,73). Early methods were based on gravimetry or the color reaction with cobalt. These methods were abandoned with the introduction of spectrophotometric methods. Different types of chromatography soon followed, first paper and thin-layer chromatography, and later, gas–liquid chromatography and high-pressure liquid chromatography. Chromatography has also been combined with mass spectrometry. This technique is known as mass fragmentography or selected ion monitoring. Recently, immunoassay techniques have also been introduced for routine monitoring of phenobarbital.

Some methods are developed for research purposes, and some are especially designed for routine analysis. Chromatographic techniques allow simultaneous quantitation of several drugs in a single run, whereas immunoassay techniques were developed for specific determination of one drug at a time.

Special precautions are necessary when metabolites or other drugs are present. For determination of phenobarbital, it is, therefore, essential that the drug can be analyzed in the presence of other antiepileptic drugs and other medication and that interference from the metabolite *p*-hydroxyphenobarbital be excluded.

Most measurements of phenobarbital concentrations are made on serum or plasma samples. For special investigations, urine, CSF, saliva, or tears may also be useful.

When spectrophotometric or chromatographic methods are used, phenobarbital is usually first extracted from an acidified sample into an organic solvent. Further solvent partitioning is then used to remove interfering substances. With immunoassay techniques, the drug is measured directly without pretreatment.

Spectrophotometry

Phenobarbital was initially measured by spectrophotometry (32,37,46,60). Separation from other drugs, especially from phenytoin, was achieved by differential extraction procedures. Quantitation of phenobarbital by these methods is based on the difference in optical density at pH 13 and at pH 10.5 or at pH 9 and at pH 1.5. The spectrophotometric methods have been optimized to achieve a better separation of phenobarbital from phenytoin through a differential back extraction into various buffers and an improved technique of separation of the aqueous and organic phases. These modifications also gave better recovery and precision. In addition, the number of operations was reduced to make the procedure more suitable for routine monitoring.

These improvements were included in a method reported by Olesen in 1967 (37). We used a slight modification of this procedure for several years in our laboratory for routine analysis of phenobarbital (and phenytoin) in patients with epilepsy.

The possibility of interfering substances still exists, and drugs such as salicylates, sulfonamides, and other barbiturates may interfere with the determination of phenobarbital. Thus, spectrophotometric methods easily give false results in inexperienced hands or when drug intake is unknown.

In 1969, Wallace (71) described a method for simultaneous determination of phenytoin and phenobarbital. After extraction with chloroform, phenytoin is converted to benzophenone by permanganate oxidation, whereas phenobarbital is determined by differential absorption at pH values of 12 and 10.5. Phenobarbital does not interfere with phenytoin or vice versa. Additional improvements of this method have been reported recently (21).

Even if spectrophotometric methods for determination of phenobarbital can give excellent results in the absence of interfering compounds, these techniques can hardly be recommended for routine monitoring of patients with epilepsy. Patients are often treated with various drugs, and these are not always reported to the laboratory. Accordingly, there is a great risk of false results as has been shown in quality control schemes (48).

About 25 years ago spectrophotometric methods based on countercurrent extraction were also reported for the metabolite p-hydroxyphenobarbital (10,70), but these methods are of little interest today.

Thin-Layer Chromatography

To avoid interfering substances and problems with spectrophotometric analysis of phenobarbital, thin-layer chromatographic systems have been useful. This technique also allows analysis of multiple antiepileptic drugs. Instead of extensive solvent partition extractions, separation is achieved on the chromatographic plate.

In 1965, Morrison and Chatten (35) reported a method for estimation of barbiturates by quantitative thin-layer chromatography. Later Olesen (36) described a chromatographic procedure for determination of phenytoin in serum in the presence of barbiturates, other antiepileptics, and various other drugs. The quantitation was based on visual inspection after staining of the plates. It was also possible to quantitate phenobarbital for clinical use by this procedure, although the visual inspection of this drug was associated with more uncertainty because of its larger and more extensive range of values. These methods were not more accurate, except at low concentrations, than spectrophotometric methods, but the specificity was considerably increased. They were used both as a check on concentrations found by spectrophotometric methods and when interfering drugs were reported.

Olesen (38) also developed a method for specific determination of phenobarbital in serum in the presence of other barbiturates, sulfonamides, salicylates, and other interfering drugs. This method was based on a rapid two-dimensional, thin-layer chromatographic procedure. The phenobarbital spots were located by means of reference spots, scraped off, and extracted with methanol. The phenobarbital content was calculated based on the difference in optical density at 240 nm between alkaline and acidic solution. Phenobarbital could be separated from 18 sulfonamides, 3 antidiabetic drugs, 17 other barbiturates, salicylic acid, salicylamide, and phenytoin.

We used a modification of this thin-layer chromatographic procedure in our laboratory for several years to complement Olesen's spectrophotometric method (37), and we found them very useful for routine purposes.

Several other semiquantitative and quantitative thin-layer chromatographic screening procedures for anticonvulsants, including phenobarbital, have also been reported (18,45).

Although many of the thin-layer chromatographic methods are specific and reproducible, they are rather complicated and time consuming, with low output. Few studies included metabolites of phenobarbital (11).

Gas–Liquid Chromatography

The determination of phenobarbital by gas–liquid chromatography soon followed thin-layer chromatography and has been widely used because of its high selectivity and sensitivity. Most of these methods also include determination of other antiepileptic drugs. In the last 10 years more than 100 papers on gas chromatographic quantitation of anticonvulsants have been published (47). However, only a few of these publications describe methods of novel character. In fact, a great many of these methods are only modifications of previous techniques. The need for publication of all of these methods is questionable, but precise and specific methods for routine application have been developed, taking the best from many of them.

It is beyond the scope of this chapter to discuss the different phenobarbital methods in detail, but some of the general principles will be outlined.

The gas chromatographic determination of phenobarbital depends on various conditions; variables include specific quantitation of phenobarbital alone or multiple drug analysis, simple or complex extraction procedures, choice of internal standards, use of derivatization, type of column, isothermal or programmed temperature, and type of detector.

Early methods were based on extraction of the drugs, usually with chloroform or ethylene dichloride, evaporation of the solvent, direct injection, and detection by flame ionization. Even though these methods were handy for routine analysis of several drugs, interfering substances often caused problems, and adsorption of the drug to the column produced peak tailing. For optimal results, a multiple-step extraction scheme able to remove normally occurring serum constituents is preferable. This also gives excellent recoveries of the drugs (52).

There are several early reports on analysis of underivatized phenobarbital under various conditions (8,43,67). One recent method, which also allows simultaneous determination of primidone and phenytoin, has been emphasized (7). The drugs are extracted from acidified serum with chloroform, back extracted into alkaline solution in order to separate them from neutral drugs, and then reextracted into chloroform. 5-Ethyl-p-tolylbarbituric acid is used as internal standard. The drugs are chromatographed isothermally on a column packed with 3% OV-17 on Chromosorp® W.H.P., using flame ionization detection.

In another method, a special column packing (2% SP-2110/1% SP-2510-DA on Supelcoport®) is used for the analysis of underivatized phenobarbital and other anticonvulsants, using flame ionization detection (62). The support surface has been deactivated to permit the analysis of nanogram quantities of drug without peak tailing. The liquid phases have been chosen to minimize interference between the antiepileptic drugs and serum components and to give separation of the more commonly used antiepileptic drugs. A single-step extraction procedure or selected extraction procedure may be used. Although isothermal separation is possible, a programmed temperature rise seems to give better results. Generally, a temperature-programmed run tends to give better peak separation.

Derivatization of phenobarbital produces peaks with little or no tailing and increases the volatility of the drug. Methylation is the most commonly used procedure and can be accomplished by various methods. Diazomethane or dimethylsulfate has been used for a methylation reaction prior to the gas chromatographic analysis (4). However, on-column or flash-heater methylation is most widely used for derivatization. Both tetramethylammonium hydroxide (TMAH) and trimethylphenylammonium hydroxide (TMPAH) used as the methyl donor produce good results (9,29,33,39,40,57,68). However, both the rapidity of the injection and the injection port temperature must be standardized. The instability of phenobarbital in strong alkaline solutions is critical, since flash-heater methylation with both TMAH and TMPAH gives decomposition products that can lead to false results. This decomposition depends on the concentration of the base and the time exposed to the base prior to injection. Low concentrations of TMPAH have been reported to decrease phenobarbital decomposition, but excessively low concentrations may give incomplete methylation of other drugs present because extraneous materials found in serum extracts are also methylated.

The controversy over the formation of multiple derivatives with phenobarbital during flash methylation has now been resolved with the introduction of 5-ethyl-5-(p-methylphenyl)-barbituric acid as an internal standard for phenobarbital (19). This compound is structurally similar to phenobarbital; it has the same extraction characteristics, and it also undergoes the same decomposition reactions.

Other alkylation reactions have also been used in the analysis of phenobarbital (15,20). Silylation is an alternative derivative formation method for analysis of antiepileptic drugs, but phenobarbital does not form stable derivatives after this procedure.

An on-column methylation technique using TMAH for determination of phenobarbital and other antiepileptic drugs has recently been emphasized (56). In this method, serum is buffered with phosphate buffer and extracted with toluene. 5-Ethyl-5-(p-methylphenyl)barbituric acid is used as internal standard for phenobarbital. The column is packed with 5% OV-17 on Gas Chrom Q®, and the drugs are detected by flame ionization following a temperature-programmed run. Alternatively, an on-column method using TMPAH has been proposed (55). Serum is extracted with chloroform, and the extracts are washed with hexane to remove normal serum constituents that could interfere with drug analysis. Internal standard, column, and detection are the same as described above, but isothermal separation is used in this method.

Kurata et al. (30) reported on the problems of decomposition by quantitative flash-methylation analysis of phenobarbital. With TMAH as the methylating agent, a small amount of water decomposes phenobarbital and interferes with the quantitative analysis. Thus, both the sample and the methylating agent must be sufficiently dehydrated to attain optimal results. Therefore, it is desirable that phenobarbital be treated with a low TMAH concentration (0.025 M). If phenytoin is also present, the drug is insufficiently methylated in 0.025 M because of contamination from biological fluids. In the simultaneous determination of phenobarbital and phenytoin, a higher concentration of TMAH (0.10–0.20 M) is required for sufficient methylation. Even if these precautions are taken, phenobarbital is frequently decomposed. The hydrolysis decomposition product of phenobarbital has been identified as N-methyl-2-phenyl-butyramide by mass spectrometry. However, the peak height ratio of the sum of these two peaks to the internal standard (cholestane) gives an accurate assay of phenobarbital.

Most gas chromatographic procedures for therapeutic monitoring have involved the use of the flame ionization detector. The sensitivity and selectivity of the nitrogen–phosphorous detector often make it possible to reduce sample size and to eliminate clean-up steps

(5,50,63,66). Thus, as shown by Bente (5), a 50-μl plasma sample can be extracted with methylene chloride, methylated with TMPAH, and run under temperature-programmed conditions with very good results.

However, there are also several problems, usually of chemical origin, in the use of the nitrogen–phosphorous detector, but this detection mode looks promising for routine analysis.

The most precise gas chromatographic method for quantitating phenobarbital is probably comparison of the dimethyl derivative of phenobarbital to a proper internal standard. Methylation seems to have several advantages over underivatized assays as also shown in quality control studies (49).

Gas chromatographic procedures are also described for determination of *p*-hydroxyphenobarbital (25,59,72). Methylation following direct extraction of the free metabolite from urine seems preferable. The conjugated metabolite is determined, following initial acid hydrolysis, to split the conjugation with glucuronic acid.

High-Pressure Liquid Chromatography

Liquid chromatographic separations are based on solubility and not on vapor pressure as in gas chromatography. Various chromatographic conditions may also be used in this method by varying flow rate, polarity of mobile phase, and oven temperature. Hence, there are several procedures for drug analysis based on ion exchange, normal phase, or reverse phase liquid chromatography. Determination of phenobarbital by liquid chromatography is a suitable alternative to gas chromatography (1–3,16,26–28,41,50).

Usually, phenobarbital and other anticonvulsants are extracted into an organic solvent which is evaporated to dryness. The residue is dissolved in a small volume of solvent and chromatographed by reverse phase. Most often, the drugs are detected by a UV detector at 240 nm.

Liquid chromatography offers several advantages over gas chromatographic methods, such as lack of derivatization, faster separation, better sample stability, and smaller sample size.

Gas Chromatography–Mass Spectrometry

The quantitation of both phenobarbital and its metabolites using selected ion detection with a gas chromatograph–mass spectrometer–computer system operated in the chemical ionization mode has been reported in several studies (22,23). By this method, the methylated compounds are separated by gas chromatography and then detected in the mass spectrometer. Alternatively, phenobarbital can be quantitated using a stable isotope-labeled internal standard and chemical ionization/mass spectrometry without prior chromatographic separation (64).

Selected ion monitoring is the most sensitive and specific method for drug analysis. Although this method can be considered as a reference procedure, the instrumentation is costly and technically difficult to operate. It is therefore limited to research laboratories.

Immunoassays

Immunoassays have been widely used in recent years as a technique for analysis of anticonvulsant drugs.

The principle of a radioimmunoassay consists of a radiolabeled ligand that binds to a specific antibody. Added unlabeled ligand competes with the label for binding sites. Measurement of the free or bound label is used for the quantitation of drug present.

Specific radioimmunoassays for determination of phenobarbital are not commercially available, but the technique has been described in several reports (12–14,17,51,58). Generally, radioimmunoassays have the advantage of excellent sensitivity, and it is possible to make the antisera highly specific. Furthermore, a large number of samples can be processed.

The disadvantages of this technique are the limited stability of the radioisotope, that a separation step is required to remove the displaced labeled substance from the antibody-bound labeled substance prior to quantitation, and that a scintillation counter is needed.

Whereas the label in radioimmunoassays is a radioactive isotope, the homogeneous enzyme immunoassays employ an enzyme as a label. In this technique, the drug concentration is quantitated by enzyme activity based on the conversion of NAD^+ to NADH, which can be measured in a spectrophotometer. No separation step is required in this assay.

Recent development of the homogeneous enzyme immunoassay (EMIT®, Syva Company, Palo Alto, California) for phenobarbital and other anticonvulsants has been a major advance in the rapid and accurate analysis of microsamples (42). The reagents are provided as a matched set for each drug. The kits also contain buffer solution and calibrators that are common for all assays. Reagent A is the antibody/substrate reagent, including the specific antibody for phenobarbital, the substrate (glucose-6-phosphate), and NAD^+, while reagent B contains the enzyme-labeled drug.

In the standard procedure, a 50-μl serum or plasma sample is mixed with reagents A and B in consecutive steps using a pipettor/dilutor so that in each step active substance is diluted with buffer. The final mixture is aspirated into a spectrophotometer flow cell thermally regulated to maintain 30°C. After a lag time of 15 sec, the reaction is followed for 30 sec at 340 nm, and the change in absorbance is automatically compared with stored calibration data with results printed in concentration units. Modified procedures for application on various instrument systems are also available. Appropriate instrumentation is essential for satisfactory performance of the assay.

The EMIT® system is designed to be accurate only within the range of calibrators supplied with the system, and optimal results are obtained within the therapeutic range. When excessively high phenobarbital concentrations are obtained, the specimen should be diluted with blank serum. It is also possible to measure low concentrations by a modified procedure including a dilution of the calibrators. Severely hemolytic, lipemic, or icteric samples may cause questionable results, and such samples should be analyzed by an alternative method, or another specimen should be obtained. The phenobarbital assay is equally sensitive to mephobarbital and heptobarbital, and the EMIT® system cannot be used to measure phenobarbital levels

in samples containing these barbiturates. Otherwise, the EMIT® phenobarbital assay is highly specific, and to date, cross reactivity of clinical significance of anticonvulsants and metabolites or other compounds in concomitant therapeutic use has not been encountered (24,54,61).

The accuracy and reproducibility are most satisfactory and of the same order as those of other relevant procedures. The standard procedure may also be modified for determination of phenobarbital and other anticonvulsants in cerebrospinal fluid, saliva, and ultrafiltrates.

The EMIT® phenobarbital assay offers several advantages. The procedure can be performed more quickly than the methods now in use because extraction and concentration are not involved. It requires less than 2 min once the calibration curve is established. Thus, it is possible for the physician to know the drug level during examination or when rapid identification, in case of intoxication, is necessary. Small samples are of most importance, both in children and adults, during intensive monitoring. Capillary samples may be used, and 50 μl of serum or plasma is sufficient for several determinations of both phenobarbital and other anticonvulsants.

However, it must be emphasized that the EMIT® system is designed for specific determination of a single drug, and therefore, simultaneous drug analysis, which is an advantage of certain chromatographic systems, is not possible.

COMPARISON OF METHODS

Numerous methods using various instrumental techniques are available for the analysis of phenobarbital. When a new method is established, it is of utmost importance to make sure that results comparable with other techniques are achieved. Several studies are available for comparison of the various techniques used for phenobarbital assays, such as spectrophotometry, gas–liquid chromatography, high-pressure liquid chromatography, mass spectrometry, radioimmunoassay, and homogeneous enzyme immunoassay (6,14,22,24,28,31,41,50,53,54, 58,65). Some of the data are summarized in

Table 1. In most cases, the comparison data are in good agreement.

The method of choice for determination of phenobarbital depends on the needs of the individual laboratory. Although spectrophotometry is an accurate and reproducible method, the lack of specificity may lead to false results from patient samples, especially when drug intake is unknown. Therefore, this method can hardly be recommended for routine analysis. Thin-layer chromatography is more specific but is too time consuming for busy laboratories. Gas chromatography is a suitable method, but highly skilled operators are needed. The choice of proper internal standard, extraction procedure, chromatographic conditions, and derivatization method is essential for optimal results. Liquid chromatography is an alternative method which offers several advantages, including faster separation, absence of need for derivatization, better sample stability, and smaller sample size. Methods involving mass spectrometers are the ultimate methods and serve as a reference source but are hardly applicable in routine laboratories because of the cost involved. Homogeneous enzyme immunoassay (EMIT®) is the method of choice in many laboratories engaged in specific routine monitoring. The EMIT® system has several advantages over other currently used methods and is a precise, reproducible, and rapid method for determination of phenobarbital in microsamples. However, this method does not

TABLE 1. *Phenobarbital analysis: comparison of methods*

Method	N	Serum PB level (μg/ml $\pm$ SD)	Slope	Intercept	r	Ref.
EMIT GLC	202	—	0.79	2.15	0.97	6
RIA GLC	56	—	0.96	1.76	0.98	14
EMIT GLC	92	21.2 $\pm$ 10.2 21.9 $\pm$ 9.1	0.840	2.40	0.940	24
EMIT Photometry	131	21.4 $\pm$ 8.3 20.7 $\pm$ 8.3	0.970	1.40	0.970	24
EMIT GLC	57	23.3 $\pm$ 10.9 24.7 $\pm$ 12.2	0.860	2.06	0.966	28
EMIT HPLC	50	22.4 $\pm$ 10.6 23.9 $\pm$ 12.3	0.844	2.29	0.976	28
HPLC GLC	140	18.7 $\pm$ 12.0 18.7 $\pm$ 11.5	1.027	−0.50	0.998	28
EMIT GLC	45	22.4 22.6	0.87	—	0.97	31
HPLC EMIT	41	23.1 21.9	1.028	−0.03	0.96	41
GLC-Nitrogen detector HPLC	130	—	0.985	0.43	0.986	50
EMIT GLC	42	37.0 $\pm$ 0.7[a] 38.0 $\pm$ 0.8[a]	0.778	7.45	0.97	54
RIA EMIT	59	—	0.867	1.19	0.909	58
RIA GLC	47	—	0.795	1.45	0.947	58
EMIT GLC	32	—	0.901	0.80	0.917	58
EMIT GLC	36	30.0 30.0	1.04	1.1	0.990	65

[a]SEM.

have the same screening potential as chromatographic methods.

No matter which method is chosen, a quality control program is mandatory.

CONVERSION

Conversion factor:

$$CF = \frac{1000}{mol.\ wt.} = \frac{1000}{232.2} = 4.31$$

Conversion:

$$(\mu g/ml) \times 4.31 = (\mu moles/liter)$$
$$(\mu moles/liter) \div 4.31 = (\mu g/ml)$$

ACKNOWLEDGMENT

The secretarial help of Ms. Trine Thommessen is gratefully acknowledged.

REFERENCES

1. Adams, R. F., Schmidt G. J., and Vandemark, F. L. (1978): A micro liquid column chromatography procedure for twelve anticonvulsants and some of their metabolites. *J. Chromatogr.*, 145:275–284.
2. Adams, R. F., and Vandemark, F. L. (1976): Simultaneous high-pressure liquid-chromatographic determination of some anticonvulsants in serum. *Clin. Chem.*, 22:25–31.
3. Atwell, S. H., Green, V. A., and Haney, W. G. (1975): Development and evaluation of method for simultaneous determination of phenobarbital and diphenylhydantoin in plasma by high pressure liquid chromatography. *J. Pharm. Sci.*, 64:806–809.
4. Baylis, E. M., Fry, D. E., and Marks, V. (1970): Micro-determination of serum phenobarbitone and diphenylhydantoin by gas–liquid chromatography. *Clin. Chim. Acta*, 30:93–103.
5. Bente, H. B. (1978): Nitrogen-selective detectors: Application to quantitation of antiepileptic drugs. In: *Antiepileptic Drugs: Quantitative Analysis and Interpretation*, edited by C. E. Pippenger, J. K. Penry, and H. Kutt, pp. 139–145. Raven Press, New York.
6. Booker, H. E., and Darcey, B. A. (1975): Enzymatic immunoassay vs. gas–liquid chromatography for determination of phenobarbital and diphenylhydantoin in serum. *Clin. Chem.*, 21:1766–1768.
7. Booker, H. E., and Darcey, B. A. (1978): Phenobarbital, primidone, and phenytoin: Simultaneous determination without derivatization. In: *Antiepileptic Drugs: Quantitative Analysis and Interpretation*, edited by C. E. Pippenger, J. K. Penry, and H. Kutt, pp. 342–345. Raven Press, New York.
8. Bredesen, J. E., and Johannessen, S. I. (1974): Simultaneous determination of some antiepileptic drugs by gas–liquid chromatography. *Epilepsia*, 15:611–617.
9. Brochmann-Hanssen, E., and Oke, T. O. (1969): Gas chromatography of barbiturates, phenolic alkaloids, and xanthine bases: Flash-heater methylation by means of trimethylanilinium hydroxide. *J. Pharm. Sci.*, 58:370–371.
10. Butler, T. C. (1956): The metabolic hydroxylation of phenobarbital. *J. Pharmacol. Exp. Ther.*, 116:326–336.
11. Christiansen, J. (1975): Determination of hydroxymetabolites of phenobarbitone and phenytoin. In: *Clinical Pharmacology of Anti-Epileptic Drugs*, edited by H. Schneider, D. Janz, C. Gardner-Thorpe, H. Meinardi, and A. L. Sherwin, pp. 131–134. Springer-Verlag, Berlin, Heidelberg, New York.
12. Cleeland, R., Davis, R., Heveran, J., and Grunberg, E. (1975): A simple ^{125}I-radioimmunoassay for the detection of barbiturates in biological fluids. *J. Forensic Sci.*, 20:45.
13. Cook, C. E., Amerson, E., Poole, W. K., Lesser, P., and O'Tuama, L. (1975): Phenytoin and phenobarbital concentrations in saliva and plasma measured by radioimmunoassay. *Clin. Pharmacol. Ther.*, 18:742–747.
14. Cook, C. E., Christensen, H. D., Amerson, E. W., Kepler, J. A., Tallent, C. R., and Taylor, G. F. (1976): Radioimmunoassay of anticonvulsant drugs: Phenytoin, phenobarbital and primidone. In: *Quantitative Analytic Studies in Epilepsy*, edited by P. Kellaway and I. Petersén, pp. 39–59. Raven Press, New York.
15. Ehrsson, H. (1974): Gas chromatographic determination of barbiturates after extractive methylation in carbon disulfide. *Anal. Chem.*, 46:922–924.
16. Evans, J. E. (1973): Simultaneous measurements of diphenylhydantoin and phenobarbitone in serum by HPLC. *Anal. Chem.*, 45:2428–2429.
17. Flynn, E. J., and Spector, S. (1972): Determination of barbiturate derivatives by radioimmunoassay. *J. Pharmacol. Exp. Ther.*, 181:547–554.
18. Gardner-Thorpe, C., Parsonage, M. J., and Toothill, C. (1971): A comprehensive scheme for the evaluation of anticonvulsant concentrations in blood using thin-layer chromatography. *Clin. Chim. Acta*, 35:29–47.
19. Gibbs, E. L., and Gibbs, T. J. (1974): Gas–liquid chromatographic determination of antiepilepsy drugs and their active metabolites in blood. In: *Gibbs Laboratory Reports, February 20*. Evanston, Illinois.
20. Greeley, R. H. (1974): New approach to derivatization and gas-chromatographic analysis of barbiturates. *Clin. Chem.*, 20:192–194.
21. Hamilton, H. E., and Wallace, J. E. (1978): Ultraviolet spectrophotometric quantitation of phenytoin and phenobarbital. In: *Antiepileptic Drugs: Quantitative Analysis and Interpretation*, edited by C. E. Pippenger, J. K. Penry, and H. Kutt, pp. 175–183. Raven Press, New York.
22. Horning, M. G., Brown, L., Nowlin, J., Lertratanangkoon, K., Kellaway, P., and Zion, T. E. (1977): Use of saliva in therapeutic drug monitoring. *Clin. Chem.*, 23:157–164.
23. Horning, M. G., Lertratanangkoon, K., Nowlin, J., Stillwell, W. G., Stillwell, R. N., Zion, T. E., Kel-

laway, P., and Hill, R. M. (1974): Anticonvulsant drug monitoring by GC–MS–COM techniques. *J. Chromatogr. Sci.,* 12:630–631.

24. Johannessen, S. I. (1977): Evaluation of enzyme multiplied immunoassay technique (EMIT) in routine analysis of antiepileptic drugs. A comparison of methods. In: *Antiepileptic Drug Monitoring,* edited by C. Gardner-Thorpe, D. Janz, H. Meinardi, and C. E. Pippenger, pp. 7–20. Pitman Medical, Kent.

25 Kållberg, N., Agurell, S., Ericsson, O., Bucht, E., Jalling, B., and Boréus, L. O. (1975): Quantitation of phenobarbital and its main metabolites in human urine. *Eur. J. Clin. Pharmacol.,* 9:161–168.

26. Kabra, P. M., Gotelli, G., Stanfill, R., and Marton, L. J. (1976): Simultaneous measurement of phenobarbital, diphenylhydantoin and primidone in blood by HPLC. *Clin. Chem.,* 22:824–827.

27. Kabra, P. M., McDonald, D. M., and Marton, L. J. (1978): A simultaneous high-pressure liquid chromatographic analysis of the most common anticonvulsants and their metabolites in serum. *J. Anal. Toxicol.,* 2:127–133.

28. Kumps, A., Mardens, Y., and Scharpé, S. (1980): Comparison between HPLC, gas–liquid chromatography, and enzyme-immunoassay for the determination of antiepileptic drugs in serum. In: *Antiepileptic Therapy: Advances in Drug Monitoring,* edited by S. I. Johannessen, P. L. Morselli, C. E. Pippenger, A. Richens, D. Schmidt, and H. Meinardi, pp. 341–347. Raven Press, New York.

29. Kupferberg, H. J. (1970): Quantitative estimation of diphenylhydantoin, primidone and phenobarbital in plasma by gas–liquid chromatography. *Clin. Chim. Acta,* 29:283–288.

30. Kurata, K., Takeuchi, M., and Yoshida, K. (1979): Quantitative flash-methylation analysis of phenobarbital. *J. Pharm. Sci.,* 68:1187–1189.

31. Legaz, M., and Raisys, V. A. (1976): Correlation of the "EMIT" antiepileptic drug assay with a gas–liquid chromatographic method. *Clin. Biochem.,* 9:35–38.

32. Lous, P. (1950): Quantitative determination of barbiturates. *Acta Pharmacol.,* 6:227–234.

33. MacGee, J. (1971): Rapid identification and quantitative determination of barbiturates and glutethimide in blood by gas chromatography. *Clin. Chem.,* 17:587–591.

34. Meijer, J. W. A., Meinardi, H., Gardner-Thorpe, C., and van der Kleijn, E. (1973): *Methods of Analysis of Antiepileptic Drugs.* Excerpta Medica, Amsterdam; American Elsevier, New York.

35. Morrison, J. C., and Chatten, L. G. (1965): Estimation of barbiturates by quantitative thin-layer chromatography. *J. Pharm. Pharmacol.,* 17:655–658.

36. Olesen, O. V. (1967): A simplified method for extracting phenytoin from serum, and a more sensitive staining reaction for quantitative determination by thin-layer chromatography. *Acta Pharmacol.,* 25:123–126.

37. Olesen, O. V. (1967): Determination of phenobarbital and phenytoin in serum by ultraviolet spectrophotometry. *Scand. J. Clin. Lab. Invest.,* 20:63–69.

38. Olesen, O. V. (1967): Determination of phenobarbital in serum in presence of other barbiturates, sulphon-

amides, salicylates and other interfering drugs. *Scand. J. Clin. Lab. Invest.,* 20:109–112.

39. Osiewicz, R., Agarwal, V., Young, R. M., and Sunshine, I. (1974): The quantitative analysis of phenobarbital with trimethylanilinium hydroxide. *J. Chromatogr.,* 88:157–164.

40. Perchalski, R. J., and Wilder, B. J. (1973): GC assay of phenobarbital. *Clin. Chem.,* 19:788–789.

41. Pesh-Imam, M., Fretthold, D. W., Sunshine, I., Kumar, S., Terrentine, S., and Willis, C. E. (1979): High pressure liquid chromatography for simultaneous analysis of anticonvulsants: Comparison with EMIT® system. *Ther. Drug. Monitor.,* 1:289–299.

42. Pippenger, C. E., Bastiani, R. J., and Schneider, R. S. (1975): Evaluation of an experimental homogenous enzyme immunoassay for the quantitation of phenytoin and phenobarbitone in serum or plasma. In: *Clinical Pharmacology of Anti-Epileptic Drugs,* edited by H. Schneider, D. Janz, C. Gardner-Thorpe, H. Meinardi, and A. L. Sherwin, pp. 331–335. Springer-Verlag, Berlin, Heidelberg, New York.

43. Pippenger, C. E., and Gillen, H. W. (1969): Gas chromatographic analysis for anticonvulsant drugs in biological fluids. *Clin. Chem.,* 16:582–590.

44. Pippenger, C. E., Penry, J. K., and Kutt, H. (1978): *Antiepileptic Drugs: Quantitative Analysis and Interpretation.* Raven Press, New York.

45. Pippenger, C. E., Scott, J. E., and Gillen, H. W. (1969): Thin-layer chromatography of anticonvulsant drugs. *Clin. Chem.,* 15:255–260.

46. Plaa, G. L., and Hine, C. H. (1956): A method for the simultaneous determination of phenobarbital and diphenylhydantoin in blood. *J. Lab. Clin. Med.,* 47:649–657.

47. Rambeck, B. (1980): Systematic review of gas chromatographic methods for the determination of antiepileptic drugs. In: *Antiepileptic Therapy: Advances in Drug Monitoring,* edited by S. I. Johannessen, P. L. Morselli, C. E. Pippenger, A. Richens, D. Schmidt, and H. Meinardi, pp. 365–372. Raven Press, New York.

48. Richens, A. (1975): Quality control of drug estimations. *Acta Neurol. Scand. [Suppl.],* 60:81–84.

49. Richens, A. (1975): Results of a phenytoin quality control scheme. In: *Clinical Pharmacology of Anti-Epileptic Drugs,* edited by H. Schneider, D. Janz, C. Gardner-Thorpe, H. Meinardi, and A. L. Sherwin, pp. 293–303. Springer-Verlag, Berlin, Heidelberg, New York.

50. Rovei, V., Sanjuan, M., and Morselli, P. L. (1980): Comparison between HPLC and GLC-ND analytical methods for the determination of AED in plasma and blood of patients. In: *Antiepileptic Therapy: Advances in Drug Monitoring,* edited by S. I. Johannessen, P. L. Morselli, C. E. Pippenger, A. Richens, D. Schmidt, and H. Meinardi, pp. 349–356. Raven Press, New York.

51. Sato, H., Kuroiwa, Y., Hamadas, A., and Uematsu, T. (1974): Radioimmunoassay for phenobarbital. *J. Biochem.,* 76:1301–1306.

52. Schäfer, H. R. (1975): Some problems concerning the quantitative assay of primidone and its metabolites. In: *Clinical Pharmacology of Antiepileptic Drugs,* edited by H. Schneider, D. Janz, C. Gardner-Thorpe,

H. Meinardi, and A. L. Sherwin, pp. 124–130. Springer-Verlag, Berlin, Heidelberg, New York.

53. Schmidt, D., Goldberg, V., Guelen, P. J. M., Johannessen, S., van der Kleijn, E., Meijer, J. W. A., Meinardi, H., Richens, A., Schneider, H., Stein-Lavie, Y., and Symann-Louette, N. (1977): Evaluation of a new immunoassay for determination of phenytoin and phenobarbital. Results of a European collaborative control study. *Epilepsia,* 18:367–374.

54. Schottelius, D. D. (1978): Homogeneous immunoassay system (EMIT) for quantitation of antiepileptic drugs in biological fluids. In: *Antiepileptic Drugs: Quantitative Analysis and Interpretation,* edited by C. E. Pippenger, J. K. Penry, and H. Kutt, pp. 95–108. Raven Press, New York.

55. Sichler, D. W., and Pippenger, C. E. (1978): Phenobarbital, carbamazepine, primidone, and phenytoin: Simultaneous determination with on-column methylation (TMPAH). In: *Antiepileptic Drugs: Quantitative Analysis and Interpretation,* edited by C. E. Pippenger, J. K. Penry, and H. Kutt, pp. 335–338. Raven Press, New York.

56. Solow, E. B. (1978): Phenytoin, phenobarbital, primidone, and ethosuximide: Simultaneous determination with on-column methylation (TMAH). In: *Antiepileptic Drugs: Quantitative Analysis and Interpretation,* edited by C. E. Pippenger, J. K. Penry, and H. Kutt, pp. 338–342. Raven Press, New York.

57. Solow, E. B., Metaxas, J. M., and Summers, T. R. (1974): A current assessment of simultaneous determination of multiple drug therapy by gas liquid chromatography. On-column methylation. *J. Chromatogr. Sci.,* 12:256–259.

58. Spiehler, V., Sun, L., Miyada, D. S., Sarandis, S. G., Walwick, E. R., Klein, M. W., Jordan, D. B., and Jessen, B. (1976): Radioimmunoassay, spectrophotometry and gas–liquid chromatography compared for determination of phenobarbital and diphenylhydantoin. *Clin. Chem.,* 22:749–753.

59. Svendsen, A. B., and Brochman-Hanssen, E. (1962): Gas chromatography of barbiturates. II. Application to the study of their metabolism and excretion in humans. *J. Pharm. Sci.,* 51:494–495.

60. Svensmark, O., and Kristensen, P. (1963): Determination of diphenylhydantoin in small amounts of serum. *J. Lab. Clin. Med.,* 61:501–507.

61. Syva (1976): *Antiepileptic Drug Assays, Syva Bulletin 6A164-1.* Syva, Palo Alto.

62. Thoma, J. J., Ewald, T., and McCoy, M. (1978): Simultaneous analysis of underivatized phenobarbital, carbamazepine, primidone and phenytoin by isothermal chromatography. *J. Anal. Toxicol.,* 2:219–225.

63. Toseland, P. A., Albani, M., and Gauchel, F. D. (1975): Organic nitrogen-selective detector used in gas-chromatographic determination of some anticonvulsant and barbiturate drugs in plasma and tissues. *Clin. Chem.,* 21:98–103.

64. Truscott, R. J. W., Burke, D. G., Korth, J., and Halpern, B. (1978): Simultaneous determination of diphenylhydantoin, mephobarbital, carbamazepine, phenobarbital and primidone in serum using direct chemical ionization mass-spectrometry. *Biomed. Mass Spectrom.,* 5:477–482.

65. Urquhart, N., Godolphin, W., and Campbell, D. J. (1979): Evaluation of automated enzyme immunoassays for five anticonvulsants and theophylline adapted to a centrifugal analyzer. *Clin. Chem.,* 25:785–787.

66. Vandemark, F. L., and Adams, R. F. (1976): Ultramicro gas-chromatographic analysis for anticonvulsants, with use of a nitrogen-selective detector. *Clin. Chem.,* 22:1062–1065.

67. Van Meter, J. C., Buckmaster, H. S., and Shelley, L. L. (1970): Concurrent assay of phenobarbital and diphenylhydantoin in plasma by vapor-phase chromatography. *Clin. Chem.,* 16:135–138.

68. Van Meter, J. C., and Gillen, H. W. (1973): A source of variation in the gas chromatographic assay of phenobarbital treated with trimethylanilinium hydroxide. *Clin. Chem.,* 19:359–360.

69. Vida, J. A., and Gerry, E. H. (1977): Cyclic ureides. In: *Anticonvulsants,* edited by J. A. Vida, pp. 151–291. Academic Press, New York.

70. Waddell, W. J., and Butler, T. C. (1957): The distribution and excretion of phenobarbital. *J. Clin. Invest.,* 36:1217–1226.

71. Wallace, J. E. (1969): Simultaneous spectrophotometric determination of diphenylhydantoin and phenobarbital in biologic specimens. *Clin. Chem.,* 15:323–330.

72. Williamson, R. A., and Kutt, H. (1978): HPPH and *p*-hydroxyphenobarbital: Determination in urine. In: *Antiepileptic Drugs: Quantitative Analysis and Interpretation,* edited by C. E. Pippenger, J. K. Penry, H. Kutt, pp. 354–355. Raven Press, New York.

73. Woodbury, D. M., Penry, J. K., and Schmidt, R. P. (1972): *Antiepileptic Drugs.* Raven Press, New York.

Antiepileptic Drugs, edited by D. M. Woodbury, J. K. Penry, and C. E. Pippenger. Raven Press, New York © 1982.

22

Phenobarbital

Absorption, Distribution, and Excretion

E. W. Maynert

ABSORPTION

Although most textbooks of pharmacology suggest that the barbiturates are rapidly and completely absorbed from the gastrointestinal tract, quantitive data to support this view are scarce. The most direct way to examine extent of absorption—analysis of the feces—has rarely been undertaken in connection with phenobarbital, mephobarbital, or metharbital. In a study in rats, Kojima et al. (28) observed that only about 1% of a 100 mg/kg dose of phenobarbital reached the large intestine.

Extent of Absorption

Indirect evidence indicates that phenobarbital administered orally to adult epileptic patients in daily doses of 2.1 to 3.2 mg/kg is nearly completely absorbed. Butler et al. (13) calculated plasma concentrations of the drug by a mathematical formula[1] requiring knowledge of the daily dose, the volume of distribution of the drug, and the proportion of the drug eliminated daily. On the basis of data collected in dogs, the volume of distribution of phenobarbital was assumed to be 75% of the body weight. The rate of elimination of the drug was measured by analysis of the plasma at various intervals over a period of at least 7 days after withdrawal of the drug. In five patients, the calculated concentration of phenobarbital averaged 26 μg/ml in comparison with 28 μg/ml actually observed.

Using similar methods, Svensmark and Buchthal (47) found excellent agreement between the calculated and observed plasma concentrations of phenobarbital in five adult patients during the accumulation of the drug over a period of 11 to 22 days of treatment. The dosage form was not specified but was probably a commercial preparation commonly used in Denmark. The doses ranged from 0.59 to 2.3 mg/kg. The volume of distribution was assumed to be 60% of the body weight. This figure may be too low, but it seems certain that at least 80% of the drug was absorbed.

Calculations based on plasma concentrations of barbiturates in three human subjects who received 0.2 g of mephobarbital (tablets) three times a day for 14 days led Butler and Waddell (14) to conclude that this drug is poorly absorbed. On the day after administration of the drug had been discontinued, the sum of the amounts of mephobarbital and phenobarbital (its

---

[1] $c = d/v(p + p^2/2)$, where c is the equilibrium plasma concentration (mg/liter), d is the daily dose (mg/kg) assumed to be given continuously at a constant rate rather than at one time, v is the volume of distribution in percent of body weight, and p is the proportion of drug eliminated daily after administration of the drug is discontinued.

primary metabolite) remaining in the body plus the amount of phenobarbital lost by metabolism and excretion were equivalent to only 50 to 60% of the total amount of drug administered. Unless mephobarbital is metabolized in man by reactions other than demethylation, incomplete absorption seems the most reasonable explanation for this result. In the dog, intravenously administered mephobarbital was almost completely converted to phenobarbital, but orally administered mephobarbital gave plasma concentrations of phenobarbital only about half those obtained from equimolar doses of phenobarbital (11). These observations are in harmony with the fact that the usual doses of mephobarbital employed for the treatment of epilepsy are about double those of phenobarbital. It is probable that the poor absorption of mephobarbital results from its insolubility in water. Phenobarbital is about 20 times more soluble.

In one human subject reported on by Butler and Waddell (14), mephobarbital appeared to be absorbed completely after the oral administration of 0.2 g three times a day. When placed on this regimen, this man experienced central depression on two occasions severe enough to require discontinuation of the treatment. Analysis of his plasma for barbiturates revealed that nearly all of the administered dose could be accounted for as mephobarbital and phenobarbital in the body and phenobarbital eliminated by metabolism and excretion. The concentration of mephobarbital achieved in the plasma was two to three times higher than that observed in other subjects on the same regimen. This finding could account for the depression, for the hypnotic activity of mephobarbital is greater than that of phenobarbital. Inasmuch as this man had no apparent defect in his capacity to demethylate mephobarbital, the accumulation of this drug was attributed to absorption at a rate exceeding that at which it could be demethylated. It is not known what proportion of the population can absorb mephobarbital completely, but whatever the incidence, individual variation in absorption is an undesirable feature of a drug.

Although plasma concentrations of metharbital and its primary metabolite, barbital, have been measured after oral administration in man (14) and the dog (12), no estimates have been published on the completeness of absorption of this barbiturate.

Rate of Absorption

The rate of absorption of barbiturates from the gastrointestinal tract depends on the preparation administered as well as on physiological factors such as gastric emptying. The rate of disintegration of tablets or capsules, the chemical form of the drug (i.e., whether free acid or salt), the crystal size, the tendency of the crystals to become wet, and the solubility of the drug in water all influence the speed of entry into the circulation. These variables have been only partially examined in connection with phenobarbital (30). An investigation (44) of other barbiturates in man demonstrated that sodium salts are absorbed more rapidly than free acids. The rate of absorption was maximal when the drug was dissolved in water prior to ingestion. The importance of wettability and/or crystal size is well illustrated by Bush (9). He found that a large dose of methanol-recrystallized hexobarbital failed to produce hypnosis in a dog when administered by stomach tube in the form of a suspension in water. A few days later, the same animal was given the same dose in the same manner, but this time the drug was dissolved in alkali and precipitated with acid immediately before administration. The dog now became anesthetized in a few minutes.

Despite the clinical impression that barbiturates are absorbed rather rapidly from the gastrointestinal tract, numerous investigations have shown that several hours may elapse before blood concentrations of the drug reach a peak. For example, in three young men given 750 mg of phenobarbital powder with 500 ml of water, Lous (31) observed the highest plasma concentrations 6 to 8 hr after intake. He suggested that the slow rate of absorption in these experiments might be partly attributable to the large dose and the insolubility of the drug. In cases of fatal poisoning, phenobarbital crystals have been observed in the stomach as long as 12 hr after ingestion of the drug. Although barbiturates can be absorbed from the stomach, under normal circumstances most of the drug enters the circulation from the small intestine (25,28). Drugs that affect the circulation or the motility of the gastrointestinal tract may influence the rate of absorption of barbiturates. In mice, Frey and Kampmann (17) showed that DL-amphetamine delayed the absorption of phenobarbital, phenytoin, and ethosuximide. In rats, Magnussen (35) found that an ethanol concentration of 1.7 mg/ml in the blood or 1 to 10% in the gastric contents expedited the absorption of phenobarbital from the stomach. This effect was attributed to the increased circulation in the gastric mucosa as measured by the secretion of the dye, neutral red. In these experiments, alcohol had no effect on the intestinal absorption of phenobarbital. Certain gastrointestinal diseases might be expected to influence the absorption of barbiturates, but there are no data on this point.

The classical studies of Schanker (42) demonstrated the importance of lipid solubility of the undissociated forms of the barbiturates in determining the rates of absorption of these drugs from the stomach, the small intestine, and the colon. These drugs can also be absorbed through the buccal mucosa (1). The pK_as of mephobarbital, metharbital, and phenobarbital are 7.70, 8.17, and 7.41, respectively (26). The $CHCl_3/H_2O$ partition coefficients for the corresponding free acids are 63.6, 20.2, and 2.33, respectively (26). From these data, it would be predicted that the rates of absorption from both the stomach and the intestines should follow the order: mephobarbital > metharbital > phenobarbital. This prediction was realized for the rat stomach, where hourly rate constants of 0.35, 0.18, and 0.14, respectively, were observed (26). This study provided evidence indicating that barbiturate ions can also be absorbed at an appreciable rate. However, the experiments involved exposure of the gastric mucosa to very alkaline solutions, and it is doubtful that the cellular barrier to diffusion remains normal under these conditions.

Investigation of the absorption of barbiturates from the rat small intestine revealed a poor correlation with the $CHCl_3/H_2O$ coefficients (27).

At pH 5.5, the hourly rate constants for mephobarbital, metharbital, and phenobarbital were 1.12, 1.01, and 1.57, respectively. Inasmuch as the drugs were administered in solution, the insolubility of the N-methyl derivatives was certainly not responsible for the unexpectedly slow absorption rates of mephobarbital and metharbital. In view of the finding that N-methylbarbiturates were distinctly inferior to oxybarbiturates in binding to intestinal mucosal suspensions, it was suggested that absorption from the small intestine depends more on protein binding than on simple diffusion through a lipoid barrier.

Routes Other than Oral

In five healthy men, Viswanathan and co-workers (48) compared serum concentrations of phenobarbital after the ingestion of commercial tablets of the free acid or injection into the deltoid muscle of the sodium salt dissolved in a mixture of 67% propylene glycol, 10% ethanol, and 23% water. The peak concentrations were slightly higher after oral administration (0.72 vs 0.67 µg/ml), but other pharmacokinetic parameters were not significantly different. The authors concluded that unless oral administration is not feasible, intramuscular phenobarbital offers no clinical advantage. An exception may be newborns treated for seizures. In such patients, Boréus and co-workers (2) observed that oral doses were absorbed at a considerably slower rate than intramuscular doses. Phenobarbital incorporated into rectal suppositories with lipophilic or hydrophilic excipients was absorbed less well in dogs than orally administered drug (3,30).

DISTRIBUTION

The pattern of localization of barbiturates in the various tissues of the body depends on the time elapsed between administration of the drug and sacrifice of the animal for dissection and analysis. Although the process of distribution can be conveniently considered as involving early (i.e., nonequilibrium) and late phases, no drug achieves true equilibrium during its sojourn in the body.

Early Distribution

Shortly after absorption, phenobarbital is present in high concentrations in the more vascular organs of the body. The outstanding exception is the brain (15). In mice, Butler (10) showed that the slow onset of anesthesia after the intravenous administration of barbital could be explained by the slow accumulation of the drug in the brain. In this species, in which most or all pharmacological effects occur more rapidly than in man, 20 to 60 min were required to achieve peak concentrations of the drug in the brain. A similar lag in the appearance of anesthesia is a prominent characteristic of phenobarbital in all laboratory animals. It may be presumed that this drug also enters the human brain slowly. When phenobarbital is used to terminate status epilepticus, immediate efficacy cannot be expected. Recently, Ramsay and colleagues (40) showed that diazepam entered the cerebral cortex of cats more rapidly than did phenobarbital.

The ability of a drug to enter the brain and accumulate in the cerebrospinal fluid is related to its oil/water partition coefficient (6). The coefficients of phenobarbital and barbital are low; those of thiopental and the N-methylbarbiturates, including metharbital, are very high. The latter group of drugs penetrates the brain more rapidly than most of the other organs. Thus, the central depressant effects, which are almost instantaneous in onset after intravenous administration of the drugs, diminish rapidly as the drugs accumulate in less vascular organs, particularly muscle, at the expense of drug removed from the brain. The research of Roth and Barlow (41) has shown that phenobarbital and thiopental differ strikingly in their distribution within the brain of the adult cat. Phenobarbital enters the gray matter more rapidly than the white. This difference appears to depend on a barrier presented by the lamination of the myelin sheaths. In the course of a few hours, the drug becomes approximately uniformly distributed throughout the brain. Unlike phenobarbital, thiopental accumulates in the brain according to the vascular supply of its various regions. Ultimately, this drug also becomes evenly distributed in the brain.

Late Distribution

A few hours after intravenous administration, phenobarbital is found in nearly equal concentrations in all the tissues of the body. Data in man derived from autopsy specimens have been collected haphazardly and are incomplete. In rabbits killed 1 hr after an intravenous dose of 50 mg/kg, Goldbaum and Smith (21) found the following concentrations (in μg/ml) of drug: whole blood, 7.5; plasma, 7.5; liver, 8.7; heart, 6.4; kidney, 6.6; lung, 5.4; brain 5.0; and muscle, 5.2. The concentration of drug in fat was not measured but would not be expected to be high. Pentobarbital, which has a higher oil/water coefficient than phenobarbital, achieves concentrations in fat about equal to those in plasma and about double those in plasma water (5). Svensmark and Buchthal (47) commented that their one serious failure in calculating plasma concentrations of phenobarbital was encountered in an obese woman. The observed values were significantly higher than the calculated, a finding that suggests that the drug was largely excluded from fat.

The cerebrospinal fluid and saliva, which contain only small amounts of protein, exhibit lower concentrations of phenobarbital than are observed in plasma. In patients receiving the drug alone or in combination with other antiepileptic medication, the CSF/plasma ratio was about 0.47, and the saliva/plasma ratio about 0.35 (43). The lower level in saliva can be explained by nonionic diffusion into a fluid with a lower pH. The concentration of phenobarbital in milk was observed to be 8 μg/ml in a woman receiving a daily dose of 225 mg (50). On the assumption of a daily intake of 100 ml/kg of this milk, an infant would receive a dose of 0.8 mg/kg of drug. Despite the slow rate of elimination of phenobarbital in neonates, the accumulation of drug would not be expected to reach levels that exert serious neurological effects.

In contrast with phenobarbital, mephobarbital and metharbital probably reach relatively high concentrations in fat. In dogs, the volumes of distribution of mephobarbital (11) and metharbital (12) were calculated to be 200% and 122% of the body weight, respectively. Comparable values for phenobarbital and barbital are 75% and 60%, respectively. These estimates are not corrected for binding of the drugs to plasma proteins. The volume of distribution of phenobarbital is larger in neonates than in children or adults (23,38). The tissue distribution of mephobarbital and metharbital has not been studied systematically. Büch et al. (8) observed that in rats the dextrorotary isomer of mephobarbital was preferentially accumulated by the brain.

Protein Binding

Phenobarbital is bound to both plasma and tissue proteins. Waddell and Butler (49) examined binding in a 4% solution of bovine serum albumin in phosphate buffers. Maximal binding amounting to 46% was observed at pH 7.6. At pH 6.1 and 8.6, binding amounted to 36% and 41%, respectively. This rather small effect of pH suggests that the intrinsic binding constants of the ionic and undissociated forms of the drug are nearly equal. Binding decreased as the albumin concentration decreased. The proportion of phenobarbital bound was almost independent of the concentration of the drug over the range of 20 to 100 μg/ml. Human serum albumin did not differ significantly from bovine albumin, and dog and human plasma were found to be equivalent to a solution of albumin of the same concentration. These findings are in fair agreement with the results of others (21,31,32). In contrast, lower binding to plasma proteins was observed in neonates: 32% versus 51% in children (19). Protein binding by mephobarbital and metharbital has apparently not received any study.

Goldbaum and Smith (21) observed that rabbit tissue homogenates were capable of binding more barbiturate than could be accounted for by their content of albumin. The extent of binding *in vitro* approximately paralleled the concentrations of drug observed in the tissue *in vivo*. These findings suggest that certain tissue proteins resemble albumin in being able to bind drugs. These workers showed that thiopental, a strongly bound barbiturate, could displace an appreciable fraction of bound pentobarbital or secobarbital from albumin. The fact that the displacement of the oxybarbiturates could not be driven to completion suggests that oxy- and thiobarbiturates do not utilize exactly the same binding sites. The possibility that drugs can displace phenobarbital from plasma and tissue binding sites and thereby accentuate toxic effects must be seriously considered. However, there is presently no evidence that this process has important clinical consequences. Whether tissue binding, like plasma protein binding, is lower in neonates than in adults is apparently unknown.

Effect of pH on Distribution

In experiments on dogs, Waddell and Butler (49) showed that decreasing the blood pH decreased the plasma concentration of phenobarbital; increasing the blood pH had the opposite effect. For example, in an animal anesthetized by a 125 mg/kg dose, the inhalation of 29% carbon dioxide caused the blood pH to fall from 7.2 to 6.8 and the plasma concentration of drug to decrease from 145 to 95 μg/ml. The intravenous infusion of sodium bicarbonate in an amount sufficient to elevate the pH from 7.3 to 7.6 raised the drug concentration from 125 to 145 μg/ml. An examination of brain, fat, liver, and muscle showed that the tissue concentrations of drug changed in the opposite direction to that of the blood pH. The normal brain/plasma concentration ratio of 0.9 rose to 1.4 in acidotic animals and fell to 0.7 in alkalotic animals.

The changes in plasma and tissue concentrations of phenobarbital result primarily from alterations in the concentration of the ionic form of the drug. The shift of drug between the tissues and plasma can be explained by assuming that the intracellular pH remains relatively constant and that the cellular membrane is permeable to the un-ionized but not the ionic form. Acidosis, whatever the cause, is accompanied by a decrease of the ionic form in the extracellular fluid and diffusion of the un-ionized form into the tissues. Alkalosis, whether respiratory or metabolic in origin, increases the concentration of the ionic form in the extracellular fluids and thereby causes the passage of drug out of the tissues.

In these experiments, alkalosis was noted to reduce the intensity of the anesthesia. This observation was supported by the measurement of median anesthetic doses (AD_{50}) in mice. Elevation of the blood pH to 7.41 from 7.23 increased the AD_{50} of phenobarbital by 20%. In contrast, alkalosis of the same degree increased the AD_{50} of barbital by only 10% and that of ether not at all. The greater effect on phenobarbital than on barbital can be attributed to its lower pK_a (7.2 versus 7.7 at 37° and ionic strength 0.16). The proportional change in the concentration of the un-ionized form resulting from a small departure from pH 7.4 is greater for phenobarbital than for the dialkylbarbiturates or N-methylbarbiturates. Inasmuch as alkalosis involves a removal of the drug from the brain, it would be expected to decrease the antiepileptic efficacy of phenobarbital. Likewise, acidosis, which increases the concentration of drug in the central nervous system, may accentuate the neurotoxicity of phenobarbital.

Distribution in the Fetus and Neonate

Barbiturates can cross the placental barrier and enter the fetus. The rate of this process has not been studied in connection with the barbiturates used for the treatment of epilepsy, but whole body autoradiography of pregnant mice demonstrated that, 30 min after the injection of ^{14}C-barbital, the fetal organs contained less drug than any maternal organ except the brain (29). The autoradiographic density of the fetal brain was comparable to that of other organs, a finding in accord with numerous other observations that the blood−brain barrier is not fully developed in the fetus. Four hours after administration of the drug, when it may be presumed that the maternal blood concentration of drug had diminished considerably (16), the uterine contents showed higher radioactivity than the maternal organs. From this study (29), it would appear that the uptake and release of barbitu-

rates by the fetus are limited in their rates by the circulation.

Ploman and Persson (39) analyzed spectrophotometrically the brains of 35 fetuses 4 to 7 months of age obtained from women who were given barbiturates prior to legal abortion. The distribution of the drug was generally uniform except for the region about the fourth ventricle which contained very high concentrations of drug. The drugs investigated were amobarbital, phenobarbital, and barbital. Earlier, Goldschmidt et al. (22) using a similar analytical method found a threefold enrichment of barbital in tissue from the rhomboid fossa of rats. It may be noted that neither of these investigations provided conclusive evidence that the substance measured was derived from the drug. Studies involving ^{14}C-phenobarbital in cats failed to reveal high concentrations of the isotope in the medulla (15).

In a study in kittens, Domek et al. (15) observed that the unmyelinated white matter of the brain accumulated ^{14}C-phenobarbital more readily than the gray matter. The difference was most apparent in newborn and 1-week-old animals examined autoradiographically 1 hr after the intraperitoneal administration of the sodium salt. In kittens 4 weeks of age, a stage of development at which histological sections revealed definite myelinization in the cerebrum, a diffuse autoradiographic pattern was seen. The brains of 8-week-old animals showed more rapid accumulation of the drug in gray than in white matter, and those of 12-week-old animals were indistinguishable from the adult. The gradually developing hindrance to drug penetration in the white matter was explained on the basis of the laying down of an increasing number of membranes in the formation of myelin. The initial greater concentration of drug in potential white matter may be related to the high water content of this tissue.

EXCRETION

Phenobarbital is partly metabolized and partly excreted unchanged in the urine. Both processes are slow. A number of studies in human adults (4,13,31,33,45) have shown that the drug disappears from the plasma at a rate of 11 to 27% per day; the corresponding range for half-life is 53 to 140 hr. The mean half-life in adults (96 hr) is shorter than that in some neonates and longer than that in children (37,38). The enhanced elimination of phenobarbital characteristic of children has been observed as early as the first month of extrauterine life (24). Between 11 and 25% of a dose, whether given singly or repeatedly, appears unchanged in the urine (36). Although no quantitative data are available, scattered clinical observations indicate that the toxicity of phenobarbital is increased in patients with renal disease (7,34). In rabbits, Fujimoto and Donnelly (18) observed a circadian rhythm in the urinary pH and the urinary excretion of phenobarbital. Whether a similar process occurs in man is unknown. Mephobarbital and metharbital are metabolized much more rapidly than phenobarbital, and only a small fraction of a dose of these drugs appears in the urine. Svendsen and Brochmann-Hanssen (46) could account for less than 1% of a 150-mg dose of mephobarbital and only 1.2% of a 200-mg dose of metharbital as unchanged drug in human urine collected over the course of 48 hr.

Waddell and Butler (49) studied the renal clearance of phenobarbital in two men who received ordinary therapeutic doses of the drug. At urinary flows of 0.8 to 1.2 ml/min, the clearance based on the concentration of unbound drug in the plasma was 2.0 to 3.0 ml/min. Diuresis produced by the ingestion of 1 liter of water increased the urine flow to 6.7 to 9.0 ml/min and the clearance to 4.3 to 7.5 ml/min. An oral dose of 50 g of sodium bicarbonate, which increased the urine flow only slightly but elevated the urine pH from 6.1 to 8.0, increased the clearance to 9.8 ml/min. After the intravenous infusion of 14 g of sodium bicarbonate, clearances as high as 29 ml/min were recorded. More extensive observations in dogs revealed that as the percent of filtered water excreted increased, the urine/plasma water concentration ratio of phenobarbital decreased and approached a limiting value of slightly over 1 for acid urine and somewhat over 2 for alkaline urine.

The relationship between water excretion and the urine/plasma water ratio can be interpreted in terms of the reabsorption of filtered phenobarbital by a process of back diffusion. The additional assumption is made that the distal tubule can absorb a small amount of water but relatively little drug (20). The influence of pH is explicable on the assumptions that the tubule is permeable only to the un-ionized form of the drug and that equilibrium of phenobarbital between the tubular urine and the plasma is achieved either in the region of the pH alteration or distal to it. For example, if equilibrium were established between tubular urine of pH 7.9 and plasma of pH 7.4, the concentration in the tubule would become 2.3 times as high as that in plasma water. Thus, the urine/plasma water ratio would approach this value at high rates of urine flow. Equilibration of tubular urine of pH 6.0 with the same plasma would yield a urine concentration ratio only 0.45 times that in plasma water. Thus, a urine/plasma ratio less than unity does not indicate an active transport system but can be accounted for by the process of nonionic diffusion. In one experiment in man, a ratio of 0.7 was actually observed.

The renal clearances of the metabolites of phenobarbital have not been measured. However, the low oil/water coefficient of p-hydroxyphenobarbital [5-(4-hydroxyphenyl)-5-phenylbarbituric acid] suggests that this compound would be poorly reabsorbed in the kidney. Glucuronide conjugates are often secreted into the tubular urine, where their high polarity impedes reabsorption. Thus, it would be predicted that the clearance of the glucuronide of p-hydroxyphenobarbital would be very high. From observations in dogs, Butler (11) recorded that the renal clearance of mephobarbital was 0.2 ml/min, whereas that of phenobarbital was 0.9 ml/min; these values are not corrected for binding to plasma proteins. No data are available for metharbital. Undoubtedly, the high oil/water coefficients of mephobarbital and metharbital dispose these compounds to very efficient reabsorption in the kidney. As mentioned above, the N-methylbarbiturates and the dialkylbarbiturates have higher pK_as than phenobarbital. Thus, their renal clearance is much less affected by alterations in the urinary pH.

REFERENCES

1. Beckett, A. H., and Moffat, A. C. (1971): Buccal absorption of some barbiturates. *J. Pharm. Pharmacol.*, 23:15–18.
2. Boréus, L. O., Jalling, B., and Kållberg, N. (1975): Clinical pharmacology of phenobarbital in the neonatal period. In: *Basic and Therapeutic Aspects of Perinatal Pharmacology*, edited by P. L. Morselli, S. Garattini, and F. Sereni, pp. 331–340. Raven Press, New York.
3. Boyd, E. M., and Singh, J. (1967): Acute toxicity following rectal thiopental, phenobarbital and leptazol. *Anesth. Analg. Curr. Res.*, 46:395–400.
4. Brilmayer, H., and Loennecken, S. J. (1962): Die Eliminationsgeschwindigkeit von Barbiturat aus dem Blut akut intoxizierter Patienten. *Arch. Int. Pharmacodyn. Ther.*, 136:137–146.
5. Brodie, B. B., Burns, J. J., Mark, L. C., Lief, P. A., Bernstein, E., and Papper, E. M. (1953): The fate of pentobarbital in man and dog and a method for its estimation in biological material. *J. Pharmacol. Exp. Ther.*, 109:26–34.
6. Brodie, B. B., Kurz, H., and Schanker, L. S. (1960): The importance of dissociation constant and lipid solubility in influencing the passage of drugs into the cerebrospinal fluid. *J. Pharmacol. Exp. Ther.*, 130:20–25.
7. Brodwall, E., and Stoa, K. F. (1956): A study of barbiturate clearance. *Acta Med. Scand.*, 154:139–144.
8. Büch, H., Buzello, W., Neurohr, O., and Rummell, W. (1968): Vergleich von Verteilung, narcotischer Wirksamkeit und metabolisher Elimination der optischen Antipoden von Methylphenobarbital. *Biochem. Pharmacol.*, 17:2391–2398.
9. Bush, M. T. (1963): Sedatives and hypnotics: Absorption, fate and excretion. In: *Physiological Pharmacology, Vol. 1*, edited by W. S. Root and F. G. Hofmann, pp. 192–218. Academic Press, New York.
10. Butler, T. C. (1950): The rate of penetration of barbituric acid derivatives into the brain. *J. Pharmacol. Exp. Ther.*, 100:219–226.
11. Butler, T. C. (1952): Quantitative studies on the metabolic fate of mephobarbital (*N*-methylphenobarbital). *J. Pharmacol. Exp. Ther.*, 106:235–245.
12. Butler, T. C. (1953): Quantitative studies of the demethylation of *N*-methylbarbital (metharbital; Gemonil). *J. Pharmacol. Exp. Ther.*, 108:474–480.
13. Butler, T. C., Mahafee, C., and Waddell, W. J. (1954): Phenobarbital: Studies of elimination, accumulation, tolerance and dosage schedules. *J. Pharmacol. Exp. Ther.*, 111:425–435.
14. Butler, T. C., and Waddell, W. J. (1958): *N*-Methylated derivatives of barbituric acid, hydantoin and oxazolidinedione used in the treatment of epilepsy. *Neurology (Minneap.)*, 8(Suppl. 1):106–112.
15. Domek, N. S., Barlow, C. F., and Roth, L. J. (1960): An ontogenetic study of phenobarbital-C^{14} in cat brain. *J. Pharmacol. Exp. Ther.*, 130:285–293.
16. Ferngren, H. (1969): Brain and blood levels of phenobarbital-2-^{14}C during postnatal development in the mouse. *Acta Pharm. Suec.*, 6:331–338.
17. Frey, H. H., and Kampmann, E. (1966): Effect of amphetamine on the absorption of anti-convulsant drugs. *Acta Pharmacol. Toxicol. (Kbh.)*, 24:310–316.
18. Fujimoto, J. M., and Donnelly, R. A. (1968): Effect of feeding and fasting on excretion of phenobarbital in the rabbit. *Clin. Toxicol.*, 1:297–307.
19. Ganshorn, A., and Kurz, H. (1968): Unterschiede zwischen der Proteinbindung Neugeborener und Erwachsener und ihre Bedeutung für die pharmakologische Wirkung. *Arch. Pharmakol. Exp. Pathol.*, 260:117–118.
20. Giotti, A., and Maynert, E. W. (1951): The renal clearance of barbital and the mechanism of its reabsorption. *J. Pharmacol. Exp. Ther.*, 101:296–309.
21. Goldbaum, L. R., and Smith, P. K. (1954): The interaction of barbiturates with serum albumin and its possible relation to their disposition and pharmacological actions. *J. Pharmacol. Exp. Ther.*, 111:197–209.
22. Goldschmidt, S., Lamprecht, W., and Helmreich, E. (1953): Die spectrophotometrische Bestimmung von Barbituraten und die Verteilung Veronal in Organismus. *Hoppe Seylers Z. Physiol. Chem.*, 292:125–137.
23. Heimann, G., and Gladtke, E. (1977): Pharmacokinetics of phenobarbital in childhood. *Eur. J. Clin. Pharmacol.*, 12:305–310.
24. Heinze, E., and Kampffmeyer, H. G. (1971): Biological half-life of phenobarbital in human babies. *Klin. Wochenschr.*, 49:1146–1147.
25. Hogben, C. A. M., Schanker, L. S., Tocco, D. J., and Brodie, B. B. (1957): Absorption of drugs from the stomach: II, The human. *J. Pharmacol. Exp. Ther.*, 120:540–545.
26. Kakemi, K., Arita, T., Hori, R., and Konishi, R. (1967): Absorption of barbituric acid derivatives from rat stomach. *Chem. Pharm. Bull. (Tokyo)*, 15:1534–1539.
27. Kakemi, K., Takaichi, A., Hori, R., and Konishi, R. (1967): Absorption of barbituric acid derivatives from rat small intestine. *Chem. Pharm. Bull. (Tokyo)*, 15:1883–1887.
28. Kojima, S., Smith, R. B., and Doluisio, J. T. (1971): Drug absorption V: Influence of food on oral absorption of phenobarbital in rats. *J. Pharm. Sci.*, 60:1639–1641.
29. Lal, H., Barlow, C. F., and Roth, L. J. (1964): Barbital-C^{14} in cat and mouse. *Arch. Int. Pharmacodyn. Ther.*, 149:25–36.
30. Leucuta, S. E., Popa, L., Ariesan, M., Popa, L., Pop, R. D., Kory, M., and Toader, S. (1977): Bioavailability of phenobarbital from different pharmaceutical forms. *Pharm. Acta Helv.*, 52:261–266.
31. Lous, P. (1954): Plasma levels and urinary excretion of three barbituric acids after oral administration to man. *Acta Pharmacol. Toxicol. (Kbh.)*, 10:147–165.
32. Lous, P. (1954): Blood serum and cerebrospinal fluid levels and renal clearance of phenemal in treated epi-

leptics. *Acta Pharmacol. Toxicol. (Kbh.),* 10:166–177.

33. Lous P. (1954): Barbituric acid concentration in serum from patients with severe acute poisoning. *Acta Pharmacol. Toxicol. (Kbh.),* 10:261–280.

34. Lous, P. (1966): Elimination of barbiturates. In: *Barbiturate Poisoning and Tetanus,* edited by S. H. Johansen, pp. 341–350. Little, Brown, Boston.

35. Magnussen, M. P. (1968): The effect of ethanol on the gastrointestinal absorption of drugs in the rat. *Acta Pharmacol. Toxicol. (Kbh.),* 26:130–144.

36. Maynert, E. W., and van Dyke, H. B. (1949): The metabolism of barbiturates. *Pharmacol. Rev.,* 1:217–242.

37. Melchior, J. C., Svensmark, O., and Trolle, D. (1967): Placental transfer of phenobarbitone in epileptic women, and elimination in newborns. *Lancet,* 2:860–861.

38. Pitlick, W., Painter, M., and Pippenger, C. (1978): Phenobarbital pharmacokinetics in neonates. *Clin. Pharmacol. Ther.,* 23:346–350.

39. Ploman, L., and Persson, B. H. (1957): The transfer of barbiturates to the human foetus and their accumulation in some of its vital organs. *J. Obstet. Gynaecol. Br. Commonw.,* 64:706–711.

40. Ramsay, R. E., Hammond, E. J., Perchalski, R. J., and Wilder, B. J. (1979): Brain uptake of phenytoin, phenobarbital, and diazepam. *Arch. Neurol.,* 36:535–539.

41. Roth, L. J., and Barlow, C. F. (1961): Drugs in the brain. *Science,* 134:22–31.

42. Schanker, L. S. (1961): Mechanisms of drug absorption and distribution. *Annu. Rev. Pharmacol.,* 1:29–44.

43. Schmidt, D., and Kupferberg, H. J. (1975): Diphenylhydantoin, phenobarbital, and primidone in saliva, plasma, and cerebrospinal fluid. *Epilepsia,* 16:735–741.

44. Sjögren, J., Sölvell, L., and Karlsson, I. (1965): Studies on the absorption rates of barbiturates in man. *Acta Med. Scand.,* 178:553–559.

45. Sunshine, I., and Hackett, E. R. (1954): Correlation between clinical condition and blood barbiturate levels. *Am. J. Clin. Pathol.,* 24:1133–1138.

46. Svendsen, A., and Brochmann-Hanssen, E. (1962): Gas chromatography of barbiturates: Application to the study of their metabolism and excretion in humans. *J. Pharm. Sci.,* 51:494–495.

47. Svensmark, O., and Buchthal, F. (1963): Accumulation of phenobarbital in man. *Epilepsia.* 4:199–206.

48. Viswanathan, C. T., Booker, H. E., and Welling, P. G. (1978): Bioavailability of oral and intramuscular phenobarbital. *J. Clin. Pharmacol.,* 18:100–105.

49. Waddell, W. J., and Butler, T. C. (1957): The distribution and excretion of phenobarbital. *J. Clin. Invest.,* 36:1217–1226.

50. Westerink, D., and Glerum, J. H. (1965): Scheiding en microbepaling van fenobarbital en fenytoin in moedermelk. *Pharm. Weekbl.,* 100:577–583.

Antiepileptic Drugs, edited by D. M. Woodbury,
J. K. Penry, and C. E. Pippenger. Raven Press,
New York © 1982.

23

Phenobarbital

Biotransformation

E. W. Maynert

EXCRETION OF UNCHANGED PHENOBARBITAL

Phenobarbital is extensively metabolized, but a substantial fraction of the drug is excreted unchanged in the urine. For quantitative studies on the excretion of single doses of phenobarbital, the collection of all the urine eliminated over a period of at least 3 weeks is needed. This requirement, a consequence of the slow elimination of phenobarbital (plasma half-life = 96 ± 12 hr), has rarely been met. Nevertheless, through the application of chromatography and ultraviolet spectrometry to the 47-day urine of an adult patient who received 6.4 g of phenobarbital over a period of 9 days, Ravn-Jonsen and colleagues (27) found about 17% of the dose in the form of unchanged drug. Utilizing gas chromatography, Whyte and Dekaban (35) observed about 23% of a 130-mg intravenous dose of phenobarbital in the 16-day urine of a healthy man. Using similar techniques, Boréus et al. (4) found 32% unchanged drug in the 30-day urine of a female volunteer given a 5.2 mg/kg oral dose and 9% unchanged drug in the 15-day urine of a male volunteer who received a 4.3 mg/kg dose.

Many investigators have published the results of phenobarbital analyses on 24-hr urine specimens obtained from patients receiving a constant daily dose of the drug for an extended time. According to pharmacokinetic theory, in the steady state, the amount of drug eliminated per unit of time equals the intake of drug in the same interval. Thus, the amount of unchanged phenobarbital found in the 24-hr urine divided by the amount of drug given daily equals the fraction of the daily dose that resists metabolism in the body. In four epileptic patients who received phenobarbital chronically, Lous (20) found 11 to 48% (average 24%) of the daily intake as unchanged drug. The more recent results of Whyte and Dekaban (35) are in good agreement. They observed 12 to 55% (average 25%) unchanged drug in the urine of eight patients, most of whom were receiving other antiepileptic drugs as well as phenobarbital.

The excretion of phenobarbital in human neonates appears to be similar to that in adults. In a comparison of 8-day urine specimens from four newborn infants and two adults given single doses of phenobarbital, Boréus et al. (4) observed that unchanged drug amounted to 17% in the infants and 16% in the adults. The urinary excretion of phenobarbital in children has apparently not received careful study. Fecal excretion appears to be of no importance in the elimination of unchanged phenobarbital in man or laboratory animals. Whyte and Dekaban (35) failed to detect the drug in the feces of any of four patients receiving daily doses of phenobarbital.

BIOTRANSFORMATION OF PHENOBARBITAL

Hydroxylation of the Phenyl Ring

Phenobarbital resembles phenytoin and many other drugs containing a phenyl ring in that it is prominently hydroxylated in the *para* position. Butler (5) isolated *p*-hydroxyphenobarbital (Fig. 1A) in pure form from the urine of man and the dog and proved its structure by synthesis. A limited amount of information is available on the urinary excretion of this compound in its unconjugated form. From the data of Whyte and Dekaban (35), it can be estimated that the quan-

tity of this metabolite in the 16-day urine of a healthy man given 130 mg of phenobarbital represented only 5 to 6% of the dose. From analyses of 8-day urine after single doses of phenobarbital, Boréus et al. (4) concluded that free *p*-hydroxyphenobarbital amounted to 10% in a healthy woman, 7% in a healthy man, and an average of 10% (range 5–19%) in four newborn infants. In a study by Alvin et al. (2), the 5-day urine from six men used as healthy controls contained about 5% of an intraduodenally administered dose of phenobarbital. These estimates are probably low because the urinary collection times were too short. The strategy of analyzing 24-hr urine specimens from patients receiving phenobarbital chronically has been utilized to estimate the conversion of the drug to free *p*-hydroxyphenobarbital. The eight subjects studied by Whyte and Dekaban (35) excreted 8% (range 2–17%) of the dose in the form of this metabolite. These investigators also ex-

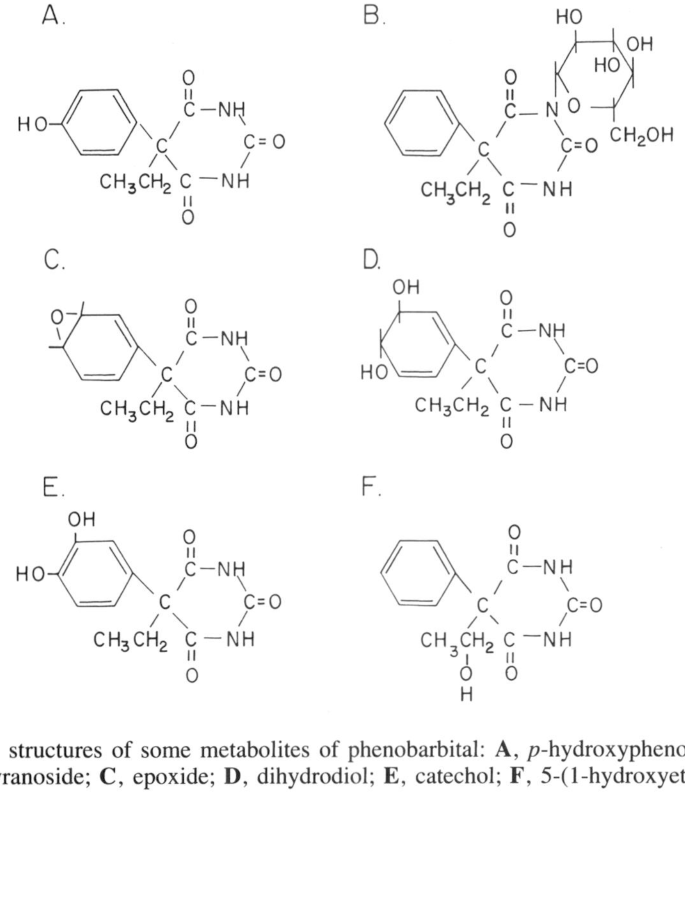

FIG. 1. Chemical structures of some metabolites of phenobarbital: **A**, *p*-hydroxyphenobarbital; **B**, phenobarbital *N*-glucopyranoside; **C**, epoxide; **D**, dihydrodiol; **E**, catechol; **F**, 5-(1-hydroxyethyl)-5-phenylbarbituric acid.

amined feces and cerebrospinal fluid for *p*-hydroxyphenobarbital, but the quantities present, if any, were below the limits of detection.

Conjugation of Phenolic Metabolites

In all species studied so far, with the possible exception of the cat, a substantial fraction of the *p*-hydroxyphenobarbital formed in the body is conjugated with glucuronic acid. In his pioneering experiments on the biotransformation of phenobarbital, Butler (5) failed to release any of the phenolic metabolite from its conjugated form by treatment of human urine with β-glucuronidase. It seems likely that this finding can be explained by inactivation of the enzyme during its passage through a fritted glass filter (21). Later workers have consistently observed the release of hydroxyphenobarbital by treatment of human urine with glucuronidase. For example, in the eight patients examined by Whyte and Dekaban (35), addition of the enzyme to urine caused hydroxyphenobarbital to increase from a level of 8%, representing free metabolite, to 17% (range 6–24%), representing free and glucuronidated metabolite. The approximate equivalence of free metabolite with conjugated metabolite observed in this study can also be seen in the average data from the two volunteers investigated by Boréus et al. (4). In the early investigation by Butler (5), the amount of free *p*-hydroxyphenobarbital found in the urine of two men was very close to that releasable by hydrolysis with hydrochloric acid. It is now believed that acid-hydrolyzable hydroxyphenobarbital is derived almost entirely from the glucuronide conjugate.

The sum of free and conjugated *p*-hydroxyphenobarbital found by Whyte and Dekaban (17%) is somewhat lower than that reported by other investigators. Kutt et al. (19) observed a value of 45% in two patients, whereas Ravn-Jonsen et al. (27) found about 33% in their patient. Glucuronide conjugates of some drugs are eliminated in the feces as well as in the urine. This mode of excretion is particularly prominent in the rat. However, inasmuch as acid hydrolysis did not reveal detectable amounts of hydroxyphenobarbital in feces (35), it may be concluded that this route of elimination of the glucuronide conjugate does not play an important role in man.

Butler's (5) failure to detect a glucuronide conjugate of *p*-hydroxyphenobarbital in human urine led him to suggest that this phenol may be conjugated with sulfuric acid in man, although he recognized that glucuronidation is the primary process in the dog. Conjugation of phenols with glucuronic acid or sulfuric acid or both has, of course, been widely observed in studies on the metabolic fate of xenobiotics. Whether the sulfuric acid ester of *p*-hydroxyphenobarbital is a metabolite of phenobarbital in any species is still somewhat uncertain. Attempts (17,35) to demonstrate the conjugate in human urine by the action of aryl sulfatase have yielded negative results. In the urine from two dogs, Butler (5) observed that 33% and 17% of the hydrochloric acid-releasable hydroxyphenobarbital was not liberated by glucuronidase. The nature of this material remains unknown. Using ^{14}C-labeled phenobarbital, Cooper and colleagues (7) reported that the urine of rats contained more of the sulfate ester than the glucuronide, but the evidence on which this conclusion was based is unknown to this reviewer. Caldwell et al. (6) subjected urine from rats given isotopic phenobarbital to thin-layer chromatography and reported the glucuronide but did not mention the sulfate. Earlier, Fujimoto et al. (11) observed that practically all the phenolic derivative of phenobarbital that appeared in the urine of rabbits was conjugated with glucuronic acid.

A reader examining the literature on *p*-hydroxyphenobarbital and its conjugated forms must be careful to distinguish among methods used to measure the conjugates. Some authors (35) have restricted attention to metabolite released by glucuronidase. Others (5) have used metabolite released by acid hydrolysis, a procedure that tends to give higher values. Some investigators (2) employing ^{14}C-labeled phenobarbital have equated isotope that resists extraction into organic solvents to conjugated drug. As will be discussed later, there is now evidence that phenobarbital is converted to polar metabolites other than conjugates of hydroxy-phenobarbital. Thus, this procedure could yield misleading results. For example, the observations of Alvin et al. (2) on normal men indicated that conjugated product exceeded that of hydroxyphenobarbital by five times (25% of the dose versus 5%). As mentioned above, the amounts of free and glucuronidated hydroxyphenobarbital are usually approximately the same when the conjugate is measured by metabolite released by glucuronidase.

Other Routes of Metabolism

The data presented above on the excretion of unchanged phenobarbital, p-hydroxyphenobarbital, and p-hydroxyphenobarbital glucuronide display wide variability but suggest that the fate of the drug cannot be fully accounted for by these three compounds. To be sure, in a few persons these metabolites have been observed to amount to 75% or more of the dose (4,5,35). On the other hand, Whyte and Dekaban (35) found that on the average the sum represented only 42% of the dose. In two patients, the three metabolites amounted to only 24 and 25% of the dose. In the single patient studied in great detail by Ravn-Jonsen et al. (27), the combined metabolites amounted to 50% of the dose. The abstract of Tang et al. (32) is of particular interest in that it reports results obtained after the administration of [^{14}C,^{15}N] phenobarbital to two healthy persons whose urine was collected for 16 days. Single doses were employed, but their size was not specified. Unchanged phenobarbital amounted to 33% of the dose, and the combined free and glucuronidated p-hydroxyphenobarbital to 17% of the dose. A new metabolite, identified as N-hydroxyphenobarbital and now presumed to be phenobarbital N-β-D-glucopyranoside, was found to account for 31% of the dose. The available information on this and other metabolites of phenobarbital not mentioned above will now be summarized.

N-*Glucosidation*

Thin-layer chromatographic separation of the urinary products of isotopically labeled pheno-

barbital led Tang et al. (32) to the recognition of a new metabolite, which they designed as the "major metabolite" of the drug. The abundance of the metabolite—31% of the dose in two persons—certainly exceeds that of p-hydroxyphenobarbital or p-hydroxyphenobarbital glucuronide reported in this study or in several others reviewed above. However, inasmuch as larger amounts of unchanged phenobarbital were observed in the same urine and have been frequently encountered in other investigations, the use of the word "major" is open to question. In the abstract, the metabolite was identified as N-hydroxyphenobarbital on the basis of its similarity to minor metabolites of amobarbital and pentobarbital previously reported by the same authors as N-hydroxy derivatives. More recent work (33) on the chemical structure of "N-hydroxyamobarbital" has provided good evidence that this substance is amobarbital N-β-D-glucopyranoside. No further reports on N-hydroxyphenobarbital have come to our attention, but it may be presumed that this metabolite is also an N-glucoside (Fig. 1B).[1] N-Glucosidation has only recently become recognized as a metabolic reaction of xenobiotics. Duggan et al. (9) observed that nitrogen atom 1 in the triazole ring of 3-(4-pyrimidinyl)-5-(4-pyridyl)-1,2,4-triazole, a xanthine oxidase inhibitor, became conjugated with glucose in rats and monkeys. A person exhibiting a genetic deficiency in the formation of the metabolite now known as amobarbital N-β-D-glucopyranoside has been reported (18). A lesion of this kind might have marked effects on the pattern of the excretory metabolites of phenobarbital.

Epoxidation and Subsequent Reactions

The probable precursor of p-hydroxyphenobarbital is the arene oxide shown in Fig. 1C. Because of its high reactivity, this substance would not be expected to appear in measureable

---

[1]B. K. Tang, W. Kalow and A. A. Grey recently compared the acetyl derivative of the "N-hydroxyphenobarbital" with synthetic N-(2,3,4,6-tetraacetyl-β-D-glucopyranosyl) phenobarbital and observed practically identical NMR and mass spectral characteristics as well as chromatographic mobilities (*Drug Metab. Dispos.*, 7:315–318, 1979).

quantities in body fluids or excreta. Such epoxides can rearrange spontaneously to phenols, and *para* orientation of the hydroxyl group is most likely. The phenobarbital expoxide would also be subject to spontaneous as well as enzyme (epoxide hydrase)-catalyzed hydrolysis to yield the corresponding dihydrodiol (Fig. 1D), which in turn could undergo dehydration to form *p*-hydroxyphenobarbital. By means of gas chromatography–mass spectrometry (GC–MS), Harvey et al. (15) were able to obtain evidence for an *N,N*-dimethylated, *bis*-trimethylsilylated derivative of this dihydrodiol [5-(3,4-dihydroxy-1,5-cyclohexadien-1-yl)-5-ethylbarbituric acid] in rat, guinea pig, and human urine. The dihydrodiol has apparently not been prepared in pure form, and the quantity formed from phenobarbital metabolism is unknown. Likewise, the question of whether conjugated forms of this compound are present in urine remains unanswered. It is worth noting that acid hydrolysis of urine would probably convert such conjugates to *p*-hydroxyphenobarbital. *In vivo* rearrangement of the epoxide or dehydration of the dihydrodiol could yield *m*-hydroxyphenobarbital as well as the *para* isomer. The former compound has been tentatively identified by GC–MS methods as a minor metabolite of phenobarbital in rats and guinea pigs (16). Searches for it in human urine with less sensitive methods failed to reveal it (5,35). Oxidation of the dihydrodiol could yield the corresponding catechol (Fig. 1E). This substance was tentatively identified in rat and human urine by GC–MS methods (16). *o*-Hydroxyphenobarbital would not be an expected product from the epoxide or dihydrodiol discussed above but conceivably could arise by epoxidation of another double bond in the phenyl ring. This phenol has apparently not been synthesized, and there are no reports on its formation as a metabolite.

Aliphatic Hydroxylation

Although ethyl groups in the 5 position of the barbituric acid ring are notoriously resistant to oxidation (22), 5-(1-hydroxyethyl)-5-phenylbarbituric acid (Fig. 1F) was detected by gas chromatographic–mass spectrometric analysis

of the urine of rats and guinea pigs treated with phenobarbital (16). No quantitative data on abundance of this metabolite are available. Earlier studies (10,14) on ^{14}C-labeled barbital revealed small quantities of a 2-hydroxyethyl derivative which was excreted in the urine partly in the form of a conjugate (probably a glucuronide).

Hydrolysis

The extent to which phenobarbital is subjected to hydrolysis in the human body is unknown. Aliprandi and Masironi (1) reported that after the administration of 2-^{14}C-phenobarbital to mice, radioactivity could be detected in exhaled carbon dioxide. Using a similar preparation in rats, Caldwell et al. (6) observed 0.14% of the dose eliminated in the breath. In contrast, Glasson and Benakis (13), who gave drugs labeled in the C-2 or C-5 position to rats, denied hydrolysis of the barbituric acid ring. Earlier work (23–25) on other barbiturates tagged with ^{15}N showed that in the dog some drugs led to the appearance in the urine of labeled ammonia and urea, whereas others did not. In rat urine, Caldwell et al. (6) encountered an acidic metabolite amounting to 4% of the dose that they considered to be ethylphenylmalonyl urea. Isotope dilution experiments with dog urine following administration of ^{15}N-labeled pentobarbital or amobarbital previously had excluded the presence of malonuric acids (23,24). It is worth noting that phenobarbital in aqueous solution is subject to spontaneous hydrolysis to a greater extent than any of the dialkylbarbiturates. In view of the excretion of rather large amounts of unchanged phenobarbital, particular care must be exercised that collected urine containing this drug is not exposed to conditions that permit hydrolysis.

ENZYMOLOGICAL CONSIDERATIONS

The hydroxylation of phenobarbital is presumed to be mediated by the cytochrome P-450 system located in the endoplasmic reticulum of the liver. Attempts to verify participation of these enzymes by incubation of the drug with hepatic microsomes and appropriate cofactors have usually resulted in at most a marginal disappearance of phenobarbital (7). This finding is not unexpected, for other long-acting barbiturates are hardly altered during the relatively short period of time that microsomes retain their hydroxylating activity. Analysis of incubation mixtures for p-hydroxyphenobarbital and its precursor epoxide and dihydrodiol offers an approach that should be superior to measurement of substrate disappearance, but no information along this line is available. Hepatic microsomes contain abundant quantities of epoxide hydrase. They also contain the enzyme (glucuronyltransferase) responsible for the formation of glucuronide conjugates of phenolic metabolites. Incubation of microsomes with p-hydroxyphenobarbital and uridinediphosphate glucuronic acid would be expected readily to yield p-hydroxyphenobarbital glucuronide, but no experiment of this kind appears to have been reported. Likewise, the enzymatic mechanisms involved in the formation of the N-glucoside of phenobarbital have not been elucidated.[2] Cooper et al. (7) have apparently had some success in demonstrating hydroxylation of phenobarbital in the isolated perfused liver of the rat. It remains unknown whether other organs of the body participate in the metabolism of phenobarbital.

The hydrolytic enzyme, β-glucuronidase, deserves some mention in relation to phenobarbital metabolism. Dog urine obtained under sterile conditions contains little, if any, free p-hydroxyphenobarbital, but this compound could be detected in urine collected in metabolism cages (5). The appearance of the metabolite in contaminated urine can be attributed to bacterial glucuronidase. As mentioned above, in man, p-hydroxyphenobarbital is usually excreted partly free and partly in the conjugated form. Inasmuch as the kidney and bladder are believed to secrete glucuronidase (2), it is possible that some or all of the free metabolite observed in urine is derived from the conjugate. In rats with biliary fistulas, Cooper et al. (7) demonstrated the appearance of large (approximately 30% of the dose of phenobarbital) amounts of p-hydroxyphenobarbital in bile, mostly in the conjugated form. Similar results were reported by Caldwell et al. (6). Inasmuch as only a small fraction of ^{14}C-labeled phenobarbital is usually eliminated in the feces of rats (6), it may be presumed that the glucuronide conjugate formed in the liver is excreted in the bile and then reabsorbed from the intestine, possibly after the action of bacterial glucuronidase. An examination of the literature on many drugs gives the impression that enterohepatic circulation of drug metabolites may be more prominent in the rat than in other species. Nevertheless, this process could occur to some extent during the sojourn of phenobarbital in the human body.

PHARMACOLOGICAL CONSIDERATIONS

The hydroxylation of phenobarbital undoubtedly plays an important role in the detoxification of the drug. p-Hydroxyphenobarbital appears to be practically devoid of hypnotic activity (5). No effects were apparent after the intravenous injection of a 100 mg/kg dose in a dog or a 500 mg/kg dose in mice. The rate of removal of p-hydroxyphenobarbital from the plasma of the dog was sufficiently rapid that only a small amount remained at 1 hr. The 24-hr urine contained 33% of the administered metabolite, mostly in the conjugated form (5). These findings are consistent with a reported failure to detect p-hydroxyphenobarbital in the plasma of patients given phenobarbital (2). The other known metabolites of phenobarbital have not been examined for pharmacological activity, but all are quite polar and, because of efficient excretion, would not be expected to contribute to the hypnotic or antiepileptic activity of phenobarbital.

As is well known, the drug-metabolizing activity of the cytochrome P-450 system can be stimulated by many drugs. For reasons that re-

---

[2]B. K. Tang and G. Carro-Ciampi have now reported that human hepatic microsomes catalyzed the formation of amobarbital-N-glycoside from the barbiturate and uridine 5′-diphosphate-D-glucose (*Biochem. Pharmacol.* 29:2085–2088, 1980).

main obscure, phenobarbital, generally recognized as the most powerful inducer of these enzymes, has rather little effect on its own metabolism. In a study of three men, Viswanathan et al. (34) observed that the serum half-life of phenobarbital was actually shorter after a single dose than after repeated doses (96 versus 150 hr). The rate constant obtained after repeated doses could be used to predict plasma concentrations of phenobarbital, but that obtained after single doses could not. The same authors reported that repeated doses did not alter the ratio of concentrations of *p*-hydroxyphenobarbital to phenobarbital in the urine. If induction of hydroxylation of the drug had occurred, an increase in the ratio during continued treatment would be expected. Butler et al. (5) found little difference in the elimination rates of the drug between six men who had been receiving the drug for months or years and five who took the drug for only 12 days. Caldwell et al. (6) used ^{14}C-phenobarbital in rats to compare the excretion of metabolites after single and repeated doses. The rates of appearance of the isotope in the urine and feces did not change, and no marked differences were detected in the pattern of metabolites. The effects of other drugs on the biotransformation of phenobarbital are discussed in Chapter 24.

CLINICAL CONSIDERATIONS

An inevitable consequence of the slow rates of biotransformation and renal clearance of phenobarbital is accumulation of the drug in the body when the dose is given repeatedly. If the average rate of elimination in man is 13.6% per day, about 20 days would be required for the plasma concentration to reach a plateau. At a low rate of elimination, e.g., 10% per day, the time would be 28 days. At a high rate, e.g., 27% per day, only 10 days would be needed. In the average adult patient placed on phenobarbital for the treatment of epilepsy, doubling the dose for 4 days is a convenient way to achieve the desired plateau in 4 days rather than 20 (29).

When children are given phenobarbital on a weight basis, they exhibit lower plasma concentrations of the drug than do adults (26,30). This difference is particularly prominent when children weighing less than 20 kg are involved. Garrettson and Dayton (12) observed half-lives in the range of 37 to 73 hr in six children ranging in age from 9 months to 9 years. The average half-life for the group was not calculated but was certainly lower than the 96-hr figure usually given for adults. The authors considered that renal function was of slight importance in the more rapid elimination of the drug, but this view is not easy to accept. Certainly, younger children have relatively greater glomerular filtration rates than adults, and phenobarbital excretion is proportional to this physiological parameter. The relatively greater mass of the liver in children, which would act to promote more rapid metabolism of the drug, constitutes the other important, probably preponderant, factor in determination of the half-life. The somewhat larger volume of distribution of the drug in children would act to diminish the rates of both hepatic metabolism and renal excretion. Svensmark and Buchthal (31) observed that, when the drug was administered on the basis of surface area, the same concentrations were observed in children and adults.

In a comparison of 8-day urine specimens from two adult volunteers and four newborn infants given single doses of phenobarbital, Boréus et al. (4) observed that both groups excreted 16 to 17% of the dose as unchanged drug and 9 to 10% as unconjugated *p*-hydroxyphenobarbital. A marked difference was noted in the output of conjugated *p*-hydroxyphenobarbital: 5% in the neonates and 15% in the adults. The authors considered deficient conjugating activity to be the main handicap in the metabolism of phenobarbital in neonates. Certainly, an impaired capacity of newborn infants to conjugate drugs with glucuronic acid is well established; disastrous effects connected with chloramphenicol administration provide a good example. However, in the absence of an increased excretion of unconjugated *p*-hydroxyphenobarbital, it would be inappropriate to assume that hydroxylation of phenobarbital proceeds at an adult rate in neonates. Deficient hydroxylating activity in the newborn is well known, and the data presented by Boréus et al. (4) do not allow an estimate of the relative importance of defects in hydroxylation and conjugation. These authors pointed out that the availability of a second route of elimination—renal excretion of unchanged drug—minimizes the clinical significance of defective metabolism of phenobarbital in neonates.

A controlled study by Alvin et al. (2) of nine men with cirrhosis and six normal subjects has supported the old clinical impression that the metabolism of phenobarbital is impaired in this form of liver disease. The average blood half-life was 130 hr in the cirrhotics and 86 hr in the controls. The 5-day excretion of unchanged drug and of unconjugated phenobarbital was not different in the two groups, but ^{14}C-labeled biotransformation products not extractable with organic solvents amounted to only 14% of the dose in the cirrhotics compared with 27% in the controls. These authors interpreted their findings as being most likely due to impaired delivery of phenobarbital into the liver because of shunting of blood around the liver and/or reduced hydroxylation of the drug. They dismissed defective conjugation as a key mechanism on the grounds that the urinary excretion of unconjugated p-hydroxyphenobarbital was not increased in the cirrhotics. It may be noted that in vitro studies by others (3) of the glucuronidation of bilirubin failed to show deficient conjugation in cirrhosis. In the investigation of Alvin et al. (2), no significant change in the mean blood half-life of phenobarbital or in the pattern of urinary metabolites was observed in eight patients with acute viral hepatitis. Wide variability in the severity of disease and in the measurements of phenobarbital metabolism in these patients was apparent. Other investigators (8,28) have shown that microsomal mixed-function oxidase activity may be depressed in severe hepatitis. Alvin et al. (2) concluded that phenobarbital is a reasonable choice as a sedative in patients with liver disease, inasmuch as elimination of unchanged drug reduces the importance of impaired hepatic function. The same argument could be applied to chronic administration of the drug in patients with epilepsy.

REFERENCES

1. Aliprandi, B., and Masironi, R. (1958): Research on radioactive barbiturates: Distribution of phenobarbital in the animal organism. *Ric. Sci.*, 28:1611–1615.
2. Alvin, J., McHorse, T., Hoyumpa, A., Bush, M. T., and Schenker, S. (1975): The effect of liver disease in man on the disposition of phenobarbital. *J. Pharmacol. Exp. Ther.*, 192:224–235.
3. Black, M., and Billing, B. (1969): Hepatic bilirubin UDP-glucuronyl transferase activity in liver disease and Gilbert's syndrome. *N. Engl. J. Med.*, 280:1266–1271.
4. Boréus, L. O., Jalling, B., and Kållberg, N. (1978): Phenobarbital metabolism in adults and in newborn infants. *Acta Paediatr. Scand.*, 67:193–200.
5. Butler, T. C. (1956): The metabolic hydroxylation of phenobarbital. *J. Pharmacol. Exp. Ther.*, 116:326–336.
6. Caldwell, J., Croft, J. E., Smith, R. L., and Snedden, W. (1977): The metabolic fate of [^{14}C]-phenobarbitone in the rat and the effect of chronic administration and dose size. *Br. J. Pharmacol.*, 60:295P–296P.
7. Cooper, D. Y., Schleyer, H., Levin, S. S., Touchstone, J. C., Eisenhardt, R. H., Vars, H. M., Rosenthal, O., Rastigar, H., and Harken, A. (1979): Biliary and urinary excretion of phenobarbital and parahydroxyphenobarbital in rats with bile fistula. In: *The Induction of Drug Metabolism*, edited by R. W. Estabrook and E. Lindenlaub, pp. 253–256. F. K. Schattauer Verlag, Stuttgart.
8. Doshi, J., Luisada-Opper, A., and Leevy, C. (1972): Microsomal pentobarbital hydroxylase activity in acute viral hepatitis. *Proc. Soc. Exp. Biol. Med.*, 140:492–495.
9. Duggan, D. E., Baldwin, J. J., Arison, B. H., and Rhodes, R. E. (1974): *N*-Glucoside formation as a detoxification mechanism in mammals. *J. Pharmacol. Exp. Ther.*, 190:563–569.
10. Ebert, A. G., Yim, G. K. W., and Miya, T. S. (1964): Distribution and metabolism of barbital-^{14}C in tolerant and nontolerant rats. *Biochem. Pharmacol.*, 13:1267–1274.
11. Fujimoto, J. M., Mason, W. H., and Murphy, M. (1968): Urinary excretion of primidone and its metabolites in rabbits. *J. Pharmacol. Exp. Ther.*, 159:379–388.
12. Garrettson, L. K., and Dayton, P. G. (1971): Disappearance of phenobarbital and diphenylhydantoin from serum of children. *Clin. Pharmacol. Ther.*, 11:674–679.
13. Glasson, B., and Benakis, A. (1961): Etude du phenobarbital C-14 dans l'organisme du rat. *Helv. Physiol. Acta*, 19:323–334.
14. Goldschmidt, S., and Wehr, R. (1957): Der Metabolismus von Veronal. *Hoppe Seylers Z. Physiol. Chem.*, 308:9–19.
15. Harvey, D. J., Glazener, L., Stratton, G., Nowlin,

J., Hill, R. M., and Horning, M. (1972): Detection of a 5-(3,4-dihydroxy-1,5-cyclohexadien-1-yl)-metabolite of phenobarbital and mephobarbital in rat, guinea pig and human. *Res. Commun. Chem. Pathol. Pharmacol.*, 3:557–565.

16. Horning, E. C., and Horning, M. G. (1971): Metabolic profiles. The study of human metabolites by gas phase analytical methods. *Clin. Chem.*, 17:802–809.

17. Kållberg, N., Agurell, S., Ericsson, O., Bucht, E., Jalling, B., and Boréus, L. O. (1975): Quantitation of phenobarbital and its main metabolites in human urine. *Eur. J. Clin. Pharmacol.*, 9:161–168.

18. Kalow, W., Kadar, D., Inaba, T., and Tang, B. K. (1977): A case of deficiency of N-hydroxylation of amobarbital. *Clin. Pharmacol. Ther.*, 21:530–535.

19. Kutt, H., Winters, W., Scherman, R., and McDowell, F. (1964): Diphenylhydantoin and phenobarbital toxicity. The role of the liver. *Arch. Neurol.*, 11:649–656.

20. Lous, P. (1954): Blood serum and cerebrospinal fluid levels and renal clearance of phenemal in treated epileptics. *Acta Pharmacol. Toxicol. (Kbh.)*, 10:261–280.

21. Maynert, E. W. (1972): Phenobarbital, mephobarbital, and metharbital: Biotransformation. In: *Antiepileptic Drugs* edited by D. M. Woodbury, J. K. Penry, and R. P. Schmidt, pp. 311–317. Raven Press, New York.

22. Maynert, E. W., and van Dyke, H. B. (1949): The metabolism of barbiturates. *Pharmacol. Rev.*, 1:217–242.

23. Maynert, E. W., and van Dyke, H. B. (1950): The metabolic fate of pentobarbital: Isotope dilution experiments with urine after the administration of labeled pentobarbital. *J. Pharmacol. Exp. Ther.*, 98:174–179.

24. Maynert, E. W., and van Dyke, H. B. (1950): The metabolism of amytal labeled with N^{15} in dogs. *J. Pharmacol. Exp. Ther.*, 98:180–183.

25. Maynert, E. W., and van Dyke, H. B. (1950): The absence of localization of barbital in divisions of the central nervous system. *J. Pharmacol. Exp. Ther.*, 98:184–187.

26. Plaa, G. L., and Hine, C. H. (1960): Hydantoin and barbiturate blood levels observed in epileptics. *Arch. Int. Pharmacodyn. Ther.*, 128:375–382.

27. Ravn-Jonsen, A., Lundin, M., and Secher, O. (1969): Excretion of phenobarbitone in urine after intake of large doses. *Acta Pharmacol. Toxicol. (Kbh)*,27:193–201.

28. Schoene, B., Fleischmann, R. A., Remmer, H., and Olderhausen, H. F. V. (1972): Determination of drug metabolizing enzymes in needle biopsies of human liver. *Eur. J. Clin. Pharmacol.*, 4:65–73.

29. Svensmark, O., and Buchthal, F. (1963): Accumulation of phenobarbital in man. *Epilepsia*, 4:199–206.

30. Svensmark, O., and Buchthal, F. (1963): Dosage of phenytoin and phenobarbital in children. *Dan. Med. Bull.*, 10:234–235.

31. Svensmark, O., and Buchthal, F. (1964): Diphenylhydantoin and phenobarbital serum levels in children. *Am. J. Dis. Child.*, 108:82–87.

32. Tang, B. K., Inaba, T., and Kalow, W. (1977): N-Hydroxyphenobarbital—The major metabolite of phenobarbital. *Fed. Proc.*, 36:966.

33. Tang, B. K., Kalow, W., and Grey, A. A. (1978): Amobarbital metabolism in man: N-Glucoside formation. *Res. Commun. Chem. Pathol. Pharmacol.*, 21:45–53.

34. Viswanathan, C. T., Booker, H. E., and Welling, P. G. (1979): Pharmacokinetics of phenobarbital following single and repeated doses. *J. Clin. Pharmacol.*, 19:282–289.

35. Whyte, M. P., and Dekaban, A. S. (1977): Metabolic fate of phenobarbital. A quantitative study of p-hydroxyphenobarbital elimination in man. *Drug Metab. Dispos.*, 5:63–70.

Antiepileptic Drugs, edited by D. M. Woodbury, J. K. Penry, and C. E. Pippenger. Raven Press, New York © 1982.

24

Phenobarbital

Interactions with Other Drugs

Henn Kutt and Helga Paris-Kutt

Interactions of phenobarbital with other drugs result in alterations of pharmacokinetic or pharmacodynamic parameters of the involved agents. Information on interactions between phenobarbital and other drugs involving alterations of pharmacodynamic parameters is rather scarce, perhaps because these are difficult to document. Observations of alterations of pharmacokinetic parameters, however, are numerous. The majority of these deal with situations in which phenobarbital has caused changes in the kinetics of other drugs. Situations where other drugs alter phenobarbital kinetics are relatively fewer. The kinetic interactions are usually documented from the measurements of plasma concentrations of the drug and sometimes confirmed by measurements of their biotransformation products.

The clinical significance of phenobarbital interactions with other drugs varies. Practically no drug combination with phenobarbital is incompatible. Only a few drug combinations with phenobarbital cause predictable changes in the majority of patients and lead to the need to adjust dosages; however, most combinations cause only minor changes in the plasma drug concentrations in most patients and do not necessitate dosage changes. Furthermore, the same drug combination with phenobarbital may lower the plasma drug concentration in some patients, cause no change in others, and raise the concentration in still others. The variability in the response is best understood by accepting the fact that not all patients are alike on genetic grounds, nor are the clinical conditions alike with regard to previous drug history and current drug dosages. Thus, it is not necessarily contradictory or conflicting if reported results of different studies disagree or point in opposite directions with the same drug combinations.

PROBABLE MECHANISMS INVOLVED IN PHARMACOKINETIC INTERACTIONS

Absorption

Phenobarbital is usually almost completely absorbed, and there have been no reports of its absorption being directly altered by other drugs through chelation. It is conceivable that drugs that greatly facilitate intestinal motility and emptying time may reduce the amount of drug absorbed. Absorption of griseofulvin (62), however, has been suspected to be reduced by phenobarbital.

Protein Binding

Phenobarbital is approximately 50% bound to plasma protein. It is unlikely that it would displace other drugs or be displaced by other drugs to any significant extent. This mechanism has not yet been implicated as a major factor in any of the reported interactions.

Altered Biotransformation

Induction and inhibition of biotransformation have been key elements in the majority of interactions between phenobarbital and other drugs, with induction being far more prevalent.

Induction of Drug Metabolism by Phenobarbital

Phenobarbital is the prototype among inducers of the hepatic mixed-function oxidase system which effects the biotransformation of numerous drugs and endogenous substances. The important components of this system effecting electron transport and oxygen transfer include cytochrome P-450 (which may exist in several subforms) and NADPH–cytochrome c reductase, contained predominantly in the smooth-membraned endoplastic reticulum of the liver cells. The heme component of membrane-bound cytochrome P-450 is ferroprotoporphyrin IX; the compound requires close association with phospholipid phosphatidylcholine for proper functioning. Several other hepatic enzymes, such as UDP–glucuronyl transferase and those involved in glucuronic acid synthesis, are utilized for conjugation of drug metabolites with glucuronic acid (6,13,68). Much of the existing knowledge about hepatic drug metabolism and the mixed-function oxidase system has been gained from animal experiments comparing phenobarbital-treated animals with control animals. There is some evidence that phenobarbital induces its own metabolism in animals to a modest extent (13). There is no clinical or laboratory evidence that autoinduction of phenobarbital metabolism occurs in humans.

Mechanism of Induction by Phenobarbital

The mode of action by which phenobarbital produces induction is complex and only partially understood. It appears that an increase of production and a decrease of degradation of enzymes both occur (6,68). Thus, actinomycin D, an inhibitor of DNA–RNA transcription, reduces or prevents induction by phenobarbital (57). There is evidence that phenobarbital stabilizes the messenger RNA, perhaps by inhibiting the ribonuclease activity (49). The changes in turnover of microsomal protein caused by phenobarbital are thought to be due to stabilization of lysosomes or inhibition of lysosomal enzymes. The increase of phospholipid concentration is thought to be due to a decrease of phospholipid degradation (27).

Induction in Animals

Treatment of rats with phenobarbital in doses of 50 to 75 mg/kg for 3 to 7 days causes an increase of total liver weight and a proliferation of endoplasmic reticulum demonstrable with electron microscopy. The content of microsomal protein per gram of liver increases as do the concentrations of cytochrome P-450, NADPH–cytochrome c reductase, and UDP–glucuronyl transferase, as well as phospholipids. The activity (V_{max}) of various steps involved in drug metabolism, such as hydroxylation and dealkylation of a number of endogenous (such as steroids) and exogenous (drugs) substrates, is considerably increased following phenobarbital treatment, as has been shown *in vitro* with isolated microsomal preparations (13,68). Figure 1 shows the increase of phenytoin hydroxylation by rat liver microsomes following phenobarbital treatment. A twofold increase of V_{max} was seen with both the washed microsomes and the 9,000 x g supernatant, the latter containing microsomes and the hepatic soluble fraction (37). Other substrates commonly used to demonstrate the induction of microsomal drug metabolism by phenobarbital are hexobarbital, aniline, benzphetamine, and ethylmorphine, among others. The activity with some of these substrates may increase up to sixfold following phenobarbital treatment (13,68).

The substrate-induced difference spectra, Type I and Type II, are both enhanced in the micro-

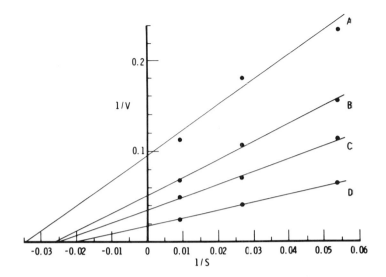

FIG. 1. Increase of phenytoin metabolism by phenobarbital in rat liver microsomal preparations. **A,** Activity in washed control microsomes; **B,** activity in control 9,000 x *g* supernatant; **C,** activity in washed microsomes following phenobarbital treatment of animals; **D,** activity in 9,000 x *g* supernatant following phenobarbital treatment of animals. Phenobarbital dose: 75 mg/kg for 7 days. Based on data of Kutt and Fouts (37).

somes from phenobarbital-treated animals, although phenobarbital itself is a Type I substrate (39).

The induced changes last for several days following discontinuation of phenobarbital administration and then slowly decline. The extent of inducibility by phenobarbital is to a degree related to its dose but is saturable (6,13,68). Furthermore, there are species differences in the extent of induction as well as differences among strains in the same animal species that are thought to be genetically determined (68,70).

Induction in Man

Changes analogous to those seen in animals have been observed in the hepatic mixed-function oxidase system of humans following treatment with phenobarbital. Thus, Lecamwasam et al. (43) gave phenobarbital in a dose of 90 mg daily for 7 days to patients with Hodgkin's disease who were scheduled to undergo laparotomy and liver biopsy. There was an increase of microsomal protein, and the cytochrome P-450 content was found in eight patients to be nearly twice that in subjects without phenobarbital

treatment. The hexobarbital oxidase activity was doubled, and the urinary excretion of D-glucaric acid had increased severalfold. Other investigators have made similar observations regarding P-450 content in liver biopsy material from patients treated sporadically with phenobarbital. With higher phenobarbital doses (180 mg daily), an increase of UDP–glucuronyl transferase was also observed (3). In an epileptic patient, needle biopsy of liver revealed an increase of P-450, NADPH–cytochrome *c* reductase, and drug-oxidizing activity (64). Thus, the biochemical parameters of induction by phenobarbital can be observed in man. It must be emphasized, however, that the hepatic P-450 content and actual enzyme activity do not always correlate well, as is often the case with animals as well.

As indirect but noninvasive indicators of induction, urinary output of D-glucaric acid (17) and 6-β-hydroxycortisol (9) as well as plasma γ-glutamyl transferase (63) concentrations have been investigated. It appears that the general trend of induction may be indicated by these parameters, but their correlation with the degree of induction in individual patients is poor if the change of the induced drug half-life or alterations of the steady-state plasma concentration are taken as criteria. Attempts have been made to utilize the rate of decline of the level of a test drug in the plasma as an indicator of the state of induction. For such half-life determinations before and after phenobarbital treatment, antipyrine, which undergoes complete hepatic biotransformation, has been recommended. Although not an ideal representative of all drugs, the changes of antipyrine half-life seem to provide some clinically useful evidence of induction of microsomal enzymes by phenobarbital (71).

It is important to realize that induction of the mixed-function oxidase system by phenobarbital in man is influenced by genetic and environmental factors as well as by the age and possibly the sex of the subject. The age may not matter so much directly, but younger subjects may have had less contact with inducing agents than older subjects. There is little evidence that sex has a great influence, but empirically, females are sometimes somewhat better inducers than males (70).

The environmental factors that influence the response of a given patient to the phenobarbital inducing effect are the lifestyle and previous drug history. Chronic consumption of alcohol has some inducing effect per se, but it also causes liver damage that may alter the response to phenobarbital induction. Other influences are tobacco smoking and probably a variety of environmental and food chemicals, all having an inducing effect to some degree. Previous and/or current contact with other drugs or medications may have some inducing effects and thus possibly reduce the phenobarbital effect (70).

Genetic Influence on Induction in Man

Genetic influence on the extent of induction by phenobarbital has been well documented. It appears that there are individuals with genetically determined high inducing capacity as well as subjects in whom only modest induction takes place. A good example is the study by Vesell and Page (72) of pairs of identical and fraternal twins (see Fig. 2). The overall induction of antipyrine metabolism by phenobarbital, evidenced by shortening of antipyrine half-life, varied in this study from 0 to 68% among individual subjects. However, the extent of induction in each of the identical twins within a pair was nearly identical despite different living habits (intrapair difference, 0 to 2.6%). In the fraternal twins, on the other hand, the intrapair differences in inducibility ranged from 8 to 31%. It has not

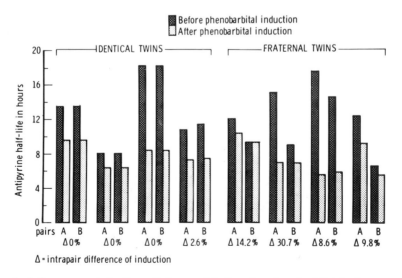

FIG. 2. Genetic influence on induction of drug metabolism by phenobarbital in humans. The intrapair difference in the extent of shortening of antipyrine half-life varied from 0 to 2.6% in identical twins in contrast with 8.6 to 31% variation in fraternal twins. Based on data of Vesell and Page (72).

yet been ascertained what genetic structures or mechanisms regulate the inducibility of the mixed-function oxidase system, but it is clear from the results with identical twins that heredity has a strong influence on the extent of inducibility by phenobarbital.

In practical terms, then, the effects of induction by phenobarbital on other drugs in individual patients are largely unpredictable. In subjects with genetically high inducing capacity and little environmental inducer contact, the phenobarbital effect may be noticeable and require adjustment of the induced drug dosage. In others with genetically low inducing capability and considerable environmental inducer contact, the effect is negligible. Empirically, only a few drug combinations with phenobarbital are predictable candidates for clinically significant interactions based on phenobarbital as an inducer of the mixed-function oxidase system. These are described below. Despite being an excellent inducer of drug metabolism in animals, in humans, phenobarbital appears to be inferior to phenytoin (a modest inducer in animals) in this respect.

Inhibition of Metabolism

Phenobarbital may also inhibit drug metabolism, particularly if it competes with another Type I drug as substrate. Thus, competitive inhibition of phenytoin hydroxylation has been demonstrated *in vitro* (38) and observed clinically in some patients (4,38).

Inhibition of phenobarbital metabolism (parahydroxylation) by other drugs also occurs, most notably that caused by valproate (31,32). These events are described in detail below.

CLINICAL INTERACTIONS MANIFESTING IN CHANGES OF PHENOBARBITAL KINETICS BY OTHER DRUGS

Valproate–Phenobarbital Interaction

The interaction between phenobarbital and valproate is probably one of the clinically most important interactions in this group, as it occurs predictably in the majority of patients taking these two drugs together. It was first noted when valproate was initially used as an adjunct in patients already taking phenobarbital. The clinical manifestation was increasing somnolence, sometimes resulting in coma, within days or weeks after the initiation of valproate administration. Plasma phenobarbital levels increased without an increase in the phenobarbital dose (8,21,32,60,73,75). This phenomenon is illustrated in Fig. 3. The rate and magnitude of phenobarbital accumulation vary among individual patients, being negligible in some but reaching double the initial value in others, and phenobarbital dosage reductions have been necessary in up to 80% of patients observed in various studies (60,73). Whether the dosage of phenobarbital needs to be reduced depends on the initial dosage, the plasma drug level, and the extent of the rise. The magnitude of the necessary reduction of the dose is best indicated by the rate of the rise of the plasma phenobarbital level.

In patients taking primidone, the plasma level of derived phenobarbital also tends to rise but not as predictably as in patients taking phenobarbital (21,60). The possibility that valproate reduces the conversion of primidone into phenobarbital has been offered as an explanation for the less predictable and sometimes

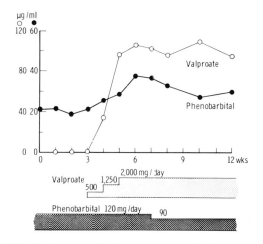

FIG. 3. Increase of plasma phenobarbital levels by valproate. (From authors' unpublished case material.)

smaller rise of the plasma level of primidone-derived phenobarbital (75).

The mechanism by which valproate causes phenobarbital accumulation is thought to involve inhibition of phenobarbital metabolism. Kapetanovic et al. (32) demonstrated that elimination of *para*-hydroxyphenobarbital in the urine declined by 30% following valproate administration, mainly because of a diminution of the output of the conjugated fraction of the metabolite, since the excretion of free *p*-hydroxyphenobarbital remained virtually unchanged after addition of valproate. No change in volume of distribution accompanied this reduction of total body clearance of phenobarbital, which led the authors to conclude that inhibition of phenobarbital metabolism had taken place. Further experiments by the same authors utilizing rat liver microsomal preparations *in vitro* provided direct evidence that valproate inhibits phenobarbital hydroxylation (31). In another study, a decrease of urinary *p*-hydroxyphenobarbital was also noted following addition of valproate (8).

Whether or not this reduction of phenobarbital biotransformation is alone sufficient to explain the accumulation of a drug which is excreted to a great extent (20–40%) unchanged remains to be clarified. Another theoretically possible mechanism that may contribute to phenobarbital accumulation is a reduction of its renal excretion by valproate lowering the pH. Measurements of plasma and urine pH of patients taking valproate, however, have not revealed drastic changes (8,32); thus, the role of pH in the mechanism of this interaction remains uncertain. It is of interest that short-chain fatty acids from another source, such as a ketogenic diet, have also caused phenobarbital accumulation (46). Most likely, the valproate-induced phenobarbital accumulation is caused by a combination of factors, some of which are still unidentified.

Phenobarbital–Phenytoin Interaction

In some patients, phenytoin has been noted to cause a rise in the plasma phenobarbital level; also, in a few patients, the phenobarbital level was noted to fall after phenytoin was discontinued (41,52,75). Eadie et al. (19) failed to find among 121 patients included in a statistical analysis any significant elevations of plasma phenobarbital levels attributable to phenytoin, which is in accordance with our experience. Thus, elevation of plasma phenobarbital levels by phenytoin is generally an infrequent manifestation occurring apparently in susceptible individuals; if it does occur, it is rarely of significant magnitude. The mechanism could be inhibition of phenobarbital biotransformation, as both drugs are hydroxylated by hepatic microsomal enzymes.

Phenobarbital–Dextropropoxyphene Interactions

Dam and co-workers (15) recently reported a study in which four epileptic patients who were stabilized on phenobarbital monotherapy were given dextropropoxyphene in a dose of 65 mg three times a day for 6 days. A modest (10–15%) elevation of plasma phenobarbital levels occurred in all patients by the sixth day. As the rise in plasma phenobarbital level was small, and dextropropoxyphene is seldom taken regularly in large amounts, it is likely that the need to change phenobarbital dosage with this drug combination would occur only rarely.

Phenobarbital–Ammonium Chloride Interaction

Accelerated elimination of phenobarbital following ammonium chloride administration has been utilized for the treatment of phenobarbital overdose. The mechanism is enhancement of renal excretion by alkalinization.

Other Observations

A number of other studies have evaluated interactions (or lack thereof) between phenobarbital and various agents that alter its kinetics. These are listed in Table 1.

Of special interest to epileptologists are probably the studies showing that a number of other antiepileptic drugs, e.g., carbamazepine, clon-

TABLE 1. *Effects of other agents on kinetics of phenobarbital*

Reference	Agent	Effect on plasma phenobarbital level
Cereghino et al. (11)	Carbamazepine	No change
Eadie et al. (19)	Carbamazepine	No change
Johannessen et al. (30)	Clonazepam	No change
Nanda et al. (55)	Clonazepam	No change
Eadie et al. (19)	Sulthiame	No change
Richens (61)	Sulthiame	Elevation
Kupferberg et al. (36)	Methylphenidate	No change
Mattson et al. (50)	Folic acid	Lowering
Eadie et al. (20)	Folic acid	Lowering
Hansson and Sillanpää (24)	Pyridoxine	Lowering
Cucinell et al. (14)	Dicoumarol	Lowering
Conney (13)	Phenylbutazone	Lowering
Ahmad et al. (2)	Frusemide	Elevation
Kelly et al. (33)	Acetazolamide	Elevation
Richens (61)	Pheneturide	Elevation
Koup et al. (35)	Chloramphenicol	Elevation

azepam, and sulthiame, usually did not alter plasma phenobarbital levels.

CLINICAL INTERACTIONS MANIFESTED IN CHANGES OF KINETICS OF OTHER AGENTS BY PHENOBARBITAL

Phenobarbital–Anticoagulant Interaction

A decline in anticoagulant effect of bishydroxycoumarin and warfarin after the start of phenobarbital administration has been reported (13,14,48). This leads to appropriate dosage adjustments of anticoagulants guided by prothrombin time determinations. Following discontinuation of phenobarbital, the anticoagulant dose is then readjusted. Thus, because of present-day controlled management routines, which include continuous monitoring of prothrombin time and anticoagulant dosage adjustments, this potentially dangerous interaction seldom leads to grave consequences (34). Although the mechanism of reduction of anticoagulant activity by phenobarbital is generally thought to be caused by induction of the anticoagulant metabolism, interference with absorption may also be partly involved. Thus, fecal excretion of bishydroxy-

coumarin after oral ingestion is doubled by barbiturates but remains unchanged when bishydroxycoumarin is administered intravenously.

Phenobarbital–Phenytoin Interaction

As mentioned earlier, phenobarbital predictably induces phenytoin metabolism in experimental animals, for example, doubling the rate in rats (37). It also acts as a competitive inhibitor with phenytoin as substrate (38), since both drugs undergo parahydroxylation and glucuronidation. It appears that the effects of these interactions in humans often balance out, leading to no change or only to minor changes in the form of decline or elevation of plasma phenytoin levels. Furthermore, humans, unlike naive laboratory animals, are likely to be at least partially induced by previous drug contacts and/or food chemicals.

In clinical studies in which groups of patients taking (a) phenytoin alone or (b) phenytoin combined with phenobarbital were compared, the maintenance plasma phenytoin levels tended to be somewhat lower in the group on combined therapy (4,38,52,67). When individual patients were studied before and after the addition of phenobarbital to phenytoin, the plasma phenytoin levels declined in some, rose in others, and remained unchanged in still others, rarely leading to a need to readjust dosages (4,14,38,52). It is fair to assume that the patients who showed a more marked decline in plasma phenytoin levels are genetically "good inducers" or had less previous contact with inducing agents. The patients in whom a rise occurred, on the other hand, may already have been fully induced and/or had a low saturation point of the hydroxylating system. It also appears that in some patients, higher phenobarbital doses cause more marked changes in plasma phenytoin levels. Similarly, the changes tend to be greater when the starting plasma phenytoin levels are higher.

Phenobarbital–Carbamazepine Interaction

Phenobarbital may cause a decline of plasma carbamazepine levels in some patients. The plasma level of 10,11-carbamazepine epoxide,

the pharmacologically active circulating carbamazepine metabolite, may remain unchanged or
decline only to a small extent. This lowers the
ratio of parent compound to metabolite in the
plasma and is thought to be caused by induction
(16,29). The extent of these changes varies from
negligible or small in the majority of patients
to considerable in some presumably good inducers, and in the latter patients, dosage read-
justments may become necessary (42). The
phenomenon is best demonstrated by monitoring plasma carbamazepine levels before and after
the initiation of phenobarbital administration.
The issue may be compounded by the decline
of plasma carbamazepine concentrations through
autoinduction. If groups of patients who are
taking carbamazepine alone and carbamazepine
together with phenobarbital are compared, the
plasma levels of carbamazepine tend to be
somewhat higher in the group on monotherapy
(11,12,29). It is worth mentioning here that
phenytoin generally causes a greater decline in
the plasma carbamazepine levels than does
phenobarbital.

Phenobarbital–Chlorpromazine Interaction

Loga et al. (47) studied the effect of phenobarbital on blood chlorpromazine levels in a
group of schizophrenic patients. After treatment
for 2 weeks with 300 mg of chlorpromazine
daily, the mean blood levels of chlorpromazine in six patients ranged from 25 to 35 ng/
ml. Then, phenobarbital (150 mg daily) was
given for 3 weeks, producing phenobarbital levels of 12 to 13 μg/ml by the end of the third
week. Soon after the onset of phenobarbital
administration, blood chlorpromazine levels declined to near 20 ng/ml (see Fig. 4). Within a
week or two following the discontinuation of
phenobarbital, the chlorpromazine levels had
risen to near the values observed before the onset of the phenobarbital administration. Considerable interindividual variation was observed in
the extent of decline of blood chlorpromazine
levels caused by phenobarbital. Antipyrine half-
lives determined before and after phenobarbital
administration paralleled the decline of blood
chlorpromazine levels, leading to the inference

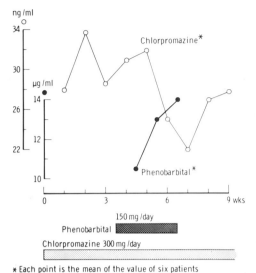

FIG. 4. Lowering of plasma chlorpromazine levels
by phenobarbital in patients. Based on data of Loga
et al. (47).

that the decline was a manifestation of induction. The clinical effectiveness of chlorpromazine evaluated by psychiatric rating scores was
not considered to be adversely influenced by
phenobarbital in these patients (40).

Phenobarbital–Tricyclic Antidepressant Interaction

Phenobarbital has been reported to cause a
decline of plasma desipramine levels. In a group
of epileptic patients whose medication included
phenobarbital or primidone, the steady-state
nortriptyline levels were lower than in nonepileptic patients (5). It thus appears that phenobarbital induction can lower the plasma levels
of tricyclic antidepressant drugs; how often this
might lead to a need to adjust dosages is unclear.

Phenobarbital–Vitamin D Interaction

Osteomalacia related to deficiency of vitamin
D has occurred in some epileptic patients. Low
plasma levels of 25-hydroxycholecalciferol, the
active metabolite of vitamin D_3, are usually seen
in these patients. Although the mechanism pro-

ducing this manifestation appears to be complex and incompletely understood, induction of microsomal enzymes may be involved as well. Studies of the rate of clearance of radioactive cholecalciferol indicated that the clearance was faster in induced (epileptic) patients than in normal subjects. Since the rate of synthesis of 25-hydroxycalciferol was the same in both groups, it was concluded that some of the calciferol was metabolized by a different route in the induced patients, perhaps producing inactive metabolites (26). Similar conclusions have been reached on the basis of animal experiments (23). Other environmental factors such as the amount of sunlight and the content of vitamin D in the diet seem to be the factors determining which patients develop clinical osteomalacia.

Phenobarbital–Oral Contraceptive Interaction

Several authors have reported contraceptive failures among epileptic women taking oral steroid contraceptives (28,53). Hempel and Klinger (25) reported that breakthrough bleeding occurred in over 50% of 52 subjects taking phenobarbital and was positively correlated with the phenobarbital dose. In the control population, the incidence of breakthrough bleeding was only 4%. Prospective studies might shed light on the clinical significance of this manifestation.

Phenobarbital Effect on Endogenous Substances

The elimination of bilirubin is enhanced by phenobarbital (69). This effect has been utilized clinically to treat Gilbert's disease as well as newborns with hyperbilirubinemia. The need to have exchange transfusions was considerably reduced by phenobarbital treatment in infants (76). The metabolism of endogenous steroids is enhanced to some extent by phenobarbital, manifested by an increase of urinary excretion of 6-β-hydroxycortisol (9). No clinical problems have been ascribed to this manifestation. Bile salts, cholesterol, and lipids in plasma can be reduced by phenobarbital (45).

Other Studies

There are further reports of phenobarbital altering, usually reducing, the plasma levels of other drugs (Table 2). The alterations are suspected to be related to induction.

INDUCTION OF DRUG METABOLISM BY PHENOBARBITAL AS A POTENTIAL CAUSE OF INCREASED DRUG TOXICITY

In most instances the induction of drug metabolism by phenobarbital is expected to result in a reduction of the effects of other drugs. With some drugs, however, increased toxicity may occur, specifically if the induction causes an increased production of a metabolite that has toxic effects (22). Thus, phenobarbital enhances the production of 2-hydroxyphenetidin from acetophenetidin, particularly in patients whose normal metabolic pathways for acetophenetidin is deficient because of their genetic makeup (65). 2-Hydroxyphenetidin is responsible for methemoglobin formation. Similarly, induction increases the hepatotoxicity of acetaminophen by increasing the production of a toxic intermediary metabolite; this is particularly relevant in cases of acetaminophen overdoses (18,51). Increase of toxicity in phenobarbital-induced subjects from fluroxene has been observed; the toxic metabolite is trifluoroethanol (54). There is also evidence that

TABLE 2. *Effects of phenobarbital on kinetics of other drugs*

Reference	Drug	Effect on plasma drug level
Brooks et al. (7)	Dexamethasone	Lowering
Padgham and Richens (58)	Quinine	Lowering
Conney (13)	Digitoxin	Lowering
Vesell and Page (72)	Antipyrine	Lowering
Sjö et al. (66)	Clonazepam	Lowering
Perucca et al. (59)	Clonazepam	Lowering
Conney (13)	Aminopyrine	Lowering
Busfield et al. (10)	Griseofulvin	Lowering
Neuvonen et al. (56)	Doxycycline	Lowering
Windorfer and Pringsheim (74)	Chloramphenicol	Lowering

induction by phenobarbital increases the toxicity of various laboratory chemicals such as carbon tetrachloride and bromobenzene, the latter via enhanced production of the 3,4-epoxide metabolite (22).

PHARMACODYNAMIC INTERACTIONS BETWEEN PHENOBARBITAL AND OTHER DRUGS

Little information is available on this subject. It has been suggested that antiepileptic drugs, including phenobarbital, reduce renal sensitivity to the diuretic action of furosemide (1). The earlier notions that phenobarbital might potentiate the effect of phenytoin at the site(s) of action probably are not true. Animal experiments evaluating the brain concentrations of these two drugs indicate that, if given together, the increase of anticonvulsant effect is additive and proportional to the sum of drug concentrations and does not demonstrate potentiation (44).

REFERENCES

1. Ahmad, S. (1974): Renal insensitivity to frusemide caused by chronic anticonvulsant therapy. *Br. Med. J.,* 2:657–659.
2. Ahmad, S., Clarke, L., Hewett, A. J., and Richens, A. (1976): Controlled trial of frusemide as an antiepileptic drug in focal epilepsy. *Br. J. Clin. Pharmacol.,* 3:621–625.
3. Black, M. Perret, R. D., and Carter, A. E. (1973): Hepatic bilirubin UDP–glucuronyl transferase activity and cytochrome P-450 content in surgical population and the effect of preoperative drug therapy. *J. Lab. Clin. Med.,* 81:704–712.
4. Booker, H. E., Tormey, A., and Toussaint, J. (1971): Concurrent administration of phenobarbital and diphenylhydantoin: Lack of an interference effect. *Neurology (Minneap.),* 21:383–385.
5. Braithwaite, R. A., Flanagan, R. A., and Richens, A. (1975): Steady state plasma nortriptyline concentrations in epileptic patients. *Br. J. Clin. Pharmacol.,* 2:469–471.
6. Bridges, J. W. (1977): The value of biochemical pharmacology in predicting drug interactions. In: *Drug Interactions (Minneap.),* edited by D. G. Grahame-Smith, pp. 101–118. University Park Press, Baltimore.
7. Brooks, S. M., Werk, E. E., Ackerman, S. J., Sullivan, I., and Thrasher, K. (1972): Adverse effects of phenobarbital on corticosteroid metabolism in patients with bronchial asthma. *N. Engl. J. Med.,* 286:1125–1128.
8. Bruni, J., Wilder, B. J., Perchalski, R. J., Hammond, E. J., and Villarreal, H. J. (1980): Valproic

acid and plasma levels of phenobarbital. *Neurology (Minneap.),* 30:94–97.
9. Burstein, S., and Klaiber, E. L. (1965): Phenobarbital induced increase in 6-betahydroxycortisol excretion: Clue to its significance in human urine. *J. Clin. Endocrinol. Metab.,* 25:293–296.
10. Busfield, D., Child, K. J., Atkinson, R. M., and Tomich, E. G. (1963): An effect of phenobarbitone on blood levels of griseofulvin in man. *Lancet,* 2:1042.
11. Cereghino, J. J., van Meter, J. C., Brock, J. T., Penry, J. K., Smith, L. D., and White, B. G. (1973): Preliminary observations of serum carbamazepine concentration in epileptic patients. *Neurology (Minneap.),* 23:357–366.
12. Christiansen, J., and Dam, M. (1973): Influence of phenobarbital and diphenylhydantoin on plasma carbamazepine levels in patients with epilepsy. *Acta Neurol. Scand.,* 49:543–546.
13. Conney, A. H. (1967): Pharmacological implications of microsomal enzyme induction. *Pharmacol. Rev.,* 19:317–366.
14. Cucinell, S. A., Conney, A. H., Sansur, M. S., and Burns, J. J. (1965): Drug interactions in man. I. Lowering effect of phenobarbital on plasma levels of bishydroxycoumarin (Dicumarol®). and diphenylhydantoin (Dilantin®). *Clin. Pharmacol. Ther.,* 6:420–429.
15. Dam, M., Christensen, J. M., Brandt, J., Hansen, B. S., Hvidberg, E. F., Angelo, H., and Lous, P. (1980): Antiepileptic Drugs: Interaction with dextropropoxyphene. In: *Antiepileptic Therapy: Advances in Drug Monitoring,* edited by S. I. Johannessen, P. L. Morselli, C. E. Pippenger, A. Richens, D. Schmidt, and H. Meinardi, pp. 299–304. Raven Press, New York.
16. Dam, M., Jensen, A., and Christiansen, J. (1975): Plasma levels and effect of carbamazepine in grand mal and psychomotor epilepsy. *Acta Neurol. Scand.* [*Suppl.*] 60:33–38.
17. Davis, M., and Labadarios, D. (1976): Urinary D-glucaric acid excretion and screening for enzyme induction. In: *Anticonvulsant Drugs and Enzyme Induction,* edited by A. Richens and F. P. Woodford, pp. 13–23. Elsevier/Excerpta Medica/North-Holland, New York.
18. Davis, M., Simmons, C., Harrison, N. G., and Williams, R. (1976): Paracetamol overdose in man: Relationship between pattern of urinary metabolites and severity of liver damage. *Q. J. Med.,* 45:181–191.
19. Eadie, M. J., Lander, C. M., Hooper, W. D., and Tyrer, J. H. (1977): Factors influencing plasma phenobarbitone levels in epileptic patients. *Br. J. Clin. Pharmacol.,* 4:541–547.
20. Eadie, M. J., Lander, C. M., and Tyrer, J. H. (1977): Plasma drug level monitoring in pregnancy. *Clin. Pharmacokinet.,* 2:427–436.
21. Flachs, H., Wurtz-Jørgensen, A., Gram, L., and Wulff, K. (1977): Sodium di-*n*-propylacetate—its interactions with other antiepileptic drugs. In: *Antiepileptic Drug Monitoring,* edited by C. Gardner-Thorpe, D. Janz, H. Meinardi, and C. E. Pippenger, pp. 165–171. Pitman Medical, Kent.
22. Gillette, J. R. (1974): A perspective on the role of chemically reactive metabolites of foreign compounds in toxicity. *Biochem. Pharmacol.,* 28:2927–2938.

23. Hahn, T. J., Birge, S. J., Shapp, C. R., and Avioli, L. V. (1972): Phenobarbital-induced alterations in vitamin D metabolism. *J. Clin. Invest.*, 51:741–748.

24. Hansson, O., and Sillanpää, M. (1976): Pyridoxine and serum concentrations of phenytoin and phenobarbitone. *Lancet*, 1:258.

25. Hempel, E., and Klinger, W. (1976): Drug stimulated biotransformation of hormonal steroid contraceptives: Clinical implications. *Drugs*, 12:442–448.

26. Hunter, J. (1976): Effects of enzyme induction on vitamin D_3 metabolism in man. In: *Anticonvulsant Drugs and Enzyme Induction*, edited by A. Richens and F. P. Woodford, pp. 77–84. Elsevier/Excerpta Medica/North-Holland, New York.

27. Infante, R., Petit, D., Polonovski, J., and Caroli, J. (1971): Microsomal phospholipid biosynthesis after phenobarbital administration. *Experientia*, 27:640–642.

28. Janz, D., and Schmidt, D. (1974): Anti-epileptic drugs and failure of oral contraceptives. *Lancet*, 1:1113.

29. Johannessen, S. I., and Strandjord, R. E. (1975): The influence of phenobarbitone and phenytoin on carbamazepine serum levels. In: *Clinical Pharmacology of Antiepileptic Drugs*, edited by H. Schneider, D. Janz, C. Gardner-Thorpe, H. Meinardi, and A. Sherwin, pp. 201–205. Springer-Verlag, Berlin.

30. Johannessen, S. I., Strandjord, R. E., and Munthe-kaas, A. W. (1977): Lack of effect of clonazepam on serum levels of diphenylhydantoin, phenobarbital and carbamazepine. *Acta Neurol. Scand.*, 55:506–512.

31. Kapetanovic, I. M., Kupferberg, H. J., Porter, R. J., Theodore, W., Schulman, E., and Penry, J. K. (1981): Mechanism of valproate- phenobarbital interaction in epileptic patients. *Clin. Pharmacol. Ther.*, 29:480–486.

32. Kapetanovic, I., Kupferberg, H. J., Porter, R. J., and Penry, J. K. (1980): Valproic acid–phenobarbital interaction: A systematic study using stable isotopically labeled phenobarbital in an epileptic patient. In: *Antiepileptic Therapy: Advances in Drug Monitoring*, edited by S. I. Johannessen, P. L. Morselli, C. E. Pippenger, A. Richens, D. Schmidt, and H. Meinardi, pp. 373–380. Raven Press, New York.

33. Kelly, W. N., Richardson, A. P., Mason, M. F., and Rector, F. C. (1966): Acetazolamide in phenobarbital intoxication. *Arch. Intern. Med.*, 117:64–69.

34. Kleinman, P. D., and Griner, P. F. (1970): Studies of the epidemiology of anticoagulant drug interactions. *Arch. Intern. Med.*, 126:522–523.

35. Koup, J. R., Gibaldi, M., McNamara, P., Hilligoss, D. M., Coburn, W. A., and Bruck, E. (1978): Interaction of chloramphenicol with phenytoin and phenobarbital. *Clin. Pharmacol. Ther.*, 24:571–575.

36. Kupferberg, H. J., Jeffrey, W., and Hunninghake, D. B. (1972): Effect of methylphenidate on plasma anticonvulsant level. *Clin. Pharmacol. Ther.*, 13:201–204.

37. Kutt, H., and Fouts, J. (1971): Diphenylhydantoin metabolism by rat liver microsomes and some of the effects of drug or chemical pretreatment on diphenylhydantoin metabolism by rat liver microsomal preparations. *J. Pharmacol. Exp. Ther.*, 176:11–26.

38. Kutt, H., Haynes, J., Verebely, K., and McDowell, F. (1969): The effect of phenobarbital on plasma diphenylhydantoin level and metabolism in man and rat liver microsomes. *Neurology (Minneap.)*, 19:611–616.

39. Kutt, H., Waters, L., and Fouts, J. R. (1971): The effects of some stimulators (inducers) of hepatic microsomal drug-metabolizing enzyme activity on substrate-induced difference spectra in rat liver microsomes. *J. Pharmacol. Exp. Ther.*, 179:101–113.

40. Lader, M. (1977): Drug interactions and the major tranquilizers. In: *Drug Interactions*, edited by D. G. Grahame-Smith, pp. 159–170. University Park Press, Baltimore.

41. Lambie, D. G., Nanda, R. M., Johnson, R. H., and Shakir, R. A. (1976): Therapeutic and pharmacokinetic effects of increasing phenytoin in chronic epileptics on multiple drug therapy. *Lancet*, 2:386–389.

42. Lander, C. M., Eadie, M. J., and Tyrer, J. H. (1977): Factors influencing plasma carbamazepine concentration. *Clin. Exp. Neurol.*, 14:184–193.

43. Leeamwasam, D. S., Franklin, C., and Turner, P. (1975): Effect of phenobarbitone on hepatic drug-metabolizing enzymes and urinary D-glucaric acid excretion in man. *Br. J. Clin. Pharmacol.*, 2:257–262.

44. Leppik, I. E., and Sherwin, A. (1977): Anticonvulsant activity of phenobarbital and phenytoin in combination. *J. Pharmacol. Exp. Ther.*, 200:570–575.

45. Linarelli, L. G., Hengstenberg, F. H., and Drash, A. L. (1973): Effect of phenobarbital on hyperlipemia in patients with intrahepatic and extrahepatic cholestasis. *J. Pediatr.*, 83:291–293.

46. Livingstone, S. (1972): *Comprehensive Management of Epilepsy in Infancy, Childhood and Adolescence*. Charles C Thomas, Springfield, Illinois.

47. Loga, S., Curry, S., and Lader, M. (1975): Interactions of orphenadrine and phenobarbitone with chlorpromazine: Plasma concentrations and effects in man. *Br. J. Clin. Pharmacol.*, 2:197–208.

48. MacDonald, M. G., and Robinson, D. S. (1968): Clinical observations of possible barbiturate interference with anticoagulation. *J.A.M.A.*, 204:97–100.

49. Matsumura, S., and Omura, T. (1973): The effects of phenobarbital on the turnover of messenger RNA's for microsomal enzymes. *Drug Metab. Dispos.*, 1:248–250.

50. Mattson, R. H., Gallagher, B. B., Reynolds, E. H., and Glass, D. (1973): Folate therapy in epilepsy. A controlled study. *Arch. Neurol.*, 29:78–81.

51. McLean, A. E. M., and Day, P. (1975): The effect of diet on the toxicity of paracetamol. *Biochem. Pharmacol.*, 23:37–42.

52. Morselli, P. L., Rizzo, M., and Garattini, S. (1971): Interaction between phenobarbital and diphenylhydantoin in animals and in epileptic patients. *Ann. N.Y. Acad. Sci.*, 179:88–107.

53. Mumford, J. P. (1974): Drugs affecting oral contraceptives. *Br. Med. J.*, 2:333–334.

54. Munson, E. S., Malagodi, M. H., Shields, R. P., Tham, M. K., Fiserova-Bergerova, V., Holaday, D. A., Perry, J. C., and Embro, W. J. (1975): Fluroxene toxicity induced by phenobarbital. *Clin. Pharmacol. Ther.*, 18:687–699.

55. Nanda, R. N., Johnson, R. H., Keogh, H. J., Lambie, D. G., and Melville, I. D. (1977): Treatment of epilepsy with clonazepam and its effect on other an-

ticonvulsants. *J. Neurol. Neurosurg. Psychiatry,* 40:538–543.

56. Neuvonen, P. J., Penttilä, O., Lehtovaara, R., and Aho, K. (1975): Effects of antiepileptic drugs on the elimination of various tetracycline derivatives. *Eur. J. Clin. Pharmacol.,* 9:147–154.

57. Orrenius, S., Ericson, J. E., and Ernster, L. (1965): Phenobarbital-induced synthesis of the microsomal drug-metabolizing enzyme system and its relationship to the proliferation of endoplasmic membranes. *J. Cell Biol.,* 25:627–639.

58. Padgham, C., and Richens, A. (1974): Quinine metabolism: A useful index of hepatic drug metabolizing capacity in man. *Br. J. Clin. Pharmacol.,* 1:352–353.

59. Perucca, E., Gatti, G., Frigo, G. M., Crema, A., Calzetti, S., and Visintini, D. (1978): Disposition of sodium valproate in epileptic patients. *Br. J. Clin. Pharmacol.,* 5:495–499.

60. Rambeck, B., Boenig, H. E., and May, T. (1979): Pharmakologische Beeinflussung der Phenobarbital und Phenytoin Serumkonzentration durch Valproate bei Epilepsie-Patienten. *Nervenarzt,* 50:743–746.

61. Richens, A. (1977): Interactions with antiepileptic drugs. *Drugs,* 13:266–275.

62. Riegelman, S., Rowland, M., and Epstein, W. L. (1970): Griseofulvin–phenobarbital interactions in man. *J.A.M.A.,* 213:426–431.

63. Rosalki, S. B. (1976): Plasma enzyme changes and their interpretation in patients receiving anticonvulsant and enzyme-inducing drugs. In: *Anticonvulsant Drugs and Enzyme Induction,* edited by A. Richens and F. P. Woodford, pp. 27–35. Elsevier/Excerpta Medica/North Holland, New York.

64. Schöne, B., Fleischmann, R. A., Remmer, H., and von Oldershausen, H. P. (1972): Determination of drug-metabolizing enzymes in needle biopsies of human liver. *Eur. J. Clin. Pharmacol.,* 4:65–73.

65. Shahidi, N. T. (1968): Acetophenetiden-induced methemoglobinemia. *Ann. N.Y. Acad. Sci.,* 151:822–831.

66. Sjö, O., Hvidberg, E. F., Naestoff, J., and Lund, M.

(1975): Pharmacokinetics and side effects of clonazepam and its 7-amino metabolite in man. *Eur. J. Clin. Pharmacol.,* 8:249–254.

67. Sotaniemi, E., Arvela, P., Hakkarainen, H., and Huhti, E. (1970): The clinical significance of microsomal enzyme induction in the therapy of epileptic patients. *Ann. Clin. Res.,* 2:223–227.

68. Testa, B., and Jenner, P. (1976): *Drug Metabolism: Chemical and Biochemical Aspects.* Marcel Dekker, New York, Basel.

69. Thompson, R. H. P., Eddleston, A. L. W. F., and Williams, R. (1969): Low plasma-billirubin in epileptics on phenobarbitone. *Lancet,* 1:21–22.

70. Vesell, E. S. (1977): Genetic and environmental factors affecting drug interactions in man. In: *Drug Interactions,* edited by D. G. Grahame-Smith, pp. 119–143. University Park Press, Baltimore.

71. Vesell, E. S. (1979): The antipyrine test in clinical pharmacology: Conceptions and misconceptions. *Clin. Pharmacol. Ther.,* 26:275–288.

72. Vesell, E. S., and Page, J. G. (1969): Genetic control of the phenobarbital-induced shortening of plasma antipyrine half-lives in man. *J. Clin. Invest.,* 48:2202–2209.

73. Wilder, B. J., Willmore, L. J., Bruni, J., and Villarreal, H. J. (1978): Valproic acid: Interaction with other anticonvulsant drugs. *Neurology (Minneap.),* 28:892–896.

74. Windorfer, A., Jr., and Pringsheim, W. (1977): Studies on the concentrations of chloramphenicol in the serum and cerebrospinal fluid of neonates, infants and small children. Reciprocal reactions between chloramphenicol, penicillin and phenobarbitone. *Eur. J. Pediatr.,* 124:129–138.

75. Windorfer, A., Jr., and Sauer, W. (1977): Drug interactions during anticonvulsant therapy in childhood: Diphenylhydantoin, primidone, phenobarbitone, clonazepam, nitrazepam, carbamazepine and dipropylacetate. *Neuropediatrie,* 8:29–41.

76. Yeung, C. Y., and Field, C. E. (1969): Phenobarbital therapy in neonatal hyperbilirubinaemia. *Lancet* 2:135–139.

Antiepileptic Drugs, edited by D. M. Woodbury, J. K. Penry, and C. E. Pippenger. Raven Press, New York © 1982.

25

Phenobarbital

Relation of Plasma Concentration to Seizure Control

Harold E. Booker

Phenobarbital was introduced in 1911, and its value as an antiepileptic drug was soon established (20). Until phenytoin was introduced some 20 years later, it was the only available drug for use against epilepsy other than the bromides. It is the most effective of all the barbiturates for long-term treatment of seizure disorders and is indicated for control of almost all kinds of seizures. However, it is only minimally effective, if at all, in absence attacks. The therapeutic effects of two other barbiturates, mephobarbital and dimethoxymethylphenobarbital, are due in large part, if not exclusively, to their *in vivo* conversion to phenobarbital. The same is true for primidone, although technically, primidone is not a barbiturate. The molecular structure of phenobarbital served as the model for many of the antiepileptic drugs subsequently developed. Few of them, however, offer any major advantage over phenobarbital, and it remains an effective, safe, and extensively used drug. Although methods for measuring the concentration of phenobarbital and its major metabolite in tissues and biologic fluids have been available for some time, the pharmacokinetics of phenobarbital in man have been explored in detail only recently. This chapter will concentrate on those aspects of its kinetics that are more relevant to

the clinical situation and on the relationship of plasma levels to control of seizures.

RELATION OF DOSE TO PLASMA LEVEL

Acute or Loading Doses

The only studies of the kinetics of phenobarbital after intravenous administration to humans both relate to the newborn (30,43). After a single intravenous loading dose, the plasma level is sustained for 12 to 24 hr. Each milligram per kilogram of dose gives a peak plasma level somewhat over 1 μg/ml.

Several studies have compared the results of single oral and intramuscular doses of phenobarbital, both in patients (4,24,44) and in volunteers (53,58). The bioavailability (the area under the curve relating plasma level to time) is the same by either route. The ratio of peak plasma level (in micrograms per milligram or milliliter) to dose (in milligrams per kilogram) is identical after either route and averages 1.5 in children (24) and 1.8 in adults (53). The peak plasma level after intramuscular injection is achieved between 1 and 3 hr independently of dose, age, or body weight.

More variance has been reported for the times of peak plasma phenobarbital levels after oral doses. Viswanathan et al. (58) found peak plasma levels between 1 and 3 hr after a 30-mg dose. Strandjord and Johannessen (53) gave 200 mg orally and found peak levels between 2 and 8 hr. In a much earlier study, higher doses were needed because the sensitivity of the then available methods of measurement was not as great. Consequently, Lous (34) gave 750 mg orally to three subjects and reported peak plasma levels between 6 and 18 hr. Thus, it appears that the time to peak plasma level after oral doses of phenobarbital is related to the dose. However, the effects of other variables such as fasting and pharmaceutical properties (crystal size, composition of tablet) are not known and were not the same in these studies. Whatever the effects of these variables, it appears that plasma levels may be higher after intramuscular injection of phenobarbital for only the first 30 to 60 min, and even these differences may not be clinically significant.

Chronic or Maintenance Doses

The relationship of the chronic dose of phenobarbital to plasma level at steady state is significantly influenced by age. In adults, the half-life of phenobarbital averages about 90 to 100 hr, so that 16 to 21 days are needed on any given dosage for steady state to be reached. When it is reached, each mg/kg per day gives a plasma level of approximately 10 μg/ml (5,9,35). This ratio may be lower in women than in men (31). However, it increases with age in women but not in men (16). These differences by sex are not marked and generally will have little practical clinical significance for the individual patient.

In children, plasma clearance is more rapid (19), the half-life averages around 50 hr (18, 24,40), and the ratio of plasma level to dose at steady state is lower. These effects are related to basal metabolic rate and, hence, indirectly to body surface area (55). Body weight or age, however, are simpler to determine and give adequate results in clinical practice. Doses in

TABLE 1. *Ratio of plasma phenobarbital level to dose*

Age (yr)	Weight (kg)	Ratio[a]
1–5	10–20	4.4
5–10	20–30	5.6
10–15	30–50	7.0
Adults	—	9.6

[a]Plasma phenobarbital level (μg/ml) produced by each mg/kg per day of dose with administration of phenobarbital alone. The values represent the average of those reported by several workers (9,31,45,55).

very young children need to be two or more times those given to adults to achieve the same steady-state plasma level; older children need about one and one-half times the adult dose (Table 1). As children reach puberty, the transition to adult values of plasma clearance is rather abrupt (19), and problems in maintaining a stable level may result (45).

Neonates present a special problem, as drug metabolism is poorly developed at birth but matures rapidly. In newborns whose mothers were treated with phenobarbital for hypertension during pregnancy, Boréus et al. (3) found half-lives averaging about 200 hr. There was marked variation, however, and the half-life was inversely proportional to the initial plasma level. The authors attributed this to the length of time the mother took phenobarbital and inferred that greater lengths of exposure decreased the half-life in the neonate. The findings of Painter et al. (43) in neonates treated postnatally for seizures support this. Half-lives of phenobarbital after 14 days of treatment averaged approximately 100 hr, whereas by 28 days of treatment the half-life had fallen to approximately 50 hr. Thus, the half-life of phenobarbital is prolonged in neonates but declines rapidly with postnatal exposure to the drug. After the initial loading dose, plasma levels were maintained for 12 to 24 hr, after which time oral doses sufficed. Oral doses of less than 4 mg/kg per day did not result in accumulation of drug, and plasma levels were low. Doses significantly over 5 mg/kg per day resulted in excessive levels and toxicity (43). In children up to 4 months of age, oral doses of phenobarbital gave lower peak plasma levels than did intramuscular doses (3). However, in children over 10 months of age the ratio was the same whether the drug was given orally or intramuscularly.

Conjoint administration of any of several other drugs can affect the kinetics of phenobarbital, generally increasing the ratio of plasma level to dose. Antiepileptic drugs implicated include phenytoin (40,45,53), valproic acid (14,31,33, 38,56), clomipramine (31), and the phenylureas (22,31). The effect of phenytoin may not be marked, however, and several workers found no significant effects for phenytoin, particularly in populations who were taking the two drugs chronically (8,9,61). The effect of valproic acid, however, is usually significant, and the plasma level of phenobarbital may be 50% or more higher than it would be if the same dose of phenobarbital were given alone. Some of the sedation initially attributed to valproic acid is due to this effect, as in early clinical trials it was common to add valproic acid to preexisting phenobarbital therapy. The major psychotropic drugs apparently do not produce any significant effect on phenobarbital metabolism or plasma levels (46).

Primidone is extensively and mephobarbital completely metabolized to phenobarbital. According to Eadie et al. (9), daily mephobarbital doses of 2, 5, or 8 mg/kg are needed to maintain plasma phenobarbital levels of 10, 20, or 30 μg/ml, respectively. The results for primidone are more variable and depend in part on whether phenytoin is also given (13,47). In general, each 1 mg/kg per day of primidone dose gives a plasma phenobarbital level at steady state of 1.5 to 2 μg/ml. This increases by 2 to 3 μg/ml when phenytoin is given concurrently (2,9,45,50,61).

Steady-state plasma levels of phenobarbital have been shown to decrease significantly in some patients during pregnancy (27), and such patients often require higher doses to maintain therapeutic effects during the pregnancy. The effect is reversible after delivery. Although the mechanism is not completely understood, this effect has been shown for several antiepileptic drugs and may account for the loss of seizure control that occurs in some patients during pregnancy. Cirrhosis, but not acute infectious hepatitis, increases the plasma half-life of phenobarbital, although renal excretion of unmetabolized phenobarbital tends to prevent major rises in the plasma level (1). Phenobarbital can apparently be given safely if cautiously to patients with renal disease (10).

RELATION OF PLASMA LEVEL TO SEIZURE CONTROL

Because of the complexities of the clinical epilepsies, it is more difficult to establish the dose−response curve for the clinical situation than it is in the experimental laboratory. Age at onset, type of seizures, etiology, and pretreatment frequency of seizures all have significant influences on the response to treatment (48), and it is difficult if not impossible to control all of these variables in clinical studies. Prospective experiments in which doses of phenobarbital are changed and the resultant changes in plasma levels correlated with changes in seizure frequency give robust data but are limited for practical and ethical reasons to small numbers of subjects. Surveys, particularly retrospective ones, allow accumulation of data on a large number of patients. However, the results tell what the plasma levels were and not necessarily what they would have been had seizure control been the only variable influencing the clinicians' prescriptions and the patients' compliance. Considering the uncontrolled variables, and the fact that some patients will not respond to phenobarbital in any dose, it is not surprising that retrospective surveys of large heterogeneous samples of patients often do not demonstrate any significant difference in the distribution of plasma levels between controlled and uncontrolled subjects. Such results should not be taken, however, to indicate that there is no relationship between plasma level and degree of control.

The original prospective study, and still the most detailed, was that of Buchthal et al. (6). These workers reported on the findings in 11 patients with frequent seizures who were hospitalized for several weeks. Although all had frequent seizures, none were on medication at the start of the study. Treatment with phenobarbital was begun with small doses that were gradually increased. In addition to careful clinical observation, frequent EEG examinations and plasma level determinations were carried out. Epileptogenic paroxysms in the EEG were reduced by 90% or more in three subjects at plasma levels of 4 μg/ml, in seven subjects at plasma levels between 8 and 15 μg/ml, and in one patient at 22 μg/ml. The average level at which the response occurred was 10 μg/ml. No grand mal attacks were noted when plasma levels were at or above 4 μg/ml, with the exception of one patient who required levels from 10 to 15 μg/ml. In three patients, phenobarbital was withdrawn after attacks were controlled. Seizures occurred in two of the three when the levels had fallen to 8 and 9 μg/ml.

Oller-Daurella and co-workers (42) took an alternative approach and gradually withdrew medication in patients who had been seizure-free for several years. The final medication for all patients was phenobarbital. When seizures recurred, they did so when the plasma phenobarbital levels averaged 9.9 μg/ml. Loiseau et al. (32) raised doses of phenobarbital in 42 uncontrolled patients so that plasma levels rose above 10 μg/ml. Twenty-three (55%) obtained seizure control. In addition, they lowered the dose of phenobarbital so that the plasma level fell to within 10 to 25 μg/ml in 27 patients in whom the plasma level was originally above 25 μg/ml. Twenty-three patients did well with no exacerbation of attacks. In the four other subjects, attacks recurred at plasma levels of 19, 22, 23, and 40 μg/ml. Most patients benefited from loss of side effects, however.

Five prospective studies of continuous phenobarbital treatment of children with febrile seizures in which plasma phenobarbital levels were monitored have been reported. Two of the studies (21,63) had concurrent control groups, whereas three (11,26,57) contrasted the results with those of a comparable sample of untreated subjects reported earlier (15). The patient sample overlapped to some degree in two of the studies (11,57). The combined population in these studies is over 450 treated patients followed from 6 months to 2 years. Plasma levels were determined in 40 patients within 12 hr or less of a recurrent convulsion. In 31 of these instances, the level was below 16 μg/ml, and in nine it was above 16 μg/ml. Average or sustained plasma levels of less than 16 μg/ml were present in 291 subjects, 49 of whom had seizure recurrences. In contrast, recurrences occurred in only 14 of the 150 subjects who had average plasma levels over 16 μg/ml. The difference for the pooled data from these five studies is significant ($\chi^2 = 6.1$, $p < 0.02$). Recurrence rates for the treated groups were significantly lower in the individual studies, although the difference did not reach conventional levels of statistical significance in one study (21). However, if one fewer recurrence had occurred in the treated group, a significant result ($p < 0.05$) would have been found in this study also. Nevertheless, the authors concluded that the data proved the lack of efficacy of phenobarbital and so titled their report (21).

The trends emerging from these prospective studies were supported by the findings in several surveys. Volanschi et al. (59) retrospectively surveyed patients with pretreatment rates of at least one seizure per month. They found no evidence of efficacy when phenobarbital plasma levels were less than 15 μg/ml. Lockman et al. (30), in a prospective survey of the efficacy of phenobarbital in controlling seizures in the neonate, found no patients controlled at less than 17 μg/ml. Feldman and Pippenger (12), however, in a retrospective survey of patients who had been completely controlled for at least 2 years, found the majority to have plasma levels below 10 μg/ml. Since a significant number of patients who have been seizure free for 2 years on treatment will continue to be seizure free when drugs are withdrawn (25,42), and the drugs were not withdrawn in this study, the proportion of patients who still needed the drugs at these low levels cannot be identified.

This last conflicting result indicates the effect of selection of patients on the results and the general limitations of retrospective surveys. Nevertheless, these limitations can to some de-

TABLE 2. *Plasma phenobarbital levels and seizure control*[a]

Plasma phenobarbital level (μg/ml)	Total no. of subjects	No. of subjects controlled	Cumulative % of controlled subjects
<10	50	14	6.5
10–14	92	23	17.2
15–19	115	50	40.6
20–24	93	50	64.0
25–29	87	29	77.6
30–34	43	12	83.2
35–39	35	16	90.7
≥40	53	20	100

[a]Based on pooled data from four studies (30,32,59,60).

gree be overcome by pooling enough data so that very large samples are accumulated. Three retrospective (32,59,60) and one prospective (30) survey gave sufficient details about plasma levels in individual subjects that the data can be pooled to give a sample of 568 patients of varied age, race, sex, and seizure type. The results are summarized in Table 2, which gives the total number of subjects and the number controlled for each range of plasma levels as well as a cumulative percentage of the number of subjects who were controlled at progressively higher plasma levels. Eighty-four percent of all subjects who were controlled had plasma levels between 10 and 40 μg/ml. Assuming that patients controlled at lower levels will continue to be controlled at higher levels, and considering that only 214 (38%) of the total were controlled, the probability of any patient being controlled and having a plasma level below 10 μg/ml is 0.025. This probability rises to 0.34 as the plasma level rises to 34 μg/ml and only increases to 0.38 when the level goes above 40 μg/ml.

Thus, although no single study is definitive, and each has some limitations, a strong consensus emerges that for individual subjects studied prospectively and for population data evaluated retrospectively, a significant increment in therapeutic efficacy is found when the plasma phenobarbital level is above 10 μg/ml. The increase in efficacy as the plasma level increases above 40 μg/ml is minimal for the population

and, in the individual subject, must be weighed against the potential for side effects. The population data surveyed suggest that approximately 84% of those subjects who do respond to treatment with phenobarbital will do so with plasma levels between 10 and 40 μg/ml. This range is frequently referred to as the "therapeutic level."

In applying the concept of a "therapeutic level" to the treatment of the individual patient, it must be remembered that this is a statistical concept and includes the mean plus and minus approximately 1.5 standard deviations of the responsive population. Some patients will be completely seizure free with plasma levels below 10 μg/ml, and there is no compelling reason to prescribe higher doses in such patients. Treatment with phenobarbital should not be abandoned as ineffective, however, until the plasma level has been at least in the upper portion of the therapeutic range for an appropriate period of time unless toxicity develops first. On the other hand, many patients who have had plasma levels above 40 μg/ml have maintained seizure control and improved from the point of toxicity when the levels have been lowered. Nevertheless, there will be some patients who require levels above this range to obtain seizure control. When experience with the individual patient indicates that such levels are needed and are not associated with significant toxicity, the patient and not the plasma level should be treated.

Data on the relative efficacy of phenobarbital for different seizure types are scanty. Although it is generally acknowledged that a smaller percentage of patients with complex partial seizures than with generalized tonic–clonic convulsions will be controlled, Schmidt (49) found no difference in the plasma phenobarbital levels in subjects with either seizure type who were controlled.

It has been argued that continuous phenobarbital treatment is ineffective for prevention of febrile seizures and that its apparent efficacy in the studies of febrile seizures discussed above was due to inclusion of many children with epileptic seizures triggered by fever rather than simple or benign febrile seizures (29). However, Wolf (62) found that phenobarbital gave better results in the group most likely to have simple febrile convulsions than in the group most likely to suffer from epilepsy. There is complete agreement, however, that intermittent treatment given at the onset of fever is ineffective. Adequate plasma levels cannot be obtained in time by this method, even when oral or intramuscular loading doses are given (11, 44,63).

Many of the subjects in the studies cited above were taking other drugs, and it is difficult if not impossible to dissect out the contribution made solely by the phenobarbital. Leppik and Sherwin (28) have shown that what had previously been interpreted as potentiation between phenytoin and phenobarbital in acute studies in the rat was actually a kinetic interaction. At the doses used and in the time course of the experiment, phenobarbital inhibited the metabolism of phenytoin. Plasma levels of phenytoin were higher in the animals given both drugs than in the animals given the same dose of phenytoin alone. When the dose–response curve was determined using brain levels, the effects of the two drugs were simply additive. In another study (51), these authors reported that the therapeutic levels on a molar basis in cerebral cortex are essentially equal. Using partition coefficients derived from human material obtained at autopsy, they have speculated that therapeutic effects in man are related to the total molar concentration in cerebral cortex of either or both drugs in a simple additive fashion. However, Volanschi et al. (59) were unable to find evidence of an additive effect, as seizure control in their retrospective survey was related to a plasma level of either phenobarbital or phenytoin within the therapeutic range but not for both drugs together.

It is generally assumed that mephobarbital is completely metabolized to phenobarbital and that the therapeutic effect is solely that of the phenobarbital. This is not the case for primidone, as both the parent drug and the other major metabolite, phenylethylmalondiamide, have antiepileptic effects. Although at steady state the plasma level of bioderived phenobarbital is greater than that of primidone, the relative contributions of primidone and its two metabolites to the overall therapeutic effect are unknown. A similar but more complex problem exists for the experimental drug dimethoxymethylphenobarbital, as it has several active metabolites including phenobarbital. Some authors have attributed the major therapeutic effect of this drug to the bioderived phenobarbital but have attributed the overall superiority of the drug to the finding of less sedation at any given plasma level of bioderived phenobarbital than when phenobarbital itself is given (17,52). Since the two phenobarbitals do not differ, the assumption is that the parent drug or another of the metabolites inhibits the sedative effect of phenobarbital without affecting the antiepileptic effect. That these two are separate pharmacologic effects is suggested by the fact that tolerance develops to the sedative but not the antiepileptic effect of phenobarbital.

TOXICITY

Although the adverse effects of phenobarbital are discussed in Chapter 26, no discussion of the therapeutic effect would be complete without considering at least those adverse effects that can be present at plasma levels within the therapeutic range. Sedation is the most common such effect and is almost universally present when treatment is started. It is difficult to relate such sedation to plasma levels in an absolute way, as some degree of tolerance usually develops, even while the plasma level is climbing to reach a higher level later at steady state (7). Such tolerance can be quite marked, and patients on chronic therapy can tolerate plasma levels that would produce loss of consciousness if they occurred as a result of a single acute dose (35). These results are often taken to indicate that if a patient does not exhibit or complain of sedation, he or she is essentially free from dose-dependent side effects of phenobarbital. Even though febrile convulsions may be prevented by phenobarbital, significant side effects other than sedation, necessitating drug withdrawal, are frequent and are often present at low doses (64). Hutt and co-workers (23) reported that performance on a variety of tests of cognitive and adaptive abilities was impaired in proportion to plasma phenobarbital levels even though the subjects had no complaints of sedation. More recently, dose-dependent differential effects on short- and long-term memory functions have been described (36). How such defects in specialized neuropsychological test performances translate into practical functional deficits for the individual patient has not been established. Even if known, they would have to be weighed against the overall benefits and the improvement in these functions that accrue from seizure control. More research should allow treatment in the future to be guided by considerations that relate plasma levels not only to the degree of seizure control but also to the subtle but definite subclinical toxicities.

SUMMARY

Phenobarbital is a relatively safe and generally effective drug for the treatment of many types of epileptic seizures. It can be given by the oral, intramuscular, or intravenous route. Because of its long half-life, it can be given in a single daily dose except in young children. Because the half-life is long, even compared with a 24-hr dosing interval, and because its kinetics are not dose dependent, the relationship between dose and plasma level at steady state is more stable than for many other antiepileptic drugs. From the figures given in Table 1, it is usually possible to calculate within 15% accuracy the dose necessary to produce a desired plasma level. When phenobarbital is given with antiepileptic drugs metabolized to phenobarbital (primidone or mephobarbital), the plasma level will be much higher and often is excessive. Conjoint administration of valproic acid and possibly phenytoin will also raise the plasma level of phenobarbital. The effects of other antiepileptic drugs on the plasma phenobarbital level are unpredictable in the individual patient. Pregnancy will probably lower the steady-state plasma level.

Oral maintenance treatment can be started with the full calculated dose, but sedation is to be expected. Although tolerance usually develops, initial sedation can be minimized by starting with a portion of the total calculated maintenance dose. In my experience, an initial dose one-third to one-half the total dose, increased by increments of one-fourth or one-third of the total maintenance dose every 5 to 7 days, will minimize patient complaints and decrease resistance to taking phenobarbital. This will, of course, prolong the time before steady state is attained at the final maintenance dose.

When the situation is urgent, and it is important to obtain a higher plasma level more rapidly, treatment can be started with loading doses. An initial oral dose of twice the desired maintenance dose for the first 3 or 4 days has been recommended (54). Significant amounts of sedation are to be expected with this procedure, and the clinician and patient must be prepared to make whatever accommodations are required. Since the bioavailability is essentially equal after oral and intramuscular administration, intramuscular doses offer no great advantage over oral doses except in the patient who cannot swallow or who might reject oral doses, and perhaps in the very young child. In truly emergent situations when high plasma phenobarbital levels are needed quickly, large doses must be given by either route, or the drug must be given intravenously. This should only be done when the clinician is prepared to manage any complications, preferably in a hospital setting. Plasma levels can be monitored by obtaining samples of blood. Saliva (37,41) or tears (39) can be used to determine the free or unbound levels.

Although not all patients will respond to treatment with phenobarbital, the literature reviewed suggests that 84% of those who do will do so when the plasma level is between 10 and 40 µg/ml. However, when experience with an individual patient indicates that higher or lower plasma levels are needed, the patient and not the plasma level should be treated. Levels above 15 µg/ml will often prevent recurrent febrile convulsions, but compliance is low, and side effects are frequent.

Recent evidence suggests that subtle but

definite effects on cognitive, adaptive, and memory functions are present even when phenobarbital plasma levels are within the therapeutic range. Although the full extent and clinical significance of these effects are unknown at present, they should be considered and weighed against the therapeutic effects to arrive at the optimum level for each patient.

REFERENCES

1. Alvin, J., McHorse, T., Hoyumpa, A., Bush, M., and Schenker, S. (1975): The effect of liver disease in man on the disposition of phenobarbital. *J. Pharmacol. Exp. Ther.*, 192:224–235.

2. Booker, H., Hosokowa, E., Burdette, R., and Darcey, B. (1970): A clinical study of serum primidone levels. *Epilepsia*, 11:395–402.

3. Boreus, L., Jalling, B., and Kallberg, N. (1975): Clinical pharmacology of phenobarbital in the neonatal period. In: *Basic and Therapeutic Aspects of Perinatal Pharmacology*, edited by P. Morselli, S. Garattini, and F. Sereni, pp. 331–340. Raven Press, New York.

4. Brachet-Liermain, A., Goutieres, F., and Aicardi, J. (1975): Absorption of phenobarbital after the intramuscular administration of single doses in infants. *J. Pediatr.*, 87:624–626.

5. Buchthal, F., and Svensmark, O. (1971): Serum concentrations of diphenylhydantoin (phenytoin) and phenobarbital and their relation to therapeutic and toxic effects. *Psychiatr. Neurol. Neurochir.*, 74:117–136.

6. Buchthal, F., Svensmark, O., and Simonsen, H. (1968): Relation of EEG and seizures to phenobarbital in serum. *Arch. Neurol.*, 19:567–572.

7. Butler, T., Mahafee, C., and Waddell, W. (1954): Phenobarbital: Studies of elimination, accumulation, tolerance and dosage schedules. *J. Pharmacol. Exp. Ther.*, 111:425–435.

8. Dekaban, A., Fugitani, K., and Constantopoulos, G. (1974): The effects of different dosages of combined antiepileptic drugs on their metabolism and their levels in body fluids. *Clin. Neurol. Neurosurg.*, 3/4:168–179.

9. Eadie, M., Lander, C., Hooper, W., and Tyrer, J. (1977): Factors influencing plasma phenibarbitone levels in epileptic patients. *Br. J. Clin. Pharmacol.*, 4:541–547.

10. Fabre, J., DeFreudenreich, J., Duckert, A., Pitton, J., Rudhardt, M., and Virieux, C. (1967): Influence of renal insufficiency in the excretion of chloroquine, phenobarbital, phenothiazines, and methacycline. *Helv. Med. Acta*, 33:307–316.

11. Faero, O., Kastrup, E., Nielsen, E., Melchior, J., and Thorn, I. (1972): Successful prophylaxis of febrile convulsions with phenobarbital. *Epilepsia*, 13:279–285.

12. Feldman, R., and Pippenger, C. (1976): The relation of anticonvulsant drug levels to complete seizure control. *J. Clin. Pharmacol.*, 16:51–59.

13. Fincham, R., Schottelius, D., and Sahs, A. (1974): The influence of diphenylhydantoin on primidone metabolism. *Arch. Neurol.*, 30:259–262.

14. Flachs, H., Wurtz-Jorgensen, A., Gram, L., and Wolff, K. (1977): Sodium di-*n*-propylacetate—its interaction with other antiepileptic drugs. In: *Antiepileptic Drug Monitoring*, edited by C. Gardner-Thorpe, D. Janz, H. Meinardi, and C. Pippenger, pp. 165–172. Pitman Medical, Tunbridge Wells, Kent.

15. Frantzen, E., Lennox-Buchthal, M., and Nygaard, A. (1968): Longitudinal EEG and clinical study of children with febrile convulsions. *Electroencephalogr. Clin. Neurophysiol.*, 24:197–212.

16. Furlanut, M., Benetello, P., Testa, G., and DaRonch, A. (1978): The effects of dose, age, and sex on the serum levels of phenobarbital and diphenylhydantoin in epileptic patients. *Pharmacol. Res. Commun.*, 10:85–89.

17. Gallagher, B., Baumel, I., Woodbury, S., and Dimicco, J. (1975): Clinical evaluation of eterobarb, a new anticonvulsant drug. *Neurology (Minneap.)*, 25:399–404.

18. Garrettson, L., and Dayton, P. (1970): Disappearance of phenobarbital and diphenylhydantoin from serum of children. *Clin. Pharmacol. Ther.*, 11:674–679.

19. Guelen, P., Van Der Kleijn, E., and Woudstra, U. (1975): Statistical analysis of pharmacokinetic parameters in epileptic patients chronically treated with antiepileptic drugs. In: *Clinical Pharmacology of Antiepileptic Drugs*, edited by H. Schnieder, D. Janz, C. Gardner-Thorpe, H. Meinardi, and A. Sherwin, pp. 2–10. Springer-Verlag, New York, Berlin.

20. Haupmann, A. (1912): Luminal bei Epilepsia. *Munch. Med. Wochenschr.*, 59:1907–1909.

21. Heckmatt, J., Houston, A., Clow, D., Stephenson, J., Dodd, E., Lealman, G., and Logan, R. (1976): Failure of phenobarbitone to prevent febrile convulsions. *Br. Med. J.*, 1:559–561.

22. Huisman, J., van Heycop ten Ham, M., and van Zijl, C. (1970): Influence of ethylphenacemide on serum levels of other anti-epileptic drugs. *Epilepsia*, 11:207–215.

23. Hutt, S., Jackson, P., Belsham, A., and Higgins, G. (1968): Perceptual-motor behaviour in relation to blood phenobarbitone level: A preliminary report. *Dev. Med. Child Neurol.*, 10:626–632.

24. Jalling, B. (1974): Plasma and cerebrospinal fluid concentrations of phenobarbital in infants given single doses. *Dev. Med. Child Neurol.*, 16:781–793.

25. Juul-Jensen, P. (1968): Frequency of recurrence after discontinuance of anticonvulsant therapy in patients with epileptic seizures. A new follow-up study after 5 years. *Epilepsia*, 9:11–16.

26. Knudsen, F., and Vestermark, S. (1978): Prophylactic diazepam or phenobarbitone in febrile convulsions: A prospective, controlled study. *Arch. Dis. Child.*, 53:660–663.

27. Lander, C., Edwards, V., Eadie, M., and Tyrer, J. (1977): Plasma anticonvulsant concentrations during pregnancy. *Neurology (Minneap.)*, 27:128–131.

28. Leppik, I., and Sherwin, A. (1977): Anticonvulsant

activity of phenobarbital and phenytoin in combination. *J. Pharmacol. Exp. Ther.*, 200:570–575.

29. Livingston, S., and Pauli, L. (1976): Treatment of "febrile seizures." *J. Pediatr.*, 89:164–165.

30. Lockman, L., Kriel, R., Zaske, D., Thompson, T., and Virnig, N. (1979): Phenobarbital dosage for control of neonatal seizures. *Neurology (Minneap.)*, 29:1445–1449.

31. Loiseau, P., Brachet, A., and Henry, P. (1975): Etude du taux serique du phenobarbital chez des epileptiques. *Encephale*, I:341–357.

32. Loiseau, P., Brachet-Liermain, A., Legroux, M., and Jogeix, M. (1977): Interet du dosage des anticonvulsivants dans le traitement des epilepsies. *Nouv. Presse Med.*, 6:813–817.

33. Loiseau, P., Orgogozo, J., Brachet-Liermain, A., and Morselli, P. (1978): Pharmacokinetic studies on the interaction between phenobarbital and valproic acid. In: *Advances in Epileptology*, edited by H. Meinardi and A. Rowan, pp. 261–265. Swets & Zeitlinger B.V., Amsterdam, Lisse.

34. Lous, P. (1954): Plasma levels and urinary excretion of three barbituric acids after oral administration to man. *Acta Pharmacol. Toxicol. (Kbh.)*, 10:147–165.

35. Lous, P. (1954): Blood serum and cerebrospinal fluid levels and renal clearance of phenemal in treated epileptics. *Acta Pharmacol. Toxicol. (Kbh.)*, 10:166–177.

36. MacLeod, C., Dekaban, A., and Hunt, E. (1978): Memory impairment in epileptic patients: Selective effects of phenobarbital concentration. *Science*, 202:1102–1104.

37. McAuliffe, J., Sherwin, A., Leppik, I., Fayle, S., and Pippinger, C. (1977): Salivary levels of anticonvulsants: A practical approach to drug monitoring. *Neurology (Minneap.)*, 27:409–413.

38. Mesdjian, E., Mesdjian, J., Bouyard, P., Dravet, C., and Roger, J. (1978): Effect of sodium valproate on phenobarbitone plasma levels in epileptic patients. In: *Advances in Epileptology*, edited by H. Meinardi and A. Rowan, pp. 266–268. Swets & Zeitlinger, B.V., Amsterdam and Lisse.

39. Monaco, F., Mutani, R., Mastropaolo, C., and Tondi, M. (1979): Tears as the best practical indicator of the unbound fraction of an anticonvulsant drug. *Epilepsia*, 20:705–710.

40. Morselli, P., Rizzo, M., and Garattini, S. (1971): Interaction between phenobarbital and diphenylhydantoin in animals and in epileptic patients. *Ann. N.Y. Acad. Sci.*, 179:88–107.

41. Nishihara, K., Uchino, K., Saitoh, Y., Honda, Y., Nakagawa, F., and Tamura, Z. (1979): Estimation of plasma unbound phenobarbital concentration by using mixed saliva. *Epilepsia*, 20:37–40.

42. Oller-Daurella, L., Oller F.-V., L., and Pamies, E. (1977): Clinical, therapeutic and social status of epileptic patients without seizures for more than 5 years. In: *Epilepsy, the Eighth International Symposium*, edited by J. Penry, pp. 69–75. Raven Press, New York.

43. Painter, M., Pippenger, C., MacDonald, H., and Pitlock, W. (1978): Phenobarbital and diphenylhydantoin levels in neonates with seizures. *J. Pediatr.*, 92:315–319.

44. Pearce, J., Sharman, J., and Forster, R. (1977): Phenobarbital in the acute management of febrile convulsions. *Pediatrics*, 60:569–572.

45. Pippenger, C. (1978): Pediatric clinical pharmacology of antiepileptic drugs: A special consideration. In: *Antiepileptic Drugs: Quantitative Analysis and Interpretation*, edited by C. Pippenger, J. Penry, and H. Kutt, pp. 315–319. Raven Press, New York.

46. Pippenger, C., Siris, J., Werner, W., and Masland, R. (1975): The effect of psychotropic drugs on serum anti-epileptic levels in psychiatric patients with seizure disorders. In: *Clinical Pharmacology of Anti-epileptic Drugs*, edited by H. Schnieder, D. Janz, C. Gardner-Thorpe, H. Meinardi, and A. Sherwin, pp. 135–144. Springer-Verlag, New York, Heidelberg, Berlin.

47. Reynolds, E. (1975): Longitudinal studies of serum anti-epileptic drug levels. In: *Clinical Pharmacology of Anti-epileptic Drugs*, edited by H. Schnieder, D. Janz, C. Gardner-Thorpe, H. Meinardi, and A. Sherwin, pp. 79–86. Springer-Verlag, New York, Heidelberg, Berlin.

48. Rodin, E. (1968): *The Prognosis of Patients with Epilepsy.* Charles C Thomas, Springfield, Illinois.

49. Schmidt, D. (1977): Variation of therapeutic plasma concentrations of phenytoin and phenobarbital with the type of seizures and comedication. In: *Epilepsy, the Eighth International Symposium*, edited by J. Penry, pp 219–221. Raven Press, New York.

50. Schottelius, D., and Fincham, R. (1978): Clinical applications of serum primidone levels. In: *Antiepileptic Drugs: Quantitative Analysis and Interpretation*, edited by C. Pippenger, J. Penry, and H. Kutt, pp. 273–282. Raven Press, New York.

51. Sherwin, A., Harvey, C., and Leppik, I. (1977): Antiepileptic drugs in human cerebral cortex: Clinical relevance of cortex : plasma ratios. In: *Epilepsy, the Eighth International Symposium*, edited by J. Penry, pp. 103–108. Raven Press, New York.

52. Smith, D., Goldstein, S., and Roomet, A. (1975): A comparison of the hypnotic effects of the anticonvulsant dimethoxymethylphenobarbital and sodium phenobarbital in normal human volunteers. *Epilepsia*, 16:201.

53. Strandjord, R., and Johannessen, S. (1977): Serum levels of phenobarbitone in healthy subjects and patients with epilepsy. In: *Antiepileptic Drug Monitoring*, edited by C. Gardner-Thorpe, D. Janz, H. Meinardi, and C. Pippenger, pp. 89–103. Pitman Medical, Tunbridge Wells, Kent.

54. Svensmark, O., and Buchthal, F. (1963): Accumulation of phenobarbital in man. *Epilepsia*, 4:199–206.

55. Svensmark, O., and Buchthal, F. (1964): Diphenylhydantoin and phenobarbital: Serum levels in children. *Am. J. Dis. Child.*, 108:82–87.

56. Taburet, A., Aymard, P., Hamar, C., Ouhab, F., and Richardet, J. (1976): Influence of combined therapy on blood phenobarbital levels. In: *Drug Interference and Drug Measurement in Clinical Chemistry*, edited by G. Siest and D. Young, pp. 170–174. S. Karger, Basel.

57. Thorn, I. (1975): A controlled study of profylactic [sic] long-term treatment of febrile convulsions with

phenobarbital. *Acta Neurol. Scand.* [*Suppl.*], 60:67–73.

58. Viswanathan, C., Booker, H., and Welling, P. (1978): Bioavailability of oral and intramuscular phenobarbital. *J. Clin. Pharmacol.,* 18:100–105.

59. Volanschi, D., Pintilie, C., Florescu, D., and Tudor, S. (1975): Therapeutic response relationship to phenobarbital and diphenylhydantoin serum and cerebrospinal fluid levels in epileptics. *Rev. Roum. Med. Neurol. Psychiatry,* 13:217–223.

60. Watanabe, S., Kuyama, C., Yokoyama, S., Kubo, S., and Iwai, H. (1977): Distribution of plasma phenobarbital, diphenylhydantoin and primidone levels in epileptic patients. *Folia Psychiatr. Neurol. Jpn.,* 31:205–217.

61. Windorfer, A., Jr., Gadeke, R., and Sauer, M. (1975): Untersuchungen uber die Medikamenten-Serumspei-gel antikonvulsiv behandelter Kinder. *Z. Kinderheilk.,* 119:15–24.

62. Wolf, S. (1977): The effectiveness of phenobarbital in the prevention of recurrent febrile convulsions in children with and without a history of pre-, peri- and postnatal abnormalities. *Acta Paediatr. Scand.,* 66:585–587.

63. Wolf, S., Carr, A., Davis, D., Davidson, S., Dale, E., Forsythe, A., Goldenberg, E., Hanson, R., Lulejian, G., Nelson, M., Treitman, P., and Weinstein, A. (1977): The value of phenobarbital in the child who has had a single febrile seizure: A controlled prospective study. *Pediatrics,* 59:378–385.

64. Wolf, S., and Forsythe, A. (1978): Behavioral disturbance, phenobarbital, and febrile seizures. *Pediatrics,* 61:728–731.

Antiepileptic Drugs, edited by D. M. Woodbury, J. K. Penry, and C. E. Pippenger. Raven Press, New York © 1982.

26

Phenobarbital

Toxicity

Richard H. Mattson and Joyce A. Cramer

Worldwide use of phenobarbital for almost a century has allowed the accumulation of considerable knowledge of its toxicity. Phenobarbital enjoys a reputation of safety because serious systemic side effects are very uncommon. Unfortunately, annoying neurological and psychological toxicity is frequent. Particular emphasis in this chapter will focus on problems associated with chronic use of the drug in doses producing serum concentrations considered effective in antiepileptic drug therapy.

NEUROTOXICITY

With the long-term use of phenobarbital, even at the usual dosage producing serum concentrations of the drug in the therapeutic range of 15 to 40 μg/ml, adverse changes in affect, behavior, and cognitive function are often encountered. High serum concentrations cause neurological signs of "drunkenness," including nystagmus, dysarthria, incoordination, and ataxia. Often, the neurotoxic side effects occur together in different degrees.

Sedation

The hallmark of barbiturate toxicity in adults is surely sedation. Complaints of fatigue and tiredness are difficult to quantify and are often variable and subtle. The patient and family may describe listlessness or lack of spontaneity even when excessive sleeping time is not observed. As dosage is increased, overt sleepiness is observable and often apparent by difficulty in arousal in the morning and naps after school or work. An associated loss of interest, particularly in social activity or playing with friends, is common. Drowsiness usually accompanies the initiation of phenobarbital and may persist for days or weeks in many patients.

Butler et al. (7) noted that patients complained of sedation at the onset of treatment when phenobarbital concentrations were only 5 μg/ml. Two weeks later, there were few complaints despite a fivefold increase in the serum levels. Others have also reported that sedation occurred primarily during the first few days of treatment and cleared rapidly as tolerance developed (5,25). Somnolence was even briefer if phenobarbital was restarted after a withdrawal period (5). It was also found that a dose that caused sedation during initiation of therapy in adults no longer caused sleepiness after 1 or 2 weeks of treatment (5). After tolerance was acquired, adverse effects of phenobarbital were not observed when the serum concentration was less than 30 μg/ml.

Mattson et al. (38), however, found many exceptions to the correlation between serum phenobarbital concentrations and complaints of tiredness. The variation among individuals was evident in that some patients were asymptomatic when serum phenobarbital levels were as high as 50 μg/ml, whereas others complained of feeling "drugged" when levels were as low as 15 μg/ml.

Neurological Side Effects

Increasing the dosage of phenobarbital eventually leads to neurological signs similar to those found with the use of other antiepileptic drugs. Dysarthria, incoordination, ataxia, and nystagmus appear as serum levels exceed 40 μg/ml. The correlation between these side effects and serum levels of phenobarbital is much less well defined than it is with the use of phenytoin (25). Since phenobarbital is usually used in combination with other drugs, it is often difficult to determine which drug is causing the side effects.

Behavior

Instead of the sedative effect of phenobarbital common in adults, a paradoxical effect of the drug in children and the elderly may produce insomnia and hyperkinetic activity. Ounsted (48) reviewing the hyperkinetic syndrome in epileptic children, found an approximately 8% incidence of overactivity in children receiving antiepileptic drug therapy. Phenobarbital commonly exacerbated aggressiveness and overactivity. The pattern of behavior included signs of distractability, shortened attention span, fluctuation of mood, and aggressive outbursts. It is of interest that 79% of the children were boys. Wolf and Forsythe (71) found a higher incidence of behavioral disturbances. Forty-two percent of 109 children receiving daily phenobarbital therapy to prevent recurrence of febrile seizures developed these problems. Surprisingly, 64% of the 38 children exhibiting hyperactivity had serum phenobarbital concentrations of less than 15 μg/ml, indicating that this is not a dose-related phenomenon. When phenobarbital therapy was stopped, behavior returned to normal in 16 children and improved in six. Only two of the improved children had a history of behavioral problems prior to the use of phenobarbital. Three of eight different children who exhibited other nonhyperkinetic behavioral disturbances during treatment also returned to normal after stopping the drug. The authors (71) concluded that behavioral disturbances associated with phenobarbital use are more likely to become evident in children in the presence of organic brain disease or deficits. Elderly patients with organic brain disease may also become agitated rather than sedated with use of phenobarbital.

Affect

Phenobarbital therapy can produce alteration of affect. For example, many patients become depressed while taking it. It is difficult to determine whether such mood changes are a reaction to the often newly diagnosed illness, the addition of another drug to treat severe seizures, or a direct neurotoxic effect of phenobarbital. Clinical observations suggest a direct effect of phenobarbital, since changes to carbamazepine therapy have been associated with improved mood scores (58).

Cognition

A side effect of phenobarbital of considerable potential importance, especially in children, is a possible disturbance in cognitive function. Problems with memory or compromised work and school performance may develop independent of sedation and hyperkinetic activity, although these factors may play a contributory role. Lennox (32) observed a marked impairment in affect and cognitive function in patients whose capacity had already been compromised: ". . . Many physicians in attempting to extinguish seizures only succeed in drowning the finer intellectual processes of their patients." Such effects are often subtle and difficult to measure despite reports by patients, families, and teachers.

Changes in cognitive function have been measured by various standardized neuropsychological tests. Interestingly, in early reports, institutionalized epileptic patients showed some improvement in intelligence testing after treatment with antiepileptic drugs. Improved test scores could be attributed to decreased seizure frequency or practice effect from repeated testing. These findings were not supported by more detailed studies, however. Lennox (32) found 58% of his patients unchanged on subjective evaluation of mentality while using phenobarbital. He separated the improvement of patients because of diminished seizure frequency from the effect of the medication on mentality. A more detailed study by Somerfeld-Ziskind and Ziskind (62) showed no overall change in I.Q. after phenobarbital therapy for a year. Twelve patients actually showed increased I.Q. scores, whereas 10 patients had lower scores (maximum change, 11 points); 79% had fewer seizures while receiving phenobarbital.

Stores (65) reviewed studies of the effect of phenobarbital on intellectual function. He commented that the educational problem for these children appears to be that their attainments fail to match their capacities as measured by standardized tests. Formal studies have not been able to assess this disparity. On careful testing, children treated with phenobarbital can perform at appropriate levels. However, in normal everyday behavior their attention and interest seem impaired. It is difficult to assess subjective concepts such as this unless the children are treated with a different medication and tested before and after the change from barbiturate therapy.

Reynolds and Travers (53) surveyed outpatients who had no signs of drug toxicity, no mental symptoms preceding their drug therapy, and no gross central nervous system lesion. They found that patients with serum phenobarbital concentrations averaging 19 µg/ml exhibited psychomotor slowing, intellectual deterioration, and psychiatric or personality change. A matched group of patients whose phenobarbital levels averaged 13 µg/ml were normal. Seizure frequency bore no relationship to these behavioral signs.

In a careful study of children receiving an average daily dose of 1.8 mg/kg of phenobarbital,

Wapner et al. (68) compared learning behavior and intelligence before therapy and 6 weeks later. Phenobarbital did not affect the function of the children in the classroom situation. Although seizure control was incomplete, there was no significant change in learning or intellect compared with a control group.

When carbamazepine was substituted for phenobarbital in children, several mental functions were improved. Schain et al. (58) found a statistically significant difference in intelligence (as measured by WISC) and results of three problem-solving tests of attentiveness and impulse control. Parents and teachers also reported a significant improvement in alertness and attentiveness. These psychotropic effects were not associated with improved seizure control but were considered to be a function of removal of the sedating drug.

Specific psychological testing has been done to sample sectors of performance thought to be more sensitive to subtle compromise by drug effects. Mirsky and Kornetsky (43) showed that barbiturates can impair performance on vigilance tests. These investigators suggested that barbiturate therapy may be related to learning difficulties in children. However, they did not take into consideration the fact that tolerance to barbiturate therapy develops very quickly. Therefore, the acute effects measured in their study could be expected to diminish with chronic administration. Other investigators (25) studied adults who had received phenobarbital for 2 weeks, allowing the development of tolerance before performance testing. They found that phenobarbital did not diminish performance on simple tasks requiring attention but did affect tasks requiring sustained effort. It is of interest to note that even the tasks requiring sustained effort showed improvement when patients were stimulated during the testing. Others also showed the difference between self-paced tests and tests in which sustained attention was necessary (31). Impaired vigilance and sensory perception during phenobarbital usage have been noted in patients of average intelligence (37).

Critical flicker fusion (CFF) has been widely used as an index of drug action on the central nervous system. Idestrom (26) evaluated CFF in chronic barbiturate usage and found that single doses of barbiturates produced a depressive effect in naive patients. In patients using barbiturates chronically, the depressive effect was weak or nonexistent. Instead, moderate doses produced a stimulating effect. With the use of CFF, it was shown that tolerance for test doses of phenobarbital developed within 1½ to 2 months.

In a comparison between phenytoin and phenobarbital, Houghton (24) defined the differences in the central actions of the two drugs by CFF threshold. As expected, phenobarbital produced significant depression of CFF compared with placebo, whereas phenytoin produced no demonstrable effect. However, these experimenters used only acute therapy (phenobarbital levels were as low as 5 µg/ml), so only acute toxicity was measured. The results may bear no relationship to those that might be found with higher serum drug concentrations during chronic therapy.

Hutt (25) tested the effects of phenobarbital after tolerance had developed. Although sedation was lessened at the time of testing compared with early acute effect, performance of perceptual–motor tests was significantly impaired in proportion to serum phenobarbital concentration. Tests requiring sustained vigilance were affected negatively. The author defined several factors that were significantly correlated with test performance: (a) serum phenobarbital concentration; (b) difficulty and duration of the task; (c) tester interaction with the subject (i.e., external stimulation).

A closely related but entirely separate issue is the question of memory impairment, which is a common complaint from epileptic patients and which might be related to the brain lesion. In detailed studies of patients tested when phenobarbital concentrations were at moderate and then high therapeutic levels, MacLeod et al. (36) compared short-term versus long-term memory storage. They found short-term memory scanning significantly impaired when phenobarbital levels were high, but retrieval of information stored in long-term memory was undiminished. Although this study was unfortunately brief in its 1-week trial at each dose, the data suggest that phenobarbital impairs access to information in short-term memory but not long-term memory. The authors suggested that impaired short-term memory may be an important influence in acquisition of new information because of impaired attention span. Oxley (49) indicated that a significant improvement in memory function can be achieved following a reduction in phenobarbital dose. This report was of interest because the patients experienced increased seizure frequency when the barbiturate level dropped, indicating that it is not seizure activity that impairs memory.

Barbiturate Overdose

Frank overdose of phenobarbital causing serum levels in excess of 50 to 60 µg/ml leads to progressive neurologic dysfunction and depression in consciousness, even in patients on chronic therapy. Excessively high doses first produce ataxia, dysarthria, nystagmus, incoordination, and uncontrollable sleepiness. As the serum level rises, these effects progress to stupor and coma. Ultimately, depression of cardiorespiratory function may lead to death. A level of 80 µg/ml is considered potentially lethal (2). The severity of CNS depression is much greater in the drug-naive patient. Because of tolerance, the occasional individual on chronic therapy may remain almost unaffected by serum levels that cause unconsciousness in the naive individual. Nonetheless, concentrations above 70 µg/ml can be expected to compromise levels of consciousness in almost all individuals. Details of treatment will be considered below.

Dependence, Habituation, and Withdrawal

Physical dependence on phenobarbital must be considered an aspect of barbiturate neurotoxicity. Phenobarbital shares the properties of other barbiturates in that chronic usage produces physical dependence: abrupt discontinuation after high dosage produces abstinence symptoms. Such symptoms include anxiety, emotional lability, insomnia, tremors, diaphoresis, confusion, and possible seizures for several days (23,27). These symptoms can be reversed by reinstituting the drug.

Isbell (27) described drug intoxication and withdrawal in terms of barbiturate abuse rather than its controlled use as an antiepileptic drug. If a decision is made to stop phenobarbital therapy, the drug should be tapered slowly to avoid withdrawal seizures.

Because phenobarbital can cross the placenta and enter the fetal system, special care must be taken during the neonatal period for children born to mothers who received phenobarbital. The neonatal withdrawal syndrome was described by Desmond et al. (16) for infants born to epileptic mothers. The infants were allowed to withdraw from phenobarbital post-partum. Hyperexcitability, tremor, irritability, and gastrointestinal upset continued for several days to several months. Although the withdrawal syndrome is similar among infants born to heroin addicts, barbiturate addicts, and epileptic mothers, the babies of women on antiepileptic doses of phenobarbital have a milder and briefer withdrawal experience with good results for all infants (3). There is no apparent residual damage after withdrawal. In order to calculate the probable length of withdrawal in neonates, it should be noted that the phenobarbital concentration in umbilical cord serum is approximately equal to the maternal serum concentration (42). The rate of elimination of phenobarbital in neonates is probably slower than in adults, possibly because neonatal liver is not fully capable of metabolizing barbiturates until induction of enzymes has occurred (19,42).

Some evidence suggests that discontinuation of phenobarbital in epileptic patients may lead to exacerbation of seizures not only because of the underlying epilepsy but also because of an additional barbiturate withdrawal mechanism (5). Even with abrupt discontinuation, the slow elimination of phenobarbital results in slowly decreasing plasma levels of the drug. Even so, gradual tapering may be advisable.

Other Aspects of Neurotoxicity

A systemic side effect of phenobarbital not documented in the literature and little appreci-

ated by treating physicians is impotence. Although primidone has been associated with this problem, there are no similar case reports of impotence caused by phenobarbital. In clinical practice, we have found that response to specific questions will reveal numerous complaints from men receiving phenobarbital. It is difficult to assess whether the problem is organic or related to psychological depression. Occasionally, dosage reduction will improve the problem. Although the effect may be on the central nervous system, we can postulate that impotence associated with antiepileptic drug therapy is the result of increased metabolism of steroids. Phenobarbital, a potent inducer of enzymes, is known to enhance metabolism of various steroids (33).

Summary of Neurotoxicity

Neurological aspects of phenobarbital toxicity include acute sedation, ataxia, dysarthria, lethargy, impaired attention and memory, as well as paradoxical hyperactivity. Excessive doses of phenobarbital can lead to coma. It is possible to adjust the dosage of barbiturates to maximum tolerance by monitoring nystagmus, dysarthria, and ataxia as well as sleepiness (39).

Because so few clinical trials of phenobarbital have been performed, reports of toxicity are minimal. The most important aspect of phenobarbital neurotoxicity is the reversibility of symptoms when the dosage is reduced or the drug is discontinued. Reports must be evaluated in terms of whether the subjects were suffering from drug intoxication acutely or after tolerance had developed or were acting idiosyncratically to drug therapy. In early studies, details of serum drug concentrations are absent. Many testing methods were inadequate and/or too insensitive to be of predictive value for measuring capacity of the children or adults to learn in school or function at home or at work. Neuropsychological problems may be marked and can be a limiting factor in the use of phenobarbital. These factors have not received sufficient attention. The extent of these side effects and the question of whether they produce long-lasting deficits have been insufficiently addressed.

HEMATOLOGICAL TOXICITY

Phenobarbital is particularly benign in its likelihood to produce serious hematological changes other than during use in combination with other antiepileptic drugs. Sole therapy with phenobarbital does not require numerous blood tests in anticipation of leukopenia, agranulocytosis, thrombocytopenia, or aplastic anemia (17).

Megaloblastic Anemia

Megaloblastic anemia has been described during treatment with phenobarbital alone or, more commonly, when it is used with other antiepileptic drugs, particularly phenytoin. Anticonvulsant megaloblastic anemia probably occurs in less than 1% of patients; the incidence was 0.15 to 0.75% in one report (21). The incidence of macrocytosis in nonanemic patients receiving antiepileptic drugs has been reported to be as high as 33% (21) to 53% (30), but these figures are much higher than those encountered in most clinical practices. The etiology and pathogenesis of macrocytosis and megaloblastic anemia during antiepileptic drug therapy are unknown, but these conditions usually respond to folate therapy.

Folate Deficiency

Frank serum and red cell folate deficiency is relatively common. Reynolds (50) surveyed 16 reports ranging from 27% to as high as 91% subnormal serum folate levels, averaging 52%, in patients receiving chronic therapy with phenytoin, phenobarbital, or primidone. The significance of low folate levels is controversial.

Reynolds and Travers (53) reported improvement in psychiatric abnormalities in patients whose low serum folate concentrations were treated with folate therapy. However, such subjective observations are difficult to assess. Controlled trials have not confirmed that replacement folate therapy in patients receiving phenobarbital or phenytoin either aggravates the disease or improves patients' psychological status (29,38).

Reynolds (51) has postulated that antiepileptic drug-induced folate deficiency diminishes seizure control and that administration of folate therapy exacerbates seizures. Mattson et al. (38) found that serum phenobarbital and phenytoin concentrations decreased when folic acid was given in very high doses. It is possible that reports of seizure exacerbation resulted in part from the decrease in drug concentration rather than from an epileptogenic activity of folate, although the mechanism of this interaction is unknown.

The significance of folate deficiency remains speculative. It is unlikely that patients taking phenobarbital or other antiepileptic drugs will develop anemia unless they suffer from inadequate dietary intake of folates (e.g., alcoholism) or excessive folate requirements (e.g., pregnancy). Other than in cases of obvious megaloblastic anemia, subnormal serum folate probably requires no therapeutic intervention. Except perhaps during pregnancy, proper nutritional balance is sufficient to maintain adequate folate levels during antiepileptic drug therapy.

Although an inverse correlation exists between folate and phenobarbital levels in both serum and cerebrospinal fluid (CSF) (52), Mattson et al. (38) found no change in CSF folate concentration during folic acid therapy. It seems unlikely that folate therapy would have any affect on brain when homeostatic mechanisms prevent elevation of CSF folate concentration to greater than three times normal during therapy with folinic acid (14). In fact, animal studies (30) show clearly that, even in severe folate deprivation, the brain maintains sufficient folate.

Vitamin K

Another hematological abnormality caused by antiepileptic drug therapy affects vitamin K. Phenobarbital and phenytoin, which enter the liver of the fetus, can compete with vitamin K to prevent production of vitamin K-dependent clotting factors. This can occur even in the presence of normal clotting factors in mothers receiving drug therapy. Mountain et al. (44) reported seven neonates with a severe coagulation defect in a series of 16 neonates whose mothers received various antiepileptic drugs (including 13 receiving barbiturates). The neonate can suffer from intraperitoneal, intrathoracic, or intracranial bleeding if vitamin K-dependent coagulation factors are deficient. These signs occur within the first day or two post-partum. Vitamin K administered to mothers prepartum or to the child after delivery will prevent this coagulation deficiency (44).

BONE DISORDERS

Antiepileptic drug therapy may affect calcium and vitamin D metabolism, leading to hypocalcemia or, rarely, osteomalacia. Reports indicate that the incidence of hypocalcemia is as high as 12% (9) to 30% (55). The incidence of increased serum alkaline phosphatase ranges from 29 to 43%, with bone mineral content averaging 80% of normal in epileptic patients (9). The degree of demineralization relates to dose and duration of drug therapy. Despite a high incidence of subnormal calcium levels, only 10% of epileptic patients were found to have osteomalacia, with these developing it only after many years of drug therapy (64). The incidence of this disorder may relate to climate (i.e., lack of sunshine) and diet.

Stamp (64) has postulated that hypocalcemia can increase seizure frequency, requiring therapy with more anticonvulsants. This can produce a further depression in calcium levels, leading to a "vicious circle." A careful study of bone mineral content, calcium, and alkaline phosphatase left Christiansen et al. (9) unable to endorse uniform prophylactic vitamin D supplementation for all epileptic patients. Whereas subnormal total body calcium can be increased by low daily doses of vitamin D supplementation, average calcium levels still do not reach normal levels.

Induction of liver enzymes leading to increased hydroxylation of vitamin D is a probable mechanism for altered calcium metabolism (55). Reversal of signs of deficiency can be accomplished with less than 125 μg of vitamin D_3 per week (46).

HEPATIC TOXICITY

Phenobarbital is a hepatotoxin only in unusually susceptible individuals. Liver disease induced by antiepileptic drugs, particularly by phenobarbital or phenytoin, appears not to be dose dependent and has a low incidence. Most drugs are indirect hepatotoxins, selectively blocking metabolic pathways and producing structural changes by precise biochemical lesions (74). Idiosyncratic acute hepatic injury may be cytotoxic, cholestatic, or mixed. Cytotoxicity can lead to liver necrosis or cholestasis. These drugs probably produce hepatocellular injury, e.g., liver necrosis or cholestasis (74) (see Hypersensitivity).

Hepatic Function

Antiepileptic drugs, particularly phenobarbital, are potent inducers of hepatic microsomal enzymes, which can lead to enhanced metabolism of other drugs or endogenous substances. Although some of these effects are considered drug interactions, the basis of these interactions must be considered a hepatic side effect of phenobarbital therapy. When metabolism of other compounds is accelerated, the end effect of drugs or substances can be diminished or negated. Phenobarbital probably affects hydroxylation pathways related to numerous endogenous and exogenous substances. Osteomalacia (see above) resulting from antiepileptic drug therapy probably results from such an effect.

Tolerance to barbiturates could result in part from increased metabolism to pharmacologically inactive metabolites. Conney et al. (11) showed that phenobarbital increased the synthesis of drug-metabolizing enzymes and stimulated liver protein synthesis. They outlined the concept of autoinduction while describing accelerated metabolism of barbiturates after pretreatment with homologous compounds; that is, phenobarbital stimulated the metabolism of other barbiturates in rats. Several examples of the clinical results of this type of unwanted phenobarbital side effect are discussed below.

Phenobarbital increases the excretion of 6β-hydroxycortisol, leading to decreased plasma cortisol half-life (6). It has also been shown to increase the rate of metabolism of dexamethasone and prednisone. The resulting lower serum concentrations of these drugs used by patients with bronchial asthma disturbed the treatment of their pulmonary disorder. Withdrawal of phenobarbital allowed reversal of these changes (4). Enhanced hormone metabolism can cause failure of oral contraceptives, particularly with low-dose pills (28,33). Interference with the anticoagulation activity of coumarin drugs has been related to phenobarbital therapy (35). Erratic control of anticoagulation with decreased prothrombin time was noted during phenobarbital therapy, and increased dosage with the anticoagulant drug was necessary. However, if phenobarbital is withdrawn, allowing decreased enzyme stimulation, the other drug also requires dosage reduction, or bleeding may occur.

Porphyria

Because phenobarbital can induce synthesis of liver enzymes, it has been shown to enhance the synthesis of aminolevulinic acid (ALA) synthetase which can cause chemical porphyria. Granick (20) hypothesized that drugs such as barbiturates may interact with heme, thereby diminishing inhibition of enzymes controlling ALA synthetase production. Hereditary acute porphyria can be exacerbated when barbiturates are used.

Thyrotoxicosis

Barbiturates were used in the management of thyrotoxicosis before the introduction of β-blocking agents. Oppenheimer et al. (47) demonstrated that phenobarbital stimulated the rate of thyroxine (T4) and triiodothyronine (T3) clearance. This resulted from increased hepatic cellular binding and stimulation of metabolism in the liver. Phenobarbital increases the rate of T4 removal, which is countered by an increase in thyroid secretion of T4 so that serum levels remain constant in euthyroid individuals. Cavalieri et al. (8) showed that hyperthyroid patients or hypothyroid patients receiving replacement doses of T4 have enhanced removal of T4. This results from a decline in circulating levels of this hormone during phenobarbital therapy (22). Untreated hyperthyroid patients without normal hypothalamic–pituitary feedback control were found to have decreased serum T4 concentration during phenobarbital therapy which reversed when the drug was stopped. The effect on T3 was inconsistent. The extent of conversion of T4 to T3 is probably not significantly altered by phenobarbital (8).

Hyperbilirubinemia

Bilirubin conjugation has been induced by phenobarbital usefully to treat neonatal hyperbilirubinemia (73). Because of induced action of hepatic microsomal enzymes, bilirubin excretion is enhanced through glucuronidation. Yeung et al. (73) showed that treatment of infants was more effective in lowering bilirubin level than treatment of their mothers. In these cases of hyperbilirubinemia, phenobarbital clearly enhanced liver function of the neonates. In addition to phenobarbital-enhanced glucuronide conjugation to reverse hyperbilirubinemia, phenobarbital also reduces the concentration of serum bile salts and increases hepatic excretion of bile salts (34). This side effect may be of importance in the treatment of hyperbiliacidemia as well as hyperbilirubinemia in cholestatic conditions.

Ethanol

Several other reports have compared the characteristics of phenobarbital with that of ethanol. Both compounds lead to hypertrophy of hepatic smooth endoplasmic reticulum, inducing a nonspecific increase in numerous hepatic drug-metabolizing enzymes and cytochrome P-450. Both compounds are oxidized by NADH microsomal systems (12,56). Barbiturate-hydroxylating enzymes are increased in men fed alcohol (57). Enzyme induction allows for increased clearance of drugs in alcoholic patients as well as in those receiving barbiturates. Conversely, barbiturates can reduce alcohol dehydrogenase activity, allowing high levels of alcohol to occur when both compounds are used concurrently. The synergy of barbiturate and ethanol toxicity can cause respiratory depression, leading to unsuspected, unanticipated suicide (23). It is interesting to note that phenobarbital used with other drugs of abuse significantly affects their metabolism. In addition to altered ethanol metabolism, phenobarbital increases the rate of heroin deacetylation. This increase in detoxification is dose related, parallel to increased enzyme induction (13).

Summary of Hepatotoxicity

Phenobarbital has often been used to study hepatic microsomal enzyme induction in animal and human experiments. The use of phenobarbital concurrently with some antibiotics, anticoagulants, antiinflammatory agents, as well as other antiepileptic drugs must be evaluated carefully for altered metabolism resulting from enzyme induction (54). If phenobarbital is discontinued while other drugs are maintained, metabolism of the other drugs and of endogenous compounds must be reevaluated.

ONCOGENICITY

Animal studies have shown liver tumors appearing with the use of phenobarbital and other drugs that activate liver enzymes. Although enzyme induction causes an increase in liver size, it may also protect against the carcinogenicity of other compounds (i.e., known chemical carcinogens) by enhancing their metabolism.

There is no evidence of an increased frequency of liver tumors in patients taking phenobarbital. In fact, Clemmesen et al. (10) found a decrease in tumor incidence in patients re-

ceiving anticonvulsants. White et al. (70) found an increase in cancer deaths for epileptic patients, but this was not statistically significant. Because epilepsy is often an early manifestation of brain tumors, it is not surprising that this survey showed a significant excess of such tumors in patients receiving antiepileptic drugs. However, the fact that liver tumors were not increased is a more important finding. It is unlikely that chronic phenobarbital therapy would cause an increase in carcinogenicity other than in the liver. White et al. (70) clearly define phenobarbital oncogenicity as a very low risk.

HYPERSENSITIVITY REACTIONS

Phenobarbital causes various types of skin reactions. These usually are mild maculopapular, morbilliform, or scarlatiniform rashes, which fade rapidly when drug administration is stopped. The incidence has been reported to be as low as 1 to 3% of all patients receiving barbiturates (59). Considering the universal usage of this drug, reports of exfoliative dermatitis, erythema multiforme, Stevens–Johnson syndrome, or toxic epidermal necrolysis are impressively rare. Welton (69) reported a case of exfoliative dermatitis with hepatitis caused by phenobarbital.

Hypersensitivity reactions, usually occurring within the first 1 to 5 weeks of therapy (74), are characterized by rash, eosinophilia, and fever. Histological changes in the liver show eosinophilic or granulomatous inflammation (74). McGeachy and Bloomer (41) reviewed 17 instances of fatal sensitivity to phenobarbital. Another half-dozen cases of acute reaction to barbiturates and details of treatment were reported by Yatzidis (72). Corticosteroids are of value in treatment (41,66). Once sensitivity has been documented, a patient should never be reexposed to any barbiturate (66).

Systemic lupus erythematosus (SLE) can develop with use of antiepileptic drugs. Alarcon-Segovia (1) suggests that the drugs elicit production of antinuclear antibodies by altering nuclear components. This may unmask SLE in predisposed individuals and can be reversed by prompt discontinuation of the drug.

TERATOGENICITY

The current awareness that some antiepileptic drugs have teratogenic effects requires counseling for the patient who wishes to become pregnant. It is difficult to correlate specific teratogenic effects with individual drug use in clinical studies of teratogenicity because of the frequent use of multiple drugs.

A variety of malformations have been observed in the offspring of six women who used only phenobarbital during their pregnancy: tracheo–esophageal fistula, ileal atresia, diaphragmatic hernia with pulmonary hypoplasia, thumb and radius aplasia, congenital heart lesion with microcephaly, mental retardation, hypospadias, and meningomyelocele (63). In this report and a similar retrospective survey by Nelson et al. (45), the lack of characteristic malformation associated with sole phenobarbital use suggests coincidence rather than causal relationship (as with phenytoin and cleft palate).

Fedrick (18) found phenytoin far more teratogenic than phenobarbital, but, when the two drugs were used in combination, teratogenicity was even more pronounced. Only 4.9% of infants born to mothers who received only phenobarbital during the first trimester were known to have birth defects. This is much lower than incidence rates of 15.2% for sole phenytoin therapy and 22% for combined phenobarbital and phenytoin therapy. Surprisingly, in the same study there was a 10.5% incidence of malformations when mothers with epilepsy took no drugs during pregnancy. A large cooperative study in the United States and Finland (60) implicated phenytoin as a teratogen but gave no evidence of an association between birth defects and phenobarbital therapy during pregnancy, whether the mothers used the drug for seizure prevention or for other indications (i.e., non-epileptic mothers). The question was raised whether fetal damage was attributable to anti-epileptic drugs or to epilepsy. Statistically sub-

tracting drug use, the malformation rate in children born to mothers with epilepsy was increased by 60%. A key factor associated with increased risk of fetal malformation may be the presence of epilepsy in either parent. The major drawback in all of these studies of antiepileptic drug teratogenicity is the difficulty in obtaining information about maternal drug use. There is some evidence that higher drug dose and serum concentration correlate with increasing risk of malformation (15).

In summary, phenobarbital when used alone has occasionally been associated with fetal malformations but is thought to potentiate teratogenic effects when used with other drugs. Whether malformations occurring in offspring of epileptic parents are caused by epilepsy, antiepileptic drug therapy, or a combination of these and other factors remains controversial. The available information suggests that phenobarbital, in comparison with phenytoin, may be considered a reasonably safe drug or, perhaps, a drug of choice during pregnancy.

TREATMENT

Many neurotoxic side effects improve with a simple reduction in dosage. Improvement is, of course, gradual because of the slow elimination of phenobarbital. Such lowering of serum concentration provides less protection against seizures (67). In the past, when seizure control could be achieved only at the cost of neurotoxic side effects, sedation and/or hyperactivity were sometimes ameliorated with concomitant administration of amphetamines. The additional complications attendant with the use of these stimulants is less necessary today. A change to treatment with an alternative antiepileptic drug may be equally effective and spare some side effects.

Recommendations for altered treatment when toxicity is apparent vary with the severity of the problem. The drug should be discontinued if a hypersensitivity reaction develops. Other acute toxicity early in the initiation of treatment should be viewed cautiously. Dosage can be held constant while symptoms abate, and increases should be slow thereafter. If decreased libido is reported, lowering the serum phenobarbital concentration might improve the problem.

In cases where reversal of side effects and lowering of serum concentration must be rapid, elimination can be accelerated by alkalinization and induction of forced diuresis (40). Approximately one-third of an oral dose of phenobarbital is found in the urine unchanged. When necessary, administration of parenteral fluids up to 5mg/kg/hr can increase clearance and excretion several-fold (7). If some of the fluid given is 1.25% sodium bicarbonate, the alkalinization of blood and urine further enhances elimination after overdose. At pH 7.4, 60% of phenobarbital is ionized. This polar compound poorly crosses cellular membranes. Penetration into and out of tissue is possible for the 40% of the drug that is un-ionized. When acidosis occurs, a higher percentage of phenobarbital is un-ionized, allowing passage into the intercellular space. This effectively increases tissue concentrations without any change in total body phenobarbital. Alkalosis has an opposite effect and leads to movement of phenobarbital out of brain and other tissues. Similarly, shifts in urinary pH can greatly modify the rate of phenobarbital elimination. Phenobarbital is cleared from the kidney and, at the usually acid pH, is largely in the un-ionized form. It is readily reabsorbed from the kidney tubule back into the circulation. In alkaline urine, the excreted phenobarbital becomes ionized and is not reabsorbed. By this mechanism alkalinization can appreciably increase elimination of phenobarbital from the body.

REFERENCES

1. Alarcón-Segovia, D. (1969): Drug-induced lupus syndromes. *Mayo Clin. Proc.*, 44:664–681.
2. Berman, L. B., Jeghers, H. J., Schreiner, G. E., and Pallotta, A. J. (1956): Hemodialysis, an effective therapy for acute barbiturate poisoning. *J.A.M.A.*, 161:820–827.
3. Bleyer, W. A., and Marshall, R. E. (1972): Barbiturate withdrawal syndrome in a passively addicted infant. *J.A.M.A.*, 221:185–186.
4. Brooks, S. M., Werk, E. E., Ackerman, S. J., Sullivan, I., and Thrasher, K. (1972): Adverse effects of phenobarbital on corticosteroid metabolism in patients with bronchial asthma. *N. Engl. J. Med.*, 286:1125–1128.
5. Buchthal, F., Svensmark, O., and Simonsen, H. (1968): Relation of EEG and seizures to phenobarbital in serum. *Arch. Neurol.*, 19:567–572.
6. Burstein, S., and Klaiber, E. (1965): Phenobarbital-induced increase in 6β-hydroxycortisol excretion: Clue to its significance in human urine. *J. Clin. Endocrinol.*, 25:293–296.
7. Butler, T. C., Mahaffee, C., and Waddell, W. J. (1954): Phenobarbital: Studies of elimination, accumulation, tolerance and dosage schedules. *J. Pharmacol. Exp. Ther.*, 111:425–435.
8. Cavalieri, R. R., Sung, L. C., and Becker, C. E. (1973): Effects of phenobarbital on thyroxine and triiodothyronine kinetics in Graves' disease. *J. Clin. Endocrinol. Metab.*, 37:308–316.
9. Christiansen, C., Rødbro, P., and Lund, M. (1973): Incidence of anticonvulsant osteomalacia and effect of vitamin D: Controlled therapeutic trial. *Br. Med. J.*, 4:695–701.
10. Clemmesen, J., Fuglsang-Frederiksen, V., and Plum, C. M. (1974): Are anticonvulsants oncogenic? *Lancet*, 1:705–707.
11. Conney, A. H., Davison, C., Gastel, R., and Burns, J. J. (1960): Adaptive increases in drug-metabolizing enzymes induced by phenobarbital and other drugs. *J. Pharmacol. Exp. Ther.*, 130:1–8.
12. Conney, A. H., Jacobson, M., Schneidman, K., and Kuntzman, R. (1965): Induction of liver microsomal cortisol 6β-hydroxylase by diphenylhydantoin or phenobarbital. An explanation for the increased excretion of 6-hydroxycortisol in humans treated with these drugs. *Life Sci.*, 4:1091–1098.
13. Cramer, J. A., Cohn, G., and Meggs, L. (1975): Effect of phenobarbital and heroin metabolism in the rat. *Fed. Proc.*, 34:814.
14. Cramer, J. A., Mattson, R. H., and Brillman, J. (1976): Folinic acid therapy in epilepsy. *Fed. Proc.*, 35:582.
15. Dansky, L., Andermann, N. C., Sherwin, A., Andermann, F., and Kinch, R. A. (1980): Maternal epilepsy and congenital malformation: A prospective study with monitoring of plasma anticonvulsant levels during pregnancy. *Neurology (Minneap.)*, 30:438.
16. Desmond, M. M., Schwanecke, R. P., Wilson, G. D., Yasunaga, S., and Burgdorff, I. (1972): Maternal barbiturate utilization and neonatal withdrawal symptomatology. *J. Pediatr.*, 80:190–197.
17. De Vries, S. I. (1965): Haematological aspects during treatment with anticonvulsant drugs. *Epilepsia*, 6:1–15.
18. Fedrick, J. (1973): Epilepsy and pregnancy: A report from the Oxford record linkage study. *Br. Med. J.*, 1:442–448.
19. Fouts, J. R., and Adamson, R. H. (1959): Drug metabolism in the newborn rabbit. *Science*, 129:897–898.
20. Granick, S. (1965): Hepatic porphyria and drug-induced or chemical porphyria. *Ann. N.Y. Acad. Sci.*, 123:188–197.
21. Hawkins, C. F., and Meynell, M. J. (1958): Macrocytosis and macrocytic anemia caused by anticonvulsant drugs. *J. Med.*, 27:45–63.

22. Hoffbrand, B. I. (1979): Barbiturate/thyroid-hormone interaction. *Lancet*, 2:903–904.

23. Hollister, L. E. (1965): Nervous system reactions to drugs. *Ann. N.Y. Acad. Sci.*, 123:342–353.

24. Houghton, G. W., Latham, A. N., and Richens, A. (1973): Difference in the central actions of phenytoin and phenobarbitone in man, measured by critical flicker fusion threshold. *Eur. J. Clin. Pharmacol.*, 6:57–60.

25. Hutt, S. J., Jackson, P. M., Belsham, A., and Higgins, G. (1968): Perceptual motor behaviour in relation to blood phenobarbitone level: A preliminary report. *Dev. Med. Child Neurol.*, 10:626–632.

26. Ideström, C. (1954): Flicker-fusion in chronic barbiturate usage: A quantitative study in the pathophysiology of drug addiction. *Acta Psychiatr. Neurol. Scand. [Suppl.]*, 91:1–93.

27. Isbell, H., and Fraser, H. F. (1950): Addiction to analgesics and barbiturates. *Pharmacol. Rev.*, 2:355–397.

28. Janz, D., and Schmidt, D. (1974): Antiepileptic drugs and failure of oral contraceptives. *Lancet*, 1:1113.

29. Jensen, O. N., and Olesen, O. V. (1970): Subnormal serum folate due to anticonvulsive therapy. *Arch. Neurol.*, 22:181–182.

30. Klipstein, F. A. (1964): Subnormal serum folate and macrocytosis associated with anticonvulsant drug therapy. *Blood*, 23:68–86.

31. Kornetsky, C., and Orzack, M. H. (1964): A research note on some of the critical factors on the dissimilar effects of chlorpromazine and secobarbital on the digit symbol substitution and continuous performance tests. *Psychopharmacology*, 6:79–86.

32. Lennox, W. G. (1942): Brain injury, drugs and environment as causes of mental decay in epilepsy. *Am. J. Psychiatry*, 99:174–180.

33. Levin, W., Kuntzman, R., and Conney, A. H. (1979): Stimulatory effect of phenobarbital on the metabolism of the oral contraceptive 17a-ethynylestradiol-3-methyl ether (Mestranol) by rat liver microsomes. *Pharmacology*, 19:249–255.

34. Linarelli, L. G., Hengstenberg, F. H., and Drash, A. L. (1973): Effect of phenobarbital on hyperlipemia in patients with intrahepatic and extrahepatic cholestasis. *Pediatr. Pharmacol. Ther.*, 83:291–298.

35. MacDonald, M. G., and Robinson, D. S. (1968): Clinical observations of possible barbiturate interference with anticoagulation. *J.A.M.A.*, 204:95–100.

36. MacLeod, C. M., Dekaban, A. S., and Hunt, E. (1978): Memory impairment in epileptic patients: Selective effects of phenobarbital concentration. *Science*, 202:1102–1104.

37. Marchesi, G. F. (1979): Effect of anticonvulsants on psychological tests in patients of normal intelligence. *Epilepsy Int., Florence, Italy* (abs).

38. Mattson, R. H., Gallagher, B. B., Reynolds, E. H., and Glass, D. (1973): Folate therapy in epilepsy: A controlled study. *Arch. Neurol.*, 29:78–81.

39. Mattson, R. H., Williamson, P. D., and Hanahan, E. (1976): Eterobarb therapy in epilepsy. *Neurology (Minneap.)*, 26:1014–1017.

40. Mawer, G. E., and Lee, H. A. (1968): Value of forced diuresis in acute barbiturate poisoning. *Br. Med. J.*, 2:790–792.

41. McGeachy, T. E., and Bloomer, W. E. (1953): The phenobarbital sensitivity syndrome. *Am. J. Med.*, 14:600–604.

42. Melchior, J. C., Svensmark, O., and Trolle, D. (1967): Placental transfer of phenobaritone in epileptic women, and elimination in newborns. *Lancet*, 2:860–861.

43. Mirsky, A. F., and Kornetsky, C. (1964): On the dissimilar effects of drugs on the digit symbol substitution and continuous performance tests: A review and preliminary integration of behavioral and physiological evidence. *Psychopharmacology*, 5:161–177.

44. Mountain, K. R., Hirsh, J., and Gallus, A. S. (1970): Neonatal coagulation defect due to anticonvulsant drug treatment in pregnancy. *Lancet*, 1:265–268.

45. Nelson, M. M., and Forfar, J. O. (1971): Associations between drugs administered during pregnancy and congenital abnormalities of the fetus. *Br. Med. J.*, 1:523–527.

46. Offermann, G., Pinto, V., and Kruse, R. (1979): Antiepileptic drugs and vitamin D supplementation. *Epilepsia*, 20:3–15.

47. Oppenheimer, J. H., Bernstein, G., and Surks, M. (1968): Increased thyroxine turnover and thyroidal function after stimulation of hepatocellular binding of thyroxine by phenobarbital. *J. Clin. Invest.*, 47:1399–1406.

48. Ounsted, C. (1955): The hyperkinetic syndrome in epileptic children. *Lancet*, 1:303–311.

49. Oxley, J. (1979): The effect of antiepileptic drugs on psychological performance. *Epilepsy Int., Florence, Italy* (abs).

50. Reynolds, E. H. (1974): Chronic antiepileptic toxicity: A review. *Epilepsia*, 16:319–352.

51. Reynolds, E. H. (1974): Folate metabolism and anticonvulsant therapy. *Proc. R. Soc. Med.*, 67:6.

52. Reynolds, E. H., Mattson, R. H., and Gallagher, B. B. (1972): Relationships between serum and cerebrospinal fluid anticonvulsant drug and folic acid concentrations in epileptic patients. *Neurology (Minneap.)*, 22:841–844.

53. Reynolds, E. H., and Travers, R. D. (1974): Serum anticonvulsant concentrations in epileptic patients with mental symptoms: A preliminary report. *Br. J. Psychiatry*, 124:440–445.

54. Richens, A. (1974): The clinical consequences of chronic hepatic enzyme induction by anticonvulsant drugs. *Br. J. Clin. Pharmacol.*, 1:185–187.

55. Richens, A., and Rowe, D. J. F. (1970): Disturbance of calcium metabolism by anticonvulsant drugs. *Br. Med. J.*, 4:73–76.

56. Rubin, E., Hutterer, F., and Lieb, C. S. (1968): Ethanol increases hepatic smooth endoplasmic reticulum and drug-metabolizing enzymes. *Science*, 159:1469–1470.

57. Rubin, E., and Lieber, C. S. (1968): Hepatic microsomal enzymes in man and rat: Induction and inhibition by ethanol. *Science*, 162:690–691.

58. Schain, R. J., Ward, J. W., and Guthrie, D. (1977): Carbamazepine as an anticonvulsant in children. *Neurology (Minneap.)*, 27:476–480.

59. Schmidt, R. P., and Wilder, B. J. (1968): *Epilepsy*. F. A. Davis, Philadelphia.

60. Shapiro, S., Hartz, S. C., Siskind, V., Mitchell, A. A., Slone, D., Rosenberg, L., Monson, R. R., and

Heinonen, O. P. (1976): Anticonvulsants and parental epilepsy in the development of birth defects. *Lancet,* 1:272–275.

61. Simpson, E., and Stewart, M. (1975): Why measure blood barbiturates? *Ann. Clin. Biochem.,* 12:156–159.
62. Somerfeld-Ziskind, E., and Ziskind, E. (1940): Effect of phenobarbital on the mentality of epileptic patients. *Arch. Neurol. Psychol.,* 43:70–79.
63. Speidel, B. D., and Meadow, S. R. (1972): Maternal epilepsy and abnormalities of the fetus and newborn. *Lancet,* 2:839–843.
64. Stamp, T. C. B. (1974): Effects of long-term anticonvulsant therapy on calcium and vitamin D metabolism. *Proc. R. Soc. Med.,* 67:64–68.
65. Stores, G. (1975): Behavioral effects of antiepileptic drugs. *Dev. Med. Child Neurol.,* 17:647–658.
66. Stüttgen, G. (1973): Toxic epidermal necrolysis provoked by barbiturates. *Br. J. Dermatol.,* 88:291–293.
67. Svensmark, O., and Buchthal, F. (1963): Accumulation of phenobarbital in man. *Epilepsia,* 4:199–206.
68. Wapner, I., Thurston, D. L., and Holowach, J. (1962): Phenobarbital: Its effect on learning in epileptic children. *J.A.M.A.,* 182:937.

69. Welton, D. G. (1950): Exfoliative dermatitis and hepatitis due to phenobarbital. *J.A.M.A.,* 143:232–234.
70. White, S. J., McLean, A. E. M., and Howland, C. (1979): Anticonvulsant drugs and cancer: A cohort study in patients with severe epilepsy. *Lancet,* 2:458–461.
71. Wolf, S. M., and Forsythe, A. (1978): Behavior disturbance, phenobarbital and febrile seizures. In: *Advances in Epileptology* (1977), *Psychology, Pharmacotherapy and New Diagnostic Approaches,* edited by H. Meinardi and A. J. Rowan, pp. 124–127. Swets & Zeitlinger, Amsterdam.
72. Yatzidis, H. (1971): The use of ion exchange resins and charcoal in acute barbiturate poisoning. In: *Acute Barbiturate Poisoning,* edited by H. Matthew, pp. 223–232. Excerpta Medica, Amsterdam.
73. Yeung, C. Y., Tam, L. S., Chan, A., and Lee, K. H. (1971): Phenobarbitone prophylaxis for neonatal hyperbilirubinemia. *Pediatrics,* 48:372–376.
74. Zimmerman, H. J. (1978): Drug-induced liver disease. *Drugs,* 16:25–45.

Antiepileptic Drugs, edited by D. M. Woodbury, J. K. Penry, and C. E. Pippenger. Raven Press, New York © 1982.

27

Phenobarbital

Mechanisms of Action

James W. Prichard

The basic mechanism(s) of antiepileptic action of phenobarbital (PB) still remain buried under two kinds of identifiable ignorance. The first is a lack of detailed understanding of epileptic pathophysiology. We know considerably more than the preceding generation did about how seizure discharge involves the major areas of the brain. Available data are numerous and precise enough to support a plausible, carefully reasoned discussion of generalized tonic–clonic and absence seizures in a single theoretical framework that invites refinement by further experimentation (38). We have acquired in the paroxysmal depolarization shift a marker of abnormal cellular behavior apparently fundamental to several kinds of seizures [for references see Gloor (38) and Ayala et al. (6)]. Nevertheless, the chain of events from cellular defect to clinical seizure is still too vaguely defined to permit discovery of where along it the critical actions of antiepileptic drugs occur. Much remains to be learned about the vulnerabilities of normal brains to epileptogenic stimuli, the properties of permanently abnormal neurons in epileptic brains, the means by which such neurons intermittently entrain normal ones to cause a clinical seizure, and, especially, the mechanisms responsible for terminating seizure discharge. These gaps in knowledge, although still important, are not hopelessly large. Experiments designed to fill them can exploit much precise information about the paroxysmal depolarization shift, postactivation potentiation, kindling, synaptic physiology, transmitter metabolism, and energy transfer among and within cells.

The second kind of missing information is detailed knowledge of the neuropharmacological differences among closely related drugs. This is a problem in the study of all antiepileptic drugs, but it is particularly clear for the barbiturates because so many of them have been studied. At present, the only abnormal phenomena that distinguish antiepileptic barbiturates as a group are the seizures used to define antiepileptic potency. It is not yet known in any detail whether the drugs can be sorted the same way by their actions on the paroxysmal depolarization shift, kindling, or other phenomena possibly intermediate between the basic cellular defects of epilepsy and their full expression in clinical seizures. In normal systems, there has been no neuropharmacological action of barbiturates yet demonstrated that is a selective property of the antiepileptic barbiturates. Further work on this problem requires no technological advances and may provide important clues to the intimate mechanisms of the antiepileptic action of PB.

However, a discussion of those mechanisms at present can be little more than a review of data that a particular author thinks might be related to them. That is what will be found on the following pages, along with mention of some barbiturate actions that excited interest earlier but now seem unlikely to be of importance in seizure control, and a proposal concerning the possible role of drug compartmentation.

ACTIONS OF PHENOBARBITAL ON ABNORMAL PHENOMENA

Seizures in Man and Animals

In man, PB is effective against generalized tonic–clonic and simple partial seizures but not against absence seizures (2,36,60,61,66,103, 139). In these respects, it resembles phenytoin and primidone. It is thought to be less effective than either of the latter drugs against complex partial seizures, although this difference has never been documented in a rigorous clinical study. The possibility of such a difference is one of the reasons for suspecting that the antiepileptic potency of primidone is independent of its conversion to PB. Primidone is also metabolized in man to phenylethylmalonamide, and both this compound and unmetabolized primidone have antiepileptic potency in animals (32,34). Thus, any of at least three compounds, or some combination of them, may be responsible for the seizure reduction observed in patients given primidone. At present, it is entirely uncertain whether one or several basic mechanisms of action are involved. Eterobarb (33, 128) presents the same problem because of its conversion to PB and monomethoxymethyl PB which may have antiepileptic potency; the unmetabolized drug does not accumulate in detectable quantities (see Chapters 70 and 71). Unmetabolized mephobarbital is antiepileptic in animals (25), but its usefulness in man is probably attributable to its conversion to PB (2,36,61,103).

In experimental animals, PB, mephobarbital, and primidone have wide spectra of antiepileptic action (13,25,32,34,39,50,59,116,119) which are qualitatively similar for particular species, ages, and types of seizure induction (94). All three drugs elevate electroshock seizure threshold and protect against pentylenetetrazol convulsions more effectively than phenytoin does. The limited data available on eterobarb (128) suggest that its spectrum of action in experimental tests resembles that of PB. As noted above, mephobarbital (25) and certain metabolites of primidone (32,34) and eterobarb (33,128) have antiepileptic potency in animals.

The overall picture presented by these data prompts two thoughts. First, the antiepileptic barbiturates must have some property not shared with phenytoin that causes elevation of threshold to electrical and chemical epileptic stimuli. This cannot be a selective effect on abnormal nervous tissue, because elevated thresholds can be demonstrated in normal animals. Second, among the barbiturates and their metabolites, the number of compounds having antiepileptic potency in animals suggests that separate mechanisms of action may be involved. However, it can also be argued that PB alone is responsible for the clinical effectiveness of mephobarbital, primidone, and eterobarb since it accumulates when any of these is given, and that experimental data on the effectiveness of other compounds, although true, are irrelevant.

Focal Epileptic Discharge

There is abundant evidence (4,16,26,35, 42,117,118,126) that subanesthetic concentrations of barbiturates can shorten the duration of and raise the threshold for epileptic afterdischarge elicited by electrical stimulation of various brain structures in normal animals. However, this effect is not limited to antiepileptic barbiturates, and quantitative differences among drugs were not defined in most studies. The work of Aston and Domino (4) is a major exception. They determined motor cortical and reticular formation afterdischarge thresholds in the monkey and showed that pentobarbital raised both equally, PB raised the cortical threshold more than the reticular one, and phenytoin raised only the cortical threshold. These findings seem quite consistent with the relative antiepileptic and hypnotic potencies of the three drugs. The depression of consciousness, elevation of thresholds for electrical and chemical seizures, and production of EEG fast activity (see below), all of which distinguish PB from phenytoin, could all be related to actions in the reticular formation. Further studies like that of Aston and Domino are necessary to extend their results and move toward a cellular explanation of them.

Studies of drug action on the electrical activity of brain areas made abnormally susceptible to epileptic discharge provide further distinctions that have important implications for mechanisms of antiepileptic action. At present, such epileptic foci define the smallest neuronal populations in which the drug sensitivities of phenomena having a known relationship to behavioral seizures can be studied. Because of this, and the fact that they can be produced in cortical and subcortical structures by several means in common laboratory animals, they offer the best opportunity currently available for bringing the techniques of cellular neurobiology to bear on epileptic events. Notable results of such efforts include definition of the paroxysmal depolarization shift characteristic of many neurons in several kinds of foci (6,38) and detection of certain biochemical differences from nearby normal tissue (43). Pharmacological studies are less advanced. Phenobarbital and other barbiturates suppress the discharge of epileptic foci (19,46,64,69,76,127). Comparison of PB and pentobarbital in the same study showed PB to be more potent against afterdischarges in isolated cortex (127) and interictal spikes in hippocampal slices exposed to penicillin (76). The latter study also included phenytoin, which was substantially less potent than PB, and diazepam, which was very slightly more potent; the authors commented on the unexpectedly strong action of PB compared with the other drugs. A study (69) on rabbits with chronic cortical freeze foci provided strong evidence that PB and phenytoin oppose epileptic discharge by different mechanisms. Phenobarbital inhibited spread of abnormal activity from the focus to adjacent cortex and diencephalon and suppressed the firing of the focus itself. Phenytoin was a better inhibitor of cortical spread but had no effect on the focus or on spread to the diencephalon.

Such data suggest that PB exerts an important part of its antiepileptic action on abnormal neurons, in contrast to phenytoin which may act primarily on normal ones. This is a plausible distinction in modes of antiepileptic action but hardly a proven one. The cellular basis for the difference is unknown. There has been little quantitative comparison of the effects of various barbiturates on epileptic foci. If sedative barbiturates in subsedative concentrations were found to suppress foci as well as antiepileptic barbiturates, interest in mechanisms of focus suppression would wane; a more selective result (76) would encourage close analysis of them. This is one of several areas in the pharmacology of antiepileptic drugs where useful data not now available could come from fairly simple experiments.

In kindled foci, one can study the development and drug sensitivities of progressively more intense epileptic responses to the same stimulus (see 129). Phenobarbital retards the kindling process more effectively than other antiepileptic drugs so far studied (3,130,133, 137), possibly for the same reasons that it suppresses other kinds of foci. Whether new data support that preeminence or not, experimental kindling seems so likely to proceed by mechanisms relevant to human epilepsy that the cellular basis of the action of PB on it is among the most promising targets for further investigation.

Hyperexcitable Axons

The abnormal firing of frog nerve caused by repetitive stimulation and low Ca was reduced by concentrations of PB below 1 mM (124); similarly, normal action potentials of squid giant axon were blocked by 100 mM PB, whereas 3 mM was sufficient to block spontaneous firing in low Ca (99). The latter observations suggest that PB is more potent against abnormal forms of excitability than normal ones. Comparable data are too few to permit a conclusion regarding the possible specificity of this action among barbiturates, but phenytoin had the same effect at lower concentration in the study on squid axon (99). Phenytoin also reduced uptake of sodium by lobster nerves (80) and, chronically administered, reduced excitability after repetitive stimulation of rabbit vagus nerve (45); PB did these things too but was less potent. In studies on frog node of Ranvier, phenytoin reduced sodium permeability and opposed the shift toward increased excitability in low Ca at concentrations less than $\frac{1}{20}$ those required for PB to exert the same effects (70, 106).

ACTIONS OF PHENOBARBITAL ON NORMAL PHENOMENA

Extraneural Tissues

Enzyme induction is the only well-defined barbiturate action outside the nervous system that has received attention as a possible antiepileptic mechanism. Barbiturates cause increased synthesis and concentration of a number of enzymes in a variety of tissues (97,98; see also Chapters 23 and 24). Phenobarbital is the most effective inducer among them, but whether this is related to any property also important for its antiepileptic potency is not known. The most thoroughly studied inductions are of hepatic microsomal enzymes, several of which have been implicated in barbiturate toxicity. Reynolds (95) has proposed that some antiepileptic drugs, including PB, act against seizures because they alter folate metabolism; the mechanisms are not completely understood but may involve hepatic enzyme induction. The relevant data as a whole do not provide strong support for this theory (see 97 for references) but do prompt reflection on the possibility that what antiepileptic drugs do in the rest of the body may influence what they do in the brain. At present, however, there is no good evidence that enzyme induction or any other extraneural action of PB is responsible for its antiepileptic potency.

Sleep and Anesthesia

Barbiturates have been used to cause sleep more frequently than for any other purpose. The exact mechanisms of their sedative action are not known, but it is known that the state they produce is not equivalent to physiological sleep.

Total time spent in the rapid eye movement phase of sleep is reduced and rebounds after barbiturate use is stopped (48,77). Prolonged use is associated with restlessness in the latter part of the night, ordinarily dominated by rapid eye movement sleep (75). Since all barbiturates and many quite different drugs have similar effects, it seems unlikely that clues to the selective anticonvulsant action of PB will be found in the mechanisms by which it can cause sleep. The same is true of barbiturate anesthesia. Behavioral and electrographic measures have provided a detailed description of how barbiturate anesthesia develops (21,100), but the basic mechanisms responsible for it are unknown. It seems probable that they, as well as mechanisms of antiepileptic action, will prove to be related to the cellular actions discussed later in this chapter, but whether to the same or different ones is unpredictable now.

Electroencephalogram and Evoked Potentials

At present, the extensive literature on barbiturates and the electroencephalogram (EEG) (83) offers few clues to the nature of barbiturate antiepileptic action. Most barbiturates appear to exert quite similar actions on the EEGs of man and common experimental animals, although their potencies and durations of action vary greatly. Electroencephalogram power spectrum analysis is beginning to reveal differences among barbiturates (37,102); however, it is too early to tell whether any of these will correlate with antiepileptic potency. All barbiturates cause widespread cortical and subcortical 20 to 30 Hz fast activity. This is seen at lower concentrations than any of their other EEG effects; it is commonly present in the EEGs of patients taking PB. Animal experiments show that it results from some action of the drugs on the mesencephalic reticular formation.

Evoked potential studies, like those on EEG, have so far shown no selective effect of antiepileptic barbiturates. In general, barbiturates depress nonspecific and neospinothalamic sensory evoked potentials at doses that spare or enhance other specific ones (see 83 for references). One study (47) found differences between antiepileptic concentrations of PB and phenytoin at several sites in cat brain, among which the mesencephalic reticular formation was the most sensitive to PB; other barbiturates were not studied.

It is not surprising that the most barbiturate-sensitive brain region detectable by EEG methods should be one known to have powerful influence over the electrical activity of the cerebrum. Nor would it be surprising if the ascending pathways that allow all barbiturates to pace fast activity in large areas of brain were also found to distribute selective effects of the antiepileptic ones. There is no evidence at present that any aspect of barbiturate antiepileptic action depends on the mesencephalic reticular formation, but experiments likely to detect such dependency have not been done.

Synaptic Transmission

The most potent neuropharmacological actions of barbiturates yet demonstrated are on synaptic transmission or phenomena plausibly related to it. At 2 mg/kg, PB increased both mono- and polysynaptic components of dorsal to ventral root transmission in the cat (28). Pentobarbital prolonged an inhibitory potential in rat olfactory cortex slices in concentrations as low as 0.01 mM (79). As little as 0.04 mM PB inhibited voltage-dependent Ca uptake by rabbit neocortical synaptosomes (111); *in vivo*, such an action would interfere with transmitter release. At 0.05 mM, PB stimulated production of free acetylcholine in brain slices (65).

However, most studies that have compared actions of various barbiturates on synaptic transmission have not revealed any selective effect of PB. Direct comparison of PB with pentobarbital showed their actions to be similar, and pentobarbital to be at least as potent as PB, on frog neuromuscular junction (86,123), sympathetic ganglia of bullfrog (72,74) and rat (14,15), cat dorsal–ventral root preparation (67), rat hippocampus (138), and rat brain slices (65). An exception of a sort was found in a study (63) on tissue-cultured neurons from mouse spinal cord: 0.2 mM PB suppressed picrotoxin-

induced intense discharge but not spontaneous activity; the latter was abolished by the same concentration of pentobarbital. Thus, PB was more selective, if not more potent, against the epileptiform activity; in other actions on the cells it was neither.

A number of the studies cited above were on postsynaptic potentials of various kinds. Phenobarbital shares the general tendency of barbiturates to depress physiological excitations (1, 8–11, 62, 68, 72, 74, 86, 92, 93, 96, 107, 112,120–123,134,135) and enhance inhibitions (7,27,67,71,73,79,81,104,105,125,138). Much evidence suggests that interactions of barbiturates with γ-aminobutyric acid (GABA) are involved in the enhanced inhibitions (11,14,15, 63,72,73,92,93,104,105,138); some of these studies (104,105,138) included PB. Reduced excitations and enhanced inhibitions are a very plausible basis for barbiturate anesthesia, which was the ultimate object of interest in most of these studies, but by themselves they cannot account for selective antiepileptic actions. Nor can such actions be attributable to the demonstrated capability of PB (111), pentobarbital (12), and phenytoin (111) to reduce Ca uptake by—and, presumably, transmitter release from—depolarized nerve terminals. Reduction of postactivation potentiation such as phenytoin causes is not seen with subanesthetic amounts of barbiturates (28,29,91,96). The selectivity of barbiturates among postsynaptic potentials is not always of the sort so far mentioned. Kleinhaus and Brand (52) described an inhibitory potential in leech ganglion that was abolished by 0.5 mM PB.

In their present state, data on the synaptic pharmacology of barbiturates do not provide any obvious clue to the specific nature of the antiepileptic action of PB. Part of the problem is simply that there are not enough data on PB itself; subtle, important differences from sedative barbiturates may yet be found.

Action Potential Mechanisms

Barbiturates affect conduction along excitable membranes only in concentrations substantially above those that affect synapses, and PB is distinguished from other barbiturates and phenytoin mainly by its lower potency. Thus, 0.8 to 2.9 mM PB produced 50% block of compound action potentials in rat nerve, and pentobarbital was equally effective at slightly lower concentrations (115). Both drugs blocked frog sciatic nerve conduction at 1 to 8 mM (57, 101,127). In the leech Retzius cell, action potentials were prolonged by six barbiturates; PB was the least potent, being effective only in the low millimolar range (53,54,82,85). Similar phenomena were seen in sensory neurons (45) and neurons of the subesophageal ganglion (44); the degree of prolongation was characteristic for each type of neuron. Calcium antagonized this action of all the barbiturates tested including PB. In bursting pacemaker neurons of *Aplysia,* voltage-clamp experiments suggested that PB, 1 to 10 mM, increased, and at higher concentrations suppressed, a slow inward calcium current responsible for controlling the normal firing pattern (44). An unusually potent action of PB and pentobarbital on action potential generation in *Aplysia* (136) did not reveal a difference between the drugs. One study (101) on axonal conduction did find a difference: in frog sciatic nerve, the blocking action of pentobarbital appeared to depend on external Ca concentration and β-adrenergic mechanisms, whereas that of PB did not.

Energy Metabolism

Barbiturates have a variety of effects measurable by chemical methods in nervous tissue. Some of these may well be related directly or through the physiological processes discussed above to mechanisms of antiepileptic action. Potentially important effects already mentioned are changes in transmitter metabolism and depression of voltage-dependent calcium entry into synaptosomes (12,111). Barbiturates can depress cerebral energy metabolism (17, 22–24,30,31,58,88,109,110), but it is not clear when this is a primary effect and when it is secondary to reduced energy demand, as would occur during periods of decreased electrophysiological activity. Primary depression of energy metabolism could be an important mechanism of antiepileptic action. A plausible theory of general anesthesia (56) suggests that an early consequence of depressed cerebral respiration would be reduced sequestration of intraneuronal free calcium, which would accumulate, with profound effects on transmitter release and membrane excitability. The same reasoning could be extended to antiepileptic mechanisms if depression of energy metabolism by barbiturates were known to occur in the antiepileptic concentration range. Most data support the general assumption that it does not. However, depressed respiration in a small part of the neuronal population might be undetectable by conventional biochemical methods, yet would have consequences as widespread as the physiological influence of the affected neurons on others. Since it is unlikely that respiration in all neurons is affected at the same drug concentration, this interesting possibility has a place in constructive speculation about antiepileptic mechanisms.

Interpretation of data on the metabolic effects of barbiturates is limited in certain ways that obscure the roles some of them may play in clinically useful seizure prevention. First, as in most physiological studies, there are too few directly comparable data on the various barbiturates to reveal any selective action the antiepileptic barbiturates may have. Much progress can be made in this area with currently available techniques. Second, the biochemical systems known to be affected by barbiturates are themselves of uncertain relation to epileptic phenomena. It is useful to know that in low concentrations PB can stimulate, and in higher ones depress, free acetylcholine production in brain slices (65), but the knowledge cannot be translated into understanding of barbiturate antiepileptic action unless one also knows how cholinergic transmission is involved in generation or control of some epileptic event. Progress here depends on better understanding of epileptic pathophysiology. Third, chemical measurements in the nervous system do not yet routinely achieve resolution at the level of the single cell. As such resolution becomes available, correlation of chemical and electrical measurements pertaining to the same identified neurons should provide substantial new insight into mechanisms of antiepileptic drug action.

CONCLUSIONS

Freud is said to have described his method of investigation as "simply staring at the facts until they make sense." Certain defects in the method could be pointed out, but Freud was a doctor, not an epistemologist. We who would understand the mechanisms of antiepileptic drug actions have much the same problem he had. Like him, we contemplate an intricate system and try to squeeze sense from whatever facts are available about it. Like him, we constantly face the seduction of the plausible. If PB is seen to depress some kind of excitation, we say we are on the right track, and so are perplexed when pentobarbital proves to do the same thing better. We next learn that PB strengthens certain inhibitions and are relieved to find such good sense in the facts, only to suffer perplexity again as barbiturates not useful in epilepsy are shown to have the same action. There is nothing wrong with this process. It is, in fact, the basis of empirical science, the means by which simple-minded assumptions about nature are molded toward understanding. It is more advanced for PB than for other antiepileptic drugs. If 2,500 hydantoins had been synthesized, and dozens of them studied in a variety of neurobiological systems, our current ideas about how phenytoin prevents seizures might seem quite naive. Because a number of simple explanations for the antiepileptic potency of PB have been eliminated by studies on related drugs, hypotheses for guiding future work can be formulated more precisely than is possible in the case of other antiepileptics.

First of all, unique actions of PB may yet be found, either in preparations already under study (87) or in new ones suggested by better knowledge of epileptic pathophysiology. Phenobarbital is distinguishable from pentobarbital by its more selective actions on motor cortex excitability (49), local electrical seizure thresholds (4),

afterdischarge of isolated cortex (127), penicillin-induced spikes in hippocampal slices (76), and picrotoxin-induced firing of tissue-cultured spinal neurons (63). Perhaps when other barbiturates are studied carefully in the same systems, these or related phenomena will indeed prove to be selectively sensitive to PB. If that happens, the mechanisms of action on the distinguishing phenomena will gain high priority as candidates for basic mechanisms of antiepileptic action. However, it may be that even after the appropriate comparisons have been made, there will be no experimental test that segregates barbiturates the way seizures do.

Second, a combination of actions in some critical proportion, rather than a single action, might be what determines the antiepileptic potency of a drug. Phenobarbital, as well as pentobarbital, depressed excitatory postsynaptic potentials in frog neuromuscular junction (86,123) and sympathetic ganglia (72,74), prolonged segmental (27,67) and cuneate (7,81) presynaptic inhibition in cat, prolonged recurrent inhibitions in rat hippocampus (138), prolonged an inhibition possibly mediated by GABA in guinea pig olfactory cortex (104,105), increased action potential duration in leech neurons (51,53–55,82,85), affected firing thresholds in *Aplysia* neurons (136), and blocked conduction in frog nerve (127). In every case, pentobarbital was of equal or greater potency. That need not mean that such actions cannot be involved in the antiepileptic action of PB. For the sake of illustration only, suppose that seizure control depends mainly on enhanced inhibition and that loss of consciousness results mainly from depressed excitation. Suppose further that pentobarbital affects excitation and inhibition equally, and that PB is more effective at prolonging inhibitions than at depressing excitations, although weaker than pentobarbital at both. If these things were so, PB would suppress seizures relatively more than consciousness, whereas pentobarbital would simply produce seizure-free anesthesia. This is essentially the kind of argument used by MacDonald and Barker (63) to interpret experiments in which both drugs enhanced GABAergic inhibition, but only pentobarbital appeared to exert another inhibitory action of uncertain nature (41).

Finally, drug distribution in nervous tissue is a possible determinant of antiepileptic potency and one that has received only occasional attention (84,89,90). Many of the actions already mentioned might suppress seizures if exerted selectively in a part of the nervous system especially important for seizure elaboration. Biochemical (108) and autoradiographic (20) measurements show that PB enters the brain in a manner reflecting blood flow patterns but in the steady state is evenly distributed in gray and white matter. Detection of some barbiturates by immunological methods (113,114) can provide a finer measure of tissue distribution. Immunofluorescent localization of PB in brains of acutely overdosed mice revealed quite uneven distribution among nuclei and among neurons within gray matter (78). The method could be used to learn more about how PB and other barbiturates to which antibodies can be made are distributed in the steady state. Such information combined with other histochemical measurements might offer a great deal of new insight into barbiturate actions.

Abnormal electrical discharge could create local conditions favoring the action of particular barbiturates. One of the most obvious of these is tissue acidosis. Generalized seizure activity lowers cortical pH (5,18,40); local cortical stimulation for 20 sec can lower local pH 0.15 unit without causing seizure activity (40). It is therefore reasonable to suppose that pH is lower in a chronically discharging epileptic focus than in surrounding tissue. At 7.3, the acid dissociation constant of PB is lower and closer to the physiologic pH range than that of any other common barbiturate; most experiments show that the uncharged form of barbiturates is active, at least for depression of membrane excitability (54,57,106). Local acidosis would shift PB into its active form proportionately more than barbiturates with more alkaline dissociation constants. Thus, PB would tend selectively to suppress firing in regions of vigorous electrical discharge such as seizure foci, while tending to spare regions better able to control hydrogen

ion activity. This would be a good arrangement for insuring that PB act in the right place at the right time. Other local or use-dependent conditions could also be important for other drugs as well as PB. The longer unique actions of antiepileptic drugs elude investigation, the more plausible such explanations will become.

ACKNOWLEDGMENTS

The leech research described in this chapter was done by the author in collaboration with Anna L. Kleinhaus, Ph.D. and with the technical assistance of Hector Goico. Various phases of it were supported by U.S.P.H.S. grants RO1-NSO8851 and P5O-NSO208 and a grant from the C. G. Swebilius Trust.

REFERENCES

1. Adams, P. (1976): Drug blockade of open end-plate channels. *J. Physiol. (Lond.)*, 260:531–552.
2. Aird, R. B., and Woodbury, D. M. (1974): *The Management of Epilepsy.* Charles C Thomas, Springfield, Illinois.
3. Albertson, T. E., Peterson, S. L., and Stark, L. G. (1978): Effects of phenobarbital and SC-13504 on partially kindled hippocampal seizures in rats. *Exp. Neurol.*, 61:270–276.
4. Aston, R., and Domino, E. F. (1961): Differential effects of phenobarbital, pentobarbital, and diphenylhydantoin on motor cortical and reticular thresholds in the rhesus monkey. *Psychopharmacologia*, 2:304–317.
5. Astrup, J., Heuser, D., Lassen, N. A., Nilsson, B., Norberg, K., and Siesjo, B. K. (1978): Evidence against H^+ and K^+ as main factors for the control of cerebral blood flow: A microelectrode study. In: *Ciba Foundation Symposium #56, Cerebrovascular Smooth Muscle and its Control*, edited by K. Elliot and M. O'Connor. pp. 313–332. Elsevier, New York.
6. Ayala, G. F., Dichter, M., Gumnit, R. J., Matsumoto, H., and Spencer, W. A. (1973): Genesis of epileptic interictal spikes. *Brain Res.*, 52:1–17.
7. Banna, N. R., and Jabbur, S. J. (1969): Pharmacological studies on inhibition in the cuneate nucleus of the cat. *Neuropharmacology*, 8:299–307.
8. Barker, J. L. (1975): CNS depressants: Effects on postsynaptic pharmacology. *Brain Res.*, 92:35–56.
9. Barker, J. L. (1975): Inhibitory and excitatory effects of CNS depressants on invertebrate synapses. *Brain Res.*, 93:77–90.
10. Barker, J. L., and Gainer, H. (1973): Pentobarbital: Selective depression of excitatory postsynaptic potentials. *Science*, 182:720–721.
11. Barker, J. L., and Ransom, B. R. (1978): Pentobarbital pharmacology of mammalian central neu-

rones grown in tissue culture. *J. Physiol. (Lond.),* 280:355–372.

12. Blaustein, M. P., and Ector, A. (1975): Inhibition of calcium uptake by depolarized nerve *in vitro. Mol. Pharmacol.,* 11:369–378.

13. Bogue, J. Y., and Carrington, H. C. (1953): The evaluation of "Mysoline"—a new anticonvulsant drug. *Br. J. Pharmacol. Chemother.,* 8:230–236.

14. Bowery, N. G., and Dray, A. (1976): Barbiturate reversal of amino acid antagonism produced by convulsant agents. *Nature,* 264:276–277.

15. Bowery, N. G., and Dray, A. (1978): Reversal of the action of amino acid antagonists by barbiturates and other hypnotic drugs. *Br. J. Pharmacol.,* 63:197–215.

16. Boyer, P. A. (1966): Anticonvulsant properties of benzodiazepines. A review. *Dis. Nerv. Syst.,* 27:35–42.

17. Bunker, J. P., and Vandam, L. D. (1965): Effect of anaesthesia on metabolism and cellular functions. *Pharmacol. Rev.,* 17:182–263.

18. Caspers, H., and Speckman, E.-J. (1969): DC potential shifts in paroxysmal states. In: *Basic Mechanisms of the Epilepsies,* edited by H. H. Jasper, A. A. Ward, Jr., and A. Pope, pp. 375–388. Little, Brown, Boston.

19. Caspers, H., and Wehmeyer, H. (1957): Die Wirkung von Diphenylhydantoin auf die Krampferregbarkeit der Hirnrinde. *Z. Gesamte Exp. Med.* 129:77–86.

20. Cassrano, G. B., Ghetti, B., Gliozzi, E., and Hansson, E. (1967): Autoradiographic distribution study of "short acting" and "long acting" barbiturates: ^{35}S-Thiopentone and ^{14}C-phenobarbitone. *Br. J. Anaesth.,* 39:11–20.

21. Clark, D. L., and Rosner, B. S. (1973): Neurophysiologic effects of general anesthetics: I. Electroencephalogram and sensory evoked responses in man. *Anesthesiology,* 38:564–582.

22. Cohen, P. J. (1973): Effect of anesthetics on mitochondrial function. *Anesthesiology,* 39:153–164.

23. Corriol, J. H., and Joanny, P. A. (1973): Oxidative and electrolytic metabolism of nervous tissue *in vitro.* In: *Anticonvulsant Drugs,* edited by J. Mercier, pp. 505–532. Pergamon Press, Oxford.

24. Cowger, M. L., and Labbe, R. F. (1967): The inhibition of terminal oxidation by porphyrinogenic drugs. *Biochem. Pharmacol.,* 18:2189–2199.

25. Craig, C. R., and Shideman, F. E. (1971): Metabolism and anticonvulsant properties of mephobarbital and phenobarbital in rats. *J. Pharmacol. Exp. Ther.,* 176:35–42.

26. Domino, E. F. (1962): Sites of action of some central nervous depressants. *Annu. Rev. Pharmacol.,* 2:215–250.

27. Eccles, J. C., Schmidt, R. F., and Willis, W. D. (1963): Pharmacological studies on presynaptic inhibition. *J. Physiol. (Lond.),* 168:500–530.

28. Esplin, D. W. (1963): Criteria for assessing effects of depressant drugs on spinal cord synaptic transmission, with examples of drug selectivity. *Arch. Int. Pharmacodyn. Ther.,* 143:479–497.

29. Esplin, D. W. (1972): Synaptic system models. In:

Experimental Models of Epilepsy, edited by D. P. Purpura, J. K. Penry, D. B. Tower, D. M. Woodbury, and R. D. Walter, pp. 223–248. Raven Press, New York.

30. Fink, B. R., and Haschke, R. H. (1973): Anesthetic effects on cerebral metabolism. *Anesthesiology,* 39:199–215.

31. Forda, O., and McIlwain, H. (1953): Anticonvulsants and electrically stimulated metabolism of separated mammalian cerebral cortex. *Br. J. Pharmacol.,* 8:225–229.

32. Frey, H.-H., and Hahn, I (1960): Untersuchungen uber die Bedeutung des durch Biotransformation gebildeten Phenobarbital fur die antikonvulsive Wirkung von Primidon. *Arch. Int. Pharmacodyn. Ther.,* 128:281–290.

33. Gallagher, B. B. (1977): Neuropharmacology and treatment of epilepsy. In: *Anticonvulsants,* edited by J. A. Vida, pp. 11–55. Academic Press, New York.

34. Gallagher, B. B., Smith, D. B., and Mattson, R. H. (1970): The relationship of the anticonvulsant properties of primidone to phenobarbital. *Epilepsia,* 11:293–301.

35. Gangloff, H. and Monnier, M. (1957): The action of anticonvulsant drugs tested by electrical stimulation of the rabbit cortex, diencephalon and rhinencephalon in the unanesthetized rabbit. *Electroencephalogr. Clin. Neurophysiol.,* 9:43–58.

36. Gastaut, H., Roger, J., and Lob, H. (1973): Medical treatment of epilepsy. In: *Anticonvulsant Drugs, Vol. 2,* edited by J. Mercier, pp. 535–598. Pergamon Press, Oxford.

37. Gehrmann, J. E., and Killam, K. F. (1976): Assessment of CNS drug activity in rhesus monkeys by analysis of the EEG. *Fed. Proc.,* 35:2258–2263.

38. Gloor, P. (1979): Generalized epilepsy with spike-and-wave discharge: A reinterpretation of its electrographic and clinical manifestations. *Epilepsia,* 20:571–588.

39. Goodman, L. S., Swinyard, E. A., Brown, W. C., Schiffman, D. O., Grewal, M. S., and Bliss, E. L. (1953): Anticonvulsant properties of 5-phenyl-5-hexahydropyrimidine-4,6-dione (Mysoline), a new antiepileptic. *J. Pharmacol. Exp. Ther.,* 108:428–436.

40. Heuser, D. (1978): The significance of H^+, K^+ and Ca^{++} activities for regulation of local cerebral blood flow under conditions of enhanced neuronal activity. In: *Ciba Foundation Symposium #56, Cerebrovascular Smooth Muscle and its Control,* pp. 339–348. Elsevier, New York.

41. Huang, L.-Y. M., and Barker, J. L. (1980): Pentobarbital: Stereospecific actions of $(+)$ and $(-)$ isomers revealed on cultured mammalian neurons. *Science,* 207:195–197.

42. Izquierdo, I. (1974): Effect of anticonvulsant drugs on the number of afferent stimuli needed to cause a hippocampal seizure discharge. *Pharmacology,* 11:146–150.

43. Jasper, H. H., Ward, A. A. Jr., and Pope, A. (1969): *Basic Mechanisms of the Epilepsies,* pp. 357–370. Little, Brown, Boston.

44. Johnston, D. (1978): Phenobarbital: Concentration-

dependent biphasic effect on *Aplysia* burst neurons. *Neurosci. Lett.*, 10:175–180.

45. Julien, R. M., and Halpern, L. M. (1970): Stabilization of excitable membrane by chronic administration of diphenylhydantoin. *J. Pharmacol. Exp. Ther.*, 175:206–213.

46. Julien, R. M., and Halpern, L. M. (1972): Effects of diphenylhydantoin and other antiepileptic drugs on epileptiform activity and Purkinje cell discharge rates. *Epilepsia*, 13:387–400.

47. Kaplan, B. J. (1977): Phenobarbital and phenytoin effects on somatosensory evoked potentials and spontaneous EEG in normal cat brain. *Epilepsia*, 18:397–403.

48. Kay, D. C., Jasinski, D. R., and Eisenstein, R. B. (1972): Quantified human sleep after pentobarbital. *Clin. Pharmacol. Ther.*, 13:221–241.

49. Keller, A. D., and Fulton, J. F. (1931): The action of anesthetic drugs on the motor cortex of monkeys. *Am. J. Physiol.*, 47:537.

50. Killam, E. K. (1976): Measurement of anticonvulsant activity in the *Papio* model of epilepsy. *Fed. Proc.*, 35:2264–2269.

51. Kleinhaus, A. L. (1975): Electrophysiological actions of convulsants and anticonvulsants on neurons of the leech subesophageal ganglion. *Comp. Biochem. Physiol.*, 52:27–34.

52. Kleinhaus, A. L., and Brand, S. (1979): A magnesium- and barbiturate-sensitive inhibitory synaptic potential in leech ganglion. *Soc. Neurosci. Abstr.*, 5:250.

53. Kleinhaus, A. L., and Prichard, J. W. (1977): A calcium-reversible action of barbiturates on the leech Retzius cell. *J. Pharmacol. Exp. Ther.*, 201:332–339.

54. Kleinhaus, A. L., and Prichard, J. W. (1977): Pentobarbital actions on a leech neuron. *Comp. Biochem. Physiol.*, 581:61–65.

55. Kleinhaus, A. L., and Prichard, J. W. (1979): Interaction of divalent cations and barbiturates on four identified leech neurons. *Comp. Biochem. Physiol. [C]*, 63:351–357.

56. Krnjevic, K. (1975): Is general anesthesia induced by neuronal asphyxia? In: *Molecular Mechanisms of Anesthesia*, edited by B. R. Fink, pp. 92–98. Raven Press, New York.

57. Krupp, P., Bianchi, C. P., and Suarez-Kurtz, G. (1969): On the local anesthetic effect of barbiturates. *J. Pharm. Pharmacol.*, 21:763–768.

58. LaManna, J. C., Cordingley, G., and Rosenthal, M. (1977): Phenobarbital actions *in vivo:* Effects on extracellular potassium activity and oxidative metabolism in cat cerebral cortex. *J. Pharmacol. Exp. Ther.*, 200:560–569.

59. Lembeck, F., and Beubler, E. (1977): Convulsions induced by hyperbaric oxygen: Inhibition by phenobarbital, diazepam and baclofen. *Naunyn Schmiedebergs Arch. Pharmacol.*, 297:47–52.

60. Lennox, W. G. (1960): *Epilepsy and Related Disorders*. Little, Brown, Boston.

61. Livingston, S. (1963): *Living With Epileptic Seizures*. Charles C Thomas, Springfield, Illinois.

62. Loyning, Y., Oshima, T., and Yokota, T. (1964):

Site of action of thiamylal sodium on the monosynaptic reflex pathway in cats. *J. Neurophysiol.*, 27:408–428.

63. MacDonald, R. L., and Barker, J. L. (1978): Different actions of anticonvulsant and anesthetic barbiturates resolved by use of cultured mammalian neurons. *Science*, 200:775–777.

64. Mares, P., Kolinova, M., and Fischer, J. (1977): The influence of pentobarbital upon cortical epileptogenic focus in rats. *Arch. Int. Pharmacodyn. Ther.*, 226:313–323.

65. McLennan, H., and Elliott, K. A. C. (1951): Effect of convulsant and narcotic drugs on acetylcholine synthesis. *J. Pharmacol. Exp. Ther.*, 103:35–43.

66. Millichap, J. G. (1973): Correlations of clinical and laboratory evaluations of anticonvulsant drugs. In: *Anticonvulsant Drugs*, edited by J. Mercier, pp. 189–202. Pergamon Press, Oxford.

67. Miyahara, J. T., Esplin, D. W., and Zablocka B. (1966): Differential effects of depressant drugs on presynaptic inhibition. *J. Pharmacol. Exp. Ther.*, 154:119–127.

68. Morgan, K. G., and Bryant, S. H. (1977): Pentobarbital—presynaptic effect in squid giant synapse. *Experientia*, 33:487–488.

69. Morrell, F., Bradley, W., and Ptashne, M. (1959): Effects of drugs on discharge characteristics of chronic epileptogenic lesions. *Neurology (Minneap.)*, 9:492–498.

70. Neuman, R. S., and Frank, G. B. (1977): Effects of diphenylhydantoin and phenobarbital on voltage-clamped myelinated nerve. *Can. J. Physiol. Pharmacol.*, 55:42–47.

71. Nicoll, R. A. (1972): The effects of anesthetics on synaptic excitation and inhibition in the olfactory bulb. *J. Physiol. (Lond.)*, 223:803–814.

72. Nicoll, R. A. (1978): Pentobarbital: Differential postsynaptic actions on sympathetic ganglion cells. *Science*, 199:451–452.

73. Nicoll, R. A., Eccles, J. C., Oshiwa, T., and Rubia, F. (1975): Prolongation of hippocampal inhibitory postsynaptic potentials by barbiturates. *Nature*, 258:265–267.

74. Nicoll, R. A., and Iwamoto, E. T. (1978): Action of pentobarbital on sympathetic ganglion cells. *J. Neurophysiol.*, 41:977–986.

75. Ogunremi, O. O., Adamson, L., Brezenova, V., Hunter, W., Maclean, A. W., Oswald, I., and Percy-Robb, I. W. (1973): Two antianxiety drugs: A psychoneuroendocrine study. *Br. Med. J.*, 2:202–205.

76. Oliver, A. P., Hoffer, B. J., and Wyatt, R. J. (1977): The hippocampal slice: A system for studying the pharmacology of seizures and for screening anticonvulsant drugs. *Epilepsia*, 18:543–548.

77. Oswald, I., and Priest, R. G. (1965): Five weeks to escape the sleeping-pill habit. *Br. Med. J.*, 2:1093–1099.

78. Pertschuk, L. P., Rainford, E., and Brigati, D. (1976): Localization of phenobarbital in mouse central nervous system by immunofluorescence. *Acta Neurol. Scand.*, 53:325–334.

79. Pickles, H. G., and Simmonds, M. A. (1978): Field potentials, inhibition and the effect of pentobarbi-

tone in the rat olfactory cortex slice. *J. Physiol. (Lond.)*, 275:135–148.

80. Pincus, J. H., Grove, I., Marino, B. B., and Glaser, G. H. (1970): Studies on the mechanism of action of diphenylhydantoin. *Arch. Neurol.*, 22:566–571.

81. Polc, P., and Haefely, W. (1976): Effects of two benzodiazepines, phenobarbitone and baclofen on synaptic transmission in the cat cuneate nucleus. *Naunyn Schmiedebergs Arch. Pharmacol.*, 294:121–132.

82. Prichard, J. W. (1972): Effect of phenobarbital on a leech neuron. *Neuropharmacology*, 11:585–590.

83. Prichard, J. W. (1980): Barbiturates: Physiological effects I. *Adv. Neurol.*, 27:505–522.

84. Prichard, J. W. (1980): Phenobarbital: Proposed mechanisms of antiepileptic action. *Adv. Neurol.*, 27:553–562.

85. Prichard, J. W., and Kleinhaus, A. L. (1974): Dual action of phenobarbital on leech ganglia. *Comp. Gen. Pharmacol.*, 5:239–250.

86. Proctor, W. R., and Weakly, J. N. (1976): A comparison of the presynaptic and postsynaptic actions of pentobarbitone and phenobarbitone on the neuromuscular junction of the frog. *J. Physiol. (Lond.)*, 258:257–258.

87. Purpura, D. P., Penry, J. K., Tower, D., Woodbury, D. M., and Walter, R. D. (1972): *Experimental Models of Epilepsy*. Raven Press, New York.

88. Quastel, J. H. (1965): Effects of drugs on the metabolism of brain *in vivo*. *Br. Med. Bull.*, 21:49–56.

89. Raines, A. (1969): Discussion of Esplin, D. W. and Zablocka, B.: Effects of tetanization on transmitter dynamics. *Epilepsia*, 10:193–210.

90. Raines, A., Blake, G. J., Richardson, B., and Gilbert, M. B. (1979): Differential selectivity of several barbiturates on experimental seizures and neurotoxicity in the mouse. *Epilepsia*, 20:105–113.

91. Raines, A., and Standaert, F. G. (1969): Effects of anticonvulsant drugs on nerve terminals. *Epilepsia*, 10:211–227.

92. Ransom, B. R., and Barker, J. L. (1975): Pentobarbital modulates transmitter effects of mouse spinal neurones grown in tissue culture. *Nature*, 254:703–705.

93. Ransom, B. R., and Barker, J. L. (1976): Pentobarbital selectively enhances GABA-mediated postsynaptic inhibition in tissue cultured mouse spinal neurons. *Brain Res.*, 114:530–535.

94. Reinhard, J. F., and Reinhard, J. F., Jr. (1977): Experimental evaluation of anticonvulsants. In: *Anticonvulsants*, edited by J. A. Vida, pp. 57–111. Academic Press, New York.

95. Reynolds, E. H. (1973): Anticonvulsants, folic acid and epilepsy. *Lancet*, 1:1376–1378.

96. Richards, C. D. (1972): On the mechanisms of barbiturate anaesthesia. *J. Physiol. (Lond.)*, 227:749–768.

97. Richens, A. (1976): *Drug Treatment of Epilepsy*. Kimpton, London.

98. Richens, A., and Woodford, F. P. (1976): *Anticonvulsant Drugs and Enzyme Induction*. Excerpta Medica, Amsterdam.

99. Rosenberg, P., and Bartels, E. (1967): Drug effects on the spontaneous electrical activity of the squid giant axon. *J. Pharmacol. Exp. Ther.*, 155:532–534.

100. Rosner, B. S., and Clark, D. L. (1973): Neurophysiologic effects of general anesthetics. II. Sequential regional actions in the brain. *Anesthesiology*, 39:59–81.

101. Sabelli, H. C., Diamond, B. I., May, J., and Havdala, H. S. (1977): Differential interactions of phenobarbital and pentobarbital with beta-adrenergic mechanisms *in vitro* and *in vivo*. *Exp. Neurol.*, 54:453–466.

102. Schallek, W., and Johnson, T. C. (1976): Spectral density analysis of the effects of barbiturates and benzodiazepines on the electrocorticogram of the squirrel monkey. *Arch. Int. Pharmacodyn. Ther.*, 233:301–310.

103. Schmidt, R. P., and Wilder, B. J. (1968): *Epilepsy*. F. A. Davis, Philadelphia.

104. Scholfield, C. N. (1978): A barbiturate induced intensification of the inhibitory potential in slices of guinea pig olfactory cortex. *J. Physiol. (Lond.)*, 275:559–566.

105. Scholfield, C. N., and Harvey, J. A. (1975): Local anesthetics and barbiturates: Effects on evoked potentials in isolated mammalian cortex. *J. Pharmacol. Exp. Ther.*, 195:522–531.

106. Schwarz, J. R. (1979): The mode of action of phenobarbital on the excitable membrane of the node of Ranvier. *Eur. J. Pharmacol.*, 56:51–60.

107. Seyama, I., and Narahashi, T. (1975): Mechanism of blockade of neuromuscular transmission by pentobarbital. *J. Pharmacol Exp. Ther.*, 192:95–104.

108. Sherwin, A. L., Harvey, C. D., and Leppik, I. E. (1976): Quantitation of antiepileptic drugs in human brain. In: *Quantitative Analytic Studies in Epilepsy*, edited by P. Kellaway and I. Petersen, pp. 172–182. Raven Press, New York.

109. Siesjo, B. K. (1978): *Brain Energy Metabolism*. John Wiley & Sons, New York.

110. Singh, P., and Huot, J. (1973): Neurochemistry of epilepsy and mechanism of action of antiepileptics. In: *Anticonvulsant Drugs*, edited by J. Mercier, pp. 427–504. Pergamon Press, Oxford.

111. Sohn, R. S., and Ferrendelli, J. A. (1976): Anticonvulsant drug mechanisms. *Arch. Neurol.*, 33:626–629.

112. Somjen, G. G. (1967): Effects of anesthetics on spinal cord of mammals. *Anesthesiology*, 28:135–143.

113. Spector, S., Berkowitz, B., Flynn, E. J., and Peskar, B. (1973): Antibodies of morphine, barbiturates and serotonin. *Pharmacol. Rev.*, 25:281–292.

114. Spector, S., and Flynn, E. J. (1971): Barbiturates: Radioimmunoassay. *Science*, 174:1036–1038.

115. Staiman, A., and Seeman, P. (1974): The impulse-blocking concentrations of anesthetics, alcohols, anticonvulsants, barbiturates and narcotics on phrenic and sciatic nerves. *Can. J. Physiol. Pharmacol.*, 52:535–557.

116. Stark, L. G., Killam, K. F., and Killam, E. K. (1970): The anticonvulsant effects of phenobarbital, diphenylhydantoin and two benzodiazapines in the

baboon, *Papio papio. J. Pharmacol. Exp. Ther.,* 173:125–133.

117. Straw, R. N., and Mitchell, C. L. (1966): Effect of phenobarbital on cortical after-discharge and overt seizure patterns in the rat. *Int. J. Neuropharmacol.,* 5:323–330.

118. Strobos, R. R. J., and Spudis, E. V. (1960): Effect of anticonvulsant drugs on cortical and subcortical seizure discharges in cats. *Arch. Neurol.,* 2:399–406.

119. Swinyard, E. A., Brown, W. C., and Goodman, L. S. (1952): Comparative assays of antiepileptic drugs in mice and rats. *J. Pharmacol. Exp. Ther.,* 106:47–59.

120. Takeuchi, H. (1968): Modifications par la phenobarbital des proprietes electriques du neurone a potentiel de membrane stable. *C. R. Soc. Biol. (Paris),* 162:488–490.

121. Takeuchi, M., and Chalazonitis, N. (1968): Effets du phenobarbital sur les neurones autactifs. *C. R. Soc. Biol. (Paris),* 162:491–493.

122. Thesleff, S. (1956): Effects of anesthetic agents on skeletal muscle membrane. *Acta Physiol. Scand.,* 37:335–349.

123. Thomson, T. D., and Turkanis, S. A. (1973): Barbiturate induced transmitter release at a frog neuromuscular junction. *Br. J. Pharmacol.,* 48:48–58.

124. Toman, J. E. P. (1952): Neuropharmacology of peripheral nerve. *Pharmacol. Rev.,* 4:168–218.

125. Tsuchiya, T., and Fukushima, H. (1978): Effects of benzodiazepines and pentobarbitone on the GABAergic recurrent inhibition of hippocampal neurons. *Eur. J. Pharmacol.,* 48:421–424.

126. Vastola, E. F., and Rosen, A. (1960): Suppression by anticonvulsants of focal electrical seizures in the neocortex. *Electroencephalogr. Clin. Neurophysiol.,* 12:237–332.

127. Vazquez, A. J., Diamond, B. I., and Sabelli, H. C. (1975): Differential effects of phenobarbital and pentobarbital on isolated nervous tissue. *Epilepsia,* 16:601–608.

128. Vida, J. A., and Gerry, E. G. (1977): Cyclic ureides. In: *Anticonvulsants,* edited by J. A. Vida, pp. 152–291. Academic Press, New York.

129. Wada, J. A. (1976): *Kindling.* Raven Press, New York.

130. Wada, J. A. (1977): Pharmacological prophylaxis in the kindling model of epilepsy. *Arch. Neurol.,* 34:389–395.

131. Wada, J. A., Osawa, T., Sato, M., Wake, A., Corcoran, M. E., and Troupin, A. S. (1976): Acute anticonvulsant effects of diphenylhydantoin, phenobarbital, and carbamazepine: A combined electroclinical and serum level study in amygdaloid kindled cats and baboons. *Epilepsia,* 17:77–88.

132. Wada, J. A., Sato, M., Wake, A., Green, J. R., and Troupin, A. S. (1976): Prophylatic effects of phenytoin, phenobarbital, and carbamazepine examined in kindling cat preparations. *Arch. Neurol.,* 33:426–434.

133. Wauquier, A., Ashton, D., and Melis, W. (1979): Behavioral analysis of amygdaloid kindling in beagle dogs and the effects of clonazepam, diazepam, phenobarbital, diphenylhydantoin and flunarizine on seizure manifestation. *Exp. Neurol.,* 64:579–586.

134. Weakly, J. N. (1969): Effect of barbiturates on quantal synaptic transmission in spinal motoneurones. *J. Physiol. (Lond.),* 204:63–77.

135. Weakly, J. N., and Proctor, W. R. (1977): Barbiturate induced changes in transmitter release independent of terminal spike configuration in the frog neuromuscular junction. *Neuropharmacology,* 16:507–510.

136. Wilson, W. A., Zbicz, K. L., and Cote, I. W. (1980): Barbiturates: Inhibition of sustained firing in *Aplysia* neurons. *Adv. Neurol.,* 27:533–540.

137. Wise, R. A., and Chinerman, J. (1974): Effects of diazepam and phenobarbital on electrically induced amygdaloid seizures and seizure development. *Exp. Neurol.,* 45:355–363.

138. Wolf, P., and Haas, H. L. (1977): Effects of diazepines and barbiturates on hippocampal recurrent inhibition. *Naunyn Schmiedebergs Arch. Pharmacol.,* 299:211–218.

139. Woodbury, D. M., and Fingl, E. (1975): Drugs effective in the therapy of the epilepsies. In: *The Pharmacological Basis of Therapeutics,* edited by L. S. Goodman and A. Gilman, pp. 201–226. MacMillan, New York.

Antiepileptic Drugs, edited by D. M. Woodbury, J. K. Penry, and C. E. Pippenger. Raven Press, New York © 1982.

28

Other Barbiturates

Methylphenobarbital and Metharbital

Mervyn J. Eadie

Over the past 30 years or longer, two *N*-methylated derivatives of barbituric acid have occasionally been employed as anticonvulsants in man. Neither drug has achieved any widespread popularity. At the present time, metharbital, which was introduced in 1948 (24), appears to be rarely used. Very little is known of its pharmacokinetics or of other aspects of its clinical pharmacology. However, methylphenobarbital, introduced in 1932 (1), is more extensively used and enjoys some popularity in certain places. Thus, in Australia, the drug is currently a little more widely prescribed than primidone and seven-eighths as widely prescribed as phenobarbital. It is reputed, at least by word of mouth, to be as effective an anticonvulsant as phenobarbital and to be less sedative. A modest amount of information has now become available about the pharmacokinetics and metabolism of methylphenobarbital in man, and it is possible to provide a coherent, although incomplete, outline of its clinical pharmacology.

CHEMISTRY AND METHODS OF DETERMINATION

Properties

Methylphenobarbital (mephobarbital, methylphenobarbitone, Mebaral®), chemically 1-methyl-5-ethyl-5-phenylbarbituric acid (Fig. 1),

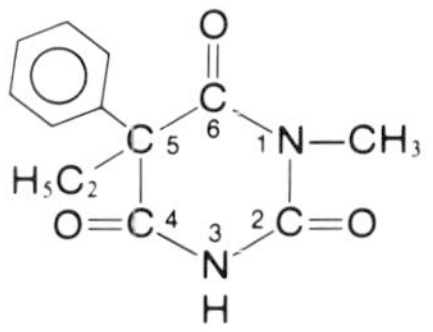

Fig. 1. Structure of methylphenobarbital.

is the *N*-methylated analog of phenobarbital. It is a white crystalline powder, weakly acidic, with a pK_c value of 7.8 and a molecular weight of 246.26. It is more lipid soluble than phenobarbital itself.

Metharbital (*N*-methylbarbitone, Gemonil®), chemically is 1-methyl-5,5-diethylbarbituric acid (Fig. 2). It also is a weak acid with a pK_a value of 8.45 and a molecular weight of 198.22. Like methylphenobarbital, it is less polar and more lipid soluble than its *N*-desmethylated analog.

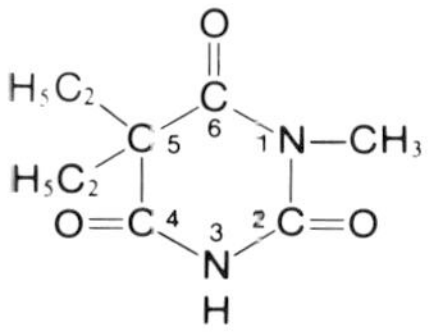

Fig. 2. Structure of metharbital.

Synthesis

The general method for barbiturate synthesis involves condensation of the appropriate malonic acid derivatives with urea (or, in the case of the N-methylbarbiturates, with methylurea) (28). The reactions may be carried out in alkaline, neutral, or acidic media. Other synthetic pathways exist, e.g., condensation of (a) cyanoacetic esters with methyl urea, (b) of malonamides with ethylcarbamate, or (c) of malonylnitrile with methylurea (3).

Methods of Determination

A number of methods have been described for the measurement of the N-methyl barbiturates and their desmethylated congeners (and metabolites) in biological material. Butler (3,4) devised ultraviolet spectrophotometric assays, first for methylphenobarbital and phenobarbital and subsequently for metharbital and barbital. The principles underlying such assays were reviewed by Bush and Sanders-Bush (2).

Nitration, followed by thin-layer chromatography, has been used to separate methylphenobarbital and phenobarbital (17). The nitrated residues were subsequently reduced, diazotized, and then diazo-coupled to yield products that were measured spectrophotometrically.

A number of gas–liquid chromatographic techniques exist for measuring methylphenobarbital and phenobarbital. The two substances can be measured without derivatization (10), but derivatization yields more satisfactory chromatographic results. However, the most commonly used derivatization technique for anticonvulsant work, i.e., formation of methyl derivatives, yields the same product from both methylphenobarbital and phenobarbital. Thus, the two substances cannot be measured individually. To overcome this difficulty, MacGee (21) formed ethyl rather than methyl derivatives. Phenobarbital forms a diethyl compound, whereas methylphenobarbital yields methylethylphenobarbital, and the two derivatives can be resolved and measured. Higher alkyl derivatives might also be made and would be expected to permit separate quantitation of methylphenobarbital and phenobarbital. Hooper et al.

(16) described a gas–liquid chromatographic assay for methylphenobarbital and phenobarbital that utilized formation of butyl derivatives of the two substances.

It is possible to measure methylphenobarbital and phenobarbital at biological concentration without derivatization by using high-pressure liquid chromatography with ultraviolet detection. This method has proved quite satisfactory for routine assays in the author's laboratory.

Various types of immunoassay methods, such as the enzyme-multiplied immune test (EMIT®) and radioimmunoassay, have been used to measure phenobarbital at biologically applicable concentrations. The antibodies used, at least for EMIT tests, are not completely specific and measure methylphenobarbital as phenobarbital. Consequently, for patients taking methylphenobarbital who are likely to have both the parent drug and phenobarbital simultaneously present in plasma, currently available EMIT assays measure only the sum of the concentrations of the two substances.

It appears likely that the methods discussed above for measuring methylphenobarbital and its desmethylated metabolite could be applied, with minor modification, to the measurement of metharbital and barbital. However, there has been little interest in the latter substances in recent years. No doubt gas chromatography–mass spectrometry could be used to measure the relevant substances specifically.

ABSORPTION, DISTRIBUTION, AND EXCRETION

Absorption

Extent of Absorption

Clinical experience shows that the dose of methylphenobarbital required to produce a given biological effect is approximately twice that of phenobarbital. Molecular weight differences cannot account for this discrepancy. Butler and Waddell (7), in studies on three humans, could account for only 50 to 60% of a methylphenobarbital dose as the parent substance plus derived phenobarbital. On this basis, it has sometimes been suggested that only about 50% of an oral methylphenobarbital dose is absorbed, although certain reports have suggested that the drug might also be excreted as an unknown metabolite or metabolites (7,22). In this case, absorption of the drug might be more complete than has been believed.

It has been suggested that the greater lipid solubility and lower aqueous solubility of methylphenobarbital, as compared with phenobarbital, would explain its incomplete absorption from the alimentary tract. One wonders whether this suggestion is valid. Methylphenobarbital is not totally insoluble in cold water, and its greater lipid solubility as compared with phenobarbital might easily mean that it is better absorbed than the latter. Work currently in progress in the author's laboratory indicates that a significant proportion of a methylphenobarbital dose in man is accounted for as a previously unmeasured *p*-hydroxyphenyl glucuronide derivative of the drug. Since no parental preparation of methylphenobarbital has been approved for administration to humans, the absolute bioavailability of the orally administered drug cannot be determined at present. However, the information now becoming available and knowledge of the physical properties of the drug both suggest that orally administered methylphenobarbital may be reasonably fully, or fully, bioavailable. A recent study in two volunteers found a 75% bioavailability for the drug (16a).

No quantitative data on the bioavailability of orally administered metharbital have been traced. It has been implied that the drug is likely to be better absorbed than methylphenobarbital because it is more water soluble, but this argument is suspect.

Rate of Absorption

With the exception of data from one patient, it has been impossible to find published information on the absorption rate constants of orally administered methylphenobarbital or metharbital. Eadie et al. (12) carried out single-dose pharmacokinetic studies on orally administered methylphenobarbital in eight human subjects. Unfortunately, in all but one subject, sufficient data points were not obtained on the rising phases of the plasma drug level curves to permit calculation of absorption rate parameters of the drug. In seven of the eight subjects, peak plasma methylphenobarbital levels occurred between 2.5 and 7 hr from the time of dosage and, in the eighth subject, after 26.5 hr. Such T_{max} values are sometimes taken as a measure of absorption rate. However, T_{max} is determined by both absorption and elimination rates, since it is the time when elimination first exceeds absorption after each drug dose. In the one subject in whom the absorption rate constant could be measured, the absorption half-time was comparatively rapid (1.4 hr).

Factors Influencing Absorption

There does not appear to be any published information concerning factors that have been shown to modify the absorption of methylphenobarbital or metharbital in man.

Distribution

Tissue Distribution

The literature does not seem to contain any experimental data on the actual distribution of methylphenobarbital or metharbital in the various tissues and body fluids of humans. Values of the apparent volume of distribution of methylphenobarbital in man (12) and dog (3) prove greater than the volume of total body water. This fact, and the known lipophilicity of the drug, suggest that it may be present in tissues (particularly adipose tissue and brain) at higher concentrations than in plasma. In rats, Craig and Shideman (10) found that brain methylphenobarbital levels were eight times simultaneously measured blood levels of the drug.

Plasma and Tissue Binding

Volume of distribution.
Eadie et al. (12) calculated that the apparent volume of distribution of methylphenobarbital in adults was between 49 and 246 liters (mean, 132 liters). These values depended on the

assumption that the orally administered drug was fully bioavailable. Butler's (3) earlier work in two dogs had provided V_d values of 1.9 and 2.1 liters kg^{-1}, which were reasonably similar to the values obtained in man. In one human subject (12), the V_d of phenobarbital (administered separately on another occasion) was 25.9 liters, whereas the V_d of methylphenobarbital was 246 liters. As mentioned above, these V_d figures suggest that methylphenobarbital appears in tissues at higher concentrations than in plasma.

There do not appear to be human data available for the V_d of metharbital. In the dog, Butler (4) found that the V_d was 1.22 liters kg^{-1}, whereas the V_d of barbital itself was 0.6 liters kg^{-1}.

Plasma protein binding.

There does not seem to be any direct or indirect information available concerning the plasma protein binding of methylphenobarbital or metharbital or on factors influencing the binding.

Elimination

Half-Life

In four subjects not pretreated with other drugs, the half-life of methylphenobarbital after the first dose of this substance was 49.0 ± 18.8 (SD) hr (12). However, in five subjects who had been pretreated with a variety of drugs, mainly anticonvulsants, the elimination half-life of methylphenobarbital was significantly shorter [19.6 ± 5.0 (SD) hr]. The latter five subjects included one member of the first group of four subjects. This patient's only pretreatment comprised the single dose of methylphenobarbital given for the initial pharmacokinetic study. In him, the half-life of methylphenobarbital fell from 35.2 hr in the first study to 18.7 hr in the second study. Since continued methylphenobarbital therapy leads to the formation of considerable amounts of phenobarbital (a known hepatic mixed-oxidase-inducing agent), and since the elimination of methylphenobarbital appears to be almost entirely by means of biotransfor-

mation, it seems likely that continued therapy with the drug would lead to autoinduction of its biotransformation capacity. Thus, in patients on chronic methylphenobarbital therapy, it might be reasonable to anticipate that the drug's half-life would be in the range of 12 to 24 hr.

In general correlation with the elimination rate constant (i.e., the half-life) data, total body clearance of methylphenobarbital averaged 1.85 ± 0.70 (SD) liters hr^{-1} in noninduced subjects and 5.8 ± 2.70 (SD) liters hr^{-1} in the presumptively induced (12). For a drug that is cleared almost exclusively by biotransformation, such clearance values do not suggest very active hepatic metabolism (in which case clearance values of the order of 90–100 liters hr^{-1} might have been obtained).

No data are available for the half-life or clearance of metharbital in man.

Routes of Elimination

Renal.

Maynert and van Dyke (23) stated that no methylphenobarbital was excreted unchanged in urine. In three human subjects, Eadie et al. (12) found that renal excretion of unchanged methylphenobarbital accounted for approximately 1.5 to 3.0% of the dose of drug administered orally. Even accepting that 50 to 60% of the drug is bioavailable, the renal excretion data suggest that methylphenobarbital is cleared from the body almost entirely by biotransformation. In the same three subjects referred to above, approximately 8 to 25% of the dose of methylphenobarbital was excreted in urine as phenobarbital.

In these subjects, the urine may not have been collected long enough to determine the full amount of phenobarbital that was excreted. Studies currently in progress indicate that, at least in the acute single-dose situation in noninduced subjects, *p*-hydroxymethylphenobarbital (1-methyl-5-ethyl-5-*p*-hydroxyphenylbarbituric acid) is a major urinary metabolite of methylphenobarbital. This hydroxy derivative is excreted mainly as its glucuronide conjugate. Small amounts of the *p*-hydroxyphenyl derivative of phenobarbital are found, as are traces of the *m*-hydroxyphenyl isomer of methylphenobarbital. However, this *m*-hydroxy isomer may occur in these circumstances as a methodological artifact.

No detailed studies of the renal mechanisms involved in handling methylphenobarbital are available. From its physical properties, one might anticipate that the drug would be filtered through the renal glomerulus and then resorbed passively as water resorbs during its passage down the renal tubules. The pK_a value of methylphenobarbital is probably high enough for changes in urine pH to have little influence on the extent of its urinary excretion. One might anticipate that *p*-hydroxymethylphenobarbital glucuronide, like other glucuronides, would be actively secreted into proximal tubular urine as well as being filtered from plasma water into the renal glomerulus. Factors influencing the renal handling of phenobarbital itself are discussed in Chapter 22.

There does not appear to be any information available regarding factors involved in the renal handling of metharbital and its metabolite, barbital. It is believed that metharbital is extensively converted to barbital, and the latter is said not to undergo further metabolic transformation (15). In dogs, barbital is filtered through the renal glomerulus and extensively resorbed during the passage of urine down the renal tubules (15). Similar considerations probably apply to man.

Hepatic.

Methylphenobarbital is cleared from the body almost exclusively by biotransformation. In rats, the demethylation of this drug, producing phenobarbital, is known to occur in the liver (6,8,27). It seems likely that the metabolism of the drug in man is also hepatic. It is not known whether disease alters the liver's capacity for biotransformation of the drug.

In the rat, metharbital is oxidatively demethylated in the liver (8,27). The analogous reaction in man is presumed to occur in the liver. No information is available regarding factors in humans that may influence the hepatic handling of the drug.

Other routes of elimination.

It is not known whether methylphenobarbital is excreted from the body in significant quantities in feces or various bodily secretions, e.g., sweat, tears, milk. Whether the drugs or their glucuronide metabolites undergo an enterohepatic circulation is also unknown.

BIOTRANSFORMATION

Chemical Aspects of Metabolism

The fact that methylphenobarbital is biotransformed to phenobarbital has been known since 1939 (5), and this has generally been thought to be the major biotransformation pathway of the drug in man. However, data now becoming available in the author's laboratory suggest that another major biotransformation pathway in man involves aromatic hydroxylation. This conclusion is based on urinary excretion findings in man. If urine from patients taking methylphenobarbital is heated with hydrochloric acid to hydrolyze any glucuronide or sulfate conjugates, both the *meta* and the *para* isomer of 1-methyl-5-ethyl-5-hydroxyphenylbarbituric acid can be identified. However, if the hydrolysis is carried out by incubation with β-glucuronidase, only the *para* isomer is found. By analogy with what happens to the aromatic hydroxylation products of phenytoin, one might infer that a dihydrodiol metabolite forms initially from methylphenobarbital (perhaps via an epoxide), and the dihydrodiol preferentially converts to the *p*-hydroxyphenyl isomer in the human liver. Although the dihydrodiol has not yet been identified in the urine of patients taking methylphenobarbital, high-pressure liquid chromatography of such urine shows an early eluting peak of unknown nature and of significant area. The identity of this peak is currently being studied. If the dihydrodiol is present in urine, acid hydrolysis might be expected to yield both *p*- and *m*-hydroxyphenyl isomers. Therefore, a tentative scheme of methylphenobarbital metabolism in man can be proposed (Fig. 3 and ref. 16b).

As far as can be ascertained, there is no direct evidence of the metabolic fate of metharbital in

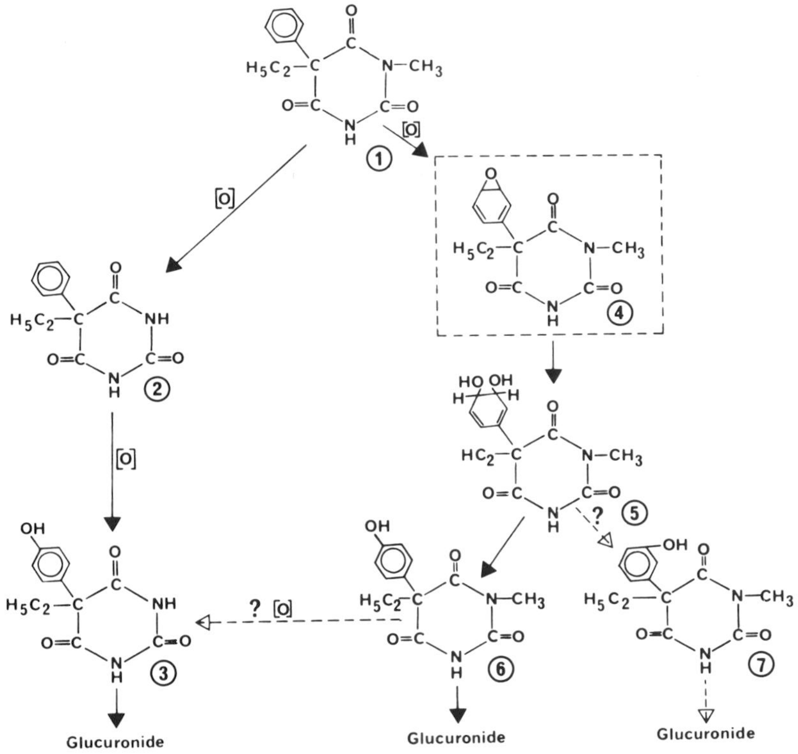

Fig. 3. Tentative scheme of methylphenobarbital biotransformation in man: **1**, methylphenobarbital; **2**, phenobarbital; **3**, *p*-hydroxyphenobarbital; **4**, presumed epoxide metabolite; **5**, dihydrodiol metabolite of methylphenobarbital; **6**, *p*-hydroxymethylphenobarbital; **7**, *m*-hydroxymethylphenobarbital.

man. It is generally assumed that the drug is oxidatively demethylated to barbital, as it is in the dog (4). The latter substance is said to probably undergo no further metabolic degradation (23).

Pharmacological Aspects of Metabolism

Some evidence now becoming available in the studies of Kunze and Hooper in the author's laboratory is consistent with the possibility that oxidative demethylation of methylphenobarbital to phenobarbital tends to increase after prolonged exposure of patients to multiple antiepileptic drugs or to methylphenobarbital itself. At the time of writing the results are incomplete. Although *p*-hydroxymethylphenobarbital may be the major urinary metabolite after the initial dose of methylphenobarbital, in patients receiving chronic anticonvulsant therapy including meth-

ylphenobarbital, phenobarbital is a quantitatively more significant metabolite. It had earlier been noticed (12) that one patient who had taken multiple anticonvulsants over several years excreted almost 25% of an initial methylphenobarbital dose as phenobarbital during the 75-hr period following the dose, whereas two subjects not previously exposed to drugs excreted 8% and 11% of their initial methylphenobarbital doses as phenobarbital in the 200 hr following dosage. Not only was methylphenobarbital cleared faster in patients on chronic anticonvulsant therapy, but in these patients, phenobarbital appeared earlier in the blood and tended to achieve higher peak plasma levels (Fig. 4).

Eadie et al. (12) studied areas under the plasma phenobarbital level–time curves in a patient who, on separate occasions, took his first dose of phenobarbital and his first dose of methylphenobarbital. By this method, it could be calcu-

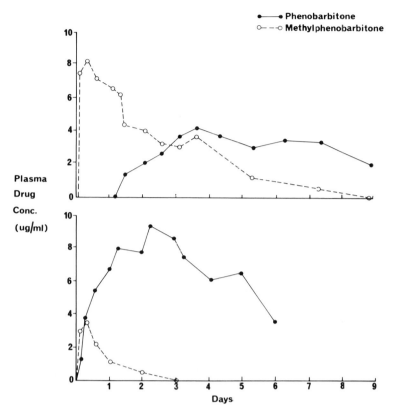

Fig. 4. Time course of plasma concentrations of methylphenobarbital and derived phenobarbital after an initial oral dose of methylphenobarbital in an untreated patient **(top panel)** and in a patient chronically treated with other antiepileptic drugs **(bottom panel)**. (From Eadie et al., ref. 12, with permission.)

lated that 52% of the methylphenobarbital dose was converted to phenobarbital. No metabolic balance studies were carried out to account for the remainder of the dose. This finding agrees very well with the widely accepted 50 to 60% conversion figure that has been derived from more indirect data, but whether it will prove more generally applicable and, in particular, applicable to patients on chronic antiepileptic therapy is uncertain.

Further work should be done to clarify its details, but the biotransformation of methylphenobarbital already appears to be a more complex process than has previously been thought and one that may provide new insights into hepatic microsomal oxidations in man.

No quantitative data on metharbital biotransformation in man are available.

INTERACTIONS WITH OTHER DRUGS

As discussed above, in man, methylphenobarbital is converted to phenobarbital. The latter is more slowly cleared than the former. Therefore, in chronic therapy, plasma phenobarbital levels (but not necessarily tissue levels) come to be almost an order of magnitude higher than plasma methylphenobarbital levels. In man, neither pharmacokinetic data nor results of plasma level monitoring are available to indicate whether similar considerations apply to metharbital. However, it seems not unreasonable to suspect that they may. Because of the presence of biologically active metabolites, unless plasma levels of all the relevant substances are measured, it may be difficult to know whether drug–drug interactions apparently involving methylphenobarbital or metharbital are related to the primary drug, to its metabolite, or to both.

It seems likely that any interaction that has been described for phenobarbital (see Chapter 24) could also occur if methylphenobarbital were the source of phenobarbital. Such interactions will not be dealt with in detail here. Methylphenobarbital itself acts as a central nervous system depressant and sedative. If combined with other drugs with sedative actions, e.g., tricyclic antidepressants, antipsychotics, benzodiazepines, or other hypnotics, it might be anticipated that the overall degree of depression of central nervous system function would be increased.

Methylphenobarbital probably is an anticonvulsant in its own right (see below) as well as by virtue of the phenobarbital it produces. It may have additive antiepileptic effects if combined with other anticonvulsants that are appropriate for the patient's type of seizure. Phenobarbital is a well-known inducer of the hepatic microsomal mixed-oxidase system. Methylphenobarbital might be expected to lead to similar induction by virtue of the phenobarbital to which it is biotransformed, if not by a direct effect.

Eadie et al. (12) carried out a multiple-variable linear-regression analysis of plasma methylphenobarbital and derived phenobarbital levels on methylphenobarbital dose in an attempt to trace interactions in which other anticonvulsants might have altered the body's handling of methylphenobarbital. Phenytoin, carbamazepine, and sulthiame, the three drugs most widely combined with methylphenobarbital in the patients studied, had no statistically significant effects on the two regressions. This failure to detect interactions in a population study does not necessarily mean that interactions do not occur in individual members of the population studied. If an interaction raises plasma drug levels in some patients and lowers them in others, the effects may cancel out to such an extent that mean plasma levels in the population do not change.

This author has not seen instances of pharmacokinetic-type interactions in individual patients taking methylphenobarbital with other antiepileptic drugs except for combinations including valproic acid. On several occasions, the introduction of valproic acid to the therapeutic regimen of a patient taking methylphenobarbital has resulted in a progressive and sustained rise of considerable magnitude in plasma phenobarbital levels and in a lesser rise in plasma methylphenobarbital levels. Such an interaction has been illustrated by Eadie and Tyrer (14). Lander et al. (19) used a multiple-variable linear-regression technique in a population of epileptic patients to see whether interactions could be detected in which methylphenobarbital altered plasma levels of concurrently taken phenytoin and carbamazepine. No such interactions were found.

There appears to be virtually nothing published on the interactions of metharbital.

RELATIONSHIP OF PLASMA CONCENTRATION TO SEIZURE CONTROL

Therapeutic Plasma Concentrations

As discussed above, when methylphenobarbital is taken on a long-term basis, steady-state plasma concentrations of phenobarbital come to exceed plasma methylphenobarbital levels. For practical purposes, it often seems sufficient to use plasma phenobarbital levels as a guide to the therapeutic situation and to ignore plasma methylphenobarbital levels. This is usually possible because the therapeutic range of plasma phenobarbital levels is wide (10–40 μg/ml), and its limits are not sharply demarcated. However, to ignore plasma methylphenobarbital levels is to overlook one active anticonvulsant substance present in the body. Further, the anticonvulsant that is being neglected is one that, because of its high V_d relative to that of phenobarbital and its lipid solubility, probably has substantially higher brain levels relative to plasma levels than has phenobarbital. This author has seen a patient receiving multiple antiepileptic drugs who failed to develop a further increase in plasma phenobarbital level beyond 20 μg/ml when his daily methylphenobarbital dose was increased from 180 to 300 mg, although he became exceedingly drowsy and ataxic. Despite the failure of his plasma phenobarbital level to increase, his plasma methylphenobarbital level rose from 2 to 8 μg/ml. Reduction in methylphenobarbital dose relieved the toxicity.

This patient almost certainly exhibited an unusual saturation of his capacity to demethylate methylphenobarbital. Nevertheless, his case history illustrates the point that methylphenobarbital is not devoid of direct biological effect. It may be sufficient to measure plasma phenobarbital levels to monitor the therapeutic situation in most patients taking methylphenobarbital and to recognize that one may be underestimating the total anticonvulsant activity present. However, the simultaneous specific measurement of methylphenobarbital and phenobarbital levels provides useful, and occasion-

ally critical, additional information. If phenobarbital is measured by a nonspecific assay that measures methylphenobarbital as phenobarbital, confusing information may occasionally be produced.

There does not appear to be any information available regarding plasma metharbital or barbital levels in man, or on the relationship of these levels to therapeutic or toxic effects. Therefore, in the remainder of this chapter, only methylphenobarbital is considered.

Relationship of Dose to Plasma Concentration

Figure 5 shows the linear relationship between simultaneous steady-state plasma concentrations of both methylphenobarbital and derived phenobarbital and methylphenobarbital dose in populations of treated patients (12). Plasma

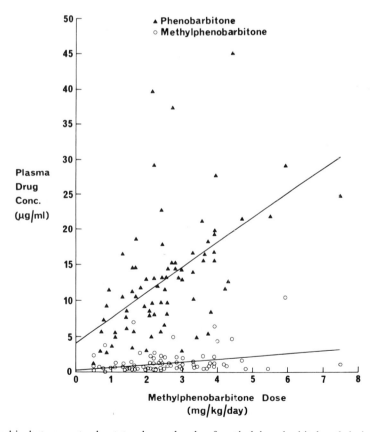

Fig. 5. Relationship between steady-state plasma levels of methylphenobarbital and derived phenobarbital and methylphenobarbital dose in a population of treated epileptic patients. (From Eadie et al., ref. 12, with permission.)

phenobarbital levels correlate more closely with methylphenobarbital dose than do plasma levels of the parent substance. However, the increased relative scatter in methylphenobarbital levels, as compared with the scatter in phenobarbital levels, is likely to have resulted from difficulty in measuring with equal precision plasma concentrations that usually differ by an order of magnitude. The assay used had been arranged to provide optional precision in measuring phenobarbital. Methylphenobarbital doses of 3 to 4 mg/kg per day produced mean plasma phenobarbital levels of 15 μg/ml, and doses of 5 mg/kg per day mean levels of 20 μg/ml.

The relationship between simultaneous plasma phenobarbital and methylphenobarbital levels in the same patients is shown in Fig. 6. Plasma phenobarbital levels tended to be 7 to 10 times those of methylphenobarbital when plasma levels of the former were between 10 and 20 μg/ml, values commonly encountered in treating epilepsy. At higher plasma methylphenobarbital levels, however, there was a tendency for plasma phenobarbital levels to be proportionately less than at lower methylphenobarbital levels. This finding raises the possibility that

the demethylation of methylphenobarbital may tend to be rate limited at the higher values of plasma concentrations of the drug that are encountered therapeutically. Kupferberg and Longacre-Shaw (18), in a small series of patients, found that plasma phenobarbital levels averaged 20 times those of methylphenobarbital.

In addition to knowing the relationships between steady-state plasma methylphenobarbital and phenobarbital levels and methylphenobarbital dose in treated populations, it is desirable to know the steady-state plasma level–dose relationship in treated individuals who have had plasma levels measured while receiving different methylphenobarbital doses at different times. As shown in Fig. 7, at least for plasma phenobarbital levels up to 30 μg/ml, the relationship between plasma phenobarbital level and methylphenobarbital dose usually appears linear (13). The relationship between methylphenobarbital plasma level and dose also appears linear (11). It should be noted that when phenobarbital itself is taken, the relationship between steady-state plasma phenobarbital level and phenobarbital dose is curvilinear (13). This difference in the

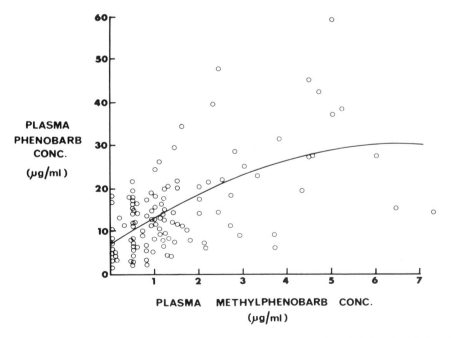

Fig. 6. Relationship between simultaneous steady-state plasma levels of methylphenobarbital and derived phenobarbital in treated patients. (From Eadie et al., ref. 12, with permission.)

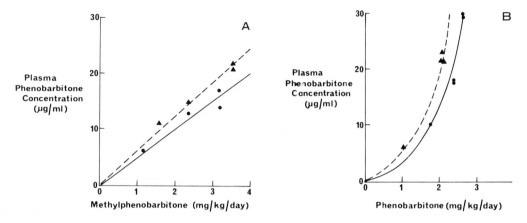

Fig. 7. Relationship between steady-state plasma level of phenobarbital and methylphenobarbital dose (**A**) and between steady-state plasma phenobarbital level and phenobarbital dose (**B**), each in two subjects who took different doses of the drugs at different times. (From Eadie et al., ref. 13, with permission.)

behavior of plasma phenobarbital levels when the drug is supplied directly or indirectly via methylphenobarbital suggests that it may be easier to manipulate plasma phenobarbital levels when using methylphenobarbital than when using phenobarbital itself.

Population studies (13) have shown that the regression for plasma phenobarbital level on drug dose changes with age. The effect of this change is such that the methylphenobarbital dose required to produce a given plasma phenobarbital level tends to decrease with age if doses are expressed relative to body weight. Thus, to achieve a plasma phenobarbital level of 15 µg/ml, a person under 15 years requires a mean daily dose of 4 mg/kg, and a person over 40 years a mean daily dose of 2 mg/kg. Regression analysis shows that the patient's sex also influences the relationship between plasma phenobarbital level and methylphenobarbital dose. For a given methylphenobarbital dose (corrected for body weight), males tend to have average plasma phenobarbital levels 5 µg/ml higher than females.

Relationship of Plasma Concentrations to Therapeutic Effect

It has already been mentioned that it is preferable to measure simultaneous plasma levels of both methylphenobarbital and phenobarbital in patients receiving methylphenobarbital. There is no information available on the therapeutic range of plasma methylphenobarbital levels. It seems that the conventional therapeutic range of plasma phenobarbital levels (15–30 or 10–40 µg/ml) usually proves a reasonable guide to the antiepileptic effects of methylphenobarbital, although it does tend to underestimate the total antiepileptic activity present.

Toxic Effects Related to Plasma Concentrations

As with anticonvulsant effects, toxic effects of methylphenobarbital tend to correlate reasonably well with plasma phenobarbital levels. Since plasma phenobarbital levels tend to parallel plasma methylphenobarbital levels, the latter are also likely to correlate with toxic effects. Toxic effects of phenobarbital (apart from idiosyncratic reactions) are mostly consequences of the central nervous depressant effects of the drug. In some individuals, such effects may appear with plasma phenobarbital levels as low as 10 to 15 µg/ml, particularly if these levels are achieved early in the course of therapy. Many patients, however, show no clinically obvious depression of nervous system functions at plasma phenobarbital levels well in excess of 40 µg/ml, particularly when these levels have been achieved slowly.

One has the impression that true pharmacological tolerance to phenobarbital, as distinct from time-related autoinduction of phenobarbital elimination, does occur, although no absolute proof of this phenomenon exists. Such tolerance would, however, explain some of the difficulty in designating any sharp toxicity threshold for phenobarbital. It is, of course, possible, and indeed likely, that refined tests of psychological function may detect a progressive impairment of performance that correlates with rising plasma levels of phenobarbital and methylphenobarbital, even though there may be no sharp toxicity threshold. Such a phenomenon has been shown to exist in the case of orally administered phenobarbital itself (26).

As mentioned above, the demethylation of methylphenobarbital may occasionally become saturated under clinical conditions. In these circumstances, significant central nervous system depression may occur at plasma phenobarbital concentrations that would usually be regarded as nontoxic but at plasma methylphenobarbital levels above perhaps 5 or 6 μg/ml.

Tolerance

The possibility of a true pharmacological tolerance developing to the effects of phenobarbital has been discussed above when we considered the determination of a therapeutic range for both phenobarbital and methylphenobarbital. Sufficient information is not yet available to determine whether a "pseudotolerance" to the effects of methylphenobarbital develops because of a time-related change in its pharmacokinetic parameters. In patients who have been on long-term therapy, methylphenobarbital clearance appears to be increased, with more of the drug being converted to phenobarbital. Thus, the effects of any "pseudotolerance" resulting from more rapid elimination of methylphenobarbital may be counterbalanced by increased concentrations of phenobarbital derived from the parent substance.

Dependence

There are reports in the psychiatric literature of dependence developing to various barbiturates, particularly in the elderly. However, there do not appear to be well-corroborated reports of dependence on methylphenobarbital or metharbital.

Pharmacological Aspects of Clinical Use

Time to Steady-State Plasma Levels

For a drug eliminated by processes following exponential kinetics, a clinically adequate approximation to a steady state is achieved after the lapse of four or five terminal elimination half-lives. Therefore, plasma levels of methylphenobarbital ($T_{1/2}$ = 2 days) should attain steady-state values some 8 to 10 days after the commencement of therapy or after the most recent dosage change. However, if autoinduction of biotransformation occurs, or if the patient's drug-metabolizing oxidative enzymes are already induced by prior exposure to other anticonvulsants, the steady state for methylphenobarbital may be achieved earlier, perhaps in as little as 4 days. From the clinical point of view, however, the plateau pharmacological effect of methylphenobarbital is determined by the time to achieve steady-state plasma levels of the phenobarbital derived from it. This substance has an elimination half-life of 3 to 4 days, and, therefore, its steady state is likely to take some 2 to 3 weeks to develop, or perhaps longer if one allows for delay in the rate of production of phenobarbital to stabilize should autoinduction of methylphenobarbital and phenobarbital biotransformation occur.

There is also a practical consideration that may determine when a plateau therapeutic state applies after methylphenobarbital therapy is commenced. If doses of the drug that is calculated likely to produce a midtherapeutic steady-state plasma level are introduced as soon as therapy is started, patients often complain of such drowsiness that they are reluctant to continue therapy. If half, or lower than half, doses are used for the first 1 or 2 weeks, this problem is usually obviated. However, there is a corresponding delay in achieving steady-state therapeutic plasma levels of derived phenobarbital.

Variation in Steady-State Plasma Levels

In view of the relatively slow elimination of both methylphenobarbital and phenobarbital, steady-state plasma levels of both primary drug and metabolite would be expected to show relatively little fluctuation over 12-hr or even 24-hr dosage intervals. This expectation is borne out in practice, as illustrated by Eadie and Tyrer (14).

Metabolism During Pregnancy

Alterations in plasma levels during pregnancy.

Lander et al. (20) showed that in women taking constant daily methylphenobarbital doses, plasma phenobarbital levels tended to fall during the course of pregnancy and to rise again in the puerperium. The mechanisms involved in this phenomenon have not yet been determined.

Teratogenesis.

It is not known whether methylphenobarbital and metharbital are teratogens in man. The evidence as to whether derived phenobarbital is a teratogen is considered in Chapter 26.

Breast milk.

It has been reported (9) that methylphenobarbital could not be found in breast milk of women taking the drug. This finding is somewhat surprising, but perhaps the assay used was not sufficiently sensitive. Phenobarbital, administered as such, also was reportedly not found in milk.

Relationship of Dose to Plasma Concentration: Interpretation

Dose Required to Achieve a Given Plasma Concentration

Loading dose.

There does not appear to be any published information on loading doses of methylphenobarbital that have proved satisfactory in practice. Although the drug is almost certainly an anticonvulsant in its own right, its therapeutic range of plasma levels when it acts as the sole antiepileptic substance present is unknown. Therefore, one has no basis on which to predict a suitable loading dose. If one aimed to attain a plasma phenobarbital level of 15 µg/ml (a reasonable initial therapeutic level), the data shown in Fig. 5 suggest that a daily methylphenobarbital dose of 3 mg/kg would suffice. However, it would take so many days for the phenobarbital to form from methylphenobarbital and achieve something approaching steady-state conditions that there seems little point in considering the question of a loading dose determined on this basis.

It seems likely that a loading dose of methylphenobarbital that would have an adequate anticonvulsant effect within a few hours could be determined empirically. However, this dose would probably make the patient very drowsy. The drowsiness might persist for several days if the usual proportion of the methylphenobarbital dose were converted to phenobarbital. By virtue of its properties and its handling by the human body, methylphenobarbital is better suited to long-term use than to acute use.

Oral therapy.

The data of Eadie et al. (13) suggest that to produce therapeutic plasma phenobarbital levels of 15 µg/ml, children require an average methylphenobarbital dose of 5 mg/kg per day, young adults an average dose of 4 mg/kg per day, and adults over 40 years of age an average dose of 2 mg/kg per day. Slightly higher doses might be used in females than in males. As mentioned above, the use of half the calculated daily methylphenobarbital dose for the first week of therapy reduces the incidence of early drowsiness, although it delays the achieving of a therapeutic effect.

When Plasma Concentrations Are Too High

When plasma concentrations of either methylphenobarbital or phenobarbital are too high, patients experience drowsiness and mental slowing. Some become irritable or depressed. Ataxia of gait, slowed speech, and nystagmus may occur.

When Plasma Concentrations Are Too Low

Subtherapeutic plasma levels of methylphenobarbital and derived phenobarbital (levels of the latter below 10 μg/ml) are likely to be associated with failure to control the types of epilepsy that might be expected to respond to the drug.

Guidelines to Dosage Adjustment

Methylphenobarbital dose may need adjustment in at least three circumstances:

1. When plasma phenobarbital levels are subtherapeutic, and the patient has a type of epilepsy in which seizures occur only at long intervals, so that it is reasonable to anticipate that the methylphenobarbital dose will ultimately prove inadequate.
2. Irrespective of plasma methylphenobarbital and phenobarbital levels, if epilepsy continues and the patient is free from toxic manifestations.
3. Irrespective of plasma methylphenobarbital and phenobarbital levels if the patient has toxic manifestations that are a greater disadvantage than the epilepsy.

In adjusting methylphenobarbital doses, at least so long as plasma phenobarbital levels are in or below the therapeutic range, changes in the plasma phenobarbital level in the individual usually occur in direct proportion to methylphenobarbital dose. Therefore, so long as the steady-state plasma phenobarbital level is known at one methylphenobarbital dose, proportionate dose changes are likely to produce proportionate changes in plasma phenobarbital levels. It is this property of methylphenobarbital that confers on it a significant advantage over phenobarbital. When phenobarbital is used, and its dose is increased, plasma phenobarbital levels tend to increase disproportionately, with consequent risk of overdosage manifestations. After the methylphenobarbital dose is al-

tered, the passage of some 2 or 3 weeks may be required for new steady-state plasma phenobarbital levels to be achieved. Earlier plasma level monitoring may provide results that are not valid for interpreting the continuing clinical situation. Making further dosage adjustments within this 2- to 3-week period risks the development of a confused therapeutic situation.

Methylphenobarbital is cleared chiefly by the liver rather than by the kidneys, and its clearance is limited by hepatic metabolic capacity rather than by hepatic blood flow. The derived phenobarbital undergoes significant renal clearance. Methylphenobarbital dosages are unlikely to need much adjustment in cardiac failure. However, dosages may need to be reduced if liver cell or renal function deteriorates.

Synergism

The possibility of synergism between methylphenobarbital and other antiepileptic drugs was mentioned in the discussion of drug–drug interactions above. Clinicians generally accept the fact that additive antiepileptic effects occur if two appropriate anticonvulsants are combined, although it is often difficult to obtain rigid proof of the phenomenon. It is even more difficult to prove that true synergism occurs in these circumstances.

It is, of course, irrational to combine methylphenobarbital with phenobarbital or primidone. Such combinations are tantamount to raising methylphenobarbital doses in a pharmacokinetically complicated way.

TOXICITY

It is difficult to make firm statements about the direct toxicity of methylphenobarbital or metharbital in man, since both drugs form biologically active metabolites. The toxic manifestations of phenobarbital are described in Chapter 26, and the account will not be repeated here. There seems to be no *a priori* reason why any of the known toxic manifestations of phenobarbital should not occur in patients taking methylphenobarbital. In practice, most of the toxic effects seen in patients taking methylphenobarbital involve depression of central nervous system function usually manifested as drowsiness, intellectual blunting, decreased concentration, and irritability. As mentioned above, such symptoms may be direct toxic effects of methylphenobarbital itself as well as consequences of the presence of excess phenobarbital. Metharbital (and probably the barbital to which it is converted) may also produce similar manifestations of central nervous system depression. There do not appear to be any characteristic toxic effects of any particular one of these four barbiturate anticonvulsants.

PHARMACODYNAMICS

As with so many aspects of the clinical pharmacology of the methylated barbiturate anticonvulsants, interpretation of studies of the pharmacodynamics of these drugs is often ambiguous, since investigators have usually not determined whether biotransformation has produced the demethylated congener of the drug in the experimental system used. The clearest investigation is that of Craig and Shideman (10) who showed that, after single doses of methylphenobarbital in rats, immediate protection against maximal electroshock seizures correlated better with brain levels of methylphenobarbital than with levels of phenobarbital.

Other studies have demonstrated anticonvulsant effects of methylphenobarbital and metharbital in various experimental preparations, although in such investigations, phenobarbital or barbital may have had a significant effect. Reinhard and Reinhard (25) tabulated the results of a number of studies in which methylphenobarbital appeared to protect against maximal electroshock seizures in the mouse, rat, and cat and against minimal electroshock seizures and pentylenetetrazol seizures in the mouse and rat. Metharbital has appeared to protect against both maximal electroshock and pentylenetetrazol seizures in the mouse (29).

There does not appear to have been any study of the actions of methylphenobarbital or metharbital in any experimental system of lesser complexity than that of the whole experimental animal. The drugs do not appear to have been studied by modern cellular electrophysiological or neurochemical techniques.

Details of the pharmacodynamics of phenobarbital are provided in Chapter 27 and elsewhere (14) and will not be considered here.

THERAPEUTIC USE

Methylphenobarbital (with the phenobarbital derived from it) appears to be a reasonably broad-spectrum anticonvulsant. It is useful in all types of partial epilepsy and in generalized epilepsy manifesting as convulsive seizures (including benign febrile convulsions of infancy) or as myoclonic attacks in adolescence or adult life. The drug does not appear to be sufficiently potent to control the more active types of myoclonic epilepsy that develop in earlier life, and it is not effective in absence (petit mal) seizures. The drug's relatively long half-life and the longer half-life of the derived phenobarbital make methylphenobarbital suitable for once- or twice-daily administration in chronic therapy. At the same time, the long half-life of phenobarbital means that there is a 2- or 3-week delay before any dosage change produces its maximal effects. Therefore, dosage adjustments usually should not be made more frequently than this.

Methylphenobarbital is thus suited to long-term therapeutic purposes and unhurried dosage manipulations, but it is less suited to clinical situations that require rapid anticonvulsant effects. Methylphenobarbital possesses the advantage that, with the exception of valproic acid, none of the other antiepileptic drugs in common use affects its plasma levels or those of the phenobarbital derived from it.

Metharbital appears to have been little used as an antiepileptic drug in recent times. Both its spectrum of activity against different types of epilepsy and its relative efficacy compared with other antiepileptic drugs are unknown.

CONCLUSIONS

Methylphenobarbital has often been regarded merely as a prodrug for phenobarbital with the disadvantages of being more expensive and less reliably absorbed after oral administration.

Pharmacokinetic and clinical pharmacological data now becoming available suggest that methylphenobarbital may be reasonably well absorbed, that it may enter the brain more readily than phenobarbital and there exert a useful anticonvulsant effect, and that it has the peculiar advantage over phenobarbital of producing plasma phenobarbital levels that vary in a simple linear fashion with drug dose. Despite the price disadvantage (which is not substantial), some might now regard methylphenobarbital as a rather advantageous way of providing phenobarbital for patients.

Little is known of metharbital. Whether it has a real role as an antiepileptic drug in contemporary practice is debatable.

ACKNOWLEDGMENTS

The writer wishes to thank Drs. W. D. Hooper and H. Kunze for providing data from their as yet unpublished studies on methylphenobarbital metabolism in man and for reviewing this manuscript. He is grateful to the editors and copyright owners of the *British Journal of Clinical Pharmacology* and *Clinical and Experimental Neurology* for permission to reproduce Figs. 4–7 from his previously published work.

CONVERSION

Methylphenobarbital

Conversion factor:

$$CF = \frac{1000}{mol.\ wt.} = \frac{1000}{246.3} = 4.06$$

Conversion:

$$(\mu g/ml) \times 4.06 = (\mu moles/liter)$$

$$(\mu moles/liter) \div 4.06 = (\mu g/ml)$$

Metharbital

Conversion factor:

$$CF = \frac{1000}{mol.\ wt.} = \frac{1000}{198.4} = 5.04$$

Conversion:

$$(\mu g/ml) \times 5.04 = (\mu moles/liter)$$

$$(\mu moles/liter) \div 5.04 = (\mu g/ml)$$

Barbital

Conversion factor:

$$CF = \frac{1000}{mol.\ wt.} = \frac{1000}{184.2} = 5.43$$

Conversion:

$$(\mu g/m) \times 5.43 = (\mu moles/liter)$$

$$(\mu moles/liter) \div 5.43 = (\mu g/ml)$$

REFERENCES

1. Blum, E. (1932): Die Bekampfung epileptischer Anfalle und iher Folgeer scheinungen mit Prominal. *Dtsch. Med. Wochenschr.*, 58:230–236.
2. Bush, M. T., and Sanders-Bush, E. (1972): Phenobarbital, mephobarbital and metharbital and their metabolites: Chemistry and methods for determination. In. *Antiepileptic Drugs,* edited by D. M. Woodbury, J. K. Penry, and R. P. Schmidt, pp. 293–302. Raven Press, New York.
3. Butler, T. C. (1952): Quantitation studies of the metabolic fate of mephobarbital (N-methylphenobarbital). *J. Pharmacol. Exp. Ther.*, 106:235–245.
4. Butler, T. C. (1953): Quantitative studies of the demethylation of N-methyl barbital (metharbital, Gemonil). *J. Pharmacol. Exp. Ther.*, 108:474–480.
5. Butler, T. C., and Bush, M. T. (1939): The metabolic fate of N-methylphenobarbituric acids. *J. Pharmacol. Exp. Ther.*, 65:205–213.
6. Butler, T. C., Mahaffee, D., and Mahaffee, C. (1952): The role of the liver in the metabolic disposition of mephabarbital. *J. Pharmacol. Exp. Ther.*, 106:364–369.
7. Butler, T. C., and Waddell, W. J. (1958): N-Methylated derivatives of barbituric acids, hydantoin and oxazolidine used in the treatment of epilepsy. *Neurology (Minneap.)*, 8(Suppl. 1):106–112.
8. Butler, T. C., Waddell, W. J., and Poole, D. T. (1965): Demethylation of trimethadione and metharbital by rat liver microsomal enzymes: Substrate concentration—yield relationships and competition between substrates. *Biochem. Pharmacol.*, 14:937–942.
9. Coradello, H. (1973): Ueber die Ausscheidung von Antiepileptika in die Muttermilch. *Wien. Klin. Wochenschr.*, 85:695–697.
10. Craig, C. R., and Shideman, F. E. (1971): Metabolism and anticonvulsant properties of mephobarbital and phenobarbital in rats. *J. Pharmacol. Exp. Ther.*, 176:35–41.

11. Eadie, M. J. (1976): Plasma level monitoring of anticonvulsants. *Clin. Pharmacokinet.*, 1:52–66.

12. Eadie, M. J., Bochner, F., Hooper, W. D., and Tyrer, J. H. (1978): Preliminary observations on the pharmacokinetics of methylphenobarbitone. *Clin. Exp. Neurol.*, 15:131–144.

13. Eadie, M. J., Lander, C. M., Hooper, W. D., and Tyrer, J. H. (1977): Factors influencing plasma phenobarbitone levels in epileptic patients. *Br. J. Clin. Pharmacol.*, 4:541–547.

14. Eadie, M. J., and Tyrer, J. H. (1980): *Anticonvulsant Therapy. Pharmacological Basis and Practice*, Second Edition. Churchill-Livingstone, London, Edinburgh, New York.

15. Giotti, A., and Maynert, E. W. (1951): The renal clearance of barbital and the mechanism of its reabsorption. *J. Pharmacol. Exp. Ther.*, 101:296–309.

16. Hooper, W. D., Dubetz, D. K., Eadie, M. J., and Tyrer, J. H. (1975): Simultaneous assay of methylphenobarbitone and phenobarbitone using gas–liquid chromatography with on-column butylation. *J. Chromatogr.*, 110:206–209.

16a. Hooper, W. D., Kunze, H. E., and Eadie, M. J. (1981): Pharmacokinetics and bioavailability of methylphenobarbital in man. *Ther. Drug Monitor.*, 3:39–44.

16b. Hooper, W. D., Kunze, H. E., and Eadie, M. J. (1981): Qualitative and quantitative studies of methylphenobarbital metabolism in man. *Drug Metab. Dispos.*, 9:381–385.

17. Huisman, J. W. (1966): The estimation of some important anticonvulsant drugs in serum. *Clin. Chim. Acta.*, 13:323–328.

18. Kupferberg, H. J., and Longacre-Shaw, J. (1979): Mephobarbital and phenobarbital plasma concentrations in epileptic patients treated with mephobarbital. *Ther. Drug Monitor.*, 1:117–122.

19. Lander, C. M., Eadie, M. J., and Tyrer, J. H. (1975): Interactions between anticonvulsants. *Proc. Aust. Assoc. Neurol.*, 12:111–116.

20. Lander, C. M., Edwards, V. E., Eadie, M. J., and Tyrer, J. H. (1977): Plasma anticonvulsant concentrations during pregnancy. *Neurology (Minneap.)*, 27:128–131.

21. MacGee, J. (1971): Rapid identification and quantitation of barbiturates and glutethimide in blood by gas–liquid chromatography. *Clin. Chem.*, 17:587–591.

22. Maynert, E. W. (1972): Phenobarbital, mephobarbital, and metharbital: Absorption, distribution and excretion. In: *Antiepileptic Drugs*, edited by D. M. Woodbury, J. K. Penry, and R. P. Schmidt, pp. 303–310. Raven Press, New York.

23. Maynert, E. W., and van Dyke, H. B. (1949): The metabolism of barbiturates. *Pharmacol. Rev.*, 1:217–242.

24. Peterman, M. G. (1948): Epilepsy in childhood: Newer methods of diagnosis and treatment. *J.A.M.A.*, 138:1012–1019.

25. Reinhard, J. F., and Reinhard, J. F., Jr. (1977): Experimental evaluation of anticonvulsants. In: *Anticonvulsants*, edited by J. A. Vida, pp. 57–111. Academic Press, New York.

26. Reynolds, E. H., and Travers, R. D. (1974): Serum anticonvulsant concentrations in epileptic patients with mental symptoms. A preliminary report. *Br. J. Psychiatry*, 124:440–445.

27. Smith, J. A., Waddell, W. J., and Butler, T. C. (1963): Demethylation of *N*-methyl derivatives of barbituric acid, hydantoin and 2,4-oxazolidinedione by rat liver microsomes. *Life Sci.*, 7:486–492.

28. Vida, J. A., and Gerry, E. H. (1977): Cyclic ureides. In: *Anticonvulsants*, edited by J. A. Vida, pp. 151–291. Academic Press, New York.

29. Vida, J. A., Hooker, M. L., Samour, C. M., and Reinhard, J. F. (1973): Anticonvulsants. 4. Metharbital and phenobarbital derivatives. *J. Med. Chem.*, 16:1378–1381.

Antiepileptic Drugs, edited by D. M. Woodbury, J. K. Penry, and C. E. Pippenger. Raven Press, New York © 1982.

29

Primidone

Chemistry and Methods of Determination

Helmut R. Schäfer

Primidone (PRM) is an important anticonvulsant used for the treatment of generalized tonic–clonic seizures and partial seizures with complex symptomatology. The pharmacological profile of PRM was first described by Bogue and Carrington (6). In man, PRM is mainly metabolized to phenylethylmalonamide (PEMA) and phenobarbital (PB) as shown in Fig. 1. Therefore, in the course of antiepileptic therapy with PRM, PEMA and PB will also be present in any body fluid. Consequently, each treatment with PRM will be a simultaneous treatment with PEMA and PB. This chapter emphasizes the chemistry and analytical aspects of PRM and PEMA. The chemical and analytical behavior of the metabolite PB will be covered in Chapter 21.

CHEMISTRY

Primidone

Primidone is 5-ethyldihydro-5-phenyl-4,6 [1H,5H]-pyrimidinedione (C.A. registry number 125-33-7), $C_{12}H_{14}N_2O_2$, and has a molecular weight of 218.25. It is a nonhygroscopic, colorless, crystalline powder with a slightly bitter taste; its melting point is 286 to 287°C, and it can be crystallized from acetone (2).

Crystal structure analysis of PRM, which shows a certain steric similarity between PRM and PB, was performed by Yeates and Palmer (68). Differences were shown in the pyrimidine parts of the molecule: the dioxopyrimidine ring of PRM is fixed in a flat boat conformation,

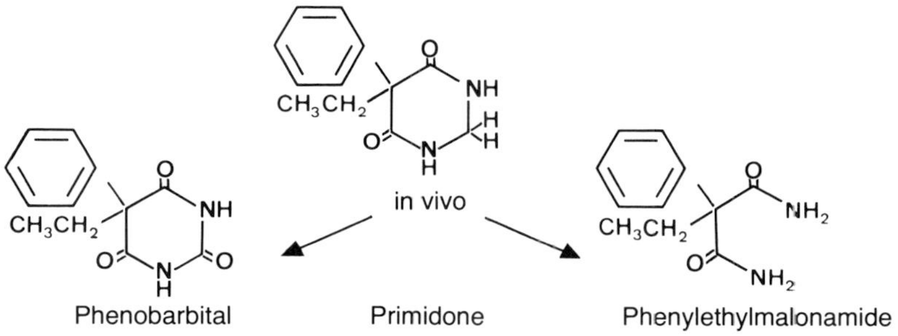

FIG. 1. Structural formulas of primidone and its main metabolites, phenylethylmalonamide and phenobarbital.

TABLE 1. *Solubility and stability of PRM, PB, and PEMA in aqueous solutions*

	Solubility (mg/liter) in				% Stability of 50 mg/liter 0.5 N NaOH after	
	H_2O (37°)	H_2O (20°)	Serum (37°)	1 N NaOH (20°)	1 hr	24 hr
PRM	0.6	0.4	0.7	4.6	100	100
PB	1.8	—[a]	—[a]	—[a]	100	79
PEMA	4.1	1.6	3.8	1.4	100	100

[a]Not determined.

whereas the trioxopyrimidine part of PB is rather planar. The fixed flat boat conformation of PRM may be the basis of its weak acidic properties: from UV data we assume that PRM has a pK_a of approximately 13.

The approximate solubility of PRM is as follows: in methanol and ethanol (95%), about 6 mg/liter; in acetone, 2 mg/liter; in chloroform, ether, and benzene, ≤ 0.1 mg/liter (13). The solubility of PRM in aqueous mixtures is shown in Table 1. As a weakly acidic cyclic amide, PRM is better soluble in 1 N NaOH than in water of pH 6.5.

The dipole moment of PRM was found to be 1.03 (67), whereas that of PB was measured as 0.73. The higher polarity of PRM (and PEMA) results in distinctly lower partition coefficients, k ($c_{lipophil}/c_{hydrophil}$), of PRM compared with that of PB (Table 2). Goedhart et al. (23), using [^{14}C]-PRM and [^{14}C]-PB (New England Nuclear, Boston, Mass.), found high partition coefficients for PRM and PB at pH 7.4 of the aqueous phase in ethyl acetate (PRM, 3.30; PB, 52.0) and lower coefficients in chloroform (PRM, 0.603; PB, 2.25) and in toluene (PRM, 0.06;

PB, 0.552). The highest partition coefficients of more than 400 were found in the system acetone/ammonium sulfate-saturated water at pH 6.6. Further values given by Alvin and Bush (2), and Schäfer (50) demonstrated that previous knowledge of these data is indispensable in developing convenient extraction procedures suitable especially for PRM and PEMA.

The UV absorption spectrum of PRM shows maxima at 264, 258, and 252 nm when scanned in a rather high concentration of about 50 mg/100 ml methanol. There are no other maxima above 210 nm (13). The IR spectrum of PRM was compared with that of PB (8). Infrared spectra of two crystal forms of PRM as mineral oil mulls between KBr plates (13) and the NMR spectrum of PRM with characteristic resonances at 3.96 and 4.12 ppm (caused by the fragment -NH-CH$_2$-NH-) are discussed by Daley (13). Mass spectra of PRM are covered in several reports (2,13,24,29,30,56). Mass spectra of PRM and 5-^{2}H$_5$-PRM recorded in the chemical ionization (CI) mode using isobutane at 65 to 133 Pa (0.5 to 1.0 torr) show the peaks of the protonated molecular ions (56). Bourgeois et al.

TABLE 2. *Partition coefficients[a] of PRM, PB, and PEMA (10 mg/liter each) in five systems*

	A[b]	B	C	D	E
PRM	2.90	2.05	0.68	0.71	<0.03
PB	49.80	10.01	2.72	2.05	<0.01
PEMA	1.004	0.822	0.64	0.64	0.17

[a]Partition coefficient = $C_{lipophilic}/C_{hydrophilic}$.
[b]Systems used: A, ethyl acetate–chloroform (210 : 40, v : v)/0.25 N HCl; B, ethyl acetate–chloroform (210 : 40, v : v)/phosphate buffer (pH 5.2); C, chloroform/phosphate buffer (pH 5.2); D, chloroform/phosphate buffer (pH 7.1); E, chloroform/1 N NaOH.

(9) discussed the electron impact (EI) mass spectra of PRM with its base peak of m/e 146 ($C_{10}H_{10}O$), which can also be observed as a minor peak during the fragmentation of PB.

Synthesis

Synthetic routes for preparation of PRM are (a) ring closure of PEMA with formamide/formic acid at 190°C (7,19) and (b) hydrogenolysis of 2-imino-(or cyanimino-)phenobarbital or of 2-thiophenobarbital with Raney nickel (7), Zn and formic acid (7), or Zn and hydrochloric acid (2,7). We believe that hydrogenolysis of 2-thiophenobarbital or its homologs with Zn and hydrochloric acid is the most convenient method of preparing PRM or its derivatives for use as internal standards (17,50) in the laboratory.

Phenylethylmalonamide

Phenylethylmalonamide is 2-ethyl-2-phenyl propandiamide (C.A. registry number 7206-76-0), $C_{11}H_{14}N_2O_2$, and has a molecular weight of 206.24. It is a colorless crystalline powder with a bitter taste, melting point 117 to 118°C, and can be crystallized from methanol/water. These crystals, dried at 50°C and 2,600 Pa (approximately 20 torr), contain about 6% crystal H_2O. Phenylethylmalonamide behaves as a nonacidic compound. Its solubility in ethanol (95%) is 125 mg/liter and in chloroform is 18 mg/liter which is greater than that of PRM. Solubilities and partition coefficients are given in Tables 1 and 2. Spectral data are available for UV (44), IR (44), NMR (44), and mass spectra (24, 29,44).

Synthesis

Phenylethylmalonamide may be synthesized from diethylphenylethylmalonate, formamide, and sodium methoxide (2). We prefer to prepare PEMA by hydrolysis of phenylethylcyanacetamide with sulfuric acid (98%). Dudley et al. (19) specified an interesting possibility for preparing PEMA and its homolog p-methyl-PEMA via the hydrogenolysis of a 4,4-disubstituted pyrazolidine-3,5-dione.

METHODS OF DETERMINATION

Procedures for the determination of PRM, PB, and other anticonvulsants partially including PEMA have been reviewed by Bente (5), Cook et al. (11), Darcey et al. (14), Gallagher and Baumel (21), Gudzinowicz and Gudzinowicz (24), Hawk and Franconi (26), Kupferberg (33), Rambeck (45), and Vogt (60). Experimental details for the gas–liquid chromatographic (GLC) determination of PRM and PB with and without on-column methylation have been given in the volume edited by Pippenger et al. (43). In this chapter we shall summarize the possibilities of quantitating PRM or PEMA, or PRM, PEMA, and PB simultaneously in body fluids and the problems concerning their determinations. Chapter 21 covers the determination procedures of PB and its metabolite p-OH-PB.

As mentioned above, one must bear in mind the content of PEMA and PB as well as PRM in body fluids when determinations of PRM are performed during treatment with this drug. This means that each method has to be specific enough to avoid any interferences among the three drugs or their metabolites. Thus, PB and PEMA were barely resolved as underivatized drugs during GLC on an OV-17 column (27). Soldin and Hill (52), however, confirmed that PRM and PEMA were not resolved by the high-performance liquid chromatographic (HPLC) method previously used.

Dijkhuis et al. (16) demonstrated that only GLC, the enzyme immunoassay EMIT®, and HPLC were the usual methods for determination of PRM used by the participants of a joint international quality control program. These methods should be discussed and judged in view of their results. In general, GLC and HPLC produce good values. The EMIT® assay also gives good results, although values were too high at subtherapeutic PRM concentrations. Pippenger et al. (42), discussing results of an antiepileptic drug level quality control program for the improvement of laboratory performance, reported that a coefficient of variation of 45% was obtained in PRM determinations of 202 laboratories. These findings clearly demonstrate that there are not only problems with the accuracy of the laboratory performance but also problems in optimizing specific determination methods.

Chromatography

Gas–Liquid Chromatography

Pippenger and Gillen (41) first described a gas–liquid chromatographic (GLC) method for simultaneous determination of free PRM, PEMA, and PB. In today's view, their results seem to be unsatisfactory. At that time, however, highly efficient columns were not available. This led to interactions between the rather polar PRM and a polar support or the liquid phase. On less polar columns, free PRM, PEMA, and PB were inadequately resolved from each other and from other drugs. Thus, on an OV-17 column, PB and PEMA were hardly separated, just as PRM and carbamazepine (CBZ) (25,49) were unsatisfactorily resolved. Therefore, derivatives of PRM, PEMA, and PB were made to decrease their polarity and to increase their volatility, resulting in sharp peaks with little or no tailing.

Determination with derivatization.

On-column or flash-heater methylation is still the most widely used derivatization technique for the routine determination of antiepileptic drugs, including PRM and PB. The drugs or metabolites being extracted from body fluids are dissolved in methanolic tetramethylammonium hydroxide (TMAH) or trimethylphenylammonium hydroxide (TMPAH) solutions. Within the high temperature of the injection port of the gas chromatograph, a rapid Hoffmann degradation reaction proceeds, yielding nearly quantitatively N,N'-dimethyl-PRM and N,N'-dimethyl-PB, for instance. Because of their instability in strong alkaline solutions such as TMAH or TMPAH, decomposition products are formed. The main decomposition product of PB is N-methyl-2-phenylbutyramide, which has a high probability of also being the on-column methylation product of PEMA. During flash-heater methylation, PRM yields about 5% of a decom-

position product, the structure of which we found not to be identical with PEMA, N,N'-dimethyl-PEMA, or N-methyl-2-phenylbutyramide. The amounts of N-methyl-2-phenylbutyramide formed during flash-heater methylation of PB are related directly to the concentration of TMAH or TMPAH and to the length of time the drug is in contact with the base prior to injection into the column.

In order to overcome this problem, the use of p-methyl-PRM and p-methyl-PB as suitable internal standards has been shown to be an important improvement (17,18). These compounds are similar in structure to PRM and PB, respectively, and therefore undergo similar decomposition. With regard to these improvements (17), the use of an automated gas chromatographic system in routine determination of antiepileptic drugs, including PRM and PB (3), may be more advantageous than supposed by Rambeck (45).

As mentioned above, the decomposition product of PB is probably identical to the methylation product of PEMA during flash-heater methylation. Therefore, the simultaneous determination of PRM, PB, and PEMA by this technique is a serious problem. Löscher and Göbel (36) solved this problem by separating PRM and PEMA from PB during the extraction procedure, using solvent–solvent partition of the extracted drugs between an alkaline aqueous phase and chloroform prior to on-column methylation. No analytical interference was observed when flash-heater methylation was used in determinations from patients who were on fluphenazine and procyclidine therapy in addition to PRM, PB, and other antiepileptic drugs (59).

Alkylation of PRM and PB before injection into the gas chromatograph offers an alternative to the on-column alkylation technique. Thus, Roseboom and Hulshoff (48) proposed the butylation of PRM and PB with butyl iodide, and Vandemark and Adams (58) methylated them with methyl iodide, with extraction into a TMPAH or TMAH solution, respectively. The alkylation of PEMA was not mentioned.

The trimethylsilylation of PRM and PEMA (4,21,35) is not suitable for PB because of the instability of its trimethylsilyl derivative (35).

Watson et al. (64) proposed the trimethylsilylation of PRM extracted from tablets. From our experience, it would be better to perform the more convenient GLC determination of underivatized PRM after its extraction from tablets using *p*-methyl-PEMA and a less polar OV-17 column. Derivatives of PRM and PEMA suitable for determination by electron-capture gas chromatography were prepared by Wallace et al. (62,63). Primidone was acylated with pentafluorobenzoyl chloride. The resulting *N,N'*-dipentafluorobenzoyl-PRM was extremely sensitive to the electron-capture detector of a gas chromatograph. Therefore, only microliter amounts of serum were required in the analysis. Phenylethylmalonamide was dehydrated by trifluoroacetic anhydride, yielding phenylethylcyanacetamide, which was also very sensitive to electron-capture detection. With *p*-methyl-PRM and *p*-methyl-PEMA used as internal standards, PRM and PEMA may be quantitated from one sample. The ethyl acetate/benzene extract is divided into separate aliquots prior to derivatization with pentafluorobenzoyl chloride and trifluoroacetic anhydride, respectively. Perchalski and Wilder (40) prepared the *N,N*-dimethylaminomethylene derivative of PEMA by its reaction with dimethylformamide dimethylacetal.

Determination without derivatization.

The simultaneous determination of PRM, PEMA, PB, and other antiepileptic drugs by GLC is best performed by injecting the free drugs into a suitable column. For this purpose, highly efficient column fillings such as 2% SP-1000 on Diatomite® CLQ (10), 1% SP-1000 on Supelcoport® (27), 3% OV-225 on Chromosorb® G-HPAW (46) or on Gas Chrom Q® (47), and GP 2% SP 2510 DA on Supelcoport® (28,34) are available. A mixed phase of 2% SP 2110/1% SP 2510 DA on Supelcoport® (55), is suitable for an efficient isothermal separation at 230°C of PEMA, PB, *p*-methyl-PB, CBZ, PRM, *p*-methyl-PRM, phenytoin (PHT), *p*-methylphenylphenyl hydantoin (MPPH) in order of increasing retention times. Cramers et al. (12) described a method to prepare high-resolution support-coated open tubular columns that may be reliable for separation of the above mentioned drugs.

Problems during extraction procedure.

With or without derivatization prior to GLC, it is imperative to develop an extraction procedure as efficient as possible with regard to absolute recovery. However, the extracts should be clean enough so that there will be no interference by extraneous peaks with peaks of the drugs in the gas chromatogram. Of the antiepileptic drugs to be determined, PRM and PEMA are usually the most difficult to extract. On the basis of their partition coefficients, acetone is the most effective solvent for extracting PRM, PEMA, PB, and other antiepileptic drugs from aqueous body fluids when saturated with ammonium sulfate (46). Ethyl acetate also appears to be a suitable solvent, resulting in excellent absolute recoveries (25,34,64). Toluene is a poor extractant. Mixtures with ethyl acetate and toluene or benzene have been proposed (62,63). They were useful because the added $(NH_4)_2SO_4$ caused a salting out effect.

In our laboratory, the PRM/PEMA/PB determination procedure includes the extraction of 1 ml of acidified body fluid with 5 ml of ethyl acetate–chloroform (210 : 40, v : v), using *p*-methyl-PRM and MPPH as internal standards. We assume that the precipitation of the protein layer will be improved by addition of some chloroform to the essential solvent ethyl acetate. Many of the published determination procedures do not include a step for purification of the extracts of the body fluids. From our experience, such a purification becomes more important the longer the time between sampling and analysis.

Primidone, PEMA, and PB in serum are stable when stored (63,66). However, degradation products from native serum contents caused by bacterial or fungal overgrowth (66) may contribute to extraneous peaks during GLC of nonpurified extracts. Furthermore, the peaks from the equipment and cholesterol from serum may interfere with the peaks of PRM, PEMA, and PB.

Ritz and Warren (47) and Davis et al. (15) proposed a double extraction to remove interfering substances by subsequently extracting the acidic drugs, such as PRM and PB, with approximately 0.5 N NaOH and reextraction into an organic solvent after acidification of the aqueous phase. Unfortunately, PEMA is lost during this procedure. We prefer a procedure similar to those described elsewhere (34, 46,50). The dried serum extract is dissolved in 0.5 ml methanol, 75 μl water is added, and the solution is twice extracted with 2 ml n-hexane. In this way, fatty acids, plasticizers, and, above all, cholesterol are removed. Primidone, PEMA, and PB, together with other antiepileptic drugs, remain almost completely in the methanolic phase. After evaporation, the residue is redissolved in methanol or acetone and injected into the gas chromatograph. Automated (39) and to-be-automated (65) extraction procedures suitable for PRM and PB have been described.

Gas–Liquid Chromatography/
Mass Spectrometry

Nitrogen-selective and electron-capture detectors substantially enhance the sensitivity and specificity of GLC procedures. However, mass spectrometry (MS) yields a significant improvement in detection of charged ions of a specific molecular weight. Depending on the MS technique, mass fragmentography, selected- or single-ion monitoring (SIM) using computer capabilities may be performed. Thus, Horning et al. (29), employing the chemical ionization mode, separated PRM, PEMA, and PB in a single analysis by SIM. The ions m/e 363, 351, and 261 corresponded, respectively, to trimethylsilyl-PRM, trimethylsilyl-PEMA, and dimethyl-PB MH^+ ions. The MH^+ of dimethyl-PB-2,4,5-^{13}C with m/e 264 was used as internal standard.

Johnson et al. (30) described SIM chromatography in a case of overdosage with PRM. Alvin and Bush (2) described mass fragmentation patterns of PRM, ethyl-1,1-^{2}D$_2$-PRM, and a mixture of the two, in preparation for GLC/

MS studies with SIM using stable isotope labeling of PRM, PEMA, and PB. Truscott et al. (56) described the determination of PRM simultaneously with PHT, CBZ, PB, and mephobarbital (MPB) in serum using direct chemical ionization MS without prior chromatographic separation. Corresponding stable-isotope-labeled drugs, e.g., 5-^{2}H$_5$-PRM, for quantitation of PRM were used as internal standards. Concentrated chloroform extracts of serum samples were transferred to a probe tip, evaporated, and admitted to the mass spectrometer. Immediately after insertion of the sample into the ion source, the instrument, operating in the CI mode, was programmed to scan repetitively for a total of 30 scans as the sample was warmed by induction from the source. During a clinical study, Nau et al (38a) evaluated the placental transfer and the neonatal disposition of PRM and its metabolites PEMA, PB and p-OH-PB by means of a new developed microassay using selected ion monitoring mass spectrometry.

High-Performance Liquid Chromatography

Although GLC is still the most widely performed chromatographic technique for the routine determination of antiepileptic drugs and their metabolites in body fluids, high-performance liquid chromatography (HPLC), especially using reversed phase (RP) columns, has gained in significance (26) and is increasingly used in drug monitoring (16). If any HPLC method reached its goal of avoiding sample preparation, analysts would decide on this technique. Although Adams et al. (1) extracted the serum sample with an organic solvent, Kabra et al. (31,32) and Soldin and Hill (52,53) approached their goal by restricting the sample preparation to a simple addition of acetonitrile. By addition of acetonitrile, serum proteins will be precipitated, and the centrifuged sample may be injected directly into the RP column.

The main problem in performing HPLC of PRM, PEMA, and PB on RP columns is the exact separation of PRM and PEMA. Because of their high polarity and their low partition coefficients in a lipophilic-stationary, hydrophilic-mobile RP system, PRM and PEMA usually appear near the beginning of the chromatogram. Thus, Soldin and Hill (52) found the HPLC retention times of PRM and PEMA to be very similar. Using the 50 : 50 (v : v) mobile phase acetonitrile–potassium phosphate buffer (10 μM, pH 8) with a flow rate of 0.8 ml/min, they obtained PRM data that may be considered to represent PRM + PEMA values. Kabra et al. (32) performed the complete separation of PRM, PEMA, and ethosuximide (ESM) utilizing a μBondapack® C_{18} column and a 21 : 79 (v : v) acetonitrile–phosphate buffer pH 4.4 mixture as mobile phase. The phosphate buffer was prepared by adding 300 μl of 1 M KH_2PO_4 to 1,800 ml of water, followed by 50 μl of 0.9 M phosphoric acid. The flow rate was 3.0 ml/min at 50°C with a column head pressure of 11 MPa (1,500 psi). Monitoring was performed at 195 nm. Background peaks appearing at elution times corresponding to PRM or PEMA ranged from 0 to 0.1 μg/ml. Hemolyzed, lipemic, and icteric samples did not interfere with the analysis.

Freeman and Rawal (20) exchanged acetonitrile in the mobile phase for methanol but did not mention a separation of PRM and PEMA. A good resolution of PRM and PEMA is obtained in our laboratory by using a LiChrosorb® RP18, 5 μm (Merck) column and a 65 : 35 (v : v) methanol–sodium/potassium phosphate buffer (6 mM, pH 5.2) mixture as mobile phase with a flow rate of 1 ml/min at 20°C. Monitoring is performed at 220 nm.

Thin-Layer Chromatography

Thin-layer chromatography (TLC) has seldom been used to quantitate PRM, PEMA, and PB simultaneously. Garceau et al. (22) separated PRM and PEMA in an ethyl acetate–benzene–acetic acid (90 : 20 : 10), developing system, whereas PB was separated from PRM + PEMA, which run together, in a benzene–ethyl acetate–acetone–acetic acid (100 : 25 : 15 : 10) system. Wad and Rosenmund (61) adapted their quantitative TLC method to the simultaneous determination of PRM, CBZ-10,11-epoxide, caffeine, CBZ, PHT, PB, and mephenytoin (MHT), specified in order of increasing R_f values. The TLC plates were developed in chloroform–acetone (85 : 15) and were scanned by measuring directly the light reflectance from the native drugs at 215 nm. Unfortunately, PEMA was not specified. Other methods of TLC, most of which are not suitable for routine determination of PRM, have been reviewed by Kupferberg (33).

Immunoassays

Immunoassay techniques for the determination of antiepileptic drugs have been reviewed elsewhere (11,51,60). Immunoassays such as the enzyme-multiplied immunoassay technique (EMIT®) or the radioimmunoassay (RIA) are based on the same principle, that is, the competitive displacement of a labeled drug from an antibody complex by the unlabeled drug in the sample. The sensitivities of the methods, especially that of RIA, are high. The basic problem is, however, that the antibody specifity for the drug to be measured be as high as possible.

In the EMIT® method, the antibody to PRM has been described as showing a cross reactivity of less than 1.25% for PB, MPB, secobarbital, PHT, ESM, CBZ, and methsuximide (MSM) (54). The specificity of PRM EMIT® relative to GLC methods was also confirmed (37,38,51). Fully mechanized EMIT® systems may increase their economy (57).

Radioimmunoassay procedures for PRM, PB, and PHT were developed by Cook et al. (11), who also described the synthetic route to PRM antigens and to the radiolabeled p-tritium-PRM used for the competitive binding assay. The cross reactivity with antibodies of 1- and 5-substituted PRM–protein conjugates, respectively, to PEMA and PB or p-hydroxyphenobarbital appears to be minimal. Immunoassays for the determination of PEMA have not yet been described.

CONVERSION

Primidone

Conversion factor:

$$CF = \frac{1000}{mol.\ wt.} = \frac{1000}{218.3} = 4.58$$

Conversion:

$$(\mu g/ml) \times 4.58 = (\mu moles/liter)$$
$$(\mu moles/liter) \div 4.58 = (\mu g/ml)$$

PEMA

Conversion factor:

$$CF = \frac{1000}{mol.\ wt.} = \frac{1000}{206.2} = 4.85$$

Conversion:

$$(\mu g/ml) \times 4.85 = (\mu moles/liter)$$
$$(\mu moles/liter) \div 4.85 = (\mu g/ml)$$

REFERENCES

1. Adams, R. F., Schmidt, G. J., and Vandemark, F. L. (1978): A micro liquid column chromatography procedure for twelve anticonvulsants and some of their metabolites. *J. Chromatogr.*, 145:275–284.
2. Alvin, J. D., and Bush, M. T. (1975): Synthesis of millimole amounts of ^{14}C- and ^{2}D-labelled primidone, phenylethylmalonamide and phenobarbital of high-sensitivity detection in biological materials. *Mikrochim. Acta (Wien)*, 1:685–696.
3. Ayers, G. J., Goudie, J. H., Reed, K., and Burnett, D. (1977): Quality control in the simultaneous assay of anticonvulsants using an automated gas chromatographic system with a nitrogen detector. *Clin. Chim. Acta*, 76:113–124.
4. Baumel, I. P., Gallagher, B. B., and Mattson, R. H. (1972): Phenylethylmalonamide (PEMA). An important metabolite of primidone. *Arch. Neurol.*, 27:34–41.
5. Bente, H. B. (1978): Nitrogen selective detectors: Application to quantitation of antiepileptic drugs. In: *Antiepileptic Drugs: Quantitative Analysis and Interpretation*, edited by C. E. Pippenger, J. K. Penry, and H. Kutt, pp. 139–146. Raven Press, New York.
6. Bogue, J. Y., and Carrington, H. C. (1953): The evaluation of "mysoline"—a new anticonvulsant drug. *Br. J. Pharmacol.*, 8:230–236.
7. Boon, W. R., Carrington, H. C., Greenhalgh, N., and Vasey, C. H. (1954): Some derivatives of tetra- and hexa-hydro-4:6-dioxopyrimidine. *J. Chem. Soc.*, 8:3263–3272.
8. Bouché, R. (1973): Proposition d'attribution des bandes d'absorption des barbituriques dans la région de 1700 cm^{-1}. *Chim. Ther.*, 6:676–681.
9. Bourgeois, G., Brachet-Liermain, A., and Ferrus, L. (1974): Etude comparée de la fragmentation de trois composés médicamenteux à structure hétérocyclique: La primaclone, le glutethimide et le phenobarbital. *Organ. Mass Spectrom.*, 9:53–57.
10. Chambers, R. E., and Cameron, J. D. (1977): *N*-Acetyltryptophan ethyl ester: A new internal standard for the gas chromatographic determination of plasma anticonvulsant levels. *Ann. Clin. Biochem.*, 14:243–244.
11. Cook, C. E., Christensen, H. D., Amerson, E. W., Kepler, J. A., Tallent, C. R., and Taylor, G. F. (1976): Radioimmunoassay of anticonvulsant drugs: Phenytoin, phenobarbital and primidone. In: *Quantitative Analytic Studies in Epilepsy*, edited by P. Kellaway and I. Petersén, pp. 39–58. Raven Press, New York.
12. Cramers, C. A., Vermeer, E. A., van Kuik, L. G., Hulsman, J. A., and Meijers, C. A. (1976): Quantitative determination of underivatized anti-convulsant drugs by high resolution gas chromatography with support-coated open tubular columns. *Clin. Chim. Acta*, 73:97–107.
13. Daley, R. D. (1973): Primidone. *Anal. Profiles Drug Subst.*, 2:409–437.
14. Darcey, B. A., Solow, E. B., and Pippenger, C. E. (1978): Gas–liquid chromatographic quantitation of phenytoin, phenobarbital, primidone and carbamazepine. In: *Antiepileptic Drugs: Quantitative Analysis and Interpretation*, edited by C. E. Pippenger, J. K. Penry, and H. Kutt, pp. 67–74. Raven Press, New York.
15. Davis, H. L., Falk, K. J., and Bailey, D. G. (1975): Improved method for the simultaneous determination of phenobarbital, primidone and diphenylhydantoin in patients' serum by gas–liquid chromatography. *J. Chromatogr.*, 107:61–66.
16. Dijkhuis, I. C., De Jong, H. J., Richens, A., Pippenger, C. E., Leskinen, E. E. A., and Nyberg, A. P. W. (1979): Joint international quality control programme on the determination of antiepileptic drugs. *Pharm. Weekbl.*, 114:151–184.
17. Dudley, K. H. (1978): Internal standards in gas–liquid chromatographic determination of antiepileptic drugs. In: *Antiepileptic Drugs: Quantitative Analysis and Interpretation*, edited by C. E. Pippenger, J. K. Penry, and H. Kutt, pp. 19–34. Raven Press, New York.
18. Dudley, K. H., Bius, D. L., Kraus, B. L., and Boyles, L. W. (1977): Gas chromatographic on-column methylation technique for the simultaneous determination of antiepileptic drugs in blood. *Epilepsia*, 18:259–275.
19. Dudley, K. H., Bius, D. L., and Maguire, J. H. (1978): Synthesis of internal standards for analytical determinations of primidone and its metabolite, phenylethylmalonamide (PEMA). *J. Heterocyclic Chem.*, 15:923–926.
20. Freeman, D. J., and Rawal, N. (1979): Serum anticonvulsant monitoring by liquid chromatography with a methanolic mobile phase. *Clin. Chem.*, 25:810–811.
21. Gallagher, B. B., and Baumel, I. P. (1972): Primi-

done, chemistry and methods for determination. In: *Antiepileptic Drugs,* edited by D. M. Woodbury, J. K. Penry, and R. P. Schmidt, pp. 353–356. Raven Press, New York.

22. Garceau, Y., Philopoulos, Y., and Hasegawa, J. (1973): Quantitative TLC determination of primidone, phenylethylmalonediamide, and phenobarbital in biological fluids. *J. Pharm. Sci.,* 62:2032–2034.

23. Goedhart, D. M., Driessen, O. M. J., and Meijer, J. W. A. (1978): The extraction of antiepileptic drugs. *Arzneim. Forsch.,* 28:19–21.

24. Gudzinowicz, B. J., and Gudzinowicz, M. J. (1977): *Analysis of Drugs and Metabolites by Gas Chromatography–Mass Spectrometry. Vol. 2: Hypnotic, Anticonvulsants and Sedatives.* Marcel Dekker, New York.

25. Gupta, R. N., Dobson, K., and Keane, P. M. (1977): Gas–liquid chromatographic determination of primidone in plasma. *J. Chromatogr.,* 132:140–144.

26. Hawk, G. L., and Franconi, L. C. (1978): High-pressure liquid chromatography in quantitation of antiepileptic drugs. In: *Antiepileptic Drugs: Quantitative Analysis and Interpretation,* edited by C. E. Pippenger, J. K. Penry, and H. Kutt, pp. 153–162. Raven Press, New York.

27. Heipertz, R., Pilz, H., and Eickhoff, K., (1977): Evaluation of a rapid gas-chromatographic method for the simultaneous quantitative determination of ethosuximide, phenylethylmalonediamide, carbamazepine, phenobarbital, primidone and diphenylhydantoin in human serum. *Clin. Chim. Acta,* 77:307–316.

28. Hewitt, T. E., Sievers, D. L., and Kessler, G. (1978): Improved gas-chromatographic analysis for anticonvulsants. *Clin. Chem.,* 24:1854–1856.

29. Horning, M. G., Lertratanangkoon, K., Nowlin, J., Stillwell, W. G., Stillwell, R. N., Zion, T. E., Kellaway, P., and Hill, R. M. (1974): Anticonvulsant drug monitoring by GC–MS–COM techniques. *J. Chromatogr. Sci.,* 12:630–635.

30. Johnson, G. F., Least, C. J., Jr., Serum, J. W., Solow, E. B., and Solomon, H. M. (1976): Monitoring drug concentrations in a case of combined overdosage with primidone and methsuximide. *Clin. Chem.,* 22:915–921.

31. Kabra, P. M., Koo, H. Y., and Marton, L. J. (1978): Simultaneous liquid-chromatographic determination of 12 common sedatives and hypnotics in serum. *Clin. Chem.,* 24:657–662.

32. Kabra, P. M., McDonald, D. M., and Marton, L. J. (1978): A simultaneous high-performance liquid chromatographic analysis of the most common anticonvulsants and their metabolites in the serum. *J. Anal. Toxicol.,* 2:127–133.

33. Kupferberg, H. J. (1978): Quantitative methods for antiepileptic drug analysis: An overview. In: *Antiepileptic Drugs: Quantitative Analysis and Interpretation,* edited by C. E. Pippenger, J. K. Penry, and H. Kutt, pp. 9–18. Raven Press, New York.

34. Leal, K. W., Lilensky, A. J., and Rapport, R. L. (1978): Simultaneous analysis of primidone, phenobarbital, and phenylethylmalonamide in plasma and brain. *J. Anal. Toxicol.,* 2:214–218.

35. Least, C. J., Jr., Johnson, G. F., and Solomon, H. M. (1975): Therapeutic monitoring of anticonvulsant

drugs: Gas chromatographic simultaneous determination of primidone, phenylethylmalonamide, carbamazepine, and diphenylhydantoin. *Clin. Chem.,* 21:1658–1662.

36. Löscher, W., and Göbel. W. (1978): Consecutive gas chromatographic determination of phenytoin, phenobarbital, primidone, phenylethylmalondiamide, carbamazepine, trimethadione, dimethadione, ethosuximide, and valproate from the same serum specimen. *Epilepsia,* 19:463–473.

37. Malkus, H., Dicesare, J. L., Meola, J. M., Pippenger, C. E., Ibanez, J., and Castro, A. (1978): Evaluation of EMIT methods for the determination of the five major antiepileptic drugs on an automated kinetic analyser. *Clin. Biochem.,* 11:139–142.

38. McClean, S. W., Young, D. S., and Yonekawa, W. (1977): Anticonvulsants in serum, determined with a fully mechanized enzyme analyzer. *Clin. Chem.,* 23:116–118.

38a. Nau, H., Jesdinsky, D., and Wittfoht, W. (1980): Microassay for primidone and its metabolites phenylethylmalondiamide, phenobarbital and p-hydroxyphenobarbital in human serum, saliva, breast milk and tissues by gas chromatography-mass spectrometry using selected ion monitoring. *J. Chromatogr.,* 182:71–79.

39. Onge, L. M. St., Dolar. E., Anglim, M. A., and Least, C. J., Jr., (1979): Improved determination of phenobarbital, primidone, and phenytoin by use of a preparative instrument for extraction, followed by gas chromatography. *Clin. Chem.,* 25:1373–1376.

40. Perchalski, R. J., and Wilder, B. J. (1978): Gas–liquid chromatographic determination of carbamazepine and phenylethylmalonamide in plasma after reaction with dimethylformamide dimethylacetal. *J. Chromatogr.,* 145:97–103.

41. Pippenger, C. E., and Gillen, H. W. (1969): Gas chromatographic analysis for anticonvulsant drugs in biologic fluids. *Clin. Chem.,* 15:582–590.

42. Pippenger, C. E., Paris-Kutt, H., and Penry, J. K. (1978): Re-appraisal of interlaboratory variability in antiepileptic drug determinations. *Clin. Chem.,* 24:1050.

43. Pippenger, C. E., Penry, J. K., and Kutt, H. (1978): *Antiepileptic Drugs: Quantitative Analysis and Interpretation.* Raven Press, New York.

44. Pirl, J. N., Spikes, J. J., and Fitzloff, J. (1977): Isolation, identification, and quantitation of 2-ethyl-2-phenylmalondiamide, a primidone metabolite. *J. Anal. Toxicol.,* 1:200–203.

45. Rambeck, B., and Meijer, J. W. A. (1980): Gas chromatographic methods for the determination of antiepileptic drugs: A systematic review. *Ther. Drug Monit.,* 2:385–396.

46. Rambeck, B., and Meijer. J. W. A. (1979): Comprehensive method for the determination of antiepileptic drugs using a novel extraction technique and a fully automatic gas chromatograph. *Arzneim. Forsch.,* 29:99–103.

47. Ritz, D. P., and Warren, C. G. (1975): Single extraction GLC analysis of six commonly prescribed antiepileptic drugs. *Clin. Toxicol.,* 8:311–324.

48. Roseboom, H., and Hulshoff, A. (1979): Rapid and simple cleanup and derivatization procedure for the

gas chromatographic determination of acidic drugs in plasma. *J. Chromatogr.*, 173:65–74.

49. Schaal, D. E., McKinley, S. L., and Chittwood, G. W. (1979): Gas–liquid chromatographic analysis of underivatized anticonvulsants on the stationary phase DC-LSX-3-0295. *J. Anal. Toxicol.*, 3:96–98.

50. Schäfer, H. R. (1975): Some problems concerning the quantitative assay of primidone and its metabolites. In: *Clinical Pharmacology of Anti-Epileptic Drugs,* edited by H. Schneider, D. Janz, C. Gardner-Thorpe, H. Meinardi, and A. L. Sherwin, pp. 124–129. Springer-Verlag, Berlin, Heidelberg, New York.

51. Schottelius, D. D. (1978): Homogeneous immunoassay system (EMIT) for quantitation of antiepileptic drugs in biological fluids. In: *Antiepileptic Drugs: Quantitative Analysis and Interpretation,* edited by C. E. Pippenger, J. K. Penry, and H. Kutt, pp. 95–108. Raven Press, New York.

52. Soldin, St. J., and Hill, J. G. (1977): Interference with column-chromatographic measurement of primidone. *Clin. Chem.*, 23:782.

53. Soldin, St. J., and Hill, J. G. (1977): Routine dual-wavelength analysis of anticonvulsant drugs by high-performance liquid chromatography. *Clin. Chem.*, 23:2352.

54. Sun, L., and Walwick, E. R. (1976): Primidone analyses: Correlation of gas-chromatographic assay with enzyme immunoassay. *Clin. Chem.*, 22:901–902.

55. Thoma, J. J., Ewald, T., and McCoy, M. (1978): Simultaneous analysis of underivatized phenobarbital, carbamazepine, primidone, and phenytoin by isothermal gas–liquid chromatography. *J. Anal. Toxicol.*, 2:219–225.

56. Truscott, R. J. W., Burke, D. G., Korth, J., Halpern, B., and Summons, R. (1978): Simultaneous determination of diphenylhydantoin, mephobarbital, carbamazepine, phenobarbital and primidone in serum using direct chemical ionization mass spectrometry. *Biomed. Mass Spectrom.*, 5:477–482.

57. Turri, J. J. (1977): Enzyme immunoassay of phenobarbital, phenytoin, and primidone with the ABA-100 bichromatic analyzer. *Clin. Chem.*, 23:1510–1512.

58. Vandemark, F. L., and Adams, R. F. (1976): Ultramicro gas-chromatographic analysis for anticonvulsants, with use of a nitrogen-selective detector. *Clin. Chem.*, 22:1062–1065.

59. Varma, R. (1978): Simultaneous gas chromatographic determination of diphenylhydantoin, carbamazepine (Tegretol), phenobarbital and primidone in presence of Kemadrin (procyclidine) and Prolixin (fluphenazine) in plasma of psychiatric patients. *J. Chromatogr.*, 155:182–186.

60. Vogt, W. (1978): *Enzymimmunoassay, Grundlagen und Praktische Anwendung.* Georg Thieme, Stuttgart.

61. Wad, N., and Rosenmund, H. (1978): Rapid quantitative method for the simultaneous determination of carbamazepine, carbamazepine-10, 11-epoxide, diphenylhydantoin, mephenytoin, phenobarbital and primidone in serum by thin-layer chromatography. *J. Chromatogr.*, 146:167–168.

62. Wallace, J. E., Hamilton, H. E., Shimek, E. L., Jr., Schwertner, H. A., and Blum, K. (1977): Determination of primidone by electron-capture gas chromatography. *Anal. Chem.*, 49:903–906.

63. Wallace, J. E., Hamilton, H. E., Shimek, E. L., Jr., Schwertner, H. A., and Haegele, C. D. (1977): Determination of phenylethylmalonamide by electron-capture gas chromatography. *Anal. Chem.*, 49:1969–1973.

64. Watson, J. R., Lawrence, R. C., and Lovering, E. G. (1978): Simple GLC analysis of anticonvulsant drugs in commercial dosage forms. *J. Pharm. Sci.*, 67:950–953.

65. Werner, M., Mohrbacher, R. J., and Riendeau, C. J. (1979): Gas–liquid chromatography of underivatized drugs after chromatographic extraction from blood. *Clin. Chem.*, 25:2020–2025.

66. Wilensky, A. J. (1978): Stability of some antiepileptic drugs in plasma. *Clin. Chem.*, 24:722–723.

67. Wollmann, H., Skaletzki, B., and Schaaf, A. (1974): Zur Bestimmung der Polarität von Arzneistoffen. *Pharmazie*, 29:708–711.

68. Yeates, D. G. R., and Palmer, R. A. (1975): The crystal structure of primidone. *Acta Crystalogr. [B]*, 31:1077–1082.

Antiepileptic Drugs, edited by D. M. Woodbury, J. K. Penry, and C. E. Pippenger. Raven Press, New York © 1982.

30

Primidone

Absorption, Distribution, and Excretion

Dorothy D. Schottelius

The pharmacokinetic parameters of absorption, distribution, and excretion of primidone are rendered more complex because of the drug's biotransformation into two metabolites—phenobarbital (PB) and phenylethylmalonamide (PEMA)—that have antiepileptic activity and complex pharmacokinetic properties (Fig. 1 of Chapter 31) (5,8). The biotransformation of primidone will be described in Chapter 31, and the pharmacokinetics of PB have been discussed in Chapters 22 and 23. This latter information will be considered with regard to the possible influence it may exert on the absorption, distribution, and excretion of primidone. The absorption, distribution, and excretion of PEMA will be considered concurrently.

ABSORPTION

Rate and Extent of Absorption

The bioavailability (30) of primidone originating from different manufacturers has not been investigated even though this information may be of importance in evaluating the therapeutic effect of this compound. Bielmann et al. (3) compared two lots of primidone (Mysoline®) obtained directly from the manufacturer (Ayerst Laboratories, Montreal, Canada) which had dif-

ferent *in vitro* disintegration and dissolution times (disintegration and dissolution time of 2 min in one lot compared with disintegration time of 16 min and dissolution time of 12 min in the other lot). The lots were compared in 12 epileptic patients who were undergoing chronic therapy with primidone. These patients received both lots as a sole medication for 2 weeks in a cross-over design. The data revealed significant between-weeks differences in the blood level of primidone and its two metabolites at 0 and 1 hr after ingestion of the drug and in the excretory phase, that is, from 8 to 24 hr after the drug was administered. There was no significant difference in mean blood levels of primidone and PEMA between the two lots, but a significant difference was found between the amounts of phenobarbital produced by each lot of primidone during the second week. Higher phenobarbital levels were found for the lot having the more rapid disintegration and dissolution time. The authors speculated that these *in vitro* chemical characteristics may have a relationship to the absorption and elimination half-life. Unfortunately, the data do not permit comparison of the two lots of primidone in specific individuals. The study, however, indicates that bioavailability of this compound may be worthy of further investigation and consideration when data on primidone are evaluated.

Other chemical characteristics of primidone that influence the rate and extent of absorption are its molecular weight (218.25), which is similar to that of several other antiepileptic drugs (phenytoin and phenobarbital), its neutral properties (in contrast to phenobarbital), and its solubility (600 μg/ml of water at 37°C). Solubility appears to be the only factor that could alter a predictably rapid rate of absorption. Concentrations of approximately 95 to 300 μg/ml have been determined in acute primidone overdosages; these concentrations have been accompanied by crystalluria (7,9,23).

Gastric and intestinal absorption of primidone have been studied directly or indirectly in a variety of laboratory animals. Prior to the development of accurate and sensitive analytical procedures for the assay of this compound, time of peak anticonvulsant effect provided the only information about a parameter composed of absorption rate and distribution time. By utilizing the maximal electroshock seizure test, Goodman et al. (15) determined that the time of peak effect of primidone was 6 hr in adult albino rats and 3 hr in adult albino mice. A peak absorption time of 1 hr was reported following a single dose of ^{14}C-primidone (40). Since the development of appropriate analytical procedures, several additional animal studies have provided more detailed pharmacokinetic data.

Baumel et al. (2) administered single doses of primidone (500, 250, 125, 62.5, 31.25, and 15.62 mg/kg) to adult male albino rats by intubation and determined plasma levels at 0.5, 1, 2, 4, 6, 12, and 24 hr after dosing. The results indicated that plasma levels of primidone peaked at 1 hr after doses of 500 mg/kg (serum level of 120 μg/ml) and 15.62 mg/kg (serum level of 5 μg/ml). Time course plots indicated a peak level at 2 hr with doses of 125 mg/kg and 62.5 mg/kg. The effects of single and multiple doses of primidone in rats were investigated by Schafer et al. (35), and the marked difference in the serum concentrations 1 hr after dosing indicated that the rate and/or the extent of absorption may be altered with multiple administration (serum level of 32.6 μg/ml with single dose of 50 mg/kg and

19.0 μg/ml with daily dose of 50 mg/kg for 5 days).

Additional studies in various strains of mice provide further evidence of the rapid absorption of primidone following oral administration of suspensions. A plasma primidone level of approximately 90 μg/ml was found 1 hr after a single oral dose of 100 mg/kg in NMRI adult mice (34). McElhatton et al. (27) administered an oral suspension of primidone in single doses of various amounts to adult female pathogen-free albino mice and measured plasma primidone levels at 1 hr and 4 hr after dosing. Higher levels were found at the 1-hr time. It is of interest to note that the ratio of plasma concentration (μg/ml) to dose (mg/kg) decreased markedly (0.96 at 25 mg/kg; 0.72 at 50 mg/kg; 0.43 at 150 mg/kg), indicating that the rate of absorption was influenced by the total amount of the dose. This group (28), using a 100-mg/kg dose, also found a peak concentration at 1 hr, and the ratio of plasma level to dose was 0.48. Single-dose pharmacokinetics in fasted adult female Swiss–Webster mice have been investigated by Leal et al. (24) who used a 50-mg/kg dose of primidone in solution delivered by transesophageal intubation. Serum concentrations peaked in 36 min at 21.6 μg/ml and remained relatively constant for 2 hr.

The rate and extent of absorption of primidone in humans has not been completely investigated. Booker et al. (6) determined sequential serum primidone levels following a 500-mg oral dose given to six fasted adult male volunteers; interpretation of the data would indicate an average peak absorption between 3 and 4 hr. Gallagher and Baumel (12) gave oral doses of 500 mg and 750 mg of primidone to 10 epileptic patients and found an average peak absorption time of 3.2 hr (range, 0.5 to 9.0 hr). The averages for each dose were 2.55 ± 0.06 hr for the 500-mg dose and 4.25 ± 2.2 hr for the 750-mg dose. Further studies (13) of 19 epileptic patients given 500 mg or 750 mg in a single dose showed that the time to peak plasma concentration was 2.7 ± 0.4 hr (range, 30 min to 7 hr) with no apparent difference in the time to peak concentration between the two doses. Multiple dosing was studied in five patients in whom the initial studies were followed by chronic administration of 750 mg daily in three equally divided doses for 2 months, and the study was repeated (500 mg was apparently given as one dose for this test). Four of these five patients showed increases in the time to peak plasma concentration that averaged 5.5 times longer than the time with single-dose administration. Initial mean time to peak concentrations increased from 1.8 hr to 4.4 hr for the five patients. Several explanations could be postulated, but insufficient data were presented to lend validity to any one. An obvious complication was the concomitant administration of other antiepileptic medications.

Kauffman et al. (22) studied absorption of primidone following single-dose administration to 12 children, 7 to 14 years of age. The total daily dose (200–700 mg) was given after a 12-hr fast and 16 hr after any previous dose of primidone. These children had been receiving a similar daily dose for more than 3 months at the time of the study. None of the 12 were receiving other barbiturate anticonvulsants; eight were receiving phenytoin. Plasma primidone concentrations peaked at 4 to 6 hr; primidone appeared to be almost completely absorbed in children under these conditions.

Factors that May Alter Rate or Extent of Absorption

Studies utilizing lower total doses of primidone in individuals with and without other medications are necessary to ascertain the rate and extent of absorption under conditions that more closely mimic the current dosing practice in patients. This information would be useful in developing a better initial dosing schedule to eliminate the side effects on initiation of therapy (14). In one case, we gave a 125-mg dose (48-kg woman) and found that 60% was absorbed in 0.5 hr (serum level, 3.6 μg/ml); the patient complained of minor side effects at this time.

Interference with primidone absorption by other drugs has been infrequently reported. Acetazolamide interference has been indicated (39). Disease- or age-related interferences in primidone absorption have not been reported.

Pregnancy has not been shown to interfere with the rate or extent of absorption of primidone in women, although it appears to occur in mice (13) where peak plasma levels (1 hr after dosing in day-14 pregnant mice) were 34%, 36%, and 43% of those in nonpregnant animals at three different doses—25, 50, and 150 mg/kg. The same effect of increase in dose resulted in a lower ratio of plasma level to dose in pregnant animals.

DISTRIBUTION

Tissue Distribution

Distribution of primidone and PEMA into tissues other than blood has not been thoroughly investigated in either man or experimental animals. The distribution of PB has been discussed in Chapter 22. Primidone has many physicochemical similarities to PB, and total-body autoradiography (16) of the squirrel monkey has been reported to reveal no particular differences in tissue and regional distribution of primidone as compared with PB.

Brain tissue levels of primidone and PEMA have been determined in mice (23,24) and rats (2) following single oral doses of primidone. In the mouse (24), maximum brain concentration (8.2 μg/g) was reached 1 hr after a dose of 50 mg/kg (maximum plasma concentration at 36 min). In the rat (2), brain levels peaked 2 hr after a single oral dose of several concentrations (peak plasma levels at 1 hr), although some variations were noted at different concentrations. The results were means of five determinations in mice and three in rats.

The graphic data showed that primidone entered the brain of the mouse and the rat rapidly (first measurement apparently about 15 min or less in mouse and 30 min in rat), and concentrations in both plasma and brain remained relatively constant up to 2 hr. In both species, the brain-to-plasma ratio remained constant over the time period measured and was 0.37 in the mouse at the time of peak concentration and 0.46 in the rat. A single oral dose of 100 mg/kg of primidone to NMRI mice (34) produced high tissue concentrations in both serum and brain (89 μg/ml and 50 μg/g, respectively) and high brain-to-serum ratios (approximately 0.56 at 1 hr; 0.59 at 4 hr; 0.69 at 7 hr and 1.0 at 10 hr). Brain tissue levels of primidone were measured in the rat (35) at 6 hr after single or multiple doses (50 mg/kg) and were found to be 5 μg/g and 3.2 μg/g, respectively. Calculations of brain-to-plasma ratios (12.5 after a single dose and 6.4 after multiple doses) were not revealing, since serum primidone levels were very low in both instances; however, these ratios do not exceed those indicated by other experiments in the rat.

Distribution of PEMA and PB as metabolites of PRM was also studied in these experiments. In the mouse (24), plasma levels of derived PEMA peaked at 6 hr and plasma levels of derived PB at 6 to 8 hr; brain levels of PEMA peaked at 4 to 6 hr and brain levels of PB at 6 to 8 hr. Brain-to-plasma ratio at peak brain concentration appeared to be ~0.5 for PEMA and ~0.6 for PB. In the rat (2), PEMA and PB were detected in plasma 30 min after 250- and 500-mg/kg doses of primidone and 1 hr after 62.5- and 125-mg/kg doses and were detected in the brain 1 hr after the higher doses (125, 250, 500 mg/kg). Brain-to-plasma ratios at different times following the various single-dose concentrations of primidone were as follows: 4 hr after 500 mg/kg: PEMA ~0.07, PB ~0.32; 6 hr after 62.5 mg/kg: PB = 0.95, with no plasma or brain concentration of PEMA. At doses below 62.5 mg/kg, no PB or PEMA were detectable in brain or plasma.

The distribution of PEMA and PB into the brain reflects not only distribution time but involves biotransformation time as well. When PB (50-mg/kg single oral dose) was administered to mice, peak plasma and brain levels occurred at 24 min and 2 hr respectively, with a brain-to-plasma ratio of 0.8 at 2 hr; PEMA (50 mg/kg single oral dose) gave peak plasma and brain levels at 36 min and 2 hr, respectively, with a

brain-to-plasma ratio of ~0.8 at 2 hr (24). In the rat (2), several doses of each metabolite were administered by intraperitoneal injection, and brain and plasma concentrations were determined 1 hr after the injection. The brain-to-plasma ratio was 0.98 ± 0.09 for PB (dose range, 5–40 mg/kg) and 0.28 ± 0.02 for PEMA (dose range, 15.6–250 mg/kg), which would indicate that PEMA does not readily enter the brain of the rat. All of the animal experiments, including those of Hunt and Miller (21) in the rabbit utilizing intravenous administration of primidone, PEMA, and PB, show a rapid disappearance from plasma of all three compounds, which indicated a rapid distribution into the tissues.

Such extensive studies have not been undertaken on the distribution of primidone, PEMA, and PB in man, and only one report exists concerning brain and plasma concentrations. Houghton et al. (20) obtained brain samples from 11 patients undergoing unilateral temporal lobe resection for intractable temporal lobe epilepsy. Patients received primidone treatment for at least 1 week before the operation, and this was continued until the day preceding surgery. Blood samples were obtained immediately after induction of anesthesia, and samples of scalp skin, muscle, bone, and temporal lobe were taken during surgery. Plasma primidone levels ranged from 1.6 to 8.6 μg/ml, and there was good correlation between brain and plasma levels of the drug (correlation coefficient = 0.96). The regression line indicated an average brain-to-plasma ratio of 0.87. This is higher than the average brain-to-serum ratio of 0.31 reported in humans (24). Primidone was present in muscle, skin, and bone, but the distribution correlated poorly with the concentration in plasma.

The distribution of primidone in cerebrospinal fluid (CSF) and saliva has been examined in humans, and the results from various studies are shown in Table 1. Our data, illustrated in Fig. 1, were collected from nine patients who had been taking primidone alone or with phenytoin for several months. For primidone, the CSF-to-serum ratio was 0.60 ± 0.05 at a dose–sample interval of 2.6 ± 0.2 hr. There was no

TABLE 1. *Primidone distribution in body fluids of humans relative to serum*

CSF/serum	Reference	Saliva/serum	Reference
1.13	12	0.99	36
1.02	32	0.97	4
0.53	29	1.08	41
0.80	36	0.73	26
0.69	41	0.85	18
0.72	4		
0.70	37		
0.81	20		

difference in this ratio between patients taking primidone alone (0.62 ± 0.08) and those taking primidone plus phenytoin (0.59 ± 0.07). There was a significant difference in this ratio when the samples were obtained at 7.2 ± 0.2 hr after dose (0.997 ± 0.18). For derived PB, the CSF-to-serum ratios for the three groups were 0.50 ± 0.06, 0.48 ± 0.02, and 0.62 ± 0.13, respectively. From these findings, the variability of CSF-to-serum ratios shown in the table may be explained by the interval between dose and sampling time. The reported saliva-to-serum ratios also vary and may well be a reflection of the same problem, but other factors (e.g., mixture of watery versus serous gland secretion) may also contribute.

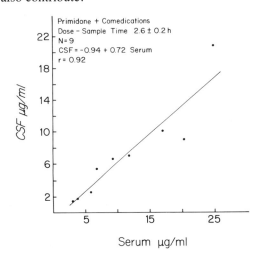

FIG. 1. Correlation of serum and cerebrospinal fluid concentration of primidone in nine patients, with both samples obtained 2.6 ± 0.2 hr after last dose of primidone. All patients had been taking medications for longer than 3 months.

Transplacental passage of primidone has been demonstrated in mothers chronically ingesting the drug (19) and in those treated with a single oral dose of 250 mg (25). The metabolites PEMA and PB are distributed through the placenta as well. Breast milk (19) has been shown to contain variable quantities of primidone (4.6–10.5 µg/ml) and PEMA (1.3–2.4 µg/ml).

Plasma and Tissue Binding

Volume of Distribution

Values of apparent volume of distribution for primidone are frequently given as 1 liter/kg (16) in humans, but relatively few data are reported. Data were obtained from several patients following the intravenous injection of ^{14}C-labeled primidone (42). The apparent volume of distribution was determined for primidone and PEMA in four patients who were not taking any additional anticonvulsants, and the mean values were 47.1 and 36.0 liters, respectively. In the group of patients taking various antiepileptic drugs, the values were 48.8 liters for primidone and 55.8 liters for PEMA.

The apparent volume of distribution was measured in rabbits (21) and found to be 0.68 liter/kg for primidone and 0.82 liter/kg for PEMA following intravenous administration of 10 mg/kg of primidone.

There have been no studies concerning age-related changes in this pharmacokinetic parameter.

Plasma Protein Binding

It has been frequently stated that primidone is not protein bound; this was based on findings of the CSF-to-serum ratio that have been discussed. Until recently, studies using ultrafiltration have been questioned because the filters either bound the drugs or permitted the passage of proteins in the long-term determinations. Utilizing ultrafiltration techniques not subject to these difficulties, we found in the plasma of 48 patients the following amounts of unbound drugs as percentage of the total drug present: PRM 76 ± 11.9% and derived PB 45 ± 11.2% (mean ± SD). Another laboratory (31) reported unbound primidone values of 80 ± 7%. This information does not support the conclusion that primidone is not bound to proteins but rather shows that a variable binding of 20 to 25% exists in plasma. Future investigations can now be undertaken to relate the effects of other drugs, disease states, and age on this binding as well as possible relationships between levels of unbound drug and seizure control.

EXCRETION

Half-Life

Various factors must be considered in evaluating reported data on the half-life of primidone and its active metabolites, PEMA and PB. Among these factors are dose and route of administration, single or chronic dose, presence of other drugs, presence of other disease processes, age of the patient, and individual variability. The half-life of primidone in humans was found to be 10 to 12 hr in six fasting normal men following a single 500-mg oral dose (6). The half-life in epileptic subjects (12,13) was investigated by giving single doses of primidone to fasting patients. These individuals had been receiving other antiepileptic medications. In the first study (12) six patients had a mean half-life of 7.2 ± 1.5 hr (range, 3.3–12.5 hr) after a 500-mg dose, and four patients had a mean half-life of 5.5 ± 0.7 hr (range, 3.5–7 hr) after a 750-mg dose. The second study (13) in 19 patients given a single dose of either 500 or 750 mg showed a mean half-life of 8.0 ± 1.1 hr (range, 3.3–19 hr). There was no consistent alteration in primidone half-life in seven subjects after administration of the drug for 2 to 4 months (half-life increased an average of 7.7 hr in three patients, decreased an average of 1.0 hr in three patients, and showed no change in one). Two patients on daily doses were followed for a period of 4 days, and increasing primidone half-lives (18–23 hr) were noted in one patient in whom PEMA remained at a con-

centration of less than 1 μg/ml and PB was not present. The other patient, in whom plasma levels of PEMA and PB increased progressively, had a primidone half-life of 19 hr. The half-lives of these compounds also were determined following acute withdrawal of primidone in two patients who had been taking 1 g of the drug in divided doses for more than 2 years. Half-lives again showed marked variation between the two individuals as follows: primidone, 7.2 and 19.2 hr; PEMA, 16.8 and 26.4 hr; PB, 48 and 84 hr.

The influence on half-lives of primidone and PEMA of prior or concurrent administration of other antiepileptic drugs was also indicated in the study utilizing ^{14}C-primidone (42). Mean primidone and PEMA half-lives were, respectively, 14.4 ± 0.55 hr and 56 ± 9.5 hr in patients not taking other antiepileptic compounds compared with 7.33 ± 0.44 hr and 41 ± 3.9 hr in subjects taking other drugs.

One report (22) of primidone half-lives in children (7–14 years of age on chronic primidone therapy, 8 of 12 concurrently taking phenytoin) gave a mean value of 8.7 hr (range, 4.5–11.0 hr). Another report (33) found a primidone half-life of 6 to 8 hr in children.

Studies in experimental animals (21,24) show a shorter half-life for primidone, PEMA, and PB than have been found in man. In the mouse and rabbit, respectively, these mean values are: primidone, 2.33 and 2.29 hr; PEMA, 2.32 and 8.83 hr; PB, 4.26 and 30.72 hr. Even though these times may reflect the differences in rate of metabolism, other factors may make it unwise to extrapolate to man pharmacokinetic information obtained in animals. Since this parameter is of importance in determining the frequency of administration of any drug, further investigations in humans are warranted to obtain a more complete picture of factors that may influence the half-lives of primidone, PEMA, and PB.

Routes of Elimination

The biotransformation (see Chapter 31) of primidone in varying degrees to PEMA and PB has complicated the investigation of elimination of this drug. There is little doubt that primidone and its metabolites are principally excreted through the renal pathway (8,11,15,38) and that PEMA, PB, and primidone are the primary compounds excreted. Three additional compounds have been identified in urine from patients taking primidone: α-phenyl-butyramide (10), α-phenyl-γ-butyrolactone (1) (Fig. 2) and hydroxyprimidone (19). The contribution of these three substances to the overall excretion pattern has not been evaluated.

The mean relative clearance of primidone per kilogram of body weight has been reported as $30.9 \pm 1.9 \times 10^{-3}$ for 10 adult patients when the drug was given alone (17). The percentage of dose excreted for the various compounds has been reported in children (22) from whom an average of 92% (72–123%) of the total daily dose was recovered in a 24-hr urine collection. A mean of 42.3% (15.2%–65.9%) was recovered as unchanged primidone, 45.2% (16.3%–65.3%) as PEMA, and 4.9% (1.1%–8.0%) as PB and PB metabolites. There was great interindividual variation in the proportion of total drug excreted as primidone and its various metabolites.

A markedly different pattern of excretion was found in adults (42) when two groups were compared: group I was not taking any concurrent medication; group II was on a variety of other drugs. During the first 24-hr period, approximately the same amount of the administered dose was excreted in both groups (46.7% and 45.5%). In group I during this period, approximately 90% was excreted as unchanged primidone; 4% as PEMA, and 2.5% as PB. Group II excreted less of the dose as primidone (70%) and more as PEMA (22%) and PB (2.8%) These groups were followed for 5 days after the dose, and the total excretion reflects a similar difference in the two groups (Group I: primidone 84.5%, PEMA 8.7%, PB 2.8%; Group II: primidone 51.2%, PEMA 36%, PB 4.3%).

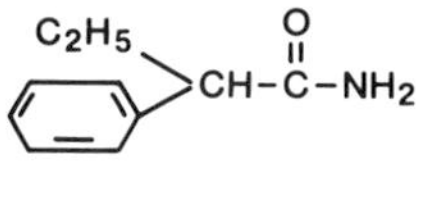

Animal experiments (21) have suggested that a four-compartment model consisting of a two-compartment model for primidone with attached one-compartment models for PEMA and PB, each with first-order formation and elimination rates, is the best kinetic model after intravenous administration in rabbits.

Since the disposal of primidone is primarily by the kidneys, one would anticipate that severe renal impairment might well present problems. Few have been reported, and no serious investigation has been conducted in humans.

As with the data on absorption and distribution, considerably more investigations are warranted in the area of excretion.

SUMMARY

The rate and extent of absorption of primidone in humans can be characterized as relatively rapid but exhibiting wide interindividual variability. Insufficient data are available to present peak absorption time with any true meaning for the clinical situation. Some studies would support the view that absorption time will increase with chronic administration.

The distribution of primidone into tissues and body fluids appears to be rapid but may not be uniform. The brain-to-plasma ratio has not been thoroughly investigated but appears to be approximately 0.8. The drug is distributed through the placenta and into breast milk in humans. Recent investigations support a conclusion that primidone is protein bound (approximately 20%), and this parameter also shows wide interindividual variability.

α-PHENYLBUTYRAMIDE

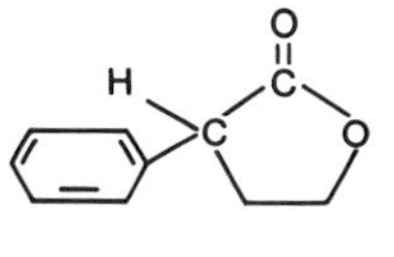

α-PHENYL-γ-BUTYROLACTONE

FIG. 2. Two minor metabolites, α-phenylbutyramide and α-phenyl-γ-butyrolactone, which, along with hydroxyprimidone, have been identified in urine from patients receiving primidone.

Plasma half-lives of primidone and PEMA exhibit variability that does not seem to be related to absorption rates or to single-dose versus chronic administration; however, they may be influenced by the presence of other medications. The relative half-lives seem consistently to be primidone $<$ PEMA $<$ PB when all three are present.

Excretion patterns have varied among the individuals investigated, and the proportions excreted as unchanged primidone, PEMA, and PB may be altered by the presence of other antiepileptic medications. A considerable percentage is excreted as unconjugated primidone, a comparable amount as unconjugated PEMA, and the least amount as PB and conjugates. The roles of concurrent medications, biotransformation, age, sex, disease, protein binding, and other variables warrant continued investigation into excretion patterns.

Although progress has been made in the understanding of this drug, future investigations are warranted to permit the most effective clinical utilization of primidone.

ACKNOWLEDGMENT

Original data presented in this chapter were obtained from studies performed at the Department of Neurology, University of Iowa Hospitals, with the assistance of Dr. R. W. Fincham and other colleagues in the Department.

REFERENCES

1. Andresen, B. D., Davis, F. T., Templeton, J. L., Hammer, R. H., and Panjik, J. L. (1976): Synthesis and characterization of *alpha*-phenyl-*gamma* butyrolactone, a metabolite of glutethimide, phenobarbital and primidone, in human urine. *Res. Commun. Chem. Pathol. Pharmacol.*, 15:21–29.
2. Baumel, I. P., Gallagher, B. B., DiMicco, J., and Goico, H. (1973): Metabolism and anticonvulsant properties of primidone in the rat. *J. Pharmacol. Exp. Ther.*, 186:305–314.
3. Bielmann, P., Levac, T. H., Langlois, Y., and Tetreault, L. (1974): Bioavailability of primidone in epileptic patients. *Int. J. Clin. Pharmacol.*, 9:132–137.
4. Blom, G. F., and Guelen, P. S. M. (1977): The distribution of antiepileptic drugs between serum, saliva, and cerebrospinal fluid. In: *Antiepileptic Drug Mon-

itoring,* edited by C. Gardener-Thorpe, D. Janz, H. Meinardi, and C. E. Pippenger, pp. 287–295. Pitman Medical Publishing, Kent.
5. Bogue, J. Y., Harrington, H. C., and Bentley, S. (1956): L'activité anticonvulsive de la mysoline. *Acta Neurol. Belg.*, 56:640–650.
6. Booker, H. E., Hosokowa, K., Burdette, R. D., and Darcey, B. (1970): A clinical study of serum primidone levels. *Epilepsia,* 11:395–402.
7. Brillman, J., Gallagher, B. B., and Mattson, R. H. (1974): Acute primidone intoxication. *Arch. Neurol.*, 30:255–258.
8. Butler, T. C., and Waddell, W. J. (1956): Metabolic conversion of primidone (Mysoline) to phenobarbital. *Proc. Soc. Exp. Biol. Med.*, 93:544–546.
9. Cate, J. C., and Tenser, R. (1975): Acute primidone overdosage with massive crystalluria. *Clin. Toxicol.*, 8:385–389.
10. Foltz, R. L., Couch, M. W., Greer, M., Scott, K. N., and Williams, C. M. (1972): Chemical ionization mass spectrometry in the identification of drug metabolites. *Biochem. Med.*, 6:294–298.
11. Fujimoto, J. M., Mason, W. H., and Murphy, M. (1968): Urinary excretion of primidone and its metabolites in rabbits. *J. Pharmacol. Exp. Ther.*, 159:379–388.
12. Gallagher, B. B., and Baumel, I. P. (1972): Primidone absorption, distribution and excretion. In: *Antiepileptic Drugs,* edited by D. M. Woodbury, J. K. Penry, and R. P. Schmidt, pp. 357–359. Raven Press, New York.
13. Gallagher, B. B., Baumel, I. P., and Mattson, R. H. (1972): Metabolic disposition of primidone and its metabolites in epileptic subjects after single and repeated administration. *Neurology (Minneap.),* 22:1186–1192.
14. Gallagher, B. B., Baumel, I. P., Mattson, R. H., and Woodbury, S. G. (1973): Primidone, diphenylhydantoin and phenobarbital. *Neurology (Minneap.),* 23:145–149.
15. Goodman, L. S., Swinyard, E. A., Brown, W. C., Schiffman, D. O., Grewal, M. S., and Bliss, E. L. (1953): Anticonvulsant properties of 5-phenyl-5-ethylhexahydropyrimidine-4,6-dione (Mysoline), a new antiepileptic. *J. Pharmacol. Exp. Ther.*, 108:428–436.
16. Guelen, P. J. M., and van der Kleijn, E. (1978): *Rational Antiepileptic Drug Therapy.* Elsevier/North-Holland, Amsterdam.
17. Guelen, P. J. M., van der Kleijn, E., and Wondstra, V. (1975): Statistical analysis of pharmacokinetic parameters in epileptic patients chronically treated with antiepileptic drugs. In: *Clinical Pharmacology of Antiepileptic Drugs,* edited by H. Schneider, D. Janz, C. Gardener-Thorpe, H. Meinardi, and A. L. Sherwin, pp. 2–33. Springer Verlag, Berlin, Heidelberg, New York.
18. Horning, M. A., Brown, L., Bowlin, J., Lertratanangkoon, K., Kellaway, P., and Zion, T. E. (1977): Use of saliva in therapeutic drug monitoring. *Clin. Chem.,* 23:157–164.
19. Horning, M. A., Nowlin, J., Butler, C. M., Lertratanangkoon, K., Sommer, K., and Hill, R. M. (1975):

Clinical applications of gas chromatography/mass spectrometer/computer systems. *Clin. Chem.*, 21:1282–1287.

20. Houghton, G. W., Richens, A., Toseland, P. A., Davidson, S., and Falconer, M. A. (1975): Brain concentrations of phenytoin, phenobarbitone, and primidone in epileptic patients. *Eur. J. Clin. Pharmacol.*, 9:73–78.

21. Hunt, R. J., and Miller, K. W. (1978): Disposition of primidone, phenylethylmalamide and phenobarbital in the rabbit. *Drug Metab. Dispos.*, 6:75–81.

22. Kauffman, R. E., Habersang, R., and Lansky, L. (1977): Kinetics of primidone metabolism and excretion in children. *Clin. Pharmacol. Ther.*, 22:200–205.

23. Lagenstein, I., Sternowsky, H. J., Iffland, E., and Blaschke, E. (1977): Intoxication with primidone: Continuous monitoring of serum primidone and its metabolites during forced diuresis. *Neuropaediatrie*, 8:190–195.

24. Leal, K. W., Rapport, R. L., Wilensky, A. J., and Friel, P. N. (1979): Single dose pharmacokinetics and anticonvulsant efficacy of primidone in mice. *Ann. Neurol.*, 5:470–474.

25. Martinez, G., and Snyder, R. D. (1973): Transplacental passage of primidone. *Neurology (Minneap.)*, 23:381–383.

26. McAuliffe, J. J., Sherwin, A. L., Leppik, I. E., Fayle, S. A., and Pippenger, C. E. (1977): Salivary levels of anticonvulsants: A practical approach to drug monitoring. *Neurology (Minneap.)*, 27:409–413.

27. McElhatton, P. R., Sullivan, F. M., and Toseland, P. A. (1977): The metabolism of primidone in nonpregnant and 14-day pregnant mice. *Xenobiotica*, 7:611–615.

28. McElhatton, P. R., Sullivan, F. M., and Toseland, P. A. (1977): Teratogenic activity and metabolism of primidone in the mouse. *Epilepsia*, 18:1–11.

29. Miyamoto, K., Seino, M., and Ikeda, Y. (1975): Consecutive determinations of the levels of twelve antiepileptic drugs in blood and cerebrospinal fluid. In: *Clinical Pharmacology of Antiepileptic Drugs*, edited by H. Schneider, D. Janz, C. Gardener-Thorpe, H. Meinardi, and A. L. Sherwin, pp. 321–329. Springer-Verlag, Berlin, Heidelberg, New York.

30. Oser, B. L., Melnick, M., and Hochberg, M. (1945): Study of methods of determining availability of vitamins in pharmaceutical products. *Indust. Eng. Chem.*, 17:405–411.

31. Pippenger, C. E., Garlock, C. M., Desaulmiers, C. W., and Sternberg, S. (1980): A rapid ultrafiltration technique for the determination of free antiepileptic drug concentrations in plasma. *Epilepsia* 21:187.

32. Reynolds, E. H., Mattson, R. H., and Gallagher, B. B. (1972): Relationships between serum and cerebrospinal fluid anticonvulsant drug and folic acid concentrations in epileptic patients. *Neurology (Minneap.)*, 22:841–844.

33. Rowan, J. A., Pippenger, C. E., McGregor, P. A., and French, J. H. (1975): Seizure activity and anticonvulsant drug concentrations. *Arch. Neurol.*, 32:281–288.

34. Schafer, H. (1976): Metabolic studies with primidone and 1,3-bis-(methoxy-methyl)-primidone. In: *Epileptology*, edited by D. Janz, pp. 139–145. George Thieme, Stuttgart.

35. Schafer, H. R., Luhrs, R., and Reith, H. (1977): Determination of phenobarbital and primidone derivatives and their metabolites in body fluid. In: *Antiepileptic Drug Monitoring*, edited by G. Gardener-Thorpe, D. Janz, H. Meinardi, and C. E. Pippenger, pp. 33–41. Pitman Medical, Tunbridge Wells, Kent.

36. Schmidt, D., and Kupferberg, H. S. (1975): Diphenylhydantoin, phenobarbital, and primidone in saliva, plasma, and cerebrospinal fluid. *Epilepsia*, 16:735–741.

37. Schottelius, D. D., and Fincham, R. W. (1977): Cerebrospinal fluid/serum ratios of primidone: Inferences to protein binding. *Epilepsia*, 18:291.

38. Swinyard, E. A., Tedeschi, D. H., and Goodman, L. S. (1954): Effect of liver damage and nephrectomy on anticonvulsant activity of mysoline and phenobarbital. *J. Am. Pharma. Assoc.*, 43:114–116.

39. Syversen, G. B., Morgan, J. P., Weintraub, M., and Myers, G. J. (1977): Acetazolamide-induced interference with primidone absorption. *Arch. Neurol.*, 34:80–84.

40. Thorpe, J. M. (1955): Physiological disposition of the anticonvulsant "Mysoline." In: *Congres Internaional de Biochimie. Resumé des Communications, Vol. 1*, p. 132. Société Belge Biochimie, Liege.

41. Troupin, A. S., and Friel, P. (1975): Anticonvulsant levels in saliva, serum and cerebrospinal fluid. *Epilepsia*, 16:223–227.

42. Zavadil, P., and Gallagher, B. B. (1976): Metabolism and excretion of ^{14}C-primidone in epileptic patients. In: *Epileptology*, edited by D. Janz, pp. 129–138. George Thieme, Stuttgart.

Antiepileptic Drugs, edited by D. M. Woodbury,
J. K. Penry, and C. E. Pippenger. Raven Press,
New York © 1982.

31

Primidone

Biotransformation

Dorothy D. Schottelius

The *in vivo* biotransformation of antiepileptic drugs has been and continues to be a subject of vital importance to the clinical utilization and therapeutic evaluation of these substances. When these compounds are converted to metabolites that possess anticonvulsant properties, the interpretation of pharmacological and clinical studies becomes more complex. Primidone is only one of the antiepileptic drugs that present us with these problems.

CHEMICAL ASPECTS OF METABOLISM

Metabolites and Metabolic Pathways

Phenylethylmalonamide (PEMA) was the first substance to be identified as a possible metabolic product of primidone when Bogue and Carrington (4) identified this compound in crystals present in rat urine. Formation of PEMA involves the opening of the pyrimidine ring and the concomitant loss of the internitrogen methylene bridge. Butler and Waddell (6), in 1956, published a report in which crystals of phenobarbital (PB) and *p*-hydroxyphenobarbital were isolated and identified from the urine of a dog who had 200 mg of primidone administered for 6 days. The same substances were identified in urine of a patient receiving 1 g of primidone. Phenobarbital was also identified in the plasma

of both dogs and humans when primidone was administered. Independently, Plaa et al. (19) had found evidence of the presence of a substance with the spectral characteristics of PB in the blood of patients and in the urine of rats receiving primidone. It was estimated (6) that the dog converted of the order of 15% of the administered dose of primidone to PB, a remarkably good approximation considering the laborious analytical techniques involved. Formation of the metabolites PEMA and PB is currently considered to represent the primary metabolic pathways in the biotransformation of primidone (Fig. 1). The substances α-phenylbutyramide, α-phenyl-γ-butyrolactone, and hydroxyprimidone have been identified in urine of patients taking primidone (see Chapter 30), but aside from the very small quantities present, no information is available concerning their importance in the metabolic pathways.

The pathway from primidone (PRM) to PB involves oxidation of the methylene group. Subsequent metabolism of PB to *p*-hydroxyphenobarbital has been discussed in Chapter 23.

PHARMACOLOGICAL ASPECTS OF METABOLISM

Swinyard et al. (21) provided the first evidence of the importance of the liver and the kidney to the metabolism of primidone when they

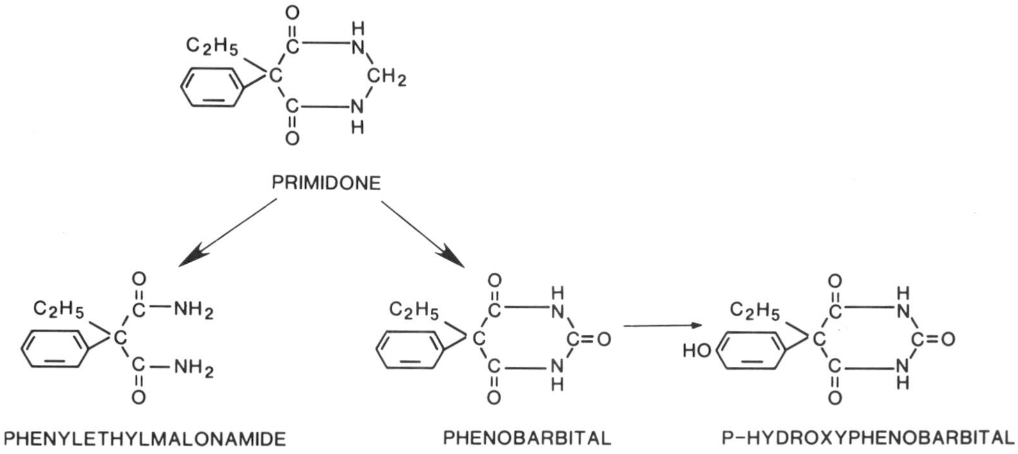

FIG. 1. Pathways of biotransformation of primidone. In addition to these pathways, there is evidence that primidone may be hydroxylated to form hydroxyprimidone. Primidone or PEMA may be further metabolized to α-phenylbutyramide.

investigated the effects of nephrectomy and liver damage on the potency and duration of anticonvulsant action. However, no suitable chemical analyses were yet available, and only PEMA was a suspected metabolite. The potency and duration of action of primidone and PB were compared in rats. The results indicated that liver damage increased the potency and duration of action of both compounds and were interpreted to mean that the liver was important for the degradation of these substances. Nephrectomy increased the potency and duration of action of primidone but not of PB. These authors concluded that the liver and the kidney appeared to be involved in the metabolism and excretion of primidone in rats.

After the finding that primidone was metabolized to PB, several studies (8,9,18) attempted to evaluate the relative importance of these pathways in man and animals, but these data are difficult to evaluate because of the analytical techniques used, the utilization of seizure control as an endpoint, and the presence of other anticonvulsant drugs. The metabolic pathways were investigated in the rabbit (9) by determining the amounts of metabolites excreted in urine following single and multiple oral doses of primidone. Approximately 20% of the single dose was excreted as unchanged primidone, 48% as PEMA, and 10% as PB (after correction for

conjugated hydroxyphenobarbital). Also, primidone was converted to PEMA more rapidly than to PB, since PEMA promptly appeared in the urine and rose to a peak at 30 hr, whereas the excretion of PB was delayed and peaked at 45 hr, well after the major part of the PRM had been excreted. This may suggest an initial delay in the formation of PB, and this conversion may be rate limited.

In six volunteers given a single 500-mg oral dose of primidone, PB could not be detected in the serum throughout a 48-hr sampling period (5). Two studies of patients (11,12) demonstrated a lag time for the appearance of PB in urine and serum and also provided evidence that PEMA was excreted in urine of man. The mean PB/PRM ratio was 2.8, and it was suggested that comedications could alter this ratio.

Another group of investigations provided further information concerning the metabolism of PRM in man and experimental animals. In man, PB increased linearly (with wide interindividual variability) with increasing primidone dosage (22). However, a 2.5-fold increase in primidone dosage resulted in a fourfold increase in serum primidone concentration and only a 50% increase in PB, which suggests a slow rate of PB formation (10). In contrast, PEMA increased directly with increments of primidone concentration. It should be noted that significant variability was present and that many of the subjects were receiving other antiepileptic medications.

In man, PEMA appeared in serum 2 hr after a single 500-mg dose of primidone, and PB was not present in the 24 hr in which two patients were studied following a first exposure to PRM (3). The appearance of PEMA and PB in the plasma of the rat occurred within 1 hr after oral dosing, and neither metabolite was detectable at doses below 62.5 mg/kg (2).

The influence of phenytoin on the metabolism of primidone to PB was shown by the finding of an enhanced conversion when these two drugs were taken concurrently (7). In steady state with regard to the pharmacokinetics of both primidone and PB and a narrow sampling time after dose, the PB/PRM ratio was 1.05 ± 0.20 when patients were taking PRM alone and was 4.35 ± 0.50 when patients were taking PRM and phenytoin. This interaction will be discussed more completely in Chapter 32. In the 15 patients taking primidone alone, there was no indication of saturability of the enzyme system responsible for the oxidation of PRM to PB. This work indicated that biotransformation studies of primidone in man and animals had been and would be complicated by the presence of other drugs.

The tissue location of the enzymes responsible for the biotransformation of PRM in man is presumed to be the liver; more definitive evidence of this was found in experimental animals. Perfusion studies of isolated rat liver showed that 98% of ^{14}C-primidone was recovered in perfusate, liver, and bile (1). The metabolites appeared before the first sample was obtained (30 min). At the end of 120 min, approximately 38% of the PRM remained; production of PB and its metabolites continued at a low rate throughout the perfusion and accounted for 15% of the PRM metabolized. The predominant metabolite was PEMA, which was equivalent to 79% of the PRM metabolized. Primidone metabolism was accelerated in the liver of rats pretreated with primidone or PB, with PB action the more potent.

The rate of disappearance of primidone from the perfusate approximated a first-order process

in each group with the following half-lives: control, 92 min; primidone-treated, 68 min; and PB treated, 28 min. The addition of PEMA (50 μg/ml) to the perfusates during the experiment caused marked breaks in the disappearance curves of PRM and half-life changes from 92 to 192 min in the control group, from 62 to 160 min in primidone-pretreated group, and from 28 to 38 min in the PB-pretreated group. The addition of PB (50 μg/ml) to the perfusate had no effect on the rate of primidone disappearance. The inhibitory effect of PEMA on primidone metabolism was rather weak, requiring addition of 65 to 75 μg/ml of PEMA to the perfusate to obtain sharp changes in the first-order decline of primidone. A later study in rabbits (13) with intravenous administration of the drugs gave somewhat different results. Again, the appearance of primidone, PEMA, and PB in the plasma was very rapid (within 5 min) after a 10 mg/kg injection, and the data for the plasma concentration were fitted with a four-compartment model consisting of a two-compartment model for primidone with attached one-compartment models each for PEMA and PB, each with first-order formation and elimination rate constants. From the data obtained in plasma and urine, it was concluded that 20% of the primidone dose was excreted unchanged, 40% was metabolized to PEMA, and 40% was metabolized to PB. Some evidence was presented that PEMA may be conjugated with glucuronide, but definitive identification was not completed.

Metabolism of PRM to PEMA and PB appears to occur very rapidly in the mouse as well (16,17), but the percentages of PRM converted to PEMA and PB cannot be estimated from the data available. From the linear portions of the log curves presented between 2 and 4 hr (16), it can be estimated that primidone disappeared at a rate of 3 μg/hr, PEMA appeared at a rate of 1.5 μg/hr, and PB appeared at a rate of 1.25 μg/hr. Therefore, approximately equivalent amounts of primidone were being converted to PEMA and PB.

Pregnancy (17) appeared to increase the rate of metabolism since the ratio of metabolites to parent compound increased with several different doses and a lesser percentage of PRM was present at 4 hr than at 1 hr in the pregnant mouse compared with the nonpregnant mouse. Domestic fowl (14) show a similar pattern to mouse, rat, and rabbit in the early appearance of PB following the intraperitoneal injection of primidone. Phenobarbital was present in the plasma 1 hr following the dose and gradually increased through 8 to 12 hr. At 12 hr, PRM had disappeared from the plasma. Only the guinea pig (8) apparently has a delay similar to man in the conversion of PRM to PB, a finding that should be pursued.

Primidone metabolism and excretion of ^{14}C-primidone were studied in adult epileptic patients to ascertain the metabolism of this compound to PEMA and PB (23). An intravenous infusion of ^{14}C-primidone was administered to two groups of subjects: group I who had no prior anticonvulsants and group II who were on daily doses of anticonvulsants. Plasma half-lives and urinary excretion of PEMA and metabolites were determined. The mean half-life of primidone in group I was approximately two times as long as that of group II. Urinary excretion of metabolites was followed by five 24-hr urine collections. During the first 24 hr, the percent of total dose excreted in each group was equivalent (I, 46.7%; II, 45.5%). However, there was a marked difference in the proportions of the three compounds excreted. In group I, unchanged PRM accounted for 90% of the total drug; PEMA, 4%; PB, 2.5%; and unidentified product 3%. In group II, unchanged primidone was 29%; PEMA, 22%; PB, 2.7%; and unidentified product, 6.1%. Primidone excretion continued throughout the entire 5 days, and the totals for the groups I and II, respectively, were as follows: percent of total dose excreted, 75.5% and 77.4%; unchanged primidone, 85% and 51.1%; PEMA, 8.7% and 36%; PB, 2.8% and 4.3%; unidentified product, 4% and 8.5%. The unidentified material was suspected to be hydroxyphenobarbital and its conjugates. This would indicate that in group I most of the primidone was excreted unchanged and the remainder was biotransformed almost equally to PEMA (8.7%) and PB (6.8%).

A study in children (15) done under markedly different experimental conditions produced somewhat different results. Twelve children who had been on the same dose of PRM for 3 months, of whom eight had been on phenytoin as well, were fasted overnight and given their last dose of primidone at least 16 hr prior to the test dose. Their entire daily dose of primidone was administered orally to determine the half-life, and urine was collected for 24 hr to determine formation of metabolites. The half-life of primidone ranged from 4.5 to 11 hr, so that the total daily dose was administered between 1.5 and 3.6 half-lives after the prior dose (primidone was not in steady-state conditions, whereas PEMA and PB probably were). The mean percent of daily dose recovered was as follows: unchanged primidone, 52.3%; PEMA, 45.2%; PB (total), 4.9%. There was great individual variation in the proportion of metabolites excreted, as indicated by the range of unchanged primidone (15.2%–65.9%), PEMA (16.5%–65.3%), and PB (1.1%–8.0%).

We have continued to investigate the biotransformation of primidone to PB in patients treated only with primidone for extended periods of time. These individuals (80 total) have been taking a mean dose of 9.7 ± 0.2 mg/kg for a mean period of 13.1 ± 2.4 months. Samples were obtained approximately 4 hr after a dose of primidone, and the mean PB/PRM ratio was 1.45 ± 0.1 (range, 0.1–5.1). Serum PB levels as a function of serum primidone levels are shown in Chapter 32 (see Fig. 1 of Chapter 32) where the linear regression equation is: serum PB level = 8.3 + 0.60 serum primidone level, with a correlation coefficient of 0.23. These 80 patients were divided into two groups based on PB concentration, and the data are shown in Fig. 2. In 49 of these patients, steady-state PB levels were less than 15 μg/ml (mean dose, 7.8 ± 0.4 mg/kg; mean time on dose, 10.3 ± 2.5 months). The mean serum primidone level was 10.9 ± 0.6 μg/ml, and serum PB level was 8.4 ± 0.06 μg/ml. The mean PB/PRM ratio was 0.87 ± 0.07. The data varied widely and showed no relationship between the serum levels of primidone and those of PB. In the 31 patients whose serum levels of PB exceeded 15 μg/ml (mean dose, 12.8 ± 0.6 mg/kg; mean

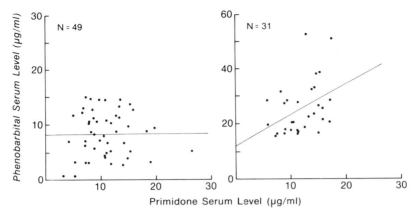

FIG. 2. Serum PB levels as a function of serum primidone levels from patients taking primidone as sole medication. Patients were maintained for a sufficient length of time to achieve steady state of both drugs. **Left:** data from individuals whose serum PB levels never exceeded 15 μg/ml: serum PB level = 8.2 + 0.02 serum primidone levels; correlation coefficient = 0.02. **Right:** data from individuals whose serum PB levels varied from 15.5 to 51.6 μg/ml; serum PB level = 12.5 + 1.08 serum primidone levels; correlation coefficient = 0.39.

time on dose, 12.6 ± 3.3 months), the situation appeared to be different. The mean serum primidone level was 11.6 ± 0.7 μg/ml and the serum PB level 25.4 ± 1.7 μg/ml. The mean PB/PRM ratio was 2.25 ± 0.1. Linear regression analysis indicated a more linear relationship between the serum levels of primidone and PB.

If one calculates regression lines of a plot of the individual ratio against the PB level (20) in these individuals, the variability is reduced, but little additional information is gained, as the slopes in both cases reflect the same trend. Because data on PEMA are lacking, the reasons for the differences in the PB/PRM ratios in these two groups are speculative. Further information about the biotransformation of primidone is indicated in view of the clinical results presented in Chapter 33.

SUMMARY

The principal site of biotransformation of primidone is, from all experimental data, the liver, as with many other drugs. The oxidation of primidone to PB is not an unusual biochemical pathway, but which enzyme system is utilized is unknown. The transformation of primidone to PEMA, which involves ring opening with the removal of a methylene bridge, also occurs by an unknown pathway. Since PEMA appears very rapidly in the serum of man and animals after an initial dose of primidone, enzyme induction apparently does not play a major role in this transformation. The considerable delay in appearance of PB in man, however, would indicate a role for enzyme induction in this pathway.

Investigations of the rate, extent, and proportion of biotransformation of primidone are complicated by differences and variability in plasma half-lives of primidone, PEMA, and PB as well as by such factors as single-dose and chronic administration, interaction among the three compounds, and enzyme induction. Experiments in animals apparently cannot be extrapolated to the situation in humans since the metabolites appear at different times in different species and the extent of biotransformation in these species is uncertain. On the basis of current information in man, it appears that a large percentage of primidone is excreted unchanged. The proportion that is transformed to either PEMA or PB is variable, but the biotransformation to PB seemingly occurs in two distinct patterns when patients have been on chronic doses of primidone as a sole drug. Further information is necessary to delineate the mechanism of this transformation since it is inferred entirely on the basis of serum levels of unchanged primidone and PB without data concerning PEMA concentrations. More complete investigations of the biotransformation of PRM would be of value in the clinical utilization of this drug.

ACKNOWLEDGMENT

Original data presented in this chapter were obtained from studies performed in the Department of Neurology, University of Iowa Hospitals, with the assistance of Dr. R. W. Fincham and other colleagues in the department.

REFERENCES

1. Alvin, J., Gohr, E., and Bush, M. T. (1975): Study of the hepatic metabolism of primidone by improved technology. *J. Pharmacol. Exp. Ther.*, 194:117–125.
2. Baumel, I. P., Gallagher, B. B., DiMicco, J., and Goico, H. (1973): Metabolism and anticonvulsant properties of primidone in the rat. *J. Pharmacol. Exp. Ther.*, 186:305–314.
3. Baumel, I. P., Gallagher, B. B., and Mattson, R. H. (1972): Phenylethylmalonamide. An important metabolite of primidone. *Arch. Neurol.*, 27:34–41.
4. Bogue, J. Y., and Carrington, H. C. (1952): Personal communication cited by Goodman, L. S., Swinyard, E. A., Brown, W. C., Schiffman, D. O., Grewal, M. S., and Bliss, E. L. (1953): Anticonvulsant properties of 5-phenyl-5-ethyl hexahydropyrimidine-4-6-dione (Mysoline), a new antiepileptic. *J. Pharmacol. Exp. Ther.*, 108:428–436.
5. Booker, H. E., Hosokowa, K., Burdette, R. D., and Darcey, B. (1970): A clinical study of serum primidone levels. *Epilepsia* 11:395–402.
6. Butler, T. C., and Waddell, W. J. (1956): Metabolic conversion of primidone (Mysoline) to phenobarbital. *Proc. Soc. Exp. Biol. Med.*, 93:544–546.
7. Fincham, R. W., Schottelius, D. D., and Sahs, A. L. (1974): The influence of diphenylhydantoin on primidone metabolism. *Arch. Neurol.*, 30:259–262.
8. Frey, H. H., and Hahn, I. (1960): Untersuchungen über die Bedentung des durch Biotransformation gebildeten Phenobarbital für die antikonvulsive Wirkung von Primidon. *Arch. Int. Pharmacodyn. Ther.*, 128:281–290.
9. Fujimoto, J. M., Mason, W. H., and Murphy, M. (1968): Urinary excretion of primidone and its metabolites in rabbits. *J. Pharmacol. Exp. Ther.*, 159:379–388.
10. Gallagher, B. B., and Baumel, I. P. (1972): Primidone—Biotransformation. In: *Antiepileptic Drugs*, edited by D. M. Woodbury, J. K. Penry, and R. D. Schmidt, pp. 361–366. Raven Press, New York.
11. Huisman, J. W. (1968): Metabolisme en werking van het anti-epilepticum primidone bij de mens. *Pharm. Weekbl.*, 103:573–600.
12. Huisman, J. W. (1969): Disposition of primidone in man: An example of autoinduction of a human enzyme system? *Pharm. Weekbl.*, 104:799–802.
13. Hunt, R. J., and Miller, K. W. (1978): Disposition of primidone phenylethylmalonamide, on phenobarbital in the rabbit. *Drug Metab. Dispos.*, 6:75–81.
14. Johnson, D. D., Davis, H. L., and Crawford, R. D. (1978): Epileptiform seizures in domestic fowl. VIII. Anticonvulsant activity of primidone and its metabolites, phenobarbital and phenylethylmalonamide. *Can. J. Physiol. Pharmacol.*, 56:630–633.
15. Kauffman, R. E., Habersang, R., and Lansky, L. (1977): Kinetics of primidone metabolism and excretion in children. *Clin. Pharmacol. Ther.*, 22:200–205.
16. Leal, K. W., Rapport, R. L., Wilensky, A. J., and Friel, P. N. (1979): Single dose pharmacokinetics and anticonvulsant efficacy of primidone in mice. *Ann. Neurol.*, 5:470–474.
17. McElhatton, P. R., Sullivan, F. M., and Toseland, P. A. (1977): The metabolism of primidone in nonpregnant and 14-day pregnant mice. *Xenobiotica*, 7:611–615.
18. Olesen, O. V., and Dam, M. (1967): The metabolic conversion of primidone (Mysoline) to phenobarbitone in patients under long-term treatment. *Acta Neurol. Scand.*, 43:348–356.
19. Plaa, G. L., Fuijimoto, J. M., and Hine, C. H. (1958): Intoxication from primidone due to its biotransformation to phenobarbital. *J.A.M.A.*, 168:1769–1770.
20. Ruf, P., and Saur, R. (1977): Influence of phenobarbital on the serum level of phenytoin and effect of phenytoin on primidone metabolism. In: *Epilepsy, the Eighth International Symposium*, edited by J. K. Penry, pp. 147–150. Raven Press, New York.
21. Swinyard, E. A., Tedeschi, D. H., and Goodman, L. S. (1954): Effects of liver damage and nephrectomy on anticonvulsant activity of Mysoline and phenobarbital. *J. Am. Pharm. Assoc.*, 43:114–116.
22. Travers, R. D., Reynolds, E. H., and Gallagher, B. B. (1972): Variation in response to anticonvulsants in a group of epileptic patients. *Arch. Neurol.*, 27:29–33.
23. Zavadil, P., and Gallagher, B. B. (1976): Metabolism and excretion of ^{14}C-primidone in epileptic patients. In: *Epileptology*, edited by D. Janz, pp. 129–139. George Thieme, Stuttgart.

Antiepileptic Drugs, edited by D. M. Woodbury,
J. K. Penry, and C. E. Pippenger. Raven Press,
New York © 1982.

32

Primidone

Interactions with Other Drugs

R. W. Fincham and Dorothy D. Schottelius

As with all other aspects of the pharmacology of primidone (PRM), the subject of drug interactions with this compound is complicated by its biotransformation to two active metabolites—phenobarbital (PB) and phenylethylmalonamide (PEMA). We must consider, therefore, the interactions among these three compounds as well as possible interactions of other drugs with these three substances. Primidone, in common with most of the other antiepileptic drugs, has a narrow therapeutic range, and in order to control seizures, it is often necessary to prescribe a dose nearly as high as one that produces dose-related toxic effects. Unlike many of the other antiepileptic drugs, primidone requires that we be concerned about the therapeutic ranges of two other substances, their toxic manifestations, and the possible contribution of these metabolites to the total therapeutic and toxic activity of the parent compound. We shall present investigations in both humans and experimental animals that provide information about drug interactions involving PRM, PB, PEMA, and other drugs that may influence this compound. We shall also consider reported instances of primidone's influence on the efficacy of other drugs. Since PRM and PB appear to be inducers of enzyme activity, their influence on other drugs may be of importance.

MANIFESTATIONS OF DRUG INTERACTIONS

Alterations in plasma drug concentrations, whether accompanied by clinical manifestations or not, are reliable indicators of drug interactions in the case of PRM. Increasing frequency of seizures when plasma PRM levels are lowered or disturbance of cortical and cerebellar function when plasma levels of the drug increase may be immediately manifested clinically or may be delayed for a variable length of time. Because of interindividual variability in all of the pharmacokinetic parameters, utilization of plasma drug level concentrations of PRM, PB, and PEMA will be assisted if base-line data are available when investigating possible drug interactions. This will enable the investigator to determine which of the three substances may be responsible for the clinical manifestations.

INTERACTIONS OF PRM, PB, AND PEMA

The possibility that the total activity of PRM might be influenced by the interaction of PB and PEMA was suggested by studies of the effect of combinations of these two substances on seizure thresholds in rats (3,9). It was noted that

PEMA in doses normally without anticonvulsant activity augmented the activity of PB on two experimental measures of seizure threshold. Since the effect was not equal, it was suggested that either separate neural mechanisms are involved or PEMA exerts quantifiably disparate effects in diverse areas of the central nervous system. Additional evidence of the possibility that PEMA has an effect on hepatic microsomal enzymes was the finding that it significantly prolonged hexabarbital sleeping time. These results suggested a possible synergistic interaction between PEMA and PB.

Studies in the rat (2) gave some indications of interaction among PRM, PEMA, and PB with respect to anticonvulsant potency.

Several findings have been reported in man that indicate the possibility of interactions of these substances. The delayed appearance of PEMA and PB in the plasma of man (3,4) and the influence of repeated administration (8,12,26) on that delay suggest that an alteration in the enzyme systems responsible for the biotransformation of PRM may be influenced by interactions among all three of these compounds. Adverse effects on the central nervous system that occur on initiation of therapy have been found to be nonexistent or greatly alleviated when the individual has had prior treatment with PRM or PB (9). Our finding of a different relationship in the PB/PRM ratio when the steady-state serum PB levels were above or below 15 μg/ml may be indicative of interactions at the level of enzyme systems responsible for biotransformation of PRM (see Fig. 2 of Chapter 31).

These findings in man are supported by the observations of Alvin et al. (1) in isolated perfused rat liver. Rats were pretreated with daily doses (50 mg/kg, intraperitoneal injection) of either PRM or PB for 4 days prior to removal of the liver for perfusion studies. Phenobarbital pretreatment greatly accelerated the rate of PRM metabolism, and pretreatment with PRM increased it to a lesser extent. There was no indication of a differential induction of the pathways. In addition, when PEMA or PB (50 μg/ml) was added directly to liver perfusates, PEMA reduced the rate of PRM metabolism, but PB

had no effect. The authors concluded that biotransformation of PRM may be simultaneously influenced by the processes of metabolite induction (PB) and metabolite inhibition (PEMA). Although it is unwise to extrapolate findings from experimental animals to man, the probability of such interactions in man is supported by the earlier findings of possible interactions. Until more definitive information is obtained in man, we can only speculate that some of the interindividual variability in half-lives, plasma concentrations, and changes in excretory patterns of PRM, PEMA, and PB is the result of the interactions of these three substances.

INTERACTIONS OF PRIMIDONE WITH OTHER DRUGS

Altered Biotransformation

Phenytoin

Fincham et al. (8) reported that phenytoin (PHT) apparently promoted the induction of the enzyme system responsible for the oxidation of PRM to PB. The possibility that PHT interfered with the hydroxylation or renal excretion of PB was also entertained. They found a significant difference in the PB/PRM ratio between patients taking only PRM (1.05 $\pm$ 0.20) and those taking PRM and PHT (4.35 $\pm$ 0.50). We have continued to examine this interaction, and our findings are illustrated in Figs. 1 and 2 and Table 1. All patients involved in these studies were in steady state with respect to PRM, PB, and PHT, having been on the same dose of drugs for many months and, in some instances, years. Blood samples were obtained 2 to 4 hr after the last dose of PRM. In contrast to the data of Reynolds and colleagues (17,18), who published similar findings concerning the PB/PRM ratios (1.57 $\pm$ 0.17, PRM only; 2.20 $\pm$ 0.12, PRM and PHT), our original data (8) did not show a correlation between the PB/PRM ratio and serum PHT levels. Unlike our patients, some of the patients in the study (17,18) were taking other anticonvulsant or psychotropic drugs, which may

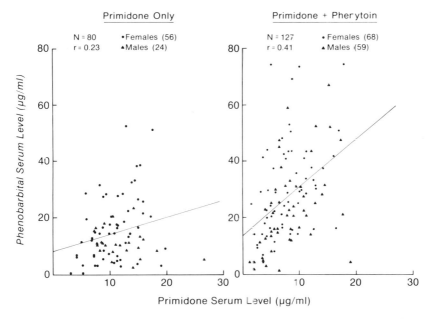

FIG. 1. Serum phenobarbital levels as a function of serum primidone levels. Linear regression analysis: for PRM only, serum PB level = 8.3 + 0.6 serum PRM level; for PRM + PHT, serum PB level = 13.6 + 1.7 serum PRM level.

have exerted an influence on the PB/PRM ratio and correlation with serum PHT levels.

In the 127 patients we have currently analyzed, there may be a weak correlation between these two. When the PB/PRM ratio was plotted versus the serum PHT level, the linear regression line indicated that PB/PRM = 3.2 + 0.05 serum PHT level, with a correlation coefficient of 0.19. This comparison, as do the comparisons illustrated in Figs. 1 and 2, shows a great deal of interindividual variability. As previously reported (8), the primidone dosage did not influence the PB/PRM ratio in either the group treated with PRM only or the group treated with PRM and PHT.

Schmidt (20) also examined the interaction of PHT and PRM in 28 patients receiving primidone alone and in 16 receiving both PRM and PHT and found a similar difference in PB/PRM ratios between the two groups (1.6 ± 0.2, PRM alone; 4.2 ± 0.7, PRM and PHT). Also undertaken was a longitudinal study of patients on PRM therapy in which PHT was added to the regimen. In both cases, serum PB levels increased with rising serum PHT levels, although

the PRM levels remained unchanged; consequently, the resulting rise in PB/PRM ratio was caused by increasing PB concentrations. This increase in PB/PRM ratio persisted during the 30 to 70 days of observation and was considered to result from an inhibition of the metabolism and/or excretion of PB and not from induction of the enzymes that oxidize PRM to PB.

There is evidence, from both patients and experimental animals (16,19), that PHT may inhibit the metabolism or impair the renal excretion of PB. This effect of PHT on PB metabolism or excretion was not confirmed in a later investigation (5) in which comparable serum PB levels were found between two groups of patients when PHT was present and when it was absent. This study found an increase in PB levels and an increase in PB/PRM ratio when comparing patients taking PRM only or PRM and PHT. There was no significant relationship between serum PHT levels and PB/PRM ratio in the patients taking both medications.

There is a contrast in urinary excretion pattern among groups taking PRM only and PRM plus a variety of comedications (26). The latter

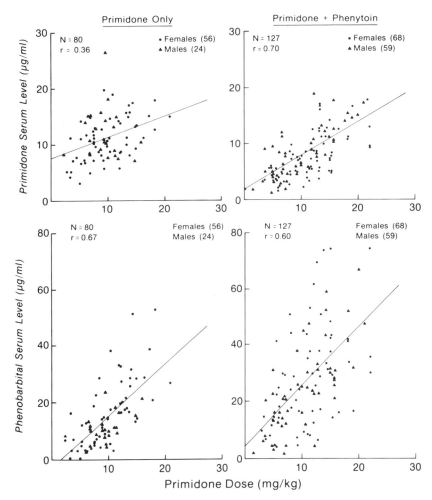

FIG. 2. Serum PB and PRM concentrations as a function of PRM dose. Primidone only: **upper left,** serum PRM level = 7.6 + 0.38 PRM dose; **lower left,** serum PB level = −3.0 + 1.8 PRM dose. PRM + PHT: **upper right,** serum PRM level = 1.6 + 0.6 PRM dose; **lower right,** serum PB level = 4.9 + 2.07 PRM dose.

TABLE 1. *Effect of phenytoin on primidone biotransformation*

	Primidone only	Primidone and phenytoin
No. of patients	80	127
PRM dose (mg/kg)	9.7 ± 0.2[a]	10.6 ± 0.4
PHT dose (mg/kg)	—	4.8 ± 0.1
Serum PHT level (μg/ml)	—	12.1 ± 0.1
Serum PRM level (μg/ml)	11.3 ± 0.2	8.1 ± 0.4
Serum PB level (μg/ml)	15.0 ± 0.4	27.2 ± 1.4
PB/PRM ratio	1.45 ± 0.10	3.82 ± 0.24

[a]Mean ± standard error.

group excreted less unchanged PRM and more PEMA and PB, and a large percentage of the dose was excreted at a later time (days 4 and 5). Both of these findings suggest that the biotransformation of PRM to PEMA and PB is enhanced by comedications and that disposal of the metabolites is not inhibited.

Only scattered reports are available concerning the interaction of PRM and PHT in children. One report (24) suggested that there is a decrease in serum PHT levels with concomitant administration of PRM and PHT; the possible alteration in PB levels in these instances was not investigated. Kauffman et al. (15) stated that this interaction between PHT and PRM was not found in children, and there was no correlation between the rate constant for metabolism and the presence or absence of concomitant PHT therapy. The calculated mean values for the children treated with PRM only or PRM and PHT are as follows: PB production, PRM only 0.0037, PRM and PHT 0.0049; PEMA production, PRM only 0.0310, PRM and PHT 0.0480. The ratio of PB/PRM in children cannot be calculated or compared to that in adults because of the difference in sampling time in relation to the last dose of PRM and lack of data.

The effects of phenytoin pretreatment on the metabolism of primidone has been investigated in the rabbit (14). Rabbits were treated for 5 days with PHT (40 mg/day, intravenous) and then with PRM (10 mg/kg intravenous), with each animal serving as its own control in a crossover fashion. Primidone was eliminated more rapidly after PHT pretreatment, and a smaller fraction was excreted unchanged in the urine. Pretreatment with PHT appeared to accelerate the rate of formation of PB and PEMA, and both were eliminated more rapidly. The total body clearance of PRM was increased almost twofold in the rabbit, a finding that would appear to be similar to that in man (5). It was thought that this finding in the rabbit conflicted with the mechanism of interaction in man in which PB levels increase and PRM levels remain constant with PHT treatment (5,8). The latter findings, however, are based on chronic administration of PRM, whereas the rabbit data are from a single intravenous injection of PRM.

From all of the evidence obtained in these various investigations under widely varying experimental conditions, the findings are somewhat more in favor of altered PRM biotransformation with PHT treatment than inhibition of metabolism or impaired renal excretion of PB or PEMA. Whichever mechanism is responsible for the increased PB/PRM ratio is not critical to ascertain before deciding that this is a clinically significant finding. We have observed several instances of PB intoxication when PRM

and PHT were used at usual or below therapeutic dosages, and the marked interindividual variability in serum drug levels indicated in Fig. 2 makes it impossible to predict a "standard" regimen when these drugs are combined. Presence of either renal or liver disease could contribute to an exaggeration of this interaction. It is possible that this interaction could be useful clinically to obtain therapeutic concentrations of three anticonvulsant substances, but it can only be achieved by careful and continuous monitoring of serum drug levels.

Ethosuximide

The combination of ethosuximide and PRM has been investigated by Schmidt (20), and no difference was found in the PB/PRM ratio.

Carbamazepine

Reports in both animals (7) and humans (5,26) have indicated that carbamazepine increases the metabolism of primidone to its metabolites. An apparent opposite effect was found with the reported increase in serum primidone levels in patients taking carbamazepine, but the study was not continued for a sufficient period to provide a definitive answer concerning increases or decreases in metabolism of primidone (6). Primidone has been reported to lower the serum level of carbamazepine (21). This interaction may be of clinical significance, since the two drugs are frequently used together. Insufficient data are available to prove an increased conversion of PRM to PB, but this possibility, along with lower carbamazepine levels than expected, indicates that monitoring of serum drug levels is necessary to achieve maximum therapeutic benefit when these drugs are used in combination.

Isoniazid

A clinical case of inhibition of PRM biotransformation by isoniazid was thoroughly studied by Sutton and Kupferberg (22). The steady-state primidone levels in this patient increased an average of 12.2 µg/ml when the two drugs were given simultaneously, and the plasma half-life of PRM increased from 8.7 hr to 14 hr. Serum levels of PB and PEMA fell during simultaneous treatment. There was some indication that sodium aminosalicylate may have potentiated the inhibition of PRM metabolism.

Valproic Acid

Windorfer et al. (25) reported that only a few days after valproic acid (VPA) was added to the medication regimen of patients, marked increases were found in serum PRM levels, which, in most cases, returned to original levels after 1 to 3 months. There was no information concerning dose–sample interval or PB levels, so it is difficult to interpret these alterations. We have examined the influence of the addition of VPA to therapeutic regimens of 16 patients in whom all medications were in steady state prior to the addition and doses of all other medications remained the same. Only two of these individuals were taking PRM as a sole medication; the other 14 were also taking PHT and/or carbamazepine. None were taking PB. Blood samples were obtained between 1.5 and 4 hr after the primidone dose, and the same dose–sample interval was utilized in the samples obtained before and after the addition of VPA to the regimen. Our results showed no significant changes in PRM or PB levels (PRM before VPA, 9.4 ± 0.7 μg/ml; PRM after VPA, 8.6 ± 0.6 μg/ml; PB before VPA, 26.7 ± 1.5 μg/ml; PB after VPA, 29.2 ± 2.0 μg/ml). The mean PB/PRM ratios were 3.01 ± 0.31 before VPA and 3.56 ± 1.4 after VPA. Interindividual variability was great: some individuals showed marked changes in serum PRM and PB levels and PB/PRM ratio, which indicated an increase in biotransformation of PRM. A greater number of patients who are taking PRM alone must be investigated to determine if this may become a clinically significant interaction.

Miscellaneous

When added to PRM therapy, ethylphenacemide (13) resulted in both an increase and a decrease in serum PRM levels in two patients, but interpretation of these findings is difficult because other medications were also used. Methylphenidate (11) was implicated in the alteration of PRM biotransformation in one child in whom serum PRM levels increased from 4.4 to 21.5 μg/ml when this drug was added to a regimen of PRM and PHT. Serum PB levels also increased from 23.0 to 34.4 μg/ml.

Altered Absorption

One report suggests that absorption may have been impaired in one of three patients tested when PRM and acetazolamide were given simultaneously (23). When these two drugs were administered together, only trace amounts of PRM and its metabolites were detectable in serum and urine; when PRM was given alone, expected levels of both were found in serum and urine.

SUMMARY

Considering the fact that polypharmacy is widespread and that many of the drugs utilized have been shown to be capable of inducing liver enzymes responsible for biotransformation, it is not surprising that more and more drug interactions are observed. Of those we have considered with PRM, the PHT interaction has had the most investigation and is clearly important clinically because of the frequency with which these two compounds have been combined in therapeutic regimens. This does not imply that the interaction will always occur to the same magnitude, and indeed it does not, as is apparent from the interindividual variability noted. It also does not imply that the other interactions are not important clinically because the frequency with which they occur may not be as prevalent as the interaction between PRM and PHT.

All of the information presented concerning the interactions of PRM, whether between the parent compound and its metabolites or between PRM and other drugs, clearly points out the necessity and benefits of serum drug level monitoring to prevent intoxications and to gain maximum therapeutic effect of this drug.

ACKNOWLEDGMENT

Original data presented in this chapter were obtained from studies performed in the Department of Neurology, University of Iowa Hospitals, with the assistance of our colleagues in that department.

REFERENCES

1. Alvin, J., Goh, E., and Bush, M. T. (1975): Study of the hepatic metabolism of primidone by improved methodology. *J. Pharmacol. Exp. Ther.*, 194:117–125.
2. Baumel, I. P., Gallagher, B. B., DiMicco, J., and Goico, H. (1973): Metabolism and anticonvulsant properties of primidone in the rat. *J. Pharmacol. Exp. Ther.*, 180:305–314.
3. Baumel, I. P., Gallagher, B. B., and Mattson, R. H. (1972): Phenylethylmalonamide (PEMA). An important metabolite of primidone. *Arch. Neurol.*, 27:34–41.
4. Booker, H. E., Hosokowa, K., Burdette, R. D., and Darcey, B. (1970): A clinical study of serum primidone levels. *Epilepsia*, 11:395–402.
5. Callaghan, N., Feeley, M., Duggan, F., O'Callaghan, M., and Sheldrup, J. (1977): The effect of anticonvulsant drugs which induce liver microsomal enzymes on derived and ingested phenobarbital levels. *Acta Neurol. Scand.*, 56:1–6.
6. Cereghino, J. J., Van Meter, J. C., Brock, J. T., Penry, J. K., Smith, L. D., and White, B. G. (1973): Preliminary observations of serum carbamazepine concentration in epileptic patients. *Neurology (Minneap.)*, 23:357–366.
7. DiMicco, J. A., and Gallagher, B. B. (1975): Induction of primidone metabolism in rat liver by anticonvulsants. *Fed. Proc.*, 34:726.
8. Fincham, R. W., Schottelius, D. D., and Sahs, A. L. (1974): The influence of diphenylhydantoin on primidone metabolism. *Arch. Neurol.*, 30:259–262.
9. Gallagher, B. B., and Baumel, I. P. (1972): Primidone—interaction with other drugs. In: *Antiepileptic Drugs*, edited by D. M. Woodbury, J. K. Penry, and R. P. Schmidt, pp. 367–371. Raven Press, New York.
10. Gallagher, B. B., Baumel, I. P., and Mattson, R. H. (1972): Metabolic disposition of primidone and its metabolites in epileptic subjects after single and repeated administration. *Neurology (Minneap.)*, 22:1186–1192.
11. Garrettson, L. K., Perel, J. M., and Dayton, P. G. (1969): Methylphenidate interaction with both anticonvulsants and ethyl biscoumacetate. *J.A.M.A.*, 207:2053–2056.
12. Huisman, J. W., (1969): Disposition of primidone in

man: An example of autoinduction of a human enzyme system? *Pharm. Weekbl.*, 104:799–802.
13. Huisman, J. W., vanHeycopten, H., and van Zijl, C. H. (1970): Influence of ethylphenacemide on serum levels of other antiepileptic drugs. *Epilepsia*, 11:207–215.
14. Hunt, R. J., and Miller, K. W. (1978): Disposition of primidone, phenylethylmalonamide, and phenobarbital in the rabbit. *Drug Metab. Dispos.*, 6:75–81.
15. Kauffman, R. E., Habersang, R., and Lansky, L. (1977): Kinetics of primidone metabolism and excretion in children. *Clin. Pharmacol. Ther.*, 22:200–205.
16. Morselli, P. L., Rizzo, M., and Garratin, S. (1971): Interaction between phenobarbital and diphenylhydantoin in animals and in epileptic patients. *Ann. N.Y. Acad. Sci.*, 179:88–107.
17. Reynolds, E. H. (1975): Longitudinal studies of antiepileptic drug levels. Preliminary observations: Interaction of phenytoin and primidone. In: *Clinical Pharmacology of Antiepileptic Drugs*, edited by H. Schneider, D. Janz, C. Gardner-Thorpe, H. Meinardi, and A. L. Sherwin. pp. 79–85. Springer-Verlag, Berlin, Heidelberg, New York.
18. Reynolds, E. H., Fenton, G., Fenwick, P., Johnson, A. L., and Laundy, M. (1975): Interaction of phenytoin and primidone. *Br. Med. J.*, 14:594–595.
19. Rizzo, M., Morselli, P. L., and Garratin, S. (1971): Further observations on the interactions between phenobarbital and diphenylhydantoin during clinical treatment in the rat. *Biochem. Pharmacol.*, 18:449–454.
20. Schmidt, D. (1975): The effect of phenytoin and ethosuximide on primidone metabolism in patients with epilepsy. *J. Neurol.*, 209:115–123.
21. Schneider, H. (1975): Carbamazepine: The influence of other antiepileptic drugs on its serum level. In: *Clinical Pharmacology of Antiepileptic Drugs*, edited by H. Schneider, D. Janz, C. Gardner-Thorpe, H. Meinardi, and A. L. Sherwin, pp. 189–196, Springer-Verlag, Berlin, Heidelberg, New York.
22. Sutton, G., and Kupferberg, H. J. (1975): Isoniazid as an inhibitor of primidone metabolism. *Neurology (Minneap.)*, 25:1179–1181.
23. Syverson, G. B., Morgan, J. P., Weintraub, M., and Myers, G. J. (1977): Acetozolamide-induced interference with primidone absorption. *Arch. Neurol.*, 34:80–84.
24. Windorfer, A., and Sauer, W. (1977): Drug interactions during anticonvulsant therapy in childhood: Diphenylhydantoin, primidone, phenobarbitone, clonazepam, nitrazepam, carbamazepine and dipropylacetate. *Neuropaediatrie*, 8:29–41.
25. Windorfer, A., Sauer, W., and Gadeke, R. (1975): Elevation of diphenylhydantoin and primidone serum concentrations by addition of dipropylacetate, a new anticonvulsant drug. *Acta Paediatr. Scand.*, 64:771–772
26. Zavadil, P., and Gallagher, B. B. (1976): Metabolism and excretion of ^{14}C-primidone in epileptic patients. In: *Epileptology*, edited by D. Janz, pp. 129–138. Georg Thieme, Stuttgart.

Antiepileptic Drugs, edited by D. M. Woodbury,
J. K. Penry, and C. E. Pippenger. Raven Press,
New York © 1982.

33

Primidone

Relation of Plasma Concentration to Seizure Control

R. W. Fincham and Dorothy D. Schottelius

STUDIES OF PRIMIDONE AS A POTENTIAL ANTICONVULSANT

Correlation of the plasma concentration of primidone (PRM) with the clinical control of seizures is complicated by a variety of unsettled issues. A primary concern centers on whether primidone itself is an effective anticonvulsant. Its metabolites including phenylethylmalonamide (PEMA) (6), which has been determined to possess at least weak anticonvulsant actions in animals (2,3,21,22), and phenobarbital (PB) (13), a well-known and potent anticonvulsant drug.

Those who doubt that primidone is an effective anticonvulsant agent emphasize that its conversion to phenobarbital accounts for its antiepileptic activity (4,30,31,40,50). However, Booker (8) has suggested that a primary anticonvulsant property not be denied for PRM simply because derived phenobarbital is present. Conflicting evidence has been cited to support each of these views in both human and animal studies.

Animal Studies

Bogue and Carrington (5) reported that PRM was more effective than PB in controlling seizures induced in rats by electroshock and pen-

tylenetetrazole stimulation. Goodman et al. (28) found PRM to be effective in treating maximal electroshock seizures (MES) in rats but less effective than PB when tested in other experimental models of epilepsy.

Swinyard et al. (62) found that the potency of PRM in preventing the tonic extensor component in the MES model was enhanced by 50% in rats with liver damage or in rats that had undergone bilateral nephrectomy. In addition, both of these procedures prolonged the anticonvulsant action of PRM fourfold. Blocking the major excretory pathway for PRM via nephrectomy and impairing hepatic function where the conversion of PRM to PB takes place suggest that the antiepileptic effect of PRM in these two experimental situations relates to PRM and not to its metabolites.

Frey and Hahn (20) found greater anticonvulsant effect on pentylenetetrazol-induced seizures in dogs and mice when they were treated with PRM and had serum levels of derived PB that were significantly lower than serum PB levels in another group of animals that had been treated with PB. They concluded that about 50% of the anticonvulsant effect of PRM related to derived PB. These same authors reported that only a trace of PB was found in the serum and none in the bile of guinea pigs 6 to 12 hr after oral doses of 150 mg/kg of PRM. The guinea pigs were noted to receive no protection from PRM against pentylenetetrazol-induced seizures, which indicated that PRM was ineffective in this model.

Gallagher et al. (25) studied seizures induced in albino rats by the volatile convulsant hexafluorodiethyl ether. The effectiveness of PRM in elevating the threshold for tonic–clonic seizures was comparable to that of a dose of PB that produced a plasma PB concentration 63% higher than the PB concentration derived from PRM. In this setting, PRM appeared to be more effective than PB as an anticonvulsant drug.

Baumel et al. (2) studied the effectiveness of PRM and its metabolites in the control of seizures in rats induced by (a) hexafluorodiethyl ether, (b) pentylenetetrazol, and (c) MES. Brain and plasma levels of PRM, PEMA, and PB were monitored. The time course of protection against the chemically induced seizures correlated best with the appearance of PB and PEMA in the brain. However, complete control of MES was achieved when brain and plasma levels of PRM were 1 μg/g or less, and PB and PEMA were not detectable.

Lockhard et al. (42) studied the effectiveness of PRM, PB, and phenytoin in controlling seizures induced in nine monkeys by injection of aluminum hydroxide gel beneath the pia in the left precentral and postcentral gyri. The effectiveness of these three drugs was evaluated for 8 months with a Latin square experimental design, and in this setting all three drugs were found to be effective. The average number of seizures in the 2-week control period was 56; in 2 weeks of PB therapy, 28; in 2 weeks of phenytoin therapy, 23; and in 2 weeks of primidone therapy, 13. Plasma primidone levels ranged between a trace and 4 μg/ml, and the plasma concentrations of derived PB were very close to plasma PB levels recorded during PB therapy.

Johnson et al. (35) found PRM to be an effective anticonvulsant against seizures induced in epileptic fowl by exposure to intermittent photic stimulation. Blockade of PRM conversion to PB by the metabolic inhibitor SKF-525A did not impair the effectiveness of PRM in this model.

Leal et al. (40), performing single-dose studies of PRM, PB, and PEMA and using the MES test in mice, concluded from the half-life, potency, peak anticonvulsant effect, and effective dose curves of these compounds that the anticonvulsant effect of short-term orally administered PRM was from derived PB.

Experimental findings of these varied studies in animal models of epilepsy do not uniformly show PRM to be an effective anticonvulsant, but, certainly, many of them do provide good evidence that PRM itself is an effective antiepileptic drug.

Human Studies

Unequivocal evidence identifying a drug as an effective anticonvulsant in humans is best supported by carefully controlled clinical trials (16,17,51,52). There are currently only a limited number of such evaluations for PRM. The clinical trials of PRM completed before 1956 did not recognize PB as a major metabolite, but they did give important insights into the toxicity and dosage of primidone. Although these studies were not carefully controlled, it seems fair to conclude that they did find PRM (or its metabolites) to be a useful antiepileptic drug. Subsequent studies in humans have often, and importantly, included measures of serum concentrations of PRM and its metabolites to clarify its pharmacokinetic properties and hence improve insights into both its mechanism of action and its clinical utilization.

An important concern was recently raised by Leal et al. (40) when they reported that "little or no" PRM was present in brain tissue obtained from six patients who were operated on for intractable epilepsy and who were reported to have been receiving long-term therapy with PRM. Houghton et al. (34) reported contrasting findings in 11 patients in whom they found a significant correlation between the concentration of PRM in brain and plasma.

Further clinical support for the action of PRM in the brain is found in instances of toxicity that may appear within 30 min to 2 hr after ingestion of the initial dose of PRM. This is indicated by such symptoms as drowsiness, ataxia, feelings of unreality, and intoxication similar to inebriation with alcohol (24,63). All of these imply that brain function is affected by PRM. Monitoring of PRM, PEMA, and PB concentrations in serum of patients when toxicity occurred showed only the presence of PRM (24,67). These clinical observations provide convincing indirect evidence that PRM does indeed rapidly gain access to the brain but that PB may not appear for 96 hr after the initial dose of PRM (23).

Handley and Stewart (32) reported the first clinical investigation of PRM in 1952. Subsequent clinical reports followed in which PRM was used alone or in conjunction with other drugs (1,7,10,12,14,15,18,26,27,29,32,36,41, 43,45,48,57–61,63,66). The possible importance of the conversion of PRM to PB was unrecognized until 1956 (13).

White et al. (65) studied the relative potency of PRM in comparison to PB and phenytoin in controlling focal motor and psychomotor seizures. Twenty patients were observed in the hospital in a double-blind study using 10 different combinations of medication administered in accordance with a schedule defined by the Latin square study design. Each medical approach was followed for 2 weeks. Serum drug levels were not measured. All three drugs were judged to be equally effective in the treatment of focal motor or psychomotor seizures.

Olesen and Dam (46) evaluated 19 patients with chronic epilepsy who had been treated with PRM. All had been receiving additional anticonvulsants (PB was stopped before this testing if it had been used previously) for at least 1 year. Drugs other than PRM or PB were not altered during this study. The patients were observed for 6 to 8 months. The evaluation was arranged so that those individuals who had been receiving PRM had this medication withdrawn over 14 days, and PB was substituted and increased in dose until the serum PB concentration was brought to the same level as that previously attained for derived PB from PRM therapy. Switching from PRM to PB in this manner, with matching of the serum concentrations of PB, produced no change in seizure control in 14 pa-

tients, improvement in one, and worsening in four. It has been noted (8) that this study indicates lessened control of seizures when PB was substituted for PRM in a small number of patients, although it was concluded "that doubt may be entertained as to the independent anticonvulsant effect of primidone."

Millichap and Aymat (44) reported a controlled evaluation of 24 children receiving PRM and phenytoin for major seizures. The authors chose not to utilize a double-blind approach or a crossover technique. Each patient served as his or her own control. Serum drug levels were not monitored. Primidone and phenytoin were judged to be equally effective in this study.

Rodin et al. (53) compared the efficacy of PRM and carbamazepine, each in combination with phenytoin, in tonic–clonic and partial seizures with complex symptomatology. Forty-five patients, serving as their own controls, completed this study. The neurologist participated in a single-blind setting, and the electroencephalographer and psychologist participated in a double-blind fashion. Three months of each combination of dual therapy (PRM and phenytoin or carbamazepine and phenytoin) were monitored. Serum drug levels were checked monthly. Compliance of these outpatients was judged to be good based on the measures of antiepileptic drug levels. The results showed no difference in effectiveness of either PRM or carbamazepine in this combined drug therapy.

A recent abstract (47) presents information obtained from a study of 21 epileptic individuals in residence at the Chalfont Center for Epilepsy. All of the subjects were taking either PRM or PB for at least 1 year, usually in conjunction with other antiepileptic drugs (doses of which were unaltered throughout the study). The doses of PRM and PB were adjusted to provide similar serum concentrations of PB. Each trial of PRM and PB was carried out for a mean duration of 12 months. Sixteen subjects took PRM, and five took PB, during the first year. A rapid changeover from PRM to PB and from PB to PRM was achieved by substituting 250 mg of PRM for 60 mg of PB. Serum PB was monitored, and drug dosage was adjusted to produce similar concentrations of PB in each group. The seizure frequency was monitored by resident staff. Fourteen of the 21 patients experienced fewer tonic seizures on PRM than on PB, four had more frequent attacks, and three showed no change. A Wilcoxon signed rank test indicated that PRM was superior to PB in control of tonic–clonic seizures ($t = 12$, $p < 0.01$). No significant difference in frequency of partial and absence attacks was observed with these two treatments.

Various conclusions have been drawn from these clinical studies with regard to the effectiveness of PRM itself as an anticonvulsant. A consideration of this issue (56) has pointed out the underlying problems leading to this uncertainty: (a) unawareness of the conversion of PRM to PB in the studies prior to 1956, (b) failure to measure serum drug concentrations in the studies between 1956 and 1970, (c) insufficient pharmacokinetic data from all antiepileptics, and (d) inadequate clinical trials utilizing available information about the pharmacodynamics of PRM. The abstract of Oxley et al. (47) is particularly interesting, as it applies to a carefully controlled clinical study of primidone. Our data correlating serum concentrations of PRM and PB with the control of seizures will give further credence to the effectiveness of PRM as an antiepileptic agent.

THERAPEUTIC PLASMA CONCENTRATION

Relation of Dose to Plasma Concentration

We have used PRM as a single drug in the treatment of 80 patients (56 females and 24 males) over the past 8 years. Their ages ranged from 16 to 68 years. These individuals were experiencing tonic–clonic and/or partial seizures with either simple or complex symptomatology. These individuals were primarily seen in the outpatient clinic, and, although this necessarily raises concerns about compliance with the recommended schedules of medication, we feel that it does not pose a major problem. This is supported by consistent measures of serum concentrations of PRM and PB obtained at intervals over months and often years and by the patient's or family's interest in successful treatment. The majority of these individuals were started on PRM as their first drug, and the rest were changed to this drug because of toxicity or ineffectiveness of the previous antiepileptic therapy. Patients who had been refractive to anticonvulsant drug therapy, including polypharmacy, were not included in our study. Etiologic substrates included brain tumors, traumatic and infectious sequelae, degenerative diseases, and, most prominently, idiopathic epilepsy. These entities were defined in part with the aid of electroencephalography, nuclide brain scan, computed tomography of the head, and, less often, cerebral angiography. Repeated clinical evaluations and measures of serum concentrations of PRM and PB with the medications in steady state were utilized in the management of drug therapy.

The relationship between the primidone dosage and serum concentrations of PRM and derived PB is summarized in Table 1. The table initially shows data from all 80 patients without regard to the serum concentrations of the derived PB. Since effective PB therapy has been reported to require a minimum serum PB level of 15 μg/ml (33), the table then shows the patients separated into two groups, one with serum concentrations of derived PB greater than 15 μg/ml and another with serum concentrations less than 15 μg/ml. The two groups are further subdivided into males and females. Figure 1 shows the serum concentrations of derived phenobarbital in these patients.

These data suggest several conclusions that also lend further support to our previous observations (56). A wide range of serum PRM and PB concentrations results from a particular dose of PRM. Therefore, adjustment of the dosage of PRM only on the basis of the derived PB is not possible, and measures of each drug must be obtained. Because of the relatively short half-life of PRM, the measurements must be obtained consistently and preferably 2 to 4 hr after

TABLE 1. *Serum PRM and PB concentrations in relation to dose of primidone*

	PRM only (mg/kg)	Serum PRM level (µg/ml)	Serum PB level (µg/ml)	PB/PRM ratio
80 patients	9.7 ± 0.2[a]	11.3 ± 0.2	15.0 ± 0.4	1.45 ± 0.1
31 patients (serum PB > 15 µg/ml)	12.8 ± 0.6	11.6 ± 3.6	25.4 ± 9.5	2.15 ± 0.9
26 females	12.8 ± 0.7	12.4 ± 0.7	26.7 ± 1.9	2.30 ± 0.2
5 males	12.5 ± 1.1	9.7 ± 1.3	18.7 ± 1.4	1.98 ± 0.01
49 patients (serum PB < 15 µg/ml)	7.8 ± 0.4	10.9 ± 0.6	8.4 ± 0.6	0.87 ± 0.07
30 females	7.5 ± 0.5	9.8 ± 0.7	7.9 ± 0.8	0.91 ± 0.1
19 males	8.3 ± 0.5	12.7 ± 1.1	9.1 ± 0.7	0.82 ± 0.08

[a]Mean ± standard error

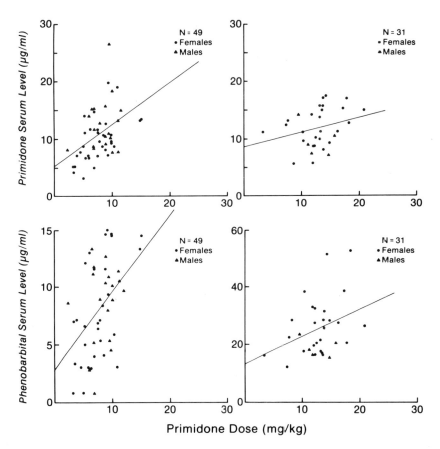

FIG. 1. Serum PRM and PB concentrations as a function of PRM dose in patients treated with PRM alone. **Left:** serum levels of derived PB < 15 µg/ml. **Right:** serum levels of derived PB > 15 µg/ml. Linear regression analyses and correlation coefficients: **Upper left,** serum PRM level = 5.2 + 0.73 PRM dose, $r = 0.45$; **lower left,** serum PB level = 2.9 + 0.68 PRM dose, $r = 0.45$; **upper right,** serum PRM level = 8.7 + 0.24 PRM dose, $r = 0.26$; **lower right,** serum PB level = 13.3 + 0.94 PRM dose, $r = 0.35$.

the dose in order to plan useful therapeutic adjustments. Lower doses of PRM are associated with lower serum concentrations of PRM and PB and with lower PB/PRM ratios. This latter finding does not support the suggestion that plasma PB levels would be proportionately higher with lower doses of PRM (21). These data also do not support the finding that females on larger doses of PRM than males achieve lower serum levels of PRM and PB (64).

Relation of Plasma Concentration to Desired Therapeutic Effect

We have analyzed the data summarized in Table 1 and Fig. 1 in relation to effectiveness of seizure control with the assumption that the serum concentration of derived PB must be at least 15 μg/ml (33) to show anticonvulsant action. Twenty-nine patients with serum PB levels of <15 μg/ml (Fig. 2B) showed excellent seizure control despite "subtherapeutic" serum concentrations of PB. Fourteen of these patients reported no seizures for more than 12-month intervals. These 29 patients had taken PRM for a mean period of 17.4 ± 5.2 months. The mean total time on dose was 16.2 ± 5.0 months. If PEMA is assumed to be of little importance as

an anticonvulsant in humans, then these findings support the concept that PRM is an effective anticonvulsant.

The range of serum PRM concentrations (10.5–13.4 μg/ml) that was associated with excellent therapeutic results (Fig. 2) is not far from the range of effectiveness (10–12 μg/ml) noted by Booker et al. (9). Additional consideration of Fig. 2 reemphasizes another observation made by Booker et al. (9)—that the serum concentrations of PRM are essentially the same in individuals with seizure control as in those without such control.

The employment of anticonvulsant drug levels to guide therapy of patients with epilepsy has identified two unique groups of patients. One attains excellent seizure control with very low serum concentrations of anticonvulsant drugs (usually a single drug), and the other, despite high serum concentrations of one and usually many drugs, fails to attain anything close to the desired therapeutic result. The severity of the epilepsies and their refractoriness to available treatments are two unexplained variables that have appropriately prompted the statement that there is "no universal therapeutic level for any anticonvulsant drug applicable to all patients" (38). Nevertheless, the concept of a "therapeutic range" of serum concentrations for various

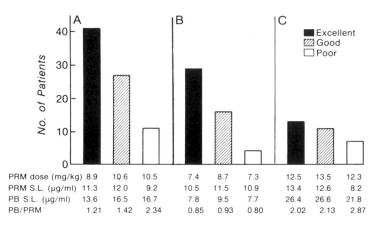

FIG. 2. The effectiveness of primidone, given as a single drug, in controlling seizures in: (**A**) 80 patients without regard to the magnitude of serum level of derived PB; (**B**) 49 patients with a serum level of derived PB (PB S.L.) <15 μg/ml; and (**C**) 31 patients with a serum level of derived PB >15 μg/ml. The serum PRM levels (PRM S.L.) and PB/PRM ratios are also shown. Seizure control: excellent, 0–2 seizures/year; good, 3–4 seizures/year; poor, >4 seizures/year.

drugs provides guidelines for treatment when applied to large populations of patients. We presently find for PRM a range of 6 to 15 μg/ml, but we shall also point out some exceptions to this range in several case summaries.

Toxic Effects Related to Plasma Concentration

Toxic Versus Therapeutic Concentrations

Booker et al. (9) expressed concern that serum concentrations of PRM in excess of 10 to 12 μg/ml are not apt to be helpful therapeutically and that the likelihood of side effects will be increased considerably if such concentrations are reached. Kutt and Penry (38) stated that serum PRM concentrations between 15 and 20 μg/ml are likely to result in continuous side effects. Primidone concentrations in excess of 15 μg/ml require that careful communication be maintained between the patient and physician in those instances where such concentrations of PRM are useful in controlling seizures.

Individual Variations in Toxic Manifestations

Clinical Variations

Case summary 1.

A 30-year-old man began experiencing tonic–clonic seizures in adolescence. Phenytoin and PB were used for a time and then discontinued. Recurrent seizures prompted the patient to seek further help. Primidone was begun as a single drug, and full control of seizures occurred in 3 weeks. This was attained with 250 mg of PRM t.i.d., which produced a serum PRM level of 18.4 μg/ml and a derived PB level of 8.9 μg/ml. The dose was subsequently increased to 250 mg q.i.d. to successfully attain control of reported auras. In 2 months, the serum PRM level was 18.8 μg/ml, and the derived PB was 24.8 μg/ml. Auras and seizures were fully controlled without toxicity.

Case summary 2.

A 20-year-old woman had experienced a mixed seizure disorder since age 3. Her seizures were now most prominently of the partial type with complex symptomatology. Poor seizure control and marked acne led to a decision to change from phenytoin and PRM to PRM alone. The dose of PRM was increased from 250 mg b.i.d. to 250 mg t.i.d. as the phenytoin was discontinued. Much improved control of seizures followed along with significant remission of the acne and no side effects to indicate PRM toxicity. The average serum concentration of PRM was 17.6 μg/ml, and the derived PB was 16.7 μg/ml over a time span of nearly 2 years.

Other case reports might include individuals with serum PRM levels in the range of 12 to 15 μg/ml who described unacceptable drowsiness and slowness that were corrected by reduction of dosage and sometimes by change to another medication. Both the patients' complaints and their antiepileptic drug concentrations must be considered in therapeutic decisions. The patients' reports are of paramount importance.

A special kind of toxicity appears so frequently with the first dose of PRM that it is imperative to forewarn the patients about its possible appearance to maintain their full confidence and cooperation in future efforts at treatment. This toxic state may appear ½ hr after the first dose of PRM and extend up to 48 hr thereafter (27,63). It prominently includes feelings of drowsiness, gastrointestinal distress, and, rarely, hallucinations and feelings of drunkenness. The difficulties, when present in the adult, can be minimized by starting with half-tablet (125 mg) doses of primidone taken at the end of the day, and, with forbearance, the distressing symptoms will disappear as small doses are repeated for several more nights before further increments are started. The use of 50-mg tablets may be appropriate for initiating treatment in some adults.

Gallagher et al. (22,24) emphasized the enhanced likelihood of this reaction appearing in individuals who were not already receiving anticonvulsant medications and commented that the use of PB prior to induction of PRM therapy seemed most helpful in mitigating against this initial state of toxicity. The doses of PRM used in their study (500 mg) must have enhanced the magnitude of the toxicity, but some degree of "toxicity," from a very slight or almost unnoticed change to intolerable states, may appear. There may be a small group of individuals who simply cannot tolerate the medication because of the development and persistence, for reasons yet unknown, of this early state of toxicity.

Clinicians who have believed that the anticonvulsant action of PRM relates to its derived PB have often added PB to PRM to increase the serum concentration of PB. We have not done this in these 80 patients. If this is done, we recommend that a thorough assessment of the clinical control and serum concentrations of PRM and PB be made prior to any addition of PB. Phenobarbital intoxication may ensue, and this comes very close to a certainty if phenytoin, PRM, and PB are combined.

Probable Causes of Individual Variations in Toxic Concentrations

Disease

Case summary 3.

A 66-year-old man with cleft palate, hypertension, a history of lacunar stroke in the previous year, recent onset of partial seizures with complex symptomatology, and polycystic kidney disease was found to have a serum PRM level of 43.8 μg/ml with a derived PB level of 27.4 μg/ml. The PRM had been gradually introduced 1 month earlier and increased to 250 mg t.i.d. 3 weeks before this evaluation. The seizures were nearly fully controlled in this month after a previous frequency of four per day. Concurrent medications included hydrochlorothiazide, hydralazine hydrochloride, propranolol hydrochloride, clonidine hydrochloride, and acetylsalicylic acid. The urinalysis was unremarkable, but the serum BUN was 35 mg/100 ml and the creatinine was 2.3 mg/100 ml.

The PRM was discontinued on the day of admission and declined to 17.8 μg/ml in 48 hr (PB increased slightly in this time to 31.9 μg/ml). Primidone was restarted at 125 mg/day, and eventually, a dose of 125 mg t.i.d. was chosen for control of seizures. Steady-state serum levels of 14.9 μg/ml for PRM and 22.5 μg/ml for PB were determined 2 months later at this dosage.

On admission, the patient's mental status (serum PRM level of 43.8 μg/ml) was marked by sleepiness, but he could always be easily aroused from this sleep by voice or gentle shake. He was oriented to person, place, and time and spoke with appropriate insights about current events. He had no difficulty recalling three items after an interval of 5 min. Gaze-evoked nystagmus was present. Assistance was required in walking to prevent falls. Moderate dysdiadochokinesia and dysmetria were present in both arms and legs. The daytime sleepiness and need for assistance in walking disappeared as the serum PRM level approached 20 μg/ml, about 36 hr after discontinuation of the PRM.

The possibility that the patient's polycystic kidney disease prevented effective excretion of PRM and hence caused the state of PRM intoxication was considered. The multiplicity of other drugs being used, however, made this conclusion less certain than it might otherwise have been. The patient's seizures were ultimately well controlled without drug toxicity by decreasing the oral dose of PRM from 11.4 mg/kg to 5.7 mg/kg.

Pregnancy and Neonatal Intoxication

The information relevant to transplacental transfer of PRM and to its presence in breast milk has been summarized in Chapter 30. We do not know of any pharmacokinetic data that have been correlated with the trimesters of pregnancy.

Rudd and Freeman (55) reported a possible embryopathy that was observed in two pregnancies of one mother. Both infants were stated to show hirsute foreheads, thick nasal roots, anteverted nares, upslanting palpebral fissures, small mandibles, juxtaductal coarctations of the aorta, tubular hyperplasia of the aortic arch and isthmus, ventricular septal defects, pulmonary artery hypertension, and biventricular hypertrophy. The mother had been taking 1.75 g of PRM per day (serum concentration was 50 μg/ml for PRM and 65 μg/ml for PB). This dose of PRM had been increased to 2.25 g per day during the third trimester of pregnancy, although serum levels were not measured at this increased dose. The authors postulated a teratogenetic effect of PRM or one of its metabolites that was related to the high drug levels in the exposed fetuses or to some undefined impairment of maternal or fetal genetic control of PRM metabolism.

Acute Intoxication

Drug Overdose

Two reports have summarized plasma concentrations of PRM, PB, and PEMA in instances of PRM overdose (11,39). Brillman et al. (11) emphasized the similarity of clinical features of PB and PRM intoxication (somnolence, lethargy, ataxia, nystagmus, dysarthria, nausea, vomiting, and, rarely, focal neurological defects). Deep coma and areflexia have been present in fatal instances. Depressed levels of consciousness were maximal at times of high concentrations of PRM in serum and cerebrospinal fluid. When these PRM levels rapidly decreased, the patients regained their alertness despite the presence of higher concentrations of PB in serum and cerebrospinal fluid than at the time of obtundation. These findings prompted the conclusion that PRM intoxication is caused by PRM itself rather than by its metabolites.

Lagenstein et al. (39) also followed the clinical course and PRM, PB, and PEMA concentrations in the serum of an 18-year-old girl as she was treated with forced diuresis for the ingestion of 15 g of PRM (330 mg/kg). Her initial serum concentration of PRM was 300 μg/ml. At this time she was found to be slow and sleepy and to have severely impaired short-term memory. She could properly identify the

day and place. Stretch reflexes were present, but abdominal reflexes were absent, and brisk pupillary light reactions were noted. She could not be wakened in another 12 hr and made only faint sounds to painful stimuli. The pupils reacted slowly to light, and the stretch reflexes were diminished. The serum PRM level was about 200 μg/ml and serum PB and PEMA levels were nearly 50 μg/ml at this time. Wakefulness with awareness of place and time returned 18 hr after admission. Cerebellar ataxia was reported to persist for 4 days.

Life-threatening symptoms appeared in this patient 9 to 13 hr after the PRM ingestion, coinciding with a decrease of serum PRM concentration (200 μg/ml) from that noted on admission (300 μg/ml) and with serum PB and PEMA values not high enough to account for the neurological changes. It was speculated that (a) the clinical conditions might relate to the combined effects of all three substances or (b) the levels of PRM in the serum might be sufficiently different from those in tissue to allow persistent elevations of tissue levels for a time, which would account for the marked state of obtundation in the presence of declining serum concentrations of PRM. The latter conclusion was favored.

The authors (39) emphasized the importance of rapid elimination of PRM via diuretic therapy, both to clear the toxic concentrations of PRM and to prevent its conversion to PB and PEMA with their additional potential for toxicity. They also observed that the presence of crystals in the urine of this girl indicated a serum PRM concentration of at least 70 to 80 μg/ml.

Relation of Dose to Plasma Concentration: Interpretation

Dose Required to Achieve a Given Plasma Concentration

The daily dosages of PRM in our 80 patients ranged from 200 to 1,250 mg (2.3–20.8 mg/kg). The average daily dose of PRM was 9.7 ± 0.2 mg/kg. Pediatric doses have been considered in relation to absorption and metabolism (37), and it has been noted that serum concentrations approach those of adulthood in early puberty and attain similar levels in adolescence (49).

The frequency with which an initial intolerance to PRM appears with the first dose makes the use of loading doses impractical. Initial treatment should begin with 50 or 125 mg given at the end of the day in order to lessen problems of sleepiness that may appear. Gradual increments to two, three, or four divided daily doses must be worked out in accordance with individual needs. Rarely, a single daily dose will suffice. Very few people in our experience have tolerated a daily dose of more than 1 g of PRM. Again, both the upper and lower limits of daily dosage must be worked out with the patient and the use of serum drug levels.

When Plasma Concentration is Too High

Excessive serum concentrations of PRM most commonly reflect excessive intake of medication. The possibility of impaired renal function leading to PRM intoxication was considered but not proved in Case summary 3. The possible role of drug interactions was discussed in Chapter 32.

When Plasma Concentration is Too Low

Inadequate PRM intake represents the most common cause of low serum concentrations of this drug. Its manifestations may include poor control of seizures and low serum concentrations of PRM. The importance of properly timing the sample for the measurement of PRM must, of course, be considered in interpreting this value. A low PRM serum level obtained 12 hr after the last dose may reflect not poor compliance but only the short half-life of PRM and perhaps a need for more frequent doses. The correlation of the EEG with serum PRM levels may be helpful in a setting of subtherapeutic serum PRM levels (54).

The effects that various diseases may have in bringing about low plasma concentrations of PRM await further investigation, and the matter of drug interaction was reviewed in Chapter 32.

Two exceptions to general rules regarding half-

life and therapeutic range for PRM are seen in the following case.

Case summary 4.

A 46-year-old housewife experienced several partial seizures with complex symptomatology and then a tonic–clonic attack. Her initial neurological examination and nuclide brain scan were unremarkable, but the EEG indicated right frontotemporal spike-and-wave activity. A right carotid arteriogram showed no abnormality. The starting dose of PRM, 250 mg/day, was not increased because of drowsiness with higher doses. The patient chose to take the drug as a single dose at bedtime. One year later, the serum PRM level 10 hr after drug ingestion was 5.1 µg/ml, and the derived PB level was 3.4 µg/ml. The patient has continued on the same dose with full control of seizures in subsequent years, including the several years that have followed surgical removal of a right frontotemporal oligodendroglioma. A seizure did recur on one occasion when the patient had discontinued the use of PRM.

Guidelines to Principles of Dose Adjustment

The most effective use of PRM as a single drug will depend on (a) careful attention to reliable information on seizure control and toxicity, (b) accurate measures of serum concentrations of primidone and its metabolites (samples should be obtained 2 to 4 hr after the preceding dose), and (c) attention to the patient's medical and social milieu (general state of health, use of additional drugs, sleep, emotional composure).

Primidone is most often used as an adjunctive anticonvulsant. The same concepts for induction of therapy and for monitoring drug effectiveness and toxicity apply to this use. Special attention needs to be given to the potential for enhanced PRM conversion to PB (19) in the presence of phenytoin therapy. The possibility of PB intoxication becomes a definite concern in this setting, and the addition of PB similarly poses a concern for this kind of toxicity. Primidone can be an effective supplementary drug when properly monitored.

ACKNOWLEDGMENTS

Original data are from studies performed in the Department of Neurology, University of Iowa Hospitals, with the assistance of our colleagues in that department. This study was supported in part by grant RR-59 from the General Clinical Research Center Program, Division of Research Resources, National Institutes of Health.

REFERENCES

1. Adderly, D. S., and Monro, A. B. (1953): Mysoline in the treatment of epilepsy. *Lancet,* 1:1154.
2. Baumel, I. P., Gallagher, B. B., DiMicco, J., and Goico, H. (1973): Metabolism and anticonvulsant properties of primidone in the rat. *J. Pharmacol. Exp. Ther.,* 186:305–314.
3. Baumel, I. P., Gallagher, B. B., and Mattson, R. H. (1972). Phenylethylmalonamide (PEMA). An important metabolite of primidone. *Arch. Neurol.,* 27:34–41.
4. Bogan, J., and Smith, H. (1968): The relation between primidone and phenobarbitone blood levels. *J. Pharm. Pharmacol.,* 20:64–67.
5. Bogue, J. Y., and Carrington, H. C. (1953). The evaluation of Mysoline—a new anticonvulsant drug. *Br. J. Pharmacol.,* 8:230–236.
6. Bogue, J. Y., Carrington, H. C., and Bentley, S. (1956): L'activité anticonvulsive de la Mysoline. *Acta Neurol. Psychiatr. Belg.,* 56:640–650.
7. Bonkalo, A., and Arthurs, R. G. S. (1953): Mysoline in the treatment of epileptic and non-epileptic psychiatric patients. *Can. Med. Assoc. J.,* 68:570–574.
8. Booker, H. E. (1972): Primidone. Relation of plasma levels to clinical control. In: *Antiepileptic Drugs,* edited by D. Woodbury, K. Penry, and R. Schmidt, pp 373–376. Raven Press, New York.
9. Booker, H. E., Hosokowa, K., Burdette, R. D., and Darcey, B. (1970): A clinical study of serum primidone levels. *Epilepsia,* 11:395–402.
10. Briggs, J. N., and Tucker, J. (1954). Primidone (Mysoline) in treatment of clinical petit mal in children. *Lancet,* 1:19–21.
11. Brillman, J., Gallagher, B. B., and Mattson, R. H. (1974). Acute primidone intoxication. *Arch. Neurol.,* 30:255–258.
12. Burton-Bradley, B. G. (1953): Report on Mysoline in treatment of mental hospital epileptics. *Med. J. Aust.,* 2:705–706.
13. Butler, T. C., and Waddell, W. J. (1956): Metabolic conversion of primidone (Mysoline) to phenobarbital. *Proc. Soc. Exp. Biol. Med.,* 93:544–546.
14. Butter, A. J. M. (1953): Mysoline in treatment of epilepsy. *Lancet,* 1:1024.
15. Calnan, W. L., and Borrell, Y. M. (1953): Mysoline in the treatment of epilepsy. *Lancet,* 2:42–43.
16. Cereghino, J. J., and Penry, J. K. (1972): General principles. Testing of anticonvulsants in man. In: *Antiepileptic Drugs,* edited by D. M. Woodbury, J. K. Penry, and R. P. Schmidt, pp. 63–73. Raven Press, New York.
17. Coatsworth, J. J., and Penry, J. K. (1972): General principles: Clinical efficacy and use. In: *Antiepileptic Drugs,* edited by D. M. Woodbury, J. K. Penry, and R. P. Schmidt, pp. 87–96. Raven Press, New York.
18. Doyle, P. J., and Livingston, S. (1953): Use of Mysoline in treatment of epilepsy. *J. Pediatr.,* 43:413–416.
19. Fincham, R. W., Schottelius, D. D., and Sahs, A. L. (1974): The influence of diphenylhydantoin on primidone metabolism. *Arch. Neurol.,* 30:259–262.
20. Frey, H. H., and Hahn, I. (1960): Untersuchungen über die Bedeutung des durch biotransformation gebildeten Phenobarbital für die antikonvulsive Wirkung von Primidon. *Arch. Int. Pharmacodyn.,* 128:281–290.
21. Gallagher, B. B., and Baumel, I. P. (1972): Primidone. Biotransformation. In: *Antiepileptic Drugs,* edited by D. M. Woodbury, J. K. Penry, and R. P. Schmidt, pp. 361–366. Raven Press, New York.
22. Gallagher, B. B., and Baumel, I. P. (1972): Primidone: Interaction with other drugs. In: *Antiepileptic Drugs,* edited by D. M. Woodbury, J. K. Penry, and R. P. Schmidt, pp. 367–371. Raven Press, New York.
23. Gallagher, B. B., Baumel, I. P., and Mattson, R. H. (1972): Metabolic disposition of primidone and its metabolites in epileptic subjects after single and repeated administration. *Neurology (Minneap.),* 22:1186–1192.
24. Gallagher, B. B., Baumel, I. P., Mattson, R. H., and Woodbury, B. S. (1973): Primidone, diphenylhydantoin and phenobarbital. Aspects of acute and chronic toxicity. *Neurology (Minneap.),* 23:145–149.
25. Gallagher, B. B., Smith, D. B., and Mattson, R. H. (1970): The relationship of the anticonvulsant properties of primidone to phenobarbital. *Epilepsia,* 11:293–301.
26. Game, J. A. (1953): Mysoline, its use in epilepsy. *Med. J. Aust.,* 2:707–709.
27. Goldin, S. (1954): Toxic effects of primidone. *Lancet,* 1:102–103.
28. Goodman, L. S., Swinyard, E. A., Brown, W. C., Schiffman, D. O., Grewal, M. S., and Bliss, E. L. (1953): Anticonvulsant properties of 5-phenyl-5-ethyl-hexahydropyrimidine-4, 6-dione (Mysoline). A new antiepileptic. *J. Pharmacol. Exp. Ther.,* 108:428–436.
29. Greenstein, L., and Sapirstein, M. R. (1953): Treatment of epilepsy with Mysoline. *Arch. Neurol. Psychiatry,* 70:469–473.
30. Gruber, C. M., Jr., Brock, J. T., and Dyken, M. (1962): Comparison of the effectiveness of phenobarbital, mephobarbital, primidone, diphenylhydantoin, ethotoin, metharbital, and methyl phenylhydantoin in motor seizures. *Clin. Pharmacol. Ther.,* 3:23–28.
31. Gruber, C. M., Jr., Mosier, J. M., and Grant, P. (1957): Objective comparison of primidone and phenobarbital in epileptics. *J. Pharmacol. Exp. Ther.,* 120:184–187.
32. Handley, R., and Stewart, A. S. R. (1952): Mysoline: A new drug in the treatment of epilepsy. *Lancet,* 1:742–744.
33. Harvey, C. D., Sherwin, A. L., and van der Kleijn, E. (1977): Distribution of anticonvulsant drugs in gray

and white matter of human brain. *Can. J. Neurol. Sci.,* 4:89–92.

34. Houghton, G. W., Richens, A., Toseland, P. A., Davidson, S., and Falconer, M. A. (1975): Brain concentrations of phenytoin, phenobarbitone and primidone in epileptic patients. *Eur. J. Clin. Pharmacol.,* 9:73–78.

35. Johnson, D. D., Davis, H. L., and Crawford, R. D. (1978): Epileptiform seizures in domestic fowl. VIII. Anticonvulsant activity of primidone and its metabolites, phenobarbital and phenylethylmalonamide. *Can. J. Physiol. Pharmacol.,* 56:630–633.

36. Jorgenson, G. (1953): Mysoline in the treatment of epilepsy. *Lancet,* 2:835.

37. Kauffman, R. E., Habersang, R., and Lansky, L. (1977): Kinetics of primidone metabolism and excretion in children. *Clin. Pharmacol. Ther.,* 22:200–205.

38. Kutt, H., and Penry, J. K. (1974): Usefulness of blood levels of antiepileptic drugs. *Arch. Neurol.,* 31:283–288.

39. Lagenstein, I., Sternowsky, H. J., Iffland, E., and Blaschke, E. (1976): Intoxication with primidone: Continuous monitoring of serum primidone and its metabolites during forced diuresis. *Neuropaediatrie,* 8:190–195.

40. Leal, K. W., Rapport, R. L., Wilenski, A. J., and Friel, B. S. (1979): Single dose pharmacokinetics and anticonvulsant efficacy of primidone in mice. *Ann. Neurol.,* 5:470–474.

41. Livingston, S., and Petersen, D. (1956): Primidone (Mysoline) in the treatment of epilepsy. *N. Engl. J. Med.,* 254:327–329.

42. Lockhard, J. S., Uhlir, V., Du Charme, L. L., Farquhar, J. A., and Huntsman, B. J. (1975): Efficacy of standard anticonvulsants in monkey model with spontaneous motor seizures. *Epilepsia,* 16:301–317.

43. Lyons, J. B., and Liversedge, L. A. (1954): Primidone in treatment of epilepsy. *Br. Med. J.,* 1:625–627.

44. Millichap, J.G., and Aymat, F. (1968): Controlled evaluation of primidone and diphenylhydantoin sodium. Comparative anticonvulsant efficacy and toxicity in children. *J.A.M.A.,* 204:738–739.

45. Nathan, P. W. (1954): Primidone in treatment of non-idiopathic epilepsy. *Lancet,* 1:21–22.

46. Olesen, O. V., and Dam, M. (1967): The metabolic conversion of primidone to phenobarbitone in patients under long-term treatment. *Acta Neurol. Scand.,* 43:348–356.

47. Oxley, J., Hebdige, S., and Richens, A. (1979): A comparison of phenobarbitone and primidone in the control of seizures in chronic epilepsy. *Br. J. Clin. Pharmacol.,* 7:414P.

48. Pence, L. M. (1954): Mysoline in epilepsy. *Tex. State J. Med.,* 50:290–292.

49. Pippenger, C. E., Pellock, J. M., and Gold, A. P. (1977): Antiepileptic drug concentrations in children on multiple therapy. In: *Antiepileptic Drug Monitoring,* edited by C. Gardner-Thorpe, D. Janz, H. Meinardi, and C. E. Pippenger, pp 282–286. Pitman Medical, Tunbridge Wells, Kent.

50. Reynolds, E. H. (1978): Drug treatment of epilepsy. *Lancet,* 2:721–725.

51. Richens, A. (1976): Clinical pharmacology and medical treatment. In: *Textbook of Epilepsy,* edited by J. Laidlaw and A. Richens, pp 234–239. Churchill Livingstone, Edinburgh, New York.

52. Rodin, E. A. (1968): *The Prognosis of Patients with Epilepsy,* p. 202. Charles C Thomas, Springfield, Illinois.

53. Rodin, E. A. Choo, S. R., Hideki, K., Lewis, R., and Rennick, P. M., (1976): A comparison of the effectiveness of primidone versus carbamazepine in epileptic outpatients. *J. Nerv. Ment. Dis.,* 163:41–46.

54. Rowan, A. J., Pippenger, C. E., McGregor, P. A., and French, J. H. (1975): Seizure activity and anticonvulsant drug concentration. 24 hour sleep waking studies. *Arch. Neurol.,* 32:281–288.

55. Rudd, N. L., and Freedman, R. M. (1979): A possible primidone embryopathy. *J. Pediatr.,* 94:835–837.

56. Schottelius, D. D., and Fincham, R. W. (1978): Clinical application of serum primidone levels. In: *Antiepileptic Drugs: Quantitative Analysis and Interpretation,* edited by C. E. Pippenger, J. K. Penry, and H. Kutt, pp. 273–282. Raven Press, New York.

57. Sciarra, D., Carter, S., Vicale, C. T., and Merritt, H. H. (1954): Clinical evaluation of primidone (Mysoline), a new anticonvulsant drug. *J.A.M.A.,* 154:827–829.

58. Selby, G. (1953): Mysoline: Clinical evaluation of new drug in treatment of refractory cases of epilepsy. *Med. J. Aust.,* 2:709–715.

59. Sharpe, D. S. (1954): Primidone in mental deficiency practice. *Br. Med. J.,* 1:627–629.

60. Smith, B., and Forster, F. M. (1954): Mysoline and Milontin: Two new medicines for epilepsy. *Neurology (Minneap.),* 4:137–142.

61. Smith, B. H., and McNaughton, F. L. (1953): Mysoline, new anticonvulsant drug: Its value in refractory cases of epilepsy. *Can. Med. Assoc. J.,* 68:464–467.

62. Swinyard, E. A., Tedeschi, D. H., and Goodman, L. S. (1954): Effect of liver damage and nephrectomy on anticonvulsant activity of Mysoline and phenobarbital. *J. Am. Pharm. Assoc.,* 43:114–116.

63. Timberlake, W. H., Abbott, J. A., and Schwab, R. S. (1955): Mysoline. An effective anticonvulsant with initial problems of adjustment. *N. Engl. J. Med.,* 252:304–307.

64. Travers, R. D., Reynolds, E. H., and Gallagher, B. B. (1972): Variation in response to anticonvulsants in a group of epileptic patients. *Arch. Neurol.,* 27:29–33.

65. White, P. T., Plott, D., and Norton, J. (1966): Relative anticonvulsant potency of primidone. A double blind comparison. *Arch. Neurol.,* 14:31–35.

66. Whitty, C. W. M. (1953): Value of primidone in epilepsy. *Br. Med. J.,* 2:540–541.

67. Zavadil, P., and Gallagher, B. B. (1975): Metabolism and excretion of ^{14}C-primidone in epileptic patients. In: *Epileptology. Proceedings of the Seventh International Symposium on Epilepsy,* edited by D. Janz, pp 129–139. Georg Thieme, Stuttgart.

Antiepileptic Drugs, edited by D. M. Woodbury,
J. K. Penry, and C. E. Pippenger. Raven Press,
New York © 1982.

34

Primidone

Toxicity

Ilo E. Leppik and James C. Cloyd

Although primidone (PRM) was rated as being less toxic than phenobarbital (PB) in the original laboratory trials (8), many patients experience symptoms of toxicity related to the use of this drug (24,34,38,56,57,60). Primidone is metabolized to PB and phenylethylmalonamide (PEMA) and is often used in combination with other antiepileptic drugs. Some side effects are attributable to the parent compound. Others may be caused by PB which can be present in high concentrations (see Chapter 31) during PRM therapy and effects of which are discussed in Chapter 26. Levels of PEMA may equal those of the parent drug, but it plays a small role, if any, in side effects (6). With comedication, some of the observed toxicity may result from the addition of another depressant drug to those already present. In discussing the adverse effects of PRM in this chapter, emphasis will be on those occurring in patients receiving only PRM or on those in which PRM could be implicated because of the reversal of toxicity with its withdrawal in the presence of continued therapy with other agents.

NERVOUS SYSTEM TOXICITY

Symptoms involving the central nervous system (CNS) were the most common side effects in patients receiving PRM; they were perceived by 209 of 486 patients reported by Livingston and Petersen (34) and ranged from 43 to 85% in other clinical studies (55–57,60). Primidone was discontinued in 9 to 32% of patients because of side effects (34,55). The most common symptom was drowsiness, which was reported by 33 to 68% of persons receiving PRM. In these patients, however, PRM was usually added to other antiepileptic drugs, and its contribution to toxicity may have been nonspecific, attributable to the addition of another centrally active drug.

Persons receiving their initial PRM dose often experience drowsiness, weakness, dizziness, and a feeling of intoxication within 1 to 2 hr after ingesting the drug. In our study of 13 patients who were hospitalized during the initiation of therapy with PRM and had regular examinations, all were affected to some degree, but symptoms were usually tolerable. Mean peak serum PRM levels were approximately 6 μg/ml. These side effects were attributable to PRM alone, as they occurred before any metabolites were present (10,24). Occasionally, these symptoms were very severe and incapacitating, with gradual improvement occurring over a few days (2,11,26).

This striking response of some patients to a dose often tolerated by others has been designated an idiosyncratic reaction to PRM (26).

However, these signs and symptoms resemble those occurring after PRM overdose (12) and may be encountered to a lesser degree in volunteers taking 500 mg and attaining peak PRM levels of approximately 10 µg/ml (10). Acute symptoms appear to be concentration related, with individual variability in degree of sensitivity to PRM accounting for the spectrum of discomfort encountered. Since these severely disturbing reactions may occur in as many as 14% of patients during initiation of therapy (60), some physicians use a test dose of 50 mg and initiate treatment according to the reaction (10). It has been reported that prior use of PB reduces symptoms on initiation of therapy with PRM (24), but in our experience, unpleasant side effects occur in most patients ingesting 250 mg of PRM regardless of history of use of other antiepileptic drugs.

Most patients develop tolerance to these side effects. In a study of the pharmacokinetics of PRM, we observed significant toxicity during the first exposure to the drug. Side effects included ataxia, nystagmus, and mental symptoms, which were rated on a four-unit scale. As shown in Fig. 1, the time course of the toxicity rating paralleled the PRM concentrations at a time when no phenobarbital was present. Symptoms decreased, and, by the next study interval, the toxicity rating was much lower, even in the presence of PB, PEMA, and PRM concentrations of 5 to 10 µg/ml.

Personality changes have been observed during use of PRM (11,34,43,56,57). In an investigation of phenytoin with comedication, patients receiving PRM had significantly higher scores on the psychopathic deviate scale of the Minnesota Multiphasic Inventory as compared with the period during which they were receiving carbamazepine (CBZ) (52). They also tended to become progressively more depressed while on PRM than while on CBZ, as judged by psychometrist's rating (52). Occasional paranoid reactions (56) have occurred; in one patient, these appeared three times as the PRM dose was increased. Acute confusional and "schizophrenia-like" psychoses have been observed with PRM in combination with phenytoin (20).

Impotence and decreased libido have been mentioned in some instances, but few details have been given regarding their severity or time of onset (52,55,60). In a report comparing CBZ with PRM, one instance of decreased libido out of a group of 60 patients was reported with PRM but none with CBZ (52).

Many persons, especially those who are active and employed, complain of nonspecific difficulties with memory, concentration, and energy during chronic PRM therapy. These effects may be documented by psychometric examina-

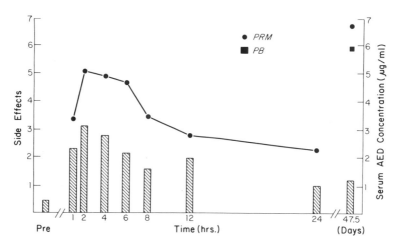

FIG. 1. Side effects (*hatched bars*) and serum PRM concentrations (*solid line*) after initial and chronic treatment with PRM. Toxicity rating is sum of ataxia, nystagmus, and mental symptoms.

tions. In an evaluation comparing PRM with CBZ when either drug was used with phenytoin, the patients had significantly more impairment on the cognitive perceptual–motor battery during the PRM phase of treatment (52). Significant negative correlations were found between PB and PRM concentrations and 11 neuropsychological subtests measuring general mental function, concentration, and fine motor performance (30).

The nystagmus described with PRM use usually does not differ from that seen with use of other antiepileptic medication (60). Three cases of partial or total external ophthalmoplegia associated with PRM and phenytoin use have been reported (45). Two cases of downbeat nystagmus during phenytoin and PRM use have been reported, and PRM was implicated by the authors as a contributing factor because phenytoin concentrations were below 20 μg/ml. However, in both patients, the abnormal ocular findings cleared after the phenytoin dose was decreased (3).

Polyradiculitis and ataxia following a single dose of PRM have been observed in two children (61). Remission of the radiculitis occurred after treatment with corticosteroids (9).

Changes in the electroencephalogram attributable to PRM consist of beta activity superimposed on alpha activity. With serum levels of 15 to 100 μg/ml attained after an overdose, slow activity was intermingled with background activity (12).

OVERDOSE

Clinical findings of PRM overdose consist of CNS depression, flaccidity, and depression of deep tendon reflexes (31). With serum PRM levels of 90 to 100 μg/ml, patients exhibit somnolence and lethargy (12,35). Symptoms correlate with plasma and CSF concentrations of PRM but not with levels of PEMA or PB which often increase as the patient improves (12). Although fatal cases of PRM overdose have been reported (7), as much as 22 g may be ingested without permanent sequelae, and PRM appears to have a wide range of safety (12). Crystalluria is a prominent feature of PRM overdose and has

been reported in most cases; it would serve to direct attention to the possibility of PRM overdose in comatose patients (4,14). Overdose should be treated with gastric lavage and supportive measures (35). Analeptic drugs have been used (18) but have been unsuccessful and are not generally recommended for treatment of PRM overdose (31).

HEMATOLOGICAL TOXICITY

Data from clinical trials conducted shortly after introduction of PRM indicated that the drug was not associated with serious hematological abnormalities (13,28,29,47,55,56,60). Subsequently, the most commonly reported disorder has been megaloblastic anemia.

Fewer than 1% of patients receiving antiepileptic drugs develop megaloblastic anemia (19), and it is most commonly observed in patients receiving phenytoin alone or in combination with other drugs. However, some cases in which PRM may be implicated as the causative agent have been reported. In one, a patient had been treated with phenytoin and PB for 4 years; PRM was substituted for phenytoin, and severe megaloblastic anemia developed 2 months later (15). Primidone was the only antiepileptic drug used in two patients who developed megaloblastic anemia; it occurred in one 4 months after substitution of PRM for PB and in the other 2 years after initiation of antiepileptic drug therapy with PRM (22). Primidone discontinuation was accompanied by a reticulocytosis of 16% and resolution of anemia in one patient whose phenytoin and PB were continued (17). In this patient, when PRM was reinstituted, the anemia recurred but this time was treated with folate and resolved without the need to stop PRM. In another individual given only PRM, a folate-responsive anemia developed in the presence of normal folic acid clearance, a state compatible with normal tissue stores of folate (16). Nevertheless, the anemia responded quickly to treatment with oral folic acid.

The mechanism by which drugs may induce folate deficiency or interfere with utilization has not been elucidated: malabsorption (49), increased hepatic clearance (58), and direct interference with folate utilization (5) have been postulated. Investigations of folate in epileptic patients revealed that usually more than 50% of all persons had subnormal concentrations, and low levels were usually associated with multiple drug therapy, often with phenytoin (50,54).

Megaloblastic changes have been reported in 38% of adult patients treated with antiepileptic drugs, with macrocytosis present in 11% (50). When present during PRM treatment, macrocytic anemia usually responds to folic acid (25); however, in some cases, it has been responsive to vitamin B_{12} (40,44).

Hemorrhagic disorders involving the use of PRM are rare. Maternal use of this drug has been linked to one case of neonatal coagulation defect (39) and suspected in others (42,59). Prophylactic use of vitamin K is indicated in women receiving PRM during pregnancy.

Well-documented thrombocytopenia has been reported in one patient who had been placed on PRM after phenytoin-induced bone marrow depression. The thrombocytopenia cleared with the discontinuation of PRM, although PB was still being given. In this patient, the PRM concentration was 10 µg/ml (46). One patient with thrombocytopenic purpura has been described (10).

Leukopenia may be an occasional complication. One patient on both PRM and mephobarbital experienced a drop in the white blood cell (WBC) count to 3,000 with 50% neutrophils, which returned to normal after both drugs were discontinued (60). Neither drug alone produced the drop in WBC count. Most studies found only transient or minor decreases in the WBC (11,33,62).

Lymphadenopathy in conjunction with folate deficiency anemia has been observed in one instance (32).

HEPATIC AND RENAL TOXICITY

No report linking primidone as the causative agent in hepatitis has been published. However, as discussed in Chapter 32, primidone is capable of inducing the hepatic enzyme system, and this must always be considered when this drug is given in combination with others.

A striking crystalluria has been reported after massive primidone overdose (4,12,35,41). No hematuria or acute or chronic renal failure developed. Occasional cases of edema with no definite renal or hepatic involvement have been reported (27).

OSTEOMALACIA

In a survey of calcium metabolism in epileptic patients in a residential center, subnormal levels of calcium were found in 22.5% of patients, and increased alkaline phosphatase in 29% (51). Although patients were receiving multiple antiepileptic drugs, there was a trend toward lower calcium values in patients receiving PRM or phenacemide as part of triple therapy. Similar results were reported in a population of institutionalized children, with patients receiving PRM having the lowest levels of calcium and 25-hydroxy vitamin D (63). Patients receiving PRM, however, also received the largest number of other antiepileptic drugs and had the longest duration of therapy, so these findings may be attributable to the total exposure to drugs rather than to PRM specifically.

TERATOGENICITY

Primidone administered to mice in doses of 100 to 250 mg/kg during days 6 to 16 of pregnancy and giving peak levels of 43 µg/ml was associated with a significant incidence of cleft palate as compared with control animals (37). Folic acid itself was not teratogenic but, when it was given in combination with PRM, there was a much higher incidence of malformations than occurred with PRM alone (36). Although PRM has been linked to human fetal malformations only occasionally (21), the number of instances in which PRM has been used as the sole agent are too few to make definitive statements regarding its ultimate teratogenicity in comparison with that of other antiepileptic drugs.

TABLE 1. *Primidone side effects
and adverse reactions*

System	Signs and symptoms
Nervous system	Acute: sedation, ataxia, nystagmus
	Chronic: decreased psychometric performance
	Personality change
	Impotence
	Polyradiculitis (R)[a]
Metabolic	Folic acid deficiency
Hematological	Megaloblastic anemia
	Leukopenia (R)
	Thrombocytopenia (R)
	Hemorrhagic disease of newborn
Hepatic and Renal	Enzyme induction
	Edema (R)
Hypersensitivity reactions	Benign maculopapular rash
	Systemic lupus erythematosus (R)
	Lymphadenopathy, malignant (R)

[a]R = rare: fewer than five well-documented cases.

HYPERSENSITIVITY REACTIONS

Dermatological side effects are infrequent and usually occur at the onset of therapy. Of 96 patients, four had transient rashes that cleared in a day or two after the drug was discontinued and did not recur when PRM was reinstituted (60). In contrast to these benign reactions, one fatal case of dermatitis bullosa has been reported (53). An unusually hypersensitive patient experienced severe mucocutaneous eruptions from PRM, PB, phenytoin, CBZ, and mephenytoin (48).

Eosinophilia of 10%, edema, and rash were observed in one patient who began taking PRM during the first month of pregnancy. Symptoms cleared when PB was substituted for PRM (23).

Primidone has been associated with systemic lupus erythematosus (SLE) in only one well-documented case (1). This occurred in a patient initially on phenytoin but later placed on primidone; symptoms of SLE developed, and LE smears were positive. Phenytoin was substituted for PRM, and symptoms cleared. The incidence of this reaction to PRM is apparently much less frequent than its appearance with the use of other antiepileptic drugs.

SUMMARY

Many patients experience side effects of drowsiness, weakness, and dizziness at the time of initiation of therapy with PRM. These symptoms are usually tolerable but occasionally may be quite severe and last for a few days. Tolerance to these symptoms usually develops, but some chronic CNS effects may be detected by psychometric testing. Primidone has only rarely been implicated in severe hematological or idiosyncratic reactions. It shares with the other antiepileptic drugs the problem of folate and vitamin D disturbance. Reported side effects of PRM are summarized in Table 1.

ACKNOWLEDGMENT

This work was supported by Contract No. 1–NS–5–2327 from the National Institute of Neurological and Communicative Disorders and Stroke, Bethesda, Maryland 20205.

REFERENCES

1. Ahuja, G. K., and Schumacher, G. A. (1966): Drug induced systemic lupus erythematosus. Primidone as a possible cause. *J.A.M.A.*, 198:669–671.
2. Ajax, E. T. (1966): An unusual case of primidone intoxication. *Dis. Nerv. Syst.*, 27:660–661.
3. Alpert, J. (1978): Downbeat nystagmus due to anticonvulsant toxicity. *Ann. Neurol.*, 4:471–473.
4. Bailey, D. N., and Jatlow, P. I. (1972): Chemical analysis of massive crystalluria following primidone overdose. *Am. J. Clin. Pathol.*, 58:583–589.
5. Baker, H., Frank, O., Huter, S., Aaronson, S., Ziffer, H., and Sobotka, H. (1962): Lesions in folic acid metabolism induced by primidone. *Experientia*, 18:224–226.
6. Baumel, I. P., Gallagher, B. B., and Mattson, R. H. (1972): Phenylethylmalonamide (PEMA). An important metabolite of primidone. *Arch. Neurol.*, 27:34–41.
7. Bogan, J., Rentoul, E., and Smith, H. (1965): Fatal poisoning by primidone. *J. Forensic Sci. Soc.*, 5:97–98.
8. Bogue, J. Y., and Carrington, H. C. (1953): Evaluation of mysoline: New anticonvulsant drug. *Br. J. Pharmacol.*, 8:230–236.
9. Booker, H. E. (1972): Primidone toxicity, In: *Anti-*

epileptic Drugs, edited by D. M. Woodbury, J. K. Penry, and R. P. Schmidt, pp. 377–383. Raven Press, New York.

10. Booker, H. E., Hosokowa, K., Burdette, R. D., and Darcy, B. (1970): A clinical study of serum primidone levels. *Epilepsia,* 11:395–402.

11. Briggs, J. N., and Tucker, J. (1954): Primidone (Mysoline®) in the treatment of clinical petit mal in children. *Lancet,* 1:19–21.

12. Brillman, J., Gallagher, B. B., and Mattson, R. (1974): Acute primidone intoxication. *Arch. Neurol.,* 30:255–258.

13. Butter, A. J. M. (1953): Mysoline® in the treatment of epilepsy. *Lancet,* 1:1024.

14. Cate, J. C., and Tenser, R. (1975): Acute primidone overdosage with massive crystalluria. *Clin. Toxicol.,* 8:385–389.

15. Chalmers, J. N. M., and Boheimer, K. (1954): Megaloblastic anemia and anticonvulsant therapy. *Lancet,* 2:920–921.

16. Chanarin, I., Elmes, P. C., and Mollin, D. L. (1958): Folic acid studies in megaloblastic anemia. *Br. Med. J.,* 2:80–82.

17. Christenson, W. N., Ultman, J. E., and Roseman, D. M. (1957): Megaloblastic anemia during primidone (Mysoline®) therapy. *J.A.M.A.,* 163:940–942.

18. Dotevall, G., and Herner, B. (1957): Treatment of acute primidone poisoning with bemegride and amiphenazole. *Br. Med. J.,* 3:451–452.

19. Flexner, J. M., and Hartmann, R. C. (1960): Megaloblastic anemia associated with anticonvulsant drugs. *Am. J. Med.,* 28:386–396.

20. Franks, R. D., and Richter, A. J. (1979): Schizophrenia-like psychosis associated with anticonvulsant toxicity. *Am. J. Psychiatry,* 136:973–974.

21. Fredrick, J. (1973): Epilepsy and pregnancy: A report from the Oxford record linkage study. *Br. Med. J.,* 1:442–448.

22. Fuld, H., and Moorhouse, E. H. (1956): Observations on megaloblastic anemias after primidone. *Br. Med. J.,* 1:1021–1023.

23. Gabriel, R. M. (1957): Delayed reaction to PRM in pregnancy. *Br. Med. J.,* 1:344.

24. Gallagher, B. B., Baumel, I. P., Mattson, R. H., and Woodbury, S. G. (1973): Primidone, diphenylhydantoin and phenobarbital: Aspects of acute and chronic toxicity. *Neurology (Minneap.),* 23:145–149.

25. Girdwood, R. H., and Lenman, J. A. R. (1956): Megaloblastic anemia occurring during primidone therapy. *Br. Med. J.,* 1:146–147.

26. Goldin, S. (1954): Toxic effects of primidone. *Lancet,* 1:102–103.

27. Goodman, L. S., Swynyard, E. A., Brown, W. C., Schiffman, D. O., Grewal, M. S., and Bliss, E. L. (1953): Anticonvulsant properties of 5-phenyl-5-ethyl-hexahydropyrimidine-4,6 dione (Mysoline®), a new anti-epileptic. *J. Pharmacol. Exp. Ther.,* 108:248–436.

28. Greenstein, L., and Sapirstein, M. R. (1953): Treatment of epilepsy with Mysoline®. *Arch. Neurol.,* 70:469–473.

29. Handley, R., and Stewart, A. S. R. (1952): Mysoline®: A new drug in the treatment of epilepsy. *Lancet,* 1:742–744.

30. Hartlage, L. C., Stovall, K., and Kocack, B. (1980): Behavioral correlates of anticonvulsant blood levels. *Epilepsia,* 21:185.

31. Kappy, M. S., and Buckley, J. (1969): Primidone intoxication in a child. *Arch. Dis. Child.,* 44:282–284.

32. Langlands, A. O., MacLean, N., Pearson, J. G., and Williamson, E. R. D. (1967): Lymphadenopathy and megaloblastic anemia in patient receiving primidone. *Br. Med. J.,* 1:215–217.

33. Livingston, S. (1966): *Drug Therapy For Epilepsy.* Charles C Thomas, Springfield, Illinois.

34. Livingston, S., and Petersen, D. (1956): Primidone (Mysoline®) in the treatment of epilepsy. *N. Engl. J. Med.,* 254:327–329.

35. Matzke, G. R., Cloyd, J. C., Sawchuk, R. J. (1981): Acute phenytoin and primidone intoxication: A pharmacokinetic analysis. *J. Clin. Pharmacol.,* 21:92–99.

36. McElhatton, P. R., and Sullivan, F. M. (1975): Teratogenic effects of primidone in mice. *Br. J. Pharmacol.,* 54:267P–268P.

37. McElhatton, P. R., Sullivan, F. M., and Toseland, P. A. (1977): Teratogenic activity and metabolism of primidone in the mouse. *Epilepsia,* 18:1–11.

38. Milletti, M. (1954): Valutazione clinica di un nuova medicamento-anticonvulsivante. I. 15-fenil-5-etiljesaidropirimidina-4,6-dione, Mysoline®. *Arch. Neurochir. (Bologna),* 2:121–151.

39. Monnet, P., Rosenberg, D., and Bovier-Lapierre, M. (1968): Therapeutique anticomitiale administrée pendant la grossesse et maladie hemorrhagique du nouveau—V^e. Remarques critiques à propos de trois observations personnelles. *Rev. Fr. Gynaecol. Obstet.,* 63:695–702.

40. Montgomery, D., and Craig, J. (1958): Megaloblastic anemia during primidone therapy. Report of a case responding to vitamin B$_{12}$. *Scott. Med. J.,* 3:460.

41. Morley, D., and Wynne, N. A. (1957): Acute primidone poisoning in a child. *Br. Med. J.,* 1:90.

42. Mountain, K. R., Hirsh, J., and Gallus, A. S. (1970): Neonatal coagulation defects due to anticonvulsant drug treatment in pregnancy. *Lancet,* 1:265–268.

43. Nathan, P. W. (1954): Primidone in treatment of nonidiopathic epilepsy. *Lancet,* 1:21.

44. Newman, M. J. D., and Sumner, D. W. (1957): Megaloblastic anemia following the use of primidone. *Blood,* 12:183–188.

45. Orth, D. N., Almedia, H., Walsh, F. B., and Honda, M. (1967): Ophthalmoplegia resulting from diphenylhydantoin and primidone intoxication. *J.A.M.A.,* 201:485–487.

46. Parker, W. A. (1974): Primidone thrombocytopenia. *Ann. Intern. Med.,* 81:559–560.

47. Poch, G. F. (1955): Estudio critico de valor de la primidona en el tratamiento de las epilepsias. *Arq. Bras. Med.,* 45:171–182.

48. Pollack, M. A., Burk, P. G., and Nathanson, G. (1979): Mucocutaneous eruptions due to antiepileptic drug therapy in children. *Ann. Neurol.,* 5:262–267.

49. Reizenstein, P., and Lund, L. (1973): Effect of anticonvulsive drugs on folate absorption and the cerebrospinal folate pump. *Scand. J. Haematol.,* 11:158–165.

50. Reynolds, E. H., Milner, G., Matthews, D. M., and Chanarin, I. (1966): Anticonvulsant therapy, mega-

loblastic haemopoiesis, and folic acid metabolism. *Q. J. Med.,* 35:521–537.

51. Richens, A., and Rowe, D. J. F. (1970): Disturbances of calcium metabolism by anticonvulsant drugs. *Br. Med. J.,* 4:73–76.

52. Rodin, E. A., Rim, C. S., Kitano, H., Lewis, R., and Rennick, P. M. (1976): A comparison of the effectiveness of primidone versus carbamazepine in epileptic outpatients. *J. Nerv. Ment. Dis.,* 163:41–46.

53. Rodriguez, V. L. E., and Oviedo, S. G. V. (1957): Dermatitis ampollosa mortal desencadenada por la primidona (Mysoline®). *Rev. Esp. Pediatr.,* 13:737–747.

54. Rose, M., and Johnson, I. (1978): Reinterpretation of the haematological effects of anticonvulsant treatment. *Lancet,* 1:1349–1350.

55. Sciarra, D., Carter, S., Vicale, C. T., and Merritt, H. H. (1954): Clinical evaluation of primidone (Mysoline®), a new anticonvulsant drug. *J.A.M.A.,* 154:827–829.

56. Smith, B., and Forster, F. M. (1954): Mysoline® and milotoin: Two new medicines for epilepsy. *Neurology (Minneap.),* 4:137–142.

57. Smith, B. H., and McNaughton, F. L. (1953): My-soline®, a new anticonvulsant drug. Its value in refractory cases of epilepsy. *Can. Med. Assoc. J.,* 68:464–467.

58. Spray, G. H., and Burns, D. G. (1972): Folate deficiency and anticonvulsant drugs. *Br. Med. J.,* 2:167–168.

59. Stevenson, M. M., and Gilbert, E. F. (1970): Anticonvulsants and hemorrhagic disease of the newborn. *J. Pediatr.,* 77:516.

60. Timberlake, W. H., Abbott, J. A., and Schwab, R. S. (1955): An effective anticonvulsant with initial problems of adjustment. *N. Engl. J. Med.,* 252:304–307.

61. Verdura, G., and Lupi, G. (1969): La prevenzione e la terapia degli effetti "neurotossici" acuti de "primicone." *Aggior. Pediatr.,* 20:81–86.

62. Wilson, W. E. J., and Hodgson, E. E. F. (1954): Mysoline® in epilepsy: A comparison with older methods of treatment. *J. Ment. Sci.,* 100:250–261.

63. Winnacker, J. L., Yeager, H., Saunders, J. A., Russell, B., and Anast, S. (1977): Rickets in children receiving anticonvulsant drugs. *Am. J. Dis. Child.,* 131:286–290.

Antiepileptic Drugs, edited by D. M. Woodbury, J. K. Penry, and C. E. Pippenger. Raven Press, New York © 1982.

35

Primidone

Mechanisms of Action

Dixon M. Woodbury and C. E. Pippenger

Although it has been recognized since its introduction into clinical use in epilepsy in 1952 (9) that primidone is an effective antiepileptic drug, particularly for complex partial seizures, and that phenobarbital is ineffective in this condition, it has not been definitively established that primidone has antiepileptic activity per se. Nor have its mechanisms of action been extensively studied. In fact, since the early studies of Butler and Waddell (4) suggested that the anticonvulsant effects of primidone with long-term administration were caused by the accumulation of phenobarbital, its principal metabolite, and not of primidone or phenylethylmalonamide (PEMA), another of its metabolites, it was assumed that primidone was not an active anticonvulsant agent. However, the subsequent studies of Gallagher and colleagues (2,3,6,7) and of Frey and Hahn (5) demonstrated anticonvulsant activity of both primidone and PEMA in laboratory animals. Hence, these researchers attempted to apply this information to the drugs' actions in humans (3,6,7).

Since many of the observed effects of primidone on chronic treatment are caused by phenobarbital, the mechanisms of action of this metabolite need not be discussed here (see Chapter 27). The objective of this chapter is to review the evidence for the anticonvulsant action of primidone and PEMA per se and to em-

phasize the differences between their effects and those of phenobarbital.

It is evident from evaluation of published reports of the effectiveness of primidone and PEMA in preventing maximal electroshock seizures (MES) and pentylenetetrazol (PTZ)-induced convulsions in experimental animals that the anticonvulsant effects of primidone and PEMA are clear and distinct from those of phenobarbital. Although this is the case, the biochemical mechanisms by which primidone and PEMA act have not been elucidated because of the difficulty in separating the effects of these two agents from those of phenobarbital. Therefore, until studies are performed at doses of primidone that affect only the MES pattern (see below) prior to the accumulation of phenobarbital and PEMA, it is not possible to delineate the biochemical mechanisms of action of primidone.

EVIDENCE FOR THE ANTICONVULSANT EFFECTS OF PRIMIDONE IN EXPERIMENTAL ANIMALS AND HUMANS

In both experimental animals and humans, primidone is metabolized by ring cleavage to yield PEMA and by oxidation at the C-2 position to produce phenobarbital (see 1, and Chapter 31). Both phenobarbital (in animals and humans) and PEMA (in animals) have been shown to have anticonvulsant activity by direct assessment of the compounds (3). However, it is not possible to assess directly the anticonvulsant effect of primidone because of the concurrent presence of both of its metabolites (PEMA and phenobarbital) following long-term administration of primidone. Therefore, to assess the anticonvulsant activity of primidone, it is necessary to evaluate its actions early in the time course of its administration, with careful monitoring of primidone, PEMA, and phenobarbital concentrations in plasma and brain. Measures of anticonvulsant activity should be performed simultaneously in conjunction with quantification of the concentrations of both primidone and its metabolites.

The only documented experiments utilizing this approach were those of Baumel et al. (2). A graphic summary of their results, derived from their work by Woodbury (13), is presented in Fig. 1. The relationship between the dose of primidone and its effects on the MES and PTZ seizure tests and the plasma and brain concentrations of primidone and its metabolites after administration of different single doses of the drug to rats is shown. Starting from the left, the first curve is the effect of primidone on MES. The ED_{50} is 2.7 mg/kg (see box). The next curve is the effect of phenobarbital on MES; the ED_{50} is 5.0 mg/kg. The next curve is the effect of phenobarbital on PTZ; the ED_{50} is 9 mg/kg. The effect of primidone on PTZ seizures is shown as the eighth curve from the left; the ED_{50} is 100 mg/kg. The next curve depicts the effects of

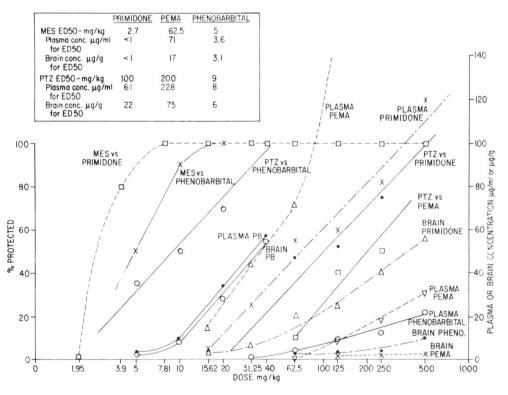

FIG. 1. Relationship between the dose (mg/kg) of primidone, phenobarbital (PB), or phenylethylmalonamide (PEMA) and their effects on the maximal electroshock (MES) and pentylenetetrazol (PTZ) seizure tests and the plasma and brain concentrations of primidone and its metabolites after administration of different single doses of the drug to rats. The graph is plotted from data presented by Baumel *et al.* (2). (From Woodbury, ref. 13, with permission.)

PEMA on PTZ seizures; the ED_{50} is 200 mg/kg. The plasma and brain concentrations of primidone and its metabolites, PEMA and phenobarbital, after various doses of primidone are shown on the right (7,10–14th curves from left), and those for phenobarbital and PEMA are given in the middle (4–6th curves from left). The plasma and brain concentrations of the three drugs at their ED_{50} values are shown in the box.

The following conclusions can be drawn from these data. (a) Primidone possesses independent anticonvulsant activity, particularly against MES. This is demonstrated by the fact that it produces protection against MES when there are no detectable concentrations of PEMA or phenobarbital in brain and plasma and primidone levels are less than 1 μg/ml or 1 μg/g. (b) Primidone seems to play no role in the body in protection against PTZ-induced seizures, since its ED_{50} is 11 times higher than that of phenobarbital, the plasma concentration for the ED_{50} value is nearly eight times higher, and the brain concentration four times higher. Since PEMA appears to play no role in either MES or PTZ protection in the body, it is apparent that phenobarbital is the active anticonvulsant against PTZ seizures when primidone is given to rats. (c) Although PEMA has anticonvulsant properties by itself, it is very weak, and following primidone administration, the levels of this metabolite are not sufficiently high to account for any of the anticonvulsant effect of primidone. However, on repeated administration of primidone, both PEMA and phenobarbital accumulate. In this case, they both contribute most of the anticonvulsant activity of primidone, as already mentioned.

Early clinical studies suggested that primidone was an effective antiepileptic drug but not more so than PB (8,12). However, these were short-term crossover studies that did not allow the achievement of steady-state drug concentrations prior to changes in dosage regimens and, therefore, must be interpreted with caution. In 1967, Vendelin-Olesen and Dam (11) described a 6-month crossover study between primidone and phenobarbital with doses designed to yield comparable serum phenobarbital concentrations. Their results, based on an evaluation of seizure frequency, suggested no difference between the anticonvulsant activity of phenobarbital and primidone.

A definitive study by Oxley et al. (10) in humans has confirmed the findings of Gallagher and colleagues in experimental animals that primidone has anticonvulsant activity that cannot be attributed to either phenobarbital or PEMA. Oxley et al. (10) performed a 12-month crossover study of primidone and phenobarbital in 21 epileptic patients. The effectiveness of each treatment regimen in the control of generalized tonic–clonic seizures was assessed by measurement of monthly seizure frequency and plasma phenobarbital concentrations. A statistically significant increase in seizure frequency was observed in those patients who were receiving phenobarbital alone as compared to the same patients who were receiving primidone. This increased seizure frequency occurred whether the patients received primidone as the first or second treatment regimen. It is to be noted that these investigators carefully controlled serum phenobarbital concentrations to assure that any change in seizure frequency could not be attributed to altered phenobarbital concentrations. The mean serum phenobarbital level in the primidone treatment period was 138 $\pm$ 69 μM and in the primidone period, 137 $\pm$ 53 μM (10).

On the basis of both the animal and clinical studies cited above, it may be concluded that primidone is an active anticonvulsant drug with pharmacodynamic properties similar to those already established for phenytoin and carbamazepine.

It has been clearly documented that phenytoin exerts its anticonvulsant effects through an alteration of Na^+ and Ca^{2+} fluxes across nerve cell membranes (see Chapter 19). On the basis of (a) the similarities among the pharmacological effects of primidone, phenytoin, and carbamazepine in experimental models of epilepsy (MES and PTZ challenges) and (b) the effectiveness of primidone, phenytoin, and carbamazepine, and the ineffectiveness of phenobarbital in complex partial seizures, we would anticipate that the mechanism of action of primidone will be established through studies of its effects on the neuronal membrane, particularly with respect to alterations of ionic fluxes. Through careful design of experimental parameters to negate potential effects of PEMA and/ or phenobarbital, the *in vivo* effects of primidone on the biochemical and electrophysiological properties of nerve cells can be established. Coupled with this *in vivo* approach should be carefully executed *in vitro* studies on the effects of primidone on ionic fluxes and other biochemical parameters in isolated nerves, synaptosomes, brain slices, and epithelial membranes, such as those found in toad bladders. *In vitro,* primidone is not metabolized to PEMA and phenobarbital; hence, its direct effects can be assessed, as has been done with phenytoin, (for example see Chapter 19).

ACKNOWLEDGMENTS

Unpublished work described in this chapter was supported by Program Project Grant Number 1 PO1-NS-15767 from the National Institute of Neurological and Communicative Disorders and Stroke. Dr. Woodbury is the recipient of a Research Career Award (5-K6-NB-13838) from NINCDS.

REFERENCES

1. Alvin, J., Goh, E., and Bush, M. T. (1975): Study of the hepatic metabolism of primidone by improved methodology. *J. Pharmacol. Exp. Ther.,* 194:117–125.
2. Baumel, I. P., Gallagher, B. B., DiMicco, H., and Goico, H. (1973): Metabolism and anticonvulsant properties of primidone in the rat. *J. Pharmacol. Ex. Ther.,* 186:305–314.
3. Baumel, I. P., Gallagher, B. B., and Mattson, R. H. (1972): Phenylethyl malonamide (PEMA). An important metabolite of primidone. *Arch. Neurol.,* 27:34–41.
4. Butler, T. C., and Waddell, W. J. (1956): Metabolic conversion of primidone (Mysoline®) to phenobarbital. *Proc. Soc. Exp. Biol. Med.,* 93:544–546.
5. Frey, H. H., and Hahn, I. (1960): Untersuchungen uber die Bedeutung des durch Biotransformation gebildeten Phenobarbital fur die antikonvulsive Wirkung von Primidon. *Arch. Int. Pharmacodyn. Ther.,* 128:281–290.
6. Gallagher, B. B., Baumel, I. P., and Mattson, R. H., (1972): Metabolic disposition of primidone and its metabolites in epileptic subjects after single and repeated administration. *Neurology (Minneap.),* 22:1186–1192.
7. Gallagher, B. B., Smith, D. B., and Mattson, R. H. (1970): The relationship of the anticonvulsant properties of primidone to phenobarbital. *Epilepsia,* 11:293–301.
8. Gruber, C. M., Brock, J. T., and Dyken, M. (1962): Comparison of the effectiveness of primidone, mephobarbital, primidone, diphenylhydantoin, ethotoin, metharbital, and methylphenylethylhydantoin in motor seizures. *Clin. Pharmacol. Ther.,* 3:23–28.
9. Handley, R., and Stewart, A. S. R. (1952): Mysoline: A new drug in the treatment of epilepsy. *Lancet,* 1:742–744.
10. Oxley, J., Hebdige, S., Laidlaw, J., Wadsworth, J., and Richens, A. (1980): A comparative study of phenobarbitone and primidone in the treatment of epilepsy. In: *Antiepileptic Therapy. Advances in Drug Monitoring,* edited by S. I. Johannessen, P. L. Morselli, C. E. Pippenger, A. Richens, D. Schmidt, and H. Meinardi, pp. 237–245. Raven Press, New York.
11. Vendelin-Olesen, O., and Dam, M. (1967): The metabolic conversion of primidone (Mysoline) to phenobarbitone in patients under long-term treatment. An attempt to estimate the independent effect of primidone. *Acta Neurol. Scand.,* 43:348–356.
12. White, P. T., Plott, D., and Norton, J. (1966): Relative anticonvulsant potency of primidone. A double blind comparison. *Arch. Neurol.,* 14:31–35.
13. Woodbury, D. M. (1978): Metabolites and the mechanisms of action of antiepileptic drugs. In: *Advances in Epileptology, 1977: Psychology, Pharmacotherapy, and New Diagnostic Approaches,* edited by H. Meinardi and A. J. Rowan, pp. 134–150. Swets & Zeitlinger, Amsterdam.

Antiepileptic Drugs, edited by D. M. Woodbury, J. K. Penry, and C. E. Pippenger. Raven Press, New York © 1982.

36

Carbamazepine

Chemistry and Methods of Determination

Henn Kutt and Helga Paris-Kutt

Carbamazepine (Tegretol®) was developed in the laboratories of J. R. Geigy AG (Basel, Switzerland) in the late 1950s. Its synthesis was described by Schindler (44) in 1961 (U.S. patent 2,948,718), and its anticonvulsant properties, demonstrated by testing in animals, were reported by Theobald and Kunz (51) in 1963.

Historically, iminodibenzyl (10,11-dihydro-5H-dibenzo[b,f]azepine), shown in Fig. 1A and first described by Thiele and Holzinger (52) in 1899, may be considered the precursor of carbamazepine. Synthesis of a number of iminodibenzyl derivatives was reported by Schindler and Häfliger (45) in 1954. These compounds possessed local anesthetic and antihistaminic properties and some modest antiepileptic activity. Considerable anticonvulsant effect, however, occurred when a carbamyl (carboxamide) group was added at the 5 position of iminodibenzyl. The carbamyl side chain combined with iminostilbene (Fig. 1B), a structure analogous to iminodibenzyl but having a double bond between the 10 and 11 positions, showed the strongest anticonvulsant properties and became known as carbamazepine (Fig. 1C). In comparison with the succinimide, hydantoin, barbiturate, and benzodiazepine anticonvulsants, carbamazepine (CBZ) lacks a saturated carbon atom, and the amide group is in the side chain rather than in the ring. It differs from imipramine only by having a double bond between positions 10 and 11 and by having a shorter side chain.

CHEMISTRY

Carbamazepine (5-carbamyl-5H-dibenzo[b,f] azepine; 5H-dibenzo[b,f]azepine-5-carboxamide) (Fig. 1C) is an iminostilbene derivative with an empirical formula $C_{15}H_{12}N_2O$ and molecular weight of 236.26. It appears as a white crystalline compound with a melting point between 190°C and 193°C. Carbamazepine can be prepared by treating iminostilbene with carbonyl chloride followed by the addition of ammonia to a boiling mixture of the latter product in absolute ethanol (44). Carbamazepine behaves as a neutral lipophilic substance; it dissolves in ethanol, chloroform, dichloromethane, and other solvents but is virtually insoluble in water. The solubility in phosphate buffer pH 7.4 is 72 mg/liter. Aqueous solution can be made with propylene glycol in which the solubility is enhanced by moderate heating.

The ultraviolet spectrum of CBZ shows a major peak at around 220 nm and a smaller one at 288 to 290 nm. Acid hydrolysis will result in a major ultraviolet absorption peak at 255 nm. Treatment with perchloric acid will render CBZ highly fluorescent (excitation max 366 nm, emission max 498 nm). The mass spectrum of

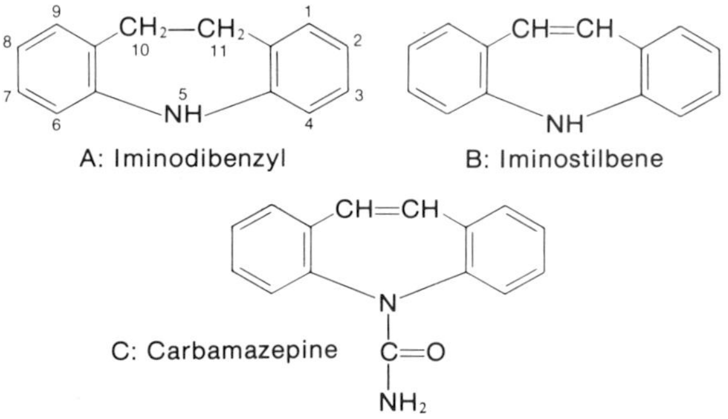

FIG. 1. Carbamazepine and its precursors.

CBZ shows a molecular ion at *m/e* 236 and a base peak at *m/e* 193 (11,33). Studies of CBZ by X-ray diffraction have revealed that in the three-dimensional structure the angle of flexure α is 53°, the angle of annelation β is 30°, and the angle of torsion γ is 3°. The distance between the centers of benzene rings measured 4.85 Å. These measurements are characteristic of tricyclic psychoactive drugs, and the similarity of CBZ to imipramine is also obvious in the steric parameters except for the torsion angle which is 20° for imipramine (13).

The double bond between positions 10 and 11 in the CBZ molecule is somewhat unstable and provides a site of action for the biotransformation enzyme(s). The metabolic products identified in man so far are a 10,11-dihydro-

10,11-epoxy compound (CBZ epoxide, Fig. 2D) and 10,11-dihydro-10,11-dihydroxy (Fig. 2E) derivatives, among others (9,11,31). Aromatic hydroxylation also takes place at positions 1, 2, or 3, resulting in OH-carbamazepines (9,31). Probably only the CBZ epoxide is of clinical significance, because it has been found to possess antiepileptic activity in animal testing (10,11) and is present in the blood of patients taking CBZ.

Separation of the carbamyl group from position 5, yielding iminostilbene, is thought to occur as a result of the action of biotransformation enzymes, since iminostilbene (Fig. 2B) has been isolated as a metabolite in rat urine (11,31). Breakdown of CBZ to iminostilbene also occurs pyrolytically as in the course of gas–liquid

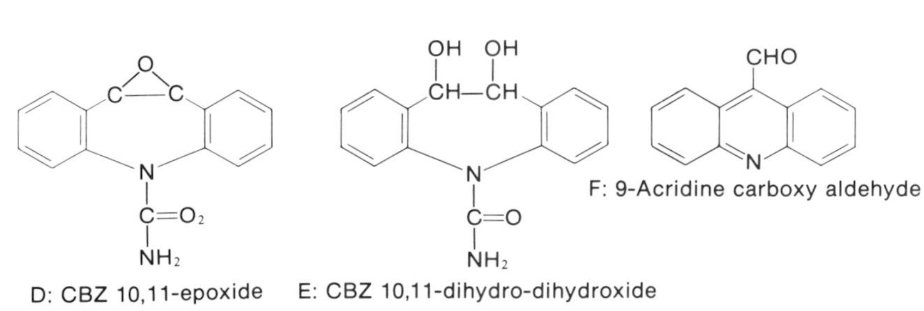

FIG. 2. Carbamazepine and its metabolites and breakdown products.

chromatography (11,21). Another pyrolysis product of CBZ is 9-methylacridine (11), shown in Fig. 2C. The pyrolytic breakdown product of CBZ epoxide and CBZ-dihydroxide is 9-acridinecarboxaldehyde (11), shown in Fig. 2F. For further details, see Chapter 38 on CBZ biotransformation.

METHODS OF DETERMINATION

Various techniques have been used to determine the concentration of CBZ in biological fluids. These include: (a) ultraviolet spectrophotometry (4,12,32), (b) spectrophotometry in the visible light spectrum (18,40), (c) fluorometry, often combined with thin-layer chromatography (TLC) (7,28,46), (d) gas–liquid chromatography (GLC) (Table 1), (e) enzyme-mediated immunoassay technique (EMIT®) (6,37,47), and (f) high-pressure liquid chromatography (HPLC) (Table 2). For an earlier review of these methods, see Kutt (22). Of 306 laboratories currently participating in an anti-epileptic drug level quality control program, 187 used immunoassay, 57 GLC, 56 HPLC, and 6 other techniques (e.g., TLC, spectrophotometry) for the determination of carbamazepine.

Extraction

Extraction of CBZ from biological materials is usually achieved with solvents such as ethyl ether, ethyl acetate, dichloromethane, dichloroethane, and chloroform. The reported recoveries range from 70% to nearly 100%. Such extracts also contain the metabolites. The concentration of CBZ in the extract can then be determined by some of the techniques mentioned above, or the extract may be submitted for further separation and isolation of CBZ and its metabolites by chromatography.

Thin-layer chromatography on silica plates was the earliest technique for separation. The spots of CBZ and its metabolites on developed TLC plates were then estimated visually under ultraviolet light, rendered fluorescent by treatment

TABLE 1. *Gas chromatographic methods for CBZ and CBZ epoxide determination*

Reference	Year	Column packing	Internal standard	Derivatization	Peak measured	CBZ epoxide	Other antiepileptic drugs
Meijer (27)	1971	QF-1-XE-60	Stigmasterol	No	CBZ	No	Yes
Kupferberg (21)	1972	OV-17	Cyheptamide	Yes	Stable derivative	No	No
Larsen et al. (23)	1972	SE-52	Diazepam	No	CBZ	No	No
Morselli and Frigerio (30)	1973	OV-17	Nordiazepam	No	CBZ	Yes	No
Roger et al. (41)	1973	OV-17	MPPH	No	Iminostilbene	No	Yes
Perchalski and Wilder (36)	1974	OV-210-OV-1	Cyheptamide	Yes	Stable derivative	No	No
Gerardin et al. (15)	1975	OV-105	10-CH$_3$-CBZ	Yes	Stable derivative	No	No
Least et al. (24)	1975	OV-17	BMMA	Yes	Stable derivative	No	Yes
Sheehan and Beam (48)	1975	OV-17	Heptabarbital	No	CBZ	No	Yes
Abraham and Joslin (1)	1976	SP-2250	MPPH	No	Iminostilbene	No	Yes
Pynnönen et al. (38)	1976	OV-1	Imipramine	No	CBZ	Yes	No
Heipertz et al. (16)	1977	SP-1000	Mephenytoin	No	CBZ	No	Yes
Thoma et al. (53)	1978	SP-2510-2110	4-CH$_3$-PRM	No	CBZ	No	Yes
Millner and Taber (29)	1979	OV-1	Besamide	Yes	Stable derivative	No	No
Rambeck and Meijer (39)	1979	OV-225	MPPH	No	CBZ	No	Yes
Schaal et al. (42)	1979	DL-LSX	Barbital	No	CBZ	No	Yes

TABLE 2. *High-pressure liquid chromatographic methods for CBZ and CBZ epoxide determination*

Reference	Year	Internal standard	Column packing	Mobile phase	CBZ epoxide	Other antiepileptic drugs
Gauchel et al. (14)	1973	Diazepam	Chromosorb A	Isooctane	No	No
Eichelbaum and Bertilson (8)	1975	CBZ-H_2	Carbowax	CH_2Cl_2	Yes	No
Westenberg and De Zeeuw (58)	1976	Nitrazepam	LiChrosorb	4-H-Furan	Yes	Yes
Soldin and Hill (49)	1976	Cyheptamide	Bondapak C_{18}	Acetonitrile	No	Yes
Adams and Vandermark (2)	1976	Phenacetin	ODS-Sil	Acetonitrile	No	Yes
Kabra et al. (19)	1978	MPPH	Bondapak C_{18}	Acetonitrile	No	Yes
Helmsing et al. (17)	1978	Diazepam	Pherisorb	Propanol	No	Yes
MacKichan (26)	1980	Lorazepam Nordiazepam	Bondapak CN	Acetonitrile	Yes	No

with acid and scanned *in situ,* or scraped off, eluted, and submitted to further quantitative procedures.

Ultraviolet Spectrophotometry

Historically, ultraviolet (UV) spectrophotometry was the earliest technique for measuring CBZ; it was first used by Führ in 1964 (12). Morselli et al. in 1971 (32) reported a technique in which the alkalinized samples were washed with *n*-heptane prior to extraction with dichloroethane. The absorbance was measured at 288 nm. Sensitivity was considered to be linear between 0.5 and 60 μg of CBZ per ml of plasma, and no interference from phenytoin or phenobarbital was seen. Absorbance of untreated CBZ is measured at the secondary absorption peak of 290 nm or 288 nm rather than at the maximum absorbance peak of 220 nm to eliminate major interference from other common anticonvulsants, which have maximum absorption in the range of 220 nm but little, if any, in the 290-nm range. Beyer and Klinge (4) reported a highly sensitive UV spectrophotometric method for determination of CBZ. The high sensitivity was obtained by heating the starting material with hydrochloric acid, which shifted the 290-nm absorption peak to 255-nm but increased the specific extinction fivefold. This resulted from an alteration of the azepine ring by acid hydrolysis and formation of 9-methylacridine (3).

Generally, direct UV spectrophotometry is not considered a highly specific method for determination of CBZ.

Spectrophotometry in the Visible Light Spectrum

A spectrophotometric method in which the measurement is carried out in the visible light spectrum was developed in the laboratory of Geigy by Herrmann in 1966 (18). Carbamazepine was extracted at neutral pH with dichloroethane and then treated with sodium nitrite and nitric acid. A yellow product formed, which was measured spectrophotometrically at 400 nm. An analogous procedure was described by Rist Nielsen and Remmer in 1969 (40). Starting material (2.5 ml sample) was extracted with dichloroethane. The color reagents were 3% sodium nitrite and 22% nitric acid; the reaction mixture was kept for 15 min at 37°C and extracted with dichloroethane for measurement at 400 nm. Since the metabolites of CBZ will also give a yellow color with this method, the measurement represents the sum total of CBZ and the metabolites unless the extract is submitted first to isolating procedures.

Fluorometry and TLC

Fluorometric determination of CBZ and its metabolites has usually been employed in combination with TLC. The use of fluorometry was first reported by Scheiffarth et al. in 1966 (43). Biological materials (CSF, plasma, urine, bile) or their dichloroethane extracts were applied to silica plates, which were then developed with carbon tetrachloride : methanol (7 : 1). The spots were visualized under UV light, scraped off, and eluted with 70% perchloric acid followed by heating at 120°C for 20 min. The resulting fluorescence was determined with a fluorescence spectrometer using excitation wavelength of 358 nm and emission wavelength of 498 nm.

An analogous but somewhat less cumbersome technique was described by Christiansen in 1973 (7). Diluted plasma (10 μl) was applied directly after 10 μl of ethanol had been placed on silica plates. The chromatograms were developed with benzene : dioxane : ethanol : ammonia (5 : 4 : 1 : 1), dried, dipped into perchloric acid reagent (70% $HClO_4$, 12 ml; ethanol, 150 ml; H_2O, 130 ml) and then heated at 108°C for 8 min. For quantitation, fluorescence was measured *in situ* by direct scanning of spots at 498 nm with a fluorescence densitometer (Vitatron TLD 100 flying spot scanner), using excitation wavelength of 366 nm. A calibration curve was made with standards.

Meilink (28) in 1974 reported a technique in which an ammonium ceric sulfate and phosphoric acid reagent was used to render CBZ and its metabolites fluorescent. Cyproheptadine, imipramine, protryptaline, and quinine, among others, were found to interfere with this method. Schneider and Berenguer (46) in 1977 used nitric acid vapors to render the CBZ spots fluorescent on thin-layer plates and scanned *in situ*. Wad and Rosenmund (57) in 1978 scanned untreated spots at 215 nm for quantitation, whereas Breyer (5) used 285 nm.

Gas–Liquid Chromatography

Gas–liquid chromatography has been one of the widely used methods for CBZ determination, as it offers high specificity and sensitivity. Numerous GLC techniques have been described, which indicates the difficulties of finding an ideal procedure. Some of the methods measure only the parent compound (21,33,36),

but others measure both the parent compound and its epoxy metabolite (30,38). Still others allow simultaneous determination of other antiepileptic drugs from the same sample preparation and application (1,16,39,41,48). The combination of GLC with mass spectrometry (GC/MS selected ion monitoring) extends the sensitivity of the procedure to the low nanogram range for CBZ determination (33,54,55).

As indicated above, the GLC determination of CBZ is not free from problems. The basic difficulty is that CBZ tends to decompose to various extents at the high temperatures necessary for gas chromatography. The decomposition is enhanced by acidic conditions and by the active sites in the chromatographic column. To deal with this problem, the following approaches have been used: (a) formation of a stable derivative of CBZ by silylation or by conversion to CBZ cyanamide prior to injection into the gas chromatograph (15,21,36); (b) creation of conditions under which it is hoped that complete and reproducible breakdown takes place and then measurement of the breakdown product, e.g., iminostilbene (1,41); (c) creation of conditions that prevent or minimize the breakdown of underivatized CBZ in the gas chromatograph (27,30,53).

To prevent the breakdown of underivatized CBZ, various steps and manipulations have been helpful. These include (a) a short column, (b) coarse mesh support, (c) high-polarity liquid phase in high concentration, (d) nonreactive injection vehicle, (e) deactivation of the column by silanizing (30) or by designing deactivated column packings (53), and/or (f) using internal standards (33,35) that should break down at the same rate as CBZ. It is of interest that a technique that works well in one laboratory may not be successful in another. Some of the reasons apparently are differences in the design of chromatographic apparatus. Common experience has shown that instruments with a metal connector between the injection port and the glass column usually perform poorly, automatic liquid injectors improve reproducibility, and U-shaped columns are preferable to coil columns in CBZ determination.

Formation of a Stable Derivative of CBZ Prior to Gas Chromatography

In the method of Kupferberg (21), cyheptamide, a structure similar to CBZ, was added to the plasma sample as an internal standard and extracted at pH 7.2 with chloroform. Other acidic drugs (barbiturates, hydantoins) were removed by intermediate extraction steps. The final extract containing CBZ was dried and reacted with TRI-SIL/BSA in pyridine or Regisil®. The column packing was OV-17. In this technique, it is important to remove phenytoin prior to derivatization and chromatography, since it has a retention time similar to that of cyheptamide. Least et al. (24) used benzylmalonate methylester monoamide (BMMA) as internal standard and Regis silylation mix to form stable derivatives. Most of the major antiepileptic drugs could be determined simultaneously by this technique, using OV-17 as column packing.

The method of Perchalski and Wilder (36) also used cyheptamide as internal standard. The plasma sample was extracted and derivatized with dimethylformamide dimethyl acetal. Just prior to injection, excess reagent was evaporated, and the residue was dissolved in carbon disulfide and injected into a column packed with OV-210 and OV-1. This time sequence is important, because the derivatized internal standard remains stable for only about 30 min; therefore, this technique is not suitable for simultaneous preparation of a large number of samples for an overnight operation with automated equipment. Millner and Taber (29) used the same system for derivatization but used benzamide as internal standard and OV-1 as column packing. The advantage of this modification is that the derivatized internal standard remains stable longer.

In the method of Gerardin et al. (15), 10-methoxycarbamazepine was used as internal standard. The alkalinized sample was extracted with ethyl ether, evaporated to dryness, and treated with triethylamine and trifluoroacetic anhydride to dehydrate CBZ into stable CBZ cyanamide which was then injected into the gas chromatograph in carbon disulfide.

Conversion of CBZ to Iminostilbene

Measuring iminostilbene as a representative of CBZ was utilized in the method of Roger et al. (41). Solvent extract of antiepileptic drugs including CBZ, to which 5-(p-methylphenyl)-5-phenylhydantoin (MPPH) is added as internal standard and which has been purified by hexane washings, is dried and reconstituted in trimethylphenylammonium hydroxide (TMPAH). This effects methylation of phenytoin, phenobarbital, and primidone, if present, and leads to nearly complete breakdown of CBZ in the column packed with OV-17. Iminostilbene is the major product, and, other conditions such as the speed of injection being stable, the iminostilbene peak is reasonably proportional to CBZ concentration. The advantage of this technique is that it allows simultaneous determination of derivatized phenytoin, phenobarbital, and primidone as well; it is essentially the method that Kupferberg (20) described for that purpose in 1970.

This technique has been used successfully for the determination of anticonvulsants, including CBZ, in clinical material in our laboratory, using a gas chromatograph equipped with an automatic liquid sampler. One of the limitations of this technique under our operating conditions is relatively low sensitivity, as the response with CBZ concentrations of less than 1 μg/ml is not linear.

Gas–Liquid Chromatography of Underivatized CBZ

The procedure of Meijer (27) required, first, the isolation of CBZ by thin-layer chromatography; it was then injected into the gas chromatograph in pentanol with stigmasterol as the internal standard. Meijer also advocated the addition of formic acid vapors to the carrier gas, which improved the resolution of peaks but added complexity to the procedure.

In Larsen's technique (23), diazepam was used as the internal standard. The sample extract was injected in ethanol into a column packed with 3% SE-52 and maintained at 290°C. The retention times are short, which allows analysis of many samples but may hamper accuracy.

The technique of Morselli et al. (30) required daily silanization of the column. A dichloroethane extract of the sample, with N-desmethyldiazepam as an internal marker, was reconstituted in acetone and injected into the gas chromatograph. The column was packed with 3% OV-17 and operated at 250°C. This procedure allows measurement of CBZ and its epoxide. We have ascertained by mass spectrometry that CBZ appears as such rather than as the breakdown product. The technique of Pynnönen et al. (38) also measures CBZ and its epoxide.

The newer commercial column packings used for CBZ determination without derivatization are SP 2510 DA or a mixture of SP 2510 DA and SP 2110 (53), and DL-LSX-3-0295 (42), among others. The breakdown of CBZ with these packings is thought not to be extensive, and reasonable accuracy and reproducibility can be achieved. All allow determination of other major antiepileptic drugs simultaneously with CBZ but not the CBZ epoxide.

Selected Ion Monitoring

The GC/MS method of Palmer et al. (33) provided high sensitivity. A linear response was seen with amounts as low as 0.05 µg/ml. As internal standard, 10,11-dihydrocarbamazepine was used in part because it breaks down at the same rate as CBZ. Samples extracted with ethyl acetate were injected into a short (35 cm) column packed with 5% SE-52 and maintained at 210°C. An LKB 9000 gas chromatograph–mass spectrometer equipped with a multiple ion detector adjusted to record the intensity of the molecular ion of carbamazepine (m/e 236) and dihydrocarbamazepine (m/e 238) was used. The peak height ratios of m/e 236 and m/e 238 were calculated and plotted against CBZ concentration. The CBZ epoxide was not measured by this technique.

Using [9-^{13}C]carboxyacridine and [10-^{13}C]-5-H-dibenz[b,f]azepine as internal standard,

Trager et al. (54) applied selected ion monitoring (SIM) to the determination of both CBZ and CBZ epoxide. The method of Pantrotto et al. (34) also measured CBZ and the epoxide. Permethylated metabolites of CBZ were determined by GC/MS by Lynn et al. (25). Truscott et al. (55) used direct chemical ionization mass spectrometry without gas chromatography for determination of CBZ simultaneously with other antiepileptic drugs.

High-Pressure Liquid Chromatography

High-pressure liquid chromatography is becoming increasingly popular for the determination of CBZ and CBZ epoxide. It circumvents the problems of thermal instability of these compounds inherent in gas chromatography and usually requires less elaborate sample preparation than is necessary for gas chromatography. Both normal-phase and reversed-phase techniques have been used successfully.

The early reports of HPLC determination of CBZ by Gauchel et al. (14) were encouraging. A practical method was described by Eichelbaum and Bertilsson (8) for measuring both CBZ and its epoxide. Purified sample extract dissolved in mobile phase was injected into the chromatograph equipped with a column packed with Durapak Carbowax 400 Corasil®. The mobile phase was n-hexane–dichloromethane–dimethyl sulfoxide, and the UV detector was set at 254 nm. At that wavelength, the detector response to CBZ epoxide, which lacks the double bond between positions 10 and 11 was more than 10 times less than the response to the parent compound, which necessitated resetting of sensitivity when the epoxide eluted. As the internal standard, 10,11-dihydrocarbamazepine (CBZ-H$_2$) was used. Other antiepileptic drugs needed to be removed, as they would interfere with the internal standard and the epoxide. The method reported by Westenberg and de Zeeuw (58) used nitrazepam as the internal standard and Li Chrosorb® SI 100 as column packing. Mobile phase was tetrahydrofuran in dichloromethane. Carbamazepine and its epoxide, along with other antiepileptic drugs, could be measured. The method of MacKichan (26) similarly measured both CBZ and the CBZ epoxide.

In the method of Adams and Vandermark (2), phenacetin was used as internal standard. Column packing was ODS-Sil XI, and the mobile phase was acetonitrile. Most major antiepileptic drugs were determined simultaneously with CBZ, but CBZ epoxide was not. Similar reversed-phase techniques have been reported by Helmsing et al. (17), Kabra et al. (19), and Soldin and Hill (49), among others, again measuring other drugs simultaneously but not the epoxide.

Recently, an HPLC technique for determining CBZ and CBZ epoxide along with other antiepileptic drugs has been adapted for use with the Technicon® autoanalyzer, which may prove practical for laboratories with high work loads.

Methods for CBZ Epoxide Determination

The need to measure CBZ epoxide concentrations has been emphasized by several investigators, since this compound was shown to possess antiepileptic activity in animal tests (10,11). Its concentration in human plasma usually ranges between 10 and 40% of that of the parent compound. It may well be that the meaningful concentration in man regarding effectiveness and toxicity is the sum total of the parent compound and the epoxide. Prospective studies with that in mind are indicated.

As indicated in the preceding discussion of assay techniques, several TLC, GLC, and HPLC methods measured both the parent compound and the epoxide. The TLC methods were those of Christiansen (7), Meilink (28), and Schneider and Berenguer (46), among others. The GLC or GC/MS SIM methods measuring both compounds are those of Morselli et al. (30), Pynnönen et al. (38), Trager et al. (54), and Pantrotto et al. (34). The HPLC techniques measuring CBZ and its epoxide are those of Eichenbaum and Bertilsson (8), Westenberg and de Zeeuw (58), and MacKichan (26). The future wide application of CBZ epoxide determination probably lies with HPLC.

Immunoassays

The enzyme-mediated immunoassay technique (EMIT®) developed by the Syva Co., Palo Alta, CA (37,47), utilizes sheep-grown antibodies specific to CBZ. The antibodies are reacted with CBZ in the test material (plasma, serum, CSF, saliva, tears), and the amount of drug–antibody complex is indicated by an enzyme (glucose-6-phosphate dehydrogenase)–substrate (glucose-6-phosphate) reaction, which in turn is quantitated by measuring spectrophotometrically the rate of cofactor (NAD) utilization.

The basic instrumentation is relatively simple, consisting of a spectrophotometer equipped with a temperature-controlled flow-through sample cell, a semiautomatic pipettor–dilutor, and a calculator–printer. The manipulative steps consist of placing the sample into a mixing cuvette with the pipettor, adding reagent A (antibody) and reagent B (enzyme), and aspirating the mixture into the spectrophotometer. The NAD utilization rate is followed for 30 sec, and the printout numbers are used to construct calibration curves. The unknown sample concentration is then interpolated from the curve. The commercial calibrators range from a concentration of 2 μg/ml to 10 μg/ml, in which the response is linear. Assay of very low (less than 2 μg/ml) concentrations is possible if one constructs a calibration curve with diluted calibrators. Samples with high concentrations need to be diluted and reassayed. Because of its relative simplicity, the technique is adaptable for routine use in laboratories lacking GLC and HPLC facilities. It can also be used in automated systems such as KA-150 (Perkin–Elmer) or centrifugal analyzers (6,56).

The advantages of EMIT® assay are that it is rapid (2–3 min for a single assay) and requires small amounts of test material (50 μl or less); thus, the samples can be obtained by fingerstick or heelstick, a distinct advantage when repeated samples are needed, particularly in children. The disadvantages are that hemolyzed, icteric, or lipemic plasma samples tend to give erroneous results and need to be analyzed by other techniques (47) and that the reagents for CBZ epoxide determination are not available. Several studies (6,47,50) evaluating different methods have shown that the values for CBZ obtained by EMIT® correlate well with those obtained by GLC or HPLC in competent hands.

CONVERSION

Carbamazepine

Conversion factor:

$$CF = \frac{1000}{mol.\ wt.} = \frac{1000}{236.3} = 4.23$$

Conversion:

$$(\mu g/ml) \times 4.23 = (\mu moles/liter)$$
$$(\mu moles/liter) \div 4.23 = (\mu g/ml)$$

Carbamazepine-10,11-epoxide

Conversion factor:

$$CF = \frac{1000}{mol.\ wt.} = \frac{1000}{252.3} = 3.96$$

Conversion:

$$(\mu g/ml) \times 3.96 = (\mu moles/liter)$$
$$(\mu moles/liter) \div 3.96 = (\mu g/ml)$$

REFERENCES

1. Abraham, C. V., and Joslin, H. D. (1976): Simultaneous gas-chromatographic analysis for phenobarbital, diphenylhydantoin, carbamazepine and primidone in serum. *Clin. Chem.*, 22:769–771.
2. Adams, R. F., and Vandermark, F. L. (1976): Simultaneous high-pressure liquid-chromatographic determination of some anticonvulsants in serum. *Clin. Chem.*, 22:25–31.
3. Beyer, K. H., Bredenstein, O., and Schenck, G. (1971): Isolierung und Identifizierung eines Carbamazepine Reaktionproduktes. *Arzneim. Forsch.*, 21:1033–1034.
4. Beyer, K. H., and Klinge, D. (1969): Zum spektrophotometrischen Nachweis von Carbamazepine. *Arzneim. Forsch.*, 19:1759–1760.
5. Breyer, U. (1975): Rapid and accurate determination of the level of carbamazepine by ultraviolet reflectance photometry on thin-layer chromatograms. *J. Chromatogr.*, 108:370–374.
6. Christensen, N. J. (1978): Study of the EMIT method

7. Christiansen, J. (1973): Assay of carbamazepine and metabolites in plasma by quantitative thin-layer chromatography. In: *Methods of Analysis of Anti-Epileptic Drugs*, edited by J. W. A. Meijer, H. Meinardi, C. Gardner-Thorpe, and E. van der Kleijn, pp. 87–90. Excerpta Medica, Amsterdam.
8. Eichelbaum, M., and Bertilsson, L. (1975): Determination of carbamazepine and its epoxide metabolite in plasma by high-speed liquid chromatography. *J. Chromatogr.*, 103:135–140.
9. Faigle, J. W., Brechbühler, S., Feldmann, K. F., and Richter, W. J. (1976): The biotransformation of carbamazepine. In: *Epileptic Seizures—Behaviour—Pain*, edited by W. Birkmayer, pp. 127–140. Huber Publishers, Bern.
10. Faigle, J. W., Feldmann, K. F., and Baltzer, V. (1977): Anticonvulsant effect of carbamazepine. An attempt to distinguish between the potency of the parent drug and its epoxide metabolite. In: *Antiepileptic Drug Monitoring*, edited by C. Gardner-Thorpe, D. Janz, H. Meinardi, and C. E. Pippenger, pp. 104–109. Pitman Medical, Tunbridge Wells, Kent.
11. Frigerio, A., and Morselli, P. L. (1975): Carbamazepine: Biotransformation. In: *Complex Partial Seizures and Their Treatment*, edited by J. K. Penry and D. D. Daly, pp. 295–308. Raven Press, New York.
12. Führ, J. (1964): Untersuchungen über die Verträglichkeit und Ausscheidung eines neuartigen Antiepilepticums. *Arzneim. Forsch.*, 14:74–75.
13. Gagneux, A. R. (1976): The chemistry of carbamazepine. In: *Epileptic Seizures—Behaviour—Pain*, edited by W. Birkmayer, pp. 120–126. Huber Publishers, Bern.
14. Gauchel, G., Gauchel, F. D., and Birkofer, L. (1973): A micromethod for the determination of carbamazepine in blood by high speed liquid chromatography. *Z. Klin. Chem. Klin. Biochem.*, 11:459–460.
15. Gerardin, A., Abadie, F., and Laffont, J. (1975): GLC determination of carbamazepine suitable for pharmacokinetic studies. *J. Pharm. Sci.*, 64:1940–1942.
16. Heipertz, R., Pilz, H., and Eickhoff, K. (1977): Evaluation of a rapid gas-chromatographic method for the simultaneous quantitative determination of ethosuximide, phenylethylmalonediamide, carbamazepine, phenobarbital, primidone and diphenylhydantoin in human serum. *Clin. Chim. Acta*, 77:307–316.
17. Helmsing, P. J., van der Woude, J., and van Eupen, O. M. (1978): A micromethod for simultaneous estimation of blood levels of some commonly used antiepileptic drugs. *Clin. Chim. Acta*, 89:301–309.
18. Herrmann, B. (1966): *Tegretol G 32883 Determination in Serum, Plasma and CSF*. Geigy Pharmaceuticals, Ardsley, New York.
19. Kabra, P. M., McDonald, D. M., and Marton, L. J. (1978): A simultaneous high-performance liquid chromatographic analysis of the most common anticonvulsants and their metabolites in serum. *J. Anal. Toxicol.*, 2:127–133.
20. Kupferberg, H. J. (1970): Quantitative estimation of diphenylhydantoin, primidone and phenobarbital in

for determination of anti-epileptic drugs in serum using an LKB 2086. *Scand. J. Clin. Lab. Invest.*, 38:781–784.

plasma by gas–liquid chromatography. *Clin. Chim. Acta*, 29:284–288.

21. Kupferberg, H. J. (1972): GLC determination of carbamazepine in plasma. *J. Pharm. Sci.*, 61:284–286.

22. Kutt, H. (1975): Carbamazepine: Chemistry and methods of determination. In: *Complex Partial Seizures and Their Treatment*, edited by J. K. Penry and D. D. Daly, pp. 249–261. Raven Press, New York.

23. Larsen, N. E., Naestoft, J., and Hvidberg, E. (1972): Rapid routine determination of some anti-epileptic drugs in serum by gas chromatography. *Clin. Chim. Acta*, 40:171–176.

24. Least, C. J., Johnson, G. F., and Solomon, H. M. (1975): Therapeutic monitoring of anticonvulsant drugs: Gas-chromatographic simultaneous determination of primidone, phenylethylmalonamide, carbamazepine and diphenylhydantoin. *Clin. Chem.*, 21:1658–1662.

25. Lynn, R. K., Smith, R. G., Thompson, R. M., Deiner, M. L., Griffin, D., and Gerber, N. (1978): Characterization of glucuronide metabolites of carbamazepine in human urine by gas chromatography and mass spectrometry. *Drug Metab. Dispos.*, 6:494–501.

26. MacKichan, J. J. (1980): Simultaneous liquid chromatographic analysis for carbamazepine and carbamazepine-10,11-epoxide in plasma and saliva by use of double internal standardization. *J. Chromatogr.*, 181:373–383.

27. Meijer, J. W. A. (1971): Simultaneous quantitative determination of anti-epileptic drugs, including carbamazepine, in body fluids. *Epilepsia*, 12:341–352.

28. Meilink, J. W. (1974): Fluorimetric assay of carbamazepine and its metabolites in blood. *Pharm. Weekbl.*, 109:22–30.

29. Millner, S. N., and Taber, C. A. (1979): Rapid gas chromatographic determination of carbamazepine for routine therapeutic monitoring. *J. Chromatogr.* 163:96–102.

30. Morselli, P. L., Biandrate, P., Frigerio, A., Gerna, M., and Tognoni, G. (1973): Gas chromatographic determination of carbamazepine and carbamazepine-10,11-epoxide in human body fluids. In: *Methods of Analysis of Anti-Epileptic Drugs*, edited by J. W. A. Meijer, H. Meinardi, C. Gardner-Thorpe, and E. van der Kleijn, pp. 169–175. Excerpta Medica, Amsterdam.

31. Morselli, P., and Frigerio, A. (1975): Metabolism and pharmacokinetics of carbamazepine. *Drug Metab. Rev.*, 1:97–113.

32. Morselli, P. L. Gerna, M., and Garattini, S. (1971): Carbamazepine plasma and tissue levels in the rat. *Biochem. Pharmacol.*, 20:2043–2047.

33. Palmer, L., Bertilsson, K., Collste, P., and Rawlins, M. (1973): Quantitative determination of carbamazepine in plasma by mass fragmentography. *Clin. Pharmacol. Ther.*, 15:827–832.

34. Pantrotto, C., Crunelli, V., Lanzoni, J., Frigerio, A., and Quattrone, A. (1979): Quantitative determination of carbamazepine and carbamazepine-10,11-epoxide in rat brain areas by multiple ion detection mass fragmentography. *Anal. Biochem.*, 93:115–123.

35. Patton, J. R., and Dudley, K. H. (1979): Synthesis of 2-methylcarbamazepine, a new internal standard for chromatographic assays of carbamazepine (Tegretol®). *J. Heterocyclic Chem.*, 16:257–262.

36. Perchalski, R. J., and Wilder, B. J. (1974): Rapid gas–liquid chromatographic determination of carbamazepine in plasma. *Clin. Chem.*, 20:492–493.

37. Pippenger, C. E., Bastiani, R. J., and Schneider, R. S. (1977): Preliminary report on the analysis of carbamazepine and ethosuximide using the EMIT system. In: *Antiepileptic Drug Monitoring*, edited by C. Gardner-Thorpe, D. Janz, H. Meinardi, and C. E. Pippenger, pp. 3–6. Pitman Medical, Tunbridge Wells, Kent.

38. Pynnönen, S., Sillanpää, M., Frey, H., and Iisalo, E. (1976): Serum concentration of carbamazepine: Comparison of Herrmann's spectrophotometric method and a new GLC method for determination of carbamazepine. *Epilepsia*, 17:67–72.

39. Rambeck, B., and Meijer, J. W. A. (1979): Comprehensive method for the determination of antiepileptic drugs using a novel extraction technique and a fully automated gas chromatograph. *Arzneim. Forsch.*, 29:99–103.

40. Rist Nielsen, H., and Remmer, H. (1969): Kvantitative bestemmelse of karbamazepin (Tegretol) i serum. *Ugeskr. Laeger*, 131:2200–2201.

41. Roger, J. C., Rodgers, G., Jr., and Soo, A. (1973): Simultaneous determination of carbamazepine (Tegretol) and other anticonvulsants in human plasma by gas–liquid chromatography. *Clin. Chem.*, 19(6):590–592.

42. Schaal, D. E., McKinley, S. L., and Chittwood, G. W. (1979): Gas–liquid chromatographic analysis of underivatized anticonvulsants on the stationary phase DL-LSX-3-0295. *J. Anal. Toxicol.*, 3:96–98.

43. Scheiffarth, F., Weist, F., and Zicha, L. (1966): Zum Nachweis von 5-Carbamyl-5H-dibenzo[b,f]azepin im Liquor cerebrospinalis mittels Dünnschichtchromatographie. *Z. Klin. Chem.*, 4:68–70.

44. Schindler, W. (1961): 5H-Dibenz[b,f]azepines. *Chem. Abstr.*, 55:1671.

45. Schindler, W. and Häfliger, F. (1954): Über Derivate des Iminodibenzyls. *Helv. Chim. Acta*, 37:472–483.

46. Schneider, H., and Berenguer, J. (1977): CSF and plasma concentrations of carbamazepine and some metabolites in steady state. In: *Antiepileptic Drug Monitoring*, edited by C. Gardner-Thorpe, D. Janz, H. Meinardi, and C. E. Pippenger, pp. 264–273. Pitman Medical, Tunbridge Wells, Kent.

47. Schottelius, D. D. (1978): Homogenous immunoassay system (EMIT) for quantitation of antiepileptic drugs in biological fluids. In: *Antiepileptic Drugs: Quantitative Analysis and Interpretation*, edited by C. E. Pippenger, J. K. Penry, and H. Kutt, pp. 95–108. Raven Press, New York.

48. Sheehan, M., and Beam, R. (1975): GLC determination of underivatized carbamazepine in whole blood. *J. Pharm. Sci.*, 64:2004–2006.

49. Soldin, S. J., and Hill, J. G. (1976): Rapid micromethod for measuring anticonvulsant drugs in serum by high-performance liquid chromatography. *Clin. Chem.*, 22:856–859.

50. Sun, L., and Szafir, I. (1977): Comparison of enzyme immunoassay and gas chromatography for determination of carbamazepine and ethosuximide in human serum. *Clin. Chem.*, 23:1753–1755.

51. Theobald, W., and Kunz, H. A. (1963): Zur Phar-

macologie des Antiepilepticums 5-Carbamyl-5H-di-benzo[b,f]azepin. *Arzneim. Forsch.*, 13:122–125.

52. Thiele and Holzinger (1899): Cited by W. Schindler and F. Häfliger (45).
53. Thoma, J. J., Ewald, T., and McCoy, M. (1978): Simultaneous analysis of underivatized phenobarbital, carbamazepine, primidone and phenytoin by isothermal gas–liquid chromatography. *J. Anal. Toxicol.*, 2:219–225.
54. Trager, W. F., Levy, H., Patel, I. H., and Neal, J. M. (1978): Simultaneous analysis of carbamazepine and carbamazepine-10,11-epoxide by GC/CI/MS stable isotope methodology. *Anal. Lett. [B]*, 11:119–133.
55. Truscott, R. J. W., Burke, D. G., Korth, J., and Halpern, B. (1978): Simultaneous determination of diphenylhydantoin, mephobarbital, carbamazepine, phenobarbital and primidone in serum using direct

chemical ionization mass spectrometry. *Biomed. Mass Spectrom.*, 5:477–482.
56. Urquhart, N., Godolphin, W., and Campbell, D. J. (1979): Evaluation of automated enzyme immunoassays for five anticonvulsants and theophylline adapted to a centrifugal analyzer. *Clin. Chem.*, 25:785–787.
57. Wad, N., and Rosenmund, H. (1978): Rapid quantitative method for simultaneous determination of carbamazepine, carbamazepine-10,11-epoxide, diphenylhydantoin, mephenytoin, phenobarbital and primidone in serum by thin layer chromatography. *J. Chromatogr.*, 146:167–168.
58. Westenberg, H. G., and De Zeeuw, R. A. (1976): Rapid and sensitive liquid chromatographic determination of carbamazepine suitable for use in monitoring multiple-drug anticonvulsant therapy. *J. Chromatogr.*, 118:217–224.

Antiepileptic Drugs, edited by D. M. Woodbury,
J. K. Penry, and C. E. Pippenger. Raven Press,
New York © 1982.

37

Carbamazepine

Absorption, Distribution, and Excretion

Paolo L. Morselli and Laura Bossi

Carbamazepine (5H-dibenzo[*b*,*f*]azepine-5-carboxamide; Tegretol®) is an iminostilbene derivative with anticonvulsant properties in animals. In man, the drug has been shown to be an effective antiepileptic agent, and at present, carbamazepine (CBZ) has found wide acceptance as a major antiepileptic drug useful in both adults and children. Best therapeutic results are obtained in patients with generalized tonic–clonic seizures and/or partial seizures with complex symptomatology (16,20,21,49,75,80,109,148). Its clinical effectiveness has been considerably improved during the last 6 to 8 years by increased information on its pharmacokinetic profile and its metabolic degradation and by a better understanding of the possible relationships between carbamazepine and carbamazepine-10,11-epoxide concentrations in body fluids and the clinical effects of the drug.

In this chapter, we shall try to review critically the available information on the absorption, distribution, and elimination of carbamazepine in both animals and man under various physiological and pathological conditions.

ABSORPTION

Experimental Animals

In rats, monkeys, and dogs, orally administered carbamazepine is absorbed relatively slowly

(38,74,101). Maximal plasma concentrations are, in fact, attained in all three species between 3 and 8 hr after dosing.

The vehicle employed for oral administration may have a significant effect on both the amount of drug absorbed and the rate of absorption. Addition of polysorbate, propylene glycol, or ethanol to the aqueous solution accelerates the absorptive process, with peak plasma concentrations attained at 1.5 to 4.0 hr after dosing and may also increase by 1.5- to 2.0-fold the area under the curve for plasma and tissue concentration over time (74,101). Also, recent data of Valli et al. (152) suggest that in the rat the time of day of drug administration may affect the absorption rate, with higher concentrations attained in the evening.

Studies in monkeys have shown that the bioavailability of orally administered carbamazepine may vary from 58 to 86%, suggesting either a modest first-pass effect or incomplete absorption (72). In the rat, peak plasma levels are proportional to the dose up to 150 mg/kg, whereas for higher doses, a reduction in peak values may be observed (26). Following intraperitoneal administration, peak plasma concentrations proportional to the dose are attained within 30 to 60 min (41,88,99). In general, peak epoxide concentrations are attained by either route 1 to 2 hr after the peak carbamazepine concentrations. The epoxide itself is well absorbed (40).

Data in Man

In man, the gastrointestinal absorption of the commercially available formulations is slow, erratic, and unpredictable (88,100–102). The absorption rate in patients seems to be more rapid than in healthy volunteers (22,61,80,88,150). Although studies performed with single doses in healthy volunteers have suggested a faster absorption rate and a better bioavailability for a suspension form containing propylene glycol (51,155), observations in patients undergoing chronic treatment with carbamazepine in tablet or syrup form do not confirm such a finding and show that the two preparations are practically equivalent, with no difference in either absorption rate or amount absorbed (102).

In general, peak plasma concentrations are attained between 4 and 8 hr after ingestion, but peaks as late as 24 to 32 hr have been reported (27, 36, 38, 50, 67, 73, 100, 101, 106, 119, 132, 142,143,150). In one case of attempted suicide in which 20 g of carbamazepine were ingested, peak plasma levels were reached during the third day after drug intake (52).

According to Diehl et al. (31), the absorptive process is slower after the evening dosing. In a recent study, however, we were unable to confirm such a finding (96). If the number of samples is increased during the absorptive phase, secondary and tertiary peaks can very frequently be observed during a chronic regimen, suggesting that the absorption of carbamazepine cannot be considered a simple first-order process. The slow and discontinuous absorption rate of the molecule following repeated treatment may

TABLE 1. *Carbamazepine pharmacokinetic parameters[a]*

	Adults	Children	Newborns
Gastrointestinal absorption	Slow and irregular	Irregular	?
Absorption T_{max} (hr)	6–12	4–8	3–6
Bioavailability (%)	75–85	?	?
Plasma protein binding (% unbound)[b]	22–30[c] 47–52[d]	?	?
CSF/plasma (%)	18–35[c] 30–60[d]	30–35[c] 40–45[d]	?
Saliva/plasma (%)	22–30[c] 30–40[d]	41–43[c]	?
Tears/plasma (%)	—	40–55[e]	?
Apparent V_d (liter/kg)	0.8–1.6	1.2–3.5	1.1–2.5
Apparent plasma $T_{1/2}$ (hr)			
Single dose	18–54[c]	25–34[c]	—
Repeated dose	10–25[c] 3–23[d]	7–20[c] —	4–27 —
Total body clearance (liter/hr per kg)			
SD	0.011–0.021[c]	0.024–0.031	0.097–0.131
RD	0.025–0.136[c]	—	—
Level/dose (%)	0.7–1.2	0.2–0.8	—
Brain/plasma (%)	0.8–1.6[c] 0.6–1.5[d]	1.0–1.4 1.0–1.1	1.0–2.0
Breast milk/plasma (%)	40–60	—	—

[a]The reported data, compiled from the literature, represent the range of values reported by the majority of authors. They are neither averages nor extreme ranges.
[b]Ultrafiltration and equilibrium dialysis.
[c]Carbamazepine only.
[d]Carbamazepine epoxide.
[e]Carbamazepine plus the epoxide.

result from a very slow dissolution rate into the gastrointestinal fluid or from the fact that the compound has an anticholinergic effect that may become evident after multiple dosing, thus modifying the gastric transit time.

Because of the lack of an injectable formulation, no precise data exist on the absolute bioavailability of carbamazepine in man. A bioavailability of 75 to 85% can, however, be expected on the basis of the data reported by Faigle and Feldmann (39) with ^{14}C-labeled carbamazepine. These results are in good agreement with more recent reports describing slightly higher bioavailability for solutions, suspensions, or new formulations with respect to the commercially available tablets (27,119,129).

According to Levy et al. (73), food may improve the absorption rate of carbamazepine without enhancing the extent of absorption. In a recent series of observations on both volunteers and patients undergoing chronic treatment with the drug, we were unable to find evidence of any effect of food on either absorption rate or amount of drug absorbed (96). It may be interesting to note that food may enhance phenytoin absorption and delay that of valproic acid (70,81). Another factor that may play a role in the rate and extent of absorption of carbamazepine in man, as it does in experimental animals, is the size of the administered dose. It is, in fact, not a rare event to encounter in either volunteers or patients a consistent delay in peak time as well as an apparent reduced absorption when daily doses higher than 20 to 25 mg/kg are employed (11,27,51,58,73,143,156). Such a finding is probably supported by a difficult or incomplete dissolution of the compound in the gastrointestinal fluid and suggests that 3 or 4 doses during the day should be preferred to twice-a-day administration.

DISTRIBUTION

Experimental Animals

Studies on mice, rats, and monkeys show that carbamazepine [as could be expected from its physicochemical properties (48)], distributes rapidly and quite uniformly to the various organs and tissues, with higher concentrations in liver, kidney, and brain (38,88,92,101,154, 158). Tissue concentrations parallel the plasma ones, and after repeated administrations, the distribution pattern is similar to that observed for a single dose, with no evident accumulation in any specific organ (41,158). In the rat, brain concentrations of carbamazepine are 1.1 to 1.6 times the plasma ones, whereas brain-to-plasma ratios for the epoxide derivative range from 0.4 to 0.8, suggesting a reduced penetration of the metabolite into the brain after single dosing (41,88,101).

An interesting observation is the parallelism that exists between brain carbamazepine concentrations and protection against maximal electroshock seizures in the rat. Threshold levels are of the order of 3.5 to 4.5 µg/g for both carbamazepine and the epoxide (40,41,101). Studies on the regional brain distribution have shown that at shorter times higher carbamazepine concentrations may be found in cortex, thalamus, and hippocampus, whereas lower levels may be observed in the cerebellum and lower brainstem (107). With time, there is a progressive leveling of drug concentrations in various areas, and at later times after dosing, subcortical structures have the highest relative drug concentrations.

Such a distribution reflects vascularity and cerebral blood flow, and it is very similar to that observed with other lipophilic drugs (95, 115,153). In contrast, the carbamazepine epoxide was found apparently to concentrate in the thalamus (107). Such data are, however, in apparent disagreement with a previous report from the same group (108) in which an even distribution was described for the epoxide, and further confirmation is needed.

In the rat, the apparent volume of distribution ranges from 1.4 to 1.7 liter/kg, and no important differences could be observed for this parameter in pregnant, young (50–100 g), or old (350–600 g) rats (41; P. L. Morselli, *unpublished data*). Similar values (0.72–1.58 liter/kg) have been computed for carbamazepine and carbamazepine epoxide in the rhesus monkey, suggesting an even distribution of the drug and of its metabolite in this species too (72,110).

No data are available in the current literature on carbamazepine plasma protein binding in mice, rats, or monkeys. It appears, however, from unpublished observations that in both rodents and monkeys the bound carbamazepine fraction is about 70 to 75% (J. W. Faigle, *personal communication*; P. L. Morselli, *unpublished data*). Recent data of Löscher (76) indicate that in the dog carbamazepine is 71 to 72% bound to serum proteins with a K_a of $2.7 \times 10^3 \, \text{M}^{-1}$

Data in Man

Limited information is available on tissue distribution in man. Reports on brain carbamazepine concentrations in patients receiving the drug chronically suggest that brain/plasma ratios (13–18 hr after last drug intake) are of the same order of magnitude as those observed in experimental animals (0.8–1.6). No difference between gray and white matter could be found in steady-state conditions. In most of the brain specimens analyzed, carbamazepine-epoxide has also been found at concentrations very close to those present in plasma, with a brain/plasma ratio of 0.6 to 1.5 (7,47,53,88,91,94,103). It may be interesting to recall that in the case of tumor patients, concentrations in gliomas were lower than in surrounding tissues, but no difference could be observed for meningiomas (91).

Cerebrospinal fluid concentrations of carbamazepine may range from 17 to 31% of those in plasma (34,58–61,80,82,139). Similar data have been reported for amniotic fluid, whereas breast milk concentrations are about 60% of total plasma drug levels (25,118). Previously, Scheiffarth et al. (136) and Weist and Zicha (157) reported concentrations of carbamazepine to be higher in CSF than in plasma. Methodological problems such as lack of specificity of the spectrophotometric method used may have been the basis of the discrepancy. Cerebrospinal fluid concentrations of carbamazepine epoxide and of carbamazepine-10,11-diol are 45 to 55% of the corresponding total plasma levels (34,59,139). All of these data on CSF concentrations of carbamazepine and its metabolite are in good agreement with what is known on the binding of the drug (see below).

Saliva concentrations of carbamazepine and carbamazepine epoxide also reflect the free fraction of the drug and may represent in steady-state conditions a useful and easy tool for measuring unbound drugs. Reported values range from 25 to 30% for carbamazepine and 30 to 40% for the carbamazepine epoxide (1, 6,14,23,78,116,135,149,151,159). Similar data have also been described for tears (85,147); however, the tears/plasma ratio for carbamazepine appears to be higher than the corresponding value for CSF or saliva. The reasons for such apparent discrepancy are not at the moment evident.

At variance with observations in animals, the biliary excretion of carbamazepine in man appears to be rather limited, since only 1% of a single 400-mg dose was eliminated as metabolites within 72 hr in the bile of patients with a T-tube drain (146). Bile/plasma ratios were found to be rather variable (0.24–0.84) and apparently related to the bile cholesterol content. These data do not exclude the possibility of a consistent biliary excretion of metabolites such as glucuronide derivatives.

Carbamazepine appears to enter the red blood cells in only limited amounts. Erythrocyte/plasma ratios of 0.15 to 0.38 have been reported, although no carbamazepine epoxide could be measured in the RBC (54,120,124).

In vitro and *in vivo* studies with healthy volunteers have shown that carbamazepine at concentrations of 5 to 30 µg/ml is 75 to 78% bound to plasma proteins (32,93,100,128). Proteins other than albumin are implicated in the binding (32). For the carbamazepine–albumin complex, only one group of binding sites is involved, and the complex has a relatively low association constant ($K = 1.30 \times 10^3 \, \text{M}^{-1}$) (32). A similar association constant has been described for the carbamazepine epoxide ($K = 0.93 \times 10^3 \, \text{M}^{-1}$), which was found to be 48 to 53% bound (100). The epoxide and other antiepileptic drugs such as phenytoin, phenobarbital, valproic acid, ethosuximide, diazepam, and N-desmethyldiazepam do not have any significant displacing effect on carbamazepine binding in an *in vitro* situation (54,100,129). The reports currently available on plasma protein binding of carbamazepine and carbamazepine epoxide indicate that in normal situations the data obtained from epileptic patients are consistent with those obtained in healthy volunteers and that the interindividual variability in carbamazepine plasma protein binding is rather limited (54,58,59,78). The lower protein binding described by Hooper et al. (54) in patients with hepatic diseases, even if significant on a statistical basis, has no practical importance considering both the low affinity constant of the molecule and the amount of the free fraction in normal conditions (20–25%). An increase of 5 to 15% in the free fraction should, in fact, not have any important clinical consequence.

In man, the apparent volume of distribution of carbamazepine, calculated in most cases assuming complete bioavailability, may range from 0.8 to 2.0 liter/kg (36,88,100,106,129,142,159). The real figures are very likely slightly lower because of possible incomplete bioavailability, as suggested by animal data. Data on the apparent V_d of carbamazepine epoxide are still unavailable.

EXCRETION AND ELIMINATION

Experimental Animals

In the rat, carbamazepine undergoes extensive metabolic degradation, and most of the injected radioactivity administered as $[^{14}C]$-CBZ is recovered in urine (~30%) and feces (~38%) within 120 hr (28,88,99). The amount of radioactivity found in stool suggests an extensive biliary excretion of either the drug or its metabolites. Significant differences in drug clearance have been reported between male (0.96 liter/kg per hr) and female (0.56 liter/kg per hr) rats as well as between young (0.72 liter/kg per hr) and old (0.32 liter/kg per hr) rats (41). The phenomenon probably reflects a higher metabolic rate constant in adult male rats and young rats, since no difference, as already noted, could be observed in apparent V_d.

In rhesus monkeys, the plasma disappearance rate of carbamazepine is of the order of 1 to 2 hr, with a total body clearance of 0.43 to 0.59 liter/kg per hr (72,133). Similar values have been

reported for the carbamazepine epoxide, whose clearance appears to be 10 to 15% faster than that of the parent compound (110).

In the dog, the apparent plasma half-life is of the order of 6 to 10 hr following a single dose of CBZ (38).

Repeated carbamazepine administration leads to a marked and significant increase (two- to fourfold) in the clearance of the drug and its metabolite, carbamazepine epoxide. This has been shown in the rat (41,92), in the dog (38; W. Löscher, *personal communication*), and in the monkey (113). The increase in carbamazepine total body clearance without a concomitant modification of the apparent volume of distribution is mainly because of increased activity of the hepatic microsomal monooxygenase systems. Following repeated carbamazepine treatment, increases in liver cytochrome P-450, in NADPH cytochrome reductase activity, as well as in N-demethylase activity have been observed (38) together with an increased formation of carbamazepine epoxide *in vitro* (35). Moreover, other recent studies indicate that not only monooxygenases but also epoxide hydrases are significantly increased and that no demonstrable rise of carbamazepine epoxide is evident during repeated treatment in animals (38,110). It may be interesting to recall that, in the monkey, the increased drug clearance has been shown to be accompanied by an increased urinary excretion of D-glucaric acid (66). All the abovementioned data indicate that carbamazepine is a strong metabolic inducer and that it induces its own metabolism; these findings are in good agreement with observations in man.

The urinary excretion of unmetabolized carbamazepine is rather limited. In rats, dogs, and monkeys, unchanged carbamazepine is present in the urine 72 to 120 hr after ingestion in amounts of the order of 1 to 2% of the administered dose (28,38,72,92,99). Several metabolic products extractable in organic solvents have been identified, and they are discussed in detail in Chapter 38. Among the major products, representing about 60% of urinary excreted material, are carbamazepine-10,11-epoxide, *trans*-carbamazepine-10,11-dihydroxide, 9-hydroxycarbamoyl acridane, iminostilbene, and the derivatives hydroxylated in the aromatic ring in either the 2, 4, or 6 position (2,3,9,28, 38,39,44,45,77,99). The remaining 35 to 39% of the urinary excreted compounds consists of very polar compounds not yet completely identified.

In the monkey, measurable amounts of carbamazepine were found in the feces after intravenous infusion (72). These data and those previously mentioned in the rat suggest the existence in animals of an enterohepatic recycling, which could partially explain some of the fluctuations in plasma carbamazepine concentrations observed by several authors during early phases of intravenous infusions.

Data in Man

In man, the elimination of carbamazepine appears to follow dose-independent kinetics and in most cases can adequately be described by a one-compartment open model. The disappearance rate may be rather variable. In healthy volunteers, half-life values of 18 to 55 hr and total body clearances of 0.011 to 0.021 liter/kg/per hr after a single dose have been reported by various authors (36,39,51,73,93,100,106,129).

Following repeated treatment in volunteers as well as in epileptic patients, the apparent plasma half-lives of carbamazepine may vary from 5 to 26 hr, with clearance values of 0.025 to 0.136 liter/kg per hr (31,35–37,67,100,114, 150,159). As discussed previously, such differences both in apparent plasma half-life and in clearance values between single doses and repeated treatment are caused by an "autoinduction" phenomenon. This autoinducing effect of carbamazepine on liver microsomal enzymes may lead to what has been defined as "time-dependent kinetics," a situation in which clearance values increase with time and higher doses are needed to maintain the same plasma concentration over time (71). It has been estimated that a certain induction may be present by 2 to 4 days of carbamazepine treatment (67,71,79). However, in order to reach a plateau for "autoinduction," the time needed is about 20 to 30 days in healthy volunteers (148). The situation and the time

course of the autoinduction of CBZ may be totally different in epileptic patients already "induced" by other antiepileptic or nonantiepileptic drugs. Reported post-steady-state apparent plasma half-lives for the carbamazepine epoxide range from 3 to 23 hr, being shorter than those of the parent compound in each individual case (36,100,159).

On the basis of these findings and on the basis of the recent experimental data of Faigle et al. (38) and Lai et al. (67), it is difficult to understand reports describing higher epoxide/carbamazepine ratios in "induced" patients (24,30,138), unless an inhibitory effect on epoxide hydrase activity is exerted by the associated drugs. Furthermore, it should be emphasized that other authors failed to note such an increase in epoxide/carbamazepine ratios or in the epoxide levels during associated treatment with other drugs such as phenytoin or phenobarbital (64,86,87). On the contrary, the carbamazepine epoxide levels may be increased by increasing the number of daily carbamazepine doses (58).

In man, as in animals, carbamazepine is almost completely metabolized. The epoxidation of the molecule followed by enzymatic hydrolysis to give *trans*-10,11-dihydrodihydroxycarbamazepine appears to be the major pathway identified so far (2,37,44). A second minor distinct pathway for the biotransformation of carbamazepine, catalyzed by hepatic oxygenases and involving the hydroxylation of the aromatic rings, has recently been described by Faigle et al. (38,39). A more detailed description of the metabolism of carbamazepine is given in Chapter 38.

In healthy volunteers, the urinary excretion of unmetabolized carbamazepine accounts for only 1% of the dose, the major portion of the urinary excreted metabolites being represented by the glycol which is present both as free and as conjugated compound (38,39,93,100). Carbamazepine, too, may be present both as free drug and as conjugated derivative (77,100). The conjugated derivative has been identified as the *N*-glucuronide (77). Other compounds identified in volunteers include the 9-hydroxy-10-car-

TABLE 2. *Urinary and fecal excretion pattern of carbamazepine in volunteers and patients*[a]

			Urine							Feces	
Ref.	Subjects	Sampling time	Carbamazepine	Carbamazepinc -10, 11-epoxide	Trans-10,11-dihydro-dihydroxy-carbamazepine	9-Hydroxy-10-carbamoylacridane	Phenolic derivatives (2,4,6-OH)	Imino-stilbene	Total identified in urine	Carbamazepine	Carbamazepine derivatives
100	Volunteers	48 hr	0.65–1.12%; 1/3 free, 2/3 conjugated	0.72–2%, free and conjugated	10–20%, free and conjugated	—	—	Traces	≈23%	—	—
39	Volunteers	296 hr [14C]-CBZ	≈2%	≈1%	10–30%; 2/3 free, 1/3 conjugated	2–10%, conjugated only	8–25%, glucuronides	None	≈40% (+30% not identified)	10–13 Total, 28%	13–15
40	Volunteers	296 hr	0.1 –2%	0.1 –2%	(trans/cis, 4/1)						
37	Patients	24 hr	0.35–0.87%	1.02–1.41%	32–60%; 2/3 free, 1/3 conjugated	5.1–8.8%, conjugated only		—	40–68%	—	
77	Not specified	Not specified	Present as free and N-glucuronide	Present as free and N-glucuronide	Present as free and O-glucuronide	Present as O-glucuronide	Present as O-glucuronide	Not found	—	—	—

[a]Data are expressed as percent of administered dose.

bamoylacridane (2–10%) present mainly in conjugated form, the carbamazepine epoxide (1–2%), and the 2-, 4-, and 6-hydroxy derivatives (6–20%) present mainly as glucuronides (38).

Following oral intake of [^{14}C]carbamazepine, about 28% of the labeled dose was found in the feces 216 hours after ingestion, suggesting both incomplete absorption and nonnegligible biliary excretion of unidentified metabolites (38,39).

In epileptic patients undergoing chronic treatment, about 32 to 61% of the daily dose is excreted as carbamazepine-*trans*-diol, 5 to 9% as 9-hydroxymethyl-10-carbomoylacridane (mainly as conjugated derivative), 1 to 1.5% as carbamazepine epoxide, and 0.5% as unmetabolized carbamazepine (37).

PREGNANCY

Experimental Animals

In pregnant rats, the absorption of carbamazepine appears to be delayed, with peak plasma levels attained 2 to 3 hr after i.p. administration (41). In this series of observations, the apparent volume of distribution was not different from that computed for control rats, whereas total body clearance was significantly lower than in nonpregnant rats, confirming the slower disposition rate during pregnancy observed for other compounds (43,65).

Equilibrium between maternal and fetal tissues was reached within 30 to 60 min, suggesting a rapid transfer of the drug across the placenta. Apparently, there was no evidence of selective accumulation in any fetal tissues, and the disappearance rate of carbamazepine from the fetal tissues followed that of maternal plasma concentrations (41,42).

Data in Man

There are no data on the absorption of carbamazepine during pregnancy in women. However, on the basis of the plasma concentrations usually observed in pregnant women, there are no reasons to support a modified absorption during the first 6 months. On the contrary, a trend toward a lowering of plasma carbamazepine concentrations during the last 3 months of pregnancy has been reported for individual cases by several authors (17,25,29,33,68). However, in a larger group of epileptic women, Bardy et al. (5) were unable to detect any significant variation in plasma carbamazepine concentrations during late pregnancy. It should be remembered that for other antiepileptic drugs there seems to be a general agreement on a consistent lowering of plasma drug concentrations in late pregnancy (4,17,29,68,69,104). Possible causes of the drop in plasma antiepileptic drug levels during the last 3 months of pregnancy have not yet been clarified, and none of the various proposed hypotheses has been proven.

Carbamazepine and carbamazepine epoxide plasma protein binding do not change significantly during pregnancy, and free fractions of 20 to 24% for carbamazepine and 27 to 38% for the epoxide have been reported (25,29).

As observed in the experimental animal, the placental transfer of carbamazepine in early pregnancy is extensive and rapid (118). The drug distributes to various fetal tissues rather homogenously, and reported brain/plasma ratios of 1 to 2 are similar to those observed in adults (47,91,118). In general, the carbamazepine epoxide is detectable in fetal tissues as well as in the amniotic fluid. Reported amniotic fluid/plasma ratios are 0.22 to 0.24 for carbamazepine and 0.28 to 0.45 for the epoxide (25,118). It may be interesting to note that human fetal livers at 15 to 21 weeks of gestation are able to metabolize carbamazepine to carbamazepine epoxide *in vitro* (112).

With regard to the possible transfer of carbamazepine from the mother to the newborn during lactation, a breast milk/plasma ratio of 0.40 to 0.60 has been reported for carbamazepine, and higher values have been described for the epoxide (63,105,118,121). Estimations of possible daily amounts transferred to the newborn in cases of lactating epileptic mothers with therapeutic plasma concentrations of carbamazepine (4–8 μg/ml) suggest that a newborn of 3 to 3.5 kg would receive about 0.5 to 0.7 mg/kg per day (90,105). Whether such a dose is totally pharmacologically inactive and has no effect on the newborn has never been evaluated.

PEDIATRIC PATIENTS

Newborns

In neonates from chronically treated epileptic mothers, the plasma carbamazepine concentrations at birth are similar to those present in mother's plasma (18,55,127).

The disappearance rate of transplacentally acquired carbamazepine appears to follow first-order kinetics. Reported plasma half-life values range from 8 to 27 hr (18,127). These values are of the same order as those reported in chronically treated adult epileptic patients, and the possibility that hepatic drug-metabolizing enzymes were induced *in utero* is very likely.

In the newborn more than 1 week of age and in the very young infant (less than 8 weeks of age), the carbamazepine absorption rate appears to be similar to that observed in adults, with peak plasma concentrations attained 3 to 6 hr after a single dose of the drug in the form of an extemporary suspension in milk (131).

No data are available on plasma protein binding of carbamazepine in the neonate. According to Rey et al. (131), the apparent volume of distribution in the neonate is 1.5 to 2 times greater than in adults. However, the reported values were estimated assuming 100% bioavailability, and on the basis of what is known about neonate absorption (89) and carbamazepine bioavailability, the figure is very probably overestimated. According to the same authors, the apparent plasma half-life of carbamazepine in the newborn 2 to 7 weeks of age may range from 4.6 to 12.6 hr. These figures are considerably smaller than those usually observed in adults after a single dose of the drug. However, they should not be surprising since, on the one hand, six out of the seven patients studied were pretreated with phenobarbital, and, on the other hand, a dramatic increase in the metabolic rate after the first week of age (and persisting up to 2–3 years) has been described for several drugs (89,90,98).

Infants

The data available on the pharmacokinetics of carbamazepine in infants are very scanty. On the basis of the available information, it seems that no major differences exist between adults and infants with regard to absorption, protein binding, and distribution. On the contrary, the disposition rate may be increased.

From autopsy observations of Pynnönen et al. (118), it appears that in infants carbamazepine is more or less evenly distributed to all tissues, with CSF concentrations of about 24% of the plasma ones. The reported apparent volume of distribution, assuming 100% bioavailability, is again 1.5 to 2 times higher than the values reported for adults (123,131).

The information available on the disappearance rate of carbamazepine in infants refers either to observations following a single administration (two cases) or to chronically treated infants also receiving other antiepileptic drugs (four cases). Reported values ranged from 12 to 36 hr (123,131).

In a more recent study conducted on a larger group of infants, children, and adolescents, Battino et al. (8) observed a significant positive correlation between age and carbamazepine level/dose ratios, with the infants showing the lowest ratios.

Children

In children, as in adults, carbamazepine (administered either as syrup or in tablet form) appears to be absorbed rather slowly and erratically. Peak plasma levels are attained about 4 to 8 hr after dosing, with wide interindividual variations and frequent secondary peaks (102,133,135). Such behavior suggests that in children, too, carbamazepine absorption is not a first-order process. Furthermore, recent observations of Battino et al. (8) seem to indicate that with high doses (>25 mg/kg), the absorption process may be impaired or reduced.

No specific data are available on plasma protein binding of carbamazepine in children. However, information on concentrations in CSF, saliva, and tears suggests that the free carbamazepine and carbamazepine epoxide fractions might be slightly higher in children than in adults, with values of 30 to 35% and 40 to 45%, respectively (6,122,134,135,147). Brain/plasma ratios of both carbamazepine and carbamazepine epoxide are of the same order as those reported for adults and the same holds true for the erythrocyte/plasma ratio (124). The apparent volume of distribution, computed from oral dose data, assuming complete bioavailability, is larger in children than in adults (12,123,131).

The findings on the apparent plasma half-life of carbamazepine are very variable, with values ranging from 3 to 32 hr (12,123,126,128,131). Such great variability depends on several factors, such as age of the children, duration of treatment, associated therapies, accuracy of the analytical method employed, and length of sampling time. In fact, in a recent paper, Bertilsson et al. (12) showed that in children of 10 to 13 years of age the apparent plasma half-life of carbamazepine may decline from 25 to 32 hr after a single dose to 18 to 22 hr after 4 to 6 days of treatment and to 10 to 14 hr after 4 weeks of therapy with the drug. These observations, indicating the presence of an autoinduction phenomenon after only a few doses of the drug, are in good agreement with observations in adult volunteers and confirm previous findings of Moller and Nielsen (84) suggesting that autoinduction in epileptic children may occur at a very early stage of the treatment.

Recent data of Battino et al. (8), however, show that in comparable groups for age the level/dose ratios tend to be lower in the case of associated treatment with phenobarbital and/or phenytoin. These observations are in good agreement with several other reports on plasma carbamazepine levels during chronic treatment, showing that, at equal daily doses, children tend to have lower carbamazepine concentrations than adults, and that they may require higher daily doses (86,87,89,94,102,123,128).

The apparent plasma half-life of carbamazepine epoxide is of the same order (13–22 hr) as that recorded in adults (123).

On the whole, the data available on pediatric patients indicate that the clearance of carbamazepine is age dependent, with highest rates during infancy and early childhood. The clearance rate then decreases progressively to reach adult values at the age of 15 to 17 years. Such an age-dependent decrease in clearance rates as well as the possible impact of associated treatment should always be considered when drug regimens are designed for infants and children.

CARBAMAZEPINE PHARMACOKINETICS IN DISEASE STATES OTHER THAN EPILEPSY

Epileptic patients may suffer from concomitant diseases that may require treatment with other drugs that may, in turn, lead to important variations of the physiological variables determining the extent of drug distribution as well as the rates of absorption and elimination.

The possible interactions of carbamazepine with other drugs are extensively treated in Chapter 39. We should like briefly to underline the possible consequences of various pathological conditions on the disposition of carbamazepine and its metabolites and hence the increased risk of either drug toxicity or loss of efficacy.

There are no specific studies available on the influence of cardiac, renal, or liver diseases on the kinetics of carbamazepine. It is, however, possible on the basis of the physicochemical properties of the molecule (see Chapter 36), of its kinetic profile in normal situations, and of the available information on other drugs to estimate with reasonable certainty the type of alteration in the disposition of the drug that could be encountered in the disease states mentioned above (97).

Cardiac Failure

In cardiac failure, reduced cardiac output is accompanied by increased filling pressure, congestion of major vital organs, edema and expansion of blood volume, tissue hypoxemia, and acidosis (10). Such a picture may easily lead to edema of intestinal epithelium, reduction of liver blood flow, impairment of microsomal hepatic enzyme activities, altered glomerular filtration and tubular resorption rates, and lower plasma and tissue protein binding. Consequently, the usual erratic and slow absorption of carbamazepine may be further reduced, and the drug will very probably be metabolized and cleared at a lower rate.

Factors such as reduced renal excretion rate and reduced plasma proteins should not play an important role for carbamazepine, but it is difficult to estimate the possible importance and significance of modified redistribution phenomena caused by differences in pH and in relative blood flow to various organs. In practical terms, depending on the prevalence of either impaired absorption or reduced clearance, we may face either a loss of efficacy or an increased risk of adverse effects. In this regard, we should remember that carbamazepine may condition an increased water and sodium retention (97, 111,125), which may further aggravate an already compromised hemodynamic situation.

Liver Diseases

No significant alterations in carbamazepine pharmacokinetics should be expected in cases of moderate alterations of liver function (117). Significant alterations may be encountered in cases of severe cirrhosis, hepatitis, and obstructive icterus. In all these situations, in fact, there may be portocaval shunts, with increased portal flow, decreased rate of protein synthesis, reduced microsomal activity, increased circulating bilirubin, diffuse edemas, and a trend toward renal failure (13,15). The consequence may be an increased drug bioavailability (reduction of intrinsic clearance) associated with reduced metabolic degradation and a possible increase in apparent volume of distribution. For carbamazepine, the reduction of metabolic liver activities appears more important than an eventual reduced plasma protein binding which, in contrast, is very important for drugs such as phenytoin and valproic acid. Because of the above-mentioned alterations in cases of severe liver disease, the risk of carbamazepine toxicity is

considerably increased, and a careful monitoring of both plasma drug levels and the clinical picture should be applied.

Renal Diseases

Because of the large variability in the clinical course of renal diseases, their effects on drug kinetics may also be very variable. In general, there may be a modified hematocrit, a reduction in glomerular and/or tubular functions, a rise in total body water with increased extracellular water, variable degrees of hypoalbuminemia, electrolyte imbalance, increased uremia, and functional changes in the gastrointestinal tract (97,98,130).

These alterations may bring about a modified drug bioavailability, reduce plasma protein binding of acidic drugs, increase the apparent V_d, cause accumulation of metabolites in body fluids, increase hepatic metabolic degradation, increase total body clearance for drugs actively metabolized by liver microsomal systems, and prolong the apparent plasma half-life of drugs depending on the kidney for their elimination.

In the case of carbamazepine, no modification in either bioavailability or clearance has been noted up to now. We should remember, however, that carbamazepine may exert a significant antidiuretic effect, thus leading to an increased danger of fluid retention. Because of this, the drug should be administered with extreme caution to patients with compromised kidney function.

Other Pathological States

Other clinical conditions that may alter the disposition of antiepileptic drugs include malnutrition syndromes, pulmonary diseases, fever, and postoperative sequelae (97). At variance with what has been described for other drugs, no alteration in the kinetics of antiepileptic drugs could be observed in thyroid disorders (83). Carbamazepine kinetics could very likely be altered in cases of malnutrition (reduced absorption), fever (increased catabolism), and pulmonary diseases (reduced catabolism). No modification should be encountered in postoperative states, in which the major modification is represented by a reduced plasma protein binding of acidic compounds.

CARBAMAZEPINE AND CARBAMAZEPINE EPOXIDE PLASMA CONCENTRATIONS IN THE COURSE OF CHRONIC TREATMENT

During chronic treatment, plasma concentrations of carbamazepine and carbamazepine epoxide show a great interindividual variability, and no evident relationship can be described between daily doses and plasma concentrations of either compound. Interindividual differences of 5 to 7 times may be observed for the same daily doses (19,21,22,34,58,80,86,87,100, 141,143).

With the currently used daily doses of 600 to 1,200 mg, morning (trough) plasma concentrations of carbamazepine plus carbamazepine epoxide may vary from 2 to 16 µg/ml without any evident relationship between concentrations of the parent compound and those of the metabolite, which may be 15 to 55% of that of carbamazepine. Furthermore, it has been shown that plasma concentrations of both compounds oscillate considerably during the dose intervals, and fluctuations of 40 to 80% for carbamazepine and of 40 to 200% for the epoxide have been described (19,31,34,56,58,59,100,143, 145).

The relationships between plasma drug concentrations and effects are treated in detail in Chapters 40 and 41. We should like, however, to briefly remember that, according to several reports, the "therapeutic" concentrations of carbamazepine are considered to range between 4 and 12 µg/ml (20,21,30,34,94,100,137, 141,143,148).

Animal data appear to be in good agreement, since minimal threshold concentrations in rat brain for protection against maximal electroshock seizures are 3.5 to 4.5 µg/ml (41,101), and similar minimal protective concentrations have been described for cats (62) and monkeys (74). Chu (26) later showed that in the rat plasma

carbamazepine concentrations of at least 3 µg/ml are necessary to protect against alcohol withdrawal seizures; furthermore, plasma levels higher than 12 to 15 µg/ml induced a strong sedation, whereas concentrations <8 µg/ml did not appear to elicit any effect on behavior.

CONCLUSIONS AND IMPLICATIONS FOR DOSAGE REGIMENS

As outlined in the previous pages, the pharmacokinetics of carbamazepine appears rather complex, and the molecule cannot be defined as one easy to handle. Furthermore, other factors such as age and concomitant drug treatment may further complicate the picture, especially with regard to the absorptive and the elimination processes.

On the basis of the evident relationships between drug concentration in body fluids and its effects, a precise dosing schedule appears to be a very important prerequisite for a correct therapeutic approach. However, because of the lack of relationship between daily doses and morning plasma levels, the wide intraindividual fluctuations in plasma concentrations, the "time-dependent" kinetics, and the variable and apparently "dose-dependent" rate of absorption, carbamazepine dose schedules are very difficult to define without the aid of plasma drug level monitoring. (This procedure should always include the measurement of the carbamazepine epoxide.)

If, in the case of associated treatment, daily doses of 14 to 20 mg/kg are apparently needed in most patients to achieve plasma levels of 6 to 12 µg/ml, then, in case of monotherapy, daily doses of 6 to 12 mg/kg may be sufficient to obtain therapeutic plasma concentrations (19–21,31,86,87,94,100,140,141,144,149,156). In practice, it may be useful to start the therapy with a dose of 200 mg given twice daily and to increase progressively to 800 to 1,200 mg/day if needed. Because of the possible "dose dependency" of the carbamazepine absorptive process, when giving doses of 800 mg or more it may be useful to administer the daily dosage in three increments, and, in selected cases, up to four daily doses may be necessary tc avoid important fluctuations in plasma carbamazepine concentrations (11,56–59).

During chronic treatment, food does not appear to have any significant influence on either the rate of absorption or the amount of carbamazepine and carbamazepine epoxide absorbed. Hence, the drug may be taken either before or after meals. Because of the possibility of autoinduction and of "time dependent" kinetics of elimination, plasma levels of carbamazepine and carbamazepine epoxide should be monitored at least twice during the first month of therapy and the dose consequently adjusted as a function of both plasma drug concentrations and clinical response.

ACKNOWLEDGMENTS

The authors wish to express their gratitude to Mme C. de Courson and Mlle E. Decor for their valuable assistance and help in the preparation of the manuscript.

REFERENCES

1. Aucamp, A. K., and Hundt, H. K. L. (1978) A study of carbamazepine and its epoxy and hydroxy-metabolites in serum and saliva of male and female epileptic patients. In: *Advances in Epileptology 1977. Psychology, Pharmacotherapy and New Diagnostic Approaches,* edited by H. Meinardi and A. J. Rowan, pp. 280–284. Swets & Zeitlinger, Amsterdam, Lisse.

2. Baker, K. M., Csetenyi, J., Frigerio, A., Morselli, P. L., Paravicini, F., and Pifferi, G. (1973): 10,11-Dihydro - 10, 11 - dihydroxy - 5H - dibenz(*b,f*)azepine-5-carboxamide, a metabolite of carbamazepine isolated from human and rat urine. *J. Med. Chem.,* 16:703–705.

3. Baker, K. M., Frigerio, A., Morselli, P. L., and Pifferi, G. (1973): Identification of a rearranged degradation product from carbamazepine-10,11-epoxide. *J. Pharm. Sci.,* 62:475–476.

4. Bardy, A. H., Hiilesmaa, V. K., and Teramo, K. (1978): Serum phenytoin during pregnancy. In: *Advances in Epileptology 1977. Psychology, Pharmacotherapy and New Diagnostic Approaches,* edited by H. Meinardi and A. J. Rowan, pp. 305–307. Swets & Zeitlinger, Amsterdam, Lisse.

5. Bardy, A. H., Hiilesmaa, V. K., and Teramo, K. (1979): Serum carbamazepine during pregnancy—Preliminary results of a prospective study. *11th Epilepsy International Symposium,* Florence 1979. Abstract 4.40.

6. Bartels, H., Oldigs, H. D., and Gunter, E. (1977): Use of saliva in monitoring carbamazepine medication in epileptic children. *Eur. J. Pediatr.,* 126:37–44.

7. Baruzzi, A., Cabrini, G. P., Gerna, M., Sironi, V. A., and Morselli, P. L. (1977): Anticonvulsant plasma level monitoring in epileptic patients undergoing stereo-EEG. In: *Antiepileptic Drug Monitoring,* edited by C. Gardner-Thorpe, D. Janz, H. Meinardi, and C. E. Pippenger, pp. 317–334. Pitman Medical, Tunbridge Wells, Kent.

8. Battino, D., Bossi, L., Croci, D., Franceschetti, S., Gomeni, C., Moise, A., Vitali, A., and Breschi, F. (1980): Carbamazepine plasma levels in children and adults: Influence of age and associated therapy. *Ther. Drug. Monit.,* 2:315–322.

9. Bauer, J. E., Gerber, N., Lynn, R. K., Smith, R. G., and Thompson, R. M. (1976): A new *N*-Glucuronide metabolite of carbamazepine. *Experientia,* 32:1032–1233.

10. Benowitz, N. L., and Meister, W. (1976): Pharmacokinetics in patients with cardiac failure. *Clin. Pharmacokinet.,* 1:389–405.

11. Bertilsson, L. (1978): Clinical pharmacokinetics of carbamazepine. *Clin. Pharmacokinet.,* 3:128–143.

12. Bertilsson, L., Höjer, B., Tybring, G., Osterloh, J., and Rane, A. (1980): Autoinduction of carbamazepine metabolism in children examined by a stable isotope technique. *Clin. Pharmacol. Ther.,* 27:83–88.

13. Blaschke, T. F. (1977): Protein binding and kinetics of drugs in liver diseases. *Clin. Pharmacokinet.,* 2:32–44.

14. Blom, G. F., and Guelen, P. J. M. (1977): The distribution of antiepileptic drugs between serum, saliva and cerebrospinal fluid. In: *Antiepileptic Drug Monitoring,* edited by C. Gardner-Thorpe, D. Janz, H. Meinardi, and C. E. Pippenger, pp. 287–296. Pitman Medical, Tunbridge Wells, Kent.

15. Bond, W. S. (1978): Clinical relevance of the effect of hepatic disease on drug disposition. *Am. J. Hosp. Pharm.,* 35:406–414.

16. Bonduelle, M., Bouygues, P., Sallou, C., Chemaly, R. (1964): Bilan de l'expérimentation clinique de l'antiépileptique, G-32-883. In: *Neuropsychopharmacology, Vol. 3,* edited by P. B. Bradley, F. Flügel, and P. H. Hoch, pp. 312–316. Elsevier, Amsterdam.

17. Bossi, L., Avanzini, G., Assael, B. M., Battino, D., Caccamo, M. L., Canger, R., Como, M. L., De Giambattista, M., Franceschetti, S., Masini, A., Pardi, G., Piffarotti, G., Porro, M. G., Rovei, V., Sanjuan, M., Soffientini, M. E., Spina, S., and Spreafico, R. (Milan Collaborative Group) (1980): Plasma levels and clinical effects of antiepileptic drugs in pregnant epileptic patients and their newborn. In: *Antiepileptic Therapy—Advances in Drug Monitoring,* edited by S. I. Johannessen, P. L. Morselli, C. E. Pippenger, A. Richens, D. Schmidt, and H. Meinardi, pp. 9–14. Raven Press, New York.

18. Bossi, L., Battino, D., Caccamo, M. L., De Giambattista, M., Latis, G. O., Oldrini, A., and Spina, S. (1981): Pharmacokinetics and clinical effects of antiepileptic drugs in newborns of chronically treated

epileptic mothers. In: *Epilepsy, Pregnancy and the Child,* edited by D. Janz, L. Bossi, M. Dam, H. Helge, A. Richens, and D. Schmidt, pp. 373–383. Raven Press, New York.

19. Callaghan, N., O'Callaghan, M., Duggan, B., and Feely, M. (1978): Carbamazepine as a single drug in the treatment of epilepsy. A prospective study of serum levels and seizure control. *J. Neurol. Neurosurg. Psychiatry,* 41:907–912.

20. Cereghino, J. J. (1975): Serum carbamazepine concentration and clinical control. *Adv. Neurol.,* 11:309–329.

21. Cereghino, J. J., Brock, J. T., Van Meter, J. C., Penry, J. K., Smith, L. D., and White, B. G. (1974): Carbamazepine for epilepsy. A controlled prospective evaluation. *Neurology (Minneap.),* 24:401–410.

22. Cereghino, J. J., Van Meter, J. C., Brock, J. T., Penry, J. K., Smith, L. D., and White, B. G. (1973): Preliminary observations of serum carbamazepine concentration in epileptic patients. *Neurology (Minneap.),* 23:357–366.

23. Chambers, R. E., Homeida, M., Hunter, K. R., and Teague, R. H. (1977): Salivary carbamazepine concentration. *Lancet,* 1:656–657.

24. Christiansen, J., and Dam, M. (1975): Drug interaction in epileptic patients. In: *Clinical Pharmacology of Antiepileptic Drug,* edited by H. Schneider, D. Janz, C. Gardner-Thorpe, H. Meinardi, and A. L. Sherwin, pp. 197–200. Springer-Verlag, Berlin.

25. Christiansen, J., and Dam, M. (1977): Plasma and salivary levels of carbamazepine and carbamazepine-10,11-epoxide during pregnancy. In: *Antiepileptic Drug Monitoring,* edited by C. Gardner-Thorpe, D. Janz, H. Meinardi, and C. E. Pippenger, pp. 128–135. Pitman Medical, Tunbridge Wells, Kent.

26. Chu, N. S. (1979): Carbamazepine: Prevention of alcohol withdrawal seizures. *Neurology (Minneap.),* 29:1397–1401.

27. Cotter, L. M., Eadie, L. J., Hooper, W. D., Lander, C. M., Smith, G. A., and Tyrer, J. H. (1977): The pharmacokinetics of carbamazepine. *Eur. J. Clin. Pharmacol.,* 12:451–456.

28. Csetenyi, J., Baker, K. M., Frigerio, A., and Morselli, P. L. (1973): Iminostilbene—a metabolite of carbamazepine isolated from rat urine. *J. Pharm. Pharmacol.,* 25:340–341.

29. Dam, M., Christiansen, J., Munck, O., and Mygind, K. I. (1979): Antiepileptic drugs: Metabolism in pregnancy. *Clin. Pharmacokinet.,* 4:53–62.

30. Dam, M., Jensen, A., and Christiansen, J. (1975): Plasma level and effect of carbamazepine in grand mal and psychomotor epilepsy. *Acta Neurol. Scand.* [*Suppl.*], 60:33–38.

31. Diehl, L. W., Müller-Oerlinghausen, B., and Riedel, E. (1976): The importance of individual pharmacokinetic data for treatment of epilepsy with carbamazepine. *Int. J. Clin. Pharmacol.,* 14:144–148.

32. Di Salle, E., Pacifici, G. M., and Morselli, P. L. (1974): Studies on plasma protein binding of carbamazepine. *Pharmacol. Res. Commun.,* 6:193–202.

33. Eadie, M. J., Lander, C. M., and Tyrer, J. H. (1977): Plasma drug level monitoring in pregnancy. *Clin. Pharmacokinet.,* 2:427–436.

34. Eichelbaum, M., Bertilsson, L., Lund, L., Palmer,

L., and Sjöqvist, F. (1976): Plasma levels of carbamazepine and carbamazepine-10,11-epoxide during treatment of epilepsy. *Eur. J. Clin. Pharmacol.,* 9:417–421.

35. Eichelbaum, M., Bertilsson, L., Rane, A., and Sjöqvist, F. (1976): Autoinduction of carbamazepine metabolism in man. In: *Anticonvulsant Drugs and Enzyme Induction,* edited by A. Richens and B. Woodford, pp. 147–158. Associated Scientific Publishers, Amsterdam.

36. Eichelbaum, M., Ekbom, K., Bertilsson, L., Ringberger, V. A., and Rane, A. (1975): Plasma kinetics of carbamazepine and its epoxide metabolite in man after single and multiple doses. *Eur. J. Clin. Pharmacol.,* 8:337–341.

37. Eichelbaum, M., Köthe, K. W., Hoffmann, F., and Von Unruh, G. E. (1979): Kinetics and metabolism of carbamazepine during combined antiepileptic drug therapy. *Clin. Pharmacol. Ther.,* 26:366–371.

38. Faigle, J. W., Brechbuher, S., Feldmann, K. F., and Richter, W. J. (1976): The biotransformation of carbamazepine. In: *Epileptic Seizure, Behaviour, Pain,* edited by W. Birkmayer, pp. 127–140. Huber Publishers, Bern.

39. Faigle, J. W., and Feldmann, K. F. (1975): Pharmacokinetic data of carbamazepine and its major metabolites in man. In: *Clinical Pharmacology of Antiepileptic Drugs,* edited by H. Schneider, D. Janz, C. Gardner-Thorpe, H. Meinardi, and H. Sherwin, pp. 159–165. Springer-Verlag, Berlin.

40. Faigle, J. W., Feldmann, K. F., and Baltzer, V. (1977): Anticonvulsant effect of carbamazepine. An attempt to distinguish between potency of the parent drug and its epoxide metabolite. In: *Antiepileptic Drug Monitoring,* edited by C. Gardner-Thorpe, D. Janz, H. Meinardi, and C. E. Pippenger, pp. 104–109. Pitman Medical, Tunbridge Wells, Kent.

41. Farghali-Hassan, Assael, B. M., Bossi, L., Garattini, S., Gerna, M., Gomeni, R., and Morselli, P. L. (1976): Carbamazepine pharmacokinetics in young, adult and pregnant rats. Relation to pharmacological effects. *Arch. Int. Pharmacodyn. Ther.,* 220:125–139.

42. Farghali-Hassan, Assael, B. M., Bossi, L., and Morselli, P. L. (1975): Placental transfer of carbamazepine in the rat. *J. Pharm. Pharmacol.,* 27:956–957.

43. Feuer, G. (1979): Action of pregnancy and various progesterones on hepatic microsomal activities. *Drug Metab. Rev.,* 9:147–169.

44. Frigerio, A., Fanelli, R., Biandrate, P., Passerini, G., Morselli, P. L., and Garattini, S. (1972): Mass spectrometric characterization of carbamazepine-10,11-epoxide, a carbamazepine metabolite isolated from human urine. *J. Pharm. Sci.,* 61:1044–1047.

45. Frigerio, A., and Morselli, P. L. (1975): Carbamazepine: Biotransformation. *Adv. Neurol.,* 11:295–308.

46. Friis, M. L., and Christiansen, J. (1978): Carbamazepine, carbamazepine-10,11-epoxide and phenytoin concentrations in brain tissue of epileptic children. *Acta Neurol. Scand.,* 58:104–108.

47. Friis, M. L., Christiansen, J., and Hvidberg, E. F. (1978): Brain concentration of carbamazepine and

carbamazepine-10,11-epoxide in epileptic patients. *Eur. J. Clin. Pharmacol.*, 14:47–51.

48. Gagneux, A. R. (1976): The chemistry of carbamazepine. In: *Epileptic Seizures, Behaviour, Pain*, edited by W. Birkmayer, pp. 120–126. Huber Publishers, Bern.

49. Gamstorp, I. (1975): Treatment with carbamazepine: Children. *Adv. Neurol.*, 11:237–246.

50. Gérardin, A. P., Abadie, F. V., Campestrini, J. A., and Theobald, W. (1976): Pharmacokinetics of carbamazepine in normal humans after single and repeated oral doses. *J. Pharmacokinet. Biopharm.*, 4:521–535.

51. Gérardin, A. P., and Hirtz, J. (1976): The quantitative assay of carbamazepine in biological material and its application to basic pharmacokinetics studies. In: *Epileptic Seizures, Behaviour, Pain*, edited by W. Birkmayer, pp. 151–164. Huber Publishers, Bern.

52. Gruska, H., Beyer, K. H., Kubicki, S., and Schneider, H. (1971): Klinik, Toxikologie und Therapie einer schweren Carbamazepine-Vergiftung. *Arch. Toxicol.*, 27:193–203.

53. Harvey, C. D., Sherwin, A. L., and Van der Kleijn, E. (1977): Distribution of anticonvulsant drugs in gray and white matter of human brain. *Can. J. Neurol. Sci.*, 4:89–92.

54. Hooper, W. D., Dubetz, D. K., Bochner, F., Cotter, L. M., Smith, G. A., Eadie, M. J., and Tyrer, J. H. (1975): Plasma protein binding of carbamazepine. *Clin. Pharmacol. Ther.*, 17:433–440.

55. Hoppel, C., Rane, A., and Sjöqvist, F. (1975): Kinetics of phenytoin and carbamazepine in the newborn. In: *Basic and Therapeutic Aspects of Perinatal Pharmacology*, edited by P. L. Morselli, S. Garattini, and F. Sereni, pp. 341–345. Raven Press, New York.

56. Höppener, R. J., and Kuyer, A. (1979): Correlations between daily fluctuations of carbamazepine serum levels and intermittent occurring side effects. *XI Epilepsy International Symposium*, Firenze. Abstract 4.78.

57. Hvidberg, E. F., and Dam, M. (1976): Clinical pharmacokinetics of anticonvulsants. *Clin. Pharmacokinet.*, 1:161–188.

58. Johannessen, S. I., Baruzzi, A., Gomeni, R., Strandjord, R. E., and Morselli, P. L. (1977): Further observations on carbamazepine and carbamazepine-10,11-epoxide kinetics in epileptic patients. In: *Antiepileptic Drug Monitoring*, edited by C. Gardner-Thorpe, D. Janz, H. Meinardi, and C. E. Pippenger, pp. 110–124. Pitman Medical, Tunbridge Wells, Kent.

59. Johannessen, S. I., Gerna, M., Bakke, J., Strandjord, R. E., and Morselli, P. L. (1976): CSF concentrations and serum protein binding of carbamazepine and carbamazepine-10,11-epoxide in epileptic patients. *Br. J. Clin. Pharmacol.*, 3:575–582.

60. Johannessen, S. I., and Strandjord, R. E. (1972): The concentration of carbamazepine (Tegretol) in serum and in cerebrospinal fluid in patients with epilepsy. *Acta Neurol. Scand. [Suppl.]*, 51:445–446.

61. Johannessen, S. I., and Strandjord, R. E. (1975): Absorption and protein binding in serum of several antiepileptic drugs. In: *Clinical Pharmacology of Antiepileptic Drugs*, edited by H. Schneider, D. Janz, C. Gardner-Thorpe, H. Meinardi, and A. L. Sherwin, pp. 262–273. Springer-Verlag, Berlin.

62. Julien, R. M., and Hollister, R. P. (1975): Carbamazepine: Mechanisms of action. *Adv. Neurol.*, 11:263–277.

63. Kaneko, S., Sato, T., and Suzuki, K. (1979): The levels of anticonvulsants in breast milk. *Br. J. Clin. Pharmacol.*, 7:624–627.

64. Korczyn, A. D., Ben-Zvi, Z., Kaplanski, J., Danon, A., and Berginer, V. V. (1978): Plasma levels of carbamazepine and metabolites: Effect of enzyme inducers. In: *Advances in Epileptology 1977. Psychology, Pharmacotherapy and New Diagnostic Approaches*, edited by H. Meinardi and A. J. Rowan, pp. 273–279. Swets & Zeitlinger, Amsterdam, Lisse.

65. Krauer, B., and Krauer, F. (1977): Drug kinetics in pregnancy. *Clin. Pharmacokinet.*, 2:167–181.

66. Lai, A. A. and Levy, R. H. (1979): Pharmacokinetic description of drug interactions by enzyme induction: Carbamazepine—Clonazepam in monkeys. *J. Pharm. Sci.*, 68:416–421.

67. Lai, A. A., Levy, R. H., and Cutler, R. E. (1978): Time course of interaction between carbamazepine and clonazepam in normal man. *Clin. Pharmacol. Ther.* 24:316–322.

68. Lander, C. M., Edwards, V. E., Eadie, M. J., and Tyrer, J. H. (1977): Plasma anticonvulsant concentrations during pregnancy. *Neurology (Minneap.)*, 27:128–131.

69. Landon, M. J., and Kirkley, M. (1979): Metabolism of diphenylhydantoin (phenytoin) during pregnancy. *Br. J. Obstet. Gynaecol.*, 86:125–132.

70. Levy, R. H., Cenraud, B., Loiseau, P., Akbaraly, R., Brachet-Liermain, A., Guyot, M., Gomeni, R., and Morselli, P. L. (1980): Meal-dependent absorption of enteric-coated sodium valproate. *Epilepsia*, 21:273–280.

71. Levy, R. H., Lane, E. A. (1978): Biological half-lives of antiepileptic drugs: Linearity and non-linearity. In: *Advances in Epileptology 1977*, edited by H. Meinardi and A. J. Rowan, pp. 186–196. Swets & Zeitlinger, Amsterdam, Lisse.

72. Levy, R. H., Lockard, J. S., Green, J. R., Friel, P., and Martis, L. (1975): Pharmacokinetics of carbamazepine in monkeys following intravenous and oral administration. *J. Pharm. Sci.*, 64:302–307.

73. Levy, R. H., Pitlick, W. H., Troupin, A. S., Green, J. R., and Neal, J. M. (1975): Pharmacokinetics of carbamazepine in normal man. *Clin. Pharmacol. Ther.*, 17:657–668.

74. Lockard, J. S., Levy, R. H., Uhlir, V., and Farmuhar, J. A. (1974): Pharmacokinetic evaluation of anticonvulsants prior to efficacy testing exemplified by carbamazepine in epileptic monkey model. *Epilepsia*, 15:351–359.

75. Lorgé, M. (1963): Etude clinique du Tégrétol (G 32833), nouvel antiépileptique avec action particulière sur l'altération épileptique de la personnalité. *Schweiz. Med. Wochenschr.*, 93:1042–1047.

76. Löscher, W. (1979): A comparative study of the protein binding of anticonvulsant drugs in serum of dog and man. *J. Pharmacol. Exp. Ther.*, 208:429–435.

77. Lynn, R. K., Smith, R. G., Thompson, R. M., Deinzer, M. L., Griffin, D., and Gerber, N. (1978): Characterization of glucuronide metabolites of carbamazepine in human urine by gas chromatography and mass spectrometry. *Drug Metab. Dispos.*, 6:494–501.

78. McAuliffe, J. J., Sherwin, A. L., Leppik, I. E., Fayle, S. A., and Pippenger, C. E. (1977): Salivary levels of anticonvulsants: A practical approach to drug monitoring. *Neurology (Minneap.)*, 27:409–413.

79. McNamara, P. J., Colburn, W. A., and Gibaldi, M. (1979): Time course of carbamazepine self-induction. *J. Pharmacokinet. Biopharm.*, 7:63–68.

80. Meinardi, H. (1972): Other antiepileptic drugs. Carbamazepine. In: *Antiepileptic Drugs,* edited by D. M. Woodbury, J. K. Penry, and R. P. Schmidt, pp. 487–496. Raven Press, New York.

81. Melander, A. (1978): Influence of food on the bioavailability of drugs. *Clin. Pharmacokinet.*, 3:337–351.

82. Miyamoto, K., Seino, M., and Ikeda, Y. (1975): Consecutive determination of the levels of twelve antiepileptic drugs·in blood and cerebrospinal fluid. In: *Clinical Pharmacology of Antiepileptic Drugs,* edited by H. Schneider, D. Janz, C. Gardner-Thorpe, H. Meinardi, and A. L. Sherwin, pp. 323–330. Springer-Verlag, Berlin.

83. Mølholm Hansen, J., Skovsted, L., Kampmann, J. P., Lumholtz, B. I., and Siersbaek-Nielsen, K. (1978): Unaltered metabolism of phenytoin in thyroid disorders. *Acta Pharmacol. Toxicol. (Kbh.)*, 42:343–346.

84. Møller, I., and Nielsen, H. R. (1972): Serum Tegretol determinations in the treatment of epileptic disorders in childhood. *Acta Paediatr. Scand.*, 61:507–510.

85. Monaco, F., Mutani, R., Mastropaolo, C., and Tondi, M. (1979): Tears as the best practical indicator of the unbound fraction of an anticonvulsant drug. *Epilepsia*, 20:705–710.

86. Monaco, F., Riccio, A., Benna, P., Covacich, A., Durelli, L., Fantini, M., Furlan, P. M., Gilli, M., Mutani, R., Troni, W., Gerna, M., and Morselli, P. L. (1976): Further observations on carbamazepine plasma levels in epileptic patients. Relationships with therapeutic and side effects. *Neurology (Minneap.)*, 26:936–943.

87. Monaco, F., Riccio, A., Fantini, M., Baruzzi, A., and Morselli, P. L. (1979): A month-by-month long-term study on carbamazepine: Clinical, EEG and pharmacological evaluation. *J. Int. Med. Res.*, 7:152–157.

88. Morselli, P. L. (1975): Carbamazepine: Absorption, distribution and excretion. *Adv. Neurol.*, 11:279–293.

89. Morselli, P. L. (1977): Antiepileptic drugs. In: *Drug Disposition During Development,* edited by P. L. Morselli, pp. 311–360. Spectrum, New York.

90. Morselli, P. L. (1978): Problems of antiepileptic drugs administration in the neonatal period. In: *Barneepilepsi,* edited by A. W. Munthe-Kass and S. I. Johannessen, pp. 173–192. Ciba Geigy, Hassle.

91. Morselli, P. L., Baruzzi, A., Gerna, M., Bossi, L., and Porta, M. (1977): Carbamazepine and carbamazepine-10,11-epoxide concentration in human brain. *Br. J. Clin. Pharmacol.*, 4:535–540.

92. Morselli, P. L., Biandrate, P., Frigerio, A., and Garattini, S. (1972): Pharmacokinetics of carbamazepine in rats and humans. *Eur. Soc. Clin. Invest.*, 2:297.

93. Morselli, P. L., Biandrate, P., Frigerio, A., Gerna, M., and Tognoni, G. (1973): Gas chromatographic determination of carbamazepine and carbamazepine-10,11-epoxide in human body fluids. In: *Methods of Analysis of Antiepileptic Drugs,* edited by J. W. A. Meijer, H. Meinardi, C. Gardner-Thorpe, and E. Van der Kleijn, pp. 169–175. Excerpta Medica, Amsterdam.

94. Morselli, P. L., Bossi, L., and Gerna, M. (1976): Pharmacokinetic studies with carbamazepine in epileptic patients. In: *Epileptic Seizures, Behaviour, Pain,* edited by W. Birkmayer, pp. 141–150. Huber Publishers, Bern.

95. Morselli, P. L., Cassano, G. B., Placidi, G. F., Muscettola, G. B., and Rizzo, M. (1973): Kinetics of the distribution of ^{14}C-diazepam and its metabolites in various areas of cat brain. In: *The Benzodiazepines,* edited by S. Garattini, E. Mussini, and O. Randall, pp. 129–143. Raven Press, New York.

96. Morselli, P. L., Cenraud, B., Tedeschi, G., Levy, R. H., and Loisseau, P. (1980): Effect of food on carbamazepine absorption. *Advances in Epileptology: XIIth Epilepsy International Symposium,* edited by M. Dam, L. Gram, and J. K. Penry, pp. 563–568. Raven Press, New York.

97. Morselli, P. L., and Franco-Morselli, R. (1980): Clinical pharmacokinetics of antiepileptic drugs in adults. *Pharmacol. Ther.*, 10:65–101.

98. Morselli, P. L., Franco-Morselli, R., and Bossi, L; (1980): Clinical pharmacokinetics in newborns and infants. *Clin. Pharmacokinet.*, 5:485–527.

99. Morselli, P. L., and Frigerio, A. (1975): Metabolism and pharmacokinetics of carbamazepine. *Drug Metab. Rev.*, 4:97–113.

100. Morselli, P. L., Gerna, M., de Mayo, D., Zanda, G., Viani, F., and Garattini, S. (1975): Pharmacokinetic studies on carbamazepine in volunteers and in epileptic patients. In: *Clinical Pharmacology of Antiepileptic Drugs,* edited by H. Schneider, D. Janz, C. Gardner-Thorpe, H. Meinardi, and A. L. Sherwin, pp. 166–180. Springer-Verlag, Berlin.

101. Morselli, P. L., Gerna, M., and Garattini, S. (1971): Carbamazepine plasma and tissue levels in the rat. *Biochem. Pharmacol.*, 20:2043–2047.

102. Morselli, P. L., Monaco, F., Gerna, M., Recchia, M., and Riccio, A. (1975): Bioavailability of two carbamazepine preparations during chronic administration to epileptic patients. *Epilepsia*, 16:759–764.

103. Munari, C., Rovei, V., Talairach, J., Sanjuan, M., Bancaud, J., and Morselli, P. L. (1978): AED concentrations in discrete brain areas of epileptic patients undergoing surgical intervention. Preliminary observations. In: *X Epilepsy International Symposium,* edited by J. A. Wada and J. K. Penry, p. 24. Raven Press, New York.

104. Mygind, K. I., Dam, M., and Christiansen, J. (1976): Phenytoin and phenobarbitone plasma clearance during pregnancy. *Acta Neurol. Scand.*, 54:160–166.

105. Niebyl, J. R., Blake, D. A., Freeman, J. M., and Luff, R. D. (1979): Carbamazepine levels in pregnancy and lactation. *Obstet. Gynecol.*, 53:139–140.

106. Palmer, L., Bertilsson, L., Collste, P., and Rawlins, M. (1973): Quantitative determination of carbamazepine in plasma by mass fragmentography. *Clin. Pharmacol. Ther.*, 14:827–832.

107. Pantarotto, C., Crunelli, V., Lanzoni, J., Frigerio, A., and Quattrone, A. (1979): Quantitative determination of carbamazepine and carbamazepine-10,11-epoxide in rat brain areas by multiple ion detection mass fragmentography, *Anal. Biochem.*, 93:115–123.

108. Pantarotto, C., Crunelli, V., Quattrone, A., Negrini, P., Frigerio, A., and Samanin, R. (1978): Distribution in brain areas of carbamazepine and carbamazepine-10,11-epoxide in 6-hydroxydopamine pretreated rats. In: *Recent Developments in Mass Spectrometry in Biochemistry and Medicine, Vol. 1*, edited by A. Frigerio, pp. 15–28. Plenum Press, New York.

109. Parsonage, M. (1975): Treatment with carbamazepine: Adults. *Adv. Neurol.*, 11:221–234.

110. Patel, I. H., Levy, R. H., and Trager, W. F. (1978): Pharmacokinetics of carbamazepine-10,11-epoxide before and after autoinduction in rhesus monkeys. *J. Pharmacol. Exp. Ther.*, 206:607–613.

111. Perucca, E., Garratt, A., Hebdige, S., and Richens, A. (1978): Water intoxication in epileptic patients receiving carbamazepine. *J. Neurol. Neurosurg. Psychiatry*, 41:713–718.

112. Piafsky, K. M., and Rane, A. (1978): Formation of carbamazepine epoxide in human fetal liver. *Drug Metab. Dispos.*, 6:502–503.

113. Pitlick, W. H., and Levy, R. H. (1977): Time-dependent kinetics I: Exponential autoinduction of carbamazepine in monkeys. *J. Pharm. Sci.*, 66 647–649.

114. Pitlick, W. H., Levy, R. H., Troupin, A. S., and Green, J. R. (1976): Pharmacokinetic model to describe self-induced decreases in steady-state concentrations of carbamazepine. *J. Pharm. Sci.*, 65:462–463.

115. Placidi, G. F., Tognoni, G., Pacifici, G. M., Cassano, G. B., and Morselli, P. L. (1976): Regional distribution of diazepam and its metabolites in the brain of cat after chronic treatment. *Psychopharmacologia*, 48:133–137.

116. Pynnönen, S. (1977): The pharmacokinetics of carbamazepine in plasma and saliva of man. *Acta Pharmacol. Toxicol. (Kbh.)*, 41:465–471.

117. Pynnönen, S., Björkquist, S. E., and Pekkarinen, A. (1978): The pharmacokinetics of carbamazepine in alcoholics. In: *Advances in Epileptology 1977. Psychology, Pharmacotherapy and New Diagnostic Approaches*, edited by H. Meinardi and A. J. Rowan, pp. 285–289. Swets & Zeitlinger, Amsterdam, Lisse.

118. Pynnönen, S., Kanto, J., Sillanpää, M., and Erkkola, R. (1977): Carbamazepine: Placental transport, tissue concentrations in foetus and newborn and level in milk. *Acta Pharmacol. Toxicol. (Kbh.)*, 41:244–253.

119. Pynnönen, S., Mäntylä, R., and Iisalo, E. (1978): Bioavailability of four different pharmaceutical preparations of carbamazepine. *Acta Pharmacol. Toxicol. (Kbh.)*, 43:306–310.

120. Pynnönen, S., Siirtola, T., Mölsä, P., and Aaltonen, L. (1978): On the distribution of carbamazepine in blood, plasma, saliva, cerebrospinal fluid and plasma water. *Acta Neurol. Scand. [Suppl.]*, 67:266–267.

121. Pynnönen, S., and Sillanpää, M. (1975): Carbamazepine and mother's milk. *Lancet*, 1:563.

122. Pynnönen, S., Sillanpää, M., Frey, H., and Iisalo, E. (1977): Carbamazepine and its 10,11-epoxide in children and adults with epilepsy. *Eur. J. Clin. Pharmacol.*, 11:129–133.

123. Pynnönen, S., Sillanpää, M., Iisalo, E., and Frey, H. (1977): Elimination of carbamazepine in children after single and multiple doses. In: *Epilepsy. the Eighth International Symposium*, edited by J. K. Penry, pp. 191–196. Raven Press, New York.

124. Pynnönen, S., and Yrjänä, T. (1977): The significance of the simultaneous determination of carbamazepine and its 10,11-epoxide from plasma and human erythrocytes. *Int. J. Clin. Pharmacol.*, 15:222–226.

125. Rado, J. P. (1973): Water intoxication during carbamazepine treatment. *Br. Med. J.*, 3:479.

126. Rane, A., and Bertilsson, L. (1980): Kinetics of carbamazepine in epileptic children. In: *Antiepileptic Therapy: Advances in Drug Monitoring*, edited by S. I. Johannessen, P. L. Morselli, C. E. Pippenger, A. Richens, D. Schmidt, and H. Meinardi, pp. 49–54. Raven Press, New York.

127. Rane, A., Bertilsson, L., and Parmér, L. (1975): Disposition of placentally transferred carbamazepine (Tegretol) in the newborn. *Eur. J. Clin. Pharmacol.*, 8:283–284.

128. Rane, A., and Wilson, J. T. (1976): Plasma level monitoring of diphenylhydantoin and carbamazepine in the pediatric patient. In: *Clinical Pharmacy and Clinical Pharmacology*, edited by W. A. Gouveia, G. Tognoni, and E. van Der Kleijn, pp. 295–302. Elsevier/North Holland Biomedical Press, Amsterdam.

129. Rawlins, M. D., Collste, P., Bertilsson, L., and Palmér, L. (1975): Distribution and elimination kinetics of carbamazepine in man. *Eur. J. Clin. Pharmacol.*, 8:91–96.

130. Reidenberg, M. M., and Drayer, D. E. (1978): Effects of renal diseases upon drug disposition. *Drug Metab. Rev.*, 8:293–302.

131. Rey, E., d'Athis, P., de Lauture, D., Dulac, O., Aicardi, J., and Olive, G. (1979): Pharmacokinetics of carbamazepine in the neonate and in the child. *Int. J. Clin. Pharmacol. Biopharm.*, 17:90–96.

132. Richter, K., and Terhaag, B. (1978): The relative bioavailability and pharmacokinetics of carbamazepine. *Int. J. Clin. Pharmacol.*, 16:377–379.

133. Ronfeld, R. A., and Benet, L. Z. (1975): Dose dependent kinetics of carbamazepine in the monkey. *Res. Commun. Chem. Pathol. Pharmacol.*, 10:303–314.

134. Rylance, G. W., Butcher, G. M., and Moreland, T. (1977): Saliva carbamazepine levels in children. *Br. Med. J.*, 3:1481.

135. Rylance, G. W., Moreland, T. A., and Butcher, G. M. (1978): Individualisation of anticonvulsant med-

ication: A new approach with carbamazepine. *Arch. Dis. Child.*, 53:690.

136. Scheiffarth, F., Weist, F., and Zicha, L. (1966): Zum Nachweiss von 5-Carbamyl-5H-dibenzo [b,f]azepin im Liquor cerebrospinalis mittels Dünnschichtchromatographie. *Z. Klin. Chem.*, 4:68–70.

137. Schneider, H. (1975): Carbamazepine: An attempt to correlate serum levels with antiepileptic and side effects. In: *Clinical Pharmacology of Antiepileptic Drugs*, edited by H. Schneider, D. Janz, C. Gardner-Thorpe, H. Meinardi, and A. L. Sherwin, pp. 151–158. Springer-Verlag, Berlin.

138. Schneider, H. (1975): Carbamazepine: The influence of other antiepileptic drugs on its serum levels. In: *Clinical Pharmacology of Antiepileptic Drugs*, edited by H. Schneider, D. Janz, C. Gardner-Thorpe, H. Meinardi, and A. L. Sherwin, pp. 189–195. Springer-Verlag, Berlin.

139. Schneider, H., and Berenguer, J. (1977): CSF and plasma concentrations of carbamazepine and some metabolites in steady state. In: *Antiepileptic Drug Monitoring*, edited by C. Gardner-Thorpe, D. Janz, H. Meinardi, and C. E. Pippenger, pp. 264–273. Pitman Medical, Tunbridge Wells, Kent.

140. Shorvon, S. D., Chadwick, D., Galbraith, A. W., and Reynolds, E. H. (1978): One drug for epilepsy, *Br. Med. J.*, 1:474–476.

141. Simonsen, N., Zander Olsen, P., Kühl, V., Lund, M., and Wendelboe, J. (1976): A comparative controlled study between carbamazepine and diphenylhydantoin in psychomotor epilepsy. *Epilepsia*, 17:169–176.

142. Smith, G. A., Hooper, W. D., Tyrer, J. H., Eadie, M. J., and Werth, B. (1979): The comparative bioavailability of carbamazepine in 100 mg and 200 mg tablets. *Clin. Exp. Pharmacol. Physiol.*, 6:37–40.

143. Strandjord, R. E., and Johannessen, S. I. (1975): A preliminary study of serum carbamazepine levels in healthy subjects and in patients with epilepsy. In: *Clinical Pharmacology of Antiepileptic Drugs*, edited by H. Schneider, D. Janz, C. Gardner-Thorpe, H. Meinardi, and A. L. Sherwin, pp. 181–188. Springer-Verlag, Berlin.

144. Strandjord, R. E., and Johannessen, S. I. (1978): Monoterapi med Karbamazepin. In: *Barneepilepsi*, edited by A. W. Munthe-Kaas and S. I. Johannessen, pp. 77–82. Ciba Geigy, Basel.

145. Suzuki, K., Kaneko, S., and Sato, T. (1978): Time-dependency of serum carbamazepine concentration. *Folia Psychiatr. Neurol. Jpn.*, 32:199–209.

146. Terhaag, B., Richter, K., and Diettrich, H. (1978): Concentration behavior of carbamazepine in bile and plasma of man. *Int. J. Clin. Pharmacol.*, 16:607–609.

147. Tondi, M., Mutani, R., Mastropaolo, C., and Mon-

148. aco, F. (1978): Greater reliability of tear versus saliva anticonvulsant levels. *Ann. Neurol.*, 4:154–155.

148. Troupin, A. S. (1978): Carbamazepine in epilepsy. In: *Clinical Neuropharmacology, Vol. 3*, edited by H. L. Klawans, pp. 15–40. Raven Press, New York.

149. Troupin, A. S., and Friel, P. (1975): Anticonvulsant level in saliva, serum and cerebrospinal fluid. *Epilepsia*, 16:223–227.

150. Troupin, A. S., Green, J. R., and Levy, R. H. (1974): Carbamazepine as an anticonvulsant: A pilot study. *Neurology (Minneap.)*, 24:863–869.

151. Troupin, A. S., Ojemann, L. M., Halpern, L., Dodrill, C., Wilkus, R., Friel, P., and Feigl, P. (1977): Carbamazepine. A double blind comparison with phenytoin. *Neurology (Minneap.)*, 27:511–519.

152. Valli, M., Gruguerolle, B., Bouyard, L., Jadot, G., and Bouyard, P. (1979): Intérêt d'une approche chronopharmacocinétique de la carbamazépine. *Therapie*, 34:393–396.

153. Van der Kleijn, E., Guelen, P. J. M., Beelen, T. C. M., Rijntjes, N. V. M., and Zuidgeest, T. L. B. (1973): Kinetics of general and regional brain distribution of closely related 7-chloro-1,4-benzodiazepines. In: *The Benzodiazepines*, edited by S. Garattini, E. Mussini, and L. O. Randall, pp. 145–164. Raven Press, New York.

154. Van der Kleijn, E., Guelen, P. J. M., Van Wijk, C., and Baars, I. (1975): Clinical pharmacokinetics in monitoring chronic medication with antiepileptic drugs. In: *Clinical Pharmacology of Antiepileptic Drugs*, edited by H. Schneider, D. Janz, C. Gardner-Thorpe, H. Meinardi, and A. L. Sherwin, pp. 11–33. Springer-Verlag, Berlin.

155. Wada, J. A., Troupin, A. S., Friel, P., Remick, R., Leal, K., and Pearmain, J. (1978): Pharmacokinetic comparison of tablet and suspension dosage forms of carbamazepine. *Epilepsia*, 19:251–255.

156. Watanabe, S., Kuyama, C., Yokoyama, S., Kubo, S., and Iwai, H. (1977): Distribution of plasma carbamazepine in epileptic patients. *Folia Psychiatr. Neurol. Jpn.*, 31:587–595.

157. Weist, F., and Zicha, L. (1967): Dünnschichtchromatographische Untersuchungen über 5-Carbamyl-5H-dibenzo[b,f]azepin in Harn and Liquor bei neunen Indikatronsgebieten. *Arzneim. Forsch.*, 17:874–875.

158. Westenberg, H. G. M., Jonkman, J. H. G., and Van der Kleijn, E. (1977): The distribution of carbamazepine and its metabolites in squirrel monkey and mouse. *Acta Pharmacol. Toxicol. [Suppl.] (Kbh.)*, 41:136–137.

159. Westenberg, H. G. M., Van der Kleijn, E., Oei, T. T., and de Zeeuw, R. (1978): Kinetics of carbamazepine and carbamazepine-epoxide, determined by use of plasma and saliva. *Clin. Pharmacol. Ther.*, 23:320–328.

Antiepileptic Drugs, edited by D. M. Woodbury, J. K. Penry, and C. E. Pippenger. Raven Press, New York © 1982.

38

Carbamazepine

Biotransformation

J. W. Faigle and K. F. Feldmann

Carbamazepine (CBZ), the active ingredient of Tegretol®, has the chemical structure of 5-carbamoyl-5H-dibenzo[*b,f*]azepine. The chemical and physical properties of CBZ are such that it can be classified as a neutral, lipophilic compound (15). The lipid solubility is attributable to the tricyclic skeleton consisting of two six-membered aromatic rings and one seven-membered (azepine) ring. The nitrogen atoms contained in the azepine ring and the carbamoyl side chain lack basic properties since they are part of a urea moiety (Fig. 1).

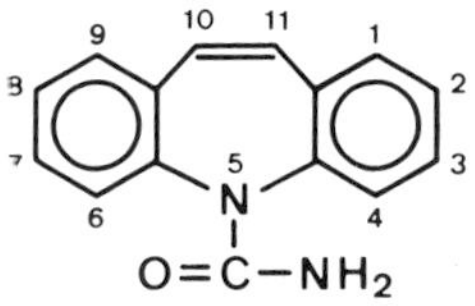

It is important to keep these properties in mind when discussing problems of biotransformation. The mammalian body possesses no mechanism by which exogenous lipophilic compounds, including especially those of a neutral character, can readily be excreted in unchanged form (56). Drug-metabolizing enzymes convert such compounds into more strongly hydrophilic products which are easily removed by the renal or hepatic–biliary system.

With CBZ, metabolic reactions are theoretically conceivable at any of the numbered positions of the tricyclic skeleton (see Fig. 1) and, in addition, at the carbamoyl side chain of the molecule. A large number of metabolites is to be expected, and efficient methods are required to separate these products and to elucidate their structures. Particular care must be taken to avoid

FIG. 1. Structural formula of CBZ, 5-carbamoyl-5H-dibenzo[*b,f*]azepine, and numbering of positions in the tricyclic skeleton of the molecule.

the formation of artifacts during work-up, since some of the structural elements of the CBZ molecule may be unstable at elevated temperature or in acid or alkaline media (6,8,19). For example, attempts to hydrolyze conjugated metabolites with mineral acid result in ring contraction of the azepine nucleus and in cleavage of the urea moiety.

CHEMICAL ASPECTS OF METABOLISM

Isolation of Metabolites from Human Urine

Numerous reports dealing with structure analysis of urinary metabolites of CBZ have appeared over the past decade. The early studies yielded qualitative information only; the fraction of a CBZ dose accounted for by any of the metabolites described could not be estimated. Moreover, some of the published structures were only speculative, and some others were based on inadequate experimental techniques. For critical reviews of the literature up to 1975, see Frigerio and Morselli (22) and Faigle et al. (15).

Quantitative data were eventually provided by a series of new experiments that were initiated in our laboratories. To insure that a mass balance could be determined, we used a radioactive CBZ preparation labeled with ^{14}C in positions 10 and 11 of the azepine ring. Urinary metabolites were separated by nondestructive methods including, in particular, liquid chromatography on high-efficiency columns. The columns were packed with silica gel for extractable metabolites (50,51) or with XAD-2 resin as a reversed-phase adsorbent for polar metabolites (11). All separations were done on a preparative scale so that the individual compounds were obtained in amounts sufficient for full structure analysis by mass spectrometry and nuclear magnetic resonance spectroscopy as well as ultraviolet and infrared spectroscopy. When possible, conjugated metabolites were isolated in their intact form, but in some cases cleavage with specific enzymes was also used to characterize the ligand of a conjugate. In addition, inverse isotope dilution methods were applied to native urine to either confirm or disprove the presence of metabolites postulated in earlier studies. The specific features of this technique, i.e., addition of an excess of unlabeled carrier substance having the same structure as the compound to be determined and reisolation of the latter in isotopically diluted form, eliminate all possibilities of artifact formation (48).

The essential findings of these radiotracer studies will be presented and discussed below. Experimental details have been published elsewhere (15,16,46).

Following single oral doses of 400 mg of ^{14}C-labeled CBZ to two healthy volunteers, the bulk of the radioactivity (72%) was recovered from the urine, with the remainder appearing in the feces (16). About half of the small ^{14}C fraction excreted in the feces was accounted for by yet unidentified metabolites, and the remainder by unchanged CBZ. The latter presumably represents nonabsorbed material, since excretion of unchanged drug in human bile was found to be insignificant (54). In the pooled urine, only about 3% of the total radioactivity present, corresponding to 2% of the dose, was identified as the original drug both by isotope dilution analysis and preparative isolation. This agrees well with the reports of other investigators who found between 0.5 and 2% of the dose as unchanged CBZ in urine (14,22,34).

Preparative liquid chromatography of the extractable and nonextractable fractions of urinary metabolites yielded a large number of biotransformation products, most of them displaying strongly polar properties. The structures identified by spectroscopic analysis of the purified metabolites (16,46) are presented in Fig. 2.

Major Pathways of Biotransformation

The metabolite structures resulting from the aforementioned radiotracer study disclose that biotransformation of CBZ in man proceeds by four major pathways (Fig. 2). Since the radioactivity recoveries were determined in the course of preparative separation, the amounts of individual metabolites present in the original urine could be estimated (46). Taking the total urinary radioactivity as 100%, the following approximate percentages are attributable to the different pathways or the corresponding metabolites: epoxidation of the 10,11 double bond of the azepine ring, 40%; hydroxylation of the six-membered aromatic rings, 25%; direct N-glucuronidation at the carbamoyl side chain, 15%; and substitution of the six-membered rings with sulfur-containing groups, 5%. Together with about 3% of intact drug in urine, these pathways cover almost 90% of the radioactivity excreted by the kidneys.

The reaction leading to 10,11-epoxycarbamazepine (epoxy-CBZ, I), which is the first intermediate of pathway 1, is catalyzed by hepatic monooxygenases (20). Only little of the epoxide is excreted as such (approximately 1%), most of it being converted to the corresponding diol, 10,11-dihydro-10,11-dihydroxycarbamazepine (10,11-di-H-10,11-di-OH-CBZ, II; approximately 35%). The hydroxy groups of this

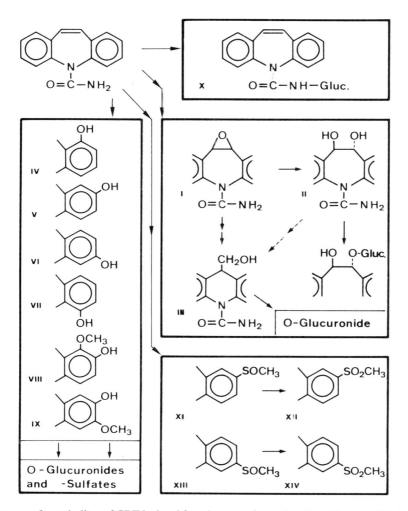

FIG. 2. Structures of metabolites of CBZ isolated from human urine and major pathways of biotransformation (15,46).

metabolite are trans to each other, as was shown by spectroscopic analysis in comparison with the synthetic cis and trans isomers (46). The *trans*-diol metabolite is formed enzymically by liver epoxide hydrase (40); accordingly, it is optically active (16). In urine, the diol is partly present as such and partly as its mono-*O*-glucuronide. A smaller portion of the epoxide intermediate is converted to a ring-contracted compound, 9-hydroxymethyl-10-carbamoyl acridan (III, approximately 5%); the reaction mechanism is still unknown. It is also unknown whether this reaction proceeds directly or via the diol. Metabolite III is almost completely

conjugated with glucuronic acid at the hydroxymethyl group before excretion (15).

Metabolites formed by the epoxide pathway have independently been described by other investigators; these include epoxy-CBZ (7,21, 28), 10,11-di-H-10,11-di-OH-CBZ (3,7,27,28), and the mono-*O*-glucuronide of the latter (36).

The second pathway by which CBZ is metabolized starts with hydroxylation at various positions of the six-membered rings; these reactions are presumably also catalyzed by monooxygenases. Single substitution results in all four possible phenols, i.e., 1-, 2-, 3-, and 4-hydroxycarbamazepine (IV to VII). Two other intermediates of this pathway carry a hydroxy group in position 2 and, additionally, a methoxy group in position 1 or 3 (46). Only trace amounts of these phenols are excreted unconjugated by the kidneys, the bulk being converted to the O-glucuronides and O-sulfates in a ratio of about 2 : 1.

Lynn et al. (35,36) have described a series of glucuronides of phenolic CBZ metabolites detected in human urine by gas chromatography and mass spectrometry. Apart from the four monohydroxy derivatives, they found three hydroxymethoxy compounds and three dihydroxy compounds. Although their method did not allow them to allocate the sites of substitution, it is evident that some additional polyfunctional phenols do exist. They may cover part of the small unidentified fraction left by the metabolites specified in Fig. 2.

Direct conjugation of CBZ with glucuronic acid is the third important route of biotransformation. In the conjugate, the ligand is bound to the amino group of the carbamoyl side chain; a possible binding to the hydroxy group of the isourea structure is ruled out by the infrared spectrum of the pure, intact metabolite (46). It can be assumed that the ligand is introduced by a hepatic glucuronyl transferase. It is interesting to note that the conjugate cannot be cleaved with β-glucuronidase. Direct glucuronidation of CBZ has also been reported by Lynn et al. (36).

The fourth pathway involves a less common type of metabolic reaction: a sulfur-containing substituent is introduced into one of the six-membered rings of the CBZ molecule. Four products resulting from this pathway were found in human urine: 2- and 3-methylsulfinylcarbamazepine (XI, XIII) and 2- and 3-methylsulfonylcarbamazepine (XII, XIV). Altogether, they account for about 5% of the urinary radioactivity. A possible substitution at the 10 or 11 position of the azepine ring was ruled out by the nuclear magnetic resonance spectra of these compounds. Comparison with synthetic XIV allowed positive identification of the binding sites (W. J. Richter, *unpublished data*).

The same type of substitution was recently reported by Goenechea et al. (26), although with incorrect placement of the substituents at position 10 of CBZ. Metabolites carrying -SOCH$_3$ or -SO$_2$CH$_3$ groups have also been described for other drugs and chemicals (32). However, the mechanism by which they are generated is still unknown. Conjugates with methionine or glutathione have been proposed as possible precursors of such metabolites (32,53).

As already mentioned, the compounds listed in Fig. 2 account for almost 90% of the total urinary metabolites of CBZ in man. The list contains only metabolites derived from single primary reactions, but it is to be expected that products from combined attack also exist. For instance, small amounts of a metabolite formed by aromatic hydroxylation of III, i.e., an intermediate of the epoxide pathway, have in fact been found in our study. Some additional products formed by pathways 1, 2, and 4 have been described by Lertratanangkoon and Horning (32a). Such products will further reduce the unidentified metabolite fraction in urine.

Minor and Questionable Pathways of Biotransformation

In various papers dealing with the metabolism of CBZ in man, products have been described that do not result from the major pathways presented above. In Table 1, these products are listed together with references and data on structure analysis and quantities. Table 1 also contains results from a specific determination of most of these compounds in urine by inverse isotope dilution analysis after administration of ^{14}C-labeled CBZ (15). For the sake of comparability, the quantities are expressed as percentage of dose. (In the radiotracer study, 1% of dose corresponded to 1.4% of total urinary ^{14}C.)

According to the data in Table 1, hydrolysis of the urea moiety of the CBZ molecule is an additional metabolic pathway. Quantitatively, however, this reaction is of only little importance. The cleavage product carrying the tricyclic skeleton, i.e., iminostilbene, comprises

TABLE 1. *Minor or postulated metabolites of CBZ in man*

Compound	Evidence for structure	Quantity[a]	Refs.
Iminostilbene	GC[b] in urine	0.1%	39
	IDA[c] in urine	≤0.1%	15
Acridone	Spectroscopic analysis after isolation from urine	No data	5
	IDA in urine	1%	15
9-Methylacridine	Spectroscopic analysis after isolation from urine	No data	5,7
	IDA in urine	≤0.1%	15
Acridine-9-carboxaldehyde	Spectroscopic analysis after isolation from urine	No data	5,7
Acridine	Spectroscopic analysis after isolation from urine	No data	5
	IDA in urine	≤0.1%	15
10,11-Dihydro-10-hydroxycarbamazepine	Spectroscopic analysis after isolation from urine	No data	3,7
	IDA in urine	≤0.1%	15

[a]Expressed in percent of dose.
[b]GC, gas chromatographic analysis.
[c]IDA, inverse isotope dilution analysis.

at most 0.1% of the dose. Acridone is an unimportant product too; it is formed by contraction of the azepine ring and cleavage of the carbamoyl group, the mechanisms still being unknown. The same basic reactions may lead to the three compounds of the acridine series listed, but there is some likelihood that these reactions actually take place artifactually during metabolite isolation. Brazier et al. (8) found that chemical hydrolysis of CBZ results in 9-methylacridine, and Frigerio et al. (19) observed that thermal degradation of CBZ and epoxy-CBZ leads to 9-methylacridine and acridine-9-carboxaldehyde, respectively. The amounts actually present in native human urine are at or below the detection limit of the inverse isotope dilution assay (≤0.1% of dose).

The last compound in Table 1 is the 10-(mono-)hydroxy derivative of 10,11-dihydrocarbamazepine. Isotope dilution analysis did not confirm its presence in urine. In the original studies, structure assignment was based on mass spectra only. Possibly, the true structure would have been that of metabolite III (9-hydroxymethyl-10-carbamoyl acridan; see Fig. 2) which is an isomer showing the same molecular ion in mass spectrometry.

PHARMACOLOGICAL ASPECTS OF METABOLISM

Metabolites Present in Blood and Brain

Knowledge of the structures and the mass balance of urinary metabolites is essential when the pathways of biotransformation of CBZ are to be deduced. As far as the pharmacological activity of the drug is concerned, however, the metabolites excreted in urine are of little direct significance. Most of them are strongly hydrophilic end products of biotransformation and are generally devoid of biological effects.

Nevertheless, biotransformation is important for both the intensity and the duration of pharmacologic effects, since the elimination of CBZ from the organism is controlled by the primary metabolic reactions rather than by renal or biliary excretion of unchanged drug. Eventually, the rate at which CBZ is eliminated depends largely on the activity of the enzymes catalyzing these reactions. One of the primary metabolites, epoxy-CBZ, possesses anticonvulsant activities similar to those of CBZ itself (see below). The kinetics of this compound are likewise under enzymic control.

When the pharmacological effects of CBZ are discussed, it is essential to consider the kinetics of the products present in blood. The radiotracer experiment mentioned earlier yielded a mass balance of CBZ and its metabolites in the plasma of two healthy volunteers after single oral doses of 400 mg (15,16). On the basis of the areas under the concentration–time curves between 0 and 96 hr, the unchanged drug accounts for about 75% of the total radioactivity present, the epoxy metabolite for 10%, and the sum of all other metabolites for only 15%. These findings suggest that the bulk of metabolites, including the strongly hydrophilic end products, is rapidly removed from the circulation by the kidneys.

Gérardin and Hirtz (25) showed that the elimination kinetics of CBZ are not dose dependent. The half-lives of elimination from plasma following single oral doses of 100, 200, and 600 mg to six healthy subjects did not differ significantly, the overall average being 37.5 hr. Accordingly, the area under the CBZ concentration curves extrapolated to infinite time ($A\infty$) and corrected for variations in body weight (W) and elimination rate constant (β) increases linearly with the dose (Fig. 3; the inset shows a plot of the dose versus the product $A\infty$ times W times β). Independent studies by Levy et al. (34) and Rawlins et al. (45) led to the same basic observations. It may therefore be concluded that, in the dose range studied, the metabolism of CBZ is not saturable.

The available plasma concentration data for the epoxy metabolite show that its area under the curve is between 5 and 15% of that of the parent drug if different single doses of CBZ are given to volunteers (12,15). There is no indication of nonlinear kinetics of this metabolic intermediate.

Carbamazepine and epoxy-CBZ pass readily from the bloodstream into the central nervous system (15). In epileptic patients under continuous treatment with CBZ, Friis et al. (23) found a brain-to-plasma concentration ratio of 1.4 to 1.6 for the parent drug and of 0.6 to 1.5 for the epoxy metabolite. Therefore, none of these compounds is preferentially taken up by the

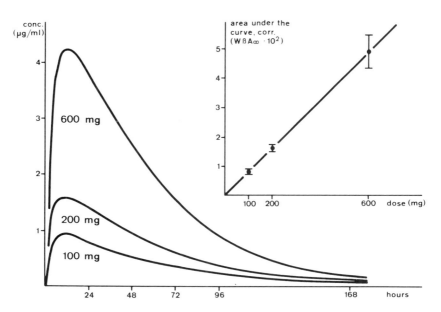

FIG. 3. Dose dependence of plasma concentrations of CBZ measured in healthy subjects following single oral doses of 100, 200, and 600 mg (25). The **inset** shows the relationship between dose and product of W times β times $A\infty$ (W, body weight; β, elimination rate constant; $A\infty$, area under the concentration–time curve extrapolated to infinite time) ($N = 6$; mean values and 95% confidence limits).

brain, and the time course of their concentrations at the site of action appears to be reflected by the time course of their concentrations in plasma.

Induction of Drug-Metabolizing Enzymes

Repeated administration of CBZ to volunteers or patients results in an accelerated elimination of the drug as was shown by several independent studies (12,15,25,38,42,55,57). In patients receiving concomitant treatment with certain other antiepileptic drugs, e.g., phenytoin, phenobarbital, primidone, ethosuximide, and methsuximide, elimination of CBZ is further accelerated (14,49,55,57). This phenomenon is explained by an induction of drug-metabolizing enzymes as a response of the organism to prolonged exposure to such drugs. The half-life by which CBZ is eliminated from plasma is reduced in these cases, but the apparent volume of distribution is about the same as that found after single doses of CBZ (14,57).

Table 2 summarizes the elimination half-lives of CBZ from plasma of volunteers and patients measured during or after various treatment regimens. The list comprises the available published data from 189 individual plasma level curves. Following single doses, the half-lives

range from 20 to 50 hr in most individuals, the overall average being 36 hr. Daily administration of CBZ for 2 to 3 weeks reduces the half-life by one-third, and long-term monotherapy with CBZ by about half. In patients receiving comedication with other antiepileptic drugs, particularly phenobarbital, phenytoin, and primidone, the average half-life is reduced to 9 to 10 hr.

The enhanced biotransformation of CBZ is important for the clinical use of the drug. In strongly induced patients under combined medication, the recommended dosage frequency, two or three times daily, may result in wide diurnal fluctuations in the plasma concentrations, with the extremes lying outside the therapeutic range (49). Such cases require more frequent dosing. From the metabolic point of view, therefore, comedication should be avoided wherever this is clinically permissible.

In animal tests it was also found that CBZ enhances its own metabolism when given repeatedly or continuously (15,18,42). As will be shown later in this chapter, the major pathways in the rat resemble those in man, although the rate of biotransformation is much higher in rat than in man. Measurement of the activity of several drug-metabolizing enzymes in the liver of rats revealed that CBZ primarily induces the

TABLE 2. *Half-lives of elimination of CBZ from plasma, measured after single and repeated oral administration of the drug to volunteers and patients*

Type and number of subjects	Measurement of plasma concentration	Elimination half-life (hr)[a]	Refs.
Healthy volunteers (N = 128)	After a single CBZ dose of 100–1,000 mg	36.0 ± 3.9	1,2,12,15,16,24,25,29,30,34, 39,41–45,52
Healthy volunteers (N = 22)	After 14–22 daily CBZ doses of 200–600 mg	23.9 ± 4.1	12,15,25,42
Patients (N = 16)	During monotherapy with CBZ, 300–1,000 mg/day	16.1 ± 2.9	38,55,57
Patients (N = 2)	After therapy with PHT[b]	12	55
Patients (N = 21)	During combined therapy with CBZ, PHT, PB, PRM, VPA, CZP, MSM, and/or ESM[b]	9.4 ± 1.2	14,49,57

[a]Mean values ± standard errors.
[b]PHT, phenytoin; PB, phenobarbital; PRM, primidone; VPA, valproate sodium; CZP, clonazepam; MSM, methsuximide; ESM, ethosuximide.

components of the microsomal monooxygenase system, e.g., cytochrome P-450 and NADPH–cytochrome c reductase (J. Wagner, *unpublished data*); UDP-glucuronyltransferase, on the other hand, is only slightly induced. The induction pattern is similar to that produced by an equimolar dose of phenobarbital, the effects of CBZ generally being lower. These findings suggest that enzyme induction accelerates especially those reactions that depend on the monooxygenase system, i.e., epoxidation of the 10,11 double bond of CBZ and hydroxylation of the six-membered rings.

In patients receiving combined antiepileptic medication, Eichelbaum et al. (14) found that the epoxide pathway is more strongly induced than are the others. Under steady-state conditions, an average of almost 60% of the daily CBZ dose appeared in urine as products of the epoxide pathway. In healthy subjects given single doses of ^{14}C-labeled drug, these products comprised only about 30% of the dose (corresponding to 40% of the urinary ^{14}C; see above). In their patients, Eichelbaum et al. observed a significant inverse correlation between the individual plasma half-lives of CBZ and the daily urinary excretion of the main product of the epoxide route, *trans*-10,11-di-H-10,11-di-OH-CBZ (II).

Accordingly, the plasma levels of the diol II and of epoxy-CBZ are increased relative to those of CBZ in strongly induced patients. Expressed as a percentage of the respective CBZ levels, most of the published values for the epoxide lie between 15 and 60% (9,37,38), and the values for the diol lie between 25 and 60% (13). After single doses, none of the metabolites exceeds 20% (16).

Anticonvulsant Activity of CBZ Metabolites

Epoxy-CBZ and several other nonconjugated metabolites were synthesized in our laboratories and tested for anticonvulsant activity in mice and rats after administration of single oral doses. The compounds are listed in Table 3 together with their ED_{50} values, i.e., the doses required to protect 50% of the animals against electroshock- or pentylenetetrazol-induced convulsions. (For structural formulas see Fig. 2.) The values for CBZ are also included in the table. In those cases where no ED_{50} was obtained, the table specifies the highest dose examined and the corresponding percentage of protected animals.

On the basis of the ED_{50}s, the efficacy of epoxy-CBZ is similar to that of the parent drug.

TABLE 3. *Anticonvulsant activity of CBZ and metabolites in animals, measured after single oral doses of the synthetic products*[a]

Compound	Anticonvulsant activity in three animal models		
	ESM[b]	ESR[b]	CSM[b]
CBZ	10–13 mg/kg	7–10 mg/kg	21–60 mg/kg
Epoxy-CBZ	12–16 mg/kg	13–15 mg/kg	8–24 mg/kg
Trans-10,11-di-H-10,11-di-OH-CBZ	100 mg/kg (0 %)	—[c]	—
9-Hydroxymethyl-10-carbamoyl acridan	17–39 mg/kg	50 mg/kg	100 mg/kg (20–40%)
2-Hydroxycarbamazepine	300 mg/kg (0%)	—	—
3-Hydroxycarbamazepine	38 mg/kg	100 mg/kg (10%)	100 mg/kg (0%)
3-Methylsulfonylcarbamazepine	300 mg/kg (0%)	—	—

[a]Data from M. Schmutz, V. Baltzer, H. Blattner, R. Heckendorn, and A. Storni (*unpublished data*).
[b]ESM, electroshock in mice; ESR, electroshock in rats; CSM, cardiazol-test in mice.
[c]not tested.

9-Hydroxymethyl-10-carbamoyl acridan, which is another product of the epoxide pathway, is considerably less active, and *trans*-10,11-di-H-10,11-di-OH-CBZ is inactive. Two products of aromatic hydroxylation, 2- and 3-hydroxycarbamazepine, show only little or no activity in the tests used. A representative of the metabolites carrying sulfur-containing substituents, 3-methylsulfonylcarbamazepine, is again devoid of anticonvulsant effects.

The activity data in Table 3 and the human plasma concentrations discussed earlier would suggest that, of all metabolites, it is only epoxy-CBZ that can significantly add to the antiepileptic effect of CBZ in patients. However, the true contribution of the metabolite cannot be reliably estimated without knowing the blood levels of the active molecules in the animal models used. Theoretically, it would even be conceivable that the pharmacological effect of CBZ is really that of the metabolite and that the parent drug is inactive.

To gain better insight, the anticonvulsant efficacy was determined in a separate experiment and compared with the blood concentrations following single oral doses of either epoxy-CBZ or CBZ to rats (17). After epoxy-CBZ, the time course of the effect, i.e., protection against electroshock-induced convulsions, was closely related to that of epoxide concentration in blood; 100% protection was reached at a concentration of about 3.5 µg/ml. After CBZ, the activity maximum coincided with the peak level of the parent drug: 100% protection required a CBZ concentration of 2.3 µg/ml, the simultaneously present concentration of the epoxy metabolite being only about 0.8 µg/ml. Therefore, it may be concluded that CBZ does possess anticonvulsant activity of its own which, on a concentration basis, is somewhat higher than that of epoxy-CBZ.

The data on the relative anticonvulsant activity of CBZ and its metabolites suggest that plasma level monitoring in epileptic patients who receive CBZ treatment should always include the epoxy metabolite. Because of their low activity or low plasma concentration or both, the other metabolites do not essentially contribute to the therapeutic effects of the drug.

SPECIES DIFFERENCES IN METABOLISM

Differences in Elimination Rates

In all animal species studied so far, CBZ is largely eliminated by metabolism. Direct excretion of CBZ is unimportant, since at most 2% of the dose can be recovered unchanged in urine or bile (33,42; W. Dieterle, *unpublished data*; K. F. Feldmann, *unpublished data*). In this respect, there is close similarity between animals and man. However, the overall rate of biotransformation in man is drastically different from that in the animal species, as reflected by the elimination half-lives of CBZ determined in plasma.

Table 4 shows that the mean half-lives in rats, dogs, rabbits, and rhesus monkeys after single CBZ doses are all in the range of 1.2 to 1.9 hr. In noninduced human volunteers, however, the half-life is 36 hr (see Table 2). Consequently, the metabolic clearance of CBZ in any of these animal species is higher by more than a power of 10 than that in man. To maintain a certain concentration of CBZ in plasma, one would need a correspondingly higher specific dose in the animals. Therefore, the same plasma concentration of CBZ, though possibly equal in pharmacological effectiveness, may toxicologically imply a higher burden to the animals than to man.

It should be noted that male rats eliminate CBZ more rapidly than females do, the half-life being about 50% longer in the latter case (see Table 4). For humans, no such comparison of half-lives exists, but the available clinical data suggest that the kinetics of CBZ in male and female patients do not differ significantly (30).

When rats and dogs are given repeated doses of CBZ, elimination of the drug from the body is enhanced (15). According to Farghali-Hassan et al. (18), administration of 14 CBZ doses of 25 mg/kg at 12-hr intervals reduced the half-life in male and female rats by about one-third and one-half, respectively. This effect is in agreement with the induction of drug-metabolizing enzymes in the liver of rats, as observed

TABLE 4. *Half-lives of elimination of CBZ from plasma in various animal species, measured after single intravenous doses of the drug*

Species, sex, and number of animals		Dose (mg/kg)	Elimination half-life (hr)[a]	Refs.
Rat	♂ (N = 4)	25	1.2 ± 0.1	18
Rat	♀ (N = 4)	25	1.9 ± 0.2	18
Dog	♂ (N = 4)	18	1.5 ± 0.4	42
Rabbit	♂[b]	10	1.2 ± 0.1	47
Rhesus monkey	♂ (N = 6)	20	1.4 ± 0.5	33

[a]Mean values ± standard deviations.
[b]Number of animals not specified.

in an independent study (J. Wagner, *unpublished data*).

Differences in Metabolic Pathways

With regard to structural identification of CBZ metabolites in animals, the rat is the only species for which results have been reported. Baker et al. (3) and Csetenyi et al. (10) described the occurrence of epoxy-CBZ (I), 10,11-di-H-10,11-di-OH-CBZ (II), and iminostilbene in the urine of rats following administration of CBZ. Bauer and others (4) identified a direct conjugate of CBZ, the *N*-glucuronide (X), in rat bile. In a later communication from the same group (35), hydroxy and hydroxymethoxy derivatives were mentioned as biliary metabolites. Horning and Lertratanangkoon (31) found that the same types of phenolic compounds are also present in the urine of rats. In most of these reports, quantitative data on metabolites or pathways are missing.

Unpublished results from a radiotracer study performed in our laboratories (W. Dieterle, *unpublished data*) revealed that rat bile and rat urine contain all metabolites of CBZ that had previously been identified in human urine (compounds I–XIV, see Fig. 2). The rat, too, excretes the bulk of metabolites in conjugated form. Therefore, in spite of the largely different rate of biotransformation in rat and man, the main pathways are qualitatively similar in both species. Some additional products were found in this rat study which are all derived from the known pathways; they include two more isomers of hydroxymethoxycarbamazepine, the 10-hydroxy-11-methylsulfonyl-10 , 11-dihydrocarbamazepine, and some compounds carrying substituents introduced by more than one pathway.

According to the data published by Baker et al. (3), conversion of CBZ into iminostilbene is another, yet minor, metabolic reaction in the rat.

The quantities and structures of the biliary and urinary metabolites in rats, as identified in our radiotracer study (W. Dieterle, *unpublished data*), imply that epoxidation of the 10,11 double bond of CBZ accounts for a higher percentage of the dose than does any of the other pathways. Unlike the situation in man, however, the epoxy intermediate is further transformed to the diol metabolite only at a comparatively low rate. This gives rise to a much higher urinary excretion of epoxy-CBZ in rat than in man, i.e., about 10% of the dose compared to 1%. Accordingly, the rat excretes less of the diol metabolite. Independent studies with styrene epoxide as a model compound in fact showed that the activity of the epoxide hydrase in liver homogenate is two times higher in human liver than in rat liver (40).

The concentration profiles of CBZ and epoxy-CBZ in plasma reflect the different rates of the metabolic reactions in rat and man (15). As shown in Fig. 4, oral administration of a single CBZ dose to the rat results in epoxide concentrations about equal to those of the original drug;

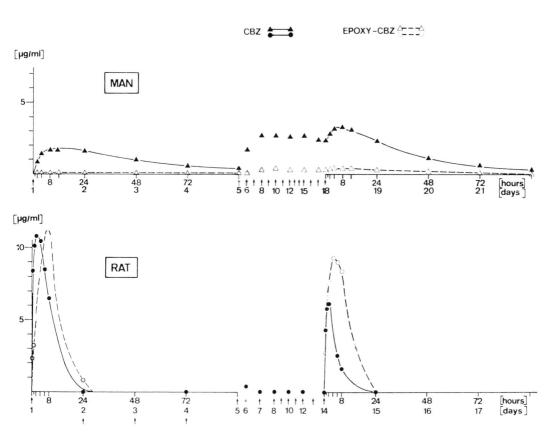

FIG. 4. Concentrations of CBZ and epoxy-CBZ in plasma of man and rat after single doses and during repeated oral administration of CBZ (15). Man: day 1, 200 mg; days 5 through 18, 200 mg daily ($N = 5$, healthy subjects). Rat: days 1 through 14, 50 mg/kg daily ($N = 5$).

after repeated administration, the epoxide reaches even higher levels than CBZ. In healthy human subjects, however, the plasma concentrations of epoxy-CBZ do not exceed 15% of those of the unchanged drug under similar experimental conditions.

Since rat and man metabolize CBZ by the same basic mechanisms, it appears permissible to extrapolate certain biochemical findings from animal models to man, for instance, findings relating to induction of drug-metabolizing enzymes. Considering the species differences in metabolic rates, however, any interpretation of pharmacological data obtained from animals should be based on the plasma concentrations of the active molecules, particularly CBZ and epoxy-CBZ.

REFERENCES

1. Anttila, M., Kahela, P., Panelius, M., Yrjänä, T., Tikkanen, R., and Aaltonen, R. (1979): Comparative bioavailability of two commercial preparations of carbamazepine tablets. *Eur. J. Clin. Pharmacol.*, 15:421–425.
2. Astier, A., Maury, M., and Barbizet, J. (1979): Simultaneous, rapid high-performance liquid chromatographic microanalysis of plasma carbamazepine and its 10,11-epoxide metabolite. *J. Chromatogr.*, 164:235–240.
3. Baker, K. M., Csetenyi, J., Frigerio, A., Morselli, P. L., Parravicini, F., and Pfifferi, G. (1973): 10,11-Dihydro-10,11-dihydroxy-5H-dibenz[b,f]azepine-5-carboxamide, a metabolite of carbamazepine isolated from human and rat urine. *J. Med. Chem.*, 16:703–705.
4. Bauer, J. E., Gerber, N., Lynn, R. K., Smith, R. G., and Thompson, R. M. (1976): A new N-glucuronide metabolite of carbamazepine. *Experientia*, 32:1032–1033.

5. Beyer, K. H., and Bredenstein, O. (1977): Untersuchungen zum Metabolismus des Antiepileptikums Carbamazepin. *Dtsch. Apoth. Z.*, 117: 1713–1717.

6. Beyer, K. H., Bredenstein, O., and Schenck, G. (1971): Isolierung und Identifizierung eines Carbamazepin-Reaktionsproduktes. *Arzneim. Forsch.*, 21:1033–1034.

7. Brazier, J. L. (1973): *Dosage de la Carbamazepine. Etude de son Metabolisme chez l'Homme.* Thesis, University of Lyons, Lyons.

8. Brazier, J. L., Deruaz, D., Rouzioux, J.-M., and Badinand, A. (1973): Etude des produits de transformation *in vitro* du Tegretol®. *Eur. J. Toxicol.*, 5:24–31.

9. Christiansen, J., and Dam, M. (1975): Drug interaction in epileptic patients. In: *Clinical Pharmacology of Anti-Epileptic Drugs*, edited by H. Schneider, D. Janz, C. Gardner-Thorpe, H. Meinardi, and A. L. Sherwin, pp. 197–200. Springer-Verlag, Berlin, Heidelberg, New York.

10. Csetenyi, J., Baker, K. M., Frigerio, A., and Morselli, P. L. (1973): Iminostilbene—a metabolite of carbamazepine isolated from rat urine. *J. Pharm. Pharmacol.*, 25:340–341.

11. Dieterle, W., Faigle, J. W., and Mory, H. (1979): Preparative reversed-phase chromatography of polar and non-polar metabolites on columns packed with micronized XAD-2 resin. *J. Chromatogr.*, 168:27–34.

12. Eichelbaum, M., Ekbom, K., Bertilsson, L., Ringberger, V. A., and Rane, A. (1975): Plasma kinetics of carbamazepine and its epoxide metabolite in man after single and multiple doses. *Eur. J. Clin. Pharmacol.*, 8:337–341.

13. Eichelbaum, M., Hoffmann, F., Köthe, K. W., and von Unruh, G. (1980): Measurement of the metabolites of the epoxide–diol pathway of carbamazepine to assess the extent of induction of carbamazepine metabolism during chronic treatment. In: *Antiepileptic Therapy. Advances in Drug Monitoring*, edited by S. I. Johannessen, P. L. Morselli, C. E. Pippenger, A. Richens, D. Schmidt, and H. Meinardi, pp. 143–148. Raven Press, New York.

14. Eichelbaum, M., Köthe, K. W., Hoffmann, F., and von Unruh, G. E. (1979): Kinetics and metabolism of carbamazepine during combined antiepileptic treatment. *Clin. Pharmacol. Ther.*, 26:366–371.

15. Faigle, J. W., Brechbühler, S., Feldmann, K. F., and Richter, W. J. (1976): The biotransformation of carbamazepine. In: *Epileptic Seizures—Behaviour—Pain*, edited by W. Birkmayer, pp. 127–140. Huber, Berne, Stuttgart, Vienna.

16. Faigle, J. W., and Feldmann, K. F. (1975): Pharmacokinetic data of carbamazepine and its major metabolites in man. In: *Clinical Pharmacology of Anti-Epileptic Drugs*, edited by H. Schneider, D. Janz, C. Gardner-Thorpe, H. Meinardi, and A. L. Sherwin, pp. 159–165. Springer-Verlag, Berlin, Heidelberg, New York.

17. Faigle, J. W., Feldmann, K. F., and Baltzer, V. (1977): Anticonvulsant effect of carbamazepine: An attempt to distinguish between the potency of the parent drug and its epoxide metabolite. In: *Antiepileptic Drug Monitoring*, edited by C. Gardner-Thorpe, D. Janz, H. Meinardi, and C. E. Pippenger, pp. 104–109. Pitman Medical, Kent.

18. Farghali-Hassan, Assael, B. M., Bossi, L., Gerna, M., Garattini, S., Gomeni, G., and Morselli, P. L. (1976): Carbamazepine pharmacokinetics in young, adult and pregnant rats. Relation to pharmacological effects. *Arch. Int. Pharmacodyn. Ther.*, 220:125–139.

19. Frigerio, A., Baker, K. M., and Belvedere, G. (1973): Gas chromatographic degradation of several drugs and their metabolites. *Anal. Chem.*, 45:1846–1851.

20. Frigerio, A., Cavo-Briones, M., and Belvedere, G. (1976): Formation of stable epoxides in the metabolism of tricyclic drugs. *Drug Metab. Rev.*, 5:197–218.

21. Frigerio, A., Fanelli, R., Biandrate, P., Passerini, G., Morselli, P. L., and Garattini, S. (1972): Mass spectrometric characterization of carbamazepine-10,11-epoxide, a carbamazepine metabolite isolated from human urine. *J. Pharm. Sci.*, 61:1144–1147.

22. Frigerio, A., and Morselli, P. L. (1975): Carbamazepine: Biotransformation. *Adv. Neurol.*, 11:295–308.

23. Friis, M. L., Christiansen, J., and Hvidberg, E. F. (1978): Brain concentrations of carbamazepine and carbamazepine-10,11-epoxide in epileptic patients. *Eur. J. Clin. Pharmacol.*, 14:47–51.

24. Gauchel, G., Gauchel, F. D., and Birkofer, L. (1973): A micromethod for the determination of carbamazepine in blood by high speed liquid chromatrography. *Z. Klin. Chem. Klin. Biochem.*, 11:459–460.

25. Gérardin, A., and Hirtz, J. (1976): The quantitative assay of carbamazepine in biological material and its application to basic pharmacokinetic studies. In: *Epileptic Seizures—Behaviour—Pain*, edited by W. Birkmayer, pp. 151–164. Huber, Berne, Stuttgart, Vienna.

26. Goenechea, S., Eckhardt, G., and Dersen, H.-D. (1976): Isolierung und Identifizierung neuer Metaboliten des Carbamazepin (Tegretal®). *Z. Anal. Chem.*, 279:113–114.

27. Goenechea, S., and Hecke-Seibicke, E. (1972): Beitrag zum Stoffwechsel von Carbamazepin. *Z. Klin. Chem. Klin. Biochem.*, 10:112–113.

28. Herrmann, B. (1971): Determination of carbamazepine in biological specimens. In: *Plasmakoncentrationsbestämningar av anti-epileptika: Metodologiska och kliniska aspecter*, edited by L. Lund, pp. 15–17. Geigy Läkemedel, Mölndal, Sweden.

29. Hooper, W. D., Cotter, L. M., Eadie, M. J., and Tyrer, J. H. (1975): The absorption and elimination of carbamazepine in man. *Clin. Exp. Pharmacol. Physiol.*, 2:428.

30. Hooper, W. D., Dubetz, D. K., Eadie, M. J., and Tyrer, J. H. (1974): Preliminary observations on the clinical pharmacology of carbamazepine (Tegretol®). *Proc. Aust. Assoc. Neurol.*, 11:189–198.

31. Horning, M. G., and Lertratanangkoon, K. (1980): High-performance liquid chromatographic separation of carbamazepine metabolites excreted in rat urine. *J. Chromatogr.*, 181:59–65.

32. Jenner, P., and Testa, B. (1978): Novel pathways in drug metabolism. *Xenobiotica*, 8:1–25.

32a. Lertratanangkoon, K., and Horning, M. G. (1981):

Metabolism of carbamazepine. *Drug. Metab. Dispos.* (*in press*).

3. Levy, R. H., Lockard, J. S., Green, J. R., Friel, P., and Martis, L. (1975): Pharmacokinetics of carbamazepine in monkeys following intravenous and oral administration. *J. Pharm. Sci.*, 64:302–307.

34. Levy, R. H., Pitlick, W. H., Troupin, A. S., Green, J. R., and Neal, J. M. (1975): Pharmacokinetics of carbamazepine in normal man. *Clin. Pharmacol. Ther.*, 17:657–668.

35. Lynn, R. K., Bowers, J. L., and Gerber, N. (1977): Identification of glucuronide metabolites of carbamazepine in human urine and in bile from the isolated perfused rat liver. *Fed. Proc.*, 36:961.

36. Lynn, R. K., Smith, R. G., Thompson, R. M., Deinzer, M. L., Griffin, D., and Gerber, N. (1978): Characterization of glucuronide metabolites of carbamazepine in human urine by gas chromatography and mass spectrometry. *Drug Metab. Dispos.*, 6:494–501.

37. Mihaly, G. W., Phillips, J. A., Louis, W. J., and Vajda, F. J. (1977): Measurement of carbamazepine and its epoxide metabolite by high performance liquid chromatography, and a comparison of assay techniques for the analysis of carbamazepine. *Clin. Chem.*, 23:2283–2287.

38. Morselli, P. L., Bossi, L., and Gerna, M. (1976): Pharmacokinetic studies with carbamazepine in epileptic patients. In: *Epileptic Seizures—Behaviour—Pain*, edited by W. Birkmayer, pp. 141–150. Huber, Berne, Stuttgart, Vienna.

39. Morselli, P. L., Gerna, M., de Maio, D., Zanda, G., Viani, F., and Garattini, S. (1975): Pharmacokinetic studies on carbamazepine in volunteers and epileptic patients. In: *Clinical Pharmacology of Anti-Epileptic Drugs*, edited by H. Schneider, D. Janz, C. Gardner-Thorpe, H. Meinardi, and A. L. Sherwin, pp. 166–180. Springer-Verlag, Berlin, Heidelberg, New York.

40. Oesch, F. (1973): Mammalian epoxide hydrase Inducible enzymes catalysing the inactivation of carcinogenic and cytotoxic metabolites derived from aromatic and olefinic compounds. *Xenobiotica*, 3:305–340.

41. Palmér, L., Bertilsson, L., Collste, P., and Rawlins, M. (1973): Quantitative determination of carbamazepine in plasma by mass fragmentography. *Clin. Pharmacol. Ther.*, 14:827–832.

42. Pitlick, W. H. (1975): *Investigation of the Pharmacokinetics of Carbamazepine, Including Dose and Time Dependency in Dogs, Monkeys and Humans*. Thesis, University of Washington, Seattle.

43. Pynnönen, S., Alihanka, J., and Pekkarinen, A. (1979): Carbamazepine concentrations in the treatment of acute alcohol withdrawal syndrome. Paper presented at: *11th Epilepsy International Symposium*, Florence.

44. Pynnönen, S., Björkquist, S.-E., and Pekkarinen, A. (1978): The pharmacokinetics of carbamazepine in alcoholics. In: *Advances in Epileptology—1977*, edited by H. Meinardi and A. J. Rowan, pp. 285–289. Swets & Zeitlinger, Amsterdam.

45. Rawlins, M. D., Collste, P., Bertilsson, L., and Palmér, L. (1975): Distribution and elimination kinetics of carbamazepine in man. *Eur. J. Clin. Pharmacol.*, 8:91–96.

46. Richter, W. J., Kriemler, P., and Faigle, J. W. (1978): Newer aspects of the biotransformation of carbamazepine: Structural characterization of highly polar metabolites. In: *Recent Developments in Mass Spectrometry in Biochemistry and Medicine, Vol. 1*, edited by A. Frigerio, pp. 1–14. Plenum Press, New York.

47. Rimerman, R. A., Taylor, S. M., Lynn, R. K., Rodgers, R. M., and Gerber, N. (1979). The excretion of carbamazepine in the semen of the rabbit and man: Comparison of the concentration in semen and plasma. *Pharmacologist*, 21:264.

48. Schmid, K., Riess, W., Egger, H.-P., and Keberle, H. (1969): Isotope dilution analysis with the aid of preparative thin-layer chromatography. In: *International Conference on Radioactive Isotopes in Pharmacology*, edited by P. G. Waser and B. Glasson, pp. 67–82. Wiley, London.

49. Schneider, H., and Stenzel, E. (1975): Carbamazepin: Tageszeitlicher Verlauf des Serumspiegels unter Langzeitmedikation. In: *Bibliotheca Psychiatrica, No. 151, Antiepileptische Langzeitmedikation*, edited by H. Helmchen and L. Diehl, pp. 32–42. S. Karger, Basel.

50. Sie, S. T., and van den Hoed, N. (1969): Preparation and performance of high-efficiency columns for liquid chromatography. *J. Chromatogr. Sci.*, 7:257–266.

51. Stierlin, H., Faigle, J. W., Sallmann, A., Küng, W., Richter, W. J., Kriemler, H.-P., Alt, K. O., and Winkler, T. (1979): Biotransformation of diclofenac sodium (Voltaren®) in animals and in man. I. Isolation and identification of principal metabolites. *Xenobiotica*, 9:601–610.

52. Strandjord, R. E., and Johannessen, S. I. (1975): A preliminary study of serum carbamazepine levels in healthy subjects and in patients with epilepsy. In: *Clinical Pharmacology of Anti-Epileptic Drugs*, edited by H. Schneider, D. Janz, C. Gardner-Thorpe, H. Meinardi, and A. L. Sherwin, pp. 181–188. Springer-Verlag, Berlin, Heidelberg, New York.

53. Tateishi, M. (1978): New pathway in drug metabolism. *Farumashia*, 14:882–887.

54. Teerhag, B., Richter, K., and Diettrich, H. (1978): Concentration behaviour of carbamazepine in bile and plasma of man. *Int. J. Clin. Pharmacol. Biopharm.*, 16:607–609.

55. Troupin, A. S., Green, J. R., and Levy, R. H. (1974): Carbamazepine as an anticonvulsant: A pilot study. *Neurology (Minneap.)*, 24:863–869.

56. Weiner, I. M. (1967): Mechanisms of drug absorption and excretion. The renal excretion of drugs and related compounds. *Annu. Rev. Pharmacol.*, 7:39–56.

57. Westenberg, H. G. M., van der Kleijn, E., Oei, T. T., and de Zeeuw, A. (1978): Kinetics of carbamazepine and carbamazepine-epoxide, determined by use of plasma and saliva. *Clin. Pharmacol. Ther.*, 23:320–328.

Antiepileptic Drugs, edited by D. M. Woodbury, J. K. Penry, and C. E. Pippenger. Raven Press, New York © 1982.

39

Carbamazepine

Interactions with Other Drugs

René H. Levy and William H. Pitlick

The clinical manifestations of interactions involving carbamazepine depend on several factors. It is necessary to consider whether carbamazepine is the affector or the affected species and whether the mechanism of the interaction involves induction or inhibition of metabolism. Carbamazepine possesses enzyme-inducing properties and generally causes decreases in steady-state levels of other drugs. Likewise, phenytoin, phenobarbital, and primidone cause decreases in carbamazepine steady-state levels. Although this type of interaction may result in breakthrough seizures, few such reports are available. In many instances, monitoring of plasma drug levels enables appropriate dosage adjustments to be made, and serious clinical manifestations are avoided. However, certain unexpected interactions associated with serious clinical manifestations still occur. Acute carbamazepine intoxication (with drowsiness, nausea, vomiting, and dizziness) was observed in epileptic patients who were treated for various infections with triacetyloleandomycin (15,43). Similarly, epileptic patients who concomitantly received carbamazepine and propoxyphene showed signs of carbamazepine intoxication (14). In all of these patients, steady-state carbamazepine levels were elevated.

The assessment of drug interactions by monitoring plasma carbamazepine levels has been complicated by two facts. First, initial clinical trials on the efficacy of carbamazepine presented a confusing array of plasma levels, which made the establishment of a therapeutic range considerably more difficult than for other drugs. Second, many studies demonstrated a poor correlation between plasma carbamazepine level and dose. Recently, however, a few findings have emerged. Efficacy of carbamazepine in the treatment of complex partial or generalized tonic–clonic seizures is associated with levels above 5 μg/ml, but side effects (drowsiness, headaches, disturbed equilibrium) often occur if the levels exceed 12 μg/ml. In addition to dose, age and concomitant therapy have been identified as the main variables affecting plasma carbamazepine levels (2).

PHARMACOKINETIC CHARACTERISTICS OF CARBAMAZEPINE AND PRINCIPLES OF INTERACTIONS

A complete discussion of the pharmacokinetic parameters of carbamazepine is presented in Chapter 37, but salient features will be reviewed here as they pertain to drug interactions. In humans, carbamazepine is readily absorbed from the gastrointestinal tract with minimal first-pass metabolism. However, bioavailability problems are possible and even suspected at high doses. Carbamazepine is completely cleared by hepatic mechanisms, in large part by conversion to hydroxylated metabolites (10,11-dihydrodiol) via a 10,11-epoxide intermediate. As with most other antiepileptic drugs, hepatic clearance of carbamazepine is small relative to liver blood flow, and its extraction ratio is less than 10%. It was pointed out in Chapter 2 that the hepatic clearance of a drug reflects the ability of the liver to extract drug from blood passing through it, and it can be affected by hepatic blood flow. Intrinsic clearance, on the other hand, represents the intrinsic ability of the eliminating organs to remove drug in the absence of any flow limitations.

For a drug with low intrinsic clearance and therefore a low extraction ratio, such as carbamazepine, hepatic clearance is relatively independent of liver blood flow (and approximates intrinsic clearance). Thus, changes in liver blood flow would not be expected to produce a change in hepatic clearance of carbamazepine. An increase in intrinsic clearance, as occurs during enzyme induction, results in an almost identical increase in hepatic clearance. Also, since carbamazepine is eliminated completely by metabolism, its hepatic and total body clearances are equal. Therefore, alterations in the intrinsic clearance of carbamazepine result in inversely proportional alterations in steady-state drug levels and in changes in half-life. The free fraction of carbamazepine in human plasma is approximately 25% and appears concentration independent within therapeutic concentrations. One binding site on albumin has been proposed. The effects of protein binding interactions on free and total drug levels are described in Chapter 2. Few such interactions have been reported for carbamazepine.

These principles can also be used to understand the effects of carbamazepine on other drugs, since the major antiepileptic drugs have low extraction ratios and are extensively metabolized. However, the characteristics of each drug (e.g., protein binding) must be taken into consideration to make accurate predictions.

EFFECTS OF CARBAMAZEPINE ON ITS OWN DISPOSITION

It has been widely reported that carbamazepine increases the total body clearance of itself and several other drugs in several species including humans (3,4,17,24,27,36,38,40,46,47, 49,51,53,54,57,60). The preponderance of evidence indicates that the increase in clearance is caused by an increased metabolic capacity of hepatic enzymes. The increased clearance is associated with shortened half-lives and a reduction in the total serum drug concentration at steady state. For example, the half-life of carbamazepine was reduced from greater than 30 hr to less than 20 hr with long-term use (53), and the average steady-state concentration of carbamazepine was reduced by 50% after 3 weeks of drug administration (18).

An early indication of the potential problem in patients came from a single-dose in eight healthy volunteers who received 3 mg/kg of carbamazepine (57). Pharmacokinetic analysis indicated that the mean half-life was approximately 36 hr. Because steady-state concentrations predicted from the results of this study were two to three times higher than those reported in patients treated chronically with carbamazepine at this dose level, the authors concluded that the pharmacokinetics of carbamazepine apparently changed during multiple dosing. In another study, carbamazepine was administered orally to four patients as a single dose, and 1 week later the drug was given three times daily for up to 3 weeks (17). After multiple doses, the half-life was approximately 21 hr in comparison with a half-life of approximately 36 hr after an initial single dose. Steady-state plasma concentrations were less than 50% of the level predicted from the single-dose studies. Maximum concentrations were observed 3 to 4 days after initiation of the multiple doses. The levels tended to decrease further during the course of the study. Similar findings were reported by Faigle et al. (20) and Gerardin et al. (24,25).

Shortly after these reports appeared, a pharmacokinetic model was developed to describe the self-induced decreases of steady-state car-bamazepine levels during long-term use of the drug (53). In six healthy volunteers given 6 mg/kg of carbamazepine daily for 3 weeks, steady-state concentrations were 50% of the level predicted from single-dose studies, and the elimination half-life at the end of the third week had decreased from 34 to 20 hr (39). Minimum concentrations decreased at an exponential rate during multiple dosing with carbamazepine, which was compatible with an increase in total body clearance. From this pharmacokinetic model, an induction half-life of 4.0 days was calculated, thus allowing an estimate of the time course of the phenomenon of autoinduction. On this basis, steady-state carbamazepine levels would be predicted to decline and reach an asymptotic level after 3 to 4 weeks of therapy. The postulated pharmacokinetic model was also tested in monkeys maintained on chronic infusions of carbamazepine (52). The findings in humans were substantiated independently in a study of six healthy humans treated with 200 mg of carbamazepine daily for 17 days (24). It was found that plasma half-lives decreased from 38 hr after single doses to approximately 21 hr after long-term treatment.

Autoinduced increases in carbamazepine clearance have also been studied in children by a stable isotope technique (3). In three children (10–13 years old), carbamazepine clearance doubled after 32 days of treatment, resulting in steady-state concentrations that were 50% less than predicted. During the next 4 months, there was no further increase in clearance or decrease in serum concentrations. These data tend to support the earlier finding that the autoinduction phenomenon is complete within 1 month.

EFFECTS OF CARBAMAZEPINE ON OTHER DRUGS

Not only does carbamazepine induct its own metabolism, but it also alters the biotransformation of other drugs, including other anticonvulsants, given concomitantly.

Carbamazepine reduces the half-life of phe-nytoin in epileptic patients when both drugs are administered simultaneously. The pharmacokinetics of phenytoin were measured in five patients before and during treatment with 600 mg of carbamazepine daily (27). The phenytoin half-life decreased from 10.6 hr to 6.4 after 9 days of carbamazepine therapy. In another seven patients, 600 mg of carbamazepine daily was added to phenytoin after steady-state levels of phenytoin were measured. In three of the patients, phenytoin levels decreased significantly following 4 to 14 days of treatment with carbamazepine. No significant changes, however, were seen in the serum phenytoin values in four of seven patients. Pretreatment with constant-rate infusion of carbamazepine resulted in a greater than 40% decrease in plasma half-life of phenytoin.

The effect of carbamazepine on primidone metabolism has also been studied. Phenobarbital, a byproduct of primidone metabolism, showed significant increases when carbamazepine was added to the dosage regimen of four patients (6). However, evidence is lacking for an effect of carbamazepine on ingested phenobarbital. In one study of 25 patients taking both phenobarbital and carbamazepine, no change in phenobarbital clearance was observed in comparison with a group taking phenobarbital alone (16).

The effects of carbamazepine on the pharmacokinetics of valproic acid have been studied in healthy subjects. Six subjects maintained on 250 mg of valproic acid twice daily for 4 weeks were given carbamazepine, 200 mg once daily, after 4 days of valproic acid therapy (4). A significant increase in clearance and a concomitant decrease in steady-state blood levels were apparent after 2 weeks of carbamazepine therapy (Fig. 1). Similar findings have also been reported in epileptic patients. In two patients receiving carbamazepine and valproic acid, steady-state valproate levels were 37 to 64% lower than predicted from a single dose of valproate (44). In another study, steady-state valproate levels were compared in two groups of adult patients, seven on valproate monotherapy and six also receiving carbamazepine. The ratio of plasma level

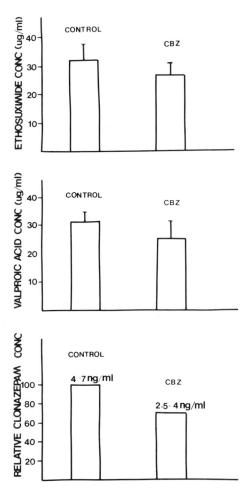

Fig. 1. Effect of carbamazepine (200 mg/day) on the steady-state concentrations of ethosuximide, valproic acid, and clonazepam. Data taken, respectively, from Warren et al. (60), Bowdle et al. (4), and Lai et al. (37).

to dose was 38% lower in the presence of carbamazepine (58).

Similar studies have been performed to determine the extent and time course of interaction between carbamazepine and clonazepam in normal subjects (37). Seven subjects receiving a 1-mg clonazepam tablet daily were given 200 mg of carbamazepine daily for up to 29 days. Fifteen days after initiation of carbamazepine, there was a marked decrease in both clonazepam and carbamazepine levels (Fig. 1). The half-life of clonazepam was reduced from 32 hr to 22 hr

after carbamazepine was added to the dosage regimen.

When carbamazepine (200 mg/day) was added to the regimen of healthy subjects maintained on 250 mg of ethosuximide a day, ethosuximide clearance increased significantly after 10 days of carbamazepine therapy with a synchronous decrease in ethosuximide half-life from 54 to 45 hr (60) (Fig. 1). Carbamazepine has also been shown to affect the half-life of the antibiotic doxycycline. In five patients on long-term carbamazepine therapy, the half-life of doxycycline (8.4 hr) was significantly shorter than its mean half-life of 15.1 hr in nine control patients (51).

Alterations in the fraction of drug bound to plasma proteins may also produce changes in total plasma drug levels. For drugs with a low extraction ratio, such as antiepileptic drugs, concentrations of free drug are independent of the free fraction, but total drug levels are inversely proportional to the free fraction. In all the above interactions, it was assumed that the mechanism involved an increase in intrinsic (metabolic) clearance. Theoretically, a protein binding displacement would also result in a decrease in steady-state levels. Such a hypothesis is unlikely for several reasons. Theoretically, carbamazepine should not behave as a displacer, since its molar concentration is very small relative to that of albumin and also its association constant is not high. In fact, the effects of carbamazepine on the protein binding of other drugs were investigated, and no displacement effect was found. In patients treated with phenytoin, addition of carbamazepine produced little or no change in the free fraction of phenytoin (28). In another study, there was no evidence of competitive binding to plasma proteins between phenytoin and carbamazepine (41). Valproic acid binding to human serum albumin was not affected by concentrations of carbamazepine within the therapeutic range (48). The ability of carbamazepine to reduce the steady-state levels of valproic acid, clonazepam, and ethosuximide was also demonstrated in controlled studies in rhesus monkeys (9,10,36). Carbamazepine and each of these anticonvulsants were administered intravenously, thereby excluding the possibility of a mechanism of interaction involving a reduction in fraction of dose absorbed.

EFFECTS OF OTHER DRUGS ON CARBAMAZEPINE

It appears that carbamazepine clearance can be altered by many other drugs including coadministered antiepileptic drugs. Both increases (metabolic inhibition) and decreases (enzymatic induction) in plasma carbamazepine levels have been reported. Reports of interactions involving carbamazepine binding have been scarce.

Inhibition

Addition of propoxyphene to a regimen containing carbamazepine (alone or with other antiepileptic drugs) was associated with signs of carbamazepine intoxication: headache, dizziness, ataxia, nausea, and tiredness (11). Dam et al. (12) have shown that propoxyphene causes an increase in plasma carbamazepine levels associated with a decrease in epoxide level.

Triacetyloleandomycin, an antibiotic widely used in France, has been shown to cause carbamazepine intoxication associated with an elevation of carbamazepine levels (15). Mesdjian et al. (43) reported that 17 epileptic subjects being treated with carbamazepine developed acute and unexpected intoxication (drowsiness, nausea, vomiting, dizziness) when triacetyloleandomycin was administered. Similar symptoms were found when erythromycin was given to two patients who were taking carbamazepine.

Reports of a possible interaction between valproic acid and carbamazepine have been conflicting. In some studies, valproic acid increased carbamazepine levels (31) as well as levels of the epoxide metabolite (26). Other studies reported no clear effects of valproic acid on carbamazepine levels (1,21,62). Further, a recent *in vitro* study has determined that high levels of valproic acid result in a small but significant increase in carbamazepine free fraction (42). This finding may explain the contradictory reports. An inhibitory effect of valproic acid

would tend to increase carbamazepine concentrations, whereas a protein binding displacement would cause a decrease. Measurement of carbamazepine free levels would allow a clearer understanding of the mechanism and significance of this interaction.

Induction

Several reports in the last decade have consistently demonstrated that carbamazepine metabolism is highly inducible by other antiepileptics. Although this effect has caused no alarming clinical findings, Hvidberg and Dam (30), underlining the clinical relevance of this interaction, point out that "patients may suffer from seizures in the morning, when plasma carbamazepine is low, and show signs and symptoms of intoxication in the evening when plasma level is high."

Christiansen and Dam (7,8) showed in 123 patients that the slope of the relationship between plasma level and dose of carbamazepine is reduced by phenytoin, by phenobarbital, and by the combination of phenytoin and phenobarbital. Similar findings were reported by Schneider (59) in 184 patients representing eight different combinations of carbamazepine and other drugs. This study showed that primidone has a significant effect in decreasing the slope of the relationship between plasma level and dose, presumably as a consequence of enzymatic induction. In 142 patients, Johannessen and Strandjord (34) found also that phenytoin, phenobarbital, or a combination of both can reduce the plasma level-to-dose ratio of carbamazepine. They emphasized the need to monitor carbamazepine levels during polytherapy, to achieve the proper dosage increments. Rane et al. (56) compared the mean carbamazepine levels in two groups of children, one on monotherapy, the other on a combination of drugs. They found that the ratio of plasma level to dose was lower in the group on polytherapy. In that same group, however, the concentration of 10,11-epoxide metabolite was significantly higher.

Using a pulse dose of stable isotope-labeled

carbamazepine, Eichelbaum et al. (19) were able to measure the half-life of carbamazepine in six patients on combined anticonvulsant therapy. Half-life ranged from 5.0 to 16 hr (mean, 8.2 hr). From those data as well as the urinary excretion of the 10,11-*trans*-diol metabolite (approximately 50% of the dose), they concluded that concomitant therapy induces the metabolism of carbamazepine. Callaghan et al. (5) confirmed the findings of others that primidone causes a significant reduction in steady-state carbamazepine levels.

Höppener et al (29) compared the daily fluctuations in carbamazepine levels in two groups, 19 patients on monotherapy and 43 patients on polytherapy. All patients received the drug three times a day (8 a.m., 12:30 p.m., and 8 p.m.). The fluctuation was 34.5 ± 10.9% in the group on monotherapy and 68.5 ± 21.2% in the group on polytherapy. The authors therefore recommended frequent administration of carbamazepine (3 to 4 times a day) in patients on multiple drug therapy.

A provocative analysis of the relationship between plasma level and dose of carbamazepine was performed by Battino et al. (2). Based on 567 determinations of plasma carbamazepine levels in 326 patients of all ages, these authors segregated the main variables in the plasma level-to-dose ratio as age, associated therapy, and carbamazepine dose. The ratio increased linearly with age between 1 and 19 years. The ratio was significantly reduced with polytherapy in several subgroups homogeneous with respect to age (0–3, 4–9, 10–15, and 19–45 years) (Fig. 2).

Numerous investigations have focused on the effects of concomitant therapy on the carbamazepine 10,11-epoxide metabolite. This metabolite is of interest because it has shown anticonvulsant activity in rats (22). Also, in cerebrospinal fluid its concentration is 40 to 60% that of carbamazepine (32,55), whereas in plasma it is 10 to 25% that of the parent drug. This difference is attributable to the lower degree of plasma protein binding of the epoxide. Several studies have found that the ratio of epoxide to carbamazepine at steady-state plasma levels was higher in patients on combined regimens (car-

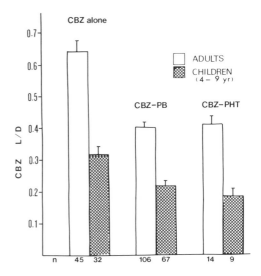

Fig. 2. Effect of phenobarbital (PB) and phenytoin (PHT) on plasma level-to-dose ratio (L/D) of carbamazepine (CBZ) in adults and children. The values of L/D represent the concentrations in μg/ml achieved for each mg/kg of daily dose. [For additional information on other associated therapy and different age groups, see Battino et al. (2)].

bamazepine with other antiepileptic drugs) than in patients taking carbamazepine alone (8,13,56,59,61).

Korczyn et al. (35) examined the plasma levels of carbamazepine and the epoxide and dihydrodiol metabolites in two groups of patients (monotherapy versus polytherapy). They concluded that heteroinduction involves the epoxidation of carbamazepine as well as the conversion of the epoxide to the dihydrodiol.

A recent study in rhesus monkeys examined the effect of phenobarbital on the ratio of epoxide to carbamazepine at steady-state levels (50). The increase in this ratio was attributed to an induction of the formation of the epoxide.

Brain-to-plasma ratios of carbamazepine and carbamazepine epoxide have been determined in two studies in epileptic patients undergoing brain surgery. In one study in 21 patients with brain tumors, the ratio was 1.1 ± 0.1 for carbamazepine and 1.1 to 1.2 for the carbamazepine epoxide (45). In the other study (23), the brain-to-plasma ratio was measured in five epileptic patients undergoing unilateral temporal lobectomy. The ratio ranged from 1.4 to 1.6 for carbamazepine and from 0.6 to 1.5 for the epoxide. It was also noted that the ratio for carbamazepine was similar in patients treated with carbamazepine alone or in combination with other anticonvulsants, but for the carbamazepine epoxide, the ratio was higher in patients on multidrug therapy. In these latter patients, the plasma and brain carbamazepine epoxide concentrations were two to three times higher than in patients receiving carbamazepine alone.

Protein Binding

The influence of several other drugs on the plasma binding of carbamazepine at a concentration of 5 μg/ml was studied by ultrafiltration. It was found that phenobarbital, phenytoin, and nortriptyline had no effect on the protein binding of carbamazepine, whereas ethosuximide and phensuximide showed a very slight increase in the percent of carbamazepine bound to protein (57). As mentioned above, valproic acid was found to cause an increase in carbamazepine free fraction (42).

In vivo studies on the protein binding of carbamazepine are relatively rare, and there are even fewer data on the effects of protein binding interactions. One study on 10 patients undergoing long-term carbamazepine therapy showed a mean CSF-to-serum ratio of 0.24 (32). In another study in 19 adult patients receiving long-term carbamazepine therapy plus other anticonvulsants, the CSF-to-serum ratio was 0.22 (33). Thus, from these data, it appears unlikely that significant interactions occur with carbamazepine as a result of alterations in protein binding.

THERAPEUTIC IMPLICATIONS

Interactions between carbamazepine and other antiepileptic drugs are prevalent. Carbamazepine tends to decrease the plasma level-to-dose ratio of other drugs. Conversely, the metabolism of carbamazepine is very sensitive to induction by other antiepileptic drugs, resulting in a decrease of the plasma carbamazepine level-to-dose ratio. This effect is found in all age groups, including infants. Monitoring of plasma carbamazepine levels in therapy-resistant patients should be useful in making optimal dosage adjustments. However, timing of blood sample collections becomes of paramount importance in view of recent reports that the carbamazepine half-life is about 6 hr. Based on currently available information, there appears to be no need to distinguish between free and total levels of carbamazepine. However, this may not be the case for other drugs affected by carbamazepine, especially when three or more drugs are administered simultaneously. Thus, a low plasma level-to-dose ratio for phenytoin may result from an increase in intrinsic clearance caused by carbamazepine induction or from a high free fraction caused by valproic acid. In such cases, monitoring of free drug levels enables a distinction to be made between the two mechanisms. Such distinction is necessary because the induction mechanism would require a dose increment, whereas the binding phenomenon would not.

A few drugs known to cause episodes of carbamazepine intoxication (by inhibition of its metabolism) should not be prescribed for patients receiving carbamazepine. These include propoxyphene, triacetyloleandomycin, and erythromycin.

ACKNOWLEDGMENTS

We thank Ms. Colleen D. Montoya and Dr. Huey-shin Lin for excellent technical assistance.

REFERENCES

1. Adams, D. J., Luders, H., and Pippenger, C. (1978): Sodium valproate in the treatment of intractable seizure disorders: A clinical and electroencephalographic study. *Neurology (Minneap.)*, 28:152–157.
2. Battino, D., Bossi, L., Croci, D., Franceschetti, S., Gomeni, C., Moise, A., and Vitali, A. (1980): Carbamazepine plasma levels in children and adults: Influence of age, dose, and associated therapy. *Ther. Drug Monit.*, 2:315–322.
3. Bertilsson, L., Höjer, B., Tybring, G., Osterloh, J., and Rane, A. (1980): Autoinduction of carbamazepine metabolism in children examined by a stable isotope technique. *Clin. Pharmacol. Ther.*, 27:83–88.
4. Bowdle, T. A., Levy, R. H., and Cutler, R. E., (1979): Effects of carbamazepine on valproic acid in normal man. *Clin. Pharmacol. Ther.*, 26:629–634.

5. Callaghan, N., Duggan, B., O'Hare, J., and O'Driscoll, D. (1980): Serum levels of phenobarbitone and phenylethylmalonamide with primidone used as a single drug and in combination with carbamazepine or phenytoin. In: Antiepileptic Therapy: Advances in Drug Monitoring, edited by S. I. Johannessen, P. L. Morselli, C. E. Pippenger, A. Richens, D. Schmidt, and H. Meinardi, pp. 307–313. Raven Press, New York.

6. Callaghan, N., Feely, M., Duggan, F., O'Callaghan, M., and Seldrup, J. (1977): The effect of anticonvulsant drugs which induce liver microsomal enzymes on derived and ingested phenobarbitone levels. Acta Neurol. Scand., 56:1–6.

7. Christiansen, J., and Dam, M. (1973): Influence of phenobarbital and diphenylhydantoin on plasma carbamazepine levels in patients with epilepsy. Acta Neurol. Scand., 49:543–546.

8. Christiansen, J., and Dam, M. (1975): Drug interaction in epileptic patients. In: Clinical Pharmacology of Anti-Epileptic Drugs, edited by H. Schneider, D. Janz, C. Gardner-Thorpe, H. Meinardi, and A. L. Sherwin, pp. 197–200. Springer-Verlag, Berlin.

9. Corbisier, P. H., and Levy, R. H. (1977): Pharmacokinetics of drug interaction by enzyme induction. I. Carbamazepine and valproic acid. APhA/Acad. Pharm. Sci. Abstr., 7:163.

10. Corbisier, P. H., and Levy, R. H. (1977): Pharmacokinetics of drug interaction by enzyme induction. III. Carbamazepine and ethosuximide. APhA/Acad. Pharm. Sci. Abstr., 7:134.

11. Dam, M., and Christiansen, J. (1977): Interaction of propoxyphene with carbamazepine. Lancet, 2:509.

12. Dam, M., Christensen, J. M., Brandt, J., Hansen, B. S., Hvidberg, E. F., Angelo, H., and Lous, P. (1980): Antiepileptic drugs: Interaction with dextropropoxyphene. In: Antiepileptic Therapy: Advances in Drug Monitoring, edited by S. I. Johannessen, P. L. Morselli, C. E. Pippenger, A. Richens, D. Schmidt, and H. Meinardi, pp. 299–306. Raven Press, New York.

13. Dam, M., Jensen, A., and Christensen, J. (1975): Plasma level and effect of carbamazepine in grand mal and psychomotor epilepsy. Acta Neurol. Scand. [Suppl.], 60:33–38.

14. Dam, M., Kristensen, C. B., Hansen, B. S., and Christiansen, J. (1977): Interaction between carbamazepine and propoxyphene in man. Acta Neurol. Scand., 56:603–607.

15. Dravet, C., Mesdjian, E., Cenraud, B., and Roger, J. (1977): Interaction between carbamazepine and triacetyloleandomycin. Lancet, 1:810–811.

16. Eadie, M. J., Lander, C. M., Hooper, W. D., and Tyrer, J. H. (1977): Factors influencing plasma phenobarbitone levels in epileptic patients. Br. J. Clin. Pharmacol., 4:541-547.

17. Eichelbaum, M., Ekbom, K., Bertilsson, L., Lund, L., Palmer, L., and Sjöqvist, F. (1976): Plasma levels of carbamazepine and carbamazepine-10,11-epoxide during treatment of epilepsy. Eur. J. Clin. Pharmacol., 9:417–421.

18. Eichelbaum, M., Ekbom, K., Bertilsson, L., Ringberger, V. A., and Rane, A. (1975): Plasma kinetics of carbamazepine and its epoxide metabolite in man after single and multiple doses. Eur. J. Clin. Pharmacol., 8:337–341.

19. Eichelbaum, M., Kothe, K. W., and Hoffman, F. (1979): Kinetics and metabolism of carbamazepine during combined antiepileptic drug therapy. Clin. Pharmacol. Ther., 26:366–371.

20. Faigle, J. W., Brechbuhler, S., Feldman, K. F., and Richter, W. J. (1976): The biotransformation of carbamazepine. In: Epileptic Seizures—Behavior—Pain, edited by W. Birkmayer, pp. 127–140. Hans Huber, Berne.

21. Flachs, H., Gram, L., Wurtz-Jorgensen, A., and Parnes, J. (1979): Drug levels of other antiepileptic drugs during concomitant treatment with sodium valproate. Epilepsia, 20:187.

22. Frigerio, A., and Morselli, P. L. (1975): Carbamazepine: Biotransformation. Adv. Neurol., 11:295–308.

23. Friis, M. L., Christiansen, J., Hvidberg, E. F. (1978): Brain concentrations of carbamazepine and carbamazepine-10,11-epoxide in epileptic patients. Eur. J. Clin. Pharmacol., 14:47–51.

24. Gerardin, A. P., Abadie, F. V., Campestrini, J. A., and Theobald, W. (1976): Pharmacokinetics of carbamazepine in normal humans after single and repeated oral doses. J. Pharmacokinet. Biopharm., 4:521.

25. Gerardin, A., and Hirtz, J. (1976): The quantitative assay of carbamazepine in biological material and its application to basic pharmacokinetic studies. In: Epileptic Seizures—Behavior—Pain, edited by W. Birkmayer, pp. 151–164. Hans Huber, Berne.

26. Gugler, R., and von Unruh, G. E. (1980): Clinical pharmacokinetics of valproic acid. Clin. Pharmacokinet., 5:67–83.

27. Hansen, J. M., Siersback-Nielsen, K., and Skovsted, L. (1971): Carbamazepine-induced acceleration of diphenylhydantoin and warfarin metabolism in man. Clin. Pharmacol. Ther., 12:539–543.

28. Hooper, W. D., Sutherland, J. M., Bochner, F., Tyrer, J. H., and Eadie, M. J. (1973): The effect of certain drugs on the plasma protein binding of phenytoin. Aust. N.Z. J. Med., 3:377–381.

29. Höppener, R. J., Kuyer, A., Meijer, J. W. A., and Hulsman, J. (1980): Correlation between daily fluctuations of carbamazepine serum levels and intermittent side effects. Epilepsia, 21:341–350.

30. Hvidberg, E. F., and Dam, M. (1976): Clinical pharmacokinetics of anticonvulsants. Clin. Pharmacokinet., 1:161–188.

31. Jeavons, P. M., and Clark, J. E. (1974): Sodium valproate in treatment of epilepsy. Br. Med. J., 2:584–586.

32. Johannessen, S. I., Gerna, M., Bakke, J., Strandjord, R. E., and Morselli, P. L. (1976): CSF concentrations and serum protein binding of carbamazepine and carbamazepine-10,11-epoxide in epileptic patients. Br. J. Clin. Pharmacol., 3:575–582.

33. Johannessen, S. I., and Strandjord, R. E. (1973): Concentration of carbamazepine (Tegretol®) in serum and in cerebrospinal fluid in patients with epilepsy. Epilepsia, 14:373–379.

34. Johannessen, S. I., and Strandjord, R. E. (1975): The influence of phenobarbitone and phenytoin on carbamazepine serum levels. In: Clinical Pharmacology of Anti-Epileptic Drugs, edited by H. Schneider, D. Janz, C. Gardner-Thorpe, H. Meinardi, and A. L. Sherwin, pp. 201–205. Springer-Verlag, Berlin.

35. Korczyn, A. D., Ben-Zvi, A., Kaplanski, J., Danon,

A., and Berginer, V. (1978): Plasma levels of car-bamazepine and metabolites: Effect of enzyme in-ducers. In: *Advances in Epileptology,* edited by H. Meinardi, and A. J. Rowan, pp. 278–279. Swets & Zeitlinger, Amsterdam.

36. Lai, A. A., and Levy, R. H. (1979): Pharmacokinetic description of drug interaction by enzyme induction: Carbamazepine–clonazepam in monkeys. *J. Pharm. Sci.,* 68:416–421.

37. Lai, A. A., Levy, R. H., and Cutler, R. E. (1978): Time-course of interaction between carbamazepine and clonzepam in normal man. *Clin. Pharmacol. Ther.,* 25:316–323.

38. Levy, R. H., and Lai, A. A. (1980): A pharmaco-kinetic model for drug interaction by enzyme induc-tion and its application to carbamazepine–clonaze-pam. In: *Antiepileptic Therapy: Advances in Drug Monitoring,* edited by S. I. Johannessen, P. L. Mor-selli, C. E. Pippenger, A. Richens, D. Schmidt, and H. Meinardi, pp. 315–323. Raven Press, New York.

39. Levy, R. H., Pitlick, W. H., Troupin, A. S., and Green, J. R. (1976): Pharmacokinetic implications of chronic drug treatment in epilepsy: Carbamazepine. In: *The Effect of Disease States on Drug Pharmaco-kinetics,* edited by L. Z. Benet, pp. 87–95. APhA/ Academy of Pharmaceutical Sciences, Washington.

40. Lindgren, S., Eeg-Olofsson, O., and Backman, E. (1980): The influence of carbamazepine on drug met-abolic capacity in children using phenazone as model. In: *Antiepileptic Therapy: Advances in Drug Moni-toring,* edited by S. I. Johannessen, P. L. Morselli, C. E., Pippenger, A. Richens, D. Schmidt, and H. Meinardi, pp. 27–36. Raven Press, New York.

41. Lunde, P. K. M., Rane, A., Yaffe, S. J., Lund, L., and Sjöqvist, F. (1970): Plasma protein binding of diphenylhydantoin in man. *Clin. Pharmacol. Ther.,* 11:846–855.

42. Mattson, G. F., Mattson, R. H., and Cramer, J. A. (1980): Valproic acid interaction with carbamazepine. *Ann. Neurol.,* 8:127.

43. Mesdjian, E., Dravet, C., Cenraud, B., and Roger, J. (1980): Carbamazepine intoxication due to triace-tyloleandomycin administration in epileptic patients. *Epilepsia,* 21:489–496.

44. Milhaly, G. W., Vajda, F. J., Miles, J. L., and Louis, W. J. (1979): Single and chronic dose pharmacoki-netic studies of sodium valproate in epileptic patients. *Eur. J. Pharmacol.,* 15:23–29.

45. Morselli, P. L., Baruzzi, A., Gerna, M., Bossi, L., and Porta, M. (1977): Carbamazepine and carbama-zepine-10,11-epoxide concentrations in human brain. *Br. J. Clin. Pharmacol.,* 4:535–540.

46. Morselli, P. L., and Frigerio, A. (1975): Metabolism and pharmacokinetics of carbamazepine. *Drug Me-tab. Rev.,* 4:97–113.

47. Neuvonen, P. J., Penttilä, O., Lehtovaara, R., and Aho, K. (1975): Effect of antiepileptic drugs on the elimination of various tetracycline derivatives. *Eur. J. Clin. Pharmacol.,* 9:147.

48. Patel, I. H., and Levy, R. H. (1979): Valproic acid binding to human serum albumin and determination of free fraction in the presence of anticonvulsants and free fatty acids. *Epilepsia,* 20:85–90.

49. Patel, I. H., Levy, R. H., and Trager, W. F. (1978): Pharmacokinetics of carbamazepine-10,11-epoxide before and after autoinduction in rhesus monkeys. *J. Pharmacol. Exp. Ther.,* 206:607–613.

50. Patel, I. H., Wedlund, P., and Levy, R. H. (1981): Induction effect of phenobarbital on the carbamaze-pine to carbamazepine-10,11-epoxide pathway in rhe-sus monkeys. *J. Pharmacol. Exp. Ther.,* 217:555–558.

51. Penttilä, O., Neuvonen, P. J., Aho, K., and Lehto-vaara, R. (1974): Interaction between doxycycline and some antiepileptic drugs. *Br. Med. J.,* 2:470–472.

52. Pitlick, W. H., and Levy, R. H. (1977): Time-de-pendent kinetics I: Exponential autoinduction of car-bamazepine in monkeys. *J. Pharm. Sci.,* 66:647–649.

53. Pitlick, W. H., Levy, R. H., Troupin, A. S., and Green, J. R. (1976): Pharmacokinetic model to de-scribe self-induced decreases in steady-state concen-trations of carbamazepine. *J. Pharm. Sci.,* 65:462.

54. Pynnönen, S., Frey, H., and Sillanpää, M. (1980): The autoinduction of carbamazepine during long-term therapy. *Int. J. Clin. Pharmacol. Ther. Toxicol.,* 18:247.

55. Pynnönen, S., Sillanpää, M., Frey, H., and Iisalo, E. (1977): Carbamazepine and its 10,11-epoxide in children and adults with epilepsy. *Eur. J. Clin. Phar-macol.,* 11:129–133.

56. Rane, A., Hojer, B., and Wilson, J. T. (1976): Ki-netics of carbamazepine and 10,11-epoxide metabo-lite in children. *Clin. Pharmacol. Ther.,* 19:276–283.

57. Rawlins, M. D., Collste, P., Bertilsson, L., and Pal-mer, L. (1975): Distribution and elimination kinetics of carbamazepine in man. *Eur. J. Clin. Pharmacol.,* 8:91–96.

58. Reunanen, M. I., Luoma, P., Myllylä, V. V., and Hokkanen, E. (1980): Low serum valproic acid con-centrations in epileptic patients on combination ther-apy. *Curr. Ther. Res.,* 28:456–462.

59. Schneider, H. (1975): Carbamazepine: The influence of other antiepileptic drugs on its serum level. In: *Clinical Pharmacology of Anti-Epileptic Drugs,* ed-ited by H. Schneider, D. Janz, C. Gardner-Thorpe, H. Meinardi, and A. L. Sherwin, pp. 189–196. Springer-Verlag, Berlin.

60. Warren, J. W., Benmaman, J. D., Wannamaker, B. B., and Levy, R. H. (1980): Kinetics of a carbama-zepine–ethosuximide interaction. *Clin. Pharmacol. Ther.,* 28:646–651.

61. Westenberg, H. G. M., van der Kleijn, E., Oei, T. T., and de Zeeuw, R. A. (1978): Kinetics of carba-mazepine and carbamazepine-epoxide, determined by use of plasma and saliva. *Clin. Pharmacol. Ther.,* 23:320–328.

62. Wilder, B. J., Willmore, I. J., Bruni, J., and Villa-real, H. J. (1978): Valproic acid: Interaction with other anticonvulsant drugs. *Neurology (Minneap.),* 28:892–896.

Antiepileptic Drugs, edited by D. M. Woodbury,
J. K. Penry, and C. E. Pippenger. Raven Press,
New York © 1982.

40

Carbamazepine

Relation of Plasma Concentration to Seizure Control

James J. Cereghino

Carbamazepine (CBZ) is one of the new generation of antiepileptic drugs developed since 1960, and its efficacy evaluation and clinical application were enhanced by the rapid parallel development of the field of clinical pharmacokinetics. The first clinical reports of this drug, after 3 years of investigational use, were presented in 1962 at the Third International Congress of Neuropsychopharmacology (6,61) By 1964, an ultraviolet spectrophotometric technique was developed to measure carbamazepine concentrations (30). As technology developed, gas–liquid chromatographic, mass spectrometric, and immunoassy methods for determination of carbamazepine and its metabolites became available (Chapter 36). Thus, for the first time in the field of epilepsy, pharmacokinetic findings from these methods could be utilized in the clinical evaluation and application of a new drug.

This chapter will discuss some of the known pharmacokinetic parameters of carbamazepine and will discuss how this information can be applied to the optimal management of the seizure patient.

THERAPEUTIC PLASMA DRUG CONCENTRATION

The role of plasma drug concentration in clinical management is controversial (23,55,

60,99), but Lasagna (55) has tersely summarized the current state of the art: ". . . blood levels of drugs can represent an important source of information, but . . . a blind, unnatural reliance on them reflects poor medical judgment." For proper interpretation of plasma drug concentrations, the physician needs to know (a) the relationship of dose to plasma drug concentration, (b) the relationship of this concentration to desired therapeutic effect, and (c) the factors that can influence the concentration.

Relation of Plasma CBZ Concentration to Dose

Single-Dose Studies

All single-dose studies on CBZ have involved orally administered drug, since an intravenous formulation is not available. Single-dose studies in volunteers have been summarized in several reports (3,8,83) and are also presented in Chapter 37. Plasma CBZ concentration curves show monoexponential decay. Peak plasma concentrations usually occur 4 to 8 hr after ingestion but have occurred as much as 30 hr afterwards. The half-life in volunteers is generally between 18 and 55 hr. Single-dose studies in patients receiving other antiepileptic drugs and in healthy volunteers receiving multiple doses reveal a shorter half-life. The concept of "autoinduction" or "self-induction" has been used to explain these differences (Chapter 37).

Prediction of steady-state plasma concentrations of CBZ and CBZ-epoxide from single dose studies has not been accurate in either adult volunteers (28,32,89), adult patients (26), or pediatric patients (86,90). Measured steady-state CBZ plasma concentrations are lower than predicted, an effect that appears to be caused by autoinduction. A self-induction, one-compartment model with a constant elimination rate constant has been proposed and has produced predictions close to observed concentrations in volunteers (58,82). The measurement of urinary metabolites has been suggested as a method of predicting steady-state plasma CBZ levels (27).

Multiple-Dose Studies

Multiple-dose studies in patients have not yielded agreement on the relationship of dose to plasma CBZ concentration. Population studies in adults (2,16,43,49,54,62,63) have shown a consistent but weak statistically significant correlation ($r = 0.2040$ to 0.396) with a wide scatter between dose and concentration. There is a stronger correlation ($r = 0.5242, p < 0.001$, $N = 295$) between CBZ dose and CBZ-epoxide concentration than between CBZ dose and CBZ concentration ($r = 0.2040$, $p < 0.01$) (63). Studies with a smaller number of patients have noted a weak to absent correlation between CBZ dose and concentration (25,46,47,51,67,68,71, 76,77,91,106). A linear correlation between dose and concentration of CBZ has been reported at low doses in patients just starting therapy (11,39,51,53). Similarly, it has been postulated that the correlation between dose and concentration may be greatest during the first 3 weeks of treatment and thereafter decline (110).

In an effort to obtain closer correlation between the individual points and the regression line, the following factors have been examined.

Body weight.
Correlation increases when dose is expressed as mg/kg rather than as g/day (43).

Age.
The effect of age on correlation is unclear. The relationship of dose to CBZ and CBZ-epoxide concentration was compared between children under 14 years of age and persons over 14 years and between adults age 21 to 31 and adults age 50 and older, but no statistically significant correlations were found (63). Similarly, no significant correlation was found between CBZ dose (2.8–53.5 mg/kg per day) and concentration (0.5–12.2 μg/ml) in 207 children and adolescents with analysis of 392 plasma samples (2). A significant linear relationship was found between the concentration-to-dose ratio and age in which the mean values of the ratio increased significantly with age up to adolescence (15 years, 11 months) (2). In 23 children receiving CBZ alone and 20 children receiving CBZ plus other antiepileptic drugs, there was a weak correlation ($r = 0.65$, $p < 0.001$) between CBZ dose (4–24 mg/kg per day) and concentration (1.7–9.9 μg/ml) for the children receiving CBZ alone and no correlation between CBZ dose (4–30 mg/kg per day) and concentration (1.4–10.7 μg/ml) for children receiving CBZ plus other drugs (88). A weak, statistically significant correlation between dose and concentration of CBZ, CBZ-epoxide, and the sum of both was found in 37 children but not in 13 adults (85). Correlation studies in the elderly have not been performed.

Sex.
Males and females show no significant difference in correlation between dose and CBZ concentration (43,63) or CBZ-epoxide concentration (63).

Concurrent medication.
The interaction of carbamazepine and other antiepileptic drugs has been well documented (Chapter 39). McKauge et al. (63) studied patients treated with CBZ alone (88 patients) and others treated with CBZ plus phenytoin (172 patients), phenobarbital (29 patients), primidone (11 patients), methylphenobarbital (16 patients), ethosuximide (5 patients), sodium valproate (37 patients), sulthiame (24 patients), or

clonazepam (26 patients). Multiple-variable linear regression analysis was used to assess the relationship of these drugs to CBZ and CBZ-epoxide concentration. There was statistically significant evidence that phenytoin lowered CBZ concentration and valproate raised CBZ-epoxide concentration. The lowering of CBZ concentration by phenobarbital as reported by others (12–14,48) was not found. An increase of CBZ-epoxide concentration when carbamazepine was given with phenytoin and phenobarbital has been reported (20). Attempts have been made to predict the influence of comedication on dose (57,117).

Autoinduction.

Plasma CBZ concentration starts to decrease after 3 days of therapy and is not accompanied by an increase in the CBZ-epoxide concentration (28,84). Autoinduction for a particular dosage appears to be maximal within 2 to 4 weeks (4,5).

Technical factors.

The technique used in determination of plasma concentration, sampling time in relation to last dose (trough versus peak versus random), duration of treatment (i.e., steady-state), degree of patient compliance, and use of single or multiple samples from the same patient have all been considered confounding factors in determining the relationship of CBZ dose to concentration.

Increasing the dosage in an individual patient already receiving carbamazepine appears to cause an increase in CBZ concentration, although the effects cannot be predicted with certainty (4,43,56,65,66,78). There appears to be a linear relationship between dose and plasma concentration, but the slope of the curve, which varies for each patient, is dependent on the degree of autoinduction (4).

Although there is a weak, statistically significant correlation between dose and both CBZ and CBZ-epoxide concentrations in either adults or children, the great interindividual variability precludes predicting the plasma concentration from the prescribed dosage. Plasma concentrations from the same daily dose may vary from

five- to sevenfold because of interindividual differences. The common adult dosage of 10 to 20 mg/kg (800–1,200 mg/day) usually produces plasma CBZ concentrations in the range of 4 to 8 μg/ml, with the epoxide concentration being about 20 to 40% of that of the parent compound.

Relation of Plasma CBZ Concentration to Desired Therapeutic Effect

To be of clinical value, a drug concentration measurement (e.g., in plasma, saliva, tears, CSF) should reflect the concentration of the drug at the site of action. Multiple factors may affect that relationship, and the roles of active metabolites, absorption, distribution (including protein binding), excretion, and associated disease have been discussed in Chapter 37. Limited information from surgical specimens suggests that the brain-to-plasma ratios are in the order of 0.8 to 1.6 (Chapter 37).

The strongest information relating plasma CBZ concentration to therapeutic efficacy comes from controlled clinical trials of the drug's efficacy and from population studies of CBZ concentrations. Several controlled clinical trials of CBZ (9,10,94,103,116) have demonstrated its efficacy in controlling complex partial or generalized tonic–clonic seizures. Absence seizures do not appear to be benefited by carbamazepine. In none of these studies has a clear-cut relationship between plasma CBZ concentration and efficacy been demonstrated because of the great interindividual variability.

Population studies relating CBZ concentration to therapeutic efficacy were reviewed in the first edition of this book (8). Since that time, Dam et al. (20) have presented an additional 117 patients. The largest population study of CBZ concentrations is that of Guelen et al. (35–37). From June, 1969, through July, 1974, data on nearly 250,000 antiepileptic drug concentrations were collected from 11 institutions in The Netherlands, Norway, England, Germany, and the United States. Data on 184,526 concentrations from 11,720 patients were utilized in the analysis. Carbamazepine, either alone or with other medications, was received by 1,361 (11.6%) of this population. (Only 43 of the patients were receiving carbamazepine alone.) The mean CBZ concentration was 4.0 ± 3.9 μg/ml. The mean CBZ dose was 14.4 ± 7.1 mg/kg.

The following study by Schneider (98) is typical of population studies of CBZ concentration and its relation to therapeutic efficacy. The study involved 75 long-term residents of an institution for epilepsy and 94 "acute" epileptic patients treated in the short-to-medium-term hospital. All but eight patients were receiving other antiepileptic drugs. Age was not specified. Clinical control was assessed historically for patients with no medication change, which ranged from 2 months for "long-term" patients to 3 to 4 weeks for "acute" patients. Clinical control was broadly classified into: Group A, worsened, unchanged, up to 49% improvement; Group B, 50 to 99% improvement; and Group C, completely controlled. Only "psychomotor attacks" (complex partial seizures) were analyzed, and trough CBZ concentrations were obtained. Mean CBZ concentrations for "long-term" patients were: Group A, 2.3 ± 1.4 μg/ml; Group B, 3.7 ± 1.9 μg/ml; and Group C, 4.6 ± 1.3 μg/ml. Mean concentrations for "acute" patients were: Group A, 2.9 ± 1.5 μg/ml; Group B, 5.2 ± 2.3 μg/ml; and Group C, 6.5 ± 3.0 μg/ml. The mean concentrations for all patients were: Group A, 2.6 ± 1.5 μg/ml; Group B, 4.6 ± 2.2 μg/ml; and Group C, 5.9 ± 2.7 μg/ml.

There is a sparse literature correlating CBZ or CBZ-epoxide concentration to either dose or therapeutic effect in patients with trigeminal neuralgia. Tomson et al. (112) reported on seven patients receiving carbamazepine and no other drugs known to interact with it. There was a correlation between dose and CBZ concentration ($r = 0.56$, $p < 0.01$) and between dose and CBZ-epoxide concentration ($r = 0.64$, $p < 0.001$). For six patients, the best therapeutic effects were seen with plasma CBZ concentrations of 5.7 to 10.0 μg/ml. Side effects were observed in two patients, both with CBZ concentrations exceeding 7.9 μg/ml.

None of these studies can be interpreted as a controlled clinical trial relating plasma CBZ level to therapeutic effect. Numerous factors can affect the relationship of reported plasma concentrations to therapeutic efficacy. Some of these factors are: (a) difference in formulations of the drug in different countries; (b) variation in methods of determination, laboratory accuracy, patient compliance, food intake, time of blood sampling, and time required to process the blood sample; (c) environmental stability of the drug; (d) intercurrent acute or chronic disease; (e) inconsistency in definitions of therapeutic efficacy and in classification of epileptic seizures; (f) inclusion of etiologically heterogeneous seizure disorders; (g) concomitant administration of both other antiepileptic drugs and other types of drugs; and (h) variation in methods of objectively assessing therapeutic efficacy.

In spite of these problems, there seems to be general agreement that a therapeutic effect is seen with concentrations in the range of 3 to 12 μg/ml (8), 6 to 12 μg/ml (113), 5 to 10 μg/ml (3), 5 to 12 μg/ml (50), 4 to 12 μg/ml (72), or 6 to 12 μg/ml (24).

The meaning of the term "therapeutic range" or "optimal range" is controversial. In one definition, "it represents a statistical summary of the best compromise between effectiveness and side effects in some groups of patients" (113). In another, "the therapeutic ranges of plasma concentrations of the various anticonvulsants cannot be derived from the pharmacokinetic parameters of these drugs. Rather, the therapeutic ranges must be determined empirically from data obtained during the course of the treatment of human epilepsy" (24). The concept that plasma concentrations in most patients come within the scope of an expected range is clinically useful in guiding therapy. The expected range cautions physicians to reevaluate those patients whose plasma concentration or clinical response exceeds or never reaches that expected. The clinician must remember that it is not the plasma concentration that is being "treated," but rather that the laboratory information should be combined with clinical judgment to obtain the best possible therapeutic results for each patient (see Guidelines for Clinical Use).

TOXIC EFFECTS AND PLASMA DRUG CONCENTRATION

Toxic effects of carbamazepine are reviewed in Chapters 41 and 42. The difference between the therapeutic and toxic plasma concentration of CBZ has not been determined with certainty.

Meinardi (66) attempted to correlate the appearance of side effects with plasma CBZ concentration. Nystagmus was observed in an appreciable number of patients with concentrations as low as 1.5 μg/ml. He has predicted that nearly half of all patients will suffer disturbance of gait, headache, feelings of inhibition, dizziness, and disturbances of vision with plasma concentrations of 8.5 to 10 μg/ml.

Troupin (113) also attempted to correlate objective side effects with plasma CBZ concentration. Clinical observations were matched to plasma concentrations within an hour of observation. The side effects did not seem to increase with increasing plasma CBZ levels. He also observed that diplopia and a subjective sensation of unsteadiness without objective ataxia are particularly likely to be related to high plasma concentrations a few hours after CBZ ingestion (114).

Case reports indicate a considerable individual variation in toxic plasma CBZ concentrations and manifestations of toxicity (11). From plasma CBZ concentrations in a double-blind study, it was not possible to predict which patients would experience persistent side effects (9,10). Many patients will develop tolerance to side effects.

Side effects during initiation of CBZ therapy are frequent. Levy et al. (59) reported that six volunteers all reported side effects of drowsiness, loss of appetite, dizziness, ataxia, loss of accommodation, and occasionally nausea at a dose of 6 mg/kg, but none of these effects were intense enough to be disturbing. In dose-dependence studies performed in this population, the incidence and intensity of side effects increased

with dose (59). Side effects were not correlated with plasma concentrations, which ranged from 5.7 to 7.9 μg/ml.

There appears to be a small but poorly documented group of patients who cannot tolerate carbamazepine, even at very low concentrations, because of side effects (113).

Many patients who receive carbamazepine also receive other antiepileptic drugs. An additive effect on toxic symptoms was reported by Kutt et al. (53). In patients with plasma phenytoin concentrations exceeding 20 μg/ml, the addition of CBZ to produce concentrations of 2 to 4 μg/ml increased disturbances of equilibrium, coordination, and vision. Decreasing the phenytoin concentration allowed for an increase in CBZ dose and concentration without producing intolerable toxicity.

The role of CBZ-epoxide or other CBZ metabolites in producing side effects is unclear. Hvidberg and Dam (45) have postulated that the epoxide might play a significant role, since the concentration of the epoxide is highest in patients receiving multiple antiepileptic drugs (14,20). In seven patients who were given propoxyphene hydrochloride (65 mg three times a day), plasma CBZ concentration increased, and symptoms and signs of drug intoxication appeared in three of the patients, but the CBZ-epoxide concentration showed no significant changes (18).

A theory has been proposed that carbamazepine has antidiuretic properties that are positively correlated with plasma concentration and that water retention might be responsible for some side effects (1,42,79,104,105). Phenytoin may reverse this effect (80).

The influence of concurrent diseases on plasma CBZ concentrations is discussed in Chapter 37, and the effects of medications received for these concurrent diseases are presented in Chapter 39.

Plasma CBZ concentrations seem to decrease during pregnancy, an effect seen with several of the antiepileptic drugs, and the CBZ-epoxide concentration increases (15,19,87). The pharmacokinetics of carbamazepine seem to be similar in infants, children, and adults, although children tend to have lower plasma concentrations than adults and may require higher daily dosages of the drug (Chapter 37; 29,70,71, 73,86).

Specific studies exploring the relationship of plasma CBZ concentrations to dose and side effects have not been done in the elderly (>70 years of age). There is a clinical impression that elderly patients tolerate the drug less well than young patients. Heathfield (41) has noted that for the elderly patient with trigeminal neuralgia, carbamazepine must be started in a very small dose that is gradually increased. Confirming plasma concentration data are not available.

The pharmacogenetics of carbamazepine remain unknown (8).

The cases of carbamazepine overdosage have been reviewed in Chapter 41. Plasma CBZ concentrations have been measured in only a few of these cases. Gruska et al. (34) reported a 41-year-old woman who ingested 20 g of carbamazepine. Peak CBZ concentration was about 22.5 μg/ml 72 hr after ingestion, and the patient regained consciousness when the concentration fell to about 10 μg/ml. Peak CBZ concentration was not obtained in a 16-year-old boy who ingested 5.8 g of carbamazepine (96). A plasma CBZ concentration determined when the patient was emerging from stupor was 10.1 μg/ml. A 23-year-old woman ingested 16 g of carbamazepine (21,22). During the first 40 hr she was "semicomatose but arousable"; CBZ concentration was about 29 μg/ml, and CBZ-epoxide concentration was about 14 μg/ml. After 45 hr, the concentrations rose abruptly to 44 μg/ml at 60 hr (CBZ) and 22 μg/ml at 60 and 72 hr (CBZ-epoxide). At 84 hr, consciousness returned when CBZ concentration was about 20 μg/ml and CBZ-epoxide concentration was about 10 μg/ml. Gülzow et al. (38) reported a 13-year-old girl who ingested 3.6 g of carbamazepine and 1.0 g of phenytoin, and they found comparable plasma concentrations. Sullivan et al. (109) reported four cases of CBZ overdosage, but the relationship of plasma concentration to state of consciousness was not specified.

An increased incidence of seizures in one patient with a CBZ concentration over 20 μg/ml

has been reported and may represent a case of "paradoxical intoxication" (115).

TOLERANCE

There is evidence for autoinduction of carbamazepine metabolism in humans, with plasma concentrations declining after a period of continuous administration. This topic is fully discussed in Chapter 37.

DEPENDENCE

Habituation, the occurrence of convulsions after medication given for several weeks or months is withdrawn, seems not to occur with carbamazepine. Even though the drug has been prescribed for a large number of nonepileptic patients with trigeminal neuralgia, there have been no reports of convulsions after abrupt withdrawal of the drug.

Rodin et al. (94) noted that 7 of 18 patients who were abruptly changed from carbamazepine (serum concentration of 5 to 7 μg/ml) to placebo experienced an exacerbation of seizures within the first 3 to 4 days. The patients were also receiving other antiepileptic medications. This was interpreted to indicate an anticonvulsant property of carbamazepine rather than a withdrawal effect because of dependence.

GUIDELINES FOR CLINICAL USE

Carbamazepine is indicated for the treatment of complex partial seizures, generalized tonic–clonic seizures, elementary partial seizures, and possibly myoclonic seizures. Absence seizures and atonic seizures do not appear to be controlled by carbamazepine.

Factors other than efficacy may influence the selection of an antiepileptic drug. In the United States, carbamazepine (Tegretol®) is expensive. In addition, the package insert in the United States recommends that "because of the necessity for frequent laboratory evaluation for potentially serious side effects, Tegretol is not recommended as the drug of first choice in seizure disorders. It should be reserved for patients whose seizures are difficult to control and/or patients experiencing marked side effects (e.g., excessive sedation)." Nevertheless, an increasing number of physicians, both in the United States and in other countries, are selecting carbamazepine as the drug for initial treatment of complex partial seizures because it does not have the sedative side effects of the barbiturates and does not induce gingival hypertrophy, hirsutism, or coarse facial features, as does phenytoin.

In previously untreated patients, monotherapy now appears to be the preferred regimen. According to Reynolds and Shorvon (92), this regimen starts with a small dose of one drug, and if seizures recur, the dose is increased in small increments, with monitoring of plasma concentrations until either seizures are controlled or the upper end of the optimum range is reached. In 42 patients treated with carbamazepine for a mean duration of 26 months, 76% were completely seizure free (92,100,102). Others have also confirmed that monotherapy with carbamazepine is feasible (107,108).

In adults, therapy with carbamazepine is usually initiated with one 200-mg tablet given twice a day on the first day (400 mg). This low dosage is recommended to minimize the possibilities of dizziness, drowsiness, unsteadiness, nausea, and vomiting frequently seen with initiation of therapy. These symptoms are seen even though the plasma concentration may be quite low (1 to 2 μg/ml); they are usually transient but may persist and become intolerable to a few patients. The dosage is then increased in 200-mg daily increments. Some prefer to administer the drug twice daily, and others three or four times a day (17). There is less daily fluctuation with a schedule of four times a day (46). A single daily dose is insufficient. If symptoms occur several hours after administration of the drug, increasing the number of times a day the drug is administered may alleviate this problem. Food may enhance peak plasma concentration, so if the drug is given before meals, the concentration may be higher. The time to peak concentration may be prolonged, and absorption may be reduced, at doses higher than 20 to 25 mg/kg per

day, so that it may be desirable to administer these doses before meals to obtain a higher plasma concentration.

Assuming that the half-life of carbamazepine is 12 $\pm$ 3 hr, the time required to reach steady-state plasma concentration will be 2 to 4 days. This relatively short half-life may be another reason to administer carbamazepine more frequently than twice a day. Seizures occurring before steady state is reached may not reflect lack of efficacy but rather lack of sufficient drug at its site of action.

Because carbamazepine autoinduces its own metabolism, a reduction of plasma concentration may be observed as early as 3 days after initiation of therapy (28,64) and is usually complete at 3 weeks (4). This effect may necessitate an increase in dosage.

Since the relationship between dose and plasma concentration is not strong, most physicians think that adjusting dosage based on plasma concentration rather than daily dosage is superior. A fasting morning plasma concentration of 5.5 to 7.5 μg/ml in the adult receiving carbamazepine monotherapy usually indicates maximal efficacy without toxicity. In a study with 16 adults and 2 children who had been treated for at least 2 years and were continuing to have seizures, the dosage of carbamazepine was modified to achieve plasma concentrations of 4 to 10 μg/ml. (No attempt was made to modify phenytoin or phenobarbital concentrations.) A 60% reduction in seizure frequency was observed after 4 to 5 weeks of plasma monitoring (68). Other studies have similarly shown treatment to be more effective when plasma concentrations are measured (111).

Studies with children (31) suggest that the seizure types most likely to respond to CBZ are the same as those controllable in adults. Gamstorp (31) considered CBZ the drug of choice in children because it provides seizure control without causing gingival hypertrophy, hypertrichosis, sedation, or hyperactivity. In the United States, the FDA did not approve the extended use of CBZ in children 6 years of age and older until 1978. The manufacturer recommends for children 6 to 12 years of age an initial dose of one-half tablet (100 mg) twice a day or 200 mg daily, gradually increasing dosage by 100 mg/day using a t.i.d. or q.i.d. schedule. The manufacturer recommends that dosage should generally not exceed 1,000 mg in this age range. Because of the differences in plasma concentrations between adults and children, concentrations are useful in monitoring therapy and must be performed before one can conclude that the drug is ineffective for a particular patient.

One very crucial but frequently overlooked factor influencing a physician's ability to utilize plasma concentration in adjusting therapy is laboratory accuracy. The carbamazepine assay presents numerous analytical problems and is prone to error if not carefully performed. In a monthly assessment of 194 U.S. laboratories performing carbamazepine assays, 122 (62.9%) showed an excellent or satisfactory performance, and 72 (37.1%) had an unsatisfactory or extremely poor performance. In comparison, 25.7% and 11.6% of the laboratories showed inaccurate phenobarbital and phenytoin assays, respectively (81).

Carbamazepine is available as a suspension, but this formulation may produce more fluctuation in the plasma concentrations (73,118). An enteric coated preparation designed to reduce the daily fluctuations is being investigated (75).

The therapeutic range for plasma concentrations must not be rigidly applied regardless of clinical inconsistencies. A patient in the upper therapeutic range who is not experiencing side effects and whose seizures are not completely controlled might reasonably be expected to have side effects if dosage and plasma concentration are increased. Some patients, however, will tolerate higher plasma concentrations without side effects and with improved seizure control, and if the treating physician arbitrarily sets an upper maximum to plasma concentration, these individuals would not receive a fair trial of the drug. Conversely, when a patient is in the lower end of the range and remains there even though dosage is increased, the physician should suspect noncompliance. These patients can be further evaluated by studies of urinary output of the drug and its metabolites (52).

Ordinarily, a fasting morning plasma speci-men is preferable to a random specimen to eliminate the possibility of a random observation that the patient is outside the therapeutic range. Since the CBZ concentration fluctuates, particularly in patients receiving other antiepileptic drugs, seizures (with low concentration) or side effects (with high concentration) may occur at a particular time of day. Measurement of plasma concentrations can document these phenomena, and alterations can be made (i.e., different dose schedule, administration with food) to correct the situation (44,95).

The use of nonprescription drugs may alter plasma CBZ concentration and must be considered if sudden loss of seizure control or side effects occur. Analgesics such as acetylsalicylic acid have no clear-cut effect on CBZ concentration when given for 3 days (40,74).

The widespread use of multiple-drug therapy (polypharmacy) has been severely questioned (92,101,102). A retrospective survey of 50 adult epileptic patients in Britain who were taking two antiepileptic drugs showed that seizure control had improved in only 36% in the 6 months after introduction of the second drug. Subsequent plasma concentration measurements showed that seizure control was significantly related to the presence of optimal plasma concentrations of at least one of the drugs (101). Before a second drug is added, an optimum plasma concentration of the first drug should be demonstrated. Once the second drug has been added and shows a sufficient plasma concentration, an effort should be made to remove the first drug. Callaghan et al. (7) successfully reduced 9 of 14 patients from polytherapy to monotherapy with carbamazepine.

Nevertheless, some patients will require therapy with multiple drugs, and seizure control may be difficult to achieve despite numerous alterations in drug therapy (93,97). The addition of carbamazepine often improves seizure control in this group of patients (9,10,33, 69,102,107,108), although it may not (25). In patients receiving carbamazepine plus other antiepileptic drugs, the possibility of an additive effect of intoxication must be considered (53).

Some authors recommend routine monitoring

of the CBZ-epoxide, but the clinical value of this information remains uncertain. Additional study of this and other metabolites are needed.

SUMMARY

Carbamazepine is a major antiepileptic drug for the treatment of complex partial, elementary partial, and generalized tonic–clonic seizures. Numerous methods are available for measurement of plasma concentrations of the drug and its epoxide metabolite, but the assay presents many technical problems and is prone to error if not carefully performed. There is a weak, statistically significant correlation between dose and CBZ and CBZ-epoxide concentrations in both adults and children. Great interindividual variability precludes prediction of the CBZ or CBZ-epoxide concentrations from the prescribed dose. Definition of the effective and toxic concentrations of the drug and its epoxide metabolite is still evolving. The common adult dosage of 10 to 20 mg/kg (800–1,200 mg/day) usually produces plasma CBZ concentrations in the range of 4 to 8 µg/ml, with the epoxide concentration being about 20 to 40% of that of the parent compound. Metabolism is autoinduced, so that a decline in plasma CBZ concentration may be seen with continuous administration. Increase in dosage usually produces a nonlinear increase in plasma concentrations of both CBZ and CBZ-epoxide. Other drugs may affect these concentrations. Phenytoin and phenobarbital, for example, appear to lower CBZ concentration and increase CBZ-epoxide concentration, whereas valproate appears to raise only the CBZ-epoxide concentration. Measurement of the plasma concentration may be of great assistance to the physician in the optimal management of the patient receiving carbamazepine.

REFERENCES

1. Ashton, M. G., Ball, S. G., Thomas, T. H., and Lee, M. R. (1977): Water intoxication associated with carbamazepine treatment. *Br. Med. J.*, 1:1134–1135.
2. Battino, D., Bossi, L., Croci, D., Franceschetti, S., Gomeni, C., Moise, A., and Vitali, A. (1980): Carbamazepine plasma levels in children and adults: Influence of age, dose, and associated therapy. *Ther. Drug Monit.*, 2:315–322.
3. Bertilsson, L. (1978): Clinical pharmacokinetics of carbamazepine. *Clin. Pharmacokinet.*, 3:128–143.
4. Bertilsson, L. (1980): Discussion. In: *Antiepileptic Therapy: Advances in Drug Monitoring*, edited by S. I. Johannessen, P. L. Morselli, C. E. Pippenger, A. Richens, D. Schmidt, and H. Meinardi, p. 235. Raven Press, New York.
5. Bertilsson, L., Höjer, B., Tybring, G., Osterloh, J., and Rane, A. (1980): Autoinduction of carbamazepine metabolism in children examined by a stable isotope technique. *Clin. Pharmacol. Ther.*, 27:83–88.
6. Bonduelle, M., Bouygues, P., Sallou, C., and Chemaly, R., (1964): Bilan de l'expérimentation clinique de l'anti-épileptique G 32 883 (5-carbomyl-5-H-dibenzo-b,f-azépine): Resultats de 89 observations. In: *International Congress of Neuropsychopharmacology, Munich 1962, Vol. 3*, edited by P. B. Bradley, F. Flugel, and P. H. Hock, pp. 312–316. Elsevier, Amsterdam.
7. Callaghan, N., O'Callaghan M., Duggan, B., and Freely, M. (1978): Carbamazepine as a single drug in the treatment of epilepsy. *J. Neurol. Neurosurg. Psychiatry*, 41:907–910.
8. Cereghino, J. J. (1975): Serum carbamazepine concentration and clinical control. *Adv. Neurol.*, 11:309–330.
9. Cereghino, J. J., Brock, J. T., Van Meter, J. C., Penry, J. K., Smith, L. D., and White B. G. (1974): Carbamazepine for epilepsy. A controlled prospective evaluation. *Neurology (Minneap.)*, 24:401–410.
10. Cereghino, J. J., Brock, J. T., Van Meter, J. C., Penry, J. K., Smith, L. D., and White, B. G. (1975): The efficacy of carbamazepine combinations in epilepsy. *Clin. Pharmacol. Ther.*, 18:733–741.
11. Cereghino, J. J., Van Meter, J. C., Brock, J. T., Penry, J. K., Smith, L. D., and White, B. G. (1973): Preliminary observations of serum carbamazepine concentration in epileptic patients. *Neurology (Minneap.)*, 23:357–366.
12. Christiansen, J., and Dam, M. (1973): Influence of phenobarbital and diphenylhydantoin on plasma carbamazepine levels in patients with epilepsy. *Acta Neurol. Scand.*, 49:543–546.
13. Christiansen, J., and Dam, M. (1974): Interaction between carbamazepine and diphenylhydantoin and/or phenobarbital in epileptic patients. In: *Drug Interactions*, edited by P. L. Morselli, S. N. Cohen, and S. Garattini, pp. 285–288. Raven Press, New York.
14. Christiansen, J., and Dam, M. (1975) Drug interaction in epileptic patients. In: *Clinical Pharmacology of Anti-Epileptic Drugs*, edited by H. Schneider, D. Janz, C. Gardner-Thorpe, H. Meinardi, and A. L. Sherwin, pp. 197–200. Springer-Verlag, Heidelberg.
15. Christiansen, J., and Dam, M. (1977): Plasma and salivary levels of carbamazepine and carbamazepine 10,11-epoxide during pregnancy. In: *Antiepileptic Drug Monitoring*, edited by C. Gardner-Thorpe, D. Janz, H. Meinardi, and C. E. Pippenger, pp. 128–137. Pitman Medical, Tunbridge Wells, Kent.

16. Cotter, L. M., Smith, G., Hooper, W. D., Tyrer, J. H., and Eadie, M. J. (1975): The bioavailability of carbamazepine. *Proc. Aust. Assoc. Neurol.*, 12: 123–128.

17. Dam, M., and Christiansen, J. (1976): Carbamazepine (Tegretol®) in the treatment of grand mal epilepsy. In: *Epileptology*, edited by D. Janz, pp. 175–179. Publishing Sciences Group, Acton, Massachusetts.

18. Dam, M., and Christiansen, J. (1977): Interaction of propoxyphene with carbamazepine. *Lancet*, 2:509.

19. Dam, M., Christiansen, J., Munck, O., and Mygind, K. I. (1979): Antiepileptic drugs: Metabolism in pregnancy. *Clin. Pharmacokinet.*, 4:53–62.

20. Dam, M., Jensen, A., and Christiansen, J. (1975): Plasma level and effect of carbamazepine in grand mal and psychomotor epilepsy. *Acta Neurol. Scand.*, 60:33–38.

21. De Zeeuw, R. A., and Westenberg, H. G. M. (1979): An unusual case of carbamazepine poisoning with a near-fatal relapse after two days. *Clin. Toxicol.*, 14:263–269.

22. De Zeeuw, R. A., Westenberg, H. G. M., van der Kleijn, E., and Gimbrere, J. S. F. (1979): An unusual case of carbamazepine poisoning with a near-fatal relapse after two days. *Vet. Hum. Toxicol.* [Suppl.], 21:95–97.

23. Dobbs, R. J., and Dobbs, S. M. (1980): Problems with the use of drug blood levels in patient management. In: *Controversies in Therapeutics*, edited by L. Lasagna, pp. 106–117. W. B. Saunders, Philadelphia.

24. Eadie, M. J. (1980): Pharmacokinetics of the anticonvulsant drugs. In: *The Treatment of Epilepsy*, edited by J. H. Tyrer, pp. 61–93. J. B. Lippincott, Philadelphia.

25. Eichelbaum, M., Bertilsson, L., Lund, L., Palmer, L., and Sjöqvist, F. (1976): Plasma levels of carbamazepine and carbamazepine-10,11-epoxide during treatment of epilepsy. *Eur. J. Clin. Pharmacol.*, 9:417–421.

26. Eichelbaum, M., Ekbom, K., Bertilsson, L., Ringberger, V. A., and Rane, A. (1975): Plasma kinetics of carbamazepine and its epoxide metabolite in man after single and multiple doses. *Eur. J. Clin. Pharmacol.*, 8:337–341.

27. Eichelbaum, M., Hoffmann, F., Kötite, K. W., and v. Unruh, G. E. (1980): Measurement of the metabolites of the epoxide–diol pathway of carbamazepine to assess the extent of induction of carbamazepine metabolism during chronic treatment. In: *Antiepileptic Therapy: Advances in Drug Monitoring*, edited by S. I. Johannessen, P. L. Morselli, C. E. Pippenger, A. Richens, D. Schmidt, and H. Meinardi, pp. 143–148. Raven Press, New York.

28. Faigle, J. W., Brechbühler, S., Feldman, K. F., and Richter, W. J. (1976): The biotransformation of carbamazepine. In: *Epileptic Seizures—Behaviour—Pain*, edited by W. Birkmayer, pp. 127–140. Hans Huber, Bern.

29. Forsythe, W. I., Prendergast, M. P., Toothill, C., and Broughton, P. M. G. (1979): Carbamazepine serum levels in children with epilepsy: A micro immuno-assay technique. *Dev. Med. Child Neurol.*, 21:441–447.

30. Führ, J. (1964): Untersuchungen über die Verträglichkeit und Ausscheidung eines neuartigen Antiepilepticums. *Arzneim. Forsch.*, 14:74–75.

31. Gamstorp, I. (1975): Treatment with carbamazepine: Children. *Adv. Neurol.*, 11:237–248.

32. Gérardin, A. P., Abadie, F. V., Campestrini, J. A., and Theobald, W. (1976): Pharmacokinetics of carbamazepine in normal humans after single and repeated oral doses. *J. Pharmacokinet. Biopharm.*, 4:521–535.

33. Grant, R. H. E. (1976): Carbamazepine in the treatment of severe epilepsy. In: *Epileptic Seizures—Behaviour—Pain*, edited by W. Birkmayer, pp. 104–110. Hans Huber, Bern.

34. Gruska, H., Beyer, K.-H., Kubicki, S., and Schneider, H. (1971): Klinik, Toxikologie und Therapie einer schweren Carbamazepin-Vergiftung. *Arch. Toxikol.*, 27:193–203.

35. Guelen, P. J. M., and van der Kleijn, E. (1978): An epidemiological study of the relative clearance. In: *Rational Anti-Epileptic Drug Therapy*, edited by P. J. M. Guelen and E. van der Kleijn, pp. 49–53. Elsevier, Amsterdam.

36. Guelen, P. J. M., and van der Kleijn, E. (1978): Plasma concentrations and relative clearances of the anti-epileptic drugs. In: *Rational Anti-Epileptic Drug Therapy*, edited by P. J. M. Guelen and E. van der Kleijn, pp. 65–72. Elsevier, Amsterdam.

37. Guelen, P. J. M., van der Kleijn, E., and Woudstra, U. (1975): Statistical analysis of pharmacokinetic parameters in epileptic patients chronically treated with anti-epileptic drugs. In: *Clinical Pharmacology of Anti-Epileptic Drugs*, edited by H. Schneider, D. Janz, C. Gardner-Thorpe, H. Meinardi, and A. L. Sherwin, pp. 2–10. Springer-Verlag, Heidelberg.

38. Gülzow, H. -U., Gottschall, S., and Hein, J. (1975): Über eine Intoxikation mit Karbamazepin und Diphenylhydantoin im Kindesalter. *Kinderaerztl. Prax.*, 43:62–66.

39. Hanke, N. F. J. (1972): Clinical tolerance of Tegretol. In: *Tegretol in Epilepsy*, edited by C. A. S. Wink, pp. 113–126. C. Nicholls, Manchester.

40. Hansen, B. S., Dam, M., Brandt, J., Hvidberg, E. F., Angelo, H., Christensen, J. M., and Lous, P. (1980): Influence of dextropropoxyphene on steady state serum levels and protein binding of three antiepileptic drugs in man. *Acta Neurol. Scand.*, 61:357–367.

41. Heathfield, K. W. G. (1972): Discussion. In: *Tegretol in Epilepsy*, edited by C. A. S. Wink, p. 125. C. Nicholls, Manchester.

42. Henry, D. A., Lawson, D. H., Reavey, P., and Renfew, S. (1977): Hyponatraemia during carbamazepine treatment. *Br. Med. J.*, 1:83–84.

43. Hooper, W. D., Dubetz, D. K., Eadie, M. J., and Tyrer, J. H. (1974): Preliminary observations on the clinical pharmacology of carbamazepine ('Tegretol'). *Proc. Aust. Assoc. Neurol.*, 11:189–198.

44. Höppener, R. J., Kuyer, A., Meijer, J. W. A., and Hulsman, J. (1980): Correlation between daily fluctuations of carbamazepine serum levels and intermittent side effects. *Epilepsia*, 21:341–350.

45. Hvidberg, E. F., and Dam, M. (1976): Clinical pharmacokinetics of anticonvulsants. *Clin. Pharmacokinet.*, 1:161–188.

46. Johannessen, S. I., Baruzzi, A., Gomeni, R., Strandjord, R. E., and Morselli, P. L. (1977): Further observations on carbamazepine and carbamazepine-10,11-epoxide kinetics in epileptic patients. In: *Antiepileptic Drug Monitoring*, edited by C. Gardner-Thorpe, D. Janz, H. Meinardi, and C. E. Pippenger, pp. 110–127. Pitman Medical, Tunbridge Wells, Kent.

47. Johannessen, S. I., Gerna, M., Bakke, J., Strandjord, R. E., and Morselli, P. L. (1976): CSF concentrations and serum protein binding of carbamazepine and carbamazepine-10,11-epoxide in epileptic patients. *Br. J. Clin. Pharmacol.*, 3:575–582.

48. Johannessen, S. I., and Strandjord, R. E. (1975): The influence of phenobarbitone and phenytoin on carbamazepine serum levels. In: *Clinical Pharmacology of Anti-Epileptic Drugs*, edited by H. Schneider, D. Janz, C. Gardner-Thorpe, H. Meinardi, and A. L. Sherwin, pp. 201–205. Springer-Verlag, Heidelberg.

49. Kristensen, O., and Larsen, H. F. (1980): Value of saliva samples in monitoring carbamazepine concentrations in epileptic patients. *Acta Neurol. Scand.*, 61:344–350.

50. Kutt, H. (1978): Anticonvulsant blood levels in the management of epileptic patients. In: *Clinical Neuropharmacology, Vol. 3*, edited by H. L. Klawans, pp. 1–13. Raven Press, New York.

51. Kutt, H. (1978): Clinical pharmacology of carbamazepine. In: *Antiepileptic Drugs: Quantitative Analysis and Interpretation*, edited by C. E. Pippenger, J. K. Penry, and H. Kutt, pp. 297–305. Raven Press, New York.

52. Kutt, H. (1978): Evaluation of unusual antiepileptic drug concentrations. In: *Antiepileptic Drugs: Quantitative Analysis and Interpretation*, edited by C. E. Pippenger, J. K. Penry, and H. Kutt, pp. 307–314. Raven Press, New York.

53. Kutt, H., Solomon, G., Wasterlain, C., Petersen, H., Louis, S., and Carruthers, R. (1975): Carbamazepine in difficult to control epileptic out-patients. *Acta Neurol. Scand. [Suppl.]*, 60:27–32.

54. Lander, C. M., Eadie, M. J., and Tyrer, J. H. (1977): Factors influencing plasma carbamazepine concentrations. *Clin. Exp. Neurol.*, 14:184–193.

55. Lasagna, L. (1980): Introduction. Is measurement of drug blood levels helpful in managing patients? In: *Controversies in Therapeutics*, edited by L. Lasagna, pp. 99. W. B. Saunders, Philadelphia.

56. Lehtovaara, R., Bardy, A., and Neuvonen, P. (1980): Effect of dose modification on the serum concentration of phenytoin and carbamazepine. In: *Antiepileptic Therapy: Advances in Drug Monitoring*, edited by S. I. Johannessen, P. L. Morselli, C. E. Pippenger, A. Richens, D. Schmidt, and H. Meinardi, pp. 287–290. Raven Press, New York.

57. Levy, R. H., and Lai, A. A. (1980): A pharmacokinetic model for drug interactions by enzyme induction and its application to carbamazepine–clonazepam. In: *Antiepileptic Therapy: Advances in Drug Monitoring*, edited by S. I. Johannessen, P. L. Morselli, C. E. Pippenger, A. Richens, D. Schmidt, and H. Meinardi, pp. 315–323. Raven Press, New York.

58. Levy R. H., Pitlick, W. H., Troupin, A. S., and Green, J. R. (1976): Pharmacokinetic implications of chronic drug treatment in epilepsy: Carbamazepine. In: *The Effect of Disease States on Drug Pharmacokinetics*, edited by L. Z. Benet, pp. 87–95. American Pharmaceutical Association, Washington.

59. Levy, R. H., Pitlick, W. H., Troupin, A. S., Green, J. R., and Neal, J. M. (1975): Pharmacokinetics of carbamazepine in normal men. *Clin. Pharmacol. Ther.*, 17:657–668.

60. Livingston, S., and Pruce, I. (1980): Clinical response is more important than measurement of blood levels in managing epileptic patients. In: *Controversies in Therapeutics*, edited by L. Lasagna, pp. 118–130. W. B. Saunders, Philadelphia.

61. Lorge, M. (1964): Ueber ein neuartiges Antiepilepticum der Iminostilbenreihe (G 32883). In: *International Congress of Neuropsychopharmacology, Munich, 1962, Vol. 3*, edited by P. B. Bradley, F. Flugel, and P. H. Hock, pp. 299–302. Elsevier, Amsterdam.

62. McKauge, L., Tyrer, J. H., and Eadie, M. J. (1979): The epoxide of carbamazepine. *Clin. Exp. Neurol.*, 16:95–104.

63. McKauge, L., Tyrer, J. H., and Eadie, M. J. (1981): Factors influencing simultaneous concentrations of carbamazepine and its epoxide in plasma. *Ther. Drug Monit.*, 3:63–70.

64. McNamara, P. J., Colburn, W. A., and Gibaldi, M. (1979): Time course of carbamazepine self-induction. *J. Pharmacokinet. Biopharm.*, 7:63–68.

65. Meinardi, H. (1971): Het verband tussen de voorgeschreven dosis anti-epileptica en de gemeten bloedspiegelwaarden. *Ned. Tijdschr. Geneeskd.*, 115:915–920.

66. Meinardi, H. (1972): Other antiepileptic drugs: Carbamazepine. In: *Antiepileptic Drugs*, edited by D. M. Woodbury, J. K. Penry, and R. P. Schmidt, pp. 487–496. Raven Press, New York.

67. Miura, H., Minagawa, K., Yagi, J., Kato, Y., and Kaneko, T. (1976): Carbamazepine (Tegretol). *Brain Dev.* 8:455–462.

68. Monaco, F., Riccio, A., Benna, P., Covacich, A., Durelli, L., Fantini, M., Furlan, P. M., Gilli, M., Mutani, R., Troni, W., Gerna, M., and Morselli, P. L. (1976): Further observations on carbamazepine plasma levels in epileptic patients. *Neurology (Minneap.)*, 26:936–943.

69. Monaco, F., Riccio, A., Fantini, M., Baruzzi, A., and Morselli, P. L. (1979): A month-by-month long-term study on carbamazepine: Clinical, EEG and pharmacological evaluation. *J. Int. Med. Res.*, 7:152–157.

70. Morselli, P. L. (1977): Antiepileptic drugs In: *Drug Disposition During Development*, edited by P. L. Morselli, pp. 311–360. Spectrum, New York.

71. Morselli, P. L., Bossi, L., and Gerna, M. (1976): Pharmacokinetic studies with carbamazepine in epileptic patients. In: *Epileptic Seizures—Behaviour—Pain*, edited by W. Birkmayer, pp. 141–150. Hans Huber, Bern.

72. Morselli, P. L., and Franco-Morselli, R. (1980): Clinical pharmacokinetics of antiepileptic drugs in adults. *Pharmacol. Ther.*, 10:65–101.

73. Morselli, P. L., Monaco, F., Gerna, M., Recchia, M., and Riccio, A. (1975): Bioavailability of two carbamazepine preparations during chronic admin-

istration to epileptic patients. *Epilepsia,* 16:759–764.

74. Neuvonen, P. J., Lehtovaara, R., Bardy, A., and Elomaa, E. (1979): Antipyretic analgesics in patients on antiepileptic drug therapy. *Eur. J. Clin. Pharmacol.,* 15:263–268.

75. Oldigs, H. D., Bartels, H., and Wallis, S. (1980): How can carbamazepine fluctuation during the day be avoided? *Acta Neurol. Scand. [Suppl.],* 79:104.

76. Oller Ferrer-Vidal, L., Sabater-Tobella, J., and Oller-Daurella, L. (1976): Preliminary report on serum carbamazepine determinations and their application to the treatment of epilepsy. In: *Epileptic Seizures—Behaviour—Pain,* edited by W. Birkmayer, pp. 165–174. Hans Huber, Bern.

77. Parsonage, M. (1972): Clinical experience with carbamazepine (Tegretol) as an anticonvulsant. In: *Tegretol in Epilepsy,* edited by C. A. S. Wink, pp. 69–79. C. Nicholls, Manchester.

78. Perucca, E., Bittencourt, P., and Richens, A. (1980): Effect of dose increments on serum carbamazepine concentration in epileptic patients. *Clin. Pharmacokinet.,* 5:576–582.

79. Perucca, E., Garratt, A., Heddige, S., and Richens, A. (1978): Water intoxication in epileptic patients receiving carbamazepine. *J. Neurol. Neurosurg. Psychiatry,* 41:713–718.

80. Perucca, E., and Richens, A. (1980): Reversal by phenytoin of carbamazepine-induced water intoxication: A pharmacokinetic interaction. *J. Neurol. Neurosurg. Psychiatry,* 43:540–545.

81. Pippenger, C. E., Paris-Kutt, H., Penry, J. K., and Daly, D. D. (1978): Antiepileptic Drug Levels Quality Control Program: Interlaboratory variability. In: *Antiepileptic Drugs: Quantitative Analysis and Interpretation,* edited by C. E. Pippenger, J. K. Penry, and H. Kutt, pp. 187–197. Raven Press, New York.

82. Pitlick, W. H., Levy, R. H., Troupin, A. S., and Green, J. R. (1976): Pharmacokinetic model to describe self-induced decreases in steady-state concentrations of carbamazepine. *J. Pharmacol. Sci.,* 65:462–463.

83. Pynnönen, S. (1979): Pharmacokinetics of carbamazepine in man: A review. *Ther. Drug Monit.,* 1:409–431.

84. Pynnönen, S., Frey, H., and Sillanpää, M. (1980): The auto-induction of carbamazepine during long-term therapy. *Int. J. Clin. Pharmacol. Ther. Toxicol.,* 18:247–252.

85. Pynnönen S., Sillanpää, M., Frey, H., and Iisalo, E. (1977): Carbamazepine and its 10,11-epoxide in children and adults with epilepsy. *Eur. J. Clin. Pharmacol.,* 11:129–133.

86. Rane, A., and Bertilsson, L. (1980): Kinetics of carbamazepine in epileptic children. In: *Antiepileptic Therapy: Advances in Drug Monitoring,* edited by S. I. Johannessen, P. L. Morselli, C. E. Pippenger, A. Richens, D. Schmidt, and H. Meinardi, pp. 49–56. Raven Press, New York.

87. Rane, A., Bertilsson, L., and Palmer, L. (1975): Disposition of placentally transferred carbamazepine (Tegretol®) in the newborn. *Eur. J. Clin. Pharmacol.,* 8:283–284.

88. Rane, A., Höjer, B., and Wilson, J. T. (1976): Ki-

netics of carbamazepine and its 10,11-epoxide metabolite in children. *Clin. Pharmacol. Ther.,* 19:276–283.

89. Rawlins, M. D., Collste, P., Bertilsson, L., and Palmer, L. (1975): Distribution and elimination kinetics of carbamazepine in man. *Eur. J. Clin. Pharmacol.,* 8:91–96.

90. Rey, E., D'Athis, P., de Lauture, D., Dulac, O., Aicardi, J., and Olive, G. (1979): Pharmacokinetics of carbamazepine in the neonate and in the child. *Int. J. Clin. Pharmacol. Biopharm.,* 17:90–96.

91. Reynolds., E. H. (1972): Discussion. In: *Tegretol in Epilepsy,* edited by C. A. S. Wink, pp. 118–126. C. Nicholls, Manchester.

92. Reynolds, E. H., and Shorvon, S. D. (1981): Monotherapy or polytherapy for epilepsy? *Epilepsia,* 22:1–10.

93. Rodin, E. A. (1968): *The Prognosis of Patients with Epilepsy.* Charles C Thomas, Springfield.

94. Rodin, E. A., Rim, C. S., and Rennick, P. M. (1974): The effects of carbamazepine on patients with psychomotor epilepsy: Results of a double-blind study. *Epilepsia,* 15:547–561.

95. Rylance, G. W., Moreland, T. A., and Butcher, G. M. (1979): Carbamazepine dose-frequency requirement in children. *Arch. Dis. Child.,* 54:454–458.

96. Salcman, M., and Pippenger, C. E. (1975): Acute carbamazepine encephalopathy. *J.A.M.A.,* 231:915.

97. Schmidt, D. (1980): One drug treatment with phenytoin in difficult-to-treat epilepsies with complex partial seizures: A preliminary report of a prospective study. In: *Antiepileptic Therapy: Advances in Drug Monitoring,* edited by S. I. Johannessen, P. L. Morselli, C. E. Pippenger, A. Richens, D. Schmidt, and H. Meinardi, pp. 221–228. Raven Press, New York.

98. Schneider, H. (1975): Carbamazepine: An attempt to correlate serum levels with anti-epileptic and side effects. In: *Clinical Pharmacology of Anti-Epileptic Drugs,* edited by H. Schneider, D. Janz, C. Gardner-Thorpe, H. Meinardi, and A. L. Sherwin, pp. 151–158. Springer-Verlag, Berlin.

99. Sheiner, L. B. (1980): Intelligent use of drug blood level data is helpful in managing patients. In: *Controversies in Therapeutics,* edited by L. Lasagna, pp. 100–105. W. B. Saunders, Philadelphia.

100. Shorvon, S. D., Galbraith, A. W., Laundy, M., Vydelingum, L., and Reynolds, E. H. (1980): Monotherapy for epilepsy. In: *Antiepileptic Therapy: Advances in Drug Monitoring,* edited by S. I. Johannessen, P. L. Morselli, C. E. Pippenger, A. Richens, D. Schmidt, and H. Meinardi, pp. 213–220. Raven Press, New York.

101. Shorvon, S. D., and Reynolds, E. H. (1977): Unnecessary polypharmacy for epilepsy. *Br. Med. J.,* 1:1635–1637.

102. Shorvon, S. D., and Reynolds, E. H. (1979): Reduction in polypharmacy for epilepsy. *Br. Med. J.,* 2:1023–1025.

103. Simonsen, N., Zander Olsen, P., Kühl, V., Lund, M., and Wendelboe, J. (1976): A comparative controlled study between carbamazepine and diphenylhydantoin in psychomotor epilepsy. *Epilepsia,* 17:169–176.

104. Smith, N. J., Espir, M. L. E., and Baylis, P. H. (1977): Raised plasma arginine vasopressin concentration in carbamazepine-induced water intoxication. *Br. Med. J.,* 2:804.

105. Stephens, W. P., Espir, M. L. E., Tattersall, R. B., Quinn, N. P., Gladwell, S. R. F., Galbraith, A. W., and Reynolds, E. H. (1977): Water intoxication due to carbamazepine. *Br. Med. J.,* 1:754–755.

106. Strandjord, R. E., and Johannessen, S. I. (1975): A preliminary study of serum carbamazepine levels in healthy subjects and in patients with epilepsy. In: *Clinical Pharmacology of Anti-Epileptic Drugs,* edited by H. Schneider, D. Janz, C. Gardner-Thorpe, H. Meinardi, and A. L. Sherwin, pp. 181–188. Springer-Verlag, Berlin.

107. Strandjord, R. E., and Johannessen, S. I. (1980): Carbamazepine as the only drug in patients with epilepsy: Serum levels and clinical effects. In: *Antiepileptic Therapy: Advances in Drug Monitoring,* edited by S. I. Johannessen, P. L. Morselli, C. E. Pippenger, A. Richens, D. Schmidt, and H. Meinardi, pp. 229–235. Raven Press, New York.

108. Strandjord, R. E., and Johannessen, S. I. (1980): Single-drug therapy with carbamazepine in patients with epilepsy: Serum levels and clinical effect. *Epilepsia,* 21:655–662.

109. Sullivan, J. B., Jr., Rumack, B. H., and Peterson, R. G. (1981): Acute carbamazepine toxicity resulting from overdose. *Neurology (NY),* 31:621–624.

110. Suzuki, K., Kaneko, S., and Sato, T. (1978): Time-dependency of serum carbamazepine concentration. *Folia Psychiatr. Neurol. Jpn.,* 32:199–209.

111. Tatzer, E., and Groh, C. (1980): Is the therapy with carbamazepine more effective when measuring blood levels? *Paediatr. Paedol.,* 15:293–296.

112. Tomson, T., Tybring, G., Bertilsson, L., Ekbom, K., and Rane, A. (1980): Carbamazepine therapy in trigeminal neuralgia: Clinical effects in relation to plasma concentration. *Arch. Neurol.,* 37:699–703.

113. Troupin, A. S. (1978): Carbamazepine in epilepsy. In: *Clinical Neuropharmacology, Vol. 3,* edited by H. L. Klawans, pp. 15–40. Raven Press, New York.

114. Troupin, A. S., Green, J. R., and Levy, R. H. (1974): Carbamazepine as an anticonvulsant: A pilot study. *Neurology (Minneap.),* 24:863–869.

115. Troupin, A. S., and Ojemann, L. M. (1975): Paradoxical intoxication—a complication of anticonvulsant administration. *Epilepsia,* 16:753–758.

116. Troupin, A., Ojemann, L. M., Halpern, L., Dodrill, C., Wilkus, R., Friel, P., and Feigl, P. (1977): Carbamazepine—a double blind comparison with phenytoin. *Neurology (Minneap.),* 27:511–519.

117. van der Kleijn, E., Vree, T. B., Guelen, P. J. M., Schobben, F., Westenberg, H., and Knop, H. J. (1978): Kinetics of drug interactions in the treatment of epilepsy. In: *Advances in Epileptology: Psychology, Pharmacotherapy and New Diagnostic Approaches,* edited by H. Meinardi and A. J. Rowan, pp. 197–210. Swets & Zeitlinger, Amsterdam.

118. Wada, J. A., Troupin, A. S., Friel, P., Remick, R., Leal, K., and Pearmain, J. (1978): Pharmacokinetic comparison of tablet and suspension dosage forms of carbamazepine. *Epilepsia,* 19:251–255.

Antiepileptic Drugs, edited by D. M. Woodbury, J. K. Penry, and C. E. Pippenger. Raven Press, New York © 1982.

41

Carbamazepine

Neurotoxicity

Richard L. Masland

An unusual feature of carbamazepine (CBZ) is that although neurological symptoms are the most common manifestations of overdosage, there are no reported instances of deaths directly attributable to neurotoxicity. Furthermore, there are no reports of irreversible neural damage from the direct neurotoxic effects of CBZ in either acute or chronic administration.

Reported forms of CBZ neurotoxicity are shown in Table 1. The commonest symptoms of overdosage are dizziness, double vision, drowsiness, headache, ataxia, and slurred speech (53,78). These symptoms can occur in almost anyone if the drug dosage is pushed to toxic levels. The tolerable level depends on the rate at which the dosage has been increased (22), the presence of other medications (41), and possibly the age of the patient (60). The tolerance level for the drug is higher when dosages are gradually increased over a 2-week period (21). In studies in which CBZ was added to preexisting medication, lower tolerance levels were observed than when it was administered as the single drug (5,41). A high incidence of neurotoxic effects has been observed in elderly patients receiving CBZ for the relief of trigeminal neuralgia. Possibly this has been because large doses have been required and dosages have been built up rapidly in order to achieve prompt relief of pain. Reports of dramatic enhancement of CBZ toxicity during concomitant administration of propoxyphene (Darvon®) (13) suggest that the toxicity that occurs when CBZ is used for relief of pain may be attributable to associated drugs.

TABLE 1. *Neurotoxic side effects of carbamazepine*

Brainstem	General(?)
Diplopia	Depression
Blurred vision	Irritability, hyperkinesis
Vertigo	Aggression
Cerebellar	Psychosis
Dizziness	Convulsions
Ataxia	Hypothalamic
Nystagmus	Water retention[a]
Extrapyramidal	Headache
Tremor	Peripheral
Chorea	Ageusia
Dystonia	Neuropathy[b]

[a]Uncertain whether origin is cerebral or renal.
[b]Not documented by individual case reports.

The variations in reported incidence of neurotoxicity are considerable. Thus, Killian and Fromm (39), reporting on 42 patients treated with CBZ for trigeminal neuralgia in a double-blind comparison, observed that 18% of the patients had vertigo and 32% were drowsy with doses of only 400 mg/day. At 600 mg/day, 43% had vertigo, and 50% were drowsy. In a similar review of 500 patients, Redpath and Gayford (57) noted drowsiness in 56%, ataxia in 46%, and gastrointestinal symptoms in 28%.

Kutt et al. (42), giving CBZ to patients already on other drugs, noted headache and drowsiness in about 25% and nystagmus and unsteadiness in about 50%. The usual dose was 1,200 mg/day with blood CBZ levels of 3.8 to 11.8 μg/ml (mean, 5.6 μg/ml). Seven patients who had some signs of ataxia on previous medication became worse when blood CBZ levels reached 4 μg/ml. In a study of 254 patients followed for 1 to 12 years, Hassan and Parsonage (31) noted the following neurotoxic side effects at the dosage ranges indicated: nausea (200–800 mg/day), blurred vision (1,000–1,200 mg/day), diplopia (800–1,000 mg/day), and dizziness (400–1,200 mg/day). No serious or irreversible changes were noted.

In a long-term follow-up (0.2–13.8 years) of 70 institutionalized patients, Schneider (67) did not report any whose CBZ was discontinued because of such side effects. Dosages ranged from 200 to 1,200 mg/day for women and 200 to 1,800 mg/day for men. Krueger (40) saw no permanent side effects in a series of patients treated for up to 10 years.

Callaghan et al. (5) found a very poor correlation among dosage, drug level, and toxic symptoms of CBZ. Among 13 patients taking CBZ as their only anticonvulsant, 11 (85%) developed some evidence of sedation, three (23%) developed diplopia or ataxia, and one (7.7%) had headache. Schneider (66) also documented the wide range of individual variation in tolerance. The average threshold for side effects was a blood CBZ level of 8.9 μg/ml; for pronounced drowsiness or ataxia, the level was 11.6 $\pm$ 4.3 μg/ml. However, the lowest blood CBZ level associated with side effects varied among individual patients from 5.9 to 22.05 μg/ml.

Meinardi (50) carried out an intensive investigation of six patients, giving progressively increasing dosages of CBZ and correlating blood levels of the drug with signs and symptoms as measured by a dexterity test and a battery of performance tests. The dexterity tests showed for each patient a high correlation coefficient with serum level of CBZ. The test that was most sensitive to increased serum levels of CBZ was simply "to place one dot in each of 100 circles scattered at random along a meandering line."

The patients were also observed for nystagmus, performance in rope walking and knee bending, diplopia, and dysarthria, and such subjective complaints as malaise, headache, feelings of inhibition, dizziness, drowsiness, disturbance of vision, and stomach discomfort. By means of probit analysis (17), a prediction was calculated of the percentage of subjects affected at serum CBZ levels ranging from 1.5 to 10 μg/ml. The results were arranged in three groups. Feelings of inhibition, stomach discomfort, diplopia, and malaise were not noted at low dosage, but these signs and complaints then increased rapidly until 40 to 50% of subjects were affected at levels of 8.5 to 10 μg/ml. Headache, disturbance of vision, and diplopia showed an almost linear rise with blood CBZ levels above 2 μg/ml. Nystagmus, drowsiness, and knee-bending and rope-walking performance were affected at very low drug levels (as low as 1.5 μg/ml) but seemed less enhanced at higher levels.

These studies and others emphasize that the neurotoxic symptoms of CBZ are diverse in nature. Whereas ataxia and incoordination are the predominant symptoms in patients with phenytoin intoxication, the commonest complaints of persons with CBZ intoxication are blurred or double vision and dizziness. These phenomena have been specifically studied (85). Incremental doses of CBZ to a total of 1,600 mg in 24 hr were given to three patients. The subjects developed drowsiness and disturbance of equilibrium, gait, and speech. Their oculomotor performance was tested for near point, gaze nystagmus, optokinetic nystagmus (OKN), and eye pursuit. On these tests, there was extension of the near point of convergence from the usual range of 30 to 40 mm to 60 to 80 mm after 800 mg of CBZ and to 180 to 250 mm after 1,600 mg. Gaze nystagmus was dysmetric and pendular on severe dosages, but these cerebellar signs disappeared on the lower doses, whereas convergence weakness and paretic gaze nystagmus persisted. Optokinetic nystagmus was depressed, a finding not true in cerebellar ataxia, and the pursuit test was mildly affected, suggesting upper brainstem involvement. It was concluded that when a cerebellar component was operative at higher dosages, the upper brainstem was also involved. Schneider (67) also noted that CBZ-induced nystagmus differs from that elicited by phenytoin and is "optokinetic" in type. Killian and Fromm (39) did nystagmography on a patient who showed slight unsteadiness while receiving CBZ (800 mg/day) and found bilateral labyrinthine abnormalities, with canal paresis on the left and hypoactivity of the right labyrinth. These effects were transitory. Hypoexcitability of the vestibular system was also noted by Warot et al. (87) and by Salcman and Pippenger (64) in cases of massive CBZ overdosage.

MASSIVE OVERDOSAGE

There are now reports of at least 15 persons who have experienced massive overdosage of CBZ, with doses ranging from 1.2 to 20 g (Table 2). No fatalities have been reported. Because of vomiting and/or gastric lavage, the exact amounts of drug retained and the corresponding blood levels of CBZ were uncertain. One patient who took 20 g had a blood CBZ level over 20 μg/ml (26). After an initial period of excitability, these patients lapsed into a period of stupor during which they were unresponsive to voice but were often hyperirritable or combative following painful stimuli.

One child was described as cyanotic (28). Respiratory impairment was noted in two other patients (26,45). In one, it followed administration of pentobarbital sodium (Nembutal®) for the control of status epilepticus. The pupils were uniformly dilated, usually sluggish to light, and, in one case, unresponsive (28). When tested, caloric responses were diminished or absent (64,87). The reflexes were weak, normally active, or overactive. In two instances, plantar responses were abnormal (27,45).

The recovery phase was generally marked by hyperirritability, hallucinations, or delirium. Myoclonic and ballistic movements were noted, and three patients experienced generalized convulsions (28,45,48). One patient developed status epilepticus. Recovery of consciousness usually occurred within 48 hr, although one patient remained unconscious for 6 days (26). Also noted were nystagmus and severe ataxia, with persistent somnolence in some cases. One patient was described as "drowsy, euphoric, uninhibited and ataxic" (29). No permanent sequelae were noted.

De Zeeuw et al. (14) reported an unusual case of CBZ intoxication in which there was a sudden worsening about 45 hr after the ingestion of 18 g of the drug. Although gastric lavage had been carried out at the time of hospitalization, the patient experienced a late rise in blood CBZ levels from an initial value of 29 μg/ml to a high of 44 μg/ml (carbamazepine 10,11-epoxide rose from 14 μg/ml to 22 μg/ml). The patient became deeply comatose and "exhibited respiratory problems requiring supportive therapy." It was postulated that the delayed rise in CBZ levels resulted from absorption of the drug from the small intestine. It was further suggested that absorption was delayed because intestinal motility was reduced by the anticholinergic action of the drug.

ENHANCEMENT OF SEIZURES

As noted above, convulsions are a clinical manifestation of acute intoxication with CBZ. It was felt that the seizure was a postasphyxic phenomenon in the 2-year-old child who became cyanotic after CBZ overdosage (28). One patient had a seizure about 12 hr after the ingestion of CBZ (48). Another developed a prolonged seizure that required the use of intravenous and intramuscular pentobarbital and was followed by severe respiratory depression requiring respiratory assist and tracheostomy (45). A patient had ballistic and convulsive movements before lapsing into coma (26), but it is doubtful that this was actually a seizure. The question arises as to whether the occurrence of seizures in some of these patients may have been, in fact, a withdrawal effect after the initial establishment of a high blood level of CBZ. However, withdrawal effects have not been a prominent feature of CBZ, and the appearance of seizures during acute intoxication in animals

TABLE 2. Case reports of massive overdosage with carbamazepine

Investigator	Age (yr)	Dose (g)	Respiration	Pupillary reaction	Labyrinth response	Tendon reflexes	Babinski reflex	Convulsion	Coma (days)	Recovery (days)
de Zeeuw et al. (14)	23	16	Respiratory support	NA	NA	NA	NA	NA	3	5
Gruska et al. (26)	41	20	Respiratory support	Slow	NA	Active	Normal	"Spasms"	6	17
Güntelberg (27)	14	17	—	Slow	NA	Absent	Abnormal	—	3	NA
Hager (28)	2	1.4	Cyanotic	Absent	NA	Weak	Abnormal	Convulsion	½	1
Hajnsek and Sartorius (29)	31	20	—	Slow	NA	Active	Normal	—	2	14
Lang-Petersen (45)	19	10-14	Respiratory support	Normal	NA	Absent	Abnormal	Status	4	?
Livingston et al. (48)	18	10-12	—	(Papilledema)	NA	Weak	?	Convulsion	2	4
Livingston et al. (48)	14	5+	—	NA	NA	NA	NA	—	2	7
Salcman and Pippenger (64)	NA	5.8	—	Normal	Absent	Active	Normal	—	1	4
Smoot and Wood (71)	15	10	—	Slow	NA	Weak	Abnormal	—	1½	2
Taghevy and Naumann (79)	16	1.2-2	—	NA	NA	NA	NA	—	0	5
Taghevy and Naumann (79)	38	10	—	NA	NA	NA	NA	—	?	4
Volmat et al. (86)	15	3	—	NA	NA	Normal	Normal	—	0	2
Volmat et al. (86)	30	10	—	NA	NA	NA	NA	—	3	9
Warot et al. (88)	28	10	—	Slow	Depressed	Normal	Normal	—	1	3

NA–not available.

given large doses of CBZ (74,86) is more suggestive of a direct effect of the drug (74).

Enhancement of seizures following the addition of CBZ to the therapeutic regimen of persons with epilepsy has been frequently reported (16,42). Most trials reported a few patients whose seizure frequency increased with the use of CBZ. In these instances, enhancement of seizures may represent random changes in seizure susceptibility. However, Troupin and Ojemann (83) reported several instances in which repeated administration of the drug caused seizure enhancement. They also noted that, like phenytoin, CBZ in overdoses (blood level greater than 20 µg/ml) can lead to seizure enhancement along with other signs of intoxication. Thus, it seems clear that CBZ in overdosage may be a convulsant drug and that dosages within the therapeutic range can cause seizure enhancement in some patients.

DYSTONIA AND MYOCLONUS

Various forms of involuntary movement disorder have been reported from the use of CBZ, most commonly in elderly or brain-damaged individuals. Crosley and Swender (9) reported severe movement disorders in three brain-damaged and severely epileptic children treated with CBZ in doses of 25 mg/kg per day. Over the course of 3 weeks, the children developed dystonia progressing to severe opisthotonus. When the drug was discontinued, the symptoms disappeared over a 3-week period. In one child, this experience was repeated a second time.

Chadwick et al. (7) compared the occurrence of three forms of movement disorder—chorea, dystonia, and asterixis—with the use of anticonvulsants and concluded that CBZ produces only asterixis, whereas phenytoin may produce chorea and dystonia.

Jacome (36) described four patients who developed transient dystonia while under treatment with CBZ. In three, this affected the axial muscles, and in one, the extremities. In each instance, symptoms occurred when the dosage exceeded 1,000 mg/day. The report does not state whether there was concomitant medication.

McLellan and Swash (49) reported a patient who developed nystagmus, ataxia, and impaired gaze and then generalized chorea enhanced by movement when CBZ (800 mg/day) was added to primidone (750 mg/day) and phenytoin (450 mg/day). The blood phenytoin level was 37 µg/ml, so the role of that drug cannot be excluded.

Wendland (88) described three patients who developed myoclonus. One was a 70-year-old woman who developed myoclonic movements of the arms 3 days after being treated with CBZ (600 mg/day). A 29-year-old man developed a similar reaction on 1,200 mg/day, and a 56-year-old woman developed severe myoclonus when CBZ (1,200 mg/day) was added to phenobarbital (45 mg/day) plus four tablets of Comital® (100 mg mephobarbital and 50 mg phenytoin) and three tablets (under 300 mg) of chlorprothixene a day. In each instance, the myoclonus disappeared within 1 to 7 days after termination of treatment.

Ironically, there are two reports of treatment of dystonia with CBZ. In a 14-year-old girl, CBZ was used to treat familial paroxysmal kinesigenic choreoathetosis, a violent movement disorder precipitated by voluntary movement (37). The violent movements were completely relieved by CBZ in a daily dose of 600 mg (133 mg/kg per day). Carbamazepine was also used in the treatment of four hereditary and four acquired cases of torsion dystonia (24). In a placebo-controlled study, significant improvement was noted with dosages of 300 to 1,200 mg/day.

PSYCHOTROPIC EFFECTS

Although coma occurs with massive overdosage of CBZ, and drowsiness is a frequent complaint during dosage within the therapeutic range, mental depression is an uncommon side effect. Patients lapsing into coma frequently pass through a phase of restless agitation, and recovery may be characterized by hyperreactive behavior, aggressiveness, and hallucinations. The close chemical resemblance of CBZ to imipramine suggests that the anticonvulsant effect of CBZ might be accompanied by a beneficial psychotropic effect. The behavioral results of CBZ therapy have been reviewed by Dalby (12). In a survey of 40 reports covering 2,500 patients, a beneficial effect was observed in half of them. However, the thesis that CBZ has a positive psychotropic effect has been difficult to prove. In a review of the literature, Trimble and Reynolds (82) found no satisfactory proof of a psychotropic effect.

Rennick et al. (58), in a controlled comparison of CBZ and phenytoin, could not confirm changes in personality, emotional adjustment, or observable behavior attributable to CBZ. Psychological effects were "minimal and unpredictable." There was a definite but small impairment of arousal and attention, suggestive of a mild sedative effect. (Patients were tested by a cognitive, perceptual–motor battery and by personality and behavior inventories.)

The unpredictable nature of this response was also documented by Rett (59) in a study of 300 children. He noted that the psychotropic effect is influenced by intelligence. Imbeciles and idiots tended to become perseverative and irritable.

Most other reported studies have been open-label and uncontrolled. Most of the controlled studies have involved comparison of CBZ with other drugs known to be depressants. Improvement with the use of CBZ may be attributable to discontinuation of the depressant drugs (81). In such studies, CBZ has been shown to be less depressant than phenobarbital, primidone, or even phenytoin (6,60,61,84). Jacobides (35) found increased alertness and scholastic achievement of epileptic school children when they were treated with CBZ. Lerman and Kivity-Ephriam (46) observed improved school performance in 80% of a group of children treated with CBZ as the sole anticonvulsant. Schain et al. (65) noted improved attention and perceptual abilities over a 4- to 6-month period in children taken off phenobarbital and primidone and placed on CBZ.

An even more significant documentation of the lack of a depressant effect of CBZ is the long-term follow-up of resident epileptic children (81), many of whom were severely retarded. Among these children were 31 whose IQ (WAIS or WISC) had fallen by 10 points or more on two tests taken a year or more apart. There were significant negative correlations between test performance and serum levels of phenobarbital, primidone, and phenytoin, but no such correlations were noted with CBZ.

That these findings are not entirely caused by withdrawal of depressant drugs is demonstrated by the effects of CBZ in patients without epilepsy who were treated for behavioral or emotional problems. In a double-blind study (25) of 20 such nonepileptic children, the treated group was significantly improved over the untreated group, as noted by observer rating scales of initiative, dysphorias, and neurotic anxiety. They also showed improved attention and perseverance on psychological testing. Improvement of behavior after treatment with CBZ has also been noted in children with psychiatric disorders who have abnormal electroencephalograms but are without overt seizures (15).

Reports vary regarding the nature and degree of psychic response to CBZ. These variations may depend on the population being studied. The "psychotropic" action is uniformly described as an increase in the psychic tempo—improvement in sluggishness, perseveration, apathy, and lack of initiative (12). There is less consistency regarding the effects on mood. Some observers report that affective changes such as irritability, aggression, impulsiveness, and depression are reduced and give way to elevation of mood. Others (73) note that emotional lability, irritability, and aggressivity were less commonly improved but sometimes worsened. These latter observations may relate especially to sluggish, severely retarded patients when sedatives are replaced by CBZ.

PSYCHOSES

Whereas most reports have emphasized the beneficial effects of CBZ on mood and behavior, there are also well-documented reports of psychoses in patients undergoing CBZ treatment (47). Among 93 patients followed for 6 years, Stores (77) noted five who developed severe mental disorders: one was schizoid, three were emotionally explosive and confused, and one was confused and had increased seizures. Berger (3) reported the case of a 76-year-old woman treated for trigeminal neuralgia who developed a toxic psychosis, including active hallucinosis, when given a daily dose of 400 mg of CBZ for 8 weeks. Symptoms disappeared in 2 days when the drug was discontinued and recurred within 2 weeks when a dose of 240 mg/day was given. This patient had previously been treated with various pain killers including propoxyphene. In view of the reported enhancement of CBZ effects by propoxyphene, one wonders whether it might have been administered concomitantly.

Franks and Richter (19) described a 23-year-old man undergoing treatment with primidone (650 mg/day), CBZ (600 mg/day), and clonazepam (10 mg/day) who developed slurred speech and bizarre behavior, then a schizophrenic-like illness with choreoathetoid movements. There was no impairment of memory or attention. These symptoms stopped when CBZ was discontinued. O'Donohoe (54) noted a schizophrenic-like withdrawal in one child among 30 treated with CBZ. Dalby (10,11), in a follow-up study of 93 epileptic children, noted four whose medication was discontinued because of severe psychic reactions. One developed severe anxiety and hallucinosis. Three developed explosive fits of rage and confusion. These manifestations ceased when CBZ was discontinued. Ganglberger (23) reported a 25-year-old postencephalitic epileptic patient taking phenytoin (300 mg/day) who developed hallucinosis when his tonic–clonic and complex partial seizures were controlled with the addition of CBZ (900 mg/day). The psychosis cleared when the CBZ was gradually discontinued but his seizures returned. This may represent an example of "forced normalization" (43,44,68).

In summary, the use of CBZ has been associated with significant improvement of alertness and of mood, especially in patients previously sedated with other more depressant drugs. In some patients it may have an additional psychotropic effect. However, in many persons it also has a depressant effect, and in a few it has caused enhanced irritability and even psychosis.

DISORDERS OF TASTE

Two observers have associated disorders of taste with the use of CBZ (30,62,63). In three instances, the drug was suspected of having caused gustatory disorders of the nature of "bitter phantageusia." In one case, progressive loss of taste was observed after 6 weeks of treatment. Taste was lost to salt, sweet, and bitter but retained to sour and to electrical stimulation. Recovery took place within 6 weeks.

PERIPHERAL NEUROPATHY

Carbamazepine has been used extensively in the treatment of trigeminal neuralgia and has been reported to benefit postherpetic neuralgia (dubious), causalgia, and various other forms of painful neuropathy. These reports do not include references to worsening that might have been attributable to CBZ. Chakrobarti and Samantary (8) treated 54 patients with diabetic neuropathy for periods of up to 1 year. Forty-nine had symptomatic relief of pain, but nerve conduction velocity was unchanged. There was no reference to worsening. However, neuropathy was named as a complication of CBZ therapy by several authors (1,51), although specific case reports were not given. This neuropathy must be extremely mild, uncommon, and reversible. In a study of 70 adults followed for periods of 5 to 7 years, polyneuropathy was listed as a cause for discontinuation of treatment in one case (67). The study also noted, however, that "the side effects mentioned were fully reversible." Five- to 10-year follow-up studies by Gamstorp (20,21) made no reference to neuropathy. Kreuger (40) followed 59 patients for periods of up to 10 years and observed no irreversible neurological complications. His study included no reference to neuropathy.

WATER RETENTION

An important but little recognized late complication of CBZ therapy is water retention. Occasionally, fluid retention and sodium loss may reach such proportions as to produce neurological symptoms, including headache, dyspnea, and mental confusion (2,18,34,38,52,69,72, 75,76). The phenomenon is reported most commonly in elderly patients being treated for trigeminal neuralgia, in patients with cardiac disease (4), and in cases of psychogenic polydipsia (56,76). Similar changes also occur in children (33). In a study of 80 persons with epilepsy and 50 control subjects, Perucca et al. (55) demonstrated grossly impaired ability to excrete a water load, with decreased plasma osmolality and lowered serum sodium in five patients. Thus, the picture very closely resembles that of the inappropriate antidiuretic hormone secretion syndrome. There are, however, opposing opinions as to whether the antidiuretic effect of CBZ is exerted on the hypothalamic osmoreceptors and depends on secretion of antidiuretic hormone, as measured by serum arginine vasopressin (AVP) levels, or whether it is the result of a direct action on the renal tubules. Some investigators (70,80) have observed significant changes in AVP and have found a normal correlation between AVP levels and urine osmolality. This suggests that it is alteration in the release of AVP rather than alteration of kidney response that accounts for the antidiuretic effect of CBZ. Other investigators (32,75,76), however, using immunoassay measurements of 8-arginine vasopressin, found a decline rather than an increase in this hormone during treatment with CBZ. Such a decline occurred in 10 of 12 CBZ-treated subjects (75). This decline occurred in spite of a water-loading test. It was concluded that the water retention cannot be a response to increased secretion of antidiuretic hormone but must represent increased renal sensitivity to normal concentrations of AVP.

Whatever the mechanism, the possibility of water retention with hyponatremia should be considered in patients developing signs of headache, mental confusion, and dyspnea after prolonged treatment with CBZ.

ELECTROENCEPHALOGRAPHIC CHANGES

The EEG changes from CBZ overdosage differ from those caused by barbiturate overdosage. Whereas fast activity is a prominent feature of the barbiturate effect, the EEG in the case of CBZ intoxication is characterized by generalized polymorphic theta and delta waves. Clinical improvement of seizure control by CBZ is not associated with diminution of epileptic activity or other abnormalities of the EEG. In fact, there may even be enhancement of preexisting abnormalities, including epileptic spike discharges (53).

SUMMARY AND CONCLUSIONS

There are no published reports of irreversible neurological effects of CBZ following either acute or chronic administration of the drug. The commonest symptoms of overdosage are diplopia and dizziness. Enhancement of seizures may occur, especially with overdosage. Various forms of CBZ-induced movement disorders, especially in elderly patients, have occurred in rare instances. Irritable and aggressive behavior sometimes occurs, especially among mentally retarded subjects. Toxic psychoses have been reported. Disturbances of taste have been noted in three reports. There are unsubstantiated reports of peripheral neuropathy. An often unrecognized complication of CBZ therapy is water retention, with high blood volume and low salt, variously attributed to inappropriate antidiuretic hormone secretion or to a direct effect of CBZ on the kidney. Among 15 reported cases of massive overdosage, there were no fatalities. Thus, from the standpoint of neurotoxicity, CBZ is a very safe drug.

REFERENCES

1. Arieff, A. J., and Mier, M. (1966): Anticonvulsant and psychotropic action of Tegretol. *J. Neurol.,* 16:107–110.
2. Ashton, M. D., Ball, S. G., Thomas, T. H., and Lee, M. R. (1977): Water intoxication associated with carbamazepine treatment. *Br. Med. J.,* 1:1134–1135.
3. Berger, H. (1971): An unusual manifestation of Tegretol (carbamazepine) toxicity. *Ann. Intern. Med.,* 74:449–450.
4. Byrne, E., Wong, C. H., Chambers, D. G., and Rice, J. P. (1979): Carbamazepine therapy complicated by nodal bradycardia and water intoxication. *Aust. N.Z. J. Med.,* 9:295–296.
5. Callaghan, N., O'Callaghan, M., Duggan, B., and Feely, M. (1978): Carbamazepine as a single drug in the treatment of epilepsy. A prospective study of serum

levels and seizure control. *J. Neurol. Neurosurg. Psychiatry*, 41:907–912.

6. Cereghino, J. J., Brock, J. T., VanMeter, J. C., Penry, J. K., Smith, L. D., and White, B. G. (1974): Carbamazepine for epilepsy: A controlled prospective evaluation. *Neurology (Minneap.)*, 24:401–410.

7. Chadwick, D., Reynolds, E. H., and Marsden, C. D. (1976): Anticonvulsant induced dyskinesias: A comparison with dyskinesias induced by neuroleptics. *J. Neurol. Neurosurg. Psychiatry*, 39:1210–1218.

8. Chakrobarti, A. K., and Samantary, S. K. (1976): Diabetic peripheral neuropathy: Nerve conduction studies before, during and after carbamazepine therapy. *Aust. N.Z. J. Med.*, 6:565–568.

9. Crosley, C. J., and Swender, P. T. (1979): Dystonia associated with carbamazepine administration: Experience in brain-damaged children. *Pediatrics*, 63:612–615.

10. Dalby, M. A. (1971): Antiepileptic and psychotropic effect of carbamazepine (Tegretol) in the treatment of psychomotor epilepsy. *Epilepsia*, 12:325–334.

11. Dalby, M. A. (1972): Antiepileptic and psychotropic effect of Tegretol in temporal lobe epilepsy. In: *Tegretol in Epilepsy*, edited by C. A. S. Wink, pp. 98–106. C. S. Nichols & Co., Manchester.

12. Dalby, M. A. (1975): Behavioral effects of carbamazepine. *Adv. Neurol.*, 11:331–344.

13. Dam, M., and Christiansen, J. (1977): Interaction of propoxyphene with carbamazepine. *Lancet*, 2:509.

14. de Zeeuw, R. A., Westenberg, H. G., Van der Kleijn, K., and Gimbrere, J. S. (1979): An unusual case of carbamazepine poisoning with a near fatal relapse after two days. *Clin. Toxicol.*, 14:263–269.

15. Donner, M., and Frisk, M. (1965): Carbamazepine treatment of epileptic and psychic symptoms in children and adolescents. *Ann. Paediatr. Fenn.*, 11:91–97.

16. Feely, M. (1977): Plasma carbamazepine levels in the control of epilepsy—a prospective study. In: *Tegretol in Epilepsy*, edited by F. D. Roberts, pp. 79–88. Geigy Pharmaceuticals, Macclesfield, England.

17. Finney, D. J. (1964): *Probit Analysis, Second Edition*. Cambridge University Press, Cambridge.

18. Flegel, K. M., and Cole, C. H. (1977): Inappropriate antidiuresis during carbamazepine treatment. *Ann. Intern. Med.*, 87:722–723.

19. Franks, R. D., and Richter, A. J. (1979): Schizophrenia-like psychosis associated with anticonvulsant toxicity. *Am. J. Psychiatry*, 131:973–974.

20. Gamstorp, I. (1970): Long-term follow-up of children with severe epilepsy treated with carbamazepine. *Acta Paediatr. Scand. [Suppl]*, 206:96–97.

21. Gamstorp, I. (1972): Nine years' experience with Tegretol in epileptic children. In: *Tegretol in Epilepsy*, edited by C. A. S. Wink, pp. 6–11. C. Nichols & Co., Manchester.

22. Gamstorp, I. (1975): Treatment with carbamazepine Children. *Adv. Neurol.*, 11:237–248.

23. Ganglberger, J. A. (1968): Erfahrungen mit dem Psychotropen Anticonvulsivum Tegretol in Neurochirurgie. *Wien Med. Wochenschr.*, 118:956–962.

24. Geller, M., Kaplan, B., and Kristoff, N. (1976): Treatment of dystonic symptoms with carbamazepine. *Adv. Neurol.*, 14:403–410.

25. Groh, C., Rosemayr, F., and Birbaumer, H. (1971):

Psychotropic effect of carbamazepine in nonepileptic children. *Med. Monatsschr.*, 25:329–333.

26. Gruska, H., Beyer, K. H., Kubucki, S., and Schneider, H. (1971): Course, toxicology and therapy of a case of severe carbamazepine poisoning. *Arch. Toxicol.*, 27:193–203.

27. Güntelberg, E. (1967): Carbamazepine (Tegretol) Forgiftning. En Oversigt og et Tilfaelde. *Ugeskr. Laeger*, 129:161–163.

28. Hager, H. (1965): Akute Tegretol-Vergiftung bei Zweizahringun Kind. *Paediatr. Prox.*, 4:241–243.

29. Hajnsek, T., and Sartorius, N. (1964): A case of intoxication with Tegretol. *Epilepsia*, 5:371–375.

30. Halbreich, U. (1974): Tegretol dependency and diversion of the sense of taste. *Isr. Ann. Psychiatry*, 12:328–332.

31. Hassan, M. N., and Parsonage, M. J. (1977): Experience in the long-term use of carbamazepine (Tegretol) in the treatment of epilepsy. In: *Epilepsy: The Eighth International Symposium*, edited by J. K. Penry, pp. 35–44. Raven Press, New York.

32. Heim, M., Conte-Devoix, B., Bonnefoy, M., and Boyard, P. (1979): Measurement of serum 8-arginine vasopressin level by radioimmunoassay in normal subjects during water loading before and during carbamazepine treatment. *Pathol. Biol.*, 27:95–98.

33. Helin, L., Nilsson, K. O., Bjerre, I., and Vegfors, P. (1977): Serum sodium and osmolality during carbamazepine treatment in children. *Br. Med. J.*, 2:558.

34. Henry, D. A., Lawson, D. H., Reavey, P., and Renfrew, S. (1977): Hyponatremia during carbamazepine treatment. *Br. Med. J.*, 1:83–84.

35. Jacobides, G. M. (1978): Alertness and scholastic achievement in young epileptics treated with carbamazepine (Tegretol). In: *Advances in Epileptology 1977: Psychology, Pharmacotherapy, and New Diagnostic Approaches* edited by H. Meinardi and A. J. Rowan, pp. 114–119. Swets & Zeitlinger, Amsterdam.

36. Jacome, D. (1979): Carbamazepine-induced dystonia. *J.A.M.A.*, 241:2263.

37. Kato, M., and Araki, S. (1969): Paroxysmal kinesigenic choreoathetosis. Report of a case relieved by carbamazepine. *Arch. Neurol.*, 20:508–513.

38. Kato, D. B. (1978): Dilutional hyponatremia and water intoxication during carbamazepine therapy: Case report and review of the literature. *Drug Intell. Clin. Pharm.*, 12:392–396.

39. Killian, J. M., and Fromm, G. H. (1968): Carbamazepine in treatment of neuralgia. Use and side effects. *Arch. Neurol.*, 19:129–136.

40. Krueger, H. J. (1972): Nine years follow up of treatment of epilepsy with carbamazepine. *Med. Welt*, 23:896–898.

41. Kutt, H. (1974): Use of blood levels of anticonvulsant drugs in clinical practice. *Pediatrics*, 53:557–560.

42. Kutt, H., Solomon, G., Wasterlain, C., Peterson, H., Louis, S., and Carruthers, R. (1975): Carbamazepine in difficult to control epileptic out-patients. *Acta Neurol. Scand. [Suppl.]*, 60:27–32.

43. Landolt, H. (1953): Some clinical electroencephalographic correlations in epileptic psychoses (twilight states). *Electroencephalogr. Clin. Neurophysiol.*, 5:121.

44. Landolt, H. (1956): L'Electroencephalogrie dans les

psychoses epileptiques et les episodes schizophre-
niques. *Rev. Neurol.* 95:597–598.

45. Lang-Petersen, J. (1969): Poisoning with carbamazepine. *Ugeskr. Laeg.,* 131:1131–1133.

46. Lerman, P., and Kivity-Ephriam, S. (1974): Carbamazepine. Sole anticonvulsant for focal epilepsy in
children. *Epilepsia,* 15:229–234.

47. Leviator, V. M., Vesclovskaia, T. D., Mar'enjo, G.
F., and Shchegoleva, A. P. (1975): Tegretol psychoses in epileptic patients. *Z. Neuropatol. Psi-
khiatr.,* 75:396–400.

48. Livingston, S., Pauli, L. I., and Berman, W. (1974):
Carbamazepine in epilepsy. *Dis. Nerv. Syst.,* 35:103–
107.

49. McLellan, D. L., and Swash, M. (1974): Choreoathetosis and encephalopathy induced by phenytoin. *Br.
Med. J.,* 2:204–205.

50. Meinardi, H. (1973): Other antiepileptic drugs: Carbamazepine. In: *Antiepileptic Drugs,* edited by D. M.
Woodbury, J. K. Penry, and R. P. Schmidt, pp. 487–
496. Raven Press, New York.

51. Meinardi, H., and Stoel, M. K. (1974): Side effects
of anticonvulsant drugs. In: *Handbook of Clinical
Neurology,* edited by P. J. Vinken and G. W. Bruyn,
pp. 705–738. North-Holland, Amsterdam.

52. Moses, A. M., and Miller, M. (1974): Drug-induced
hyponatremia. *N. Engl. J. Med.,* 291:1234–1237.

53. Muller, J., and Muller, D. (1972): Correlation between brain electric activity and overdose of anticonvulsants. *Nervenarzt,* 43:270–272.

54. O'Donohoe, N. V. (1973): A series of epileptic children treated with Tegretol. In: *Tegretol in Epilepsy,*
edited by C. A. S. Wink, pp. 25–29. C. S. Nichols
& Co., Manchester.

55. Perucca, E., Garrott, A., Hebdige, S., and Richens,
A. (1978): Water intoxication in epileptic patients receiving carbamazepine. *J. Neurol. Neurosurg. Psychiatry,* 41:713–718.

56. Rado, J. P. (1973): Water intoxication during carbamazepine treatment. *Br. Med. J.,* 3:479.

57. Redpath, T. H., and Gayford, T. J. (1968): The side
effects of carbamazepine therapy. *Oral Surg.,* 26:299–
303.

58. Rennick, P., Keiser, T., and Rodin, E. (1975): Carbamazepine (Tegretol): Behavioral side effects in
temporal lobe epilepsy during a short term comparison with placebo. *Epilepsia,* 16:198.

59. Rett, A. (1973): Tegretol therapy of epileptic children. In: *Tegretol in Epilepsy,* edited by C. A. S.
Wink, pp. 12–15. C. Nichols & Co., Manchester.

60. Reynolds, E. H. (1975): Neurotoxicity of carbamazepine. *Adv. Neurol.,* 11:345–353.

61. Rodin, E. A., Kim, C. S., Ketano, H., Lewis, R.,
and Rennick, P. M. (1975): A comparison of the effectiveness of primidone vs. carbamazepine in epileptic out-patients. *J. Nerv. Ment. Dis.,* 163:41
–46.

62. Rollin, H. (1976): Gustatory disturbances as side effects of medical treatment. *Laryngol. Rhinol. Otol.
(Stuttg.),* 55:873–878.

63. Rollin, H. (1978): Drug-related gustatory disorders.
Ann. Otol. Rhinol. Laryngol., 87:37–42.

64. Salcman, M., and Pippenger, C. E. (1975): Acute
carbamazepine encephalopathy. *J.A.M.A.,* 231:915.

65. Schain, R. J., Ward, J. W., and Guthrie, D. (1977):
Carbamazepine as an anticonvulsant in children. *Neurology (Minneap.),* 27:476–480.

66. Schneider, H. (1975): Carbamazepine: An attempt to
correlate serum levels with anti-epileptic and side effects. In: *Clinical Pharmacology of Anti-epileptic
Drugs,* edited by H. Schneider, D. Janz, C. Gardner-
Thorpe, H. Meinardi, and A. L. Sherwin, pp. 151–
158. Springer-Verlag, New York.

67. Schneider, H. (1977): Long-term treatment in severe
epilepsy (institutionalized patients): II. Retrospective
Evaluation of Carbamazepine. In: *Epilepsy: The Eighth
International Symposium,* edited by J. K. Penry, pp.
57–62. Raven Press, New York.

68. Scott, J. S., and Masland, R. L. (1953): Occurrence
of "continuous symptoms" in epilepsy patients. *Neurology (Minneap.),* 3:297–301.

69. Singh, A. N. (1978): Fluid retention during treatment
with carbamazepine. *Can. Med. Assoc. J.,* 118:24.

70. Smith, N. J., Espir, M. L., and Bayles, P. N. (1977):
Raised plasma arginine vasopressin concentration in
carbamazepine-induced water retention. *Br. Med. J.,*
2:804.

71. Smoot, C. A., and Wood, D. L. (1977): Carbamazepine toxicity: Report of a case. *J. Am. Osteopath.
Assoc.,* 76:758–760.

72. Sordello, P., Sagransky, D. M., Mercado, R. M.,
and Michelis, M. F. (1978): Carbamazepine-induced
syndrome of inappropriate ADH secretion. Reversal
by concomitant phenyton therapy. *Arch. Intern. Med.,*
138:299–300.

73. Steinbrecher, W. (1966): Therapie zerebraler Ansfal-
laformen mit Tegretol. *Med. Welt,* 25:1381–1385.

74. Stenger, E. G., and Roulet, F. C. (1964): On the
toxicity of the antiepileptic agent Tegretol. *Med. Exp.
(Basel),* 11:191–201.

75. Stephens, W. P., Coe, J. Y., and Baylis, P. H. (1978):
Plasma arginine vasopressin concentration and antidiuretic action of carbamazepine. *Br. Med. J.,* 1:1445–
1447.

76. Stephens, W. P., Espir, M. L. E., Tattersall, R. B.,
Quinn, N. P., Gladwell, S. R. F., Galbreith, A. W.,
and Reynolds, E. H. (1977): Water intoxication due
to carbamazepine. *Br. Med. J.,* 1:754–755.

77. Stores, G. (1975): Behavioural effects of anti-epileptic drugs. *Dev. Med. Child Neurol.,* 17:647–658.

78. Strandjord, R. E., and Johannessen, S. I. (1975): A
preliminary study of serum carbamazepine levels in
healthy subjects and in patients with epilepsy. In:
Clinical Pharmacology of Anti-Epileptic Drugs. Edited by H. Schneider, D. Janz, C. Gardner-Thorpe,
H. Meinardi, and A. L. Sherwin, pp. 181–187. Springer-Verlag, New York.

79. Taghevy, A., and Naumann, L. (1971): Tegretol intoxication. *Electroencephalogr. Clin. Neurophysiol.,*
30:264.

80. Thomas, T. H., Ball, S. G., Wales, J. K., and Lee,
M. R. (1978): Effect of carbamazepine on plasma and
urine arginine-vasopressin. *Clin. Sci. Mol. Med.,*
54:419–424.

81. Trimble, M. R., Thompson, P. J. and Huppert, F.
(1980): Anticonvulsant Drugs and Cognitive Abilities. In: *Advances in Epileptology: XIth Epilepsy
International Symposium,* edited by R. Canger, F.

Angeleri, and J. K. Penry, pp. 199–204. Raven Press, New York.

82. Trimble, M. R., and Reynolds, E. H. (1976) Anticonvulsant drugs and mental symptoms: A review: *Psychol. Med.*, 6:169–178.

83. Troupin, A. S., and Ojemann, L. M. (1968): Paradoxical intoxication: A complication of anticonvulsant administration. *Epilepsia*, 16:753–758.

84. Troupin, A., Ojemann, L. M., Halpern, L., Dodrill, C., Wilkus, R., Friel, P., and Feigl, P. (1977): Carbamazepine—a double-blind comparison with phenytoin. *Neurology (Minneap.)*, 27:511–519.

85. Umida, Y., and Sakata, E. (1977): Equilibrium disorders in carbamazepine toxicity. *Ann. Otol. Rhinol. Laryngol.*, 86:318–322.

86. Volmat, R., Beaudouin, J. L., Collin, J., Nicolas-Charles, P. J., and Allers, G. (1964): Experimentation clinique du Tegretol dans l'epilepsie grave et les syndromes douloureux rebelles. *Centre-Est Med.*, 40:1395–1405.

87. Warot, P., Arnott, G., Delahousse, J., and Pettit, H. (1967): Acute ataxia after massive ingestion of Tegretol: Favorable development. *Lille Med.*, 12:601–604.

88. Wendland, K. I. (1968): Myoclonus following doses of carbamazepine. *Nervenarzt*, 39:231–233.

Antiepileptic Drugs, edited by D. M. Woodbury, J. K. Penry, and C. E. Pippenger. Raven Press, New York © 1982.

42

Carbamazepine

Hematological Toxicity

Anthony V. Pisciotta

Carbamazepine (CBZ) is a tricyclic compound derived from an iminostilbene derivative, 5H-dibenz(*b*,*f*)azepine-5-carboxamide, and related to imipramine and nortriptyline. It has found extensive clinical use in the treatment of epilepsy, trigeminal neuralgia, migraine, and various psychoses.

A clear warning has been issued of the possible hematological toxicity of carbamazepine, which requires that clinical and hematological surveillance be carried out during treatment. Adverse reactions that may affect hematopoietic, hepatic, genitourinary, nervous, skin, digestive, cardiovascular, ophthalmological, musculoskeletal, and metabolic systems are described in the package insert that accompanies CBZ (3). A wide variety of possible toxic effects are mentioned; whether any of these have actually occurred is not known. Mention of all possible adverse reactions may be an expression of caution, covering the use of a relatively new compound for which a toxic spectrum has not yet been established.

Although adverse hematological reactions to CBZ are very rare, their importance is paramount because of the serious, protracted, or even fatal consequences of bone marrow depression. The question remains whether early identification of hematological toxicity is sufficiently protective, especially if serious reactions turn out to be irreversible or rapidly fatal. Since presently existing data do not permit a definitive decision, these points can only be clarified by experience and careful record keeping.

CLINICAL DATA

This chapter covers the total experience, brought up to date, concerning the types of hematological disorders that have been attributed to CBZ. It is suggested that the reader consult an earlier review (12) for definitions and descriptions of various types of hematological disorders that could be produced by drugs. To the 13 cases of aplastic anemia and 5 of miscellaneous blood disorders reported in that review, added here are 9 additional cases of aplastic anemia, 15 of leukopenia and agranulocytosis, and 3 of lymphadenopathy. Most of these are brief reports submitted to Dr. Gibney of the Ciba-Geigy Corporation (P. Gibney, *personal communication,* 1979) without details or documentation. The others represent case reports obtained from a search of the current literature. Details of hematological criteria, pathological findings, and clinical data were not provided. However, the persistent listing of diseases continues to offer a warning as to the possible hematological toxicity of CBZ.

Table 1 provides an updated summary of

TABLE 1. *Summary of aplastic anemia in patients treated with carbamazepine*

Age	Sex	CBZ (mg/day)	Days of treatment	Outcome	Reference
59	M	200–600	>90	Died	Fellows and Knighton (6)
32	M	500	120	Died	A. Peters (*unpublished data*, 1972)
75	F	600	18	Died	A. Colinet (*unpublished data*, 1967)
52	F	300–1,200	180	Died	S. H. Davies (*unpublished data*, 1964)
69	F	400–800	240	Died	Donaldson and Graham (4)
48	F	600–800	270	Recovered	Dyer et al. (5)
45	F	800	330	Died	A.E.C. Salek and D.E. Mendes de Leon (*unpublished data*, 1968)
44	F	800	180	Died	V. Silingardi (*unpublished data*, 1969)
18	F	200–400	16	Died	LeDez, LeBol, and LaCroix-Herpin (*unpublished data*, 1968)
54	M	?	20	Died	Naets (*unpublished data*, 1967)
51	M	600	30	Died	A. Poy Serradall (*unpublished data*, 1968)
?	?	?	?	Recovered	Subirana et al. (16)
90	F	800	40	Recovered	Van der Beken (*unpublished data*, 1966)
32	M	500	30–90	Died	P. Gibney (*personal communication*, 1979)
62	F	?	15	Died	P. Gibney (*personal communication*, 1979)
30	F	?	Months	On treatment	P. Gibney (*personal communication*, 1979)
15	F	600	120	Died	P. Gibney (*personal communication*, 1979)
63	F	?	4	Recovered	P. Gibney (*personal communication*, 1979)
32	M	600	120	On treatment	P. Gibney (*personal communication*, 1979)
17	F	100–300	120	Recovered	P. Gibney (*personal communication*, 1979)
21	F	200	>1,500	Recovered	P. Gibney (*personal communication*, 1979)
2	F	?	90	?	P. Gibney (*personal communication*, 1979)

"aplastic anemia" reported in patients given CBZ either alone or together with other drugs. Of 22 patients with aplastic anemia, 15 women and 6 men (1 sex unknown), ranging in age from 2 to 90 years, 13 died, 8 recovered, and 1 outcome is unknown. Of the eight that recovered, two are still being treated with CBZ. This group developed bone marrow toxicity while being treated with CBZ for a period of 11 to more than 1,500 days.

Sixteen patients, seven women and eight men (one sex unknown), ranging in age from 2 to 62 years, developed leukopenia and agranulocytosis (Table 2). Of this number, one died, one

TABLE 2. *Summary of leukopenia and agranulocytosis in patients treated with carbamazepine*

Age	Sex	CBZ (mg/day)	Days of treatment	Outcome	Reference
62	M	600	60	Recovered	B.H. Dessel (*unpublished data*, 1973)
11	F	15 mg/kg	30	Recovered	Prieur et al. (13)
47	M	400–600	56	Recovered	Al-Ubairy and Nally (1)
31	M	400–900	34	Recovered	Gerber et al. (7)
2	?	?	90	Recovered	P. Gibney (*personal communication*, 1979)
59	M	300	120	Recovered	P. Gibney (*personal communication*, 1979)
57	F	?	?	Recovered	P. Gibney (*personal communication*, 1979)
9	M	1,400	120	Recovered	P. Gibney (*personal communication*, 1979)
40	F	600	75	Died	P. Gibney (*personal communication*, 1979)
7	M	400	150	Recovered	P. Gibney (*personal communication*, 1979)
29	F	800	?	On treatment	P. Gibney (*personal communication*, 1979)
13	F	400	1100	On treatment	P. Gibney (*personal communication*, 1979)
42	F	200–600	7	Recovered	P. Gibney (*personal communication*, 1979)
5	F	700	?	?	P. Gibney (*personal communication*, 1979)
31	M	900	30	Recovered	P. Gibney (*personal communication*, 1979)
2	M	200	6	Recovered	P. Gibney (*personal communication*, 1979)

outcome is unknown, and the rest recovered. Two are back on treatment with CBZ, apparently without redevelopment of the disease.

Few details are available on the clinical or hematological characteristics of agranulocytosis attributed to CBZ. Only three reports were available for review. Prieur et al. (13) reported the case of an 11-year-old girl who developed multiple abnormalities suggestive of hypersensitivity following 14 days of continuous therapy with CBZ. These consisted of rash, purpura, edema, and eosinophilia. She also developed splenomegaly and lymphadenopathy 1 week later. Agranulocytosis was noted at the same time. All of these manifestations regressed when CBZ was discontinued about a month later. Al-Ubairy and Nally (1) described a 47-year-old man who experienced a mild and asymptomatic drop in leukocytes over 84 months, which regressed when the drug was stopped. Gerber et al. (7) described a 31-year-old man who developed leukopenia 1 month after CBZ was started and who returned to normal only after this drug was stopped. This event seemed independent of treatment with other drugs also capable of producing bone marrow suppression, since he recovered while still taking phenytoin, and the leukopenia developed 1 month after azathio-

prine and cyclophosphamide were stopped. The 12 additional reports provided by Gibney (P. Gibney, *personal communication,* 1979) offered no further details other than those given in Table 2.

Table 3 shows a variety of hematological and related reactions that occurred in patients during treatment with CBZ. Reported in the original review (12) were two patients with megaloblastic anemia, one with eosinophilia, and one with hemolytic anemia. To these are added 3 patients with lymphadenopathy (one later developed lymphoma), 2 with thrombocytopenia, and 10 with a "hypersensitivity reaction" consisting of chills, fever, arthralgia, myalgia, skin rash, eosinophilia, and lymphadenopathy. In several of these patients, atypical reactive lymphocytes were present. This histological picture of the lymph nodes was not described. However, one patient reported to Gibney developed a lymphoma at a later date (P. Gibney, *personal communication,* 1979), which probably minimizes the role of the drug in this case. The two cases of thrombocytopenia cleared up following cessation of treatment with CBZ.

The clinical indications for which CBZ was given are listed in Table 4. The cases added since the first review (12) showed no unusual

TABLE 3. *Summary of miscellaneous hematological reactions in patients treated with carbamazepine*

Reaction	Age	Sex	CBZ (mg/day)	Days of treatment	Outcome	Reference
Megaloblastic anemia	42	M	100–200	>250	Recovered	H.W. Kienast (*unpublished data,* 1968)
	20	F	600	900	Recovered	Germano and Scholer (8)
Lymphadenopathy	?	M	?	?	Lymphoma	P. Gibney (*personal communication,* 1979)
	44	M	500	21	Recovered	P. Gibney (*personal communication,* 1979)
	12	F	?	200	?	P. Gibney (*personal communication,* 1979)
Eosinophilia, skin eruption, splenomegaly, reactive lymphocytes, etc.	11	F	200	3	Recovered	Steen-Johnson (15)
	70	M	200–800	?	Recovered	Al-Ubairy and Nally (1)
	11	F	15 mg/kg	30	Recovered	Prieur et al. (13) Houwerzijl et al. (9)
	Seven patients reported; age, sex, dosage, and duration of treatment unknown.					
Hemolytic anemia/RBC	43	M	?	?	Recovered	Boivin et al. (2)
Thrombocytopenia	16	F	600	14	Recovered	Rutman (14)
	79	F	800	120	Recovered	Pearce and Ron (10)

TABLE 4. *Relationship of blood dyscrasias to underlying nervous system disorder*

Blood disorder	Trigeminal neuralgia	Epilepsy	Migraine	Psychosis
Aplastic anemia	10	11	1	0
Agranulocytosis	4	8	0	0
Lymphadenopathy	0	2	0	0
Thrombocytopenia	0	1	0	0
Leukocytosis	0	1	0	0
Megaloblastic anemia	0[a]	2[a]	0	0
Eosinophilia	?	?	0	1
Hemolytic anemia	0	0	1	0

[a]Seven patients reported, but the number in each category was not given.

association of hematological disorders with any specific neurological disease. Ten patients with trigeminal neuralgia and 11 with epilepsy developed aplastic anemia. Four patients with trigeminal neuralgia and eight with epilepsy developed agranulocytosis. The two patients who developed megaloblastic anemia were epileptics who were also being treated with phenytoin, a drug implicated as an etiological factor in megaloblastic anemia. Although seven patients with trigeminal neuralgia and epilepsy developed a skin and lymph node sensitivity while on CBZ, the number in each diagnostic category was not stated.

Through the courtesy of the drug's manufacturer, we have received information on the number of CBZ tablets dispensed and the number of patients at risk from 1972 to 1979 (Table 5). The number of hematological disorders of various types reported to Dr. Gibney during this time is listed at yearly intervals. Assuming that all patients enumerated took all the CBZ that was prescribed and that all cases of blood disorders that developed were known to the manufacturer, there was a progressive increase in the number of blood disorders as the number of patients at risk increased. This amounted to a ratio ranging from 1 : 10,800 to 1 : 38,000. If these figures are accurate, then the likelihood of a patient developing a hematological disorder during treatment with CBZ is low, indeed. A great deal of confirmatory data are required before this relationship can be established.

The association between a toxic drug reaction and a given drug rests only on circumstantial evidence. Therefore, it is necessary to examine the conditions under which the disorder occurs, as well as the disorder itself, in order to come to an arbitrary decision whether CBZ could be implicated in producing a given hematological reaction. It is necessary, first of all, to identify the hematological disorder accurately to be sure

TABLE 5. *Number of cases of CBZ-associated blood disorders per tablets dispensed and patients at risk*

Year	Number of tablets dispensed ($\times 10^6$)	Number of patients treated ($\times 10^3$)	Number of blood dyscrasias	Ratio of toxicity to patients at risk
1972	15	25	—	—
1973	17	30	1	1 : 30,000
1974	23	38	1	1 : 38,000
1975	37	54	5	1 : 10,800
1976	53	77	5	1 : 15,400
1977	69	101	4	1 : 25,250
1978	95	138	8	1 : 17,250
1979[a]	113	350	14	1 : 25,000

[a]Projected.

that it does indeed fit the disease category related to the drug and is not something else which it closely resembles. For example, aplastic anemia and agranulocytosis are frequently confused with aleukemic or preleukemic leukemia, myelofibrosis, congestive splenomegaly, systemic lupus erythematosus, paroxysmal nocturnal hemoglobinuria, metastasis, radiotherapy, or disseminated tuberculosis, all unrelated to drug toxicity. Second, the association between drugs and the development of a blood reaction must be temporally related. For example, if the onset of the reaction occurs before the administration of a drug, that would rule out the drug as a causative agent. In addition, one must be sure that the patient has, in fact, taken the drug, that the identifying label corresponds to the drug itself, and that the patient has not been given simultaneously any other drug(s) that might similarly affect the blood or bone marrow.

The association between a drug and toxicity may be identified as certain if the diagnosis of the blood dyscrasia is accurate, if the drug is the only one given during or before the reaction, and if the reaction recurs each time the patient is given that drug alone. It seems clear that moral and ethical principles preclude the last condition, so that very few drug-induced blood dyscrasias may be shown to be certain.

By such criteria only three patients were adjudged probably to have sustained aplastic anemia induced by CBZ (Table 6). The other 19 instances of aplastic anemia could only be considered as possibly induced by CBZ because of

coincidental disease that may have produced or simulated the aplastic state (hepatitis, lupus, tuberculosis, leukemia) or because of simultaneous treatment with other drugs capable of producing a similar reaction (e.g., phenytoin, mephenytoin, ethotoin, aminopyrine, primaquine). In six cases, the diagnosis of aplastic anemia was uncertain because adequate data were lacking.

Carbamazepine-induced agranulocytosis was adjudged probable in seven cases and possible in seven (Table 6). In the possible category, one patient had splenomegaly, four were simultaneously treated with other toxic drugs, and in two patients the diagnosis of agranulocytosis was uncertain.

The greatest degree of certainty concerning the toxicity of CBZ was in the category of hypersensitivity reaction (dermatitis, eosinophilia, reactive lymphocytes, lymphadenopathy, and splenomegaly). This reaction was reported nine times in patients who were treated with no other potentially harmful drugs (Table 6). Furthermore, in this group, lymphocyte blastogenesis and a positive skin patch test were produced when the drug was used as test antigen. In controls who were treated with CBZ without developing such a reaction, blastogenesis and skin reactivity to patch test did not occur. In six patients with aplastic anemia and two with agranulocytosis, we were not assured of the diagnosis because the clinical, hematological, or bone marrow criteria used to establish the diagnosis were inadequate.

TABLE 6. *Probabilities of CBZ-induced hematological toxicity*

Probability	Aplastic anemia	Agranulo-cytosis	Hypersensitivity; dermatitis, eosinophilia, lymphadenopathy	Hemolytic anemia	Megalo-blastic anemia	Thrombo-cyto-penia
Certain	0	0	0	0	0	0
Probable						
Other drugs (nontoxic)	2	6	1	0	0	0
No other drugs	1	1	8	0	0	0
Possible						
Coincidental						
Similar disease	5	1	0	1	0	0
Other drugs (toxic)	8	4	3	0	2	2
Diagnosis uncertain	6	2	1	0	0	0

Assuming the validity of the diagnosis, a number of ancillary clinical findings cast some doubt on the role of CBZ in producing blood disorders. In two patients, aplastic anemia developed concomitantly with hepatitis. The association between these disorders is well known. Nevertheless, the possibility exists that CBZ could have produced not only aplastic anemia but hepatitis as well. One patient had tuberculosis and chondrosarcoma, the latter treated with irradiation. Either of these disturbances can be characterized by pancytopenia, which can be erroneously attributed to CBZ. In this patient, however, no evidence for disseminated tuberculosis or metastatic carcinoma could be elicited. The possibility that aplasia could be secondary to irradiation could not be ruled out. In one patient, the mention of an increased number of "blasts" in the bone marrow brings up the question of acute leukemia; unfortunately, no further details were given. In another patient, the positive antinuclear antibody test together with a positive Coombs' antiglobulin test suggested possible systemic lupus erythematosus, another disorder frequently confused with aplastic anemia. In a single instance, the presence of congestive splenomegaly and cirrhosis in a heavy-drinking man suggested splenic sequestration as a possible cause of leukopenia rather than drug sensitivity. In this group of patients, the toxic role of CBZ is doubtful because of the simultaneous administration of other drugs known to produce marrow suppression. This list includes phenytoin, mephenytoin, primidone, chlorpropamide, ethotoin, ethosuximide, and aminopyrine. Accordingly, any patient with aplastic anemia or agranulocytosis who has taken CBZ as well as one of the above drugs cannot be accurately judged as far as etiology of the reaction is concerned. Three patients, however, developed pancytopenia while taking no other concomitant medication or while taking other drugs judged to be innocent of inducing hematological toxicity, such as ethosuximide, hydroxyzine, prednisone, digitalis, spironolactone, phenobarbital, primidone, and penicillin. Of particular interest are two patients who developed megaloblastic anemia while taking CBZ and phenytoin simultaneously. Since phenytoin has been well documented as an important etiological factor in development of megaloblastic anemia, and since there have been no new cases of this type, the possibility that CBZ might do the same thing remains doubtful.

In most of the patients reported to the manufacturer, so few details were given regarding the bone marrow or peripheral blood morphology, diagnosis, clinical course, or autopsy that the relationship of CBZ to bone marrow depression remains doubtful. In the single case of hemolytic anemia with Heinz bodies, the large number of drugs received by the patient whose erythrocytes were deficient in glutathione peroxidase made etiological assessment impossible. It is clear that firm, published data are required before the role of CBZ in producing hematological disorders can be fully appreciated.

DISCUSSION

The question of whether routine periodic hematological examinations will be useful as a safeguard in predicting marrow susceptibility is best answered in terms of the frequency of CBZ-induced suppression. If this complication of treatment occurs frequently (i.e., in about 10% of those treated), then the likelihood of identifying an idiosyncratic patient by doing routine blood counts during treatment is enhanced. However, if this reaction is as rare as it seems to be, then it is demanding a great deal of chance to identify a sensitive patient by doing weekly blood counts. For example, between 1960 and 1969, we tried to identify phenothiazine-sensitive patients by doing a total of six white counts between weeks 2 and 10 after initiating treatment (11). During this time, almost 40,000 leukocyte counts were made to identify five new cases of agranulocytosis and about 500 instances of transient leukopenia. With respect to chloramphenicol, where the incidence of marrow suppression was calculated by Wallerstein et al. (17) to be one case in 20,000 to 40,000 patients, the extreme rarity of this situation precludes its identification by routine blood counts. Furthermore, the occurrence of aplastic anemia is not necessarily dose related, and it may not occur concomitantly with treatment. However, a universally reversible bone marrow suppression that is different from aplastic anemia has been associated with chloramphenicol and can be identified by doing erythrocyte, leukocyte, platelet, and reticulocyte counts during treatment. In addition, ferrokinetic studies with ^{59}Fe and serum iron and iron-binding capacity studies have been useful for identifying transient marrow suppression. The occurrence of this transient reaction is not necessarily followed by aplastic anemia, nor has such a reaction been identified with carbamazepine.

Despite detailed routine laboratory surveillance, our experience with carbamazepine to date does not permit us to make an accurate statement on the incidence of marrow suppression, either transient or permanent. For this reason, all physicians who use this drug should be admonished to obtain complete blood counts, including platelets and reticulocytes, and possibly serum iron and total iron-binding capacity from the second to 12th week of therapy. Together with this, careful clinical checks should be conducted weekly for signs of hematological suppression such as pallor, infection, fever, sore throat, purpura, ecchymosis, and bleeding from mucous membranes.

There are no specific routine laboratory examinations that enable one to make an early diagnosis of aplastic anemia. However, serum iron and ferrokinetic studies have been of some value with the use of chloramphenicol and may be helpful here, too. In the event of depression of peripheral blood values, bone marrow should be examined without delay. The description of blastogenesis in lymphocytes coincubated with CBZ may provide a satisfactory means of monitoring treatment in CBZ-sensitive patients.

If a patient has developed hematological suppression during treatment with CBZ, it would not be morally or ethically justifiable to rechallenge with the same drug. There have been instances in which patients who had had agranulocytosis were rechallenged with a suspected drug after recovery. In the case of phenothiazines, recurrence turned out to be dose related and was invariably followed by prompt recovery. However, since aplastic anemia is protracted, permanent, or fatal, there is no justification for retreating a patient who has recovered from pancytopenia with any drug suspected of playing an etiological role.

The point at which CBZ must be discontinued to prevent permanent marrow damage is unknown. In general, any suspected myelotoxic drug should be discontinued if a patient sustains evidence of marrow suppression as follows: erythrocytes less than $4.0 \times 10^6/\text{mm}^3$; hematocrit less than 32%; hemoglobin less than 11 g/100 ml; leukocytes less than 4,000/mm^3; platelets less than 100,000/mm^3; reticulocytes less than 0.3% (20,000/mm^3); serum iron greater than 150 μg/100 ml. Should evidence of bone marrow suppression develop after treatment with CBZ, it is necessary to stop the drug and to do a daily CBC, platelet, and reticulocyte count. A bone marrow aspiration and trephine biopsy should be performed immediately and repeated with sufficient frequency to monitor recovery. Special studies might be helpful, including white cell and platelet antibodies, ^{59}Fe ferrokinetic studies, cytogenetic studies on marrow and peripheral blood, bone marrow culture studies for colony-forming units, hemoglobin electrophoresis for A$_2$ and F hemoglobin, and serum folic acid and vitamin B$_{12}$ levels. Treatment of fully developed aplastic anemia includes transfusion of packed erythrocytes, leukocytes, and platelets as indicated; intramuscular injection of androgens, e.g., testosterone enanthate and administration of folic acid in case of megaloblastosis or diminished blood folic acid.

Because of the importance of fully assessing and documenting hematological reactions attributed to CBZ, all physicians who use this drug should order appropriate laboratory studies to establish the disorder. Any case of fully documented hematological toxicity should be promptly published.

MECHANISMS OF HEMATOLOGICAL TOXICITY

It is not possible to generalize on the mechanisms or predictability of drug-induced hematological toxicity because these vary with the pharmacological and toxicological properties of the drug itself. From a broad point of view, idiosyncratic drug reactions might be mediated through immune, toxicological, or biochemical mechanisms. In the first of these, the drug stimulates the formation of antibodies which, either alone or in conjunction with the drug, inflict immune damage on a target cell, generally leading to its rapid destruction. Only limited data are available concerning relation of antibodies to immune destruction of leukocytes leading to agranulocytosis or aplastic anemia associated with CBZ. The single instance that came under my observation was a patient with a large liver and spleen who developed leukopenia following treatment with chlordiazepoxide, phenytoin, and CBZ. Search of his serum for substances that inhibit leukocyte function failed to disclose any such activity, either alone or in conjunction with CBZ.

However, some findings do indicate an immune mediation of CBZ-associated dermatitis, eosinophilia, lymphadenopathy, and splenomegaly. Houwerzijl et al. (9) have convincingly shown that lymphocytes obtained from these sensitized patients undergo transformation to reactive "blast" cells and synthesize DNA when incubated with CBZ. Furthermore, a patch test with CBZ produced an erythematous skin reaction in six sensitized patients. Such changes were not observed with lymphocytes or skin of patients who were not sensitized to CBZ.

There is no convincing evidence that CBZ acts by suppressing cell proliferation or cellular function in a manner comparable to chlorpromazine. Concentrations of CBZ as high as 10^{-4} M failed to elicit any significant suppression of postphagocytosis respiratory burst (Fig. 1), phagocytic index (Fig. 2), DNA synthesis in a BeWo cell line in culture (Fig. 3), or development of granulocyte-forming units in tissue culture (Fig. 4).

SUMMARY AND CONCLUSIONS

In a review of the literature and unpublished data obtained from the manufacturer, carbamazepine was found to be rarely associated with aplastic anemia, agranulocytosis, leukopenia,

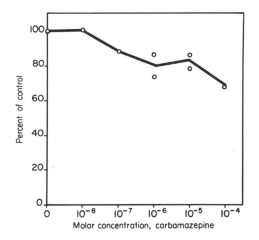

FIG. 1. Effect of carbamazepine on postphagocytosis respiratory burst.

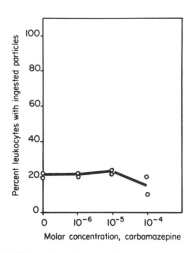

FIG. 2. Effect of carbamazepine on phagocytosis of latex particles (phagocytic index).

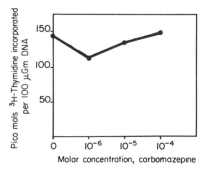

FIG. 3. Effect of carbamazepine on DNA synthesis in BeWo trophoblastic cells.

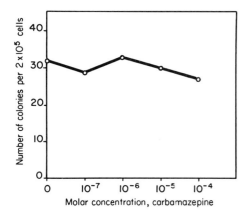

FIG. 4. Effect of carbamazepine on granulocyte colony-forming units.

thrombocytopenia, and a hypersensitivity syndrome consisting of dermatitis, eosinophilia, lymphadenopathy, and splenomegaly. The mechanisms and predictability of such reactions are unexplained, but published data indicate an immune-mediated lymphocyte reactivity in connection with the hypersensitivity reaction. Because of the limited number of reports of CBZ-induced blood dyscrasias, such cases should be critically documented and reported if convincing data can be elicited.

ACKNOWLEDGMENT

This work was aided by grant CA-05524 from the National Institutes of Health and by the Ciba-Geigy Pharmaceutical Corp.

REFERENCES

1. Al-Ubaidy, S. S., and Nally, F. F. (1976): Adverse reactions to carbamazepine (Tegretol). *Br. J. Oral Surg.*, 13:289–293.

2. Boivin, P., Galand, C., Hakim, J., and Blery, M. (1970): Déficit en glutathion-peroxydase érythrocytaire et anémie hémolytique médicamentense. Une nouvelle observation. *Presse Med.*, 78:171–174.

3. Ciba-Geigy Pharmaceutical Corp. (1979): Package insert for Tegretol®.

4. Donaldson, G. W. K., and Graham, J. G. (1965): Aplastic anemia following the administration of Tegretol. *Br. J. Clin. Pract.*, 19:699–702.

5. Dyer, N. H., Hughes, D. T. D., and Jenkins, G. C. (1966): Hypoplastic anemia following treatment with carbamazepine. *Clin. Trials*, 8:52–57.

6. Fellows, W. R. (1969): A case of aplastic anemia and pancytopenia with Tegretol therapy. *Headache*, 9:92–95.

7. Gerber, J. G., Stiles, G., and Niles, A. S. (1979): Severe leukopenia secondary to carbamazepine administration. *South Med. J.*, 72:81–83.

8. Germano, G., and Scholer, Y. (1968): Erythroblastopénie non mégalocytaire et sensible à l'acide folique chez une épileptique. *Acta Haematol. (Basel)*, 39:159–166.

9. Houwerzijl, J., DeGast, G. C., Nater, J. P., Esselink, M. T., and Nieweg, H. O. (1977): Lymphocyte stimulation tests and patch tests to carbamazepine hypersensitivity. *Clin. Exp. Immunol.*, 29:272–277.

10. Pearce, J., and Ron, M. A. (1968): Thrombocytopenia after carbamazepine [letter]. *Lancet*, 2:223.

11. Pisciotta, A. V. (1974): The effect of chlorpromazine on peripheral leukocytes. In: *Drugs and Hematologic Reactions,* edited by N. V. Dimitrov and J. H. Nodine, pp. 233–247. Grune & Stratton, New York.

12. Pisciotta, A. V. (1975): Hematologic toxicity of carbamazepine. *Adv. Neurol.* 11:355–368.

13. Prieur, A. M., LeBovar, Y., Griscelli, C., and Mozziconacci, F. (1973): Agranulocytose a la carbamazépine. *Ann. Pediatr.* (Paris), 20:909–912.

14. Rutman, J. Y. (1978): Effect of carbamazepine on blood elements [letter]. *Ann. Neurol.*, 3:373–379.

15. Steen-Johnson, J. (1970): Alvorlige bivirkninger ved bruk av karbamazepin (Tegretol). *Tidsskr. Nor. Laegeforen.*, 90:1631–1632.

16. Subirana, A., Oller-Daurella, L., and Chillon, D. (1967): Dos años de experiencia del tratamiento de la epilepsia con Tegretol. *Rev. Clin. Esp.*, 104:336–342.

17. Wallerstein, R. O., Condit, P. K., Kasper, C. K., Brown, J. W., and Morrison, F. R. (1969): Statewide study of chloramphenicol therapy and fatal aplastic anemia. *J.A.M.A.* 208:2045–2050.

Antiepileptic Drugs, edited by D. M. Woodbury, J. K. Penry, and C. E. Pippenger. Raven Press, New York © 1982.

43

Carbamazepine

Mechanisms of Action

Robert M. Julien

Before the possible mechanisms of the anti-epileptic action of carbamazepine (CBZ) are discussed, at least two caveats must be stated. First, CBZ has very limited solubility, making it unattractive for study in a variety of simple systems. This also limits the observations of acute drug action, since chronic exposure to the drug may be necessary in order to achieve a therapeutic intracellular concentration despite a presumed therapeutic concentration in bathing media. This limited solubility also introduces a time dependence to drug action, as illustrated by Hershkowitz and Raines (14). The second caveat concerning CBZ is that although the therapeutic clinical concentrations of the drug are usually below 10 μg/ml (2), many of the studies on the mechanisms of action of this drug have derived conclusions from experiments utilizing drug concentrations far in excess of this therapeutic range. Therapeutic implications derived from such data must therefore be interpreted with extreme caution. This chapter will attempt not only to summarize the work to date but to interpret these works in light of the above-stated caveats. An earlier review (18) is available.

ANTIEPILEPTIC ACTIONS IN ANIMALS

Carbamazepine was synthesized in 1954 (27) and was later found to possess marked anti-epileptic activity in animals (8,10,17,22,30). Hernandez-Peón (12) demonstrated in cats that CBZ (15 mg/kg i.p.) depressed synaptic transmission of trigeminal pain impulses, especially of potentials recorded from n. centrum medianum of the thalamus. In contrast, Dolce (5) reported that CBZ (5 mg/kg) exerted no significant effect on recruitment responses elicited by stimulation of the centrum medianum. Fromm and Killian (9) reported that CBZ (6 mg/kg i.v.) depressed synaptic transmission in the spinal trigeminal nucleus of cats anesthetized with chloralose (75 mg/kg) or pentobarbital (40 mg/kg). This effect was similar to that obtained with phenytoin (3–5 mg/kg i.v.). Additional depressant action of CBZ (15–32 mg/kg i.v. in propylene glycol) on polysynaptic pathways (hindlimb flexors of the cat) was demonstrated by Theobald and Kunz (30). None of these studies correlated antiepileptic effectiveness with serum concentrations of the drug.

Correlation of antiepileptic effectiveness with serum levels of CBZ was first reported by Holm et al. (15). They reported in cats (encephale isolé) a rather specific depressant action of CBZ on the n. ventralis anterior of the thalamus at doses (20 mg/kg i.p.) and blood levels (5–9 μg/ml) below those required to depress the n. centrum medianum, reticular formation, amygdala, hypothalamus, hippocampus, caudate, or pallidum. Since the n. ventralis anterior has been

543

implicated in the generalization and spread of epileptiform discharge (31,32), such action may be important in the therapeutic usefulness of this compound.

Since Esplin (7) demonstrated that phenytoin depresses posttetanic potentiation (PTP) in cat spinal cord, this preparation has been a popular model for the evaluation of antiepileptic actions of various compounds. Several investigators (13,18,19,29) have all reported various degrees of PTP depression by CBZ. However, whether the results of any of the studies can be related to the clinical effectiveness of CBZ can be seriously questioned. Carbamazepine suppresses PTP only after doses in excess of 20 mg/kg i.v. or, in some reports, after doses as large as 300 mg/kg i.p. In addition, significant suppression of PTP is seen only at blood CBZ levels greater than 20 μg/ml. A time-dependent action with onset as late as 90 min has also been noted (13). Thus, the relationship of CBZ-induced suppression of PTP to the prevention of seizure spread and to the drug's therapeutic effectiveness in man has not been demonstrated.

Schauf et al. (26) studied the effects of CBZ on ionic conductances of voltage-clamped *Myxicola* giant axons. Concentrations of 0.10 to 1.0 mM were utilized (23.6 to 236.3 μg/ml). At 0.1 mM (23.6 μg/ml), CBZ exerted no effect on any membrane parameter. At 0.5 mM (118 μg/ml), sodium and potassium conductances were decreased by 50 and 40%, respectively, membrane leakage conductance was decreased, and transmembrane potentials were depolarized by 4 to 9 mV. Although these effects of the drug occurred at concentrations well above the therapeutic range, they may provide an explanation for the depressant effects of very high doses of CBZ on the compound action potential of mammalian sciatic nerves (16,19). In the heart, CBZ (5 mg/kg i.v.) terminates digitalis-induced ventricular arrhythmias, decreases the time course of repolarization, and shortens action potential duration (28).

Julien and Hollister (18) studied the spectrum of antiepileptic actions of CBZ in a variety of experimental models of epilepsy. In mice, the drug was effective against both maximal and minimal electroshock seizures and also against seizures induced by pentylenetetrazol. The therapeutic indices for CBZ in mice were in the range of 16 to 26, values considerably greater than those for phenytoin and other antiepileptic drugs. In acute experiments on locally anesthetized, curarized, and mechanically ventilated cats, CBZ (2.5–5 mg/kg i.v.; blood levels of 4–9 μg/ml) reduced or abolished penicillin-induced epileptiform discharge and estrogen-induced spike-and-wave epileptiform discharge and elevated the threshold for induction of electrically induced cortical afterdischarges while shortening the duration of prolonged afterdischarge episodes. This afterdischarge data verified the earlier reports of Hernandez-Peón (10,11), Dolce (5), and Holm et al. (15). In three rhesus monkeys with aluminum oxide-induced behavioral and electrographic seizures, CBZ (20 mg/kg i.m. daily; blood levels of 4–8 μg/ml) suppressed all convulsant activity in each of the animals and returned EEG patterns to normal (18). When drug administration was discontinued, the seizures returned only after 10 to 16 days. These observations were verified and extended by David and Grewal (4) who demonstrated that CBZ administered to rhesus monkeys with epileptogenic foci in the sensorimotor cortex or hippocampus effectively arrested spontaneous and/or stress-induced seizures, elevated the pentylenetetrazol threshold severalfold, and significantly reduced interictal EEG abnormalities. Such action was accompanied by a reduction of aggressivity and temporal lobe phenomena in monkeys with hippocampal foci. No side effects were observed during this period of antiepileptic effectiveness.

In amygdaloid-kindled cats and baboons, Wada et al. (33) demonstrated that CBZ at serum levels of 10 μg/ml either significantly reduced or abolished both electrographic afterdischarges and clinical seizures following amygdalar stimulation.

Hershkowitz and Raines (14) demonstrated that CBZ (200–300 mg/kg i.p. in 1% methylcellulose in saline) produced depression of muscle spindle activity in spinal and α-chloralose-anesthetized cats at serum CBZ concentrations of 9 to 45 μg/ml. The relationship of this peripheral influence on the muscle spindle to the central antiepileptic actions of CBZ is unclear, although Anderson and Raines (1) have demonstrated a similar action for phenytoin.

NEUROCHEMICAL STUDIES

Cholinergic Mechanisms

Consolo et al. (3) studied the action of CBZ on acetylcholine, choline, choline O-acetyltransferase, and cholinesterase in selected areas of rat brain. CBZ (7.5–50 mg/kg) was dissolved in propylene glycol and administered i.p. in a volume of 0.2 ml/100 g body weight. Brain levels of CBZ and carbamazepine-10,11-epoxide were measured by gas chromotography. Acetylcholine levels were increased in the corpus striatum by 66% at a dose of 25 mg/kg and by a lesser amount following 15 mg/kg. Acetylcholine levels were unaltered in the cerebellum, diencephalon, mesencephalon, and hippocampus. Choline levels were significantly decreased in the striatum. This increase in acetylcholine and decrease in choline were also observed in the cerebral hemispheres. The increase in striatal acetylcholine by CBZ was apparently not mediated through a dopaminergic system since pretreatment with pimozide (1 mg/kg), a dopaminergic antagonist, did not prevent the effect. Striatal choline O-acetyltransferase and cholinesterase were not affected by either CBZ or its metabolite (carbamazepine-10,11-epoxide) after *in vitro* incubation.

The authors postulated that CBZ does not induce its effect on acetylcholine via a direct action on the metabolism of acetylcholine. This study did not report the blood CBZ levels achieved and did not correlate biochemical data with antiepileptic action. Although these data are intriguing, the correlation between acetylcholine levels and the mechanisms of the epilepsies remains speculative.

Catecholamine Mechanisms

Quattrone and Samanin (25) studied the antiepileptic action of CBZ in rats pretreated with 6-hydroxydopamine. Forebrain levels of norepinephrine and dopamine were markedly lower in control animals treated with 6-hydroxydopamine, but levels of 5-hydroxytryptamine were not affected. The electroconvulsive threshold (defined as the amperage necessary to induce a tonic hindlimb extension in 50% of rats following stimulation through ear-clip electrodes) was lowered in 6-hydroxydopamine-treated animals. A significantly reduced antiepileptic effect of CBZ (10 mg/kg i.p. in propylene glycol) was noted in treated animals compared with nontreated controls. Blood levels of CBZ were not determined. The authors concluded that brain catecholamines may play a role in the control of seizure susceptibility in rats and that brain catecholamines may also, at least partially, mediate the antiepileptic activity of CBZ.

Purdy et al. (24) studied the effect of CBZ on the *in vitro* uptake and release of norepinephrine in adrenergic nerves of rabbit aorta and in whole brain synaptosomes. Carbamazepine (10^{-5} M) significantly inhibited the uptake of tritiated norepinephrine in rat synaptosomes. This concentration of CBZ is within the drug's therapeutic range in both man (2) and animals (23). However, this CBZ blockade of norepinephrine uptake was only approximately 25% of that induced by imipramine at equimolar concentrations. Although imipramine is an effective antiepileptic compound (20), it is a much less effective anticonvulsant agent than is CBZ. It was therefore concluded that uptake blockade is not likely to be the major mechanism underlying the anticonvulsant activity of CBZ. Such an action, however, may be involved in the analeptic effect of the drug.

Lewin and Bleck (21) studied the effects of CBZ, phenobarbital, and phenytoin on cyclic AMP accumulation in rat cerebral cortical slices stimulated by ouabain, adenosine, and norepinephrine. Carbamazepine in a concentration of 10^{-1} mM decreased by 56% the ouabain-induced cyclic AMP accumulation, whereas lower concentrations had no effect. Similarly, 1.0 mM CBZ reduced by 76% and 63% the cyclic AMP accumulation induced by adenosine and norepinephrine, respectively. The effects of lower concentrations were not reported. The proposed role of increased cyclic AMP in epileptogenesis was discussed. However, the fact that concentrations of CBZ in the range of 0.1 to 1.0 mM were necessary to elicit depression of cyclic AMP accumulation indicates that this action of CBZ may not be an important phenomenon at therapeutically effective serum concentrations of the drug. Additional experimentation is necessary in order to answer this objection before the data may be regarded with more interest.

On a more speculative note, Dretchen et al. (6), in a study of the cat soleus nerve–muscle preparation, concluded that phenytoin blocks a cyclic AMP-mediated calcium influx that is associated both with transmitter release and with the control of a slow potassium current. The latter is thought to be responsible for both posttetanic hyperpolarization and posttetanic repetitive activity in the preparation. Although CBZ has not been examined in this system (because of technical difficulty associated with the limited solubility of the drug) (A. Raines, *personal communication*), it is felt that the effects of CBZ on this system would be qualitatively similar to those of phenytoin. Should the technical difficulties be overcome, studies on this model might provide exciting new insights into the molecular action of CBZ. Should cyclic AMP be involved in the regulation of calcium fluxes and therefore in membrane responsiveness, CBZ-induced alteration in cyclic nucleotides may account for the antiepileptic action of the drug. As demonstrated by the above reports, however, such studies are still in their infancy.

REFERENCES

1. Anderson, R. J., and Raines, A. (1974): Suppression by diphenylhydantoin of afferent discharges arising in muscle spindles of the triceps surae of the cat. *J. Pharmacol. Exp. Ther.*, 191:290–299.
2. Cereghino, J. J., Van Meter, J. C., Brock, J. T., Penry, J. K., Smith, L. D., and White, B. G. (1973): Preliminary observations of serum carbamazepine concentration in epileptic patients. *Neurology (Minneap.)*, 23:357–366.
3. Consolo, S., Bianchi, S., and Ladinsky, H. (1976): Effect of carbamazepine on cholinergic parameters in rat brain areas. *Neuropharmacology*, 35:653–657.
4. David, J., and Grewal, R. S. (1976): Effect of car-

5. Dolce, G. (1969): Ueber den antiepileptisken Aktions-Mechanismus von 5-Carbamyl-5H-dibenzo (b,F) azepin—Neuro-physiologische Untersuchunger on Katzen. *Arzneim. Forsch.*, 19:1257–1263.
6. Dretchen, K. L., Standaert, F. G., and Raines, A. (1977): Effects of phenytoin on the cyclic nucleotide system in the motor nerve terminal. *Epilepsia*, 18:337–347.
7. Esplin, D. W. (1957): Effects of diphenylhydantoin on synaptic transmission in the cat spinal cord and stellate ganglion. *J. Pharmacol. Exp. Ther.*, 120:301–323.
8. Fernandez, E. (1967): Farmacologia de la carbamazepine. *Rev. Neuropsiquiatr.*, 30:273–289.
9. Fromm, G. H., and Killian, J. M. (1967): Effect of some anticonvulsant drugs on the spinal trigeminal nucleus. *Neurology (Minneap.)*, 17:275–280.
10. Hernandez-Peón, R. (1962): Anticonvulsant action of G32883. In: *Third Proceedings of the Collegium Internationale Neuro-psychopharmacologicum*, pp. 303–311. Elsevier, Amsterdam.
11. Hernandez-Peón, R. (1964): Anticonvulsant action of G32883. In: *Neuropsychopharmacology*, edited by P. B. Bradley, F. Flugel, and P. H. Hock, pp. 303–311. Elsevier, Amsterdam.
12. Hernandez-Peón, R. (1965): Central action of G32883 upon transmission of trigeminal pain impulses. *Med. Pharmacol. Exp. (Basel)*, 12:73–80.
13. Hershkowitz, N., Dretchen, K. L., and Raines, A. (1978): Carbamazepine suppression of post-tetanic potentiation at the neuromuscular junction. *J. Pharmacol. Exp. Ther.*, 207:810–816.
14. Hershkowitz, N., and Raines, A. (1978): Effects of carbamazepine on muscle spindle discharges. *J. Pharmacol. Exp. Ther.*, 204:581–591.
15. Holm, E., Kelleter, R., Heinemann, H., and Hamann, K. F., (1970): Elektrophysiologische Analyse der Wirkungen von Carbamazepine auf das Behirn der Katze. *Pharmakopsychiatr. Neuropsychopharmakol.*, 3:187–200.
16. Honda, H., and Allen, M. (1973): The effect of an iminostilbene derivative (G32883) on peripheral nerve. *J. Med. Assoc. Ga.*, 62:38–42.
17. Jongmans, J. W. M. (1964): Report on the antiepileptic action of tegretol. *Epilepsia*, 5:74–82.
18. Julien, R. M., and Hollister, R. P., (1975): Carbamazepine: Mechanisms of action. *Adv. Neurol.*, 11:263–276.
19. Krupp, P. (1969): The effect of Tegretol on some elementary neuronal mechanisms. *Headache*, 9:42–46.
20. Lange, S. C., Julien, R. M., and Fowler, G. W. (1976): Biphasic effects of imipramine in experimental models of epilepsy. *Epilepsia*, 17:183–196.
21. Lewin, E., and Bleck, V. (1977): Cyclic AMP accumulation in cerebral cortical slices: Effect of carbamazepine, phenobarbital, and phenytoin. *Epilepsia*, 18:237–242.
22. Lorge, M. (1963): Klinische Erfahrungen mit einem neuen Antiepilepticum Tegretol (G32883) mit besonderer Wirkung auf de epileptische Wesensveranderung. *Schweiz. Med. Wochenschr.*, 93:1042–1047.
23. Masuda, Y., Utsui, Y., Shiraishi, Y., Karasawa, T.,

Yoshida, K., and Shimizu, M. (1979): Relationships between plasma concentrations of diphenylhydantoin, phenobarbital, carbamazepine, and 3-sulfamoylmethyl-1,2-benzisoxozole (AD-810), new anticonvulsant agent, and their anticonvulsant or neurotoxic effect in experimental animals. *Epilepsia*, 20:623–633.

24. Purdy, R. E., Julien, R. M., Fairhurst, A. S., and Terry, M. D. (1977): Effect of carbamazepine on the *in vitro* uptake and release of norepinephrine in adrenergic nerves of rabbit aorta and in whole brain synaptosomes. *Epilepsia*, 18:251–257.

25. Quattrone, A., and Samanin, R. (1977): Decreased anticonvulsant activity of carbamazepine in 6-hydroxydopamine-treated rats. *Eur. J. Pharmacol.*, 41:333–336.

26. Schauf, C. L., Davis, F. A., and Marder, J. (1974): Effects of carbamazepine on the ionic conductances of *Myxicola* giant axons. *J. Pharmacol. Exp. Ther.*, 189:538–543.

27. Schindler, W., and Häflinger, F. (1954): Ueber Derivate des Imino-dibenzyls. *Helv. Chim. Acta*, 37:472–483.

28. Steiner, C. A., Wit, A. L., Weiss, M. B., and Damato, A. N. (1970): The antiarrhythmic actions of carbamazepine (Tegretol). *J. Pharmacol. Exp. Ther.*, 173:323–335.

29. Theobald, W., Krupp, P., and Levin, P. (1970): Neuropharmacologic aspects of the therapeutic action of carbamazepine in trigeminal neuralgia. In: *Trigeminal Neuralgia; Pathogenesis and Pathophysiology*, edited by R. Hassler and A. E. Walker, pp. 107–114. Georg Thieme, Stuttgart.

30. Theobald, W., and Kunz, H. A. (1963): Zur Pharmakologie des Antiepilepticums 5-Carbamyl-5H-dibenzo (B,f) azepin. *Arzneim. Forsch.*, 13:122–125.

31. Verzeano, M. (1972): Pacemakers, synchronization and epilepsy. In: *Synchronization of EEG Activity in Epilepsies*, edited by H. Petsche and Mary A. B. Brazier, pp. 154–188. Springer-Verlag, New York.

32. Verzeano, M., Laufer, M., Spear, P., and McDonald, S. (1970): The activity of neuronal networks in the thalamus of the monkey. In: *Biology of Memory*, edited by K. Pribram and D. E. Broadbent, pp. 239–271. Academic Press, New York.

33. Wada, J. A., Osawa, T., Sato, M., Wake, A., Corcoran, M. E., and Troupin, A. S. (1976): Acute anticonvulsant effects of diphenylhydantoin, phenobarbital, and carbamazepine: A combined electroclinical and serum level study in amygdaloid kindled cats and baboons. *Epilepsia*, 17:77–88.

Antiepileptic Drugs, edited by D. M. Woodbury,
J. K. Penry, and C. E. Pippenger. Raven Press,
New York © 1982.

44

Valproate

Chemistry and Methods of Determination

Harvey J. Kupferberg

Valproic acid (2-propylpentanoic acid; dipro-pylacetic acid; Depakene®) was synthesized by Burton in 1882 (6). Its anticonvulsant properties, discovered by chance in mice, were described nearly a century later (32). After its first clinical trial in 1964 (7), valproic acid was introduced into the armamentarium of antiepileptic therapy. As it became accepted as a useful therapeutic agent, various attempts were made to predict the efficacy of valproic acid from its serum concentration. It appeared that serum valproic acid concentrations must exceed 50 μg/ml to provide a therapeutic response. Once this relationship had been established, numerous analytical methods for therapeutic monitoring of valproic acid were developed.

The majority of these methods use gas–liquid chromatography (GLC) to separate and quantitate valproic acid in biological fluids. Newer quantitative methods include high-performance liquid chromatography (HPLC) and mass spectrometry.

The GLC methods usually entail the extraction of valproic acid from acidified samples into an organic solvent, such as chloroform, before quantitation. In a few GLC methods, nonextracted plasma samples are injected directly into the gas chromatograph.

PHYSICOCHEMICAL PROPERTIES

The physical and chemical properties of valproic acid have been reviewed by Chang (8). Valproic acid, with a molecular weight of 144, is a colorless, slightly viscous liquid with a boiling point of 221 to 222°C at 1 atm. It is soluble in most organic solvents (e.g., methanol, chloroform, diethyl ether, hexane). The solubility is 1.27 mg/ml in water, 1.15 mg/ml in 0.1 N HCl, and >10% (v/v) in 1 N NaOH. The specific gravity of valproic acid is 0.904 g/ml at 25°C.

The sodium salt of valproic acid is a white crystalline powder that does not melt when heated. It is extremely hygroscopic when the relative humidity is above 50%. The compound liquefies when allowed to stand overnight. Sodium valproate is very soluble in water (2.5 g/ml), somewhat less soluble in methanol or ethanol, and practically insoluble in most organic solvents. The magnesium and calcium salts are insoluble in water.

SYNTHESIS

The synthetic pathways of valproic acid and sodium valproate are shown in Fig. 1.

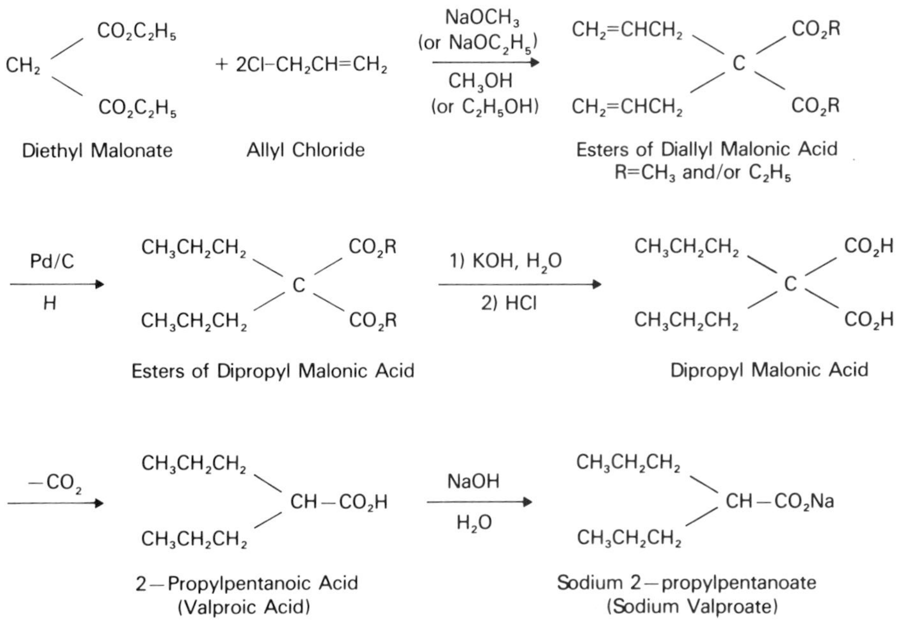

FIG. 1. Synthetic pathways of valproic acid and sodium valproate. (From Chang, ref. 8, with permission.)

METHODS OF ANALYSIS

Gas–Liquid Chromatography

The majority of GLC methods for analysis of valproic acid differ mainly in the analytical conditions (e.g., liquid phase, oven temperature, internal standard, extraction solvents). The first method used for the quantitative analysis of valproic acid was described by Meijer and Hessing-Brand (31). This method was unique because a microdiffusion technique, rather than a conventional organic solvent extraction procedure, was used to remove the drug from plasma. Only volatile components of the biological sample were transferred by the diffusion technique. The usefulness of this elegant method, however, was limited by the lengthy diffusion process. Thus, more conventional types of extraction procedures were developed for the analysis of valproic acid.

Extraction Methods

Because valproic acid has a pK_a of 4.95, biological specimens containing the drug must be acidified in order to extract the valproic acid into organic solvents. Mineral acids such as sulfuric, hydrochloric, and perchloric acid have been used in a variety of volumes and concentrations. The extractability of valproic acid does not appear to be influenced by the acidifying reagent. Levy et al. (28), however, suggested that strong mineral acid causes hydrolysis of valproic acid conjugates. If the plasma contains large amounts of valproic acid conjugates during chronic therapy, quantitation could be in error if the drug were liberated by hydrolysis during extraction with a strong mineral acid. To avoid this possibility, they recommended that plasma be buffered to pH 4.5 before extraction with diethyl ether.

A variety of organic solvents have been used to extract valproic acid from acidified biological samples. Chloroform (3,4,17,24,25,27,28,30, 33,36,37,39,42,45,47), diethyl ether (5,14, 21,26,40,46), methylene chloride (1,2), carbon tetrachloride (10), heptane (13), butyl acetate (15), toluene (22,44), carbon disulfide (29,41), hexane (43), and pentane (18) have been used in the extraction step. Here, two approaches have been taken: (a) large-volume extraction (1 to 5 ml of organic solvent), or (b) small-volume extraction (100 to 300 μl of organic solvent). The large volume of organic solvent must be reduced before the drug is quantitated. In some cases, the volume reduction is carried out at atmospheric pressure at elevated temperatures. Care must be taken under these conditions not to reduce the volume too rapidly or too near to dryness. Valproic acid and/or the internal standard may be lost during volume reduction, giving erroneous results. This error may be minimized by adding a small amount of solvent with higher boiling point (e.g., 100 μl of isoamyl acetate) to the organic phase prior to volume reduction. The solvent with lower boiling point is then removed, leaving the smaller volume of solvent with higher boiling point. When small volumes of solvent are used, 1 to 3 μl of the organic solvent can be injected into the gas chromatograph. In this case, the choice of organic solvent is important because the volume of acidified plasma is equal to or greater than the volume of organic solvent. A favorable partition coefficient for extraction of valproic acid is desired.

Nonextraction Methods

Dacremont and Cocquyt (9), followed by Jakobs et al. (23), described methods of analysis for valproic acid that did not require an extraction step. Small volumes of plasma or serum (20 to 100 μl) were acidified with 10 to 20 μl of 1 N HCl. The mixture was allowed to stand for a few minutes, and 1 μl of supernatant was then injected into the gas chromatograph. Pileire (35) did not use acidified samples but instead injected the sample directly into the column and created the volatile valproic acid by saturating the carrier gas with formic acid. Nonextraction methods must use column packing that is compatible with aqueous injections. Problems may also arise from serum proteins either clogging the syringe or precipitating into the injection port of the column. Columns can be rejuvenated by replacing the first 10 cm of the column packing. As the column deteriorates, irregular peak shape and peak tailing become evident, with the loss of precision and sensitivity.

Internal Standards

Proper quantitation of valproic acid, as well as other antiepileptic drugs, requires the use of an internal standard. An internal standard has been used in every method developed for the quantitation of valproic acid. Most commonly used as internal standards are the carboxylic acids: hexanoic acid or its analogs (3,28,34, 36,40), octanoic acid or its analogs (13,17, 22,24,33,35,41,44), heptanoic acid (14,20,21), nonanoic acid derivatives (9,10,21,23,29–31,42), or cyclohexaneacetic acid (4,15, 18, 21,27,43,45,46). Nonacids used as internal standards are thymol (37), acetophenone (25,39), paramethadione (1,2), or succinic anhydride (26). The use of carboxylic acids with physical properties similar to valproic acid assures a more suitable extraction and chromatographic scheme.

Hershey et al. (21) studied the stability of the standard curve for valproic acid when cyclohexanecarboxylic acid (CHCA), 2-ethylpentanoic acid (EPA), and 2-propylhexanoic acid (PHA) were used as internal standards. They used a 10% SP-1000 column. As the column "aged," the data varied according to specific characteristics of the internal standards. During the early lifetime of the column, the peak height ratios based on EPA remained essentially constant, those based on PHA varied slightly, and those based on CHCA drifted characteristically. Three weeks later, the ratios based on EPA and PHA became less predictable and continued to deteriorate. Those based on CHCA, however, became constant over the lifetime of the column. These findings indicate that standard curves should be run periodically to assure that the column characteristics have not changed.

Derivative Formation

Several methods of analysis for valproic acid use derivative formation following extraction of the drug from plasma. A more volatile product with excellent chromatographic characteristics is formed. Ferrandes and Eymard (14) formed trimethylsilyl (TMS) derivatives of valproic acid and the internal standard, methylpentylacetic acid, following their extraction from acidified plasma into ether. Trimethylchlorosilane and hexamethyldisilane in anhydrous pyridine were added to the ether residue and allowed to react for 30 min. The TMS derivative appeared to be stable for 2 hr. Both compounds tended to elute on the pyridine solvent front.

Willox and Foote (46) extracted valproic acid and cyclohexanecarboxylic acid from acidified plasma into ether. The ether extract was evaporated, and the residue was dissolved in a methanolic solution of trimethylphenylammonium hydroxide (0.1 M). The carboxylic acid was methylated by "on column" flash methylation in a manner similar to that described by Kupferberg (27) and others for the analysis of other antiepileptic drugs.

Tupper et al. (43) esterified valproic acid following extraction into hexane. Hydrochloric acid in methanol was added to the hexane extract and heated for 30 min at 60°C. The resulting methyl ester of valproic acid was quantitated by gas chromatography.

Hulshoff and Roseboom (22) determined valproic acid by forming its butyl ester. The derivatization technique is based on that of Greeley (16). Acidic drugs can be alkylated when a base such as tetramethylammonium hydroxide (2 M) is combined with *N,N*-dimethylacetamide and 1-iodobutane. Valproic acid was extracted into toluene and then back-extracted into tetramethylammonium hydroxide in methanol.

Gyllenhaal and Albinsson (20) developed a method of analysis for valproic acid involving its partition, as an ion pair with tetrabutylammonium as counter ion, into dichloromethane containing iodomethane. Complete methylation occurred after 35 min.

Gupta et al. (18) converted valproic acid and the internal standard, cyclohexanecarboxylic acid, to their corresponding phenylacyl esters. Valproic acid extracts were reacted with α-bromoacetophenone for 60 min at 55°C. The resulting stable esters were chromatographed on 3% OV-17 at 205°C. Nitrophenacyl esters, for analysis with a nitrogen–phosphorous detector, can be made by using α-bromo-*p*-nitroacetophenone as the derivatizing agent.

Derivative formation should be used if interfering materials produce irreproducible results.

Column Packings

Various types of column packings have been used in the analysis of valproic acid. The majority of methods use polar liquid stationary phases: polyethylene glycol (PEG) or modified PEG (3,4,9–11,15,17,20,21,24,27–31,34–37, 42,44,45) or polyesters (5,13,23,25,33,39, 41,47). These phases have been modified with substituted terephthalic acid or phosphoric acid to reduce tailing of carboxylic acid peaks and improve the thermal stability of the polyesters.

The phase load on the solid support varies from 5 to 10%. Column temperature ranges from 150°C (polyesters) to 180°C (PEG). Retention time for valproic acid varies from 3 to 5 min. Because these phases have limited thermal stability, care must be taken to insure that injection port temperatures do not exceed the manufacturer's specifications. When the peak shape of valproic acid and the internal standard appears to deteriorate, removal of the initial 10 cm of column packing and repacking with stationary phase will renew the column performance. Care must be taken to flush oxygen from the column before elevating the oven temperature.

Silicone phases, such as SE-30, OV-17, or OV-225, are sometimes used (1,2,14,18,22, 26,43,46). In this case, oven temperatures are much lower, in the range of 90 to 110°C, depending on the length of the column or percent coating of the liquid phase.

Sensitivity and Specificity

All methods for the analysis of valproic acid are sensitive enough to allow its quantitation in patients receiving either a single dose or multiple doses of the drug. At least 85% of valproic acid is recovered by the majority of extraction procedures. Five micrograms of valproic acid extracted from a plasma sample can be quantitated with good precision.

Other antiepileptic drugs do not interfere with any of these methods. However, metabolites of valproic acid or other endogenous materials may, under certain conditions, cause erroneous results (see section on Extraction).

High-Performance Liquid Chromatography

Since valproic acid has no ultraviolet maximum between 205 and 400 nm, alternative methods of detection are required. In one HPLC method, the detection of valproic acid involved a colorimetric procedure based on variation in color of a solution of bromocresol purple (12). Gupta et al. (19) applied the phenacyl derivative technique described above to reverse-phase liquid chromatography.

Gas Chromatography–Mass Spectrometry

Balkon (2) adapted a gas chromatographic method for valproic acid to chemical ionization mass spectrometry. The quasimolecular ion, m/z 145 for valproic acid, was used in the determination with methane as the reagent gas. Schier et al. (38) have also developed a similar method.

CONCLUSIONS

Over 40 methods of analysis for the determination of valproic acid have been published since Meijer and Hessing-Brand's original report in 1973. The methods are similar, and each is sensitive and rapid enough to meet the needs of most therapeutic monitoring programs. Therefore, the choice of a method for determination of valproic acid should be based on available equipment and personnel and an understanding of the pitfalls that can occur.

CONVERSION

Conversion factor:

$$CF = \frac{1000}{mol. \ wt.} = \frac{1000}{144.0} = 6.94$$

Conversion:

$$(\mu g/ml) \times 6.94 = (\mu moles/liter)$$
$$(\mu moles/liter) \div 6.94 = (\mu g/ml)$$

REFERENCES

1. Balkon, J. (1978): Rapid determination of valproic acid in biological specimens. *J. Anal. Toxicol.*, 2:207–209.
2. Balkon, J. (1979): Rapid CI–MS determination of valproic acid; adaptation of a gas chromatographic assay. *J. Anal. Toxicol.*, 3:78–79.
3. Berry, D. J., and Clarke, L. A. (1978): Determination of valproic acid (dipropylacetic acid) in plasma by gas–liquid chromatography. *J. Chromatogr.*, 156:301–307.
4. Blom, G. F. (1977): Evaluation of routine gas liquid chromatographic methods for the determination of antiepileptic drugs. In: *Antiepileptic Drug Monitoring*, edited by C. Gardner-Thorpe, D. Janz, H. Meinardi, and C. E. Pippenger, pp. 21–32. Pitman Medical, Tunbridge Wells.
5. Bruni, J., Wilder, B. J., Willmore, L. J., Perchalski, R. J., and Villarreal, H. J. (1978): Steady-state kinetics of valproic acid in epileptic patients. *Clin. Pharmacol. Ther.*, 24:324–332.
6. Burton, B. S. (1882): On the propyl derivatives and decomposition products of ethyl acetoacetate. *Am. Chem. J.*, 3:385–395.
7. Carraz, G., Fau, R., Chateau, R., and Bonnin, J. (1964): First clinical trials of the antiepileptic activity of *n*-dipropylacetic acid (sodium salt). *Ann. Med. Psychol. (Paris)*, 122:577–585.
8. Chang, Z. L. (1979): Sodium valproate and valproic acid. In: *Analytical Profiles of Drug Substances, Vol. 8*, edited by K. Florey, pp. 529–556. Academic Press, New York.
9. Dacremont, G., and Cocquyt, G. (1977): Simple method for the determination of di-*n*-propylacetic acid in serum. *Acta Paediatr. Belg.*, 30:41–44.
10. Dijkhuis, I. C., and Vervloet, E. (1977): Rapid determination of the antiepileptic drug di-*n*-propylacetic acid in serum. In: *Pharmacokinetics and Metabolism of the Antiepileptic Drug Sodium Valproate (Depakine, Epilim)*, edited by T. B. Vree and E. van der Kleijn, pp. 4–6. Bohn, Scheltema & Holkema, Utrecht.
11. Dusci, D. J., and Hackett, L. P. (1977): Gas chromatographic determination of valproic acid in human plasma. *J. Chromatogr.*, 132:145–147.
12. Farinotti, R., Pfaff, M. C., and Mahuzier, G. (1978): Dosage simultané du phénobarbital et de l'acide valproïque dans le plasma par chromatographie liquide haute performance. *Ann. Biol. Clin. (Paris)*, 36:347–353.
13. Fellenberg, A. J., and Pollard, A. C. (1977): A rapid and sensitive gas–liquid chromatographic procedure for the micro determination of sodium valproate (sodium di-*n*-propylacetate) in plasma or serum. *Clin. Chim. Acta*, 81:203–208.
14. Ferrandes, B., and Eymard, P. (1973): Méthode rapide d'analyse quantitative du dipropylacétate de sodium dans le sérum ou le plasma. *Ann. Pharm. Fr.*, 31:279–282.
15. Friel, P. N., Leal, K. W., and Wilensky, A. J. (1979): Valproic acid–phenytoin interaction. *Ther. Drug Monitor.*, 1:243–248.
16. Greeley, R. H. (1974): New approach to derivatization and gas-chromatographic analysis of barbiturates. *Clin. Chem.*, 20:192–194.
17. Grgurinovich, N., and Miners, J. O. (1980): Simple, rapid procedure for the determination of valproate and ethosuximide in plasma by gas–liquid chromatography. *J. Chromatogr.*, 182:237–240.
18. Gupta, R. N., Eng, F., and Gupta, M. L. (1979): Gas-chromatographic analysis for valproic acid as phenacyl esters. *Clin. Chem.*, 25:1303–1305.

19. Gupta, T. N., Keane, P. M., and Gupta, M. L. (1979): Valproic acid in plasma, as determined by liquid chromatography. *Clin. Chem.*, 25:1984–1985.

20. Gyllenhaal, O., and Albinsson, A. (1978): Gas chromatographic determination of valproate in minute serum samples after extractive methylation. *J. Chromatogr.*, 161:343–346.

21. Hershey, A. E., Patton, J. R., and Dudley, K. H. (1979): Gas chromatographic method for the determination of valproic acid in human plasma. *Ther. Drug Monitor.*, 1:217–241.

22. Hulshoff, A., and Roseboom, H. (1979): Determination of valproic acid (di-*n*-propyl acetic acid) in plasma by gas–liquid chromatography with pre-column butylation. *Clin. Chim. Acta*, 93:9–13.

23. Jakobs, C., Bojasch, M., and Hanefeld, F. (1978): New direct micro-method for determination of valproic acid in serum by gas chromatography. *J. Chromatogr.*, 146:494–497.

24. Jensen, C. J., and Gugler, R. (1977): Sensitive gas–liquid chromatographic method for determination of valproic acid in biological fluids. *J. Chromatogr.*, 137:188–193.

25. Johannessen, S. I. (1977): Preliminary observations on valproic acid kinetics in patients with epilepsy. *Arzneim. Forsch.*, 27:1083–1085.

26. Klotz, U. (1977): Pharmacokinetic studies with valproic acid in man. *Arzneim. Forsch.*, 27:1085–1088.

27. Kupferberg, H. J. (1978): Gas–liquid chromatographic quantitation of valproic acid. In: *Antiepileptic Drugs: Quantitative Analysis and Interpretation*, edited by C. E. Pippenger, J. K. Penry, and H. Kutt, pp. 147–151. Raven Press, New York.

28. Levy, R. H., Martis, L., and Lai, A. A. (1978): GLC determination of valproic acid in plasma. *Anal. Lett.*, B11:257–267.

29. Libeer, J.-C., Scharpé, S., Schepens, P., and Verkerk, R. (1978): Gas chromatographic analysis of sodium di-*n*-propylacetate in human plasma. *J. Chromatogr.*, 160:285–287.

30. Löscher, W. and Göbel, W. (1978): Consecutive gas chromatographic determination of phenytoin, phenobarbital, primidone, phenylethylmalondiamide, carbamazepine, trimethadione, dimethadione, ethosuximide, and valproate from the same serum specimen. *Epilepsia*, 19:463–473.

31. Meijer, J. W. A., and Hessing-Brand, L. (1973): Determination of lower fatty acids, particularly the antiepileptic dipropyl-acetic acid, in biological materials by means of micro diffusion and gas chromatography. *Clin. Chim. Acta*, 43:215–222.

32. Meunier, H., Carraz, G., Meunier, Y., Eymard, P., and Aimard, M. (1963): Propriétés pharmacodynamiques de l'acide *n*-dipropylacétique. I. Propriétés antiepileptiques. *Therapie*, 18:435–438.

33. Mihaly, G. W., Vajda, F. J., Miles, J. L., and Louis, W. J. (1979): Single and chronic dose pharmacokinetic studies of sodium valproate in epileptic patients. *Eur. J. Clin. Pharmacol.*, 16:23–29.

34. Peyton, G. A., Harris, S. C., and Wallace, J. E. (1979): Determination of valproic acid by flame-ionization gas–liquid chromatography. *J. Anal. Toxicol.*, 3:108–110.

35. Pileire, B. (1979): Use of formic acid in carrier gas: A rapid method to quantitate dipropylacetate in plasma by gas–liquid chromatography. *J. Chromatogr.*, 162:446–450.

36. Puukka, M., Reunanen, M., Lamminsivu, U., and Puukka, R. (1978): Determination of sodium valproate (sodium di-*n*-propylacetate) in serum by gas–liquid chromatography. *Acta Neurol. Scand.*, 57:286–287.

37. Runci, F. M., and Segre, G. (1979): Simultaneous determination of di-*n*-propylacetic acid and ethosuximide in plasma by gas–liquid chromatography. *Farmaco [Prat.]*, 34:261–265.

38. Schier, G. M., Gan, I. E., Halpern, B., Korth, J. (1980): Measurement of sodium valproate in serum by direct-insertion chemical-ionization/mass spectrometry. *Clin. Chem.*, 26:147–149.

39. Schobben, F., and van der Kleijn, E. (1977): Determination of sodium di-*n*-propylacetate in plasma by gas–liquid chromatography. In: *Pharmacokinetics and Metabolism of the Antiepileptic Drug Sodium Valproate (Depakine, Epilim)*, edited by T. B. Vree and E. van der Kleijn, pp. 7–9. Bohn, Scheltema & Holkema, Utrecht.

40. Schulz, H.-U., and Toseland, P. A. (1977): Determination of the anticonvulsant drug—dipropyl acetate (Epilim) in human plasma by gas chromatography. *Ann. Clin. Biochem.*, 14:240–242.

41. Sioufi, A., Colussi, D., and Marfil, F. (1980): Gas chromatographic determination of valproic acid in human plasma. *J. Chromatogr.*, 182:241–245.

42. Swanson, B. N., Harland, R. C., Dickinson, R. G., and Gerber, N. (1978): Excretion of valproic acid into semen of rabbits and man. *Epilepsia*, 19:541–546.

43. Tupper, N. L., Solow, E. B., and Kenfield, C. P. (1978): A method for esterfication of valproic acid for gas–liquid chromatography: Clinical data from epileptic patients. *J. Anal. Toxicol.*, 2:203–206.

44. Vajda, F. J. E., Drummer, O. H., Morris, P. M., McNeil, J. J., and Bladin, P. F. (1978): Gas chromatographic measurement of plasma levels of sodium valproate: Tentative therapeutic range of a new anticonvulsant in the treatment of refractory epileptics. *Clin. Exp. Pharmacol. Physiol.*, 5:67–73.

45. Vree, T. B., van der Kleijn, E., and Knop, H. J. (1976): Rapid determination of 4-hydroxybutyric acid (gamma OH) and 2-propylpentanoate (Depakine) in human plasma by means of gas–liquid chromatography. *J. Chromatogr.*, 121:150–152.

46. Willox, S., and Foote, S. E. (1978): Simple method for measuring valproate (Epilim) in biological fluids. *J. Chromatogr.*, 151:67–70.

47. Wood, M. H., Sampson, D. C., and Hensley, W. J. (1977): The estimation of plasma valproate by gas–liquid chromatography. *Clin. Chim. Acta*, 77:343–347.

Antiepileptic Drugs, edited by D. M. Woodbury, J. K. Penry, and C. E. Pippenger. Raven Press, New York © 1982.

45

Valproate

Absorption, Distribution, and Excretion

René H. Levy and Allen A. Lai

The pharmacokinetic characteristics of valproic acid (VPA) are in many ways related to the physicochemical properties of the drug (see Chapter 44). As is the case for most aliphatic carboxylic acids, VPA is highly plasma protein bound in humans and has a relatively small volume of distribution. Its fatty acid structure explains the existence of metabolic routes of elimination involving α and β oxidation and of competitive protein binding interactions with endogenous fatty acids. The physicochemical properties of VPA can also account for its unusual nonlinear plasma level–dose relationship. At plasma levels above 80 μg/ml, its binding becomes saturable both *in vitro* and *in vivo.* Consequently, clearance becomes dose dependent, and, as dose increases, total drug levels increase in a less-than-proportional fashion. The literature on the disposition of VPA has expanded significantly in the last few years, and the early reviews on this drug have become outdated. In this chapter, more emphasis has been placed on recent literature. For additional information, the reader is referred to a recent review on the clinical pharmacokinetics of VPA (18).

ABSORPTION

Extent and Rate of Absorption

Most of the early studies of the absorption of VPA were single-dose studies. The extent of absorption or absolute bioavailability was recently determined using classical pharmacokinetic techniques, i.e., by comparison of the areas under the plasma concentration–time curves following single oral and intravenous bolus administration. Table 1 summarizes the absorption parameters for VPA obtained from studies in which the absolute bioavailability was determined. The sodium salt of valproic acid was used in these four studies. Despite differences in population (healthy volunteers and epileptic patients) and formulation (oral solution, immediate release tablet, and enteric-coated tablet), the absolute bioavailability of VPA was consistently found close to unity. These findings indicate that the absorption of VPA in the form of sodium salt is essentially complete. Although the literature does not contain any absolute bioavailability study on the acid itself, the absorption of the acid could be considered complete, since bioequivalence between the acid (capsules) and the sodium salt has been demonstrated (38).

There are no quantitative studies on the absorption kinetics of VPA. However, several studies provide qualitative absorption parameters such as peak time and latency time. Representative examples of peak times are listed in Table 1. In general, the rapid release formulations, regardless of chemical entity (acid or sodium salt) or dosage form (solution, syrup, or tablet), were absorbed with peak times of less

TABLE 1. *Rate and extent of valproate absorption (mean ± SD) from single-dose studies*

No. of subjects	Population	Dosage form[a]	Peak time (hr)	Absolute bioavailability[b]	Reference
6	Healthy adults	Immediate release tablets[c]	1.8 ± 1.3	1.00 ± 0.10	41
6	Epileptic adults	Immediate release tablets[c]	1.2 ± 0.6	0.96 ± 0.09	42
6	Healthy adults	Enteric coated tablets[d]	4.8 ± 2.0	0.90 ± 0.14	23
		Solution[e]	1.3 ± 0.6	0.95 ± 0.06	27
6	Healthy adults	Enteric coated tablets[f]	8.2 ± 4.1	1.08 ± 0.07	27

[a]The sodium salt of valproic acid was used in all four studies.
[b]Measured as AUC_o/AUC_{iv}.
[c]Depakene®.
[d]Orfiril®.
[e]Engenyl®.
[f]Depakene® 500R.

than 2 hr (1,9,17,23,29,42). In view of the high incidence of gastric discomfort following oral intake of VPA, enteric-coated tablets became available in several countries. These tablets exhibited much longer peak times than regular tablets, generally between 3 and 8 hr (17,23, 27,38). The long peak times actually represent delayed absorption and not prolonged absorption, since latency periods of 1 to 6 hr were observed following the ingestion of the enteric-coated tablet. The latency period is related to gastric emptying time as well as other factors, including tablet disintegration. It appears that once the absorption process began, the enteric-coated tablet attained peak concentrations as fast as the immediate-release formulation (17,23,27). These studies suggest that VPA has no site specificity for absorption and is probably absorbed throughout the intestine.

Factors Altering Absorption

The bioavailability of VPA appeared to be similar regardless of when the drug was taken: in a fasting state, immediately before, during, or after a meal (1,9,23,27,33). However, the same cannot be said about the rate of absorption. For immediate release formulations, peak concentrations were generally attained within 2 hr when the drug was taken under a fasting regimen or immediately before a meal. When the drug was ingested after a meal, peak concentrations were not reached until 3 to 8 hr after dosing (9). For enteric-coated tablets, peak concentrations were attained within 3 to 8 hr under a fasting regimen. However, when this formulation was ingested during or after a meal, peak concentrations were delayed by a few more hours (23,27).

These observations suggest that absorption profiles may be affected by meals. This source of variability should be taken into consideration in selecting optimum times for blood level monitoring (27; P. Loiseau, B. Centraud, R. H. Levy, R. Akbaraly, A. Brachet-Liermain, M. Guyot, and P. L. Morselli, *unpublished data*).

Effect of Disease State on Absorption

The absorption of VPA in epileptic patients was also found to be complete (Table 1). Epileptic patients appeared to have shorter peak times than did normal adults (42,44). However, the difference (0.5 to 1.0 hr) is probably not of any clinical significance. Patients with liver disease also appeared to absorb VPA as rapidly as epileptic patients (24).

DISTRIBUTION

Whole-Body Distribution

Whole-body autoradiograms of a pregnant squirrel monkey taken following short intravenous infusions of ^{14}C-VPA showed that the labeled drug crossed the placental barrier freely (47). The majority of the dose was found in blood, liver, kidney, and intestines of both the fetus and the mother. Valproic acid also appeared to accumulate in growing bones and to enter the brain rapidly. In the brain, redistribution of VPA and/or its metabolites was thought to take place. Initially, the labeled material was found predominantly in the white matter, especially in the cerebellar fiber tracts. Subsequently, radioactivity was found predominantly in the gray matter. Substantial accumulation of radioactivity in yellow ligaments of the brain was also observed.

Relation of Concentration in Other Body Fluids to Serum Concentration

Valproic acid penetrates into breast milk. In one nursing mother, the ratio of milk valproate concentration to serum concentration was approximately 7% (10). The cerebrospinal fluid VPA concentrations in over 700 epileptic patients receiving chronic VPA therapy were about 10% of those in serum (32). This finding is in agreement with the determination of a subsequent study (3). However, studies in dogs (12) and monkeys (25) suggest that VPA is actively transported out of cerebrospinal fluid. In rhesus monkey, there appears to be little or no blood–brain barrier for VPA. Continuous monitoring of valproate concentration in cerebrospinal fluid (fourth ventricle) showed that upswing and decay curves in cerebrospinal fluid closely followed the corresponding plasma curves (25,28). The ratio of saliva to serum VPA concentration was reported to range from 0.4 to 6% (3,17) with a poor correlation between saliva and plasma free concentration (15). These authors concluded that monitoring of valproic acid in saliva is not useful. It should be noted that the extent of penetration of VPA from plasma into other body fluids should be assessed with respect to the plasma free concentration. Valproic acid is extensively bound to plasma proteins, and it will be shown in the next section that the free fraction is nonlinear with respect to total plasma concentration.

Plasma Protein Binding

Fraction Bound

Since the binding of drugs to plasma protein can influence both volume of distribution and clearance of drugs in the body, the protein binding of VPA was extensively examined by many investigators. Studies were conducted in healthy volunteers and in patients with different diseases and/or at various total plasma concentrations. Table 2 summarizes the results of equilibrium dialysis studies reported in the literature. Within therapeutic plasma concentrations (50–100 µg/ml), valproate is highly bound (~90%) to plasma proteins in subjects with normal renal and hepatic function. The mean free (or unbound) fraction ranged from 5 to 13% (5,16,17,23,30,39,48).

In studies investigating the concentration dependence of valproate binding (5,23,39), the free fraction was shown to increase as the total plasma VPA concentration increased (Fig. 1). This phenomenon has profound effects on VPA clearance and volume of distribution as well as on the interpretation of VPA total levels during therapeutic monitoring. The relationship of nonlinear protein binding to VPA elimination will be taken up in a later section.

Binding Sites and Binding Constants

Valproic acid can be considered to bind mainly to albumin. It was found that the binding of valproate to α- and γ-globulin was minimal (22). Two different groups of albumin binding sites were found (16,43). The existence of one of these groups could have been overlooked by some investigators (39,48). One study reported that the number of binding sites was 1.5 for the primary

TABLE 2. *The binding of valproate to human plasma protein[a] (mean ± SD)*

Nature of plasma/ serum samples	Valproate concentration (μg/ml)	Free fraction	Reference
Spiked samples: plasma from six healthy adults	80	0.11	23
	~150	~0.30	
	~300	~0.65	
Spiked samples: plasma from seven patients with alcoholic cirrhosis	80	0.29	24
Spiked samples: plasma from four patients recovering from acute hepatitis	80	0.22	24
Spiked samples: plasma from blood bank	50–100	0.12–0.25	48
Plasma samples from six healthy adults dosed with valproate	60–90	0.07	17
Spiked samples: plasma from 24 patients with renal disease	50	0.18	16
Spiked samples: plasma from 16 healthy volunteers	50	0.08	16
Spiked samples: serum from three healthy volunteers	56 ± 3	0.05	30
Spiked reconstituted human serum albumin	27	0.13	39
	103	0.49	
Spiked samples: plasma from six healthy volunteers	47	0.07	5
	95	0.10	

[a]Equilibrium dialysis was used by all investigators.

group of albumin ($k = 6.9 \times 10^4$ liter/mole) and 6.8 sites for the secondary group ($k = 6.7 \times 10^2$ liter/mole) (16). A subsequent study found 2.1 sites for the primary group ($k = 2.7 \times 10^4$ liter/mole) (39).

Effect of Other Agents on Valproate– Albumin Binding

A significant proportion of epileptic patients are maintained on multiple drugs. Since other antiepileptic drugs are also highly bound, the effect of concomitant medications on VPA–albumin binding was investigated. It was found that the major anticonvulsant drugs, including phenytoin, carbamazepine, ethosuximide, and phenobarbital, had no effect on VPA–albumin binding (34,39,43,48,53). There are several reasons for this lack of effect on the valproate free fraction. Valproic acid is more tightly bound to serum albumin than other protein-bound antiepileptic drugs such as phenytoin ($n = 1.0$ and $k = 1.3 \times 10^4$ liter/mole) (13) and carbamazepine ($n = 1.1$ and $k = 1.4 \times 10^3$ liter/mole) (36). The molar concentrations of other antiepileptic drugs are smaller than those of valproic

acid and of albumin (600 μM). Also, since valproate has more than one type of site and more than one site of each type, displacement effects would not be readily apparent.

Salicylic acid (a tightly and highly protein-bound drug) was found to decrease valproate binding to plasma or human serum albumin *in vitro* (11,47). This interaction was evaluated *in vivo* in the rhesus monkey. Valproate free fraction and clearance increased with no change in valproate free fraction (50). It should not be surprising that free fatty acids are also able to competitively decrease valproate binding to human serum albumin (35,39) and human serum (35) (Fig. 1). This effect was demonstrated in the sera of patients treated with Intralipid® (53).

The competitive binding relationship between free fatty acids and VPA may have consequences at two levels. Endogenous free fatty acid levels oscillate during the diurnal period and result in concomitant oscillations in valproate free fraction (40). Also, the level of free fatty acids in serum increases during equilibrium dialysis, especially in samples obtained from fed (rather than fasted) subjects (T.A. Bowdle, I.H. Patel, R.H. Levy, and A.J. Wil-

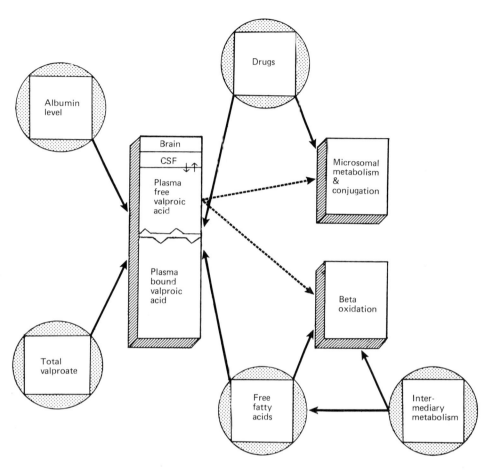

FIG. 1. Valproate binding and metabolism can be affected by a number of exogenous and endogenous factors.

ensky, *unpublished data*). This phenomenon could result in experimental artifacts in the determination of valproate free fraction by equilibrium dialysis.

Effect of Disease States on Valproate–Albumin Binding

In patients with alcoholic cirrhosis (23), acute hepatitis (23), or renal disease (7,16), the free fraction of VPA was found to increase two- to threefold. This difference in fraction unbound is associated with corresponding increases in clearance and volume of distribution of VPA. These are examined further in the description of the pharmacokinetics of VPA in disease states.

Apparent Volume of Distribution

The plasma VPA concentration–time curve after single-dose intravenous administration fits a two-compartment open model with first-order elimination (23,27,41). The mean apparent volume of distribution $(V_d\text{area})$[1] determined in those studies was consistent and ranged from 0.13 to 0.23 liter/kg (Table 3). A number of studies in which VPA was administered orally report volumes of distribution. Those values also range between 0.12 and 0.25 liter/kg (5,17,23, 27,41) which is not surprising, since VPA generally

---

[1]The volume of distribution at steady state was not different from $V_{d\text{ area}}$ in one study (23).

TABLE 3. *Pharmacokinetic parameters for valproate (mean ± SD)*

Population	Dose (mg) and route	$(V_d)_{area}$[a] (liter/kg)	$t_{1/2}\beta$ (hr)	Clearance (ml/hr per kg)	Reference
Six epileptic children	150–300 mg p.o. (tablet)	0.25 ± 0.10	9.4 ± 1.4	19 ± 10	46
One adult with Parkinson's disease	600 mg p.o. (tablet)	0.15	15.3	7	
Six healthy adults	400 mg i.v.	0.14 ± 0.05	12.2 ± 3.7	7 ± 3	23
	400 mg p.o. (solution)	0.12 ± 0.04	12.3 ± 4.6	8 ± 3	
	400 mg p.o. (enteric coated tablets)	0.14 ± 0.03	12.2 ± 2.5	7 ± 3	
Six healthy adults	600 mg p.o. (enteric coated tablets)	0.15 ± 0.02	15.9 ± 2.6	6 ± 1	17
Six healthy adults	800 mg i.v.	0.15 ± 0.00	12.8 ± 1.6	8 ± 1	41
	800 mg p.o. (tablets)	0.15 ± 0.02	12.7 ± 2.0	8 ± 1	
Six epileptic adults	800 mg i.v.	0.18 ± 0.03	9.0 ± 1.4	14 ± 4	13
	800 mg p.o. (tablets)	0.18 ± 0.03	9.0 ± 1.2	15 ± 4	
Seven patients with alcoholic cirrhosis	450 mg p.o. (solution)	0.22 ± 0.09	18.9 ± 5.1	8 ± 2	24
Four patients recovering from acute hepatitis	450 mg p.o. (solution)	0.20 ± 0.07	17.0 ± 3.7	9 ± 5	24
Six healthy adults	400 mg i.v.	0.23 ± 0.07	17.7 ± 6.5	11 ± 2	27
	500 mg p.o. (enteric coated tablets)	0.22 ± 0.10	15.8 ± 8.3	10 ± 2	
Six healthy adults	250 mg p.o. (capsule)	0.13 ± 0.01	9.8 ± 2.3	8 ± 2	5
Five healthy adults	600 mg p.o. (tablets)	0.16	12.0		21
	600 mg p.o. (solution)	0.16	15.7		

[a] In the calculation of $(V_d)_{area}$ and clearance following oral administration, complete absorption is assumed.

exhibits complete bioavailability. The relatively small value of the volume of distribution of VPA suggests that the distribution of this drug is restricted to the systemic circulation and rapidly exchangeable extracellular water. This restricted distribution is consistent with the physicochemical properties ($pK_a = 4.95$) of VPA and its protein-binding characteristics. However, this drug must also exhibit some tissue binding since the volume of distribution of free drug is larger than total body water.

The volumes of distribution of VPA for both epileptic children and adults were larger than that of healthy volunteers (Table 3). The mean volume of distribution for epileptic adults was 0.18 liter/kg (42), and the mean for epileptic children was 0.25 liter/kg (46). Patients with alcoholic cirrhosis and patients recovering from acute hepatitis also had volume terms larger than that of healthy volunteers (Table 3); the mean

volumes of distribution for these two groups of patients with liver disease were 0.22 and 0.20 liter/kg, respectively (24). The larger volume of distribution observed in patients with hepatic disease was probably caused by the increase in free fraction.

ELIMINATION

Clearance

Clearance in Healthy Volunteers

Mean values for plasma clearance of VPA in healthy volunteers are presented in Table 3. Within an intravenous dosage range of 400 to 800 mg, the mean plasma clearance ranged from 7 to 11 ml/hr per kg (24,28,43). As was the case for volume of distribution, valproate clearance values obtained from oral studies were very close to the intravenous values (6 to 11 ml/hr per kg) (5,17,23,27,41). Using a blood-to-plasma VPA concentration ratio of 0.28 (23), the blood clearance of valproate was calculated to range from 25 to 46 ml/min for a 70-kg person. This range of blood clearance represents only a small fraction (≤ 0.03) of the average hepatic blood flow (1,500 ml/min). Thus, VPA may be classified as a low-extraction drug with a clearance independent of blood flow (see Chapter 2). Furthermore, since the free fraction of VPA in plasma ($\alpha \simeq 0.1$) is larger than the extraction ratio ($E \leq 0.03$), the clearance is of the restrictive type, and only unbound VPA is cleared (51).

Effect of Disease States on Valproate Clearance

Disease states that change the plasma protein binding of VPA should affect the clearance of this drug, since an increase in free fraction should theoretically result in a proportional increase in clearance (see Chapter 2). As mentioned previously, valproate free fraction is increased at least twofold in patients with liver disease (24) and in patients with renal impairment (16) (Table 2). However, the clearance of VPA in patients with liver disease was not different from that in healthy volunteers (Table 3). This was because valproate intrinsic clearance (reflecting drug-metabolizing activity) was reduced, presumably as a consequence of liver cell damage (24). Thus, hepatic disease causes two opposing effects resulting in no apparent change in total clearance. As a result, valproate total steady-state levels would not change, whereas valproate free levels would be increased in such a situation (26). For additional information on this pharmacokinetic concept, the reader is referred to Chapter 2 (equation 27).

Effect of Concomitant Medications on Valproate Clearance

Valproic acid clearance in epileptic patients was larger than that in healthy volunteers (Table 3). The increase in clearance was attributed to liver enzyme induction caused by concurrent antiepileptic medications (2,19,21,42,44–46). The increase in VPA clearance as reflected by decrease in steady-state concentration has been seen in patients on phenobarbital, phenytoin, or carbamazepine (Fig. 1). Thus, higher doses of VPA may be required to maintain therapeutic concentrations in patients receiving concurrent antiepileptic drugs. Some reports indicate that these interactions are so pronounced that therapeutic levels of VPA cannot be achieved in some patients (19,21). The induction of VPA clearance by carbamazepine was verified in a study in healthy volunteers (4).

Nonlinearity in Valproate Clearance

A lack of correlation between plasma valproate level and dose during chronic administration was reported in several studies (2,8, 14,21,29,49,52) (Fig. 2). However, a linear relationship between these two parameters has also been reported (37). The mechanism of nonlinearity in VPA clearance was examined in a multiple-dose study in healthy volunteers (5). Each volunteer received 500, 1,000, and 1,500 mg/day in three consecutive steps. The nonlinearity in clearance was attributed principally to an increase in free fraction (as VPA concentration increases) and perhaps to a decrease in intrinsic clearance (5). The hypothesis that increases in free fraction lead to increases in plasma clearance of VPA explains why the nonlinearity in the level–dose relationship is of a convex nature (decrease in slope with an increase in dose) (Fig. 2) (see also Fig. 3 in Chapter 2).

Half-Life

The mean half-life of VPA in healthy volunteers as determined in several studies (5, 17,21,23,27,41) ranged from 9.5 to 17.7 hr (Table 3). Epileptic patients exhibited shorter half-lives, consistent with the inducibility of valproate metabolism by other antiepileptic drugs. The mean half-life in epileptic adults was approximately 9.0 hr (31,42). The relatively short

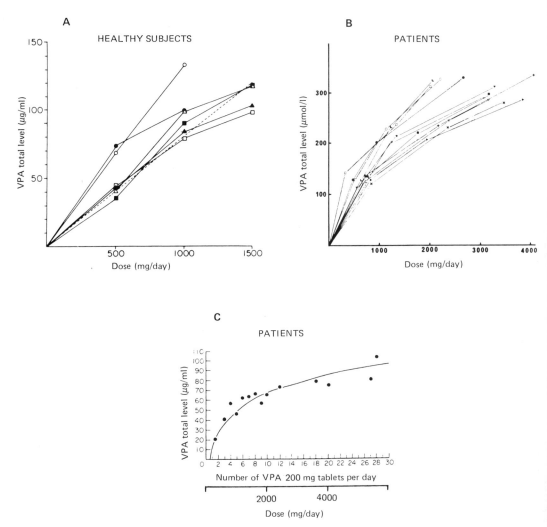

FIG. 2. Hyperbolic plasma level–dose relationship for valproic acid in epileptic patients and healthy subjects. **A:** Bowdle et al. (5); **B:** Gram et al. (14); **C:** Vajda et al. (49).

half-life of VPA explains (at least in part) the frequently reported oscillations in valproate levels during chronic therapy.

The VPA half-life appeared to be correlated with age in newborns and infants (6). Within the first 10 days after birth, half-lives ranged between 10 and 67 hr. Half-lives of infants between 10 and 60 days of age are longer in adults and reach adult values after 2 months of age (6). The mean half-life in epileptic children under 12 years of age was reported in two studies as 9.4 hr (46) and 12 hr (20), respectively.

The half-lives of VPA in patients with liver diseases have also been determined. The mean half-life in seven patients with alcoholic cirrhosis was 18.9 hr, and that in patients recovering from acute hepatitis was 17.0 hr (24). The increase in valproate free fraction associated with hepatic disease should have no effect on its half-life since it increases both clearance and volume of distribution. However, the decrease in intrinsic metabolic clearance of VPA (liver cell damage) explains the longer half-life of VPA in patients with hepatic disease (24).

Urinary Excretion

Valproic acid is extensively metabolized in man. The mean fraction of dose of VPA excreted unchanged in urine was 1.8% after a single dose and 3.2% at steady state in six healthy volunteers (17).

The renal clearance of free VPA (2–4 ml/min) is very small relative to glomerular filtration rate, suggesting that VPA is significantly reabsorbed. It can also be inferred that renal insufficiency should not affect the levels of VPA, although it could result in retention of metabolites.

CONCLUSION

Valproic acid is a relatively new antiepileptic drug in many ways different from the other members of this class of drugs. In terms of drug disposition, it exhibits some peculiar properties that must be taken into consideration to enhance the therapeutic management of patients on this drug. Its rapid absorption, short half-life, and saturable plasma binding result in extensive variations in serum level during chronic therapy. As a result, several issues pertaining to the serum level monitoring of valproate remain unresolved.

ACKNOWLEDGMENT

The authors acknowledge the excellent technical assistance provided by Ms. Colleen D. Montoya.

REFERENCES

1. Abbott Laboratories (1978): Drug Monograph on Depakene (Valproic Acid). Abbott Laboratories, Chicago.
2. Baruzzi, B., Bondo, B., Bossi, L., Castelli, D., Gerna, M., Tognoni, G., and Zagnoni, P. (1977): Plasma levels of di-*n*-propylacetate and clonazepam in epileptic patients. *Int. J. Clin. Pharmacol.*, 15:403–408.
3. Blom, G. F., and Guelen, P. J. M. (1977): The distribution of antiepileptic drugs between serum, saliva, and cerebrospinal fluid. In: *Antiepileptic Drug Monitoring*, edited by C. Gardner-Thorpe, D. Janz, H. Meinardi, and C. E. Pippinger, pp. 287–297. Pitman Medical, Tunbridge Wells, Kent.
4. Bowdle, T. A., Levy, R. H., and Cutler, R. E. (1979): Effects of carbamazepine on valproic acid kinetics in normal subjects. *Clin. Pharmacol. Ther.*, 26:629–634.
5. Bowdle, T. A., Patel, I. H., Levy, R. H., and Wilensky, A. J. (1980): Valproic acid dosage and plasma protein binding and clearance. *Clin. Pharmacol. Ther.*, 28:486–492.
6. Brachet-Liermain, A., and Demarquez, J. L. (1977): Pharmacokinetics of dipropyl acetate in infants and young children. *Pharm. Weekbl.*, 112:293–297.
7. Brewster, D., and Muir, N. D. (1980): Valproate plasma protein binding in the uremic condition. *Clin. Pharmacol. Ther.*, 27:76–82.
8. Bruni, J., Wilder, B. J., Willmore, L. J., Perchalski, R. J., and Villarreal, H. J. (1978): Steady-state kinetics of valproic acid in epileptic patients. *Clin. Pharmacol. Ther.*, 24:324–332.
9. Chun, A. H. C., Hoffman, D. J., Friedmann, N., and Carrijan, P. J. (1980): Bioavailability of valproic acid under fasting/nonfasting regimens. *J. Clin. Pharm.*, 20:30–36.
10. Espin, M. L. E., Benton, P., Will, E., Hayes, M. J., and Walker, G. (1979): Sodium valproate (Epilim)—Some clinical and pharmacological aspects. In: *Clinical and Pharmacological Aspects of Sodium Valproate (Epilim) in the Treatment of Epilepsy*, edited by N. J. Legg, pp. 145–151. MCS Consultants, Tunbridge Wells, Kent.
11. Fleitman, J. S., Bruni, J., Perrin, T. H., and Wilder, B. J. (1980): Albumin-binding interactions of sodium valproate. *J. Clin. Pharmacol.*, 20:514–517.
12. Frey, H. H., and Löshen, W. (1978): Distribution of valproate across the interface between blood and cerebrospinal fluid. *Neuropharmacology*, 17:637–642.
13. Goldstein, A. (1949): The interaction of drugs and plasma proteins. *J. Pharmacol. Exp. Ther.*, 95:102–165.
14. Gram, L., Flachs, H., Würtz-Jørgensen, A., Parnes, J., and Anderson, B. (1980): Sodium valproate, relationship between serum levels and therapeutic effect: A controlled study. In: *Antiepileptic Therapy: Advances in Drug Monitoring*, edited by S. I. Johannessen, P. L. Morselli, C. E. Pippenger, A. Richens, D. Schmidt, and H. Meinardi, pp. 247–252. Raven Press, New York.
15. Gugler, R., Eichelbaum, M., Schell, A., Fröscher, W., Kiefer, H., Schulz, H. U., and Müller, G. (1980): The disposition of valproic acid. In: *Antiepileptic Therapy: Advances in Drug Monitoring*, edited by S. I. Johannessen, P. L. Morselli, C. E. Pippenger, A. Richens, D. Schmidt, and H. Meinardi, pp. 121–129. Raven Press, New York.
16. Gugler, R., and Mueller, G. (1978): Plasma protein binding of valproic acid in healthy subjects and in patients with renal disease. *Br. J. Clin. Pharmacol.*, 5:441–446.
17. Gugler, R., Schell, A., Eichelbaum, M., Fröscher, W., and Schulz, H. U. (1977): Disposition of valproic acid in man. *Eur. J. Clin. Pharmacol.*, 12:125–132.
18. Gugler, R., and von Unruh, G. E. (1980): Clinical pharmacokinetics of valproic acid. *Clin. Pharmacokinet.*, 5:67–83.
19. Henriksen, O., and Johannessen, S. I. (1980): Clinical observations of sodium valproate in children: An

evaluation of therapeutic serum levels. In: *Antiepileptic Therapy: Advances in Drug Monitoring,* edited by S. I. Johannessen, P. L. Morselli, C. E. Pippenger, A. Richens, D. Schmidt, and H. Meinardi, pp. 253–261. Raven Press, New York.

20. Johannessen, S. I., and Henriksen, O. (1980): Pharmacokinetic observations of dipropylacetate in children. In: *Xth International Symposium on Epilepsy,* edited by J. A. Wada and J. K. Penry, p. 353. Raven Press, New York.

21. Johannessen, S. I., and Henriksen, O. (1980): Pharmacokinetic observations of sodium valproate in healthy subjects and in patients with epilepsy. In: *Antiepileptic Therapy: Advances in Drug Monitoring,* edited by S. I. Johannessen, P. L. Morselli, C. E. Pippenger, A. Richens, D. Schmidt, and H. Meinardi, pp. 131–137. Raven Press, New York.

22. Jordan, B. J., Shillingford, J. S., and Steed, K. P. (1976): Preliminary observations on the protein-binding and enzyme-inducing properties of sodium valproate (Epilim). In: *Clinical and Pharmacological Aspects of Sodium Valproate (Epilim) in the Treatment of Epilepsy,* edited by N. J. Legg, pp. 112–118. MCS Consultants, Tunbridge Wells, Kent.

23. Klotz, U., and Antonin, K. H. (1977): Pharmacokinetics and bioavailability of sodium valproate. *Clin. Pharmacol. Ther.,* 21:736–743.

24. Klotz, U., Rapp, T., and Müller, W. A. (1978): Disposition of valproic acid in patients with liver disease. *Eur. J. Clin. Pharmacol.,* 13:55–60.

25. Levy, R. H. (1980): CSF and plasma pharmacokinetics: Relationship to mechanisms of action as exemplified by valproic acid in monkey. In: *Epilepsy: A Window to Brain Mechanisms,* edited by J. S. Lockard and A. A. Ward, pp. 191–200. Raven Press, New York.

26. Levy, R. H. (1980): Monitoring of free valproic acid levels? *Ther. Drug Monit.,* 2:199–201.

27. Levy, R. H., Cenraud, B., Loiseau, P., Akbaraly, R., Brachet-Liermain, A., Guyot, M., Gomeni, R., and Morselli, P. L. (1980): Meal-dependent absorption of enteric-coated sodium valproate. *Epilepsia,* 21:273–280.

28. Levy, R. H., Lockard, J. S., and Ludwick, B. T. (1981): Nonlinear plasma protein binding and CSF concentration of valproic acid in monkey. *Epilepsia,* 22:229.

29. Loiseau, P., Brachet, A., and Henry, P. (1975): Concentration of dipropylacetate in plasma. *Epilepsia,* 16:609–615.

30. Löscher, W. (1978): Serum protein binding and pharmacokinetics of valproate in man, dog, rat and mouse. *J. Pharmacol. Exp. Ther.,* 204:255–261.

31. Mattson, R. H., Cramer, J. A., Williamson, P. D., and Novelly, R. A. (1978): Valproic acid in epilepsy: Clinical and pharmacological effects. *Ann. Neurol.,* 3:20–25.

32. Meijer, J. W. A., and Hessing-Brand, L. (1973): Determination of lower fatty acids, particularly the antiepileptic dipropyl-acetic acid, in biological materials by means of microdiffusion and gas chromatography. *Clin. Chim. Acta,* 43:215–222.

33. Meinardi, H., van der Kleijn, E., Meijer, J. W. A.,

and van Rees, H. (1975): Absorption and distribution of antiepileptic drugs. *Epilepsia,* 16:353.

34. Monks, A., Boobis, S., Wadsworth, J., and Richens, A. (1978): Plasma protein binding interaction between phenytoin and valproic acid in vitro. *Br. J. Clin. Pharmacol.,* 6:487–492.

35. Monks, A., and Richens, A. (1979): Serum protein binding of valproic acid and its displacement by palmitic acid *in vitro. Br. J. Clin. Pharmacol.,* 8:187–188.

36. Morselli, P. L., Genna, M., DeMaio, D., Zanda, G., Vaini, F., and Garattini, S. (1975): Pharmacokinetic studies on carbamazepine in volunteers and in epileptic patients. In: *Clinical Pharmacology of Anti-Epileptic Drugs,* edited by H. Schneider, D. Janz, C. Gardner-Thorpe, H. Meinardi, and A. L. Sherwin, pp. 166–180. Springer-Verlag, New York.

37. Nutt, J. G., and Kupferberg, H. J. (1979): Linear relationship between plasma concentration and dosage of sodium valproate. *Epilepsia,* 20:589–592.

38. Oelkers, V. W., Stoffels, G., Schafer, H., and Reith, H. (1977): Enteral absorption of valproic acid. *Arzneim. Forsch.,* 27:1088–1090.

39. Patel, I. H., and Levy, R. H. (1979): Valproic acid binding to human serum albumin and determination of free fraction in the presence of anticonvulsants and free fatty acids. *Epilepsia,* 20:85–90.

40. Patel, I. H., Levy, R. H., Venkataramanan, R., Viswanathan, C. T., and Moretti-Ojemann, L. (1980): Diurnal variation in protein binding of valproic acid and phenytoin and the role of free fatty acids. *Clin. Pharmacol. Ther.,* 27:277.

41. Perucca, E., Gatti, G., Frigo, G. M., and Crema, A. (1978): Pharmacokinetics of valproic acid after oral and intravenous administration. *Br. J. Clin. Pharmacol.,* 5:313–318.

42. Perucca, E., Gatti, G., Frigo, G. M., Crema, A., Calzetti, S., and Visintini, D. (1978): Disposition of sodium valproate in epileptic patients. *Br. J. Clin. Pharmacol.,* 5:495–499.

43. Potratz, J., and Schulz, H.-U. (1976): Protein binding of dipropylacetate (DPA) in human plasma. *Naunyn Schmiedebergs Arch. Pharmacol.,* 294:9R.

44. Richens, S. A., Scoular, I. T., Ahmad, S., and Jordan, B. J. (1976): Pharmacokinetics and efficacy of Epilim in patients receiving long-term therapy with other antiepileptic drugs. In: *Clinical and Pharmacological Treatment of Epilepsy,* edited by N. J. Legg, pp. 78–88. MCS Consultants, Tunbridge Wells, Kent.

45. Sackellares, C., Sato, S., Dreifuss, F. E., and Penry, J. K. (1981): Reduction of steady-state valproate levels by other antiepileptic drugs. *Epilepsia,* 22:437–441.

46. Schobben, F., van der Kleijn, E., and Gabreëls, F. J. M. (1975): Pharmacokinetics of di-*n*-propylacetate in epileptic patients. *Eur. J. Clin. Pharmacol.,* 8:97–105.

47. Schobben, F., Vree, T. B., and van der Kleijn, E. (1978): Pharmacokinetics, metabolism and distribution of 2-*n*-propyl-pentanoate (sodium valproate) and the influence of salicylate co-medication. In: *Advances in Epileptology, 1977,* edited by H. Meinardi

and A. J. Rowan, pp. 271–277. Swets & Zeitlinger, Amsterdam.

48. Taburet, A. M., and van der Kleijn, E. (1977): Plasma protein binding of 2-*n*-propyl pentanoate. *Pharm. Weekbl.*, 112:356–361.

49. Vajda, F. J. E., Drummer, O. H., Morries, P. M., McNeil, J. J. and Bladin, P. F. (1978): Gas chromatographic measurement of plasma levels of sodium valproate: Tentative therapeutic range of a new anticonvulsant in the treatment of refactory epileptics. *Clin. Exp. Pharmacol. Physiol.*, 5:67–73.

50. Viswanathan, C. T., and Levy, R. H.: Plasma protein binding interaction between valproic and salicylic acid in rhesus monkey. *J. Pharm. Sci. (in press.)*

51. Wilkinson, G. R., and Shand, D. G. (1975): A physiological approach to hepatic drug clearance. *Clin. Pharmacol. Ther.*, 18:377–390.

52. Wulff, K., Flachs, H., Würtz-Jørgensen, A., and Gram, L. (1977): Clinical pharmacological aspects of valproate sodium. *Epilepsia*, 18:149–157.

53. Zimmerman, C. L., Patel, I. H., Levy, R. H., Edwards, D., Nelson, S. D., and Hutchinson, M. (1981): Protein binding of valproic acid in the presence of elevated free fatty acids in patient and normal human serum. *Epilepsia*, 20:11–17.

Antiepileptic Drugs, edited by D. M. Woodbury, J. K. Penry, and C. E. Pippenger. Raven Press, New York © 1982.

46

Valproate

Biotransformation

Fred Schobben and Eppo van der Kleijn

Although valproic acid (VPA) has been known chemically for almost a century (1), interest in its *in vivo* fate has arisen only since the discovery of its anticonvulsant properties in 1963 (16). The only previous data, obtained by Keil (7) in 1947, indicated that this compound may be partially excreted unchanged in urine.

The mechanism of action of valproic acid has not been elucidated. In view of the delayed onset and sustained duration of therapeutic effects, which are incompatible with the short half-life of the drug itself, accumulation of metabolites may help to explain these effects.

Being a branched-chain fatty acid, valproic acid is subject to several oxidative processes that may lead to a series of metabolic products. Because of the physicochemical properties of the drug and derived substances, only a few analytical detection methods are appropriate. Gas–liquid chromatography (GLC) can be considered the only practical possibility for the analysis of nonradioactive material. However, the search for metabolites by the usual nonspecific detection methods is impaired by the natural occurrence of closely related substances in body fluids and tissues. Major advances in increased specificity of detection have recently been made by the use of mass spectrometry. The earliest information on the metabolism of valproic acid was obtained by the use of the radioactively labeled drug.

DETECTION OF METABOLITES IN TRACER STUDIES

After administration of [1 - ^{14}C] valproic acid to rats, Eymard et al. (2) found a marked excretion of radioactivity in bile. By thin-layer chromatography, they demonstrated the presence of unchanged valproic acid and six other radioactive components. Thirty-four percent of total radioactivity could be extracted by a lipophilic solvent, the major fraction of this representing unchanged valproic acid. Because substantial enterohepatic cycling was demonstrated, the authors suggested that valproic acid or its metabolites could be found in bile in conjugated form. Indeed, Kukino et al. (12) demonstrated in similar animal experiments that both bile and urine contained valproic acid and large amounts of its glucuronide.

According to Eymard et al. (2), a small percentage of the administered amount of radioactivity was recovered as $^{14}CO_2$ in expired air. Kukino et al. (12) and Kochen et al. (8) estimated that 10 to 20% of the total dose would be excreted in this way. Kukino et al. (12) demonstrated the origin of the labeled CO_2 to be the mitochondrial fraction of liver homogenates. The influence of various physical and chemical factors on the production of $^{14}CO_2$ led them to conclude that an oxidative enzymatic reaction involving coenzyme-A (CoA) was the principal factor. Beta-oxidation was suggested as the metabolic pathway.

In the urine of rats treated with valproic acid for a few weeks, Kochen et al. (8) found as many as 10 different radioactive components. Without hydrolysis, only four components could be separated. This indicates the presence of conjugated or esterified substances. However, the formation of artifacts by their procedure cannot be ruled out. Two compounds could not be detected during the first week of treatment. This observation deserves special attention, as it indicates that the metabolite pattern of the drug is not yet in equilibrium when the parent drug reaches steady state.

Similar conclusions can be drawn from pharmacokinetic studies in dog and monkey in which the radioactively labeled drug was used. The elimination of total radioactivity from plasma was considerably slower than the disappearance of the drug itself. In dog, the half-life for total radioactivity was found to be 17 times as long as that of valproic acid (22). In monkeys, smaller but still significant differences have been found. Single-compartment kinetics were found during intravenous infusion for a few hours. Half-lives of about 60 min were found for valproic acid, whereas the half-lives for total radioactivity averaged 100 min (23).

After infusion of labeled valproic acid into monkeys for 0.5–9 hours, the distribution pattern of metabolites could be shown by analysis of blood and tissue homogenates for composition of radioactive compounds. A representative chromatogram is shown in Fig. 1. Metabolites were present in urine and intestinal fluid containing bile as well as in blood and brain tissue (24). Although the total amount of radioactivity in brain was low, small amounts of pharmacologically active metabolites could be one explanation for the therapeutic effects of valproic acid.

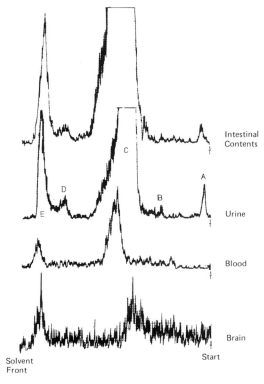

2- PROPYL- PENTANOATE-CARBOXY-^{14}C IN SQUIRREL MONKEY

T.L.C.-separation of radioactive compounds

FIG. 1. Distribution of radioactive compounds in squirrel monkey after 4-hr i.v. infusion of [1-^{14}C] valproic acid. Body fluids and tissue homogenates were hydrolyzed with alkali prior to acidic extraction. Radioscans show separation by thin-layer chromatography. The R_f value of valproic acid corresponds to peak C. (From Schobben et al., ref. 24, with permission.)

METABOLITES AND METABOLIC PATHWAYS

Urinary Metabolites

Products of Oxidative Reactions

Only during recent years have the structures of a number of metabolites of valproic acid been discovered by means of gas chromatographic/mass spectrometric (GC/MS) techniques. In 1974, Kuhara and Matsumoto (11) searched for metabolites by this technique in the urine of rats treated with valproic acid. Extracts of urine were screened for drug-specific peaks after formation of trimethylsilyl derivatives. They identified 2-propylglutaric acid (PGA) by comparison with the authentic compound. Another peak was thought to represent the intermediate oxidation product, 2-propyl-5-hydroxyvaleric acid (5-OH-VPA). In this way they proved ω-oxidation to be a metabolic pathway (see Fig. 2, left column).

Two years later, the same authors reported the presence of several additional metabolites (14). The mass spectra of the drug-specific peaks were interpreted as belonging to the trimethylsilyl derivatives of 2-propyl-3-hydroxyvaleric acid (3-OH-VPA), 2-propyl-4-hydroxyvaleric acid (4-OH-VPA), and 2-propyl-3-ketovaleric

acid (3-oxo-VPA). Although no comparison was made with synthetic products, the oxidation of valproic acid at the β, γ, and δ atoms was considered likely. With ethyl acetate as the extracting agent, the presence of valproic acid glucuronide could be confirmed by GC/MS. Previous evidence had been based on the liberation of valproic acid by treatment of urine with β-glucuronidase. In addition to the metabolites mentioned above, the excretion of a number of hydroxy acids was increased in comparison with control animals. However, there is no evidence

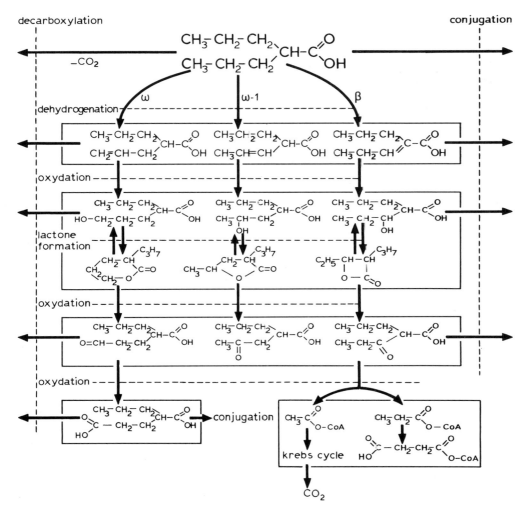

FIG. 2. Metabolic pathways of valproic acid. For the sake of clarity, the three oxidative routes are supposed to proceed by identical steps, including some hypothetical ones. The metabolism of 3-oxo-VPA (**lower right**) has been proposed by Matsumoto et al. (14). At most intermediate levels decarboxylation and formation of conjugates are possible. Almost all compounds shown have been detected *in vivo*.

that these substances are actual metabolites of valproic acid.

In 1977, Gompertz et al. (4) proved the presence of 3-oxo-VPA in the urine of patients treated with valproic acid by comparison with the synthetic product. This compound was accidently discovered when the urines of two patients were screened for organic acids. After methylation, in gas chromatographic analysis on a diethyleneglycolsuccinate column, a major peak was observed at the position of the benzoic acid methyl ester. Further investigation showed that this peak represented a major urinary metabolite of valproic acid, accounting for approximately 20% of the administered dose. In addition, minor amounts of 2-propylglutaric acid appeared to be present. Besides these substances, Kochen et al. (8) suggested that 5-OH-VPA and 2-propylmalonic acid may be found in human urine. The analysis of some 24-hr urine specimens of two patients receiving valproic acid showed that 6 to 24% of the daily dose was excreted as 3-oxo-VPA, 1 to 4% as 5-OH-VPA, and 1 to 5% as PGA. Kuhara et al. (10) detected in human urine the same metabolites they had found in rats. In this way, the series of human metabolites was enlarged with 3-OH-VPA and 4-OH-VPA.

In addition, Kochen and Scheffner (9a) have detected some unsaturated metabolites in the urine of patients chronically treated with VPA. In patients on multiple antiepileptic drug therapy, almost 100% of the daily dose could be recovered in 24-hr urine samples as VPA and 10 metabolites. The urinary concentrations of unstaturated metabolites were found remarkably high in a patient during the terminal stage of a fatal liver disease.

Products of Conjugation Reactions

Valproic acid glucuronide is the major urinary metabolite, accounting for about 40% of the dose during chronic administration (8,19). Treatment of urine with β-glucuronidase or heating with strong alkali did not liberate equal amounts of valproic acid (27). Therefore, valproic acid is present in other chemical combinations that are susceptible to hydrolysis. The formation of the glycine conjugate has been denied by Gompertz et al. (4). Treatment with sulfatase did not set free valproic acid (18). Apparently, the amide of valproic acid has not been found after the administration of the drug (17). Thus, the observed differences in liberated amounts of valproic acid will have to be explained by the presence of esters or substituted amides of the drug unless they are caused by artifacts generated by boiling with alkali. Conjugation with glutamates is a remaining possibility.

Metabolites in Plasma

In 1978, Kuhara et al. (10) reported the presence of a metabolite of valproic acid in human plasma. The mass spectrum of the silylated compound suggested the presence of a double bond in the valproic acid molecule. The same compound had been demonstrated before in human urine by Kochen et al. (8) who suggested subsequently that it might have been an artifact (9). Under the acidic conditions chosen for extraction and the high temperatures required for GC/MS, some of the hydroxy acids found to be metabolites may undergo dehydration to form unsaturated derivatives of valproic acid. At acidic pH values, hydroxy acids tend to form lactones, losing a water molecule as well. Therefore, a molecular weight of 142, which has been observed for several underivatized metabolites of the drug, can be attributed either to a monounsaturated valproic acid or to a lactone of 4-OH-VPA or 5-OH-VPA. 2-Propyl-3-hydroxyvaleric acid would not react in a similar way, as β-lactones are generally unstable. This compound would preferentially form an unsaturated acid, even under mild conditions. Because valproic acid and its metabolites are usually extracted at acidic pH values, 4-OH-VPA and 5-OH-VPA are analyzed as their lactones.

Jakobs and Löscher (6) screened sera of epileptic patients and of several animal species for metabolites of valproic acid without derivatization of the serum extracts. Using a similar technique, Pfaff et al. (17) had discovered two peaks in extracts of patient urine that were specific for treatment with valproic acid. The former authors discovered four metabolites in serum (Fig. 3); three of them had a molecular weight of 142. After obtaining the reference compounds from Schäfer and Lührs (19), they proved that two of these compounds were identical to 4-OH-VPA-lactone and 5-OH-VPA-lactone. The mass spectrum of a third compound suggested the structure 2-propyl-2-pentenoic acid (α,β-unsaturated VPA). According to the authors, this would be an artifact generated from 3-OH-VPA under their analytical conditions. The fourth metabolite apparently had a molecular weight of 140. Both Pfaff et al. (17) and Jakobs and Löscher (6) formulated the hypothesis that the mass spectrum obtained was derived from dihydroxyvalproic acid by loss of two molecules of water.

Comparison with Synthetic References

As mentioned before, the hydroxy acids may undergo dehydration to form the respective unsaturated compounds. The unsaturated acids, however, may be hydrolyzed to the hydroxy acids under other conditions. Thus, it was difficult to prove which of these compounds were the real metabolites until all related substances had become available by chemical synthesis. Schäfer and colleagues (19,20) have provided a substantial number of reference compounds. In their first paper (19), they described the synthesis of 3-OH-VPA, 4-OH-VPA, and 3-oxo-VPA and the analysis of these compounds in urine. The last-named compound could not be analyzed by GLC until it was hydrolyzed to form 3-heptanone. Although the absolute specificity of this method is still unproven, it was confirmed that 3-oxo-VPA is a major urinary metabolite in man. Smaller amounts of 4-OH-VPA and 5-OH-VPA were also present. In a subsequent publication, Schäfer et al. (20) also reported on 3-OH-VPA. This substance appeared to decompose during GLC analysis, and, therefore, acetylation was carried out before quantitation. Special precautions had to be taken to prevent dehydration to α,β-unsaturated VPA. 2-Propyl-3-hydroxyvaleric acid was found in the serum and cerebrospinal fluid of two patients on valproic acid

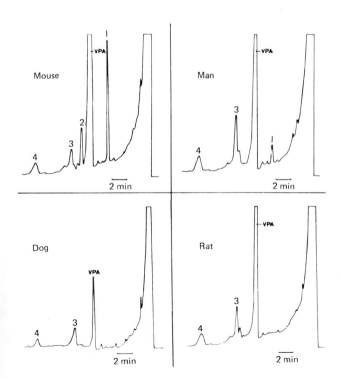

FIG. 3. Gas–liquid chromatographic separation of valproic acid and four metabolites on a Carbowax® 6000 column in serum of an epileptic patient and three animal species. Detection was achieved by electron ionization (GC/MS total ion current). Peak 1 corresponds to 4-OH-VPA, peak 2 is 5-OH-VPA, and peak 3 is considered α,β-unsaturated VPA. Peak 4 is ascribed to a dihydroxy metabolite. (From Jakobs and Löscher, ref. 6, with permission.)

treatment. The authors reported that 3-oxo-VPA is often found in patient serum, sometimes at high concentrations. In serum of mice, 3-OH-VPA and 4-OH-VPA but not the ketone were found. In brain tissue of these mice, only 3-OH-VPA could be detected.

Kochen and Scheffner (9) also have synthesized several potential metabolites, including two of the three possible monounsaturated derivatives. By capillary GLC, they were able to separate the trimethylsilyl derivatives of these compounds. In plasma of patients on chronic valproate treatment, they could detect both stereoisomers of α,β-unsaturated VPA. According to their interpretation, two isomers of the β,γ analog (2-propyl-3-pentenoic acid) were also present. γ,δ-Unsaturated valproic acid (2-propyl-4-pentenoic acid) was difficult to separate from valproic acid itself, but its presence was likely. Thus, all three monounsaturated derivatives of valproic acid may be found in patient plasma. The existence of doubly unsaturated valproate metabolites was also made plausible (9,9a).

Schobben (21) synthesized the missing metabolite, β,γ-unsaturated valproic acid. Analysis of plasma of man, monkey, and dog showed the presence of a similar compound, although a very small difference between the native product and the pure compound was observed. Monitoring of plasma concentrations by frequent sampling showed that the corresponding plasma component had a longer half-life than valproic acid in all species tested. In contrast to the method of Kochen and Scheffner (9), analyses were carried out by direct extraction of plasma and GLC separation on a packed column without derivatization. Since then, the GLC properties of the three unsaturated compounds have been compared by this method, and separation appeared to be possible (Fig. 4). The mass spectra of the three compounds showed only slight quantitative differences. The major metabolite peak in serum was attributed to α,β-unsaturated VPA while only a minor amount of the β,γ analog was present. The third unsaturated compound could not be detected. It could be determined that the unsaturated compounds were not artifacts formed from the corresponding hy-

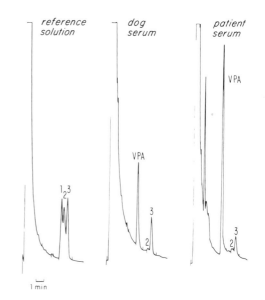

FIG. 4. Gas–liquid chromatographic separation of the three monounsaturated forms of valproic acid on an SP 1000 column. Peak 1 represents γ,δ-unsaturated VPA, peak 2 the β,γ analog, and peak 3 the α,β isomer. The last-named compound appeared to be the most important one in serum, as shown for a dog sample taken 8 hr after a single dose and for a sample from an epileptic child chronically treated with valproate and carbamazepine.

droxy acids during analysis, as similar treatment of plasma samples spiked with the three available hydroxy acids gave blank results in this respect.

Combining elements of the aforementioned analytical procedures, Löscher (13a) has developed an assay for VPA and its most important metabolites in blood plasma by GLC with simple flame ionization detection: After the hydrolysis of 3-oxo-VPA to 3-heptanone as described above (19), a dual extraction procedure is employed. One extract is used without derivatization, the other one is analyzed after trimethylsilylation. Two different stationary phases are used for GLC separation. In patients on chronic treatment with VPA the following amounts of metabolites have been found by this method (mean $\pm$ SD): α,β unsaturated VPA, 8.4 $\pm$ 3.7 mg/liter; 3-keto VPA, 5.4 $\pm$ 2.9; 3-OH-VPA, 2.1 $\pm$ 1.7; 5-OH-VPA, 1.7 $\pm$ 0.9; and 4-OH-VPA, 0.7 $\pm$ 0.6 mg/liter ($N = 26$).

MECHANISM AND PRINCIPAL SITES OF METABOLISM

β-Oxidation

As may be concluded from the presence of the metabolites mentioned above, valproic acid undergoes β-, ω-, and (ω–1)-oxidation. Although β-oxidation is theoretically the most obvious way of metabolism for straight-chain fatty acids, the other pathways may be favored in the case of branched fatty acids. However, the relatively high concentrations of α,β-unsaturated VPA in plasma and of 3-oxo-VPA in urine suggest that β-oxidation is the main route.

According to Matsumoto et al. (14), the oxidation steps of valproic acid resemble those of isoleucine, which include the oxidation of the intermediate 2-methylbutyryl-CoA to 2-methyl-3-hydroxybutyryl-CoA. In agreement with this theory, they were able to show that the urinary excretion of products of β-oxidation of both valproic acid and isoleucine was decreased when the two substances were administered to rats concomitantly. As the oxidation of branched-chain amino acids mainly takes place in extrahepatic tissues, the same might be true for the β-oxidation of valproic acid.

The presence of α,β-unsaturated VPA is in accordance with the mechanism of the β-oxidation of fatty acids, the first step of which is the dehydrogenation of the CoA ester. This step is catalyzed by the enzyme acyl-CoA-dehydrogenase. Under the influence of enoylhydratase, 3-OH-VPA-CoA then could be formed; this would, in turn, be dehydrogenated to form 3-oxo-VPA-CoA (Fig. 2, right column).

High concentrations of α,β-unsaturated VPA are found in dog plasma and are even further increased by pretreatment with carbamazepine (21). Apparently, the enzymes involved in the β-oxidation of valproic acid are susceptible to enzyme induction.

Decarboxylation

Several authors have reported the expiration of $^{14}CO_2$ after administration of [1-^{14}C] valproic acid to experimental animals. Kukino et al. (12) demonstrated that the formation of the labeled carbon dioxide mainly takes place in liver mitochondria by an enzymatic reaction requiring oxygen and coenzyme-A. Matsumoto et al. (14) pointed out a hypothetical metabolic pathway to explain the formation of the labeled CO_2 by β-oxidation: 3-oxo-VPA-CoA would be cleaved to propionyl-CoA and pentanoyl-CoA, the latter substance being further oxidized to acetyl-CoA and propionyl-CoA. Both acetyl-CoA and propionyl-CoA can enter the Krebs' cycle—the latter via methylmalonyl-CoA and succinyl-CoA—and can be completely oxidized to carbon dioxide in this way (Fig. 2).

Comparison of the formation of $^{14}CO_2$ after administration of [1-^{14}C] valproic acid and [3-^{14}C] valproic acid to the same monkey showed that the proposed mechanism is not likely to be the most important one (25). About 8% of the dose of [1-^{14}C] valproic acid was rapidly expired as $^{14}CO_2$. In contrast, the formation of labeled carbon dioxide was very slow in the case of the alternative label and amounted to less than 1% of the dose. These findings suggest that an almost complete breakdown of the drug molecule plays only a minor role. Decarboxylation of valproic acid or intermediate metabolic products may be the major mechanism in the formation of carbon dioxide (Fig. 2).

The part of the molecule left after decarboxylation will have to be identified in order to prove the exact mechanism. As shown by Schäfer and Lührs (19), 3-oxo-VPA can easily be hydrolyzed to 3-heptanone. The latter substance has been demonstrated in rat urine by Matsumoto et al. (14). However, it is not unlikely that the substance was formed in urine during storage or analysis.

ω-Oxidation

Fatty acids may undergo ω-hydroxylation involving liver microsomal enzymes. Alcohol dehydrogenase and aldehyde dehydrogenase are responsible for the subsequent formation of dicarboxylic acids. In the case of linear fatty acids, no unsaturated intermediates could be traced (5). The metabolite pattern of valproic acid may be similar inasmuch as the concentrations of the γ,δ-unsaturated compound that have been determined are extremely low. Another explanation for the formation of this unsaturated compound and for its β,γ-unsaturated analog may be found in a desaturase reaction in liver microsomes (9).

Conjugation

Although valproic acid is metabolized by oxidative processes to a large extent, the most important urinary metabolite in all species is the glucuronide of the drug. Glucuronidation takes place in liver, and the conjugate can be recovered in bile and urine. Apparently, all biliary glucuronide is hydrolyzed in the intestines, and the free drug is reabsorbed. Depending on the site of sampling in the intestines, varying fractions of the drug appear to be conjugated (21,23). No glucuronide and only small amounts of free valproic acid have been found in feces.

Vree and van der Kleijn (27) studied the excretion of valproic acid glucuronide after single oral doses of sodium valproate. Increasing doses were administered to the same volunteer, and the urinary pH was strictly controlled. The excretion of glucuronide relative to the administered dose appeared to depend on urinary pH and on the dose. Higher doses resulted in significantly increased excretion of the glucuronide. The findings even suggested that with a dose below 4 mg/kg no glucuronide would be formed at all. The amount of free valproic acid in urine was negligible in all cases. As no bioavailability or first-pass problems have been described for the drug, these results suggest that other pathways for the elimination of valproic acid, i.e., oxidative metabolism, may be capacity limited. To investigate this possibility, the excretion of valproic acid at several dose levels will have to be studied again but with inclusion of the analysis of a number of metabolites.

SPECIES DIFFERENCES IN METABOLISM

In some of the abovementioned investigations, metabolite patterns have been compared in several species. However, only a few species have been screened for all known metabolites. Quantitative data are lacking in general. Therefore, information on this topic will be fragmentary.

Ferrandes and Eymard (3) quantitated propylglutaric acid in the urine of rabbit, rat, dog, and man after administration of valproic acid. The highest recovery was found in rabbit (17%), whereas less than 2% of the dose was recovered in rats and in a human volunteer. In the dog, the metabolite could hardly be detected. Surprisingly, they found an almost 100% recovery of unchanged valproic acid in two dogs after hydrolysis of the urine samples. This result is in contrast with that of other studies in dogs in which significant amounts of oxidation products have been found (6,15,21).

Jakobs and Löscher (6) compared some metabolites in serum of mouse, rat, and dog after a single dose of valproic acid and in serum of some patients on chronic therapy. The α,β-unsaturated VPA, thought by the authors to be derived from 3-OH-VPA, was found in all species; 4-OH-VPA was found in mice and in a relatively low concentration in human plasma, but it appeared to be absent in other species. The presence of 5-OH-VPA could be clearly demonstrated only in mouse plasma. Using a similar analytical technique for urine, Schobben (21) found 4-OH-VPA and 5-OH-VPA in man and monkey. Only traces of these substances could be found in dog. The latter species appeared to be unique in excreting α,β-unsaturated VPA. The largest fraction of the compound was present as glucuronic acid conjugate.

Metabolism of valproic acid in man and monkey appears to be rather similar (21). After a single dose of the drug to rhesus monkey and after termination of valproate treatment in epileptic patients, similar plasma curves for α,β-unsaturated VPA and 4-OH-VPA were observed (Figs. 5 and 6). The similarity does not hold for all types of monkey, as in squirrel monkey the first metabolite was lacking (21). Merits (15) compared the excretion of [2-^{14}C] valproic acid in man and four animal species. Details of their experiments are too scarce for proper judgment. Nevertheless, their findings

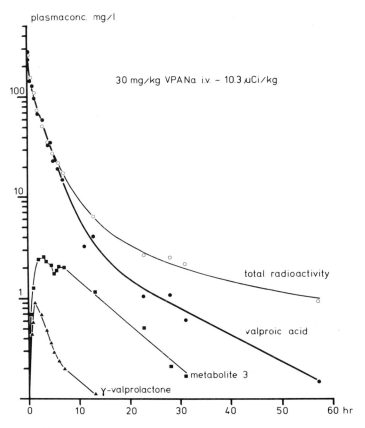

FIG. 5. Elimination of ^{14}C activity, valproic acid, and two metabolites from plasma of a rhesus monkey after rapid i.v. injection of the 1-^{14}C-labeled drug. Metabolite 3 represents α,β-unsaturated VPA; from the linear part of the curve, a half-life of 7 hr is estimated. γ-Valprolactone is the lactone of 4-OH-VPA. The concentrations of valproic acid are fitted to a three-exponential function with half-lives for the β and γ phases of 102 min and 11.3 hr, respectively. (From Schobben et al., ref. 25, with permission.)

give a rough indication of the relative importance of conjugation and oxidation reactions in the species tested. The excretion of the glucuronide of valproic acid accounts for 75 to 90% of the administered dose in dog, monkey, and rabbit but for only about 50% in rat and man.

In order to complete the information from comparative studies given above, all available qualitative data on the presence of metabolites of valproic acid in several species have been summarized in Table 1. From the data presented, β-oxidation appears to occur in all species. In dog, glucuronidation and β-oxidation seem to be the exclusive pathways. In rabbit, however, ω-oxidation appears to be the preferred alternative to conjugation. Rat and monkey appear to be the best models for the me-

tabolism of valproic acid in man, as β-oxidation is preferred over ω- and (ω–1)-oxidation in these species. In mouse, all three pathways might be equally important.

SIGNIFICANCE OF METABOLISM TO PHARMACOLOGICAL EFFECTS

Information on the pharmacological activities of the metabolites that have been detected is scarce and preliminary. Schäfer et al. (20) reported results of pharmacological testing of 3-OH-VPA, 4-OH-VPA, and 3-oxo-VPA in rats. These substances appeared to offer protection against maximal electroshock seizures, but their potencies were less than that of valproic acid itself. However, 4-OH-VPA significantly

TABLE 1. *Occurrence of valproic acid metabolites in several species*[a]

Species	3-OH-VPA	4-OH-VPA	5-OH-VPA	Unsaturated VPA α,β	β,γ	γ,δ	3-oxo-VPA	PGA[b]	VPA glucuronide	References
Man										
Blood	+	+	+	+ +	+	?	+			6,9,13a,20,21
Urine	+	+	+	+			+ +	+	+ +	8,9a,10,20,21
CSF	+						+			20
Monkey										
Blood		+		+						21
Urine		+	+	−					+ +	21
Brain		+		−						21
Rat										
Blood		−	−	+						6
Urine	+	+	+				+	+ +	+ +	11,14,20
Mouse										
Blood	+	+ +	+	+			−			6,20
Brain	+	−								20
Dog										
Blood		−	−	+	+					6,21
Urine		−	−	+				−	+ +	3,21
Rabbit										
Urine		+						+ +	+ +	3,15

[a]Symbols used: +, present; + +, relatively important concentration; −, absent or very low concentration; ?, conflicting results reported.
[b]2-Propylglutaric acid.

decreased mortality in the pentylenetetrazol test and was as effective as the parent drug.

Testing of the unsaturated metabolites has produced conflicting results. Kochen and Scheffner (9) reported the preliminary observation that α,β- and γ,δ-unsaturated VPA had much lower anticonvulsant activity than valproic acid in kindled cats. Taillandier et al. (26), however, found both substances almost as effective as valproic acid in the pentylenetetrazol test in mice. Recently Löscher (13a) has tested the effects of a couple of VPA metabolites on the chemo- and electroconvulsive threshold in mice. Among the compounds, mentioned in Table 1, α,β- and γ, d-unsaturated VPA appeared to be the most active compounds, accounting for 50 to 90% of the potency of VPA. Starting from these results, VPA metabolites would add less than 10% to the therapeutic effect of VPA in epileptic patients. However, this opinion is based only on comparison of plasma concentrations in different species and does not account for differences in tissue distribution.

As long as more information is not available, no conclusions can be drawn about the significance of valproic acid metabolism on the therapeutic effect. Some compounds, however, deserve special attention. α,β-Unsaturated VPA has a long half-life in man in comparison with the parent drug (Fig. 6). If this substance contributes to the therapeutic effects of the drug, it might explain to some extent the lack of a temporal relationship between plasma valproate concentrations and the protection against seizures. Moreover, the concentrations of the compound in plasma of patients on valproate treatment are high enough to monitor in a routine analysis, which enables the correlation with seizure frequency. Other compounds may be of interest because their presence has been demonstrated in brain tissue of animals: 3-OH-VPA in mice and 4-OH-VPA in monkeys; also, 3-oxo-VPA has been found in human cerebrospinal fluid.

A search for the mechanism of action of valproic acid will have to include pharmacological screening of the relevant metabolites and the study of their pharmacokinetic behavior. As long

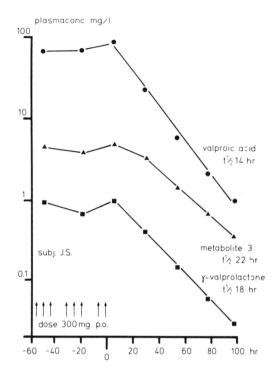

plasmaconc mg/l

valproic acid
t½ 14 hr

subj. J.S.

metabolite 3
t½ 22 hr

γ-valprolactone
t½ 18 hr

dose 300 mg p.o.

FIG. 6. Plasma concentrations of valproic acid and two metabolites in an epileptic patient during treatment and after discontinuation of treatment. Valproate monotherapy was replaced by phenytoin. Metabolite 3 represents α,β-unsaturated VPA. (From Schobben et al., ref. 25, with permission.)

as it is still uncertain whether valproic acid itself or one or more of its metabolites is responsible for the therapeutic effects, the experiments by Lockard et al. (13) in rhesus monkeys may be considered the best test for the anticonvulsant activity of valproic acid in man, in view of the close resemblance of the metabolic disposition of valproic acid in both species. From a metabolic point of view, testing in rats seems to be an appropriate alternative.

ACKNOWLEDGMENTS

Some of the original data presented in this chapter were obtained from studies performed at the Saint Paul-Ramsey Medical Center and the School of Pharmacy, University of Minnesota, Saint Paul/Minneapolis, Minnesota. The authors wish to express their appreciation to their colleagues, Dr. Ilo E. Leppik and Dr. Ronald J. Sawchuk.

The authors are very grateful to Dr. H. Schäfer, Desitin Werk, Hamburg, West Germany, for the supply of several synthetic valproic acid metabolites.

This research was supported in part by the Foundation for Medical Research FUNGO, which is subsidized by the Netherlands Organisation for the Advancement of Pure Research ZWO, and by NINCDS contract NO1-NS-5-2327 administered through the Comprehensive Epilepsy Program for the State of Minnesota.

REFERENCES

1. Burton, B. S. (1881): On the propyl derivatives and decomposition products of ethyl acetoacetate. *Am. Chem. J.*, 3:389.
2. Eymard, P., Simiand, J., Teoule, R., Polverelli, M., Werbenec, J. P., and Broll, M. (1971): Etude de la répartition et de la résorption du dipropylacetate de sodium marqué au ^{14}C chez le rat. *J. Pharmacol. (Paris)*, 2:359–368.
3. Ferrandes, B., and Eymard, P. (1977): Metabolism of valproate sodium in rabbit, rat, dog and man. *Epilepsia*, 18:169–182.
4. Gompertz, D., Tippett, P., Barlett, K., and Baillie, T. (1977): Identification of urinary metabolites of sodium dipropylacetate in man; potential sources of interference in organic acid screening procedures. *Clin. Chim. Acta*, 74:153–160.
5. Hamberg, M., and Björkheim, I. (1971): ω-Oxidation of fatty acids. *J. Biol. Chem.*, 246:7411–7416.
6. Jakobs, C., and Löscher, W. (1978): Identification of metabolites of valproic acid in serum of humans, dog, rat and mouse. *Epilepsia*, 19:591–602.
7. Keil, W. (1947): Zur Kenntnis der Fette aus Fettsäuren mit ungerader Kohlenstoffatomzahle. *Hoppe Seylers Z. Physiol. Chem.*, 282:137–142.
8. Kochen, W., Imbeck, H., and Jakobs, C. (1977): Untersuchungen über die Ausscheidung von Metaboliten der Valproinsäure im Urin der Ratte und des Menschen. *Arzneim. Forsch.*, 27:1090–1099.
9. Kochen, W., and Scheffner, H. (1980): On unsaturated metabolites of valproic acid in serum of epileptic children. In: *Antiepileptic Therapy: Advances in Drug Monitoring*, edited by S. I. Johannessen, P. L. Morselli, C. E. Pippenger, A. Richens, D. Schmidt, and H. Meinardi, pp. 111–117. Raven Press, New York.
9a. Kochen, W., and Scheffner, D. (1981): The metabolism of valproic acid in chronically treated patients. Presented at the Epilepsy International Congress, 1981, Kyoto.
10. Kuhara, T., Hirohata, Y., Yamada, S., and Matsumoto, I. (1978): Metabolism of sodium dipropylacetate in human. *Eur. J. Drug Metab. Pharmacokinet.*, 3:171–177.

11. Kuhara, T., and Matsumoto, I. (1974): Metabolism of branched medium chain length fatty acid: I. ω-Oxidation of sodium dipropylacetate in rats. *Biomed. Mass Spectrom.,* 1:291–294.

12. Kukino, K., Mineura, K., Deguchi, T., Ishii, A., and Takahira, H. (1972): Studies on a new anticonvulsant drug, sodium dipropylacetate: Assay for metabolites and metabolic pathway. *J. Pharm. Soc. Jpn.,* 92:896–900.

13. Lockard, J. S., Levy, R. H., Congdon, W. C., Ducharme, L. L., and Patel, I. H. (1977): Efficacy testing of valproic acid compared to ethosuximide in monkey model: II. Seizure, EEG, and diurnal variations. *Epilepsia,* 18:205–221.

13a. Löscher, W. (1981): Concentration of metabolites of valproic acid in plasma of epileptic patients. *Epilepsia,* 22:169–178.

14. Matsumoto, I., Kuhara, T., and Yoshino, M. (1976): Metabolism of branched medium chain fatty acid: II. β-Oxidation of sodium dipropylacetate in rats. *Biomed. Mass Spectrom.,* 3:235–240.

15. Merits, I. (1977): Metabolic fate of valproate sodium in dog, rat, rabbit, monkey and human. *Epilepsia,* 18:289–290.

16. Meunier, H., Carraz, G., Meunier, Y., Eymard, P., and Aimard, M. (1963): Propriétés pharmacodynamiques de l'acide *n*-dipropylacetique. *Therapie,* 18:435–438.

17. Pfaff, M. C., Mahuzier, G., Pousset, J. L., and Preaux, N. (1975): Study of urinary elimination of dipropylacetic acid and dipropylacetamide. In: *Drug Interference and Drug Measurement in Clinical Chemistry,* edited by G. Siest and D. S. Young, pp. 186–192. Karger, Basel.

18. Regazzi Bonora, M., Schobben, F., Taburet, A. M., and van der Kleijn, E. (1979): Preliminary pharmacokinetics and metabolism of sodium 2-*n*-propylpentanoate in pig and human. *Arzneim. Forsch.,* 29:1161–1163.

19. Schäfer, H., and Lührs, R. (1978): Metabolite pattern of valproic acid. *Arzneim. Forsch.,* 28:657–662.

20. Schäfer, H., Lührs, R., and Reith, H. (1980): Chemistry, pharmacokinetics and biological activity of some metabolites of valproic acid. In: *Antiepileptic Therapy: Advances in Drug Monitoring,* edited by S. I. Johannessen, P. L. Morselli, C. E. Pippenger, A. Richens, D. Schmidt, and H. Meinardi, pp. 103–110. Raven Press, New York.

21. Schobben, A. F. A. M. (1979): *Pharmacokinetics and Therapeutics in Epilepsy.* Thesis, Catholic University, Nijmegen, the Netherlands.

22. Schobben, F., and van der Kleijn, E. (1974): Pharmacokinetics of distribution and elimination of sodium di-*n*-propylacetate in mouse and dog. *Pharm. Weekbl.,* 109:33–42.

23. Schobben, F., van der Kleijn, E., Vree, T. B., and Guelen, P. J. M. (1977): Pharmacokinetics of di-propylacetate (2-*n*-propyl-pentanoate) in man and laboratory animals. In: *Antiepileptic Drug Monitoring,* edited by C. Gardner-Thorpe, D. Janz, H. Meinardi, and C. E. Pippenger, pp. 147–163. Pitman Medical, Tunbridge Wells, Kent.

24. Schobben, F., Vree, T. B., and van der Kleijn, E. (1978): Pharmacokinetics, metabolism and distribution of 2-*n*-propyl-pentanoate and the influence of salicylate comedication. In: *Advances in Epileptology—1977,* edited by H. Meinardi and A. J. Rowan, pp. 271–277. Swets & Zeitlinger, Amsterdam.

25. Schobben, F., Vree, T. B., van der Kleijn, E., Claessens, R., and Renier, W. O. (1980): Metabolism of valproic acid in monkey and man. In: *Antiepileptic Therapy: Advances in Drug Monitoring,* edited by S. I. Johannessen, P. L. Morselli, C. E. Pippenger, A. Richens, D. Schmidt, and H. Meinardi, pp. 91–102. Raven Press, New York.

26. Taillandier, G., Benoit-Guyod, J. L., Boucherle, A., Broll, M., and Eymard, P. (1975): Recherches dans la serie dipropylacetique XII. Acides et alcools aliphatiques ramifiés anticonvulsivants. *Eur. J. Med. Chem.,* 10:453–462.

27. Vree, T. B., and van der Kleijn, E. (1977): Pharmacokinetics and renal excretion of 2-*n*-propyl-pentanoate in man, dog and rhesus monkey. In: *Pharmacokinetics and Metabolism of the Antiepileptic Drug Sodium Valproate,* edited by T. B. Vree and E. van der Kleijn, pp. 37–39, Bohn, Utrecht.

Antiepileptic Drugs, edited by Ɔ. M. Woodbury,
J. K. Penry, and C. E. Pippenger. Raven Press,
New York © 1982.

47

Valproate

Interactions with Other Drugs

Richard H. Mattson

Valproic acid (VPA) frequently interacts with other antiepileptic drugs. The extent of such interactions often is sufficient to alter the pharmacokinetics of both VPA and the interacting drugs in clinically significant ways. Available evidence not only indicates the probability of an interaction between VPA and phenobarbital and phenytoin but also the mechanisms responsible for the interaction (38,68). This understanding should allow prediction of similar changes in pharmacokinetics when VPA is used in combination with other drugs for which fewer observations and studies have been done. Not only does VPA affect the pharmacokinetics of other drugs, but these in turn have interactions with VPA, leading to more rapid elimination and lower blood levels of VPA. Endogenous substances and disease states may also at times alter VPA pharmacokinetics.

VALPROIC ACID-INDUCED CHANGES IN THE PHARMACOKINETICS OF OTHER DRUGS

Phenobarbital

In many early clinical trials, sedation often appeared when VPA was given to patients already receiving phenobarbital and/or other antiepileptic drugs (3,23,24,28,54,66). An interaction was suspected because sedative side effects

eased with a decrease in phenobarbital dosage. Also, sedation was much less, even on higher VPA dosage, when VPA was given as the sole drug. Subsequent clinical trials confirmed that serum phenobarbital levels rose when valproic acid therapy was initiated: Schobben et al. (60) reported three patients who had increases ranging from 35% to 200%. Later reports confirmed these changes (Table 1). The increases usually have ranged from 15 to 70%, but at times have been much higher.

Such an interaction has not occurred in all patients, and evidence is insufficient to allow prediction of who will be affected. The dose of VPA used does not seem to be a critical factor, but perhaps high serum levels of phenobarbital before the initiation of VPA make interaction more probable. We (40) found no significant changes in serum phenobarbital levels in adult patients on a mean phenobarbital dose of 90 mg/day, whereas Vakil et al. (64) noted increased levels of phenobarbital in six patients, all of whom were receiving a phenobarbital dose of 200 mg/day.

Mechanism

There are four possible mechanisms by which VPA might alter the pharmacokinetics and elevate the serum levels of phenobarbital.

First, the use of VPA might theoretically

TABLE 1. *Serum phenobarbital (PB) increases after initiation of valproic acid therapy*

Patients (No.)	Affected (%)	Increase in serum PB level (%)	Ref.
3	100	35–200	60
7	100	17–48	55
6	100	34–71	64
—	33	30	23
—	—	66	50
—	—	30[a]	21
11	87	46[a]	68
1 (4[b])	70	10–25	1
6 (1[b])	50	30–59	65
5	39	34–126	51

[a]Percent that PB dosage had to be decreased to avoid elevation of serum levels.

[b]Phenobarbital derived from primidone.

increase gastrointestinal absorption of phenobarbital. The possibility of such an effect seems quite unlikely, although it has not been investigated. Phenobarbital absorption is essentially complete, and any change could only decrease rather than increase serum phenobarbital levels (67).

Second, VPA is highly protein bound (95%) and might competitively displace phenobarbital. However, any alterations in protein binding would not be expected to elevate phenobarbital levels. Only 40 to 50% of phenobarbital is protein bound, and displacement would produce minor changes in free drug distribution. In fact, any such change would be likely to lower total serum levels.

Third, acidification of the urine by VPA might facilitate resorption of phenobarbital and cause its accumulation. Unchanged phenobarbital is cleared from the kidney in variable amounts depending on blood flow and urinary pH. Shifts from ionized to un-ionized (dissociated to undissociated) forms of phenobarbital (pK_a 7.3) occur readily with any change in the normal serum pH of 7.4 (see Chapter 26). A decrease in urinary pH caused by VPA might produce a shift to un-ionized phenobarbital and lead to increased reabsorption of drug. In the usually acidic urine, however, phenobarbital is already pri-

marily in the un-ionized form. Further acidification should have little effect. Indeed, a study of pH in urine and blood after administration of VPA to both cats and humans failed to reveal any change (9). No decrease in phenobarbital excretion, suggesting increased renal reabsorption (9,31), has been found after initiation of VPA therapy (9,31,36,45) (Table 2).

Fourth, VPA may inhibit biotransformation of phenobarbital to oxidated metabolites. Wilson (69) pointed out that fatty acids bind to hepatic microsomes including the phenobarbital site. Because VPA is chemically similar to these fatty acids, he suggested that a blockade of phenobarbital metabolism in the liver would cause secondary accumulation of phenobarbital and elevated serum levels. The possibility that VPA could inhibit phenobarbital metabolism was further studied by Loiseau et al. (36). They noted elevation of serum phenobarbital levels and an increase in phenobarbital half-life from a mean of 83 to 105 hr after administering VPA. At the same time, they observed a decrease in urinary output of hydroxyphenobarbital but no change in phenobarbital excretion. Bruni et al. (9) reported similar results in four patients whose serum phenobarbital levels rose after addition of VPA. The 24-hr urinary output of hydroxyphenobarbital and the ratio of hydroxyphenobarbital to phenobarbital decreased simultaneously. Patel et al. (45) studied six volunteers given phenobarbital followed by a second phase in which the same subjects received both phenobarbital and VPA. The phenobarbital half-

TABLE 2. *Changes in half-life and urinary excretion of phenobarbital (PB) and p-hydroxyphenobarbital (p-OHPB) following addition of valproic acid (VPA)*

T½ (hr)		Urinary excretion			
PB	PB + VPA	PB	p-OHPB	Ratio of p-OHPB/PB	Ref.
83	105	NC[a]	↓	↓	36
		↑	↓	↓	9
100	144	NC[a]	↓	↓	45
126	181	↑	↓	↓	31

[a]NC, no change.

life increased from 100 to 144 hr. Plasma clearance decreased while renal excretion of phenobarbital remained unchanged. Kapetanovic et al. (31) carried out an especially careful study of VPA–phenobarbital interaction. After giving a single pulse dose of phenobarbital containing a stable isotope, they observed the patient at steady state for a month and established the drug's elimination half-life to be 126 hr. After addition of VPA, phenobarbital levels rose 25% without change in dosage. A second pulse dose of isotope-containing phenobarbital allowed repeated half-life determination. An increase from 126 to 181 hr occurred. The daily urinary excretion of phenobarbital actually increased somewhat, whereas output of the metabolite, hydroxyphenobarbital, decreased from 60 to 40 mg/day.

In summary, evidence converging from many studies indicates that the coadministration of VPA and phenobarbital inhibits the biotransformation and hydroxylation of phenobarbital to hydroxyphenobarbital, increases its elimination half-life, and ultimately causes elevation of serum phenobarbital levels.

Phenytoin

Early reports provided conflicting evidence of interaction between VPA and phenytoin. Richens et al. (55) noted no consistent change in phenytoin levels when VPA was begun, but other investigators found an increase in serum phenytoin concentrations (24,29,63,70). Bardy et al. (2), however, found a rise in serum phenytoin levels when VPA was discontinued in six patients and inferred that VPA therapy actually had lowered the phenytoin levels. Vakil et al. (64) observed a small and transient, but statistically significant, decrease in serum phenytoin levels in 10 patients after initiating VPA therapy. Subsequent reports have consistently noted a fall in phenytoin levels (1,10,14,18,35,40,43,46, 47,50,59). We (40) found a decrease in mean serum phenytoin levels in 21 patients: the levels dropped from 19.4 μg/ml to 14.6 μg/ml after a week of VPA therapy. After 2 to 3 months and higher dosages of VPA, phenytoin levels declined further to 11.1 μg/ml. The changes were

highly significant ($p < 0.001$). Vakil et al. (64) reported an initial fall in phenytoin levels after administration of VPA but a later rise to pre-VPA levels. Bruni et al. (10) observed a decrease in plasma phenytoin levels in seven of eight patients but also noted a return to higher levels after a year of therapy without any change in phenytoin dosage.

Mechanism

The mechanism by which VPA causes a fall in total plasma phenytoin levels appears to be well established. Valproic acid is highly protein bound in plasma (95%) and displaces phenytoin from binding sites (30). Lascelles, in the discussion of the report by Vakil et al. (64), postulated that such an effect might cause increased free phenytoin levels in blood and produce acute neurotoxicity. Confirming this possibility was the finding of increased phenytoin levels in brains of rats when VPA was administered after pretreatment with phenytoin (46). Evidence of toxicity was observed, which was not seen after giving either drug alone. Mattson et al. (40) first reported in clinical studies that a rise in the percentage of free phenytoin accompanied the fall in total serum phenytoin levels when VPA therapy was initiated. Yet, total free or unbound phenytoin concentrations in blood did not change significantly. Valproic acid apparently displaces phenytoin from plasma protein, but the increased free levels are cleared by the liver.

In addition, another study reported an increase in the volume of distribution of phenytoin resulting from increased concentration of unbound phenytoin (19). Figure 1 illustrates these changes in one patient. The rise in percentage of free phenytoin was associated with a transient increase in urinary excretion of hydroxyphenylphenylhydantoin (HPPH), a primary phenytoin metabolite. Increased hepatic clearance established a new steady state with free phenytoin levels unchanged from those present prior to initiation of VPA therapy, even though total serum levels were lower (40). Bruni et al. (10) confirmed these changes in HPPH excretion. They also noted a later rise in total serum

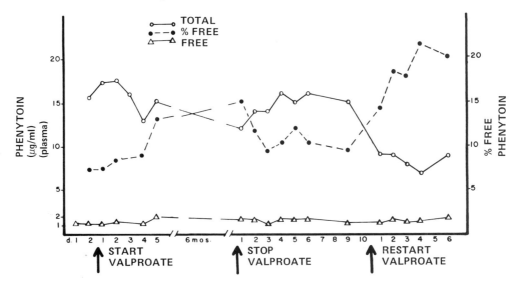

FIG. 1. Characteristic changes in total, percent free, and free phenytoin with initiation and discontinuation of VPA therapy in one patient. (From Mattson et al., ref. 40, with permission.)

phenytoin to levels similar to those present before VPA was given, even though dosage was not changed. Percentage of free phenytoin remained high throughout the period of observation. They concluded that a secondary inhibition of hydroxylation of phenytoin had occurred comparable to the mechanism producing elevated phenobarbital levels. These dual interactions have been confirmed by others (48) and may explain some early reports that failed to note decreased phenytoin levels.

Initial *in vitro* studies of VPA–phenytoin interaction reported displacement of phenytoin but only at very high levels of VPA (30). Patsalos and Lascelles (46) found evidence of decreased protein binding of phenytoin when it was combined with VPA in defatted plasma but not in normal untreated human plasma. Subsequent studies (7,13,33,42) reported more marked changes at VPA levels well within the therapeutic range (50–150 μg/ml). The percentage of free phenytoin rises increasingly at higher concentrations of VPA (Table 3).

Interactions with Other Drugs

Reports of VPA interactions with other drugs have been much less frequent or consistent than those with phenobarbital and phenytoin. This may be a consequence of less interaction as well as fewer opportunities for careful observations because of less frequent use of the other drugs.

Other Barbiturates

An increase in sedation has been observed when VPA was added to primidone therapy (23,54). Windorfer et al. (70) reported that mean serum primidone levels more than doubled (7.0 to 15.7 μg/ml) in seven patients, but Adams et al. (1) found only a modest 17% increase in five patients after addition of VPA. The variability between peak and predose blood levels of primidone or of other drugs with a relatively short half-life makes interpretation and recognition of

TABLE 3. *Percent free phenytoin when combined with different concentrations of valproic acid in vitro*[a]

Valproic acid (μg/ml)	Percent free PHT
0	19.6
45	21.5
90	26.1

[a]Adapted from Cramer and Mattson (13).

interaction difficult unless the time of sampling has been carefully controlled.

Not surprisingly, levels of phenobarbital metabolically derived from primidone have been observed to rise in some patients after administration of VPA (Table 1). A few patients have been receiving mephobarbital when VPA was initiated, but effects have not been reported. Phenobarbital derived from biotransformation of mephobarbital also may be expected to rise with addition of VPA.

Ethosuximide

Despite the frequent combined use of VPA and ethosuximide, only one study found evidence of an interaction (39). Five of six patients had a mean increase of 53% in ethosuximide levels when VPA was added to the regimen. All patients were taking multiple drugs, and the mechanism of action was suspected to be an inhibition of oxidation similar to the VPA–phenobarbital interaction.

Carbamazepine

Evidence of an effect of VPA on carbamazepine has been reported infrequently. Some patients have developed sedation, nausea, diplopia, and/or a confusional state when VPA was added to carbamazepine therapy. Toxic symptoms cleared only with reduction or discontinuation of carbamazepine (1,24,28,34). These anecdotal case reports suggested an interaction, but none was proved with blood level changes. The considerable variation in carbamazepine levels between doses would make analysis difficult unless determinations were consistently made both predose and at times of clinical toxicity.

Because carbamazepine is moderately protein bound (75%) (15,25), it may be postulated that displacement by VPA analogous to the VPA–phenytoin interaction could occur clinically. We found that when VPA was added *in vitro* to plasma samples containing carbamazepine in concentrations of 12 μg/ml, the free, pharmacologically active fraction of carbamazepine increased 25% (37). In clinical use, such an increase might produce toxicity without evidence of increased total carbamazepine levels. Hoppener et al. (26) have shown that periodic diurnal carbamazepine toxicity does occur. This effect may be compounded with VPA therapy. Carbamazepine toxicity likely would occur particularly at times of peak concentrations of both drugs, but would be transient and recurrent. The interaction might easily escape detection by predose determination of total drug levels. Serum samples obtained at times of side effects and analyzed specifically for free carbamazepine levels would be most useful. Further clinical studies are needed to clarify this possible interaction between VPA and carbamazepine.

Clonazepam

The combined use of VPA with benzodiazepines (diazepam, nitrazepam, clorazepate, clonazepam) is not unusual because there is considerable overlap in the indication for their use in treatment of seizures. There is no evidence of a change in serum levels of the benzodiazepines when used in combination with VPA. However, a clinical interaction between clonazepam and VPA was reported by Jeavons and Clark (27). Absence status developed in 5 of 12 patients placed on the two drugs. In total, 9 of the 12 patients had unwanted side effects leading to discontinuation of the clonazepam. The observation is unexplained, and the mechanism of the suspected interaction is unknown. After careful review, Browne (5) concluded that the interaction was uncommon and should not preclude the use of the drugs together when otherwise indicated.

CHANGES IN VPA PHARMACOKINETICS INDUCED BY OTHER DRUGS

Antiepileptic Drugs

Other drugs have important effects on the pharmacokinetics of VPA. Coulthard (12) noted increasing serum levels of VPA and improved seizure control in one patient only after discontinuation of phenytoin. He postulated that other drugs caused hepatic enzyme induction and increased metabolism of VPA. Subsequent studies lend strong support to this observation. Reunanen et al. (53) reported the serum concentration of VPA found in patients treated with single or combined drugs and found that for those on VPA alone, the concentration in blood was 22.4 μmole/liter per mg/kg, whereas for those on carbamazepine or phenytoin it was 13.8 and 14.4 μmole/liter per mg/kg, respectively. Mihaly et al. (41) similarly found that average doses of 25.4 mg/kg of VPA in patients receiving VPA alone produced plasma VPA levels of 90.3 μg/ml, whereas patients concomitantly receiving other antiepileptic drugs took a higher average dose of 41.6 mg/kg of VPA and yet achieved mean VPA levels of only 73.5 μg/ml.

Sackellares et al. (58) noted similar effects in a group of children treated with VPA alone or in combination with phenytoin and/or phenobarbital. Despite a comparable dosage per unit body weight, the mean plasma VPA levels were much higher in the patients receiving VPA alone (99.3 versus 63.0 μg/ml).

Mechanism

Richens et al. (55) reported a VPA half-life of 5.88 hr in patients treated with VPA combined with other drugs, whereas the half-life was 9.21 hr in those patients receiving only VPA. Other studies have confirmed that report (16,49) (Table 4). An increase in the VPA elimination rate constant and clearance was found in patients concomitantly receiving other drugs. When administered with VPA, carbamazepine (4,41,53), phenobarbital (58), and phenytoin

(41,53,58), each altered VPA pharmacokinetics in the same manner. Sufficient data are not available to know if other drugs have similar effects. The mechanism of action has not been fully studied, but hepatic microsomal enzyme induction and a secondary increased clearance are very likely. The lower serum levels might also result if phenytoin displaced VPA from albumin (48). The increased free fraction would be expected to increase the volume of distribution and hepatic clearance, leading to a new lower total serum VPA level (see VPA–phenytoin interaction above). However, VPA binding changes induced by phenytoin are modest (Table 5) and, indeed, have not been confirmed by other studies (7,21,42). Furthermore, such changes in binding alone cannot explain low VPA levels when carbamazepine or phenobarbital are administered, since neither drug significantly affects VPA binding (25,37).

Nonantiepileptic Drugs

Occasions are few that allow clinical observations of VPA interactions with nonantiepileptic drugs, but the potential for a competitive effect with other highly protein bound drugs has been tested in vitro (17,42). Salicylic acid, in particular, displaced VPA from protein, resulting in higher free levels of drug. Schobben et al. (61) noted a significant rise in urinary excretion of VPA after daily administration of 1 to 2 g of aspirin daily to two human volunteers. They suggested that salicylic acid had displaced VPA from protein, resulting in an increased volume of distribution and subsequent hepatic clearance. Studies indicate lesser interaction with

TABLE 4. *Half-life of valproic acid in patients receiving VPA only or VPA plus other antiepileptic drugs*

VPA only (hr)	VPA plus other drugs (hr)	Ref.
9.2	5.9	55
12.5	9.0	49
12.0	8.1	16

TABLE 5. *Percent free valproic acid at varied concentrations of phenytoin* in vitro

Phenytoin (μg/ml)	Percent free VPA
0	7.8
10	8.4
20	10.7

[a]Adapted from Cramer and Mattson (13).

phenylbutazone and no effect of warfarin on VPA protein binding (17,42). The likelihood is low that patients treated with VPA will also take regular high doses of salicylates as may be used in rheumatoid arthritis, but in these rare cases, changes in binding might be clinically significant.

With the exception of aspirin, the changes in VPA protein binding caused by exogenous displacers are relatively small compared to endogenous effects. Saturation of binding sites at higher levels of VPA (80–90 µg/ml) (13,44) leads to a rapid increase in free VPA many times greater than that induced by phenytoin or other drugs (Fig. 2). Interaction with endogenous free fatty acids can also produce a marked change in VPA binding and percentage of free drug (44).

DISEASES ALTERING VPA LEVELS

The extensive binding of VPA to serum albumin can be changed not only by aspirin and endogenous fatty acid displacers but also by disease. *In vitro* studies have shown twice as much free VPA available in low-protein plasma (18% less albumin) (Fig. 2) (13,46). Lower levels of serum albumin may be found in association with malnutrition, impaired synthesis in hepatic disease and malignancy, or associated with protein loss secondary to burns and renal or gastrointestinal disease. In such cases, total VPA concentration will decrease although quantities of free pharmacologically active drug will remain unchanged (8,22,32,52,56).

Decreased binding is found in uremia and can only partly be attributed to decreased protein concentration (56). Allosteric changes in plasma protein have been suggested (48) and may explain increased levels of free VPA. Endogenous "toxic" uremic displacers also may be responsible for the decrease in VPA binding (8). In either case, the result is a lower total serum VPA concentration and an increase in percentage of free VPA without any change in the amount of free drug. Consequently, dosage need not be increased (48,56).

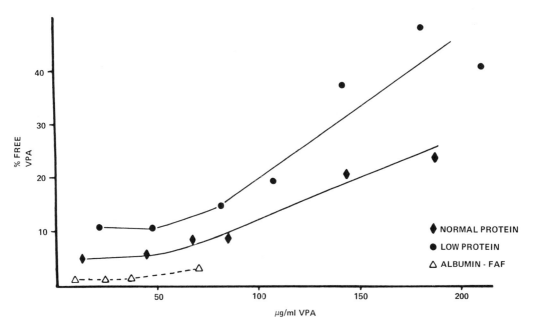

FIG. 2. Valproic acid binding to plasma proteins *in vitro*. Binding is maximal with fatty acid free (FAF) albumin and least with low concentration of protein. Modified from Cramer and Mattson (13).

CONCLUSIONS AND CLINICAL IMPLICATIONS

Interactions between VPA and other drugs are frequent and potentially important. Accumulating evidence suggests not only the areas of interaction but also the mechanisms responsible for these interactions.

Valproic acid is metabolized almost completely in the liver and can interfere with the usual biotransformation of other antiepileptic drugs. Specifically, VPA slows hydroxylation and elimination of other antiepileptic drugs, causing a rise of serum levels. Such an effect has been well demonstrated with phenobarbital and consequently is likely to occur with use of mephobarbital or primidone as well. Some evidence suggests a similar effect on phenytoin metabolism which is masked by changes in protein binding that produce opposite results. The interaction of VPA with ethosuximide and other drugs that undergo oxidative biotransformation may be expected, even though evidence of such an effect is not extensive. The increase in levels of other drugs may lead to neurotoxicity and require a reduction in their dosage.

The appearance of sedation or other neurotoxicity cannot be assumed to be entirely or even partly caused by phenobarbital because occasionally VPA can independently cause dramatic hypnotic side effects (11,57). Monitoring of serum phenobarbital levels helps to establish the cause of side effects. Unless this information is readily available it can be inferred that sedation appearing in the first few hours or even the first day is caused by VPA. Phenobarbital levels should not rise in clinically important amounts for days or weeks until the drug accumulates. The assessment can be confounded if other drugs such as phenytoin, carbamazepine, primidone, or ethosuximide are being taken concurrently.

Valproic acid has a strong affinity for protein and is highly bound to serum albumin (95%). When VPA is taken together with phenytoin, the competitive displacement produces an increase in the percentage of free phenytoin. The acute change may produce paradoxical neuro-toxicity with redistribution of free drug. Brain levels rise while total plasma levels are decreasing. After clearance and reequilibration, total phenytoin concentrations are lowered, while free levels remain unchanged. Changes in phenytoin dosage to bring total levels back to the usual therapeutic range (10–20 μg/ml) may raise free phenytoin to toxic levels. In general, changes in total levels induced by binding changes do not affect pharmacologically active drug and are not important if understood and anticipated (56). Carbamazepine binding can also be affected by VPA, especially at high concentrations of both drugs. Such effects may be transient but recurrent and easily escape detection if total rather than free drug concentrations are used to assess efficacy and toxicity.

· Valproic acid induces neither its own metabolism nor that of other drugs (30,40) Evidence strongly suggests, however, that many other drugs induce hepatic enzymatic activity to accelerate VPA metabolism and clearance. This results in lower plasma VPA concentrations per dose and a shorter VPA half-life. The effect of lower VPA concentrations in the presence of other drugs can be clinically important. Valproic acid given as the sole drug has a slower clearance and longer half-life, leading to higher plasma levels per dose of VPA. This allows smaller (and less costly) amounts of drug to be taken at less frequent dosing intervals. The high levels achieved with VPA as the sole drug often exceed 80 to 90 μg/ml, at which point a much higher percent of free, pharmacologically active drug becomes available. Conversely, the lower VPA levels achieved with the combined use of VPA and other antiepileptic drugs may prevent the patient from obtaining maximal therapeutic effect from the VPA.

When other drugs that are highly bound to protein, such as aspirin, are taken in combination with VPA, the VPA may be displaced. Significantly increased levels of free VPA are also caused by disease states that alter or lower plasma protein concentration.

The prevalence of VPA interactions calls for clinical awareness and frequent determinations of blood levels of both VPA and other drugs.

Free drug levels should be determined for drugs that are significantly bound to protein.

REFERENCES

1. Adams, D. J., Luders, H., and Pippenger, C. (1978): Sodium valproate in the treatment of intractable seizure disorders: A clinical and electroencephalographic study. *Neurology (Minneap.)*, 28:152–157.
2. Bardy, A., Hari, R., Lehtovaara, R., and Majuri, H. (1977): Valproate may lower serum phenytoin. *Lancet*, 1:1256–1257.
3. Barnes, S. E., and Bower, B. D. (1975): Sodium valproate in the treatment of intractable childhood epilepsy. *Dev. Med. Child. Neurol.*, 17:175–181.
4. Bowdle, T. A., Levy, R. H., and Cutler, R. E. (1979): Effects of carbamazepine on valproic acid kinetics in normal subjects. *Clin. Pharmacol. Ther.*, 26:629–634.
5. Browne, T. R. (1980): Valproic acid. Medical intelligence. *N. Engl. J. Med.*, 302:661–666.
6. Bruni, J., Gallo, J. M., Lee, C. S., Perchalski, R. J., and Wilder, B. J. (1980): Interactions of valproic acid with phenytoin. *Neurology (Minneap.)*, 30:1233–1236.
7. Bruni, J., Gallo, J. M., and Wilder, B. J. (1979): Effect of phenytoin on protein binding of valproic acid. *Can. J. Neurol. Sci.*, 6:433–434.
8. Bruni, J., Wang, L. H., Marburt, T. C., Lee, C. S., and Wilder, B. J. (1980): Protein binding of valproic acid in uremic patients. *Neurology (Minneap.)*, 30:557–559.
9. Bruni, J., Wilder, B. J., Perchalski, R. J., Hammond, E. J., and Villareal, H. J. (1980): Valproic acid and plasma levels of phenobarbital. *Neurology (Minneap.)*, 30:94–97.
10. Bruni, J., Wilder, B. J., Willmore, L. J., and Barbour, B. (1979): Valproic acid and plasma levels of serum phenytoin. *Neurology (Minneap.)*, 29:904–905.
11. Chadwick, D. W., Cumming, W. J. K., Livingstone, I., and Cartlidge, N. E. F. (1979): Acute intoxication with sodium valproate. *Ann. Neurol.*, 6:552–553.
12. Coulthard, M. G. (1975): Sodium valproate in the treatment of intractable childhood epilepsy. *Dev. Med. Child. Neurol.*, 17:534.
13. Cramer, J. A., and Mattson, R. H. (1979): Valproic acid: *In vitro* plasma protein binding and interactions with phenytoin. *Ther. Drug Monitor.* 1:105–116.
14. Dahlqvist, R., Borga, O., Rane, A., Walsh, Z., and Sjoqvist, F. (1979): Decreased plasma protein binding of phenytoin in patients on valproic acid. *Br. J. Clin. Pharmacol.*, 8:547–552.
15. Disalle, E., Pacifici, G. M., and Morselli, P. L. (1974): Studies on plasma protein binding of carbamazepine. *Pharmacol. Res. Commun.*, 6:193–202.
16. Fisher, J. H., Cloyd, J. C., Kriel, R. L., Eggreth, R., and Sawchuck, R. J. (1981): The effect of concomitant antiepileptic therapy on valproic acid pharmacokinetics. *Epilepsia (in press)*.
17. Fleitman, J. S., Bruni, J., Perrin, J. H., and Wilder, B. J. (1980): Albumin binding interactions of sodium valproate. *J. Clin. Pharmacol.*, 20:314–317.
18. Friel, P. N., Leal, K. W., and Wilensky, A. J. (1979):

19. Frigo, G. M., Lecchini, S., Gatti, G., Perucca, E., and Crema, A. (1979): Modification of phenytoin clearance by valproic acid in normal subjects. *Br. J. Clin. Pharmacol.*, 8:553–556.
20. Gallo, J. M., Bruni, J., Lee, C. S., Fleittman, J., and Wilder, B. J. (1981): Protein binding and salivary concentrations of valproic acid in epileptic patients. *Eur. J. Clin. Pharmacol. (in press)*.
21. Gram, L., Wulff, K., Rasmussen, K. E., Flachs, H., Wurtz-Jorgensen, A., Sommerbeck, K. W., and Lohren, V. (1977): Valproate sodium: A controlled clinical trial including monitoring of drug levels. *Epilepsia*, 18:141–148.
22. Gugler, R., and Mueller, G. (1978): Plasma protein binding of valproic acid in healthy patients and in patients with renal disease. *Br. J. Clin. Pharmacol.*, 5:441–446.
23. Harwood, G., and Harvey, P. K. P. (1976): Results of a clinical trial on the use of Epilim in convulsive disorders, with special reference to its efficacy in temporal lobe attacks with focal features. In: *Clinical and Pharmacological Aspects of Sodium Valproate (Epilim) in the Treatment of Epilepsy*, edited by N. J. Legg, pp. 40–43. MCS Consultants, Tunbridge Wells, Kent.
24. Hassan, M. N., Laljee, H. C. K., and Parsonage, M. J. (1976): Sodium valproate in the treatment of resistant epilepsy. *Acta Neurol. Scand.*, 54:209–218.
25. Hooper, W. D., Dubetz, D. K., Bochner, F., Cotter, L. M., Smith, G. A., Eadie, M. J., and Tyrer, J. H. (1975): Plasma protein binding of carbamazepine. *Clin. Pharmacol. Ther.*, 17:433–440.
26. Hoppener, R. J., Kuyer, A., Meijer, J. W. A., and Hulsman, J. (1980): Correlation between daily fluctuations of carbamazepine serum levels and intermittent side effects. *Epilepsia*, 21:341–350.
27. Jeavons, P. M., and Clark, J. E. (1974): Sodium valproate in treatment of epilepsy. *Br. Med. J.*, 2:584–586.
28. Jeavons, P. M., Clark, J. E., and Maheswari, M. C. (1977): Treatment of generalized epilepsies of childhood and adolescence with sodium valproate ('Epilim'). *Dev. Med. Child. Neurol.*, 19:9–25.
29. Johannessen, S. (1977): Preliminary observations on valproic acid kinetics in patients with epilepsy. *Arzneim. Forsch.*, 27:1083–1085.
30. Jordan, B. J., Shillingford, J. S., and Steed, K. P. (1976): Preliminary observations on the protein binding and enzyme-inducing properties of sodium valproate (Epilim). In: *Clinical and Pharmacological Aspects of Sodium Valproate (Epilim) in the Treatment of Epilepsy*, edited by N. J. Legg, pp. 112–116. MCS Consultants, Tunbridge Wells, Kent.
31. Kapetanovic, I., Kupferberg, H. J., Porter, R. J., and Penry, J. K. (1980): Valproic acid–phenobarbital interaction: A systematic study using stable isotopically labeled phenobarbital in an epileptic patient. In: *Antiepileptic Therapy: Advances in Drug Monitoring*, edited by P. L. Morselli, C. E. Pippenger, A. Richens, D. Schmidt, and H. Meinardi, pp. 373–380. Raven Press, New York.
32. Klotz, U., Rapp, T., and Mueller, W. A. (1978):

Valproic acid–phenytoin interaction. *Ther. Drug Monitor.*, 1:243–248.

Disposition of valproic acid in patients with liver disease. *Eur. J. Clin. Pharmacol.,* 13:55–60.

33. Lecchini, S., Gatti, G., DeBernardi, M., Caravaggi, M., Frigo, G., Calzetti, S., and Visinitini, D. (1978): Serum protein binding of diphenylhydantoin in man. I. Interaction with sodium valproate. *Farmaco,* 33:80–82.

34. l'Hermitte, F., Marteau, R., and Serdaru, M. (1978): Dipropylacetate (valproate de sodium) et carbamazepine: Une association antiepileptique suspecte. *Presse Med.,* 7:3780.

35. Lines, D. R. (1978): Sodium valproate (Epilim) in the treatment of refractory epilepsy. *N.Z. Med. J.,* 87:9–12.

36. Loiseau, P., Orgogozo, J. M., Centaud, B., and Brachet-Liermain A. (1980): Further pharmacokinetic observations on the interaction between phenobarbital and valproic acid in epileptic patients. In: *Advances in Epileptology: The Xth Epilepsy International Symposium,* edited by J. A. Wada and J. K. Penry, pp. 353–354, New York, Raven Press.

37. Mattson, G. F., Mattson, R. H., and Cramer, J. A. (1982): Interaction between valproic acid and carbamazepine: An *in vitro* study of protein binding. *Ther. Drug Monit. (in press).*

38. Mattson, R. H. (1979): Valproate and the management of seizures. In: *Current Neurology, Vol. 2,* edited by R. Tyler and D. Dawson, pp. 233–234, Houghton Mifflin, Boston.

39. Mattson, R. H., and Cramer, J. A. (1980): Valproic acid and ethosuximide interaction. *Ann. Neurol.,* 7:583–584.

40. Mattson, R. H., Cramer, J. A., Williamson, P. D., and Novelly, R. (1978): Valproic acid in epilepsy: Clinical and pharmacological effects. *Ann. Neurol.,* 3:20–25.

41. Mihaly, G. W., Vajda, F. J., Miles, J. L., and Louis, W. J. (1979): Single and chronic dose pharmacokinetic studies of sodium valproate in epileptic patients. *Eur. J. Pharmacol.,* 15:23–29.

42. Monks, A., Boobis, S., Wadsworth, J., and Richens, A. (1978): Plasma protein binding interaction between phenytoin and valproic acid in vitro. *Br. J. Clin. Pharmacol.,* 6:487–492.

43. Monks, A., and Richens, A. (1980): Effect of single doses of sodium valproate on serum phenytoin concentration and protein binding in epileptic patients. *Clin. Pharmacol. Ther.,* 27:89–95.

44. Patel, I. H., and Levy, R. H. (1979): Valproic acid binding to human serum albumin and determination of free fraction in the presence of anticonvulsants and free fatty acids. *Epilepsia,* 20:85–90.

45. Patel, I. H., Levy, R. H., and Cutler, R. E. (1980): Phenobarbital–valproic acid interaction in normal man. *Clin. Pharmacol. Ther.,* 27:515–521.

46. Patsalos, P. N., and Lascelles, P. T. (1977): Effect of sodium valproate on plasma protein binding of diphenylhydantoin. *J. Neurol. Neurosurg. Psychiatry,* 50:570–574.

47. Penry, J. K., Porter, R. J., Sato, S., Redenbaugh, J., and Dreifuss, F. E. (1976): Effect of sodium valproate on generalized spike-wave paroxysms in the electroencephalogram. In: *Clinical and Pharmacological Aspects of Sodium Valproate (Epilim) in the*

Treatment of Epilepsy, edited by N. J. Legg, pp. 158–164. MCS Consultants, Tunbridge Wells, Kent.

48. Perucca, E. (1980): Plasma protein binding of phenytoin in health and disease: Relevance to therapeutic drug monitoring. *Ther. Drug Monitor.,* 2:331–344.

49. Perucca, E., Gatti, G., Frigo, G. M., Crema, A., Calzetti, S., and Visintini, D. (1978): Sodium valproate in epileptic patients. *Br. J. Pharmacol.,* 5:495–499.

50. Potolicchio, S. J., Jr. (1977): *L'Efficacite du di-n-Propylacetate de Sodium (Depakine) en Monotherapie dans les Absences Simples et Complexes.* These Medecine, Université de Génève, Geneva.

51. Redenbaugh, J. E., Sata, S., Penry, J. K., Dreifuss, F. E., and Kupferberg, H. J. (1980): Sodium valproate: Pharmacokinetics and effectiveness in treating intractable seizures. *Neurology (Minneap.),* 30:1–6.

52. Reidenberg, M. M. (1977): The binding of drugs to plasma proteins and the interpretation of measurements of plasma concentrations of drugs in patients with poor renal function. *Am. J. Med.,* 62:466–470.

53. Reunanen, M. I., Luoma, P., Myllyla, V. V., and Hokkanen, E. (1980): Low serum valproic acid concentrations in epileptic patients on combination therapy. *Curr. Ther. Res.,* 28:455–462.

54. Richens, A., and Ahmad, S. (1975): Controlled trial of sodium valproate in severe epilepsy. *Br. Med. J.,* 4:255–256.

55. Richens, A., Scoular, I. T., Ahmad, S., and Jordan, B. J. (1976): Pharmacokinetics and efficacy of Epilim in patients receiving long-term therapy with other antiepileptic drugs. In: *Clinical and Pharmacological Aspects of Sodium Valproate (Epilim) in the Treatment of Epilepsy,* edited by N. J. Legg, pp. 78–88. MCS Consultants, Tunbridge Wells, Kent.

56. Rowland, M. (1980): Plasma protein binding and therapeutic drug monitoring. *Ther. Drug Monitor.,* 2:29–37.

57. Sackellares, J. C., Lee, S. I., and Dreifuss, F. E. (1979): Stupor following administration of valproic acid to patients receiving other antiepileptic drugs. *Epilepsia,* 20:697–703.

58. Sackellares, J. C., Sato, S., Dreifuss, F. E., and Penry, J. K. (1981): Reduction of steady state valproate levels by other antiepileptic drugs. *Epilepsia,* 22:437–441.

59. Sansom, L. N., Beran, R. C., and Schapel, G. J. (1980): Interaction between phenytoin and valproate. *Med. J. Aust.,* 2:212.

60. Schobben, F., van der Kleijn, E., and Gabreels, F. J. M. (1975): Pharmacokinetics of di-*N*-propylacetate in epileptic patients. *Eur. J. Clin. Pharmacol.,* 8:97–105.

61. Schobben, F., Vree, T. B., and van der Kleijn, E. (1978): Pharmacokinetics, metabolism and distribution of 2-*N*-propyl pentanoate (sodium valproate) and the influence of salicylate comedication. In: *Advances in Epileptology, 1977,* edited by H. Meinardi and A. J. Rowan, pp. 271–277. Swets & Zeitlinger, Amsterdam.

62. Taburet, A. M., Aymard, P., and Richardet, J. M. (1975): Influence of joint therapy on phenobarbital blood levels. *Ann. Biol. Clin.,* 33:231.

63. Vajda, F. J., McNeil, J. J., Morris, P., Drummer,

O., and Bladin, P. F. (1978): Sodium valproate (Epilim) in refractory epilepsy. *Aust. N.Z. J. Med.*, 8:46–51.

64. Vakil, S. D., Critchley, E. M. R., Philips, J. C., Haydock, C., Cocks, A., and Dyer, T. (1976): The effect of sodium valproate (Epilim) on phenytoin and phenobarbitone blood levels. In: *Clinical and Pharmacological Aspects of Sodium Valproate (Epilim) in the Treatment of Epilepsy,* edited by N. J. Legg, pp. 75–77. MCS Consultants, Tunbridge Wells, Kent.

65. Varma, R., and Hoshimo, A. (1979): Simultaneous gas-chromatographic measurement of valproic acid in psychiatric patients: Effect on levels of other simultaneously administered anticonvulsants. *Neurosci. Lett.*, 11:353–356.

66. Voelzke, E., and Doose, H. (1973): Dipropylacetate (Depakine, Ergenyl) in the treatment of epilepsy. *Epilepsia*, 14:185–193.

67. Whyte, M. P., and Dekaban, A. S. (1977): Metabolic fate of phenobarbital. A quantitative study of *p*-hydroxyphenobarbital in man. *Drug Metab. Dispos.*, 5:63–70.

68. Wilder, B. J., Willmore, L. J., Bruni, J., and Villareal, H. J. (1978): Valproic acid: Interaction with other anticonvulsant drugs. *Neurology (Minneap.)*, 28:892–896.

69. Wilson, A. (1976): Discussion of Vakil, S. D., Critchley, E. M. R., Philips, J. C., Haydock, C., Cocks, A., and Dyer, T. (1976): The effect of sodium valproate (Epilim) on phenytoin and phenobarbitone blood levels. In: *Clinical and Pharmacological Aspects of Sodium Valproate (Epilim) in the Treatment of Epilepsy,* edited by N. J. Legg, p. 77. MCS Consultants, Tunbridge Wells, Kent.

70. Windorfer, A., Sauer, W., and Gadeke, R. (1972): Elevation of diphenylhydantoin and primidone serum concentration by addition of dipropylacetate, a new anticonvulsant drug. *Acta Paediatr. Scand.*, 64:771–772.

Antiepileptic Drugs, edited by D. M. Woodbury,
J. K. Penry, and C. E. Pippenger. Raven Press,
New York © 1982.

48

Valproate

Relation of Plasma Concentration to Seizure Control

B. J. Wilder and B. J. Karas

Valproic acid (VPA) is also marketed as sodium valproate, magnesium valproate, and an amide of valproic acid. A new preparation, sodium hydrogen divalproate, will soon be marketed in an enteric-coated formulation in the United States. Immediate release formulations, enteric coated tablets, and oral syrups are available for use in most parts of the world. A variety of proprietary names are used worldwide: Depakene®, Epilim®, Ergenyl®, Labazene®, Deprakine®, Orfiril®, and Atemperator®, to mention a few.

CLINICAL EFFICACY IN VARIOUS SEIZURE TYPES

The first clinical trial of VPA was reported by Carraz and co-workers in 1964 (12); following this report, the drug rapidly gained acceptance as an effective antiepileptic agent. The drug was first used in France in 1964 and subsequently in Holland and Germany in 1968, the United Kingdom in 1973, and, finally, in North America in 1978. The rapidity of its worldwide acceptance attests to its clinical efficacy, which has been demonstrated in a wide variety of seizure types. Valproic acid is a major drug for the treatment of primary generalized seizure disorders. These include absence, generalized tonic–

clonic, myoclonic, atonic, and akinetic seizures and other less well-defined seizure types often characterized by generalized spike, spike-and-wave, or other paroxysmal abnormalities in the EEG (1,8,10,17,22,26,30,47,49,56,67,69). Henriksen and Johannessen (27,28) reported on a 5-year follow-up of 100 children 3 to 16 years of age with intractable epilepsy. After the institution of VPA therapy, 50% of the patients obtained a greater than 75% reduction in seizure frequency, with 33% becoming seizure-free. The authors concluded that VPA is the drug of choice in patients with absence and atonic seizures and that it is also effective in all seizure types regardless of the EEG findings, although patients with generalized paroxysmal spike and slow wave abnormalities in the EEG respond best.

Karas and Wilder (37) reported on the efficacy of VPA in comparison with phenytoin in the treatment of patients with newly diagnosed generalized tonic–clonic seizures who had not received prior therapy. Patients received either VPA or phenytoin as monotherapy. Both drugs were judged to be equally effective in preventing generalized tonic–clonic seizure recurrence. Cavazzuti (13) reported that VPA is as effective as phenobarbital in preventing febrile seizures.

Valproic acid has generally been found to be

less effective than other anticonvulsants in patients with simple and complex partial seizures, but the response of patients with complex partial attacks is often favorable (70).

PLASMA VPA LEVELS AND CLINICAL PHARMACOKINETICS

Absorption

Both the acid and VPA salts are rapidly absorbed following oral ingestion (27,28,43). The non-enteric-coated VPA preparations are rapidly absorbed, and peak plasma levels of the drug occur within 2 hr following ingestion (14). Enteric-coated preparations delay absorption, and plasma VPA levels reach a peak 3 to 8 hr after ingestion (B. J. Wilder and B. J. Karas, *unpublished data*) (33,43). Ingestion of either rapid-release or enteric-coated preparations with meals generally delays and may or may not slow absorption of VPA. Thus, the type of formulation and time of ingestion in relation to meals alter absorption. Plasma sampling to determine trough or peak plasma levels of valproate should be varied depending on the formulation given the patient.

The bioavailabilities of the various preparations are equal and approach unity (35,43).

Distribution

Valproic acid is distributed mainly in the extracellular space, but both one- and two-compartment models are used to describe the kinetics of VPA (7,39,61,62). After injection of ^{14}C-VPA into pregnant monkeys, the drug rapidly crosses the placenta and is found in highest concentration in the blood, liver, kidney, and intestines of mother and fetus. Valproic acid accumulates in growing bone, and high concentrations are found in brain (61,62,64). The drug is found in breast milk of mothers in a plasma-to-milk ratio of approximately 12 (18) (B. J. Wilder, *unpublished data*). Unbound VPA freely moves into and out of the cerebrospinal fluid (CSF), and a plasma-to-CSF ratio of 1 is maintained. Continuous monitoring of VPA concentration in CSF and plasma of monkeys shows that the CSF concentration closely follows the total plasma concentration in a ratio of approximatley 0.1 (44), which closely parallels the ratio of unbound, or free, VPA to total VPA (19,52). In higher concentrations, the binding of VPA is nonlinear, with the free fraction increasing in relationship to the total VPA present (4,6,46). This variation of free to protein-bound VPA results in changes in tissue distribution, metabolism, and drug clearance that can affect the interpretation of plasma VPA levels in therapeutic monitoring (see Plasma VPA Levels and Seizure Control).

Elimination

The elimination of VPA and its metabolites occurs principally via renal excretion with minor amounts being excreted in feces and expired air (24,70). In humans, 1 to 3% is excreted unchanged, 10 to 30% is excreted as the glucuronic acid conjugate, and the remainder is metabolized in the liver by β-oxidation with the formation of 3-hydroxy-2-propylpentanoic acid. A second metabolic route involves ω-oxidation with the formation of 4-hydroxy-2-propylpentanoic acid (29). Minor quantities of other metabolites are also found in humans. Metabolism is rapid, and the half-life ($T_{1/2}$) of the drug ranges from 6 to 12 hr (7) in epileptic patients on long-term polytherapy and from 9 to 18 hr in healthy volunteers (34,39,43,53,54).

In epileptic patients receiving VPA along with other anticonvulsant drugs, the $T_{1/2}$ is shorter, and the dose-to-plasma level ratio is higher than in patients receiving VPA only. Patients on long-term therapy with only VPA show $T_{1/2}$ and dose-to-plasma level ratios similar to those of normal volunteers (B. J. Wilder and B. J. Karas, *unpublished data*). Half-lives of 9 to 12 hr have been reported in preteenage children (34,63). Thus, VPA does not appear to induce its own metabolism. Other antiepileptic drugs such as phenobarbital, carbamazepine, and phenytoin, however, enhance the metabolism of VPA by their enzyme-inducing effects (3,55,58). When patients are changed from multiple-drug therapy to monotherapy, the dose of VPA can usually be reduced.

In neonates (<1 to 10 days) the $T_{1/2}$ ranges

between 10 and 67 hr. In infants between 10 and 60 days, the $T_{1/2}$ is longer than that in adults. After 2 months of age, the $T_{1/2}$ approximates that of adults (5). Redenbaugh et al. (57) also showed that the $T_{1/2}$ is similar in adults and children.

PLASMA VPA LEVELS AND SEIZURE CONTROL

The relationship between control of epileptic seizures and the achievement of certain plasma levels of antiepileptic drugs is well established as a principal of anticonvulsant drug therapy (11,41,66). It can rightly be argued, however, that the plasma drug levels do not truly represent the amount of bioactive drug in the plasma. This is certainly true. Only un-ionized drug that is not protein bound is free to cross membranes, penetrate the brain, and exert a pharmacological effect. Valproic acid has a pK_a of 4.95, indicating that it is highly ionized in plasma and would therefore not be available for penetration of cellular membranes. This factor is not significant, however, because VPA is similar to endogenous fatty acids which undergo transmembrane migration and may be actively transported into and out of the brain and spinal fluid (20).

Most studies report that VPA is 90 to 95% protein bound, a limiting factor in its penetration into the brain. *In vitro* and *in vivo* studies, however, have shown the protein binding of VPA to be concentration dependent with significant increases in unbound drug at high plasma concentrations (6,23,52). Furthermore, other compounds (e.g., aspirin and phenylbutazone) have been shown to displace VPA from protein binding sites and raise the levels of free drug. Increases in endogenous plasma fatty acids also reduce VPA binding (6,19).

At least two disease states may affect protein binding of VPA. Renal and liver disease with hypoproteinemia may result in a marked increase in the free (unbound) fraction of VPA (23,40). In these conditions, the measurement of free (unbound) drug is desirable for therapeutic monitoring.

Data on the concentration-dependent protein binding of VPA have been reported by Bowdle

and co-workers (4) who showed *in vivo* a 44% increase in unbound VPA when total plasma levels increased from 47 to 100 μg/ml, corresponding to a dosage increase from 500 to 1,500 mg/day. Bruni et al. (6) reported an *in vitro* increase in free VPA of 300% as the total plasma level increased from 40 to 160 μg/ml. These data provide a kinetic basis for the therapeutic range of plasma VPA levels, generally accepted to be between 50 and 100 μg/ml (9).

Clinical studies that have attempted to correlate plasma VPA levels with the onset of clinical response have generally found 40 to 50 μg/ml to be the lowest level at which efficacy can be demonstrated. Furthermore, efficacy in the various populations of patients studied increased as plasma VPA levels increased to approximately 100 μg/ml (1,2,9,21,22,27,28,37, 45,57,63,67). The lowest clinically effective plasma level of VPA occurs when protein binding becomes saturated and the ratio of free (unbound) VPA to total VPA begins to increase. Although the upper limit of therapeutic effectiveness is generally accepted to be 100 μg/ml, some patients may not experience seizure control until levels exceed that limit (59). Bruni et al. (9), for example, reported two patients who achieved optimal control only when trough plasma VPA levels of 136 μg/ml had been reached.

The wide variation in clinical response coupled with the known changes in protein binding at different concentrations and in the presence of other compounds indicate that the measurement of free drug levels is superior to measurement of total drug levels in assessing clinical response and toxicity.

PLASMA VPA LEVELS AND DOSE

Loiseau et al. (45) reported a linear relationship between dose and plasma VPA levels in epileptic patients receiving single doses of 400, 600, or 800 mg of VPA. Mean peak levels of 24, 44, and 75 μg/ml, respectively, were obtained. In long-term therapy with VPA, they obtained plasma VPA levels of 29 and 37 μg/ml from patients on average daily doses of 16.2 and 22.2 mg/kg, respectively. These patients were concomitantly receiving other anticonvulsant drugs.

Nutt and Kupferberg (51) also reported a linear relationship between plasma concentration and dose of VPA in individual patients who were not receiving other anticonvulsant drugs. Interpretation of their graphic data shows that mean steady-state trough levels of 66 μg/ml were obtained at a total daily dose of 20 mg/kg. Increasing the dose to as much as 60 mg/kg resulted in a linear increase in plasma VPA levels in individual patients, although the slopes of the regression lines in different patients, which reflected clearance rates, varied as much as twofold. These authors concluded that if the plasma VPA concentration is known at two different dose levels, the concentration that would result from further dose increases could be predicted.

Karas and Wilder (37) found that daily doses of 5 to 35 mg/kg of VPA produced trough levels of 30 to 124 μg/ml in 18 patients receiving no other medication (Fig. 1). Notice the curvilinear dose response with flattening of the curve occurring at a daily dose of approximately 25 mg/kg. The curvilinear response suggests an increase in the free fraction of VPA made available for metabolism by saturation of protein binding. The resulting trough levels are lower than would be predicted by a direct linear dose-versus-plasma concentration plot. Rarely, some patients showed the opposite effects, indicating a rate-limited metabolism or inhibition of metabolism. Bowdle et al. (3) found a dose-related decline in intrinsic clearance at low dose levels, suggesting autoinhibition or saturation kinetics, but patients at higher dose levels showed an increase in clearance.

Gram et al. (22) reported a curvilinear rela-

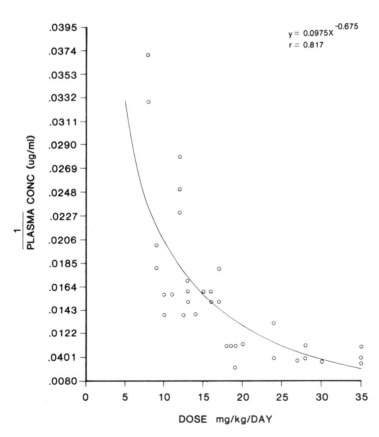

FIG. 1. Dose–response curve from 18 patients on VPA monotherapy. Curve derived from a least-square fit to a power function given by the equation $Y = 0.0975\,X^{-0.675}$. Correlation coefficient is 0.817; standard error 0.208.

tionship between dose and plasma levels of VPA. Their data were obtained from adults receiving constant daily doses of 300 to 4,000 mg of VPA in addition to other anticonvulsant drugs. Trough plasma VPA levels ranged from 113 to 344 μM or 16.2 to 49.5 $\mu g/ml$.

The plasma VPA levels obtained by Loiseau et al. (45) and Gram et al. (22) were considerably lower than those obtained by Nutt and Kupferberg (51) and Karas and Wilder (37) at roughly equivalent daily doses. The enzyme-inducing effects of concomitantly administered anticonvulsant drugs, leading to increased clearance of VPA, probably accounted for the difference. In regard to the curvilinear relationship between dose and plasma VPA levels found by Gram et al. (22) and Karas and Wilder (37), the former give three explanations: (a) autoinduction of VPA, (b) reduction in the amount of VPA absorbed, and (c) lower protein binding at increased concentrations of VPA, resulting in redistribution in body tissues and more free drug being available for metabolism and elimination. The latter explanation seems most likely in view of experimental data on protein binding (6).

Various other reports have shown a poor correlation between dose and plasma concentration of VPA. Meijer and Hessing-Brand (48) reported plasma VPA levels of 10 to 166 $\mu g/ml$ in patients receiving doses of 300 to 2,400 mg per day. Other studies have also shown a poor relationship between dose and plasma concentrations of the drug in different populations of patients. Interpatient variation in plasma VPA levels is great (2,9,21,25,32,60,65,67). Much of the variation can be attributed to the rapid absorption, variation in dosage, and short $T_{1/2}$ of the drug. Furthermore, many studies have not separated patients receiving only VPA from patients taking both VPA and other anticonvulsant drugs.

Henriksen and Johannessen (28) reported plasma drug levels in 36 patients who had been on multiple-drug therapy when VPA was begun. After VPA monotherapy was achieved, plasma VPA levels increased significantly, and in many patients, when the dose of VPA was reduced, plasma VPA levels remained as high as those obtained when the patients were taking multiple anticonvulsant drugs or even became higher.

PLASMA VPA LEVELS AND TOXICITY

Laljee and Parsonage (42), in reviewing side effects associated with VPA therapy, correlated toxicity with high doses of the drug and recommended that the daily dose for adults should not exceed 2.5 g. Clark et al. (15) concluded that serious side effects in children do not occur with doses of less than 30 mg/kg per day. Jeavons and co-workers (31) reported that side effects occur more commonly when plasma VPA levels exceed 120 $\mu g/ml$, and serious side effects occur much more commonly when VPA is administered concurrently with other anticonvulsants.

The toxic effects of VPA are generally unrelated to the plasma level of the drug. Some of these effects, however, do appear to have some correlation with plasma levels of the drug and are discussed below (the toxic effects of VPA are fully discussed in Chapter 49).

The enteric-coated formulation of sodium hydrogen divalproate has been used in some of our patients and produces few of the usual gastrointestinal complaints. Nausea and vomiting in some of these patients, however, correlate with peak plasma VPA levels which occur after the delayed absorption of the enteric-coated preparation (B. J. Wilder and B. J. Karas, *unpublished data*).

The clinically significant, but rare, hematological toxicity in patients receiving VPA usually occurs when the daily dose exceeds 50 mg/kg (15,30).

Mild, clinically insignificant tremors may occur in patients receiving VPA alone or with other drugs. The tremors increase as the dose of VPA increases (38) and respond favorably to low doses of propranolol (36). Accidental overdoses of VPA, resulting in mild stupor, have occurred in two of our patients in whom plasma VPA levels of 95 and 162 $\mu g/ml$ were obtained (B. J. Wilder, *unpublished data*). Both patients recovered uneventfully.

The most serious, although uncommon, toxic effect of VPA is hepatotoxicity (68,71). Usually, hepatotoxicity is suspected because of hepatic enzyme elevations that spontaneously return to normal without reduction in dosage of the drug or, if persistent, return to normal after a modest reduction in dosage. Willmore et al. (71) correlated a fall in SGOT and SGPT levels and other parameters of liver function in two cases of clinically apparent hepatotoxicity after withdrawal of VPA. B. J. Wilder and B. J. Karas (*unpublished data*) have observed sudden elevations of trough plasma levels of VPA in patients on stable doses and receiving no other drugs. In three patients, such VPA plasma level increases occurred at the same time SGOT levels rose. In these patients no adverse clinical effects were observed, and SGOT levels subsequently returned to normal. Fatal cases of liver failure which did not respond to withdrawal of VPA have been reported (68). In these cases, there was no consistent correlation between the clinical picture and daily dosage or plasma levels of VPA. Most patients were infants and children receiving multiple anticonvulsant drugs.

Hyperammonemia occurring during VPA therapy may be a sign of hepatic toxicity. Coulter and Allen (16) reported hyperammonemia and altered states of consciousness in some patients taking VPA in addition to other anticonvulsant drugs. They recommended reduction of VPA dosage if ammonia levels exceed 60 μM. Murphy and Marquardt (50) reported ammonia level increases in 29 of 55 children receiving VPA alone or in combination with other drugs. Clinical abnormalities did not correlate with elevated ammonia levels. Fifty percent of the patients taking only VPA had ammonia levels exceeding 35 μM, whereas more than 80% of the patients taking a combination of VPA and phenytoin or phenobarbital had similar elevations. The authors concluded that closer biochemical surveillance is warranted in individuals receiving VPA and other anticonvulsants, especially phenytoin.

SUMMARY

Valproic acid is an effective anticonvulsant drug with a broad spectrum of activity against primary generalized seizure disorders. It is less effective against partial seizures. It is chemically and structurally unrelated to the traditional antiepileptic drugs. Valproic acid is highly protein bound at lower plasma levels (<50 μg/ml), but free (unbound) drug increases disproportionately to total drug as plasma concentration increases. Clinical efficacy of VPA has been correlated with plasma levels of total drug exceeding 50 μg/ml, the level at which drug saturation of plasma proteins begins. Drug clearance is curvilinear and increases at higher plasma concentrations. Good correlation exists between daily dose and plasma levels of VPA in individual patients, but considerable interpatient variation occurs. The ratio of plasma VPA level to dose is higher in patients receiving VPA monotherapy than in patients receiving VPA plus other antiepileptic drugs.

With the exception of VPA-induced tremors, no clear-cut relationship between dose and toxicity has been established.

The measurement of free (unbound) VPA in plasma will improve the assessment of clinical response.

ACKNOWLEDGMENTS

This work was supported by the Medical Research Service of the Veterans Administration Medical Center and the Epilepsy Research Foundation of Florida, Inc. We thank Ms. Millie Walden for her assistance in the preparation of this manuscript.

REFERENCES

1. Adams, D. J., Luders, H., and Pippenger, C., (1978): Sodium valproate in the treatment of intractable seizure disorders: A clinical and electroencephalographic study. *Neurology (Minneap.)*, 28:152–157.
2. Baruzzi, A., Bordo, B., Bossi, L., Castelli, D., Gerna, M., Togononi, G., and Zagnoni, P. (1977): Plasma levels of di-*n*-propylacetate and clonazepam in epileptic patients. *Int. J. Clin. Pharmacol. Biopharm.*, 15:403–408.
3. Bowdle, T. A., Levy, R. H., and Cutler, R. E. (1979): Effects of carbamazepine on valproic acid kinetics in normal subjects. *Clin. Pharmacol. Ther.*, 26:629–634.
4. Bowdle, T. A., Patel, I. H., Levy, R. H., and Wilensky, A. J. (1980): Valproic acid dosage and plasma

protein binding and clearance. *Clin. Pharmacol. Ther.*, 28:486–492.

5. Brachet-Liermain, A., and Demarquez, J. L. (1977): Pharmacokinetics of dipropylacetate in infants and young children. *Pharm. Weekbl.*, 112:293–297.

6. Bruni, J., Gallo, J. M., and Wilder, B. J. (1979): Effect of phenytoin on protein binding of valproic acid. *Can. J. Neurol. Sci.*, 6:453–454.

7. Bruni, J., and Wilder, B. J. (1979): Valproic acid. Review of a new antiepileptic drug. *Arch. Neurol.*, 36:393–398.

8. Bruni, J., Wilder, B. J., Willmore, L. J., Perchalski, R. J., and Villarreal, H. J. (1978): Steady state kinetics of valproic acid in epileptic patients. *Clin. Pharmacol. Ther.*, 24:324–332.

9. Bruni, J., Wilder, B. J., Bauman, A. W., and Willmore, L. J. (1980): Clinical efficacy and long-term effects of valproic acid therapy on spike and wave discharges. *Neurology*, 30:42–46.

10. Bruni, J., Wilder, B. J., Willmore, L. J., Villarreal, H. J., Thomas, M., and Crawford, L. E. M. (1978): Clinical efficacy of valproic acid in relation to plasma levels. *Can. J. Neurol. Sci.*, 5:385–387.

11. Buchthal, F., and Lennon-Buchthal, M. (1972): Diphenylhydantoin. Relation of anticonvulsant effect to concentration in serum. In: *Antiepileptic Drugs*, edited by D. M. Woodbury, J. K. Penry, and R. P. Schmidt, pp. 193–209. Raven Press, New York.

12. Carraz, G., Gau, R., Chateau, R., and Bonnin, J. (1964): Communication a propos des premiers essais clinics sur l'activite anti-epileptique de l'acide *n*-dipropylacetique (sel de Na⁺). *Ann. Med. Psychol.*, 122:577–585.

13. Cavazzuti, G. B. (1975): Prevention of febrile convulsions with dipropyl acetate (Depakene). *Epilepsia*, 16:647–648.

14. Chun, A. H. C., Hoffman, D. J., Friedmann, N., and Carrijan, P. J. (1980): Bioavailability of valproic acid under fasting/nonfasting regimens. *J. Clin. Pharm.*, 20:30–36.

15. Clark, J. E., Covanis, A., Gupta, A. K., and Jeavons, P. M. (1980): Unwanted effects of sodium valproate in children and adolescents. In: *The Place of Sodium Valproate in the Treatment of Children*, edited by M. J. Parsonage and A. D. S. Caldwell, pp. 223–233. Royal Society of Medicine, London.

16. Coulter, D. L., and Allen, R. J. (1980): Secondary hyperammonaemia: A possible mechanism for valproate encephalopathy. *Lancet*, 2:1310–1311.

17. Coulthard, M. G. (1975): Sodium valproate in the treatment of intractable childhood epilepsy. *Dev. Med Child Neurol.*, 17:543.

18. Espir, M. L. E., Benton, P., Will, E., Hayes, M. J., and Walker, G. (1976): Sodium valproate (Epilim): Some clinical and pharmacological aspects. In: *Clinical and Pharmacological Aspects of Sodium Valproate (Epilim) in the Treatment of Epilepsy*, edited by N. J. Legg, pp. 145–151. MCS Consultants, Tunbridge Wells, Kent.

19. Fleitman, J. S., Bruni, J., Perrin, J. H., and Wilder, B. J. (1980): Albumin binding interaction of sodium valproate. *J. Pharmacol.*, 20:514–517.

20. Frey, H. H., and Loescher, W. (1978): Distribution of valproate across the interface between blood and cerebrospinal fluid. *Neuropharmacology*, 17:637–642

21. Gram, L., Wulff, K., Rasmussen, K. E., Flachs, H., Wurtz-Jorgensen, A., Sommerbeck, K. W., and Lohren, V. (1977): Valproate sodium: A controlled clinical trial including monitoring of drug levels. *Epilepsia*, 18:141–148.

22. Gram, L., Flachs, H., Wurtz-Jorgensen, A., Parnas, J., and Andersen, B. (1979): Sodium valproate, serum level and clinical effect in epilepsy: A controlled study. *Epilepsia*, 20:303–312.

23. Gugler, R., and Mueller, G. (1978): Plasma protein binding of valproic acid in healthy subjects and in patients with renal disease. *Br. J. Clin. Pharmacol.*, 5:441–446.

24. Gugler, R., Schell, A., Eichelbaum, M., Froscher, W., and Schultz, H. U. (1977): Disposition of valproic acid in man. *Eur. J. Clin. Pharmacol.*, 12:125–132.

25. Haigh, D., and Forsyth, W. I. (1975): The treatment of childhood epilepsy with sodium valproate. *Dev. Med. Child. Neurol.*, 17:743–748.

26. Hassan, M. N., Laljee, H. C. K., and Parsonage, M. J. (1976): Sodium valproate in the treatment of resistant epilepsy. *Acta Neurol. Scand.*, 54:209–218.

27. Henriksen, O., and Johannessen, S. I. (1980): Treatment with valproate in children with epilepsy—a five-year follow-up based on serum levels. *Dev. Med. Child Neurol.*, 22:253–254.

28. Henriksen, O., and Johannessen, S. I. (1982): Clinical and pharmacokinetic observations on sodium valproate—a five year follow-up study in 100 children with epilepsy. *Epilepsia, (in press)* (abs).

29. Jacobs, C., and Loscher, W. (1978): Identification of metabolites of valproic acid in serum of humans, dogs, rats, and mice. *Epilepsia*, 19:591–602.

30. Jeavons, P. M., Clark, J. E., and Maheshwari, M. C. (1977): Treatment of generalized epilepsies of childhood and adolescence with sodium valproate (Epilim). *Dev. Med. Child Neurol.*, 19:9–25.

31. Jeavons, P. M., Covanis, A., Gupta, A. K., and Clark, J. E. (1980): Monotherapy with sodium valproate in childhood epilepsy. In: *The Place of Sodium Valproate in the Treatment of Epilepsy*, edited by M. J. Parsonage and A. D. S. Caldwell, pp. 53–60. Royal Society of Medicine, London.

32. Jensen, I. (1977): Preliminary investigations of valproic acid plasma levels in epileptic patients controlled on valproate sodium. *Epilepsia*, 18:293.

33. Johannessen, S. I., and Henriksen, O. (1979): Comparative steady state serum levels of valproic acid administered as two different formulations—Deprakine and Orfiril. *Acta Neurol. Scand.*, 60:371–374.

34. Johannessen, S. I., and Henriksen, O. (1980): Pharmacokinetic observations of dipropylacetate in children. In: *Advances in Epileptology: X Epilepsy International Symposium*, edited by J. A. Wada and J. K. Penry, p. 353. Raven Press, New York.

35. Johannessen, S. I., and Henriksen, O. (1980): Pharmacokinetic observations of sodium valproate in healthy subjects and in patients with epilepsy. In: *Antiepileptic Therapy: Advances in Drug Monitoring*, edited by S. I. Johannessen, P. L. Morselli, C. L. Pippenger, A. Richens, D. Schmidt, and H. Meinardi, pp. 131–137. Raven Press, New York.

36. Karas, B. J., Hammond, E. J., Wilder, B. J., and Bauman, A. W. (1982): An analysis and treatment

approach of valproic acid in epileptic patients. *Epilepsia, (in press)* (abs).

37. Karas, B. J., and Wilder, B. J. (1982): The efficacy of valproic acid as compared with phenytoin in the treatment of patients with newly diagnosed tonic–clonic seizures. *Epilepsia (in press)* (abs).

38. Karas, B. J., Wilder, B. J., Hammond, E. J., and Bauman, A. W. (1982): Valproate tremors. *Neurology (Minneap.) (in press)*.

39. Klotz, R., and Antonin, K. E. (1977): Pharmacokinetics and bioavailability of sodium valproate. *Clin. Pharmacol. Ther.*, 21:736–743.

40. Klotz, V., Rapp, T., and Muller, W. A. (1978): Disposition of valproic acid in patients with liver disease. *Eur. J. Clin. Pharmacol.*, 13:55–60.

41. Kutt, H., and Penry, J. K. (1974): Usefulness of blood levels of antiepileptic drugs. *Arch. Neurol.*, 31:283–288.

42. Laljee, H. C. K., and Parsonage, M. J. (1980): Unwanted side effects of sodium valproate (Epilim) in the treatment of adult patients with epilepsy. In: *The Place of Sodium Valproate in the Treatment of Epilepsy,* edited by M. J. Parsonage and A. D. S. Caldwell, pp. 234–274. Royal Society of Medicine, London.

43. Levy, R. H., Cenraud, B., Loiseau, P., Akbaraly, R., Brachet-Liermain, A., Guyot, M., Gomeni, R., and Morselli, P. L. (1980): Meal-dependent absorption of enteric-coated sodium valproate. *Epilepsia,* 21:273–280.

44. Levy, R. H., Lockard, J. S., and Ludwick, B. T. (1981): Non-linear plasma protein binding and cerebrospinal fluid concentration of valproic acid in monkey. *Epilepsia,* 22:229.

45. Loiseau, P., Brachet, A., and Henry, P. (1975): Concentration of dipropylacetate in plasma. *Epilepsia,* 16:609–615.

46. Loscher, W. (1978): Serum protein binding and pharmacokinetics of valproate in man, dog, rat, and mouse. *J. Pharmacol. Exp. Ther.*, 204:255–261.

47. Mattson, R. H. (1979): Valproate and the management of seizures. In: *Current Neurology,* edited by H. R. Tyler and D. M. Dawson, pp. 229–248. Houghton Mifflin, Boston.

48. Meijer, J. W. A., and Hessing-Brand, L. (1973): Determination of lower fatty acids, particularly the antiepileptic dipropyl acetic acid in biological materials by means of microdiffusion and gas chromatography. *Clin. Chim. Acta,* 43:215–222.

49. Meinardi, H. (1971): Clinical trials on anti-epileptic drugs. *Psychiatry Neurol. Neurochir.*, 74:141–151.

50. Murphy, J. V., and Marquardt, K., (1982): Asymptomatic hyperammonemia in patients receiving valproic acid. *Arch. Neurol., (in press)*.

51. Nutt, J. G., and Kupferberg, H. J. (1979): Linear relationship between plasma concentration and dosage of sodium valproate. *Epilepsia,* 20:589–592.

52. Patel, I. H., and Levy, R. H. (1979): Valproic acid binding to human serum albumin and determination of free fraction in the presence of anticonvulsants and free fatty acids. *Epilepsia,* 20:85–90.

53. Perucca, E., Gatti, G., Frigo, G. M., and Crema, A. (1978): Pharmacokinetics of valproic acid after oral and intravenous administration. *Br. J. Clin. Pharmacol.*, 5:313–318.

54. Perucca, E., Gatti, G., Frigo, G. M., Crema, A., Calzetti, S., and Visintini, D. (1978): Disposition of sodium valproate in epileptic patients. *Br. J. Clin. Pharmacol.*, 5:495–499.

55. Perucca, E., Gatti, G., Frigo, G. M., Crema, A., Calzetti, S., and Visintini, D. (1978): Pharmacokinetics of sodium valproate in epileptic patients and normal volunteers. In: *Advances in Epileptology, 1977: Psychology, Pharmacotherapy, and New Diagnostic Approaches,* edited by H. Meinardi and A. J. Rowan, pp. 245–248. Swets & Zeitlinger, Amsterdam.

56. Pinder, R. M., Brodgen, R. N., and Speight, T. M. (1977): Sodium valproate: A review of its pharmacological properties and therapeutic efficacy in epilepsy. *Drugs,* 13:81–123.

57. Redenbaugh, J. E., Sato, S., Penry, J. K., Dreifuss, F. E., and Kupferberg, H. J. (1980): Sodium valproate: Pharmacokinetics and effectiveness in treating intractable seizures. *Neurology (Minneap.),* 30:1–6.

58. Richens, A., Scoular, I., Ahmad, S., and Jordan, B. J. (1976): Pharmacokinetics and efficacy of Epilim in patients receiving long-term therapy with other antiepileptic drugs. In: *Clinical and Pharmacological Aspects of Sodium Valproate (Epilim) in the Treatment of Epilepsy,* edited by N. J. Legg, pp. 78–88. MCS Consultants, Tunbridge Wells, Kent.

59. Rowan, A. J., Binnie, C. D., De Beer-Pawlikowski, N. K. B., Goedhart, D. M., Gutter, T., Van Der Geest, P., Meinardi, H., and Meijer, J. W. A. (1979): Sodium valproate: Serial monitoring of EEG and serum levels. *Neurology (Minneap.),* 29:1450–1459.

60. Schmidt, D. (1977): Variation in plasma levels of dipropylacetate (DPA) given three times daily. In: *Posttraumatic Epilepsy and Pharmacological Prophylaxis,* edited by J. Majkowski, pp. 306–313. Polfa, Warsaw.

61. Schobben, F., and van der Kleijn, E. (1974): Determination of sodium di-*n*-propylacetate in plasma by gas–liquid chromatography. *Pharm. Weekbl.,* 109:30–33.

62. Schobben, F., and van der Kleijn, E. (1974): Pharmacokinetics of distribution and elimination of sodium di-*n*-propylacetate in mouse and dog. *Pharm. Weekbl.,* 109:33–41.

63. Schobben, F., van der Kleijn, E., and Gabreels, F. J. M. (1975): Pharmacokinetics of di-*n*-propylacetate in epileptic patients. *Eur. J. Clin. Pharmacol.,* 8:97–107.

64. Schobben, F., Vree, T. B., and van der Kleijn, E. (1977): Pharmacokinetics, metabolism and distribution of 2-*n*-propyl pentanoate (sodium valproate) and the influence of salicylate comedication. In: *Advances in Epileptology, 1977: Psychology, Pharmacotherapy, and New Diagnostic Approaches,* edited by H. Meinardi and A. J. Rowan, pp. 271–277. Swets & Zeitlinger, Amsterdam.

65. Schulz, H. U., Froscher, W., Gugler, R., and Eichelbaum, M. (1979): Untersuchungen zum "therapeutischen Bereich" der Valproinsaure. *Med. Welt.,* 30:59–61.

66. Sherwin, A. L., and Robb, J. P. (1972): Ethosuximide: Relation to plasma levels to clinical control. In: *Antiepileptic Drugs,* edited by D. M. Woodbury, J. K. Penry, and R. P. Schmidt, pp. 443–448. Raven Press, New York.

67. Simon, D., and Penry, J. K. (1975): Sodium di-*n*-propylacetate (DPA) in the treatment of epilepsy: A review. *Epilepsia,* 22:1701–1708.

68. Suchy, F. J., Balistreri, W. F., Buchino, J. J., Sondheimer, J. M., Bates, S. R., Kearns, G. L., Stull, J. D., and Bove, K. E. (1979): Acute hepatic failure associated with the use of sodium valproate. *N. Engl. J. Med.,* 300:962–966.

69. Villarreal, H. J., Wilder, B. J., Willmore, L. J., Bauman, A. W., Hammond, E. J., and Bruni, J. (1978): Effect of valproic acid on spike and wave discharges in patients with absence seizures. *Neurology (Minneap.),* 28:886–891.

70. Wilder, B. J., and Bruni, J. (1981): *Seizure Disorders: A Pharmacological Approach to Treatment,* pp. 83–92. Raven Press, New York.

71. Willmore, L. J., Wilder, B. J., Bruni, J., and Villarreal, H. J. (1978): Effect of valproic acid on hepatic function. *Neurology (Minneap.),* 28:961–964.

Antiepileptic Drugs, edited by D. M. Woodbury, J. K. Penry, and C. E. Pippenger. Raven Press, New York © 1982.

49

Valproate

Toxicity

Peter M. Jeavons

Sodium valproate (Epilim®, Depakine®, Ergenyl®) has been used in France since 1964, in Holland and Germany since 1968, and in the United Kingdom since 1973 and has proved to be singularly free from serious side effects, especially if given as a sole antiepileptic drug. Valproic acid (Depakene®) has been available for restricted use in the United States since 1978. Different formulations are available and may possibly influence the incidence of gastrointestinal side effects. Some side effects, such as sedation, appear to result from drug interaction. In general, side effects are less common on low daily dosage. For 6 years, we have used a relatively low daily dosage (mean dose of 20–26 mg/kg) and have not encountered any serious side effects. We have treated more than 500 patients for a minimum period of 6 months and have never seen an idiosyncratic response. In fact, there exists only a single report of valproate-induced skin rash (51). The toxic effects of the drug have been reviewed by Simon and Penry (76), Noronha and Bevan (60), and Pinder et al. (62).

Some of the information in this chapter is based on information supplied by clinicians to the manufacturer of VPA in the United Kingdom and has not been previously published (48; Reckitt and Colman, *unpublished results*).

GASTROINTESTINAL SYMPTOMS

Anorexia, indigestion, heartburn, and nausea are more common than vomiting and are usually temporary; diarrhea is very rare. Gastrointestinal symptoms were reported in 9 to 22% of patients by Noronha and Bevan (60), the higher mean figure being in children. Symptoms can be avoided or reduced by taking medication with or after food, by gradual introduction of the drug, and by avoiding carbonated beverages. Gastrointestinal symptoms occurred in 6% of our patients who were taking valproate alone, and this was before the introduction of enteric-coated tablets. The formulation of the drug appears to be a factor in gastrointestinal disturbances, and symptoms seem to be more commonly reported with the use of oral drops of sodium valproate than with the syrup. Also, valproic acid seems to cause more symptoms than sodium valproate; one study reported a 45% incidence of side effects with the use of valproic acid (71), a higher figure than ever reported for sodium valproate. Gastrointestinal side effects are not a problem with enteric-coated tablets.

Although appetite may be reduced occasionally, it is more commonly increased (2,40,86), and there may be an increase in weight (29, 71,86), which may be as great as 20 kg in a matter of months (63). It is often difficult to evaluate the cause and degree of weight gain in children, adolescents, and women taking oral contraceptives, but allowing for these factors, we found that weight increased in 18% of 392 patients (10). Weight gain can be a considerable problem in females, who are more likely than males to put on weight (25% compared to 11% in males). Some female patients were unable to reduce weight even on a strict 1,000-calorie diet, and we had to withdraw the VPA and substitute carbamazepine.

Pancreatitis has been reported in 6 children (3,8,15,70) and in two adults (53,58). Four of the patients received a daily dose of VPA in excess of 45 mg/kg, and seven were on comedication. Two patients died, both having had a laparotomy. In three cases VPA was reintroduced after recovery from pancreatitis, and the pancreatitis recurred. Symptoms had appeared after a period of therapy with VPA lasting between 5 weeks and 6 months, most commonly after 3 months.

Temporary gastrointestinal symptoms, usually nausea, are common during the first month of therapy in patients taking VPA unless an enteric-coated tablet is used. If vomiting occurs after the first 5 or 6 weeks of therapy, and especially if there is marked pain, serum amylase should be measured, but routine measurements are not justified, because pancreatitis is very rare.

NEUROLOGICAL TOXICITY

Noronha and Bevan (60) found that drowsiness was reported in 4 to 5% of patients taking VPA and other drugs, but the incidence was only 0.2% for patients on VPA alone. We observed drowsiness in 22% of 152 VPA-treated patients on polytherapy, but the drowsiness was often temporary and most commonly occurred in those also on barbiturates, as noted in many other reports (2,28,40,41,86). Raised serum levels of barbiturates during VPA therapy have been widely reported (Chapter 47).

About 18 cases of stupor with the use of VPA have been reported (28,40,46,55,64,67,86), and in all cases the patients were also receiving bar-

biturates before being given VPA. There is one case of coma following an accidental overdose of the drug in a patient on VPA monotherapy (79).

Seventeen of our patients received a combination of VPA and clonazepam, and five (all with Lennox syndrome) developed an absence status on this combination of drugs (42), although Lance and Anthony (51) did not encounter this problem. Ten other patients became so sedated that clonazepam had to be withdrawn (10). This combination of drugs was noted to lead to deterioration of "psychomotor tempo" by Sommerbeck et al. (77).

Sedation with the use of sodium valproate alone is rare. It occurred in 2% of our 240 patients. In four there was some drowsiness in the morning after once daily administration of VPA at night, using the enteric-coated tablets (20–25 mg/kg). One patient was drowsy on a daily dosage of 39 mg/kg (10). Sedation in normal subjects has rarely been reported (6,7).

Noronha and Bevan (60) found reports of "worsened behavior" in 0.9% of patients, with an incidence of 2.4% in children. Most reports of increased aggression or hyperactivity have involved children who were also on barbiturates (2,17,26,28,40). Hyperactivity rarely occurs in children who are on VPA alone.

Increased alertness and liveliness are common and occur in patients on sodium valproate alone and also before other drugs are reduced (17,29,40,47,51,71,85). Clinical observations of a shortened reaction time in patients and controls have been confirmed by laboratory findings (27). Despite the numerous clinical reports of altered behavior with the use of VPA, Sonnen et al. (78) found no influence of VPA on behavior in a double-blind trial, possibly because their subjects were treated for only 3 weeks. Two cases of acute behavioral disturbance have been attributed to VPA (4,9).

Valproate-induced tremor was first reported in 1976 (21,28,63). It is fine to medium (21), static (63), or benign essential (34). Only 35 cases of tremor have been published, the incidence being 0.5% to 12% (mean, 3%). The most detailed account is that of Hyman et al. (34)

who noted that tremor may not appear for a year after the initiation of therapy. There is only one report of tremor occurring with monotherapy (21). There is no clear relationship of tremor to total daily dose, mg/kg dosage level, or serum VPA level. Tremor has occurred with daily doses of 600 mg (50), 1 to 2 g (34), 40 and 57 mg/kg (10), and with serum VPA levels of 33 to 154 mg/liter (34). Price (63) reported tremor in patients with serum VPA levels above 120 mg/liter. It is probable that this rare side effect is more likely with high dosages of the drug.

HAIR CHANGES

Temporary thinning of the hair after the use of VPA was first noted in 1973 (47,86), and we reported an incidence of 9.5% in 1974 (40). Subsequently, an incidence of 2.6% to 5% was reported (2,21,26,28,29,49–51,69). In 1977 we noted the occurrence of waviness or curliness in previously straight hair (41). Hair changes have occurred in 12% of our 392 patients, being found equally in those on VPA alone or combined with other drugs, and equally in children and adults, males and females. Sometimes thinning was followed by curly or wavy regrowth; at other times, the waviness was the sole change. In all cases the loss has been temporary, and in none has the drug been withdrawn. There is one report of prolonged or persistent hair loss, necessitating the wearing of a wig (50).

The increased hair fall associated with VPA is probably telogen shedding and is likely to appear after about 3 months of drug administration. It is probably not dose related. Hair loss has been associated with serum VPA levels about 600 μmole/liter (30), but we have not found any relationship to serum levels of the drug. We have one case among our patients (10). There is a tendency for adults with hair loss also to gain weight, although this does not occur in children (10).

HEMATOLOGICAL TOXICITY

Published reports of VPA-induced blood disorders are rare. Transient (51) and persistent (38) neutropenia has been noted. Fibrinogen depletion or abnormality in the erythrocyte sedimentation rate has been reported (18,61,81) but not confirmed (33,71).

The most numerous reports of blood disorders are on the effect of VPA on platelets. Abnormalities of coagulation and bleeding time were reported by Sutor and Jesdinsky-Buscher (82,83), von Voss et al. (87), and Gadner et al. (22). They were not confirmed by Richardson et al. (66), who did find inhibition of the secondary phase of platelet aggregation. Thrombocytopenia with or without bruising was reported by Espir et al. (21), and there were further reports (65,91) that have not been confirmed in a number of larger studies (49,51,71). An antiimmune factor has been implicated in the reaction (68,69). Hill (32) found a significant correlation between the VIIIR:WF and serum levels. Thrombocytopenia may occur transiently with infections, and withdrawal of the drug may be unnecessary (13).

Neophytides et al. (59) found a platelet count of less than 145,000/mm^3 in 10 of 30 patients treated with VPA and found that the incidence of reduced platelet count was higher in association with doses of 2 to 3 g daily. Monnet et al. (56) reported coagulation defects in 20 patients, but 14 of them were receiving a daily dose of VPA greater than 50 mg/kg, and only 5 were on a daily dose of 40 mg/kg or less. Laljee and Parsonage (50) found thrombocytopenia in 4 of 320 patients on VPA, and there was one death associated with daily dosage up to 4 g (72 mg/kg). Clark et al. (10) compared platelet counts in 125 patients on VPA alone, 105 on VPA combined with carbamazepine, and 81 on carbamazepine alone. Counts below 130,000/mm^3 were found in eight, six, and two patients, respectively. The mean count for those on VPA alone was 190,000/mm^3 for males and 200,000/mm^3 for females; for those on combined therapy, it was 210,000/mm^3 for both sexes; and for patients on carbamazepine only, it was 250,000/mm^3 for males and 240,000/mm^3 for females. None of the patients had any clinical signs or symptoms. The mean daily dosage of VPA was 23 mg/kg (range, 15–31 mg/kg). There was no correlation between platelet count and serum VPA levels. A significant difference in mean platelet count between epileptic patients on VPA and those not on this drug has been reported (20).

I have studied 56 reports from clinicians to the manufacturer of VPA, most of which have not been published (48; Reckitt and Colman, *unpublished results*). The information supplied by the clinicians was not always complete, but it seems that in 12 cases of thrombocytopenia the patients were asymptomatic, with the mean daily dose of VPA being 35 mg/kg (range, 16 – 46 mg/kg). In 10 cases there was evidence of an infective illness, commonly viral, and in five of these cases the daily dose exceeded 50 mg/kg (mean, 77 mg/kg). In 21 cases, the daily dose exceeded 50 mg/kg; seven patients were asymptomatic on a mean daily dose of 74 mg/kg (range, 50 – 105 mg/kg). The mean daily dose of VPA in those with symptoms was 106 mg/kg (range, 55 – 181 mg/kg). One patient had thrombocytopenia in association with liver disease. In 12 patients with some clinical symptoms, there was no evidence of high dosage or associated illness or infection, and their daily dose of VPA was less than 50 mg/kg (mean, 38 mg/kg).

Clinical symptoms were present in 28 of the 56 patients, 15 showing bruising. Of these, seven were on a high dosage of VPA (mean, 76 mg/kg), and one had a viral infection. Rarer symptoms were epistaxis (three cases), hematomata (two cases), prolonged bleeding on venipuncture (two cases), and bleeding gums (one case). Five patients had more severe symptoms: bleeding from gums combined with epistaxis and bruising, or rectal bleeding. Four of these patients were on a very high daily dosage (120, 160, 166, 181 mg/kg). One patient with purpura had a viral infection.

Although VPA may affect platelet levels and reduce the mean count, thrombocytopenia is rare, often asymptomatic, and most likely to occur and cause symptoms if the daily dosage exceeds 50 mg/kg. There is no clear evidence that thrombocytopenia is related to serum levels of VPA.

HEPATIC DISORDERS

Raised levels of serum glutamic oxalacetic transaminase (SGOT) and serum glutamic pyruvic transaminase (SGPT) have been widely reported and are usually transient or respond to reduction in dosage of VPA. Kingsley et al. (45), from a study of rat hepatocyte cultures, concluded that VPA was a dose-related hepatotoxin. The incidence varies from 2.4% to 44% (17,25,71,80,86,90), although in one study abnormal levels of SGOT and SGPT were reported in four of nine patients (81). However, no such abnormality was found in two large series (49,51). In one study of 19 patients (5) there was no evidence of abnormal hepatic function in eight patients on monotherapy, and four who showed deteriorating function were on comedication with phenytoin. We found a raised aspartate or SGOT level in 3% of 109 patients on sodium valproate alone, with 8% having an abnormal alkaline phosphatase level (10). Most of the latter group were children, none of whom had levels more than twice the upper limit of normal. In only 1 of 73 patients was the γ-glutamyl transpeptidase abnormal. This test is frequently abnormal in patients receiving enzyme-inducing antiepileptic drugs. None of our patients had any signs or symptoms of hepatic disorder, and there has been no evidence of any liver disorder in more than 500 patients whom we have treated for more than 6 months. In a large series of 320 adults (50), no clinical abnormalities of liver function were found.

Up to March 1981, 43 deaths with hepatic involvement had been reported to the pharmaceutical suppliers. The amount of information which had been made available varied considerably, and it is by no means certain that VPA was a causative factor in all 43 cases. I have compared the information that has been given to the pharmaceutical suppliers or the regulatory authorities (e.g., Committee on Safety of Medicines) with that that has been published on the same cases in various journals and have found that the details (e.g., dose, duration of therapy, comedication) sometimes differed. This makes it difficult to make a reliable evaluation in some cases. I have excluded six patients either because the details were inadequate or the patients had received VPA for less than 1 week. There are 14 published cases (1,11,19,23,35,54, 56,80,88,92) and 23 unpublished (48; Reckitt and Colman, *unpublished results*). Nineteen of these 37 cases are from the United States, where VPA can only be used as an adjuvant drug (apart from absences) and where it has only been available for about 3 years. There are seven cases from the United Kingdom, four from West Germany, three from France, two from Belgium, and two from Australia. It is interesting that no case has been reported in the Netherlands, where VPA has been used for over 12 years.

Thirty-three of the 37 patients had received comedication, 22 having received barbiturates, 19 phenytoin, 13 clonazepam, 8 carbamazepine, and others a wide variety of antiepileptic and other drugs.

Information on age, daily dosage, and duration of therapy prior to the onset of symptoms of hepatic disorder is summarized in Table 1. Only eight patients were aged 16 years or more; 15 patients were aged less than 3 years. There are many factors in the eight adult cases that must raise some doubt as to whether VPA is really implicated, and if these adults are excluded, the mean age of onset of hepatic symptoms is 4.7 ± 3.9 years.

In 9 of the 14 published cases, mention is made of mental retardation, but unfortunately this information is lacking in most of the unpublished cases. The seizure patterns are known in 35 cases, of whom 15 had myoclonic, akinetic,

or drop attacks, 7 had focal seizures, 3 had generalized status epilepticus, 3 had "a chronic seizure disorder," 3 had tonic–clonic seizures, 3 had absences, and 1 had febrile seizures.

Among the associated conditions were "multiple congenital deformities," "severe metabolic disease with developmental delay," Friedreichs ataxia, "progressive heredo-familial degenerative disease," adrenal hypoplasia, and neuronal ceroid lipofuschinosis.

Among the unpublished cases, it is of interest that there have been multiple deaths in two families. In the United Kingdom, two brothers died following treatment with VPA, phenytoin, and phenobarbital. Both showed similar brain pathology with "general astrocytic proliferation usually seen in cases of hepatic coma and also occurring in other metabolic disturbances, e.g., hyperammonemia; many Alzheimer-type 2 cells in cerebral hemispheres." These changes are similar to those shown in Case 1 of Sills et al. (72), diagnosed as having hyperammonemia (R. H. T. Jones, *personal communication*). In Germany, a brother and sister died, both being treated with VPA and clonazepam, and another sister who was treated with a barbiturate but not VPA died in hepatic coma 13 days after contracting mumps. The autopsies of the brother and sister treated with VPA showed similar changes of "subacute hepatic dystrophy" said to be like those reported by Suchy et al. (80).

Ware and Millward-Sadler (88) pointed out that centrilobular necrosis with severe fatty change was a constant feature in their own and other cases (23,35,80), and they interpreted these findings as indicating primary damage to the

TABLE 1. *Data on 37 fatal cases of hepatic disorder in VPA therapy*

	Male	Female	Age (yr)	Daily dose (mg/kg)	Total daily dose (mg)	Duration of therapy before symptoms (days)
Patients on whom data were available (N)	18	19	37	25	11[a]	34
Mean ± SD			8.4 ± 8.2	40 ± 23	925 ± 562	62 ± 37
Range			<1 – 30	13 – 128	99 – 1,800	15 – 180

[a]Body weight not given.

centrilobular hepatocytes rather than to the bile secretory apparatus, as suggested by Suchy et al. (80). The autopsy or liver biopsy reports in 16 of the unpublished cases are scanty and vary as follows: "hepatic necrosis (6 cases), hepatitis (4 cases), centrilobular necrosis (1 case), cirrhosis (1 case), hepatomegaly with fatty infiltration (1 case), cholestasis and inflammation (1 case), end-stage liver disease with multinodular changes (1 case), fibrosis (1 case)."

Hyperammonemia has been reported in patients receiving VPA and has been associated with symptoms of lethargy, although the problem is still poorly understood. Coulter and Allen (16) suggested that secondary hyperammonemia not caused by liver disease could occur in patients taking VPA and account for some cases of stupor and coma. This was doubted by Jaeken et al. (36). Further cases were reported by Coulter (14), and Sills et al. (72) reported two patients, one of whom died. In this latter case, the gross liver histology was normal, but cerebral changes suggested hepatic encephalopathy of the type associated with hyperammonemia. The other child had normal liver function tests with serum VPA levels within the therapeutic range. These authors suggested that the plasma ammonia should be measured if a child receiving VPA showed deterioration, increased seizure activity, or signs of toxic encephalopathy.

A recent review of hepatic disorders (52) stated:

Fatal liver disease seems to be a rare complication of what is otherwise a fairly non-toxic drug. There is no case at present for curtailing its use, except in patients with pre-existing liver disease in whom other anticonvulsants are probably safer. Routine measurement of liver function is not necessary in all patients but is a sensible precaution in those who seem to be most at risk, i.e., children with severe epilepsy associated with mental retardation or structural damage, in the first 6 months of sodium valproate.

This statement was based on the published data.

Although full information is still lacking from much of the unpublished data, certain factors appear to be sufficiently common in the 37 cases of hepatic disorder that I have analyzed, and in the published cases of pancreatitis, to act as pointers to the clinician.

1. Toxic hepatitis and pancreatitis have occurred most commonly within 3 months of the start of VPA therapy, rarely before 1 month, and all before 6 months. The mean onset of hepatic disorder was 62 days.
2. In all but five cases the patient was receiving comedication, most commonly including phenytoin.
3. Most fatalities occurred in children and in patients with intractable epilepsy, often with associated mental retardation.
4. In the published cases the patients showed prodromal clinical symptoms such as loss of seizure control, malaise, lethargy, drowsiness, weakness, vomiting, anorexia, or jaundice.
5. In general, VPA dosage has been within the recommended range and serum VPA levels within the "optimum" range.

The present evidence therefore suggests that deaths result from an idiosyncratic response.

If any patient shows clinical symptoms, and liver function tests (especially SGOT) are abnormal, VPA should be withdrawn immediately. On the other hand, there is no scientific evidence that the finding of a raised SGOT or SGPT level in a patient who has no clinical symptoms of liver dysfunction is an indication for withdrawing VPA, since abnormal laboratory findings are often transient. Clinical monitoring is more important than laboratory tests, and patients should be reviewed every 2 weeks for the first 2 months of VPA therapy and every month for the subsequent 4 months. It is wise to assess liver function and establish a hematological profile before starting therapy with VPA, but if every patient who shows a raised SGOT level has VPA reduced or withdrawn, although the doctor may be protected from the medico–legal viewpoint, the patients may suffer (39).

TERATOGENICITY AND REPRODUCTIVE FUNCTION

There have been no reports of human fetal or reproductive abnormalities; teratogenic effects have been shown in animals, however, and these have been summarized by Whittle (89). In rabbits, defects of kidney or vertebrae occurred in 31% at a dosage of 315 mg/kg. In rats, there were skeletal or kidney defects in 27% at 150 mg/kg, in 29% at 300 mg/kg, and in 67% at 600 mg/kg. In mice, 15% showed defects at 600 mg/kg, mostly encephaloceles. Animal studies have shown that testicular damage may occur [Dejong quoted by Swanson et al. (84)], but sperm motility is not affected in animals or man (84). Cohn et al. (12) found that VPA had no influence on the maturation of the sex organs of the male rat.

Unpublished reports (Reckitt and Colman, *unpublished results*) on 49 pregnancies in women who had received sodium valproate showed that 17 women had received no other drugs apart from iron or vitamins and had produced 14 normal babies. Three had spontaneous abortions. Of the remaining 32 women, three had received VPA during the last trimester only but had taken phenytoin throughout the pregnancy. One of these three women had a baby with sacral agenesis who died on the first day; the other two babies were normal. There were 23 normal babies of mothers who had received VPA throughout pregnancy. One baby had spina bifida, the mother having been on phenobarbital as well as VPA. The dosage of VPA was 600 mg daily. This woman had previously had a normal baby and one stillborn child. One baby who died had gross congenital abnormalities, including cleft palate and cleft lip, imperforate anus, and renal agenesis. The pregnant mother had received VPA, phenytoin, and primidone. Another child whose mother had been on the same combination of drugs had an obstructive hernia. One child with a family history of mental retardation and seizures was also retarded and had convulsions; the mother had taken a combination of phenobarbital and VPA during pregnancy. One baby had "visual problems, strabismus, retrogeniculate defect, attentional defect, and developmental delay." His mother had also received sodium pentobarbital, promazine, and flurazepan during pregnancy. No malformations were found in the babies of 12 women in Finland who had taken VPA throughout pregnancy (31).

OTHER EFFECTS

Hyperglycinemia, hyperglycinuria, and hyperaminoaciduria have been reported rarely (37,44,57,73–75), without associated clinical problems.

Nine cases of accidental and 14 cases of suicidal overdosage have been reported to the pharmaceutical suppliers (48). Full recovery occurred in 22; the only fatality followed a massive unsuspected suicidal overdose with a serum level of 1,970 mg/liter (24).

There have been unpublished reports of irregular menses and secondary amenorrhea (48; Reckitt and Colman, *unpublished results*).

CONCLUSION

A daily dosage of 2.5 g of VPA should not be exceeded in an adult, since there appears to be no therapeutic gain, and the incidence of side effects increases (50). At a mean daily dosage of less than 30 mg/kg, serious side effects have not been encountered (10).

In infants with severe epilepsy, dosage may be as high as 50 mg/kg, but if such a dosage is used it is essential to monitor SGOT, platelets, and serum VPA levels. Side effects are likely to be more common and more severe if the serum level of VPA is higher than 120 mg/liter. When VPA is the sole drug, a daily dose between 20 and 30 mg/kg is usually adequate to achieve control of seizures (43). With comedication, higher doses may be necessary because of hepatic enzyme induction by other antiepileptic drugs. With once daily administration of VPA, even lower daily dosage is effective (43).

REFERENCES

1. Addison, G. M., and Gordon, N. S. (1980): Sodium valproate and acute hepatic failure. *Dev. Med. Child Neurol.*, 22:248–249.
2. Barnes, S. E., and Bower, B. D. (1975): Sodium valproate in the treatment of intractable childhood epilepsy. *Dev. Med. Child Neurol.*, 17:175–181.
3. Batalden, P. B., Van Dyne, B. J., and Cloyd, J. C. (1979): Pancreatitis associated with valproic acid therapy. *Pediatrics*, 64:520–522.
4. Bellman, M. H., and Ross, E. M. (1977): Side effects of sodium valproate. *Br. Med. J.*, 2:1662.
5. Beran, R. G., and Rischbieth, R. H. C. (1979): Sodium valproate and hepatoxicity in epileptics. *Med. J. Aust.*, 2:603.
6. Bowdle, T. A., Patel, I. H., Wilensky, A. J., and Comfort, C. (1979): Hepatic failure from valproic acid. *N. Engl. J. Med.*, 301:435–436.
7. Boxer, C. M., Herzberg, J. L., and Scott, D. F. (1976): Has sodium valproate hypnotic effects? *Epilepsia*, 17:367–370.
8. Camfield, P. R., Bagnell, P., Camfield, C. S., and Tibbles, J. A. R. (1979): Pancreatitis due to valproic acid. *Lancet*, 1:1198–1199.
9. Chadwick, D. W., Cumming, W. J. K., Livingstone, I., and Cartlidge, N. E. F. (1979): Acute intoxication with sodium valproate. *Ann. Neurol.*, 6:552–553.
10. Clark, J. E., Covanis, A., Gupta, A. K., and Jeavons, P. M. (1980): Unwanted effects of sodium valproate in children and adolescents. In: *The Place of Sodium Valproate in the Treatment of Epilepsy*, edited by M. J. Parsonage and A. D. S. Caldwell, pp. 223–233. Royal Society of Medicine, London.
11. Coeckelberghs, M., Van Caillie-Bertrand, M., Bultinck, J., and Clara, R. (1980): Ernstige leverbeschadiging na gebruik van valproinezuur (Depakine). *Ned. Tijdsch. Geneeskd.*, 124:1428–1431.
12. Cohn, D. F., Paz, G., Hommonai, Z. T., Hammawi, D., and Streifler, M. (1980): The effect of anticonvulsive drugs on the maturation of the sex organs of the male rat. *Acta Neurol. Scand. [Suppl. 79]*, 62:91–92.
13. Cole, A. P. (1978): Transient thrombocytopenia in a child on sodium valproate. *Dev. Med. Child Neurol.*, 20:482–490.
14. Coulter, D. L. (1980): Valproate, hyperammonaemia, hyperglycinaemia. *Lancet*, 2:260.
15. Coulter, D. L., and Allen, R. J. (1980): Pancreatitis associated with valproic acid therapy for epilepsy. *Ann. Neurol.*, 7:92.
16. Coulter, D. L., and Allen, R. J. (1980): Secondary hyperammonaemia: A possible mechanism for valproate encephalopathy. *Lancet*, 2:1310–1311.
17. Coulter, D. L., Wu, H., and Allen, R. J. (1980): Valproic acid therapy in childhood epilepsy. *J.A.M.A.*, 244:785–788.
18. Dale, B. M., Purdie, G. H., and Rischbieth, R. H. (1978): Fibrinogen depletion with sodium valproate. *Lancet*, 1:1316–1317.
19. Donat, J. F., Bocchini, J. A., Gonzalez, E., and Schwendimann, R. N. (1979): Valproic acid and fatal hepatitis. *Neurology (Minneap.)*, 29:273–274.
20. Eastham, R. D., and Jancar, J. (1980): Sodium valproate and platelet counts. *Br. Med. J.*, 1:186.
21. Espir, M. L. E., Benton, P., Will, E., Hayes, M. J., and Walker, G. (1976): Sodium valproate (Epilim)—some clinical and pharmacological aspects. In: *Clinical and Pharmacological Aspects of Sodium Valproate (Epilim) in the Treatment of Epilepsy*, edited by N. J. Legg, pp. 145–151. MCS Consultants, Tunbridge Wells, Kent.
22. Gadner, H., Bensel, I., Grimm, B., and Riehm, H. (1976): Beeinflussung der Haemostase durch Dipropylessigsäure. *Monatsschr. Kinderheilkd.*, 124:448–449.
23. Gerber, N., Dickinson, R. G., Harland, R. C., Lynn, R. K., Houghton, D., Antonias, J. I., and Schimschock, J. C. (1979): Reye-like syndrome associated with valproic acid therapy. *J. Pediatr.*, 95:142–144.
24. Gourru, J.-L. (1980): *Intoxication Aigue Massive par le Valproate de Sodium. A Propos d'une Observation d'Intoxication Volontaire Mortelle.* Thesis, Claude-Bernard University, Lyon.
25. Hagen, N., Frelander, A., Verjee, S., and Vance, J. (1979): Valproic acid in epilepsy. Presented at the *11th Epilepsy International Symposium, Florence*.
26. Haigh, D., and Forsyth, W. I. (1975): The treatment of childhood epilepsy with sodium valproate. *Dev. Med. Child Neurol.*, 17:743–748.
27. Harding, G. F. A., and Pullan, J. J. (1977): Effect of sodium valproate on the EEG, the photosensitive range, the CNV and reaction time. *Electroencephalogr. Clin. Neurophysiol.*, 43:465.
28. Harwood, G., and Harvey, P. K. P. (1976): Results of a clinical trial on the use of Epilim in convulsive disorders, with special reference to its efficacy in temporal lobe attacks with focal features. In: *Clinical and Pharmacological Aspects of Sodium Valproate (Epilim) in the Treatment of Epilepsy*, edited by N. J. Legg, pp. 40–49. MCS Consultants, Tunbridge Wells, Kent.
29. Hassan, M. N., Laljee, H. C. K., and Parsonage, M. J. (1976): Sodium valproate in the treatment of resistant epilepsy. *Acta Neurol. Scand.*, 54:209–218.
30. Henriksen, O., and Johannessen, S. I. (1979): Monotherapy with sodium valproate. Presented at the *11th Epilepsy International Symposium, Florence*.
31. Hiilesmaa, V. K., Bardy, A. H., Granström, M.-L, and Teramoa, K. A. W. (1980): Valproic acid during pregnancy. *Lancet*, 1:883.
32. Hill, F. G. H. (1980): Haematological side-effects of sodium valproate. In: *The Place of Sodium Valproate in the Treatment of Epilepsy*, edited by M. J. Parsonage and A. D. S. Caldwell, pp. 165–167. Royal Society of Medicine, London.
33. Hutchinson, R. M., Clay, C.M., Simpson, M. R., and Wood, J. K. (1978): Lowered erythrocyte-sedimentation rate with sodium valproate. *Lancet*, 2:1309.
34. Hyman, N. M., Dennis, P. D., and Sinclair, K. G. A. (1979): Tremor due to sodium valproate. *Neurology (Minneap.)*, 29:1177–1180.
35. Jacobi, G., Thorbeck, R., Ritz, A., Janssen, W., and Schmidts, H.-L. (1980): Fatal hepatotoxicity in child on phenobarbitone and sodium valproate. *Lancet*, 1:712–713.

36. Jaeken, J., Casaer, P., and Corbeel, L. (1980): Valproate, hyperammonaemia and hyperglycinaemia. *Lancet*, 2:260.

37. Jaeken, J., Corbeel, L., Casaer, P., Carchon, H., Eggermont, E., and Eeckels, R. (1977): Dipropylacetate (valproate) and glycine metabolism. *Lancet*, 2:617.

38. Jaeken, J., van Goethem, C., Casaer, P., Devlieger, H., and Eggermont, E. (1979): Neutropenia during sodium valproate treatment. *Arch. Dis. Child.*, 54:985–986.

39. Jeavons, P. M. (1980): Sodium valproate and acute hepatic failure. *Dev. Med. Child Neurol.*, 22:547–548.

40. Jeavons, P. M., and Clark, J. E. (1974): Sodium valproate in treatment of epilepsy. *Br. Med. J.*, 2:584–586.

41. Jeavons, P. M., Clark, J. E., and Harding, G. F. A. (1977): Valproate and curly hair. *Lancet*, 1:359.

42. Jeavons, P. M., Clark, J. E., and Maheshwari, M. C. (1977): Treatment of generalized epilepsies of childhood and adolescence with sodium valproate (Epilim). *Dev. Med. Child Neurol.*, 19:9–25.

43. Jeavons, P. M., Covanis, A., Gupta, A. K., and Clark, J. E. (1980): Monotherapy with sodium valproate in childhood epilepsy. In: *The Place of Sodium Valproate in the Treatment of Epilepsy*, edited by M. J. Parsonage and A. D. S. Caldwell, pp. 53–60. Royal Society of Medicine, London.

44. Kamoun, P., and Parvy, P. (1978): Effet du *n*-dipropyl acétate sur l'élimination urinaire des acides aminés. *Helv. Paediat Acta*, 33:379–383.

45. Kingsley, E. Tweedale, R., and Tolman, K. G. (1980): Hepatotoxicity of sodium valproate and other anticonvulsants in rat hepatocyte cultures. *Epilepsia*, 21:699–704.

46. Koskiniemi, M., and Hakamies, L. (1979): Valproic acid and coma. *Neurology (Minneap.)*, 29:1430.

47. Kugler, J., Knörl, G., and Empt, J. (1973): Die Behandlung therapieresistenter Epilepsien mit Dipropylacetat. *Munch. Med. Wochenschr.*, 115:1103–1108.

48. Labaz (1981): *Data Sheet—Epilim*; and unpublished reports. Labaz, Basel.

49. Lagenstein, I., Sternowsky, H. J., Blaschke, E., Rothe, M., and Fehr, R. (1978): Treatment of childhood epilepsy with dipropylacetic acid (DPA). *Arch. Psychiatr. Nervenkr.*, 226:43–55.

50. Laljee, H. C. K., and Parsonage, M. J. (1980): Unwanted effects of sodium valproate (Epilim) in the treatment of adult patients with epilepsy. In: *The Place of Sodium Valproate in the Treatment of Epilepsy*, edited by M. J. Parsonage and A. D. S. Caldwell, pp. 234–274. Royal Society of Medicine, London.

51. Lance, J. W., and Anthony, M. (1977): The anticonvulsant action of sodium valproate (Epilim) in 100 patients with various forms of epilepsy. *Med. J. Aust.*, 1:911–915.

52. *Lancet* (1980): Sodium valproate and the liver. *Lancet*, 2:1119–1120.

53. Lankisch, P. G., Criée, C. P., and Winkler, K. (1980): Akute Pankreatitis unter antikonvulsiver Therapie mit Natriumvalprionat (Ergenyl). *Dtsch. Med. Wochenschr.*, 105:905

54. Le Bihan, G., Bourreille, J., Sampson, M., Leroy, J., Szekely, A. M., and Coquerel, A. (1980): Fatal hepatic failure and sodium valproate. *Lancet*, 2:1298–1299.

55. Meinardi, H., Hanke, N. F. J., and van Beveren, J. (1974): Sodium di-*N*-propylacetate: Estimation of effective serum levels. *Pharm. Weekbl.*, 109:45–47.

56. Monnet, P., David, M., Philippe, N., Dechavanne, M., Floret, D., Renaud, H., Trezeciak, M. C., Brazier, J. L., and Bourdillon, D. (1979): Altérations de l'hemostase lors des traitments au dipropylacetate de sodium (Depakine). *Pediatrie*, 34:603–620.

57. Mortensen, P. B., Køluraa, S., and Christensen, E. (1980): Inhibition of the glycine cleavage system: Hyperglycinemia and hyperglycinuria caused by valproic acid. *Epilepsia*, 21:563–569.

58. Murphy, M. J., Lyon, L. W., Taylor, J. W., and Mitts, G. (1981): Valproic acid associated pancreatitis in an adult. *Lancet*, 1:41–42.

59. Neophytides, A. N., Nutt, J. G., and Lodish, J. R. (1979): Thrombocytopenia associated with sodium valproate treatment. *Ann. Neurol.*, 5:389–390.

60. Noronha, M. J., and Bevan, P. L. T. (1976): A literature review of unwanted effects of treatment with Epilim. In: *Clinical and Pharmacological Aspects of Sodium Valproate (Epilim) in the Treatment of Epilepsy*, edited by N. J. Legg, pp. 61–67. MCS Consultants, Tunbridge Wells, Kent.

61. Nutt, J. G., Neophytides, A. N., and Lodish, J. R. (1978): Lowered erythrocyte-sedimentation rate with sodium valproate. *Lancet*, 2:636.

62. Pinder, R. M., Brogden, R. N., Speight, T. M., and Avery, G. S. (1977): Sodium valproate: A review of its pharmacological properties and therapeutic efficacy in epilepsy. *Drugs*, 13:81–123.

63. Price, D. J. E. (1976): The advantages of sodium valproate in neurosurgical practice. In: *Clinical and Pharmacological Aspects of Sodium Valproate (Epilim) in the Treatment of Epilepsy*, edited by N. J. Legg, pp. 44–49. MCS Consultants, Tunbridge Wells, Kent.

64. Rai, P. V. (1978): Acute intoxication during a combined treatment of sodium valproate and phenobarbitone. In: *Advances in Epileptology—1977*, edited by H. Meinardi and A. J. Rowan, pp. 366–369. Swets & Zeitlinger, Amsterdam.

65. Raworth, R. E., and Birchall, G. (1978): Sodium valproate and platelet count. *Lancet*, 1:670–671.

66. Richardson, S. G. N., Fletcher, D. J., Jeavons, P. M., and Stuart, J. (1976): Sodium valproate and platelet function. *Br. Med. J.*, 1:221–222.

67. Sackellares, J. C., Lee, S. I., and Dreifuss, F. E. (1979): Stupor following administration of valproic acid to patients receiving other antiepileptic drugs. *Epilepsia*, 20:697–703.

68. Sandler, R. M., Bevan, P. C., Roberts, G. E., Emberson, C., Voak, D., Darnborough, J., and Heeley, A. F. (1979): Interaction between sodium valproate and platelets. A further study. *Br. Med. J.*, 2:1476.

69. Sandler, R. M., Emberson, C., Roberts, G. E., Voak, D., Darnborough, J., and Heeley, A. F. (1978): IgM platelet antibody due to sodium valproate. *Br. Med. J.*, 2:1683–1684.

70. Sasaki, M., Tonoda, S., Aoki, Y., and Katsumi, M. (1980): Pancreatitis due to valproic acid. *Lancet,* 1:1196.

71. Sherard, E. S., Steiman, G. S., and Couri, D. (1980): Treatment of childhood epilepsy with valproic acid: Results of the first 100 patients in a 6-month trial. *Neurology (Minneap.),* 30:31–35.

72. Sills, J. A., Jones, R. H. T., and Taylor, W. H. (1980): Valproate, hyperammonaemia, and hyperglycinaemia. *Lancet,* 2:260–261.

73. Similä, S., von Wendt, L., Hartikainen-Sorri, A.-L., Kääpä, P., and Saukkonen, A.-L. (1979): Sodium valproate, pregnancy, and neonatal hyperglycinaemia. *Arch. Dis. Child.,* 54:985–986.

74. Similä, S., von Wendt, L., and Linna, S.-L. (1980): Dipropylacetate and aminoaciduria. *J. Neurol. Sci.,* 45:83–86.

75. Similä, S., von Wendt, L., Linna, S.-L., Saukkonen, A.-L., and Huhtaniemi, I. (1979): Dipropylacetate and hyperglycinemia. *Neuropaediatrie,* 10:158–160.

76. Simon, D., and Penry, J. K. (1975): Sodium di-*N*-propylacetate (DPA) in the treatment of epilepsy. A review. *Epilepsia,* 16:549–573.

77. Sommerbeck, K. W., Theilgaard, A., Rasmussen, K. E., Løhrne, V., Gran, I., and Wulff, K. (1977): Valproate sodium: Evaluation of so-called psychotropic effect. A controlled study. *Epilepsia,* 18:159–167.

78. Sonnen, A. E. H., Zelweder, W. H., and Bruens, J. H. (1975): A double blind study of the influence of dipropylacetate on behavior. *Acta Neurol. Scand.,* 52:43–47.

79. Steiman, G. S., Woerpel, R. W., and Sherard, E. S. (1979): Treatment of accidental sodium valproate overdose with an opiate antagonist. *Ann. Neurol.,* 6:274.

80. Suchy, F. J., Balistreri, W. F., Buchino, J. J., Sondheimer, J. M., Bates, S. R., Kearns, G. L., Stull, J. D., and Bove, K. E. (1979): Acute hepatic failure associated with the use of sodium valproate. *N. Engl. J. Med.,* 300:962–966.

81. Sussman, N. M., and McLain, L. W. (1979): A direct hepatoxic effect of valproic acid. *J.A.M.A.,* 242:1173–1174.

82. Sutor, A. H., and Jesdinsky-Buscher, C. (1974): Gerinnungsveränderungen durch Dipropylessigsäure (Ergenyl). *Med. Welt.,* 25:447–449.

83. Sutor, A. H., and Jesdinsky-Buscher, C. (1976): Veränderungen der Haemostase bei Epilepsie-behandlung mit Dipropylessigsäure erweiterte Untersuchung. *Fortschr. Med.,* 94:411–414.

84. Swanson, B. N., Harland, R. C., Dickenson, R. G., and Gerber, N. (1978): Excretion of valproic acid into semen of rabbits and man. *Epilepsia,* 19:541–546.

85. Vining, E. P. G., Botsford, E., and Freeman, J. M. (1979): Valproate sodium in refractory seizures. A study of efficacy. *Am. J. Dis. Child.,* 133:274–276.

86. Völzke, E., and Doose, H. (1973): Dipropylacetate (Dépakine, Ergenyl) in the treatment of epilepsy. *Epilepsia,* 14:185–193.

87. Von Voss, H., Petrich, C., Karch, D., Schulz, H.-U., and Göbel, U. (1976): Sodium valproate and platelet function. *Br. Med. J.,* 2:179.

88. Ware, S., and Millward-Sadler, G. H. (1980): Acute liver disease associated with sodium valproate. *Lancet,* 2:1110–1113.

89. Whittle, B. A. (1976): Pre-clinical teratological studies on sodium valproate (Epilim) and other anticonvulsants. In: *Clinical and Pharmacological Aspects of Sodium Valproate (Epilim) in the Treatment of Epilepsy,* edited by N. J. Legg, pp. 105–111. MCS Consultants, Tunbridge Wells, Kent.

90. Willmore, L. J., Wilder, B. J., Bruni, J., and Villareal, H. J. (1978): Effect of valproic acid on hepatic function. *Neurology (Minneap.),* 28:961–964.

91. Winfield, D. A., Benton, P., Espir, M. L. E., and Arthur, L. J. H. (1976): Sodium valproate and thrombocytopenia. *Br. Med. J.,* 2:981.

92. Young, R. S. K., Bergman, I., Gang, D. L., and Richardson, E. P. (1980): Fatal Reye-like syndrome associated with valproic acid. *Ann. Neurol.,* 7:389.

Antiepileptic Drugs, edited by D. M. Woodbury,
J. K. Penry, and C. E. Pippenger. Raven Press,
New York © 1982.

50

Valproate

Mechanisms of Action

Daniel Johnston and Gerald E. Slater

Since Meunier et al. (19) first reported in 1963 that the compound *n*-dipropylacetate (VPA; sodium valproate) had anticonvulsant properties, it has been widely used as an antiepileptic agent. Despite an accumulating literature on the metabolic and neurophysiological effects of sodium valproate, however, the basic mechanism of action remains obscure.

Three major hypotheses based on quite different experimental studies exist for the mechanisms of action of VPA. The first suggests that VPA increases γ-aminobutyric acid (GABA) levels in the brain, thereby exerting its anticonvulsant action by increasing neuronal inhibition. Most of the literature on VPA uses this hypothesis as a reference point. The second hypothesis suggests that VPA has a direct membrane effect that reduces the excitability of neurons. The third hypothesis suggests that VPA potentiates the GABA receptor such that, in the presence of VPA, a given release of GABA exerts a greater inhibitory action on the postsynaptic neuron. In this review, we shall attempt to summarize the available evidence for each of these hypotheses and outline areas for further research.

SODIUM VALPROATE INCREASES BRAIN GABA

The pioneering work of Elliott and Florey (7) and much subsequent work (for reviews, see 16 and 21) have established GABA as a major inhibitory transmitter candidate in mammalian brain. Godin et al. (12) studied the effects of sodium valproate on GABA metabolism in rats, both *in vitro*, using brain homogenates, and *in vivo*. In both studies, the biosynthesis of GABA from glutamic acid did not change significantly after the administration of VPA, even though there was a significant increase in GABA brain content without a change in other amino acids. However, the authors demonstrated that the activity of the enzymes glutamate decarboxylase (GAD) and γ-aminobutyrate transaminase (GABA-T) was inhibited *in vitro*. A 25 mM concentration of VPA had a more pronounced inhibitory effect on GABA-T (37.6%) than a 50 mM concentration had on GAD activity (22.6%).

The authors suggested that the anticonvulsant effect of VPA can be related to an increased GABA level in the brain, perhaps by decreasing the activity of the catabolic enzyme GABA-T.

However, their enzymatic findings on the reduction of GABA-T, even though GABA levels were elevated, could not be confirmed *in vivo* after the intraperitoneal administration to rats of sodium valproate in large doses (400 mg/kg).

Additional evidence for the action of VPA on brain GABA levels was provided by Simler et al. (24). Previously, this group had demonstrated that VPA protects genetically susceptible mice from audiogenic seizures (25) in a dose-related fashion. They noted that there was no difference between the brain GABA levels of genetically susceptible and normal mice. Furthermore, after an audiogenic seizure, the brain GABA level decreased by approximately 18% (24).

After intramuscular injection of VPA, the GABA level in the brain of audiogenic-sensitive mice was shown to increase significantly. This increase in GABA was correlated to the degree of protection against seizures. Simler's group provided additional evidence that VPA may competitively inhibit GABA-T.

In 1975, Fowler et al. (10) compared the binding properties of other carboxylic acids in regard to GABA. Butyric, valeric, and propionic acids were shown to be potent inhibitors of GABA-T. Dipropylacetate and α-ketoglutarate also inhibited the binding of GABA-T to GABA but were relatively weak inhibitors. The different binding capacities are perhaps explained by the fact that the simple acids are closer analogs of the substrate than VPA. Furthermore, it was suggested that massive doses of VPA would be required *in vivo* to effect a significant inhibition of GABA-T (9).

Other researchers have noted that VPA has even more potent inhibitory effects on other degradative enzymes of the GABA cycle (13). Specifically, VPA has been shown to be a potent competitive inhibitor of succinic semialdehyde dehydrogenase (SSAD), the enzyme that catalyzes the reaction of succinic semialdehyde to succinate, thus retarding the catabolism of GABA. The effect of VPA on GABA-T reported by Simler et al. (24) and by Fowler (9) may be secondary to the effect of VPA on SSAD. Harvey et al. (13) suggested that although

GABA-T was initially present in excess in Fowler's assay, it may have become a rate-limiting factor following its inhibition by VPA.

In 1976, Anlezark et al. (3) compared the effects of ethanolamine-*O*-sulfate (EOS) and VPA on GABA using mice with audiogenic seizures. Ethanolamine-*O*-sulfate is known to inhibit GABA-T irreversibly, with a concomitant increase in brain GABA content, when injected into the cerebral ventricles of mice (11). Treatment with EOS protected 50% of mice at 7.5 mg/kg and 80% at 15 mg/kg from audiogenic seizures in comparison to a saline-treated control group. Behavior changes were also noted in both groups treated with EOS. Mice treated with VPA at a dose of 200 mg/kg did not differ from controls in terms of behavior or seizure response. However, at doses of 400 mg/kg and 600 mg/kg, VPA-treated mice were protected against seizures induced by auditory stimulation. At the higher doses of VPA, intermittent ataxia was also noted in the mice.

In all mice treated with EOS, the GABA concentration in homogenized brain extracts increased from fourfold to 10-fold, compared with control animals. The activity of GABA-T was also significantly inhibited (54–68%) at both concentrations of EOS. The low dose of EOS did not change SSAD activity, and with the higher dose, the activity was activated by only 12%.

Only the highest dose of VPA (600 mg/kg) significantly increased the concentration of GABA. There was no change in SSAD activity after VPA treatment in any of the mice in comparison to the control group. However, with *in vitro* experiments, VPA at concentrations of 5 mM did produce a significant competitive inhibition of SSAD activity. There was weak or absent inhibition of GABA-T in the same set of *in vitro* experiments with concentrations of VPA up to 20 mM. The inhibition of GABA-T noted by Godin et al. (12) required a 25 mM concentration of VPA.

Both Harvey et al. (13) and Anlezark et al. (3) concluded that VPA *in vitro* is probably not a competitive inhibitor of GABA-T. This erroneous observation is more in the nature of an epiphenomenon and probably arose because the assay system employed a linked reaction including SSAD. Extremely large doses of VPA produce a competition with succinic semialdehyde, inhibiting SSAD. Current evidence indicates that other anticonvulsants, such as phenobarbital, phenytoin, and ethosuximide, also have an inhibitory effect on SSAD (22).

The coincidence of peak GABA levels with the maximum anticonvulsant effect of VPA certainly suggests a direct causal link between the two. However, as both Roberts and Hammerschlag (21) and Harvey et al. (13) point out, caution should be exercised in correlating measurements of GABA levels in whole brain to global phenomena such as seizures, since raised GABA concentrations will not necessarily lead to raised GABA levels at inhibitory receptors. Changes in GABA turnover rates or GABA concentrations at nerve terminals and an increased GABA release in response to physiological stimuli must be demonstrated before the suggested causal link is strengthened. There are other problems with accepting the hypothesis that the anticonvulsant action of VPA is mediated solely through brain GABA elevation and enzyme inhibition. First, the concentration of VPA required to produce significant inhibition of the GABA-degradative enzymes is much greater than the concentration of VPA in brain that will provide an anticonvulsant effect. Second, there is the interesting paradox expressed by Anlezark et al. (3). They demonstrated that VPA does not inhibit GABA-T significantly *in vitro* but does inhibit SSAD. *In vivo,* in pretreated rats, there is a significant increase in brain GABA. Although this increase does not correlate with the inhibition of SSAD, it does appear to correlate with the inhibition of GABA-T. Third, it has not been demonstrated that raised GABA levels lead to an increased inhibition. Recent studies with *in vitro* brain slices have shown that GABA iontophoresis has a biphasic effect and suggest that large GABA concentrations might actually provide an excitatory influence (2,27).

Other investigators have contributed data that also put the GABA hypothesis in question. Emson (8) compared the effects of VPA and ami-

nooxyacetic acid (AOAA) on cobalt-induced epileptic foci in the rat. Aminooxyacetic acid has been shown to be an *in vivo* inhibitor of GABA-T by combining with the GABA-T coenzyme, pyridoxal phosphate to form an inactive oxime (4). In moderate doses, AOAA has also been shown to be a potent anticonvulsant (28). Chronic treatment of cobalt-epileptic rats with intraperitoneal VPA (100–400 mg/kg) or AOAA (20–60 mg/kg) produced significantly increased levels of brain GABA in both groups. However, only AOAA produced a marked reduction in epileptic spike frequency. Sodium valproate had no suppressive effect on the spike foci. In addition, Emson failed to demonstrate any effect of VPA on GABA-T activity in either the primary or the secondary spike foci, whereas AOAA produced a substantial reduction in GABA-T activity.

One problem, however, with these and other studies in which the effects of VPA and AOAA are compared is that no attempt was made to account for regional variations in the brain with respect to either GABA turnover or steady-state GABA concentrations. Regional differences might result in differential GABA levels after treatment with VPA or AOAA. Iadarola et al. (15) investigated this possibility and indeed found significant regional differences in the brain between VPA- and AOAA-induced increases in GABA levels. Moreover, Iadarola and Gale (14) presented data that suggested that the GABA increase produced by VPA is associated with nerve terminals, whereas AOAA elevates GABA in glia and neural perikarya.

The data thus far would suggest that there is no simple relationship between the elevation of brain GABA and the anticonvulsant effect of VPA. This gives rise to another speculation that VPA may act by limiting the spread of seizure activity rather than by directly suppressing the seizure focus. If found to be true, this conjecture may explain why, in clinical trials, VPA has not been an effective anticonvulsant in complex partial seizures with focal temporal spikes (1,20).

It might also be pointed out that the doses of VPA required to produce an anticonvulsant effect in humans (20–60 mg/kg) are an order of magnitude smaller than the doses of VPA required to demonstrate an elevated brain GABA level in most animal model systems. The conclusions proposed by many investigators are not necessarily invalidated because of this difference in drug dosage. The difference in required concentrations may reflect species differences, differences in cellular metabolism and drug binding, effects of acute versus chronic application of the drug, or regional variations of increased GABA in the brain.

DIRECT MEMBRANE EFFECTS OF VPA

Slater and Johnston (26) performed the first experiments examining the effect of VPA at the neuronal level in single-cell studies using the abdominal ganglion of the mollusk, *Aplysia californica*. With doses of VPA ranging from 5 to 20 mM, they demonstrated a concentration-dependent hyperpolarization of the membrane potential in certain identified neurons of *Aplysia* using standard electrophysiological procedures. They also demonstrated a decrease in the input resistance. Both of these effects were dose dependent, and both were easily reversible with rinsing.

When individual cells were exposed to an increased extracellular potassium concentration, the VPA-induced hyperpolarization diminished markedly. By varying the external concentration of potassium in the presence of a fixed concentration of VPA (15 mM), the authors demonstrated that the observed hyperpolarization resulted from an increased membrane conductance to potassium. The authors performed other experiments to rule out an increase in activity of the electrogenic sodium pump in the presence of VPA.

The authors also noted that VPA caused inhibitory effects on the membrane properties of other cells in the abdominal ganglion. Specifically, VPA decreased the repetitive firing of pacemaker cells and decreased the duration of excitatory postsynaptic potentials, thus reducing the effects of temporal summation. Although VPA appeared to be a potent inhibitor of neural activity in these experiments, the relationship, if any, between the increased membrane conductance and elevated GABA levels suggested by other experiments in mammals remains unknown.

In stark contrast to these *Aplysia* studies, Blume et al. (5) found that the iontophoretic application of VPA to cortical neurons increased their firing rate. These authors suggested that VPA may enhance neuronal excitability by an action involving the excitatory amino acids glutamate and aspartate. However, high concentrations of VPA were used in the study (0.5 M), and, therefore, the results are difficult to interpret and correlate with those of other studies.

SODIUM VALPROATE MODULATES GABA ACTION

Macdonald and Bergey (18) examined the effects of VPA on inhibitory synaptic mechanisms in cultured mammalian neurons. Using cultured mouse spinal cord neurons, they studied the postsynaptic action of VPA on responses to GABA, glycine, and glutamate. With iontophoretic application of VPA, there was a selective augmentation of postsynaptic GABA-mediated inhibition. The effect of VPA on glycine and glutamate responses was negligible. When VPA was directly applied to the cell soma via a large extracellular pipette, there was no effect on neuronal membrane potential or input resistance with 0.5 M VPA in the iontophoretic pipette. However, in an analogous although less direct study using extracellular recordings in rats, Schmutz et al. (23) could find no significant effect on GABAergic inhibition using iontophoretic application of VPA or intraperitoneal injections.

CONCLUSIONS

Despite a growing literature, which was briefly reviewed in the preceding pages, the mechanism of action of VPA, in our opinion, has not been established. Although there is considerable evidence for a VPA-induced increase in

GABA levels, a link between this finding and an anticonvulsant action, or even an increased GABAergic inhibition, has not been made. To support this hypothesis for the mechanism of action of VPA, for example, it must be established that increased amounts of GABA are released in response to stimulation and that an increased release leads to an increased inhibition of the postsynaptic neuron.

Since there is yet no clearly defined cellular abnormality that can be isolated as the cause of seizures, there is therefore no known primary action that an ideal anticonvulsant drug should possess. Certainly, the well-known convulsant compounds, such as penicillin, picrotoxin, and bicuculline, all decrease inhibition. A reasonable conclusion would be that an agent that increases inhibition should have anticonvulsant properties. However, an action on other neuronal properties may prove to be more effective in seizure control. For example, phenytoin, one of the most widely used anticonvulsants, has not been shown to affect inhibition in mammalian systems (6; N. Hershkowitz, *personal communication*); therefore, its anticonvulsant action may not be through effects on inhibitory mechanisms.

The study of Macdonald and Bergey (18) on cultured spinal cord neurons in which they found that VPA can modulate a postsynaptic GABA response is extremely interesting, but the results must be confirmed at lower concentrations with continuous perfusion of the drug and in other mammalian systems before they can be accepted as a possible mechanism of action of VPA. This is especially important because of the negative results of Schmutz et al. (23). Slater's and Johnston's study (26) points to the need for further evaluation of the possible direct membrane effects of VPA in a mammalian system in which lower concentrations can be used but careful intracellular measurements can still be made. Possible direct membrane effects of VPA should not be ignored, especially since the "membrane-stabilizing" effect of phenytoin seems to be the more important action of that compound in suppressing seizures.

Few cellular neurophysiological investigations of the effects of VPA have been made, in contrast to numerous such studies on phenytoin and phenobarbital. In part this is because of the relatively recent licensure of the drug in this country. Also, it has been difficult to obtain the drug in pure form for research purposes. Since VPA is readily soluble, stable in solution, and may be completely reversible in action, it is hoped that as the effectiveness of VPA is expanded and reconfirmed clinically, further neurophysiological research will be motivated and will ultimately provide a firmer basis for defining its mechanism of action. It is worth remembering, however, that care must be taken in extrapolating data from simple systems to humans, since the acute, direct effect of VPA applied to an isolated neuronal system may be quite different from, and unrelated to, the effect of chronic administration of VPA to humans, where the drug is metabolized into several different compounds (17).

ACKNOWLEDGMENT

The preparation of this manuscript was supported by grants NS 11535 and NS 15772 from the National Institute of Neurological and Communicative Disorders and Stroke, National Institutes of Health, Bethesda, Maryland.

REFERENCES

1. Adams, D. J., Luders, H., and Pippenger, C. (1978): Sodium valproate in the treatment of intractable seizure disorders: A clinical and electroencephalographic study. *Neurology (Minneap.)*, 28:152–157.
2. Alger, B. E., and Nicoll, R. A. (1979): GABA-mediated biphasic response in hippocampus. *Nature*, 281:315–317.
3. Anlezark, G., Horton, R. W., Meldrum, B. S., and Sawaya, M. C. B. (1976): Anticonvulsant action of ethanolamine-O-sulfate and di-n-propylacetate and the metabolism of gamma-aminobutyric acid (GABA) in mice with audiogenic seizures. *Biochem. Pharmacol.*, 25:413–417.
4. Baxter, C. F., and Roberts, E. (1961): Elevation of gamma-aminobutyric acid in brain: Selective inhibition of gamma-aminobutyric–alpha-ketoglutaric acid transaminase. *J. Biol. Chem.*, 236:3287–3294.
5. Blume, H. W., Lamour, Y., Arnauld, E., Layton, B. S., and Renaud, L. P. (1979): Sodium di-n-propyl-acetate (valproate) action on single neurons in rat

cerebral cortex and hippocampus. *Brain Res.*, 171:182–185.

6. Connors, B. W. (1979): Pentobarbital and diphenylhydantoin effects on the excitability and GABA sensitivity of rat dorsal ganglion cells. *Soc. Neurosci. Abstr.*, 5:587.

7. Elliott, K. A. C., and Florey, E. (1956): Factor I—Inhibitory factor from brain. *J. Neurochem.*, 1:181–191.

8. Emson, P. C. (1976): Effects of chronic treatment with aminooxyacetic acid or sodium *n*-dipropylacetate on brain GABA levels and the development and regression of cobalt epileptic foci in rats. *J. Neurochem.*, 27:1489–1494.

9. Fowler, L. J. (1973): Analysis of the major amino acids of rat brain after *in vivo* inhibition of GABA transaminase by ethanolamine-*O*-sulfate. *J. Neurochem.*, 21:437–440.

10. Fowler, L. J., Beckford, J., and John, R. A. (1975): An analysis of the kinetics of the inhibition of rabbit brain gamma-aminobutyrate aminotransferase by sodium *n*-dipropylacetate and some other simple carboxylic acids. *Biochem. Pharmacol.*, 24:1267–1270.

11. Fowler, L. J., and John, R. A. (1972): Active-site directed irreversible inhibition of rat brain 4-aminobutrate aminotransferase by ethanolamine-*O*-sulfate *in vitro* and *in vivo*. *Biochem. J.*, 130:569–573.

12. Godin, Y., Heiner, L., Mark, J., and Mandel, P. (1969): Effects of di-*n*-propylacetate, an anticonvulsive compound, on GABA metabolism. *J. Neurochem.*, 16:869–873.

13. Harvey, P. K. P., Bradford, H. F., and Davison, A. N. (1975): The inhibitory effect of sodium *n*-dipropylacetate on the degradative enzymes of the GABA shunt. *FEBS Lett.*, 52:251–254.

14. Iadarola, M. J., and Gale, K. (1979): Dissociation between drug-induced increase in nerve terminal and non-nerve terminal pools of GABA *in vivo*. *Eur. J. Pharmacol.*, 59:125–129.

15. Iadarola, M. J., Raines, A., and Gale, K. (1979): Differential effects of *n*-dipropylacetate and aminooxyacetic acid on γ-aminobutyric acid levels in discrete areas of rat brain. *J. Neurochem.*, 33:1119–1123.

16. Krnjevic, K. (1974): Chemical nature of synaptic transmission in vertebrates. *Physiol. Rev.*, 54:418–540.

17. Kupferberg, H. J. (1980): Sodium valproate. In: *An-tiepileptic Drugs: Mechanisms of Action,* edited by G. H. Glaser, J. K. Penry, and D. M. Woodbury, pp. 643–654. Raven Press, New York.

18. Macdonald, R. L., and Bergey, G. K. (1979): Valproic acid augments GABA-mediated postsynaptic inhibition in cultured mammalia neurons. *Brain Res.*, 170:558–562.

19. Meunier, H., Carray, G., Meunier, Y., Eymard, P., and Aimard, M. (1963): Pharmacology of 2-propylvaleric acid. *Therapie*, 18:435–483.

20. Pinder, R. M., Brogden, R. N., Speight, T. M., and Avery, G. S. (1977): Sodium valproate: A review of its pharmacological properties and therapeutic efficacy in epilepsy. *Drugs*, 13:81–123.

21. Roberts, E., and Hammerschlag, R. (1976): Amino acid transmitters. In: *Basic Neurochemistry*, edited by G. J. Siegel, R. W. Albers, R. Katzman, and B. W. Agranoff, pp. 218–245. Little, Brown, Boston.

22. Sawaya, M. C. B., Horton, R. W., and Meldrum, B. S. (1975): Effects of anticonvulsant drugs on the cerebral enzymes metabolizing GABA. *Epilepsia*, 16:649–655.

23. Schmutz, M., Olpe, H.-R., and Koella, W. P. (1979): Central actions of valproate sodium. *J. Pharm. Pharmacol.*, 31:413–414.

24. Simler, S., Ciesielski, L., Maitre, M., Randrianariosa, H., and Mandel, P. (1973): Effect of sodium *n*-dipropylacetate on audiogenic seizures and brain gamma-aminobutyric acid level. *Biochem. Pharmacol.*, 22:1701–1708.

25. Simler, S., Randrianariosa, H., Lehmann, A., and Mandel, P. (1968): Effets du di-*n*-propylacetate sur les crises audiogénes de la souris. *J. Physiol. (Paris)*, 60:547.

26. Slater, G. E., and Johnston, D. (1978): Sodium valproate increases potassium conductance in *Aplysia* neurons. *Epilepsia*, 19:379–384.

27. Thalmann, R. H., Peck, E. J., and Ayala, G. F. (1979): Biphasic response of pyramidal neurons to GABA iontophoresis in hippocampal slices. *Soc. Neurosci. Abstr.*, 5:747.

28. Wood, J. D., and Pesker, S. J. (1973): The role of GABA metabolism in the convulsant and anticonvulsant actions of aminooxyacetic acid. *J. Neurochem.*, 20:379–387.

Antiepileptic Drugs, edited by D. M. Woodbury,
... K. Penry, and C. E. Pippenger. Raven Press,
New York © 1982.

51

Ethosuximide

Chemistry and Methods of Determination

Anthony J. Glazko

The first clinical reports on ethosuximide (Zarontin®, Parke–Davis) in 1958 by Vossen (42) and by Zimmerman and Burgmeister (45) indicated a high and dramatic effectiveness against pure petit mal epilepsy with a low incidence of undesirable side effects. It still remains an outstanding, widely used drug for this indication.

Ethosuximide is the generic name for 2-ethyl-2-methylsuccinimide, which has the structure shown in Fig. 1. Its molecular weight is 141.17; the melting point is 64 to 65°C. This drug is highly soluble in water (about 190 mg/ml at 25°C). Its low melting point and high volatility may result in losses during the concentration of organic solvent extracts by evaporation. The LD_{50} in mice has been reported to be $1,530 \pm 40$ mg/kg perorally (6). Methods of chemical synthesis have been reported by Miller and Long (25).

SPECTROPHOTOMETRIC AND THIN-LAYER CHROMATOGRAPHIC METHODS

The first attempts to quantitate ethosuximide using a spectrophotometric procedure were reported by Hansen (12). Extensive interference was encountered with barbiturates, and the method lacked the sensitivity and specificity needed for clinical use. Thin-layer chromatography (TLC) was employed by Wechselburg and

Hübel (44) and later by Vedso et al. (41). Although these procedures are suitable for qualitative estimates, much better procedures are now available for quantitative work.

GAS–LIQUID CHROMATOGRAPHY

Nonderivatized Ethosuximide

In 1965, Dill et al. (8) described a gas–liquid chromatographic (GLC) procedure for nonderivatized ethosuximide that was used in the first definitive studies on plasma and tissue levels and excretion characteristics of the drug in laboratory animals and in man. A more detailed description of the assay procedure appeared in the first edition of *Antiepileptic Drugs* (11) and included a microassay procedure for 0.2-ml samples of finger blood. Several points were established in this work: (a) the use of α,α-dimethyl-β-methylsuccinimide as an internal standard (now available from Aldrich Chemical

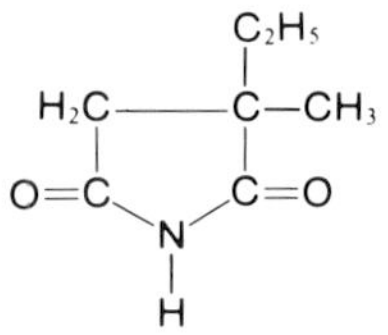

FIG. 1. Structure of ethosuximide.

Co., Milwaukee, WI) and (b) the need for the addition of a higher-boiling solvent such as amyl acetate to the chloroform extract during the evaporation step to reduce losses of ethosuximide resulting from its volatility. This procedure was modified slightly by Buchanan et al. (4), also in the Parke–Davis Laboratories, by filtration of the chloroform extract through phase-separating paper for the removal of water and by using isoamyl acetate in place of amyl acetate during the evaporation step. A similar technique has been described by Sherwin and co-workers (13,31).

Very little additional work was done with ethosuximide until the early 1970s. Meijer (23) described GLC systems for various underivatized anticonvulsant drugs including ethosuximide but did not report any quantitative data. Van der Kleijn et al. (40) acidified plasma (0.5 ml) with KH_2PO_4 and extracted with small volumes of chloroform (0.2 ml), using naphthalene as an internal standard. Gas–liquid chromatography was carried out without derivatization using a 3% OV-17 column at 125°C. Ritz and Warren (29) used single extraction techniques for temperature-programmed GLC analysis of six anticonvulsant drugs (underivatized) including ethosuximide. Chloroform extracts were back-extracted into alkali and then reextracted into chloroform to eliminate interfering substances. Gas–liquid chromatography was carried out with a 3% OV-225 column. Bonitati (3) obtained good separation of ethosuximide, phensuximide, methsuximide, and its dealkylated metabolite by temperature programming on a 5% OV-17 column, again without derivative formation. Assays were scaled down to 10 to 100 μl of plasma, and fluorene was used as the internal standard.

Heipertz et al. (14) used a highly polar phase in GLC columns, following the suggestion of Toseland et al. (39), for assay of ethosuximide, carbamazepine, phenobarbital, and phenytoin without derivative formation. The use of a nitrogen-sensitive detector, also introduced by Toseland et al. (38), improved the sensitivity of the assay. Berry and Clarke (2) used a 4% OV-225 column with nonderivatized ethosuximide,

extracting 100-μl samples of plasma with chloroform.

Derivatized Ethosuximide

Although ethosuximide produces sharp peaks at low column temperatures, and assay procedures are perfectly satisfactory without derivatization, current trends are in the direction of multiple-drug determinations. Cremers and Verheesen (7) assayed ethosuximide underivatized and then used flash methylation or silylation for determination of the other anticonvulsant drugs, using the same column (3% OV-225) at elevated temperatures. Latham and Varlow (20) and Hill and Latham (15) assayed nonderivatized ethosuximide followed by on-column methylation of phenobarbital, primidone, and phenytoin at higher column temperatures. Solow and Green (33) used on-column methylation of ethosuximide with tetramethylammonium hydroxide reagent and a 5% OV-17 column. This was later modified to include multiple anticonvulsant drugs (34), using temperature programming. Further improvements in multidrug analyses have been described by Solow et al. (35), including a micro adaptation for 200-μl serum samples. Typical results are shown in Chapter 12 (see Fig. 1 of Chapter 12). Dudley et al. (9) described on-column methylation techniques in some detail, using trimethylanilinium hydroxide as the methylating agent for multiple drug assays.

Disadvantages of the on-column alkylation technique include the need for high injection port temperatures and, in some cases, the need for slow injection of the sample to reduce pyrolysis of the reagent, which contributes to the background. Least et al. (21) prepared the N-butyl derivative of ethosuximide, using butyl iodide as the alkylating reagent, before injection of the sample into the column. They also were successful in using on-column alkylation with tetrabutylammonium hydroxide but preferred to prepare the derivative prior to GLC. The butyl iodide reagent produced rapid and complete derivatization at room temperature, and the product was stable. Menyharth et al. (24) combined a simplified butylation procedure with a rapid extraction technique and used a nitrogen-sensitive detector. Solow et al. (36) recommended the use of α-methyl-α-propylsuccinimide as an internal standard for on-column methylation procedures with ethosuximide because of its greater elution time. Wallace et al. (43) prepared derivatives of ethosuximide and desalkyl-methsuximide by reaction with pentafluorobenzoyl chloride, permitting the use of electron-capture detection. They also used the internal standard proposed by Solow et al. (36).

Combined GLC–mass spectrometer–computer systems have been used most successfully by Horning et al. (16,17) for the assay of ethosuximide as well as other anticonvulsant drugs. The ethosuximide was first converted to the trimethylsilyl derivative before assay. Studies were carried out with a Finnigan 1015 quadrupole mass spectrometer operated in the chemical ionization mode with selective ion monitoring (MH + = 214).

HIGH-PERFORMANCE LIQUID CHROMATOGRAPHY

No reference was made to high-performance liquid chromatography (HPLC) techniques in the first edition of *Antiepileptic Drugs* (11) because methods were just being developed. The HPLC detection of ethosuximide was briefly described by Riedel et al. (28) at the 1972 Workshop on Determination of Antiepileptic Drugs in Body Fluids in The Netherlands. Columns of silica gel were used, and it was immediately evident that large numbers of samples could be assayed before the column packing deteriorated. Adams and Vandemark (1) used a reverse-phase column and a mobile phase consisting of acetonitrile and water (17 : 83). The procedure was sensitive to 0.5 μg/ml using 0.5 ml of serum. Other anticonvulsant drugs measured in the same run included phenobarbital, phenytoin, methsuximide, and carbamazepine. Assays showed good correlation with GLC procedures.

Soldin and Hill (32) used a similar system with the reverse-phase packing μBondapack®-C$_{18}$. Proteins were precipitated with acetoni-trile, and a pH 8 phosphate buffer (0.01 M) with acetonitrile (1 : 1) was used as the mobile phase. Up to 1,200 assays could be run on each column, with proper care, before replacement became necessary. Kabra et al. (19) improved this assay procedure by using an acidic buffer (pH 4.4 phosphate) with acetonitrile, reducing the interference caused by salicylates, phenacetin, and caffeine. Typical results are shown in Fig. 2. Because of the excellent separations achieved by HPLC, the relative shortness of the assay, lack of need for derivative formation, and applicability to multi-drug assays, the HPLC procedures appear to be just as satisfactory for routine clinical use as the GLC procedures.

IMMUNOASSAY PROCEDURES

Most of the early work with immunoassay procedures for anticonvulsant drugs was limited to phenytoin, primidone, and phenobarbital. Reagents for the assay of ethosuximide are now available for the EMIT system, described briefly in Chapter 12. Sun and Szafir (37) compared ethosuximide assays in sera from 30 patients using the EMIT system and a nonderivatized GLC procedure and found no statistically significant differences between the two procedures. Malkus et al. (22) evaluated the performance of the EMIT procedure for five major antiepileptic drugs including ethosuximide using an automated kinetic analyzer (Perkin–Elmer Model KA-150, Norwalk, CT). The assays showed good correlation with GLC procedures. Schottelius (30) also compared assay data in 265 patients using EMIT and GLC assay procedures for ethosuximide. The average time for EMIT assays was about 8 min, and the accuracy was generally good. However, reagent costs were high. Some difficulties were encountered with ethosuximide levels greater than 50 μg/ml, and appropriate dilution of the serum was recommended. Pippenger and Kutt (26) have observed some cross reactivity of the EMIT reagents for ethosuximide with the active desalkyl metabolite of methsuximide. The response was linear, and they suggested that the ethosuximide reagents could be used to assay desmethylmethsuximide.

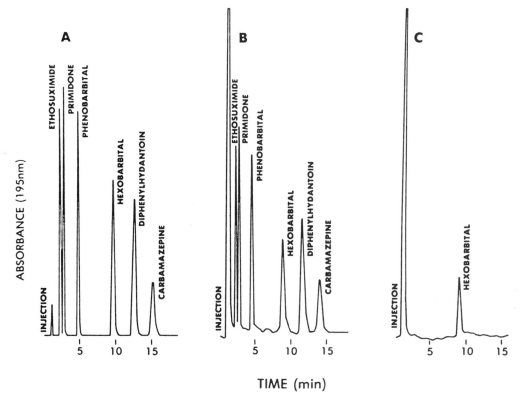

FIG. 2. High-performance liquid chromatography of anticonvulsant drugs on a reverse-phase μBondapack®-C₁₈ column with mobile phase of 95 ml acetonitrile in 405 ml of pH 4.4 phosphate buffer. **A,** standard mixture of drugs (750 ng); **B,** drugs added to serum (20 μg/ml); **C,** drug-free serum plus internal standard (50 μg/ml). (From Kabra et al., ref. 19, with permission of authors and publisher. Copyright © 1977, *Clinical Chemistry*.)

METABOLITES OF ETHOSUXIMIDE

Chang et al. (5) identified 2-(1-hydroxyethyl)-2-methylsuccinimide as a major metabolite of ethosuximide in human urine. This is formed by hydroxylation of the carbon next to the ring in the ethyl side chain. The metabolite is present in the form of two isomers, partly conjugated with glucuronic acid, that give two separate GLC peaks when chromatographed as the trimethylsilyl derivatives. Details of an assay procedure developed for this metabolite by T. Chang have been described elsewhere (10). The procedure involves hydrolysis of the conjugates with β-glucuronidase (Glusulase®), extraction with ethyl acetate, and oxidation with

chromic acid to form the 2-acetyl derivative. This in turn was extracted from the reaction mixture and measured by GLC against an internal standard. Later, it was found that the 3-hydroxy metabolite, unknown at that time, could interfere with the assay. Corrections can be made by running a second assay omitting the chromic acid oxidation step to determine the extent of interference. Assays of human urine over a 10-day period following single 1-g doses of ethosuximide indicated that 31 to 41% of the dose was recovered in the form of the hydroxyethyl metabolites, whereas unchanged ethosuximide accounted for 17 to 35% of the dose (10).

Horning et al. (18) confirmed the presence of the 1-hydroxyethyl metabolite in urine and reported a number of other metabolites including the ring-hydroxylated 3-hydroxyethosuximide (2-ethyl-2-methyl-3-hydroxysuccinimide). Preste et al. (27) also identified the ring-hydroxylated metabolite and indicated that the amount present in urine could be close to that of the hydroxyethyl metabolites. However, no additional progress has been made in this area.

CONVERSION

Conversion factor:

$$CF = \frac{1000}{mol.\ wt.} = \frac{1000}{141.2} = 7.08$$

Conversion:

$$(\mu g/ml) \times 7.08 = (\mu moles/liter)$$
$$(\mu moles/liter) \div 7.08 = (\mu g/ml)$$

REFERENCES

1. Adams, R. F., and Vandemark, F. L. (1976): Simultaneous high-pressure liquid-chromatographic determination of some anticonvulsants in serum. *Clin. Chem.,* 22:25–31.
2. Berry, D. J., and Clarke, L. A. (1978): Gas chromatographic analysis of ethosuximide (2-ethyl-2-methyl succinimide) in plasma at therapeutic concentrations. *J. Chromatogr.,* 150:537–541.
3. Bonitati, J. (1976): Gas–chromatographic analysis for succinimide anticonvulsants in serum: Macro- and micro-scale methods. *Clin. Chem.,* 22:341–345.
4. Buchanan, R. A., Fernandez, L., and Kinkel, A. W. (1969): Absorption and elimination of ethosuximide in children. *J. Clin. Pharmacol.,* 9:393–398.
5. Chang, T., Burkett, A. R., and Glazko, A. J. (1972): Ethosuximide, biotransformation. In: *Antiepileptic Drugs,* edited by D. M. Woodbury, J. K. Penry, and R. P. Schmidt, pp. 425–429. Raven Press, New York.
6. Chen, G., Weston, J. K., and Bratton, A. C. (1963): Anticonvulsant activity and toxicity of phensuximide, methsuximide and ethosuximide. *Epilepsia,* 4:66–76.
7. Cremers, H. M. H. G., and Verheesen, P. E. (1973): A rapid method for the estimation of anti-epileptic drugs in blood serum by gas–liquid chromatography. *Clin. Chim. Acta,* 48:413–420.
8. Dill, W. A., Peterson, L., Chang, T., and Glazko, A. J. (1965): Physiological disposition of α-methyl-α-ethylsuccinimide (ethosuximide, Zarontin®) in animals and in man. *Abstracts of Papers, 149th National Meeting, American Chemical Society, Detroit, Michigan,* p. 30N. American Chemical Society, Washington.
9. Dudley, K. H., Bius, D. L., Kraus, B. L., and Boyles,

10. L. W. (1977): Gas chromatographic on-column methylation technique for the simultaneous determination of antiepileptic drugs in blood. *Epilepsia,* 18:259–276.
10. Glazko, A. J. (1975): Antiepileptic drugs: Biotransformation, metabolism and serum half-life. *Epilepsia,* 16:367–391.
11. Glazko, A. J., and Dill, W. A. (1972): Ethosuximide: Chemistry and methods for determination. In: *Antiepileptic Drugs,* edited by D. M. Woodbury, J. K. Penry, and R. P. Schmidt, pp. 413–415. Raven Press, New York.
12. Hansen, S. E. (1963): Quantitative determination of ethosuximide. *Acta Pharmacol. Toxicol. (Kbh.),* 20:286–290.
13. Harvey, C. D., and Sherwin, A. L. (1978): Gas–liquid chromatographic quantitation of ethosuximide. In: *Antiepileptic Drugs: Quantitative Analysis and Interpretation,* edited by C. E. Pippenger, J. K. Penry, and H. Kutt, pp. 87–93. Raven Press, New York.
14. Heipertz, R., Pilz, H., and Eickhoff, K. (1977): Evaluation of a rapid gas–chromatographic method for the simultaneous quantitative determination of ethosuximide, phenylethylmalonediamide, carbamazepine, phenobarbital, primidone and diphenylhydantoin in human serum. *Clin. Chim. Acta,* 77:307–316.
15. Hill, R. E., and Latham, A. N. (1977): Simultaneous determination of anticonvulsant drugs by gas–liquid chromatography. *J. Chromatogr.,* 131:341–346.
16. Horning, M. G., Brown, L., Nowlin, J., Lertratanangkoon, K. Kellaway, P., and Zion, T. E. (1977): Use of saliva in therapeutic drug monitoring. *Clin. Chem.,* 23:157–164.
17. Horning, M. G., Lertratanangkoon, K., Nowlin, J., Stillwell, W. G., Zion, T. E., Kellaway, P., and Hill, R. M. (1974): Anticonvulsant drug monitoring by GC–MS–COM techniques. *J. Chromatogr. Sci.,* 12:630–635.
18. Horning, M. G., Stratton, C., Nowlin, J., Harvey, D. J., and Hill, R. M. (1973): Metabolism of 2-ethyl-2-methylsuccinimide (ethosuximide) in the rat and human. *Drug Metab. Dispos.,* 1:569–576.
19. Kabra, P. M., Stafford, B. E., and Marton, L. J. (1977): Simultaneous measurement of phenobarbital, phenytoin, primidone, ethosuximide and carbamazepine in serum by high-pressure liquid chromatography. *Clin. Chem.,* 23:1284–1288.
20. Latham, A. N., and Varlow, G. (1976): Simultaneous quantitative gas–chromatographic analysis of ethosuximide, phenobarbitone, primidone and diphenylhydantoin. *Br. J. Clin. Pharmacol.,* 3:145–150.
21. Least, C. J., Johnson, G. F., and Solomon, H. M. (1975): A quantitative gas chromatography determination of ethosuximide based on N-butylation. *Clin. Chim. Acta,* 60:285–292.
22. Malkus, H., Dicesare, J. L., Meola, J. M., Pippenger, C. E., Ibanez, J., and Castro, A. (1978): Evaluation of EMIT methods for the determination of the five major antiepileptic drugs on an automated kinetic analyzer. *Clin. Biochem.,* 11:139–142.
23. Meijer, J. W. A. (1971): Simultaneous quantitative determination of antiepileptic drugs, including carbamazepine, in body fluids. *Epilepsia,* 12:341–352.
24. Menyharth, P., Lehane, D. P., and Levy, A. L. (1977): Rapid gas chromatographic method for the determi-

nation of ethosuximide in serum. *Clin. Chem.*, 23:1795–1796.

25. Miller, C. A., and Long, L. M. (1953): Anticonvulsants. III. A study of *N*,alpha,beta-alkylsuccinimides. *J. Am. Chem. Soc.*, 75:373–375.

26. Pippenger, C. E., and Kutt, H. (1978): Common errors in the analysis of antiepileptic drugs. In: *Antiepileptic Drugs: Quantitative Analysis and Interpretation,* edited by C. E. Pippenger, J. K. Penry, and H. Kutt, pp. 199–208. Raven Press, New York.

27. Preste, P. G., Westerman, C. E., Das, N. P., Wilder, B. J., and Duncan, J. H. (1974): Identification of 2-ethyl-2-methyl-3-hydroxysuccinimide as a major metabolite of ethosuximide in humans. *J. Pharm. Sci.*, 63:467–469.

28. Riedel, E., Klocke, H., and Bayer, H. (1973): Separation of drugs by gas–liquid chromatography (GLC) and high-pressure liquid chromatography (HPLC). In: *Methods of Analysis of Anti-Epileptic Drugs,* edited by J. W. A. Meijer, H. Meinardi, C. Gardner-Thorpe, and E. van der Kleijn, pp. 194–197. Excerpta Medica, Amsterdam; American Elsevier, New York.

29. Ritz, D. P., and Warren, C. G. (1975): Single extraction of six commonly prescribed antiepileptic drugs. *Clin. Toxicol.*, 8:311–324.

30. Schottelius, D. D. (1978): Homogeneous immunoassay system (EMIT) for quantitation of antiepileptic drugs in biological fluids. In: *Antiepileptic Drugs: Quantitative Analysis and Interpretation,* edited by C. E. Pippenger, J. K. Penry, and H. Kutt, pp. 95–108. Raven Press, New York.

31. Sherwin, A. L., Robb, J. P., and Lecher, M. (1973): Improved control of epilepsy by monitoring plasma ethosuximide. *Arch. Neurol.*, 28:178–181.

32. Soldin, S. J., and Hill, J. G. (1976): Rapid micromethod for measuring anticonvulsant drugs in serum by high-performance liquid chromatography. *Clin. Chem.*, 22:856–859.

33. Solow, E. B., and Green, J. B. (1971): The determination of ethosuximide in serum by gas chromatography. *Clin. Chim. Acta,* 33:87–90.

34. Solow, E. B., and Green, J. B. (1972): The simultaneous determination of multiple anticonvulsant drug levels by gas–liquid chromatography. *Neurology (Minneap.),* 22:540–550.

35. Solow, E. B., Metaxas, J. M., and Summers, T. R.

(1974): Antiepileptic drugs: A current assessment of simultaneous determination of multiple drug therapy by gas liquid chromatography–on column methylation. *J. Chromatogr. Sci.,* 12:256–260.

36. Solow, E. B., Tupper, N. L., and Kenfield, C. P. (1978): An alternative internal standard for analysis of ethosuximide by on-column methylation and gas chromatography. *J. Anal. Toxicol.,* 2:39–40.

37. Sun, L., and Szafir, I. (1977): Comparison of enzyme immunoassay and gas chromatography for determination of carbamazepine and ethosuximide in human serum. *Clin. Chem.*, 23:1753–1756.

38. Toseland, P. A., Albani, M., and Gauchei, F. D. (1975): Organic nitrogen-selective detector used in gas–chromatographic determination of some anticonvulsant and barbiturate drugs in plasma and tissues. *Clin. Chem.*, 21:98–103.

39. Toseland, P. A., Grove, J., and Berry, D. J. (1972): An isothermal GLC determination of the plasma levels of carbamazepine, diphenylhydantoin, phenobarbitone and primidone. *Clin. Chim. Acta,* 38:321–328.

40. Van der Kleijn, E., Collste, P., Norlander, B., Agurell, S., and Sjöqvist, F. (1973): Gas chromatographic determination of ethosuximide and phensuximide in plasma and urine of man. *J. Pharm. Pharmacol.,* 25:324–327.

41. Vedso, S., Rud, C., and Place, J. F. (1969): Determination of phenytoin in serum in the presence of barbiturates, sulthiame and ethosuximide by thin-layer chromatography. *Scand. J. Clin. Lab. Invest.,* 23:175–180.

42. Vossen, R. (1958): On the anticonvulsant effect of succinimides. *Dtsch. Med. Wochenschr.,* 83:1227–1230.

43. Wallace, J. E., Schwertner, H. A., Hamilton, H. E., and Shimek, E. L. (1979): Electron-capture gas–liquid chromatographic determination of ethosuximide and desmethylmethsuximide in plasma and serum. *Clin. Chem.*, 25:252–255.

44. Wechselburg, K., and Hübel, G. (1967): Zur Resorption und Verteilung von Methyl-ethyl-succinimid (MAS) im Serum und Liquor bei Kindern. *Z. Kinderheilkd.,* 100:10–19.

45. Zimmerman, F. T., and Burgmeister, B. B. (1958): A new drug for petit mal epilepsy. *Neurology (Minneap.),* 8:769–775.

Antiepileptic Drugs, edited by D. M. Woodbury, J. K. Penry, and C. E. Pippenger. Raven Press, New York © 1982.

52

Ethosuximide

Absorption, Distribution, and Excretion

Anthony J. Glazko and Tsun Chang

HISTORICAL PERIOD (1963–1967)

Our knowledge concerning the absorption, tissue distribution, and elimination of ethosuximide has been dependent on the development of sensitive and specific assay procedures. Hansen and Feldberg (16), using a spectrophotometric procedure (15), measured plasma ethosuximide levels in two normal subjects receiving single 750-mg oral doses of the drug. The concentration of drug rose to 15 μg/ml in 2 to 4 hr and remained elevated over a 24-hr period. Repeated doses of 250 mg given three times each day for 12 days in two additional subjects produced a steady increase in plasma levels over a 4-day period, with plateau levels of 37 to 53 μg/ml appearing thereafter. Following termination of dosage, the plasma levels fell slowly with a half-life of 3 to 4 days. These observations were uncertain because of the lack of specificity in the assay procedure. Wechselburg and Hübel (33), using a thin-layer chromatographic procedure, administered 250-mg oral doses of ethosuximide to epileptic children and detected plasma levels of 25 to 50 μg/ml 1 to 2 hr after dosing. These levels persisted for 24 hr and then fell slowly. Assay of ventricular and lumbar cerebrospinal fluid (CSF) in the same patients indicated rapid appearance of drug, with peak levels appearing in 12 to 15 hr, followed by slow elimination.

The first gas–liquid chromatographic (GLC) assays were reported by Dill et al. (7) in 1965, using α, α-dimethyl-β-methylsuccinimide as an internal standard. The plasma levels obtained in albino rats, Rhesus monkeys, and normal human subjects are shown in Fig. 1. Peak levels were attained within a few hours after dosing, with apparent plasma half-lives of 12 hr in the rat, 22 hr in the monkey, and 60 hr in man. The drug concentrations in rat tissues were extremely uniform with the exception of body fat, where concentrations were lower than in the other tissues. This was supported by the data of Chang et al. (5) who used ^{14}C-labeled ethosuximide in their studies. Unchanged ethosuximide was identified in the urine, bile, and feces, and a number of metabolites were detected in rat and monkey urine after enzymatic hydrolysis of conjugates (7).

EARLY STUDIES IN MAN (1969–1973)

With a modification of the GLC procedure described by Dill et al. (7), plasma level studies were carried out in children by Buchanan et al. (2) with single 0.5-g oral doses of ethosuximide. The plasma half-lives were found to be about

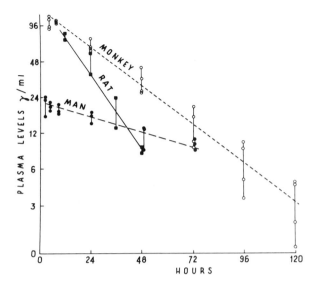

FIG. 1. Plasma ethosuximide levels in rat, monkey, and man. Single oral doses: man, 1 g = 14 mg/kg; monkey and rat, 100 mg/kg. Individual GLC assays are shown for three adult human subjects, four rhesus monkeys, and two rats. (From Chang et al., ref. 5, with permission.)

30 hr in contrast with previously observed half-lives of 60 hr in adults. Additional work by the Parke–Davis group established an average plasma level of 40 ± 14.9 μg/ml in children and young adults with average daily doses of 20.7 ± 5.8 mg/kg body weight (14). However, there was considerable individual variation among the subjects (29). This dose/plasma level relationship was confirmed by the work of Sherwin et al. (29,31) and by Browne and colleagues (1,27) who also demonstrated a direct relationship between plasma levels and dosage.

In other trials, Buchanan et al. (3) administered 0.5-g oral doses of ethosuximide once daily to normal adult males over a period of 21 days, followed by a 1-g daily dose for 7 additional days. The 0.5-g daily dose produced mean steady-state plasma levels of 34 μg/ml about 9 days after the start of dosing, with a mean maximum-to-minimum variation of 8 μg/ml. The duration of the 1-g dosing was too short to reach steady-state levels. The plasma half-life averaged about 56 hr, and the volume of distribution was 0.7 liters/kg, indicating a uniform distribution of ethosuximide in the body water. The mean urinary excretion of unchanged drug accounted for 19% of the dose.

RECENT STUDIES IN MAN (1975–1979)

During the past 5 years, clinical pharmacology studies have become more sophisticated, with increasing emphasis on pharmacokinetic measurements. Browne et al. (1) demonstrated a statistically significant relationship between dosage and plasma ethosuximide levels in children with absence seizures who had not received antiabsence medication previously. However, the rise in plasma levels with increased dosage was lower in children under 10 years of age than in older children (Fig. 2). Plasma half-lives ranged from 15 hr to 68 hr (mean, 36–39 hr) with no significant changes between the first and eighth week of dosing. The half-lives did not vary significantly with age in the 5- to 15-year age bracket, with increasing plasma levels, or with dosage. The authors concluded that there was no evidence of microsomal enzyme induction. However, because of the wide variations noted among individual subjects, it was impossible to predict the plasma ethosuximide levels that might result from any given dose.

Clinical trials in the Parke–Davis laboratories by Buchanan et al. (4) involved a compari-

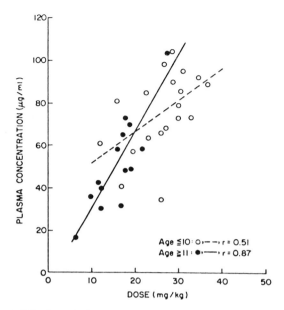

FIG. 2. Relationship of plasma ethosuximide concentration to ethosuximide dose after 8 weeks of treatment for patients age 10 years or younger and 11 years or older. (From Browne et al., ref. 1, with permission.)

son of plasma ethosuximide levels in children resulting from single daily doses versus equally divided doses of the drug given twice daily in the same total amount. In both cases, the mean plasma levels remained within the therapeutic range. Goulet et al. (13) ran the same type of trial in 10 normal adult subjects with single daily doses of 500 mg of ethosuximide given once daily for 14 days and in 10 additional subjects with 250-mg doses given twice daily over the same time period. Both groups then received 750 mg daily for an additional 14 days, either as single daily doses or 250 mg given three times daily. Absorption was rapid in both groups, and plasma ethosuximide levels were directly proportional to dosage. The mean half-lives were nearly identical for the two groups, and the mean steady-state levels were quite similar. Renal excretion of unchanged drug reached a plateau by day 12, and the excretion patterns were similar for both dosage schedules. Using advanced pharmacokinetic treatment of data, Colburn and

Gibaldi (6) reexamined the data of Goulet et al. (13) and came to essentially the same conclusions.

An assay procedure for measuring the urinary excretion of metabolite II [2-(1-hydroxyethyl)-2-methylsuccinimide] was used in a study with six adult subjects who received single 1-g oral doses of ethosuximide; the results are shown in Fig. 3 (12). Peak excretion rates for unchanged ethosuximide were found in the first 12-hr period after dosing, but the excretion rate for metabolite II was greatest in the 24- to 48-hr period, indicating a delay in the oxidation and conjugation of this metabolite with glucuronic acid. The total amount of unchanged ethosuximide plus metabolite II excreted in the urine accounted for 50 to 76% of the administered dose. The same assay procedure was used by Goulet et al. (13) for metabolite II, with similar excretion patterns being found for the single-versus divided-dose study. However, with the smaller dose employed in this study (500 mg daily), up to 80% of the dose was accounted for by the urinary excretion of unchanged drug plus metabolite II.

A number of excellent papers have appeared in the past several years summarizing extensive work on the pharmacokinetics of ethosuximide in human subjects. Eadie et al. (8) in Australia reported peak plasma levels of ethosuximide in adult subjects within 3 hr after dosing. The apparent volume of distribution was 0.67 ± 0.04 liter/kg, and the elimination rate was 0.015 ± 0.006 hr^{-1}, corresponding to a mean half-life of 52.7 ± 24.5 hr. Clearance was 0.010 ± 0.004 liter/kg per hr, considerably below the hepatic plasma flow (0.9 liter/kg per hr). Sherwin (28) confirmed the observations of Browne et al. (1) regarding dose/plasma level differences in children 3 to 10 years of age versus older children. Smith et al. (32) summarized factors affecting plasma levels of ethosuximide based on their experience with steady-state plasma levels in 46 patients over a 3-year period. No significant differences were found in the dose/plasma level relationship for children under 10 years of age (14 subjects) and those

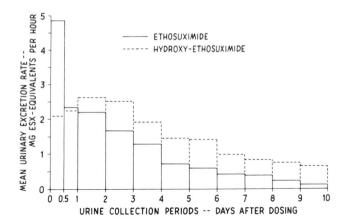

FIG. 3. Mean urinary excretion of ethosuximide and hydroxyethosuximide in six normal adult males receiving 1-g oral doses of ethosuximide. (From Glazko, ref. 12, with permission.)

over 15 years of age (20 subjects). However, a significant sex difference was found, with the plasma levels rising more sharply with increasing doses in the females. They also found that successive dose increments of equal size produced progressively greater increments in the steady-state plasma levels, leading to the suggestion that the dose/plasma level relationship might not be linear.

Koup et al. (20) studied ethosuximide levels in pregnant women near term who were receiving daily doses of ethosuximide. Plasma levels of 40 to 50 μg/ml prior to delivery rose to 60 to 70 μg/ml after delivery although the dose schedule remained unchanged. The ethosuximide concentration in milk was about 94% of the plasma levels, confirming earlier reports of Hill et al. (17). The cord blood level of ethosuximide at parturition was 61.9 μg/ml, confirming evidence for placental transfer reported earlier by Horning et al. (19). The serum half-life in the neonate was 41.3 hr.

The ease with which ethosuximide passes through membrane barriers such as the placenta is in part because of its nonionized form at physiological pH (10) and its poor protein-binding characteristics (5,9,30). Consequently, it appears rapidly in the cerebrospinal fluid (30,33), milk (17,20), and saliva (18,21). The latter is of particular interest, since the levels of ethosuximide in saliva are close to those observed in blood plasma, and samples can easily be obtained for assay.

RECENT ANIMAL STUDIES

Early metabolic work with animals has been mentioned above. Plasma levels, tissue distribution, and excretion studies with [¹⁴C] ethosuximide were carried out by Chang et al. (5). The establishment of external bile duct fistulas in the monkey did not reduce the plasma half-life of ethosuximide, and parenteral doses of ethosuximide did not result in appreciable biliary excretion, indicating that this is not an important route of ethosuximide excretion in this species. Tissue distribution data obtained with ¹⁴C-labeled drug in the rat confirmed our earlier GLC assay data. We also established that maternal/fetal transfer of drug occurred in rats (5).

Patel et al. (23,24) carried out an extensive series of experiments in rhesus monkeys at the University of Washington using single and multiple doses of ethosuximide administered perorally and intravenously. Single i.v. doses of 30, 60, and 90 mg/kg showed a very short distribution phase followed by a first-order decline in plasma levels. The volume of distribution averaged 0.8 liter/kg, and plasma half-lives averaged 29 to 30 hr at each dose level. Similar oral doses produced data on volume of distribution and on plasma half-lives that were very close to those obtained in the i.v. series. Absorption appeared to be complete as evaluated from a comparison of data on plasma levels in the i.v. and oral dose studies. A one-compartment open model with first-order elimination adequately described the kinetic behavior of ethosuximide in the monkey. However, the peak plasma levels and time required to reach the peak were not strictly proportional to dosage at the higher dose levels.

Patel and Levy (23) then applied the pharmacokinetic parameters developed in the single-dose study to multiple-dose trials in the monkey. Continuous i.v. infusion of ethosuximide at a fixed rate over a 10-day period produced plasma levels that were within 12% of theoretical values, on the average, and the half-lives after termination of dosage showed good agreement with the single-dose data. When initial priming doses were used, followed by i.v. infusion, the plasma levels showed excellent agreement with theoretical values at three different dose levels. In contrast to the single-dose studies, there was no indication of dose dependence in the multidose trials. However, plasma ethosuximide levels were somewhat higher in the morning than in the evening, suggesting a diurnal variation. Subsequent work by Patel et al. (25) confirmed these observations and suggested a circadian rhythm in total body clearance. This could result from a number of factors such as variation in the volume of distribution, renal excretion, or metabolic disposition (biotransformation).

El Sayed et al. (9) compared the pharmacokinetics of ethosuximide in dogs with reported observations in man. Intravenous doses of 40 mg/kg in nine animals produced serum levels that were adequately described by the one-compartment open model. At doses of 20 to 60 mg/kg, the half-lives ranged from 11 to 25 hr (mean, 17–18 hr), about one-third to one-half as great as in man. The volumes of distribution indicated primary association with body water and no extensive accumulation in the tissues. Peroral doses were rapidly absorbed, with peak plasma levels occurring 1 to 4 hr after dosing.

The CSF levels of ethosuximide rose rapidly and were equal to the plasma levels within 20 to 30 min. Protein binding measurements by equilibrium dialysis techniques indicated no significant binding with dog or rat serum at drug concentrations up to 150 μg/ml. There was some evidence of dose dependence, indicating possible saturation of the drug-metabolizing enzyme systems at high doses.

Earlier work on the tissue distribution of ethosuximide in animals showed remarkably uniform concentrations in most tissues with the exception of body fat (5,7). Ethosuximide levels in rat brain were found to be nearly identical with the plasma levels. Patel et al. (26) examined different areas of rat brain with GLC techniques following 4.5 days of i.p. dosing, twice daily, at four different dose levels. The area distribution ratio for midbrain appeared to be about 3% higher than that for the cerebellum. However, this difference was not great enough to justify any firm conclusions. It would be of interest to run an autoradiographic study with tritium-labeled drug to establish possible sites of intracellular localization.

Orton and Nicholls (22) reported that 70 mg/kg peroral doses of ethosuximide administered to rats in two equally divided doses each day for 3 days produced a slight increase in the hepatic microsomal enzyme activity which was not considered to be significant. However, doses of 282 mg/kg per day produced a significant decrease in hexobarbital sleeping time, increased the oxidation of hexobarbital and hydroxylation of aniline, increased liver weight, microsomal cytochrome P-450, and δ-aminolevulinic acid synthetase, and produced a proliferation of the hepatic smooth endoplasmic reticulum. The significance of these observations is not clear in terms of human use, since the dosage was far greater than any normally encountered. Gilbert et al. (11) found that the injection of ethosuximide into guinea pigs twice daily (10 mg/kg per day) for 5 to 10 days did not significantly affect the protein content or microsomal cytochrome P-450 content of the liver. In another series of experiments, guinea pigs receiving 50 mg/kg per day for 5 and 10 days showed more variability in hepatic protein and cytochrome P-450 content, but they were not significantly different from the controls. Rats receiving a higher dose (100 mg/kg per day) by i.p. administration showed significant increases in both hepatic protein and microsomal P-450. The excretion of glucaric acid was also measured in animals and in man, but the use of this parameter as a measure of microsomal enzyme induction is open to question.

REFERENCES

1. Browne, T. R., Dreifuss, F. E., Dyken, P. R., Goode, D. J., Penry, J. K., Porter, R. J., White, B. G., and White, P. T. (1975): Ethosuximide in the treatment of absence (petit mal) seizures. *Neurology (Minneap.)*, 25:515–524.
2. Buchanan, R. A., Fernandez, L., and Kinkel, A. W. (1969): Absorption and elimination of ethosuximide in children. *J. Clin. Pharmacol.*, 9:393–398.
3. Buchanan, R. A., Kinkel, A. W., and Smith, T. C. (1973): The absorption and excretion of ethosuximide. *Int. J. Clin. Pharmacol.*, 7:213–218.
4. Buchanan, R. A., Kinkel, A. W., Turner, J. L., and Heffelfinger, J. C. (1976): Ethosuximide dosage regimens. *Clin. Pharmacol. Ther.*, 19:143–147.
5. Chang, T., Dill, W. A., and Glazko, A. J. (1972): Ethosuximide: Absorption, distribution and excretion. In: *Antiepileptic Drugs*, edited by D. M. Woodbury, J. K. Penry, and R. P. Schmidt, pp. 417–423. Raven Press, New York.
6. Colburn, W. A., and Gibaldi, M. (1978): Use of MULTDOS for pharmacokinetic analysis of ethosuximide data during repetitive administration of single or divided daily doses. *J. Pharm. Sci.*, 67:574–575.
7. Dill, W. A., Peterson, L., Chang, T., and Glazko, A. J. (1965): Physiologic disposition of α-methyl-α-ethylsuccinimide (ethosuximide; Zarontin®) in animals and man. *Abstracts, 149th National Meeting, American Chemical Society, Detroit, Michigan*, p. 30N. American Chemical Society, Washington.
8. Eadie, M. J., Tyrer, J. H., Smith, G. A., and Mc-Kauge, L. (1977): Pharmacokinetics of drugs used for petit mal "absence" epilepsy. *Clin. Exp. Neurol.*, 14:172–183.
9. El Sayed, M. A., Löscher, W., and Frey, H.-H. (1978): Pharmacokinetics of ethosuximide in the dog. *Arch. Int. Pharmacodyn.*, 234:180–192.
10. Erwin, V. G., and Deltrich, R. A. (1973): Inhibition of bovine brain aldehyde reductase by anticonvulsant compounds *in vitro. Biochem. Pharmacol.*, 22:2615–2624.
11. Gilbert, J. C., Scott, A. K., Galloway, D. B., and Petrie, J. C. (1974): Ethosuximide: Liver enzyme induction and D-glucaric acid excretion. *Br. J. Pharmacol.*, 1:249–252.
12. Glazko, A. J. (1975): Antiepileptic drugs: Biotrans-

13. formation, metabolism and serum half-life. *Epilepsia*, 16:367–391.
Goulet, J. R., Kinkel, A. W., and Smith, T. C. (1976): Metabolism of ethosuximide. *Clin. Pharmacol. Ther.*, 20:213–218.
14. Haerer, A. F., Buchanan, R. A., and Wiygul, F. M. (1970): Ethosuximide blood levels in epileptics. *J. Clin. Pharmacol.*, 10:370–374.
15. Hansen, S. E. (1963): Quantitative determination of ethosuximide (Zarontin®, α-methyl, α-ethylsuccinimide) in serum. *Acta Pharmacol. Toxicol. (Kbh.)*, 20:286–290.
16. Hansen, S. E., and Feldberg, L. (1964): Absorption and elimination of Zarontin. *Dan. Med. Bull.*, 11:54–55.
17. Hill, R., Horning, M., and Horning, E. (1973): Identification of transplacentally acquired anticonvulsant agents in the neonate. In: *Methods of Analysis of Antiepileptic Drugs*, edited by J. W. A. Meijer, H. Meinardi, C. Gardner-Thorp, and E. van der Kleijn, pp. 14–147. American Elsevier, New York.
18. Horning, M. G., Brown, L., Nowlin, J., Lertratanangkoon, K., Kellaway, P., and Zion, T. E. (1977): Use of saliva in therapeutic drug monitoring. *Clin. Chem.*, 23:157–164.
19. Horning, M. G., Stratton, C., Nowlin, J., Harvey, D. J., and Hill, R. M. (1973): Metabolism of 2-ethyl-2-methyl succinimide in the rat and human. *Drug Metab. Dispos.*, 1:569–576.
20. Koup, J. R., Rose, J. Q., and Cohen, M. E. (1978): Ethosuximide pharmacokinetics in a pregnant patient and her newborn. *Epilepsia*, 19:535–539.
21. McCauliffe, J. J., Sherwin, A. L., Leppick, I. E., Fayle, S. A., and Pippenger, C. E. (1977): Salivary levels of anticonvulsants: A practical approach to drug monitoring. *Neurology (Minneap.)*, 27:409–413.
22. Orton, T. C., and Nicholls, P. J. (1972): Effect in rats of subacute administration of ethosuximide, methsuximide and phensuximide on hepatic microsomal enzymes and porphyrin turnover. *Biochem. Pharmacol.*, 21:2253–2261.
23. Patel, I. H., and Levy, R. H. (1975): Pharmacokinetic properties of ethosuximide in monkeys. II. Chronic intravenous and oral administration. *Epilepsia*, 16:717–730.
24. Patel, I. H., Levy, R. H., and Bauer, T. G. (1975): Pharmacokinetic properties of ethosuximide in monkeys. I. Single-dose intravenous and oral administration. *Epilepsia*, 16:705–716.
25. Patel, I. H., Levy, R. H., and Lockard, J. S. (1977): Time-dependent kinetics II: Diurnal oscillations in steady-state plasma ethosuximide levels in rhesus monkeys. *J. Pharm. Sci.*, 66:650–653.
26. Patel, I. H., Levy, R. H., and Rapport, R. L. (1977): Distribution characteristics of ethosuximide in discrete areas of rat brain. *Epilepsia*, 18:533–540.
27. Penry, J. K., Browne, T. R., Porter, R. J., Dreifuss, F. E., Dyken, P. R., and White, P. T. (1972): Determinations of plasma ethosuximide (Zarontin®) concentration and the management of absence (petit mal) seizures. *Neurology (Minneap.)*, 22:410.
28. Sherwin, A. L. (1978): Clinical pharmacology of ethosuximide. In: *Antiepileptic Drugs: Quantitative Analysis and Interpretation*, edited by C. E. Pippen-

ger, J. K. Penry, and H. Kutt, pp. 283–295. Raven Press, New York.

29. Sherwin, A. L., Lechter, M., Marlin, A. E., and Robb, J. P. (1971): Plasma ethosuximide (Zarontin®) levels: As new aid in the management of epilepsy. *Ann. R. Coll. Physicians Surg. Can., 4*:48–49.

30. Sherwin, A. L., and Robb, J. P. (1972): Ethosuximide: Relation of plasma levels to clinical control. In: *Antiepileptic Drugs,* edited by D. M. Woodbury, J. K. Penry, and R. P. Schmidt, pp. 443–448. Raven Press, New York.

31. Sherwin, A. L., Robb, J. P., and Lechter, M. (1973): Improved control of epilepsy by monitoring plasma ethosuximide. *Arch. Neurol., 28*:178–181.

32. Smith, G. A., McKauge, L., Dubetz, D., Tyrer, J. H., and Eadie, M. J. (1979): Factors influencing plasma concentrations of ethosuximide. *Clin. Pharmacokinet. 4*:38–52.

33. Wechselburg, K., and Hübel, G. (1967): Zur resorption und Verteilung von Methyl-äthyl-succinimid (MAS) im serum und liquor bei kindern. *Z. Kinderheilkd., 100*:10–19.

Antiepileptic Drugs, edited by D. M. Woodbury, J. K. Penry, and C. E. Pippenger. Raven Press, New York © 1982.

53

Ethosuximide

Biotransformation

Tsun Chang and Anthony J. Glazko

Using gas–liquid chromatography (GLC), Dill et al. (4) identified unchanged ethosuximide[1] in the urine, bile, and feces of albino rats and rhesus monkeys, representing some 15 to 20% of the administered dose. Normal human subjects receiving a single 1-g dose of ethosuximide excreted 10 to 20% in the urine as unchanged drug. Following treatment of rat and monkey urine with β-glucuronidase, GLC of chloroform extracts revealed the presence of several metabolic products.

Biotransformation studies with ethosuximide were greatly facilitated by the synthesis of [1-^{14}C]ethosuximide (2). This involved the preparation of 2-ethyl-2-methylsuccinic acid (9) and ring closure with ammonia. The resulting product was labeled in the C-1 position of the succinimide ring and had a specific activity of 1.22 μCi/mg (Fig. 1).

Thin-layer chromatography (TLC) of urine specimens from rats dosed with [^{14}C]ethosuximide clearly indicated the presence of unchanged drug plus two major radioactive fractions. A typical TLC chromatogram is shown in Fig. 2. In this system, ethosuximide had the highest R_f value, metabolite II had an intermediate value, and metabolite I was closest to the

*Location of ^{14}C label

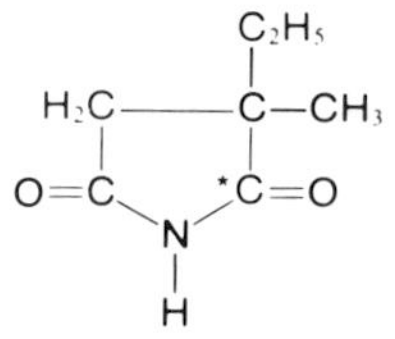

FIG. 1. Structure of ethosuximide showing the location of the ^{14}C label (*asterisk*). This is the C-1 location in the 2-ethyl-2-methylsuccinimide nomenclature.

origin, representing the most polar metabolites or water-soluble conjugates.

ETHOSUXIMIDE FRACTION

The synthetic ethosuximide used in clinical practice has one asymmetric carbon atom and consists of a racemic mixture of two optical isomers. Consequently, the optical rotation of this preparation is zero. If the two isomers are metabolized by different pathways at different rates, as occurs with glutethimide (7), the residual ethosuximide excreted in the urine should be optically active.

To examine this possibility, unchanged ethosuximide was isolated from rat urine using solvent extraction and preparative TLC techniques. Urine collected from rats dosed perorally with ethosuximide (100 mg/kg) was adjusted to

---

[1] Usual chemical name, 2-ethyl-2-methylsuccinimide; *Chemical Abstracts* name, 3-ethyl-3-methyl-2,5-pyrrolidinedione.

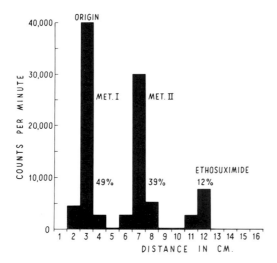

FIG. 2. Thin-layer chromatogram of rat urine following a 66-mg/kg peroral dose of [1-^{14}C]ethosuximide. Silica gel GF; ethyl acetate : carbon tetrachloride (2 : 1).

pH 5 to 6 and extracted twice with chloroform. The combined extracts were evaporated to dryness. The residue was dissolved in a small amount of chloroform and chromatographed on silica gel GF$_{254}$ TLC plates using chloroform : ethyl acetate (2 : 1) as the developing solvent. The band corresponding to ethosuximide was eluted, and the solution was evaporated to dryness, leaving about 9 mg of a crystalline solid. Subsequent GLC of this material indicated that the retention time was the same as that of ethosuximide and that the preparation was free of impurities. The optical rotation of the purified material was zero, indicating that in the rat the two isomers were metabolized at the same rate.

2-(1-HYDROXYETHYL)-2-METHYLSUCCINIMIDE

Metabolite II shown in Fig. 2 was isolated from rat urine and identified as 2-(1-hydroxyethyl)-2-methylsuccinimide[2] (1). Hydroxyla-

tion of the ethyl side chain at the C-1 position results in the formation of a new asymmetric center. Optical rotation measurements indicated that the isolated material was levorotatory ($[\alpha]_D^{25} = -7.9°$). The diastereoisomers were readily separated by GLC as their trimethylsilyl (TMS) derivatives, and metabolite II was found to be a 40 : 60 mixture of the diastereoisomers. Oxidation of metabolite II with chromic acid produced the corresponding ketone derivative, 2-acetyl-2-methylsuccinimide.[3] A GLC method for quantitative assay of metabolite II based on this oxidation procedure was developed later (see Chapter 51).

A small amount of 2-(1-hydroxyethyl)-2-methylsuccinimide (metabolite II) was synthesized for use as reference standard (2). Comparison of the synthetic material with the isolated metabolite showed that the two compounds were identical in their infrared absorbance characteristics and GLC retention times, supporting the proposed structure. The nuclear magnetic resonance (NMR) spectrum of the synthetic compound was slightly different from that of the urinary metabolite because of differences in the proportions of the diastereoisomers in the two preparations. The structure of metabolite II was confirmed later by Horning et al. (6) and Preste et al. (8) using gas chromatography–mass spectrometry (GC–MS).

Urine from a human subject receiving repeated doses of ethosuximide was incubated overnight with β-glucuronidase (Glusulase®) to hydrolyze any conjugates. It was then passed through an Amberlite® XAD-2 column to retain ethosuximide and its metabolites. These were eluted with methanol, which was then evaporated to dryness. The residue was derivatized with bis-(trimethylsilyl)acetamide and subjected to gas chromatography. The results shown in Fig. 3 indicated a double peak with retention times of 7.1 min and 8.1 min caused by the diastereoisomers of metabolite II. Un-

---

[2]*Chemical Abstracts* name, 3-(1-hydroxyethyl)-3-methyl-2,5-pyrrolidinedione.

[3]*Chemical Abstracts* name, 3-acetyl-3-methyl-2,5-pyrrolidinedione.

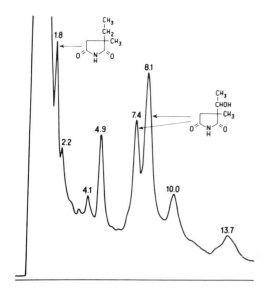

FIG. 3. Ethosuximide metabolites: gas–liquid chromatography of trimethylsilyl derivatives. Human urine from a subject receiving 0.5 g ethosuximide once a day for 21 days was treated with β-glucuronidase overnight; metabolites were separated on a column of Amberlite® XAD-2, eluted with methanol, evaporated to dryness, and treated with bis-(trimethylsilyl)acetamide. The GLC was accomplished on a 6-foot column of OV-1 (GasChrom Q®) at 110°C.

changed ethosuximide (1.8 min) and a metabolite with a retention time of 4.9 min were also detected. This metabolite (4.9 min) was originally thought to be 2-acetyl-2-methylsuccinimide, since the retention time was close to that of a synthetic reference standard (2). However, the ring-hydroxylated metabolite 2-ethyl-3-hydroxy-2-methylsuccinimide[4] reported by other investigators (6,8) has a similar retention time, and the peak is probably caused by this metabolite.

The possible presence of a glucuronide conjugate of metabolite II was examined in animals and in man. Rats weighing 250 g were dosed with 10 mg of [14C]ethosuximide, and urine was collected over a 24-hr period. Thin-layer chromatography of the urine on silica gel with chlo-

roform : methanol : water (3 : 2 : 1, lower phase) resulted in the appearance of three peaks similar to those seen in Fig. 2. In this case, the radioactivity in the ethosuximide fraction represented about 10% of the total ^{14}C on the plate; the intermediate peak corresponding to metabolite II had 54% of the total radioactivity, and the area near the origin had 36% of the radioactivity. The latter peak was eluted from the silica gel with methanol, evaporated to dryness, and redissolved in 6 ml of pH 5 acetate buffer (0.1 M). Half of this was incubated at 37°C for 24 hr with β-glucuronidase plus 1 drop of chloroform; the other half served as a control without β-glucuronidase. Thin-layer chromatography of the two preparations resulted in most of the radioactivity (88%) remaining at the origin, with a small amount of activity (12%) appearing in the location of metabolite II. However, the chromatographic patterns were identical in the control and enzyme-treated preparations, indicating that metabolite II probably was not conjugated to any great extent in the rat. Horning et al. (6) later reported the presence of several glucuronides of hydroxyethosuximides in rat urine. When we repeated the same experiment with urine from a monkey dosed with ethosuximide, treatment of the TLC fraction near the origin with β-glucuronidase resulted in the release of material with the same chromatographic characteristics as metabolite II. These observations indicate that significant amounts of a glucuronic acid conjugate of metabolite II are present in monkey urine.

Similar observations were made with human urine specimens obtained from subjects receiving a single 1-g oral dose of ethosuximide. The urine was saturated with sodium chloride and extracted with *n*-butanol, concentrated by evaporation, and chromatographed (GLC). When direct extraction without enzymatic hydrolysis was employed, 14% of the dose was recovered as free metabolite II. Treatment of the urine with β-glucuronidase before extraction resulted in 39% of the dose being recovered in the form of metabolite II, indicating that much of this metabolite was conjugated. Quantitative data obtained in the Parke-Davis laboratories, reported

---

[4]*Chemical Abstracts* name, 3-ethyl-4-hydroxy-3-methyl-2,5-pyrrolidinedione.

TABLE 1. *Anticonvulsant effect of ethosuximide and metabolite II against pentylenetetrazol-induced clonic seizures in mice*

Ethosuximide		Metabolite II	
Dose (mg/kg)[a]	Protected/ dosed (N)	Dose (mg/kg)[a]	Protected/ dosed (N)
125	5/5	250	2/5
62.5	3/5	125	0/5

[a]Drug was given intraperitoneally 30 min prior to pentylenetetrazol.

by Glazko (5), indicated that the excretion of metabolite II in human urine accounted for 33 to 41% of the administered dose.

The possible anticonvulsant effect of metabolite II was tested in mice, using pentylenetetrazol to induce clonic seizures (3). Groups of five mice were predosed with ethosuximide or with metabolite II (isolated from rat urine). These compounds were administered intraperitoneally as aqueous solutions 30 min before the test dose of pentylenetetrazol. The results shown in Table 1 indicate no significant anticonvulsant activity of metabolite II at a dose of 125 mg/kg, whereas ethosuximide gave complete protection at the same dose level.

2-ETHYL-3-HYDROXY-2-METHYLSUCCINIMIDE AND 2-(2-HYDROXYETHYL)-2-METHYLSUCCINIMIDE

Using GC–MS techniques, Horning et al. (6) identified two minor metabolites, 2-ethyl-3-hydroxy-2-methylsuccinimide and 2-(2-hydroxyethyl)-2-methylsuccinimide,[5] in rat urine and human urine. Male rats receiving a single intraperitoneal dose (83 mg) of ethosuximide excreted approximately 5.7 mg and 1.9 mg of the 3-hydroxy- and 2-hydroxyethyl metabolites, respectively, in 48-hr urine (6). However, the

diastereoisomers of the 1-hydroxyethyl metabolite accounted for a total of 44.2 mg in the same collection period. Assuming an area response factor of unity relative to the internal standard, Horning et al. (6) estimated that as much as 16 mg was excreted as glucuronide conjugates of the hydroxyethosuximides in rat urine. A dihydroxy metabolite of unknown structure was also detected in rat urine. In rat plasma, unchanged ethosuximide was the predominant component, but only trace amounts of the isomeric 1-hydroxyethyl metabolites were found. In human adult and infant plasma, the hydroxyethosuximides were the major products.

In a subsequent report, Preste et al. (8) confirmed the structure of 2-ethyl-3-hydroxy-2-methylsuccinimide by low- and high-resolution mass spectrometry as well as by NMR spectroscopy. Gas–liquid chromatography of urine from patients receiving ethosuximide suggested that nearly as much of the 3-hydroxy metabolite might be present as the stereoisomeric 1-hydroxyethylethosuximide.[6] However, quantitative data were not obtained (8).

METABOLIC PATHWAYS

Previous work with urine from rats and rhesus monkeys receiving [^{14}C]-ethosuximide demonstrated the presence of a polar fraction that did not migrate far from the origin of TLC plates (Fig. 2). This appears to be a mixture of metabolites including the glucuronic acid conjugate of 2-(1-hydroxyethyl)-2-methylsuccinimide. However, after enzymatic hydrolysis, TLC indicated that a polar residue remained at the origin. On heating in strong hydrochloric acid, the succinimide ring appeared to open, forming an insoluble product whose structure has not been established.

On the basis of the limited information we have on the metabolic disposition of ethosuximide, the biotransformation pathways can be summarized as shown in Fig. 4.

---

[5]*Chemical Abstracts* name, 3-(2-hydroxyethyl)-3-methyl-2,5-pyrrolidinedione.

[6]*Chemical Abstracts* name, 2-(1-hydroxyethyl)-2-methylsuccinimide.

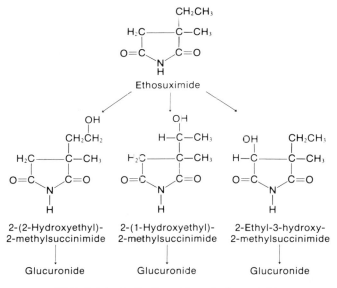

FIG. 4. Metabolic disposition of ethosuximide.

REFERENCES

1. Burkett, A. R., Chang, T., and Glazko, A. J. (1971): A hydroxylated metabolite of ethosuximide (Zarontin®) in rat urine. *Fed. Proc.*, 30:391.
2. Chang, T., Burkett, A. R., and Glazko, A. J. (1972): Ethosuximide. Biotransformation. In: *Antiepileptic Drugs,* edited by D. M. Woodbury, J. K. Penry, and R. P. Schmidt, pp. 425–429. Raven Press, New York.
3. Chen, G., and Portman, R. (1952): Titration of central nervous system depression. *Arch. Neurol. Psychiatry.*, 68:498–505.
4. Dill, W. A., Peterson, L., Chang, T., and Glazko, A. J. (1965): Physiologic disposition of α-methyl-α-ethyl-succinimide (ethosuximide; Zarontin®) in animals and in man. In: *Abstracts of papers, 149th National Meeting, American Chemical Society, Detroit, Michigan,* p. 30N. American Chemical Society, Washington.
5. Glazko, A. J. (1975): Antiepileptic drugs: Biotransformation, metabolism, and serum half-life. *Epilepsia,* 16:367–391.
6. Horning, M. G., Stratton, J., Nowlin, D. J., Harvey, D. J., and Hill, R. M. (1973): Metabolism of 2-ethyl-2-methyl succinimide (ethosuximide) in the rat and human. *Drug Metab. Dispos.*, 3:569–576.
7. Kerberle, H., Hoffman, K., and Bernhard, K. (1962): The metabolism of glutethimide (Doriden®). *Experientia,* 18:105–162.
8. Preste, P. G., Westerman, C. E., Das, N. P., Wilder, B. J., and Duncan, J. H. (1974): Identification of 2-ethyl-2-methyl-3-hydroxysuccinimide as a major metabolite of ethosuximide in humans. *J. Pharm. Sci.,* 63:467–469.
9. Smith, P. A. S., and Horwitz, J. P. (1949): A synthesis of unsymmetrically substituted succinic acids. *J. Am. Chem. Soc.*, 71:3418–3419.

Antiepileptic Drugs, edited by D. M. Woodbury, J. K. Penry, and C. E. Pippenger. Raven Press, New York © 1982.

54

Ethosuximide

Relation of Plasma Concentration to Seizure Control

Allan L. Sherwin

Ethosuximide is particularly effective in the control of absence seizures of both the typical and atypical types which almost invariably commence during childhood (4,27,30). It can be employed as monotherapy in the majority of patients with absence attacks without a history of tonic–clonic seizures, although the parents should be warned that their child is at risk for such attacks. If tonic–clonic seizures have occurred, ethosuximide can be readily combined with carbamazepine, phenytoin, or other agents, as clinically significant drug interactions are rare. Ethosuximide is clearly the contemporary drug of choice for children with typical absence seizures when the potential hepatotoxicity of valproic acid is of particular concern.

TYPICAL ABSENCE SEIZURES

Absence seizures are characterized by brief episodes of transient loss of awareness without gross convulsive movements. There may be blinking of the eyes, loss of postural tone, simple automatisms, or other minor movements. Sweating and changes in color are unusual, and although the body may sway, patients seldom fall. The attacks usually last a few seconds, seldom more than half a minute, and usually terminate abruptly without after-effects. Seizures occur on a daily basis, especially in the morning, ranging in frequency from five to 50 or more per day. The children are usually unaware of them. Absence seizures are relatively uncommon, accounting for 5 to 10% of seizure patterns observed in childhood. Fortunately, in the majority of cases where absence is the only seizure pattern, they cease to be a clinical problem by 20 years of age. The prognosis is less favorable in the presence of tonic–clonic seizures which occur at some time in 40 to 50% of absence patients (6,18).

The first clinical and EEG manifestations in this group of seizures indicate that both cerebral hemispheres are involved; they are accordingly classified as a form of generalized seizures (9). This is presumably a reflection of widespread neuronal discharge, usually with impaired consciousness as the initial manifestation. Seizures lasting more than a few seconds are commonly associated with other manifestations such as mild clonic movements of the eyelids or corners of the mouth or transient alterations of tone in postural muscles, resulting in drooping of the head or some movement of the extremities. Automatisms consisting of quasipurposeful movements like licking of the lips, swallowing, or fumbling with clothes may be observed. Autonomic features include incontinence, which is fortunately infrequent. The ictal EEG in patients with typical absence seizures reveals regular and symmetrical 2.5 to 3.5 Hz spike-and-wave complexes or multiple spike-and-slow-wave complexes which emerge abruptly from a normal background activity. The neurological examination, intelligence, and computerized tomographic (CT) scan of the brain are usually normal.

ATYPICAL ABSENCE SEIZURES

Patients with atypical absence seizures have a somewhat similar seizure pattern but often exhibit more pronounced changes in tone, including drop attacks. Both the onset and cessation of the seizures may be more gradual. The EEG findings in this group of patients are more heterogeneous, with slow-spike-and-slow-wave complexes that, in this case, arise out of an abnormal background activity which can be asymmetrical. The neurological examination, psychological tests and CT scan usually reveal some degree of abnormality. Although these patients also respond to ethosuximide therapy, they frequently exhibit other types of seizures including tonic–clonic attacks, and the outlook for the eventual complete cessation of the seizure disorder is more guarded (25).

DIAGNOSIS OF ABSENCE SEIZURES

Absence seizures constitute a distinct clinical entity readily diagnosed on the basis of a sound history. Attacks can frequently be elicited by prolonged voluntary hyperventilation and, in some patients, by photic stimulation. Although clear descriptions of absence attacks date from the 18th century, modern progress stems from the recognition of the characteristic 3 Hz spike-and-wave EEG pattern (10). This important discovery revealed that absence seizures differ from other types of nonconvulsive attacks, such as complex partial seizures, not only in degree but also in kind. Genetic analysis of this pattern in patients and near relatives showed that the EEG trait, but not the epilepsy, was inherited as an autosomal dominant with age-related penetrance (17). Absence seizures now appear to fit the genetic model of multifactorial inheritance in which environmental factors are also considered to be important in determining whether clinical seizures occur (1).

The differential diagnosis of absence seizures includes brief, complex partial seizures originating in the temporal or frontal lobe. These can usually be distinguished by the presence of an aura, the longer duration of the attacks, and the presence of postictal confusion. Careful analysis of the EEG provides a more precise electro-clinical correlation. Nonepileptic states like tics, daydreaming, and psychiatric disorders can usually be readily eliminated by a careful history and ancillary data.

ABSENCE STATUS

Absence status refers to an almost continuous state of abnormal behavior and response that ranges from mild confusion to stupor (9). It differs from absence attacks in that patients do not blink or stare but instead appear to be inattentive and disorientated. The EEG abnormalities (2) consist of near-continuous spike-and-wave discharges, but in some cases the tracing may bear only a faint resemblance to the classical pattern. The episodes usually last just a few minutes but occasionally persist for hours or even days. The differential diagnosis includes complex partial status, which can be distinguished by the presence of continuously recurring cycles of the clinical stages of the individual seizures, amnestic states resembling posttraumatic amnesia, hysterical behavior, and schizophrenic reactions. Absence status can be prevented or controlled by ethosuximide therapy (3).

PATHOPHYSIOLOGICAL CHARACTERISTICS OF ABSENCE SEIZURES

Absence seizures result from a generalized epileptic disturbance that is somewhat different from the focal epileptic spike discharge characteristic of partial seizures. Generalized and bilaterally synchronous spike-and-wave discharges begin in the cerebral cortex and result from the development of a markedly increased excitation of neurons (23). This excitation appears to be the major event and is followed by inhibition, which increases in response to the excitation. The spike-and-wave complex results from a remarkable oscillation between periods of increased excitation of cortical neurons corresponding to the spike and periods of decreased firing, corresponding to the wave. Thalamocortical volleys may help pace and synchronize the bilateral 3 Hz spike-and-wave activity which, however, is generated at the level of the cerebral cortex (11,24). Ethosuximide acts on low-frequency inhibitory pathways to prevent or reduce the duration of 3 Hz spike-and-wave discharges which are the electrographic manifestation of absence seizures (8,12).

PLASMA ETHOSUXIMIDE LEVELS AND CLINICAL CONTROL OF ABSENCE SEIZURES

Despite their brevity, frequent absence seizures require treatment because of their disruptive effect on the child's normal activities. Often they lead to embarrassment at school or interference with work, and the possibility of accidental injury is always present. There is also evidence that the generalized 3 Hz spike-and-wave epileptic discharge, the hallmark of this seizure pattern, causes impairment in sustained attention (5,22). Because absence seizures can usually be precipitated by hyperventilation, the physician is nearly always able to make a direct observation and improve the accuracy of diagnosis. Moreover, absence seizures are accompanied by quantifiable EEG spike-and-wave discharges (21). Consequently, this type of epilepsy permits accurate assessment of the relationship of plasma ethosuximide levels to clinical control, particularly since ethosuximide is a reversibly acting drug with inactive metabolites.

Comparison of plasma ethosuximide levels with clinical control was first reported by Haerer et al. (13) in a study of 21 outpatients. The patients ranged from 4 to 27 years with an average age of 12.4 years. Eight patients had only absence seizures, whereas 13 had other types of seizures as well as absences; the latter patients were taking other antiepileptic drugs in addition to ethosuximide. Seizure frequency was not reported, and clinical control was reported only as "improvement on drug." Ten patients were found to be markedly improved, seven moderately improved, and four either slightly or less than 50% improved. Plasma ethosuximide levels ranged from 10.8 to 55.2 µg/ml with an average of 40 µg/ml. The authors concluded that ethosuximide levels could be useful in the evaluation of problem patients who had not exhibited the expected clinical response after taking the drug. Solow and Green (29) recorded the range of ethosuximide levels in 50 patients with controlled absence seizures as 25 to 168 µg/ml. The average plasma level was 63.2 µg/ml, with an average dose 20.6 mg/kg. However, control was not defined, and the presence of other anticonvulsant drugs was not stated. Eadie and Tyrer (7) reported that absence attacks could be fully controlled with plasma ethosuximide levels ranging between 26 and 180 µg/ml and that these levels have been well tolerated by the majority of patients concerned.

There is no single satisfactory definition of clinical control; disagreement exists among neurologists concerning the meaning of "satisfactory control" and "complete control." In general, reduction of seizure frequency is the most satisfactory indication. When control is incomplete, any change in the character and/or duration of the seizure becomes important. For example, in absence seizures, several isolated brief staring episodes will be less likely to impair performance than a prolonged attack associated with automatisms. General difficulties in defining control and additional nonpharmacological factors that influence the frequency of seizures have been discussed in Chapters 9 and 11.

Brown et al. and Penry et al. (4,20) were the first to carry out a comprehensive prospective study of the efficacy of ethosuximide in controlling absence attacks. Measurements to quantitate the degree of seizure control in patients were developed. Moreover, the characteristics of absence seizures were clearly described in general accordance with the International Classification of Epileptic Seizures (9). Each patient was admitted to their study only after an absence seizure, as defined above, was observed by the principal investigator. Most patients had several absence attacks a day. Patients who had other types of seizures in addition to absence attacks were not excluded unless they had been treated with antiabsence medication before the other seizures. Patients were continued on their other routine anticonvulsants. All patients were admitted to the hospital for a 2-week period, discharged home for 6 weeks, and then readmitted for another week of study. During the first hospital week, patients were given one placebo capsule three times a day, and this was followed by three 250-mg capsules of ethosuximide on the second week of the study. However, if the seizure frequency was not reduced by 50% on this dosage, it was increased to as much as 1,500 mg daily.

The frequency of seizures in each patient was measured by (a) observation by a trained observer, (b) observation by the ward staff, (c) mother's history of seizure frequency before and during ethosuximide administration, (d) examination by a physician, which included hyperventilation, and (e) standardized video tape–EEG recording. The complete physical examinations included careful recording of even minor neurological deficits indicative of brain injury that might have occurred at birth or in the early years of life. The examining physician was instructed to note all absence seizures and to describe two absence attacks in detail. If the patient did not have two spontaneous attacks during the examination, the physician had the patient hyperventilate for 3 min twice in an effort to elicit two absence attacks. The five types of data on the seizure frequency were combined into a "seizure index." Psychometric examinations consisted of the Wechsler Intelligence Scale for Children and a modified Halstead–Reitan Battery prepared for this study and age group. Plasma ethosuximide concentrations were determined by gas–liquid chromatography.

Analysis of the detailed data on absence seizure control revealed that seven of 37 patients

(19%) had a 100% reduction in seizure index, that is, were seizure-free during the eighth treatment week. Eighteen patients (49%) had a 90% or greater reduction in seizure index, and 35 (95%) had a 50% or greater reduction in seizure index. The difference in seizure index between the placebo week and the eighth treatment week were statistically significant ($p < 0.005$) by the Wilcoxon Matched Pairs Signed Rank Test. The antiabsence effect of a given dose of ethosuximide appeared to be almost fully achieved during the first week of oral administration. The doses of ethosuximide ranged from 6.5 to 36.7 mg/kg; plasma concentrations ranged from 16.6 to 104.0 µg/ml with a statistically significant relationship between an increased ethosuximide dose and an increased plasma concentration ($r = 0.76; p < 0.01$). The mean ratio of plasma ethosuximide concentration (µg/ml) to dose (mg/kg) was 2.95. However, it is important to note that for any given dose, there was such a wide variability in the plasma-to-dose ratio among patients that it was impossible to predict a given patient's plasma concentration from the ethosuximide dose. The optimal range of plasma ethosuximide concentration as determined with the aid of the seizure index showed a 100% decrease for seven patients and a 75% or greater decrease for 23 of 29 patients (79%) when the plasma concentrations ranged from 41 to 99 µg/ml. Only three of six patients with plasma concentrations less than 41 µg/ml had 75% or greater reduction in seizure index. The estimated optimal range of plasma ethosuximide concentration was 40 to 100 µg/ml in this study (Fig. 1).

Sherwin et al. (27) carried out a prospective study of 70 patients with absence seizures selected using clinical and electrographic criteria similar to those of the Collaborative Study of Epilepsy (4,19). This group of patients had been treated with the aid of therapeutic monitoring of plasma ethosuximide levels for up to 2½ years, 75% of the group being evaluated for periods greater than 1½ years. The group comprised 38 females and 32 males ranging in age from 4 to 28 years (median 12 years). Absence attacks were the sole manifestation of epilepsy in 38 of the patients (54%). Tonic–clonic seizures were also

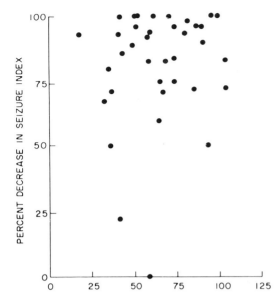

FIG. 1. Relationship of decrease in seizure index (as described in text) to plasma ethosuximide concentration (μg/ml, *abscissa*) after 8 weeks of treatment. (From Browne et al., ref. 4, with permission.)

present in 21 patients (30%), and an additional 11 patients (16%) had a past history of one or more generalized seizures prior to entering the study. The dosage of ethosuximide employed ranged from 0.5 to 1.75 g/day (9.4 to 73.5 mg/kg). Other drugs administered concurrently to some patients included phenytoin (30 patients), phenobarbital (six patients), and various minor psychotropic drugs (five patients). All patients were examined at 6-month intervals, and more frequently if necessary, with detailed recording of seizure frequency and plasma antiepileptic drug levels. In the group of 33 completely controlled patients, only 9% were found to have levels below 40 μg/ml, with none below 30 μg/ml. Thus, efforts were directed toward achieving levels greater than 40 μg/ml in patients with uncontrolled seizures.

These efforts resulted in a significant improvement in the clinical control of absence seizures within the first 2½ years (Fig. 2). Only three of the 70 patients had an increased seizure frequency compared with their status at the onset of the study. Nineteen patients had a significant increase in plasma ethosuximide concen-

tration. In seven, this resulted from a prescribed increase in dosage, whereas in 10 it was because of better cooperation. Both factors operated in the remaining two patients. Thirteen of the 19 patients with increased levels improved clinically; 10 achieved complete control. Patients with absence seizures tend to cease having attacks with advancing age (6), although some studies have reported a more guarded prognosis (18). Janz (15) observed that the rate of spontaneous arrest of absence attacks over 2-year periods was in the order of 3%. This gradual rate of improvement could not account for the marked increase in the number of controlled patients (13 of 37 uncontrolled patients) observed during the first 2½-year period. During this time, the mean plasma ethosuximide levels in the newly controlled patients rose from 57.2 μg/ml to 76.1 μg/ml, a significant increase ($p < 0.05$) which was not observed in those patients who continued to have frequent attacks. This improvement was continued in the second half of the 5-year study (26).

PLASMA ETHOSUXIMIDE LEVEL AND DOSE

The relationship of plasma ethosuximide level to administered dose is illustrated in Fig. 3. Plasma levels were obtained on single blood samples in patients known to be receiving constant dosages of ethosuximide either alone or in combination with other anticonvulsants. In agreement with the data of Browne et al. (4), the slope of the linear regression line of ethosuximide dose to plasma level was significantly less ($p < 0.01$) in children from 3 to 10 years than in patients 11 years of age and over. Thus, daily administration of 20 mg/kg ethosuximide in children 11 years of age or less will result in mean plasma levels of 50 μg/ml, whereas in older patients the administration of approximately 15 mg/kg will result in similar levels. The generally accepted maximum daily dosage is 30 mg/kg for adults and 40 mg/kg for children. The daily dose may be increased every 4 to 7 days until seizure control and the desired plasma concentration are achieved. In a study of plasma

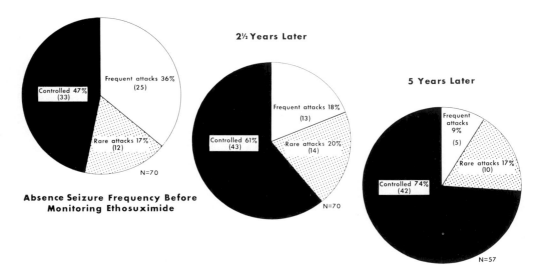

FIG. 2. Control of absence attacks before and after commencing regular plasma level monitoring with titration of ethosuximide dosage. There is a highly significant alteration in the distribution of clinical control. (X^2 test, $p < 0.005$). The improvement noted in the first 2½ years is far greater than would be expected from the natural course of absence seizures (see ref. 15). Approximately two-thirds of the patients were managed on ethosuximide monotherapy.

ethosuximide levels examined at 3-month intervals in 245 patients receiving stable doses, there was a highly significant variation in the dose plasma level relationship of ethosuximide with increasing age ($p < 0.001$). No significant differences were demonstrated between the mean plasma levels of males and females in any age group. This is in contrast to sex differences observed by Smith et al. (28) in a group of 36 patients ranging in age for 1.5 to 38 years.

Plasma ethosuximide levels remain extremely stable on successive examination of patients when the medication is taken regularly. Although trough levels are theoretically more accurate, it appears that the time of day that the blood sample is obtained is not likely to significantly alter the therapeutic implications of the plasma level. Saliva and plasma ethosuximide levels are very similar, and salivary levels can be used to monitor therapy providing controls of pooled normal saliva spiked with ethosuximide are utilized to determine the standard curve used in the assay (14,16).

PROGNOSTIC FACTORS IN ABSENCE SEIZURES

The relationship of plasma ethosuximide levels to clinical control is profoundly influenced by the natural history observed in children with absence seizures. Sato et al. (25) reported a longitudinal, long-term, prospective follow-up study of patients selected solely on the basis of clinical observations but all meeting the clinical and EEG classification of epileptic seizures. The data strongly illustrated the point that patients presenting initially with absence seizures alone have a significantly better outcome for the eventual cessation of seizures than do patients presenting with both absence and generalized tonic–clonic seizures. The two most important factors favoring natural cessation of absence attacks were the presence of normal EEG background activity and a normal or above normal intelligence quotient. There was also a more favorable prognosis for seizure cessation in males. The authors suggested that effective treatment should be insti-

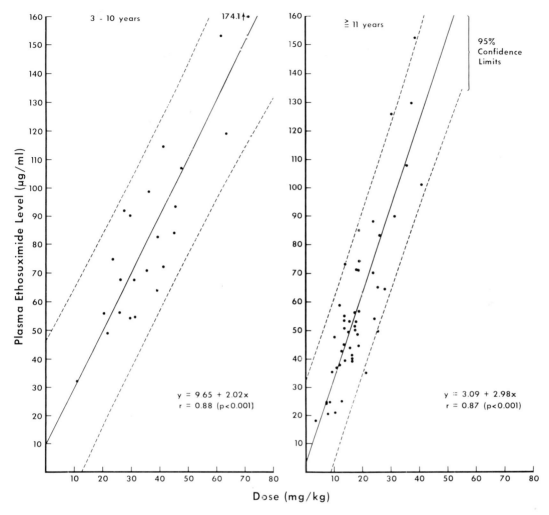

FIG. 3. Relationship of plasma ethosuximide level to dose at steady state. The slope of the regression line for patients ranging in age from 2 to 10 years ($N = 23$) is significantly less than that for patients 11 years of age and older ($N = 49$) ($p < 0.01$). These regression lines are useful in selecting appropriate dosage.

tuted early in the course of the illness. The presence of a normal neurological examination and a shorter duration of illness tended to favor cessation of seizures. For any seizure type, significant prognostic factors were a negative history of generalized tonic–clonic seizures, normal or above normal intelligence, and a negative family history of seizure disorders. Nearly 90% of the patients with all significant prognostic factors for both absence seizures and seizures of all types became seizure-free. In contrast, the patients who lacked all significant prognostic factors had a poor outlook for seizure relief.

CONCLUSION

Monitoring of plasma ethosuximide levels is helpful in individualizing drug regimens and identifying noncompliant patients. Some important considerations of such monitoring are summarized in Table 1. Maintenance of plasma ethosuximide at levels from 40 to 100 µg/ml

TABLE 1. *Monitoring plasma ethosuximide concentrations*

Optimal range
  40 to 100 μg/ml
Indications
  Subtherapeutic response
  Noncompliance
  Suboptimal dose
  Maintenance of optimal levels
Occasional patients may need > 100 μg/ml
  Establish optimal individual levels
Dosage adjustments
  Necessitate plasma concentration determinations
    (after steady-state levels achieved)
  Concomitant drug therapy: whenever another drug is
    added to or deleted from drug regimen
Maintenance monitoring
  4- to 6-month intervals, provided therapeutic response is
    good
Time to achieve steady state
  Children, 6 days
  Adults, 12 days
Obtaining sample
  Ethosuximide's long half-life permits samples to be
    drawn at any time, although trough samples insure
    reproducibility when comparing plasma concentrations.
    Level in saliva equivalent to plasma level.

---

will be associated with practical control in 80% of patients, 60% becoming seizure-free. The starting dosage should be 20 mg/kg per day to anticipate a plasma level of 50 to 60 μg/ml to be adjusted after repeated plasma level monitoring. Plasma ethosuximide levels ranging from 40 to 100 μg/ml are considered optimal for effective seizure control. Very occasionally, levels of up to 150 μg/ml may be required. Ethosuximide is particularly indicated as monotherapy in patients with absence seizures as the sole seizure type when both the IQ and EEG background activity are within the normal range. However, ethosuximide is also effective in atypical absence seizures and if necessary can be readily combined with other antiepileptic drugs.

When absence seizures have been controlled for a period of 2 years, consideration may be given to the discontinuation of ethosuximide therapy, particularly if EEG examination including 3 min of forceful hyperventilation fails to reveal evidence of 3 Hz spike-and-wave discharges. The dosage of ethosuximide should be gradually tapered over a period of 1 or more months following which the patient can be reexamined and the EEG repeated.

ACKNOWLEDGMENTS

This investigation was supported by a grant from the Medical Research Council of Canada. The work would not have been possible without the encouragement and wholehearted support of Dr. J. Preston Robb.

REFERENCES

1. Andermann, E. (1980): Multifactorial inheritance in the epilepsies. In: *Advances in Epileptology: XIth Epilepsy International Symposium,* edited by R. Canger, F. Angeleri, and J. K. Penry, pp. 297–309. Raven Press, New York.
2. Andermann, F., and Robb, J. P. (1972): Absence status. *Epilepsia,* 13:177–187.
3. Browne, T. R. (1978): Drug therapy of status epilepticus. *J. Maine Med. Assoc.,* 69:199–204.
4. Browne, T. R., Dreifuss, F. E., Dyken, P. R., Goode, D. J., Penry, J. K., Porter, R. J., White, B. G., and White, P. T. (1975): Ethosuximide in the treatment of absence (petit mal) seizures. *Neurology (Minneap.),* 25:515–524.
5. Browne, T. R., Penry, J. K., Porter, R. J., and Dreifuss, F. E. (1974): Responsiveness before, during and after spike–wave paroxysms. *Neurology (Minneap.),* 24:659–665.
6. Dalby, M. A. (1969): Epilepsy and 3 per second spike-and-wave rhythms. *Acta Neurol. Scand.,* 45(Suppl. 40):1–83.
7. Eadie, M. J., and Tyrer, J. H. (1980): *Anticonvulsant Therapy. Pharmacological Basis and Practice,* Second Edition, pp. 211–223. Churchill Livingstone, Edinburgh.
8. Fromm, G. H., Glass, J. D., Chattha, A. S., and Martinez, A. J. (1981): Effect of anticonvulsant drugs on inhibitory and excitatory pathways. *Epilepsia,* 22:65–73.
9. Gastaut, H. (1970): Clinical and electroencephalographic classification of epileptic seizures. *Epilepsia,* 13:121–131.
10. Gibbs, F., Davis, H., and Lennox, W. (1935): The electroencephalogram in epilepsy and in conditions of impaired consciousness. *Arch. Neurol. Psychiatry,* 3:1133–1148.
11. Gloor, P. (1979): Generalized epilepsy with spike-and-wave discharge: A reinterpretation of its electrographic and clinical manifestations. *Epilepsia,* 20:571–588.
12. Guberman, A., Gloor, P., and Sherwin, A. L. (1975): Response of generalized penicillin epilepsy in the cat to ethosuximide and diphenylhydantoin. *Neurology (Minneap.),* 25:758–764.
13. Haerer, A. F., Buchanan, R. A., and Wiygul, F. M.

(1970): Ethosuximide blood levels in epileptics. *J. Clin. Pharmacol.*, 10:370–374.

14. Horning, M. G., Brown, L., Nowlin, J., Lertratanangkoon, L., Kellaway, P., and Zion, T. E. (1977): Use of saliva in therapeutic drug monitoring. *Clin. Chem.*, 23:157–164.

15. Janz, D. (1969): *Die Epilepsien-Spezielle Pathologie und Therapie*, p. 94. Georg Thieme, Stuttgart.

16. McAuliff, J. J., Sherwin, A. L., Leppik, I. E., Fayle, S. A., and Pippenger, C. E. (1970): Salivary levels of anticonvulsants: A practical approach to drug monitoring. *Neurology (Minneap.)*, 27:409–413.

17. Metrakos, K., and Metrakos, J. D. (1961): Genetic and electroencephalographic studies in centrencephalic epilepsy. *Neurology (Minneap.)*, 11:474–483.

18. Okuma, T., and Kumashiro, H. (1981): Natural history and prognosis of epilepsy: Report of a multi-institutional study in Japan. *Epilepsia*, 22:35–53.

19. Penry, J. K., Porter, R. J., and Dreifuss, F. E. (1971): Quantitation of paroxysmal abnormal discharge in the EEG's of patients with absence (petit mal) seizures for evaluation of antiepileptic drugs. *Epilepsia*, 12:278–279.

20. Penry, J. K., Porter, R. J., and Dreifuss, F. E. (1972): Ethosuximide: Relation of plasma levels to clinical control. In: *Antiepileptic Drugs*, First Edition, edited by D. M. Woodbury, J. K. Penry, and R. P. Schmidt, pp. 431–441. Raven Press, New York.

21. Penry, J. K., Porter, R. J., and Dreifuss, F. E. (1975): Simultaneous recording of absence seizures with video tape and electroencephalography: A study of 374 seizures in 48 patients. *Brain*, 98:427–440.

22. Porter, R. J., Penry, J. K., and Dreifuss, F. E. (1973): Responsiveness at the onset of spike-wave bursts. *Electroencephalogr. Clin. Neurophysiol.*, 34:239–245.

23. Quesney, L. F. (1977): *Pathophysiology of Generalized Penicillin Epilepsy in the Cat: The Role of Cortical and Subcortical Structures*. Ph.D. Thesis, McGill University, Montreal.

24. Quesney, L. F., and Gloor, P. (1978): Generalized penicillin epilepsy in the cat: Correlation between electrophysiological data and distribution of ^{14}C-penicillin in the brain. *Epilepsia*, 19:35–45.

25. Sato, S., Dreifuss, F. E., and Penry, J. K. (1976): Prognostic factors in absence seizures. *Neurology (Minneap.)*, 26:788–796.

26. Sherwin, A. L. (1978): Clinical Pharmacology of ethosuximide. In: *Antiepileptic Drugs: Quantitative Analysis and Interpretation*, edited by C. E. Pippenger, J. K. Penry, and H. Kutt, pp. 283–295. Raven Press, New York.

27. Sherwin, A. L., Robb, J. P., and Lechter, M. (1973): Improved control of epilepsy by monitoring plasma ethosuximide. *Arch. Neurol.*, 28:178–181.

28. Smith, G. A., McKauge, L., Dubetz, D., Tyrer, J. H., and Eadie, M. J. (1979): Factors influencing plasma concentrations of ethosuximide. *Clin. Pharmacokinet.*, 4:38–52.

29. Solow, E. B., and Green, J. B. (1972): The simultaneous determination of multiple anticonvulsant drug levels by gas–liquid chromatography. *Neurology (Minneap.)* 22:540–550.

30. Suzuki, M., Maruyama, H., Ishibashi, Y., Ogawa, S., Seki, T., Hoshino, M., Mackawa, K., Yo, T., and Sato, Y. (1972): A double-blind comparative trial of sodium dipropylacetate and ethosuximide in children, with special emphasis on pure petit mal seizures. *Med Prog. (Jpn)*, 82:470–488.

Antiepileptic Drugs, edited by D. M. Woodbury,
J. K. Penry, and C. E. Pippenger. Raven Press,
New York © 1982.

55

Ethosuximide

Toxicity

F. E. Dreifuss

"All things are poisons, for there is nothing without poisonous qualities. It is only the dose which makes a thing a poison." Paracelsus (1493–1541)

As early as 1857, when Charles Locock introduced potassium bromide to the treatment of epilepsy, physicians were confronted with a dilemma: namely, the need to temper therapeutic enthusiasm with an acknowledgment of the risks of adverse effects. Potassium bromide frequently resulted in the development of severe skin eruptions such as acne vulgaris, intellectual sluggishness, and, particularly in older people, the development of a progressive psychosis. William Hammond, in 1874, presenting a patient, stated: "As you see, he is broken down in appearance, has large abscesses in his neck, and is altogether in a bad condition. But this is better than to have epilepsy" (20).

All drugs are toxic in overdose, and there is great variation in sensitivity to drugs from person to person, so that a safe dose for one person may be an excessive dose for another. Even a therapeutic dose may have unavoidable side effects.

Adverse effects of ethosuximide may be divided into (a) toxic effects that are the result of overdose or unwanted reactions that may accompany a dose in the therapeutic range—these effects usually occur soon after administration

of the drug and fall into the general category of acute toxicity; (b) specific organ effects, including dermatological and most hematological complications, and alterations of the immune system with the appearance of immunologic disturbances such as systemic lupus erythematosus and drug allergies; (c) drug interactions; and (d) teratogenetic effects. The latter three reactions may be considered chronic drug toxicity in that they rarely occur with acute administration but may be observed after weeks, months, or even years of use.

The incidence of adverse drug effects varies greatly, ranging in different studies from none (18,30) to 9% (55), 31% (16), 33% (4), and 44% (54). Most of these are associated with direct dose-related problems.

ACUTE TOXICITY

Dose-Related Side Effects

The majority of toxic effects of ethosuximide as reported in different series are accounted for by relatively few symptoms, including nausea, abdominal discomfort, drowsiness, anorexia, hiccups, and headache. Nausea, the commonest side effect, usually occurs within the first few days of ethosuximide administration and frequently responds to reduction of the dose. Drowsiness likewise responds to reduction in ethosuximide dosage, as does anorexia. Headache often proves rather more persistent and falls into the category of unwanted accompanying reactions rather than being strictly dose related and amenable to dose reduction. In the study by Browne et al. (4), 13 of 39 patients experienced side effects. Nausea was described in nine instances, and drowsiness five times, indicating that most of the side effects were of a benign, dose-related nature. This was also the experience in other reports (5,10,16,21,54,55).

Side Effects Unrelated to Dose

Ethosuximide has been reported to cause the exacerbation of various types of seizures. DeHaas and Kuilman, in a study of 107 patients, noted exacerbation of seizures, except for absence attacks in seven patients (9). Gordon (18) reported that of four patients with myoclonus, two became worse after ethosuximide administration, and Friedel and Lempp (14) described the transformation of absence seizures into "grand mal" during the course of treatment with trimethadione, methsuximide, and ethosuximide in 22 out of 85 patients. Todorov et al. (50) reported that exacerbation of absence seizures in a patient undergoing treatment with ethosuximide was ameliorated with phenobarbital. Most authors, however, specifically noted no instances of exacerbation of any seizure type during administration of ethosuximide (4,5,21, 52,55). In view of the occurrence of generalized tonic–clonic seizures at some time during the course of absence seizures in some 25% of patients, it would not be surprising to find the emergence of generalized tonic–clonic seizures coincidentally with ethosuximide therapy in a certain number of patients, and this is the probable explanation for some, if not most, of the reported events.

Behavioral changes have been reported in persons taking ethosuximide. The psychopharmacology of antiepileptic drugs is in an unsatisfactory state because of inadequate and unsophisticated evaluation of behavior. Most reports deal with persons who are taking several drugs, and most contain no mention of antiepileptic drug blood levels. Many of the reports do not adequately distinguish between mental or behavioral changes that may result from seizures and those that may be related to drug effects.

One of the first reports was that of Fischer et al. (13) who reported on five psychotic episodes in three adult patients occurring within a few days of starting treatment with ethosuximide. The report dealt with a total of 105 patients, and the seizure types were not clearly distinguished. The psychotic episodes consisted of intermittent impairment of consciousness, anxiety, depression, and visual and auditory hallucinations which improved following cessation of treatment with ethosuximide. All had a history of mental disorder. Individual cases of psychotic behavior were noted by Cohadon et al. (6), Lairy (27), and Sato et al. (40). Roger et al. (39) and Soulayrol and Roger (45) described the falling-off of school performance and efficiency and, on occasions, the appearance of hallucinations and ideas of persecution. The symptoms remitted when ethosuximide was discontinued and recurred on reinstitution of treatment.

There appeared to be a reciprocal relationship between the epilepsy and the psychosis in that when seizures were controlled the psychosis remitted and vice versa. A similar phenomenon in complex partial seizures was described by Landolt (29). Guey et al. (19) reported on 25 children with absence attacks who were assessed before and after the administration of ethosuximide. They found disturbances of memory and speech, particularly in the older patients and in those who were receiving large doses of the drug. Fifteen of the patients were mentally retarded, no control group was included in the study, and antiepileptic drug levels were not monitored. As pointed out by Trimble and Reynolds (51), such studies should have control groups for comparison, as it has been shown that the EEG spike-and-wave activity of absence seizures may be related to impaired visual–motor performance (17,37).

Smith et al. (43) described a double-blind study

in which verbal and full-scale IQ scores improved in nonepileptic children given ethosuximide. Browne et al. (4) studied psychometric performance in 39 children, using matched controls, and found that performance improved significantly in 17 patients treated with ethosuximide. Only one showed diminished ability because of a decrease in alertness. This group was more homogeneous than that reported by Guey et al. (19); mental retardation was less prevalent, and barbiturate administration less pervasive. Also, the blood levels of ethosuximide were within the therapeutic range. None of the other studies included data on blood ethosuximide levels, and some of the mental symptoms may have stemmed from drug intoxication.

DELAYED SPECIFIC ORGAN EFFECTS

An idiosyncratic reaction has been defined as a peculiar and therefore unusual or rare drug reaction (3). Reasons for this may be multifactorial. Strictly speaking, pharmacologists tend to regard an idiosyncratic reaction as a genetically determined abnormal reactivity to drugs, and a complete understanding of such a reaction requires knowledge of the mechanisms by which the usual drug effect is altered in the genetically variant person, of the biochemical abnormality involved, and of the pattern of inheritance. Thus, for example, prolonged apnea occurring after succinylcholine administration, primaquine-induced hemolytic anemia, and acute intermittent porphyria enhanced by drugs are true genetically determined idiosyncrasies on the basis of individual genotypes. In this context, the reactions described below are not truly idiosyncratic, although further study may show them to be related to a genetic trait at least as one of a number of factors.

Skin rashes have been frequently described, as have erythema multiforme and the Stevens–Johnson syndrome (36,48), in the course of treatment with ethosuximide. The dermatological complications usually remit after discontinuation of the drug, but steroid therapy is sometimes indicated, especially in the more severe

cases. Teoh and Chan (49) reported that lupus erythematosus and scleroderma were reversed after withdrawal of medication. Readministration of ethosuximide for the treatment of persistent seizures resulted in a relapse with predominant sclerodermatous features that again resolved after ethosuximide withdrawal.

Systemic lupus erythematosus (SLE) or a lupus-like syndrome as an adverse reaction to antiepileptic drugs has been the subject of many reports (1,2,5,8,22,31,35,41,43,49). It is likely that the SLE-activating properties of anticonvulsant drugs reside in their potential to induce antinuclear antibodies. Drugs that activate SLE may do so by pharmacological properties of their own or by causing allergic reactions which in turn bring about SLE (1). Many persons develop antinuclear antibodies without developing SLE, and it may be that only predisposed individuals among those with antinuclear antibodies will become symptomatic. Most anticonvulsants elicit antibodies primarily directed to soluble nucleoprotein, but each may do so by altering different sites in the nucleoprotein molecule. Development of DNA antibodies may result from action of the drugs on an antigenic site of nucleoprotein closely related to the nucleic acid or from the fact that patients who develop anti-DNA antibodies have underlying SLE as a basis for their seizures (1). The lupus-like illness consists of fever, malar rash, arthritis, lymphadenopathy, and, on occasions, pleural effusions, myocarditis, and pericarditis. Most patients developing a lupus-like syndrome have a relatively benign, albeit prolonged, course after cessation of the medication. Singsen et al. (41) reported no improvement in one of five affected children after discontinuation of ethosuximide, and this patient had renal involvement, which is an unusual organ involvement in drug-induced lupus.

Three types of lupus-like reactions have been described. In one type, the patients develop only antinuclear antibodies. These asymptomatic children with antinuclear antibodies should be carefully observed, but they do not usually develop evidence of lupus. In the second type, a classical lupus-like illness develops. Silverman et al. (44) described a third type in which clinical and chemical evidence of an immunologic disorder, including a nephrotic syndrome, occurs. Lupus preparations and antinuclear antibodies are negative, and the apparent immunologic disorder abates on cessation of ethosuximide.

There is one report of adverse effects of anticonvulsant therapy, including ethosuximide, on renal allograft survival (53). This may occur through interference with the immune system or alteration of metabolism of administered corticosteroids, leading to less effective immunosuppression and hence a higher incidence of graft failure.

Basal ganglia involvement has been reported several times. Some of these have been acute reactions to the administration of ethosuximide similar to those seen after administration of some phenothiazines (12,25). The symptoms respond to the discontinuation of the drug or to the administration of diphenhydramine hydrochloride. More severe bradykinesia as a manifestation of ethosuximide toxicity (among other drugs administered) and occurring after several years of treatment has been described (38) as has a parkinsonian syndrome (16).

Blood dyscrasias are among the most serious side effects of treatment with antiepileptic drugs (4,5,7,11,24,26,33,46,54). Damage may be to mature cell lines, in which case often only one element is involved, resulting in a disorder such as thrombocytopenia. In more severe cases of bone marrow hypoplasia with involvement of less differentiated cell types, pancytopenia or aplastic anemia is the result. Bone marrow depression may be the result of an allergic phenomenon or of a toxic effect. In the former, the platelets have been implicated as targets of allergic drug reactions, and antibodies to the drug have been demonstrated in the serum of patients developing thrombocytopenic purpura. In chloramphenicol toxicity and in the case of the anticonvulsant drugs, it would appear that bone marrow toxicity is a more likely explanation than an allergic phenomenon.

Depression of blood-forming elements has been mentioned sporadically in many of the larger studies of patients treated with ethosuximide (4,5,24,54). Further, specific cases were reported by Koutsoulieris (26), who described a 9-year-old child who developed pancytopenia 10 weeks after starting ethosuximide and who recovered after the drug was stopped; by Mann and Habenicht (33), who reported a case of fatal bone marrow aplasia; and by Spittler (46), who reported a fatal case of agranulocytosis in a 7-year-old patient who had been treated for 9 weeks when the condition was diagnosed and who subsequently succumbed to complications. Cohn (7) reported a child who died approximately 6 months after the institution of ethosuximide therapy. Buchanan (5) noted two fatal cases, an 11-year-old child who developed pancytopenia some 7 months after beginning treatment and a 6-year-old who developed an aplastic bone marrow some 6 weeks after the addition of ethosuximide to the regimen.

In the hope of detecting bone marrow depression early, it is generally recommended that periodic blood counts be performed at no greater than monthly intervals for the duration of treatment with ethosuximide and that the dosage be reduced or the drug discontinued should the total white blood count fall below 3,500 or the proportion of granulocytes below 25% of the total white blood count. Prescribing physicians are advised to observe patients for the development of fever, sore throat, or cutaneous and other hemorrhages, in addition to periodic hematological monitoring.

In the author's experience, ethosuximide-related granulocytopenia frequently responds to reduction of the dose and does not always require cessation of therapy, indicating that to some extent, at least, this may be a dose-related phenomenon.

DRUG INTERACTIONS

No significant drug interactions between ethosuximide and other antiepileptic drugs have been reported. Enzyme induction does not appear to occur to any significant degree (15). There is no significant increase in the plasma concentration of phenobarbital derived from primidone with the addition of ethosuximide as there is with phenytoin (37), but one report suggests that some increase does occur (42). Another report suggests that some increase in plasma concentration of phenytoin occurs with administration of ethosuximide (28).

TERATOGENIC EFFECTS

It is generally accepted that birth defects occur with increased frequency among children born of mothers with epilepsy who were exposed to anticonvulsant drugs in pregnancy and that this frequency exceeds that occurring in children born of mothers with epilepsy who did not take drugs during pregnancy (23,32,34). The drugs most often implicated are phenytoin and phenobarbital, and these are, of course, the most commonly used drugs. Trimethadione, although now rarely used, carries by far the greatest risk of teratogenicity.

Little information is available concerning the risk to the fetus exposed to ethosuximide. The primary indication for the administration of ethosuximide is absence seizures, and these rarely persist into child-bearing age. It appears to be a largely age-limited condition which tends to go into abeyance in the teen-age years and no longer requires treatment with the drug. Experimental data (47), however, suggest that ethosuximide is considerably less teratogenic than phenytoin, carbamazepine, phenobarbital, or primidone.

Teratogenic effects must be distinguished from mutagenic or genetic effects. The former are more likely to result from toxic affliction or organogenesis, either directly or through metabolic changes (folic acid metabolism abnormalities have come under scrutiny). Certain agents, of course, have mutagenic and carcinogenic effects as well as teratogenic activity, but most teratogens are neither mutagenic nor carcinogenic. The latter actions require heritable alteration in a cell line such as cytogenetic abnormalities of the translocation type.

In general, it is recommended that the medication regimen be kept as simple as possible during pregnancy, with administration of the smallest possible number of agents. Only rarely will it be necessary to continue antiabsence drugs in the child-bearing age group.

SUMMARY

The side effects associated with the administration of ethosuximide include dose-related reactions such as nausea, gastrointestinal discomfort, drowsiness, and anorexia. These are common, relatively trivial in the context of overall patient management, and usually respond to dosage reduction.

Side effects not related to the dose include exacerbation of various types of seizures. This is a rare complication and more likely represents the natural history of epilepsy than a cause-and-effect relationship. Behavioral changes, including transient psychoses, and interference with cognitive function, apart from some idiosyncratic phenomena, may be related to drug intoxication, as they have not been prominent when blood ethosuximide levels have been within the therapeutic range.

Delayed specific organ sensitivities, including hematological, dermatological, and immunologic disorders, represent the most serious and potentially lethal complications. These are rare and, in some degree, avoidable by careful monitoring and ameliorable by early intervention.

Neither drug interactions nor teratogenicity is believed to play a significant role in ethosuximide pharmacotherapy.

REFERENCES

1. Alarcon-Segovia, D., Fishbein, E., Reyes, P. A., Dies, H., and Shwadsky, S. (1972): Antinuclear antibodies in patients on anticonvulsant therapy. *Clin. Exp. Immunol.*, 12:39–47.
2. Beernink, D. H., and Miller, J. J. (1973): Anticonvulsant induced antinuclear antibodies and lupus like disease in children. *J. Pediatr.*, 82:113–117.
3. Booker, H. E. (1975): Idiosyncratic reactions to the antiepileptic drugs. *Epilepsia*, 16:171–181.
4. Browne, T. R., Dreifuss, F. E., Dyken, P. R., Goode, D. J., Penry, J. K., Porter, R. J., White, P. T., and White, B. G. (1975): Ethosuximide in the treatment of absence (petil mal) epilepsy. *Neurology (Minneap.)*, 25:515–525.
5. Buchanan, R. A. (1972): Ethosuximide: Toxicity. In: *Antiepileptic Drugs*, edited by D. M. Woodbury,

J. K. Penry, and R. P. Schmidt, pp. 449–454. Raven Press, New York.

6. Cohadon, F., Loiseau, P., and Cohadon, S. (1964): Results of treatment of certain forms of epilepsy of the petit mal type by ethosuximide. *Rev. Neurol.,* 110:201–207.

7. Cohn, R. (1968): A neuropathological study of a case of petit mal epilepsy. *Electroencephalogr. Clin. Neurophysiol.,* 24:282.

8. Dabbous, I. A., and Idriss, H. M. (1970): Occurrence of systemic lupus erythematosus in association with ethosuximide therapy. *J. Pediatr.,* 76:617–620.

9. deHaas, A. M. L., and Kuilman, M. (1964): Ethosuximide (α-ethyl-α-methylsuccinimide) and grand mal. *Epilepsia,* 5:90–96.

10. deHaas, A. M. L., and Stoel, L. M. K. (1959): Experiences with α-ethyl-α-methylsuccinimide in the treatment of epilepsy. *Epilepsia,* 1:501–511.

11. DeVries, S. I. (1965): Haematological aspects during treatment with anticonvulsant drugs. *Epilepsia,* 6:1–15.

12. Ehyai, A., Kilroy, A. W., and Fenichel, G. M. (1978): Dyskinesia and akathisia induced by ethosuximide. *Am. J. Dis. Child.,* 132:527–528.

13. Fischer, M., Korskjeer, G., and Pederson, E. (1965): Psychotic episodes in Zarondan treatment. *Epilepsia,* 6:325–334.

14. Friedel, B., and Lempp, R. (1962): Grand-mal Provokation bei der Behandlung Kindlicher petit-mal mit Oxazolidinen oder Succinimiden und ihre therapeutischen Konsequenzen. *Z. Kinderheilkd.,* 87:42–51.

15. Gilbert, J. C., Scott, A. K., Galloway, D. B., and Petrie, J. C. (1974): Ethosuximide: Liver enzyme induction and D-glucaric acid excretion. *Br. J. Clin. Pharmacol.,* 1:249–252.

16. Goldensohn, E. S., Hardie, J., and Borea, E. (1962): Ethosuximide in the treatment of epilepsy. *J.A.M.A.,* 180:840–842.

17. Goode, D. J., Penry, J. K., and Dreifuss, F. E. (1970): Effects of paroxysmal spike-wave on continuous motor performance. *Epilepsia,* 11:241–254.

18. Gordon, N. (1961): Treatment of epilepsy with α-ethyl-α-methylsuccinimide (P.M. 671). *Neurology (Minneap.),* 11:266–268.

19. Guey, J., Charles, C., Coquery, C., Roger, J., and Soulayrol, R. (1967): Study of psychological effects of ethosuximide (Zarontin) on 25 children suffering from petit mal epilepsy. *Epilepsia,* 8:129–141.

20. Hammond, W. A. (1874): *Clinical Lectures on Diseases of the Nervous System.* T. M. B. Cross, New York.

21. Heathfield, K. W. G., and Jewesbury, E. C. O. (1964): Treatment of petit mal with ethosuximide: Follow-up report. *Br. Med. J.,* 3:616.

22. Jacobs, J. C. (1963): Systemic lupus erythematosus in childhood. Report of 35 cases, with discussion of seven apparently induced by anticonvulsant medication, and of prognosis and treatment. *Pediatrics,* 32:257.

23. Janz, D. (1975): The teratogenic risk of antiepileptic drugs. *Epilepsia,* 16:159–169.

24. Kiorboe, E., Paludan, J., Trolle, E., and Overvad, E. (1964): Zarontin (ethosuximide) in the treatment of petit mal and related disorders. *Epilepsia,* 5:83–89.

25. Kirschberg, G. J. (1975): Dyskinesia—an unusual reaction to ethosuximide. *Arch. Neurol.,* 32:137–138.

26. Koutsoulieris, E. (1967): Granulopenia and thrombocytopenia after ethosuximide. *Lancet,* 2:310–311.

27. Lairy, C. C. (1964): Psychotic signs in epileptics during treatment with ethosuximide. *Rev. Neurol.,* 110:225–226.

28. Lander, C. M., Eadie, M. J., and Tyrer, J. H. (1975): Interactions between anticonvulsants. *Proc. Aust. Assoc. Neurol.,* 12:111–116.

29. Landolt, H. (1958): Serial electroencephalographic investigations during psychotic episodes in epileptic patients and during schizophrenic attacks. In: *Lectures on Epilepsy,* edited by A. M. L. deHaas. Elsevier, Amsterdam.

30. Livingstone, S., Pauli, L., and Najmabadi, A. (1952): Ethosuximide in the treatment of epilepsy. *J.A.M.A.,* 180:104–107.

31. Livingstone, S., Rodriguez, H., Greene, C. A., and Pauli, L. (1968): Systemic lupus erythematosus. Occurrence in association with ethosuximide therapy. *J.A.M.A.,* 203:731–732.

32. Lowe, C. R., (1973): Congenital malformations among infants born to epileptic women. *Obstet. Gynecol. Surv.,* 28:493–494.

33. Mann, L. B., and Habenicht, H. A. (1962): Fatal bone marrow aplasia associated with administration of ethosuximide (Zarontin) for petit mal epilepsy. *Bull. Los Angeles Neurol. Soc.,* 27:173–176.

34. Meyer, J. G. (1973): Teratological effects of anticonvulsants and the effects on pregnancy and birth. *Eur. Neurol.,* 10:179–190.

35. Monnet, P., Salle, B., Poncet, J., Gauthier, J., Philippe, N., and Germain, D. (1967): Disseminated lupus erythematosus induced by ethosuximide in a girl aged 6. *Rev. Med. Dijon,* 2:319–330.

36. Mueller, K. (1963): Erythema exudativum multiforme majus (Stevens–Johnson syndrome) infolge Suxinutin-Ueberempfindlichkeit. *Z. Kinderheilkd.,* 88:548–563.

37. Porter, R. J., Penry, J. K., and Dreifuss, F. E. (1973): Responsiveness at the onset of spike-wave bursts. *Electroencephalogr. Clin. Neurophysiol.,* 34:239–245.

38. Prensky, A. L., DeVivo, D. C., and Palkes, H. (1971): Severe bradykinesia as a manifestation of toxicity to antiepileptic medications. *J. Pediatr.,* 78:700–704.

39. Roger, J., Grangeon, H., Guey, J., and Lob, H. (1968): Psychiatric and psychological complications of ethosuximide treatment in epileptics. *Encephale,* 57:407–438.

40. Sato, T., Kondo, Y., Matsuo, T., Iwata, H., Okuyama, Y., and Aoki, Y. (1965): Clinical experiences of ethosuximide (Zarontin) in therapy-resident epileptics. *Brain Nerve (Tokyo),* 17:958–964.

41. Singsen, B. H., Fishman, L., and Hanson, V. (1976): Antinuclear antibodies and lupus-like syndromes in children receiving anticonvulsants. *Pediatrics,* 57:529–534.

42. Schmidt. D. (1975): The effect of phenytoin and ethosuximide on primidone metabolism in patients with epilepsy. *J. Neurol.,* 209:115–123.

43. Smith, L. W., Phillipus, M. J., and Guard, H. L. (1968): Psychometric study of children with learning problems and 14-6 positive spike EEG patterns, treated

with ethosuximide (Zarontin) and placebo. *Arch. Dis. Child.*, 43:616–619.

44. Silverman, S. H., Gribetz, D., and Rausen, A. R. (1978): Nephrotic syndrome associated with ethosuccimide. *Am. J. Dis. Child.*, 132:99.

45. Soulayrol, R., and Roger, J. (1970): Adverse psychiatric effects of antiepileptic drugs. *Rev. Neuropsychiatr. Infant,* 18:591.

46. Spittler, J. F. (1974): Agranulocytosis due to ethosuximide with a fatal outcome. *Klin. Paediatr.,* 186:364–366.

47. Sullivan, F. M., and McElhatton, P. R. (1977): A comparison of the teratogenic activity of the antiepileptic drugs carbamazepine, clonazepam, ethosuximide, phenobarbital, phenytoin and primidone in mice. *Toxicol. Appl. Pharmacol.,* 40:365–378.

48. Taaffe, A., and O'Brien, C. (1975): A case of Stevens–Johnson syndrome associated with the anticonvulsants sulthiame and ethosuximide. *Br. Dent. J.,* 138:172–174.

49. Teoh, P. C., and Chan, H. L. (1975): Lupus-scleroderma syndrome induced by ethosuximide. *Arch. Dis. Child.,* 50:658–661.

50. Todorov, A. B., Lenn, N. J., and Gabor, A. J. (1978): Exacerbation of generalized non-convulsive seizures with ethosuximide therapy. *Arch. Neurol.,* 35:389–391.

51. Trimble, M. R., and Reynolds, E. H. (1976): Anticonvulsant drugs and mental symptoms. *Psychol. Med.,* 6:169–178.

52. Vossen, R. (1958): The anticonvulsive effect of succinimides. *Dtsch. Med. Wochenschr.,* 83:1227–1230.

53. Wassner, S. J., Pennisi, A. J., Malekzadeh, M. H., and Fine, R. N. (1976): The adverse effect of anticonvulsant therapy on renal allograft survival. A preliminary report. *J. Pediatr.,* 88:134–137.

54. Weinstein, A. W., and Allen, R. J. (1966): Ethosuximide treatment of petit mal seizures. A study of 87 pediatric patients. *Am. J. Dis. Child.,* 111:63–67.

55. Zimmerman, F. T., and Burgemeister, B. B. (1958): A new drug for petit mal epilepsy. *Neurology (Minneap.),* 8:769–776.

Antiepileptic Drugs, edited by D. M. Woodbury,
J. K. Penry, and C. E. Pippenger. Raven Press,
New York © 1982.

56

Ethosuximide

Mechanisms of Action

James A. Ferrendelli and William E. Klunk

Ethosuximide (ESM), α-ethyl-α-methyl-suc-cinimide, has been used extensively for the treatment of absence (petit mal) seizures for more than 20 years. Despite its frequent use, the site(s) and mechanism(s) of action of ESM are still unexplained. In this chapter, we review the available published data on basic pharmacological actions of ESM. To facilitate presentation, this information is divided into three categories: effects on clinical and experimental seizure activity, effects on biochemical processes in nervous tissue, and neurophysiologic effects. Finally, a hypothesis is presented that attempts to explain the antiepileptic action of ESM.

EFFECTS ON CLINICAL AND EXPERIMENTAL SEIZURES

One of the most intriguing facts about ESM is its highly selective effect on clinical and experimental seizures. It completely, or almost completely, prevents absence seizures in about 50% of patients with petit mal epilepsy and reduces their frequency in another 40 to 45% (2). In contrast, it has no apparent effect against generalized tonic–clonic convulsions or partial seizures.

The high degree of therapeutic specificity of ESM in human seizure disorders is reflected by its selective anticonvulsant action against ex-perimental seizures. It is well known that ESM prevents pentylenetetrazol (Metrazol®) seizures at nontoxic doses in experimental animals but has no effect on maximal electroshock seizures except at very high, toxic concentrations (4). Ethosuximide has also been reported to have an anticonvulsant action on seizures induced by implantation of cobalt into the cerebral cortex (6,17,31), systemic administration of γ-hy-droxybutyrate (13,32,33), application of conjugated estrogen to the brain (16), inhalation of fluorothyl (1) or enflurane (30), barbiturate withdrawal (26), and systemic administration of penicillin (15). However, it seems to be inactive against allylglycine seizures in photosensitive baboons (24), stroboscopic seizures in epileptic fowl (5), and seizures produced by application of aluminum hydroxide (22) to the cerebral cortex.

The fact that ESM prevents several seemingly different experimental seizures suggests either that the drug may have more than one anticonvulsant action or that the several types of seizures prevented by ESM have a common epileptogenic mechanism. In either case, the observation that it is effective against only certain types of clinical and experimental seizures clearly indicates that this drug must have fairly selective actions in the CNS. It probably does not have a widespread depressant effect on nervous tissue as do some other anticonvulsant drugs such as barbiturates, which can suppress most seizures.

An interesting and pertinent fact is that the effects of ESM on clinical seizures are almost exactly opposite to those of phenytoin. Thus, phenytoin is effective in the treatment of tonic–clonic convulsions and partial seizures but does not prevent absence seizures and, in fact, may precipitate motor convulsions in patients with petit mal epilepsy. Phenytoin and ESM have very different effects on experimental seizures as well (Table 1). Phenytoin is effective against many of the experimental seizures that are not prevented by ESM. In contrast, those that are prevented by ESM are either unaffected by phenytoin or changed in character and sometimes made more severe. For example, convulsant doses of pentylenetetrazol in rodents produce intermittent myoclonic and clonic seizures, often followed after several minutes by a tonic convulsion that is usually fatal. All seizure activity may be prevented by pretreatment of animals with ESM, but phenytoin pretreatment results in continuous and long-lasting clonic seizure activity, although no tonic convulsion occurs. The marked difference between the effects of ESM and phenytoin on seizure activity strongly indicates that the mechanism of action of ESM, although still uncertain, must be very different from that of phenytoin.

EFFECTS ON NEUROCHEMICAL PROCESSES

Brain Enzyme Activity

Two laboratories have reported that ESM inhibits (Na^+,K^+)-ATPase, but not Mg-ATPase, activity in broken cell preparations of brain (11,12,21). The studies of Gilbert and colleagues (11,12) indicate that the inhibitory effect of ESM may be selective for (Na^+,K^+)-ATPase existing in the plasma membranes of nerve terminals. Unfortunately, they found effects only at drug concentrations of 2.5 and 25 mM, levels that are considerably greater than those producing antiepileptic effects. Most other assessments of the effects of ESM on enzyme activities in nervous tissue have only been screening studies. Nevertheless, it has been reported that ESM also inhibits GABA transaminase (29) and succinic dehydrogenase (21). Succinic semialdehyde dehydrogenase activity is stimulated by high levels of ESM but unaffected by therapeutic concentrations (29). Ethosuximide has been reported to have no effect on Mg-ATPase, glutamic acid decarboxylase, monoamine oxidase, acetylcholinesterase, and arylsulfatase (21).

Ethosuximide has also been reported to inhibit (noncompetitively) NADPH-linked aldehyde reductase from bovine brain (8). This en-

TABLE 1. *Comparison of anticonvulsant effects of ethosuximide and phenytoin on experimental seizures*

Experimental seizure	Anticonvulsant efficacy		Reference
	Ethosuximide	Phenytoin	
Pentylenetetrazol	Effective	Ineffective	4
Cobalt implantation	Effective	Ineffective	6
γ-Hydroxybutyrate	Effective	Ineffective	13,32,33
Estrogen application	Effective	Ineffective	16
Fluorothyl	Effective	?	1
Enflurane dysrhythmias	Effective	Ineffective	30
Penicillin	Effective	Partially effective	15
Allylglycine in photosensitive baboons	Ineffective	Effective	24
Stroboscopic seizures in epileptic fowl	Ineffective	Effective	5
Al(OH)$_3$ application	Ineffective	Effective	22
Maximal electroshock	Ineffective	Effective	4

zyme is capable of converting succinic semialdehyde to γ-hydroxybutyrate (36). This may be the biochemical mechanism of the recently reported ability of ESM to decrease endogenous levels of the latter compound after chronic treatment (34). In view of the fact that exogenously administered γ-hydroxybutyrate induces behavioral and EEG abnormalities resembling absence seizures (13,32,38), this property of ESM may have a direct relation to its anticonvulsant effect.

Cerebral Metabolism

Nahorski (25) compared the effects of trimethadione, ESM, and chlordiazepoxide on *in vivo* levels of energy and carbohydrate reserves, glycolytic and citric acid cycle intermediates, and some amino acids in rat brain. He reported that ESM elevated brain glucose levels and increased the brain/blood glucose ratio. Decreased levels of fructose-1,6-bisphosphate, pyruvate, and glutamate and increased levels of malate were also found, but there were no changes in the concentration of any of the other substances measured in this study. He concluded that the observed effects probably resulted from a depression of metabolic rate. In support of this idea is the observation that ESM reduces oxygen consumption of brain tissue, *in vivo* and *in vitro* (21). However, it is unlikely that ESM depresses brain metabolism as generally or to the same extent as do many other antiepileptic drugs, hypnotics and sedatives, or general anesthetics.

Membrane Transport Functions

Gray and Gilbert (14) reported that ESM stimulated uptake of xylose into brain slices, probably by increasing the affinity of the carrier for xylose. We have examined the effect of several anticonvulsant drugs on calcium accumulation in isolated nerve terminals (synaptosomes) (35). Ethosuximide has no effect on passive "leak" of calcium into unstimulated synaptosomes. It also has no effect on stimulated calcium accumulation in synaptosomes depolarized with veratridine or high levels of

K^+, except at very high concentrations, 10 mM or greater. This is in contrast to drugs such as phenytoin and carbamazepine which inhibit Ca^{2+} accumulation in synaptosomes at therapeutic concentrations.

Cyclic Nucleotide Regulation

As do most other anticonvulsant drugs, ESM treatment has been observed to reduce basal cyclic GMP levels in rodent cerebellum (23). However, none of the anticonvulsant drugs tested has any effect on cyclic GMP levels in cerebral cortex or any consistent effect on cyclic AMP levels in either region of brain. Experimental seizures elevate brain levels of both cyclic AMP and cyclic GMP. Anticonvulsant drugs, including ESM, prevent seizure-induced elevations of cyclic nucleotides, but only to the extent that they prevent seizures. Agents that cause cellular depolarization (i.e., veratridine, ouabain, K^+) produce marked elevations of levels of cyclic AMP and cyclic GMP in incubated brain slices. Several anticonvulsant drugs inhibit these depolarization-induced elevations of cyclic nucleotides, but with the exception of phenytoin and carbamazepine, concentrations much higher than therapeutic levels are necessary to produce an effect (9). Ethosuximide, as well as other drugs highly effective in the treatment of absence seizures, are the least potent.

Neurotransmitter Systems

At present, there are no data that unequivocally demonstrate a direct effect of ESM on a specific neurotransmitter system in the brain. However, there are several bits of information that indirectly indicate relationships between ESM and CNS neurotransmitters. For example, Čapek and Esplin (3) found that ESM augmented the decline of monosynaptic response amplitude evoked by trains of stimuli in spinal cord. They suggested that this effect was a result of ESM causing an increased fractional release of neurotransmitter per volley and, as a result of this, partially depleting transmitter stores in presynaptic terminals. Unfortunately, the neurotransmitter mediating the spinal monosynaptic reflex has not been identified. Furthermore, it is unclear how this effect of ESM in spinal cord relates to its antiepileptic action.

A relationship between ESM and dopamine, primarily an inhibitory neurotransmitter in CNS, has been suggested by studies of experimental seizures in animals. Several laboratories have determined that γ-hydroxybutyrate produces seizures in experimental animals (13,32,38). Although the mechanisms responsible for the epileptogenic action of γ-hydroxybutyrate have not been defined, it has been established that it is capable of blocking impulse flow in dopaminergic pathways in the brain (28). As noted above, ESM is highly effective in preventing γ-hydroxybutyrate-induced seizures. Recently, we observed that the anticonvulsant effect of ESM in this seizure model can be reversed by pretreatment of animals with fluphenazine, a dopamine receptor antagonist, or α-methylparatyrosine, an agent that inhibits synthesis of dopamine (19). These data may indicate that the antiepileptic action of ESM, at least in the γ-hydroxybutyrate seizure model, is related to some effect on CNS dopamine neurotransmission, possibly augmentation of dopaminergic influence in CNS. In support of this idea is the finding that treatment of animals with L-DOPA, a dopamine precursor, prevents cobalt-induced seizures, which are also prevented by ESM (31). Likewise, cortical spikes produced by topical application of penicillin are prevented by systemic L-DOPA and by topical dopamine but not by topical norepinephrine (20). As previously mentioned, seizures produced by systemic administration of penicillin are prevented by ESM (15).

It is possible that a relationship between ESM and GABA may also exist, since valproic acid and benzodiazepines, drugs with antiepileptic effects similar to ESM, have been shown to have effects on GABA neurotransmitter systems.

NEUROPHYSIOLOGICAL EFFECTS

Fromm and Kohli (10) reported that ESM (and trimethadione) preferentially depresses corticofugal inhibition of afferent activity in the spinal trigeminal nucleus, whereas phenytoin and carbamazepine have the opposite effect. Ethosuximide has also been shown to fully suppress pentylenetetrazol-induced spindle activity and significantly reduce photic recruitment and photic afterdischarges (37). These rhythmic activities are considered to be an expression of synchronized afterdischarges of the thalamocortical system, and the effect of ESM is thought to be on ascending reticular activation or directly on inhibitory cells in the thalamic relays. The lateral geniculate body is probably not the site of action of ESM in preventing photically evoked afterdischarges because whereas i.p. administration abolishes the effect, injection into the lateral geniculate body has no effect (18). Some studies have presented very interesting data on the effects of anticonvulsant drugs on thalamocortical excitability (7,27). Paired stimuli were administered to the ventrolateral thalamus, and evoked responses were recorded from the cortex. Phenytoin and diazepam depressed the evoked responses at all frequencies equally, but ESM and valproic acid were disproportionately effective at reducing potentials evoked by stimuli in the 3/sec range. These data suggest a basis for the effectiveness of ESM and valproic acid in controlling 3/sec repetitive activity in absence seizures.

POSSIBLE MECHANISMS OF ACTION OF ESM

Any complete description of the mechanisms of action of an antiepileptic drug would require a full understanding of the pathophysiological mechanisms of epilepsy and an explanation of how the drug modifies these to prevent seizures. Since the pathophysiological mechanisms of epilepsy are still incompletely understood, one can only speculate about the mechanisms of action of antiepileptic drugs.

We propose that a drug may produce an anticonvulsant effect by two general mechanisms: direct modification of membrane function in excitable cells and/or alteration of chemically mediated neurotransmission. Decreasing membrane excitability by the first mechanism may be accomplished in any of the following ways: (a) nonspecific alteration of the membrane bilayers so as to disrupt ionic channels; (b) specific blockade of Na^+ and/or Ca^{2+} conductances; (c) enhanced efflux of Na^+ by increased active pumping mechanisms; and (d) enhanced ionic conductance of Cl^- and/or K^+. To achieve an anticonvulsant effect by the second mechanism would require decreasing the influence of excitatory neurotransmitters and/or increasing the influence of inhibitory transmitters. This could occur anywhere in the complex process responsible for synthesis, packaging, transport, release, reuptake, and interaction with pre- and postsynaptic receptors of individual neurotransmitters. Obviously, an anticonvulsant drug could act at more than one site and have both direct membrane effects and direct actions on neurotransmitter processes. Moreover, an action on neurotransmission would indirectly modify membrane excitability and vice versa.

With regard to ESM, there is no evidence that it nonspecifically alters membrane structure, thereby disrupting ionic channels. It is highly water soluble, so it is unlikely that much of it inserts into cellular membranes which have a high lipid content. Furthermore, it has none of the properties of general anesthetics which are believed to exert their effects by a direct action on cellular membranes. It is apparent that ESM does not inhibit calcium conductance in nervous tissues, and it probably also does not affect sodium conductance. The observation that ESM inhibits (Na^+, K^+)-ATPase activity in plasma membranes in vitro does not explain its antiepileptic effects. On the contrary, inhibition of the sodium pump would cause accumulation of intracellular sodium, make the membrane potential more positive, increase excitability, and thus perhaps produce seizures rather than prevent them. There are no data indicating that ESM has any effect on Cl^- or K^+ conductances.

The above considerations lead to the conclusion that the antiepileptic action of ESM is probably not a result of some direct effect on membrane function. This contention is further supported by the fact that ESM has effects on seizure activity which are very different from the effects of phenytoin. Much evidence now indicates that the anticonvulsant action of phenytoin is, at least partially, a result of its ability to directly "stabilize" membranes by altering ionic fluxes (39).

If, indeed, the antiepileptic effect of ESM does not result from an action on cellular membranes, it may be a result of some effect on neurotransmission. There is indirect evidence to indicate that it may deplete excitatory neurotransmitter stores mediating the spinal monosynaptic reflex. This is thought to occur by an increase in fractional release per stimulus without resultant increase in synthesis. Although a similar effect in brain might selectively depress repetitive impulses, thereby preventing seizures, it is not likely because the increased release of excitatory neurotransmitters on initial impulses might be enough to potentiate seizure activity. In addition, direct measurements of neurotransmitters indicate that, in many systems, synthesis can more than compensate for increased release even at the highest firing rates attainable. Perhaps a more plausible explanation is that ESM may increase the influence of inhibitory neurotransmitters. The suggested depressant effects of ESM on corticofugal inhibition of the spinal trigeminal nucleus, thalamocortical excitability (especially that produced by pulse-pair interval stimuli longer than 3/sec), and pentylenetetrazol-induced spindle activity may well be a result of some action on neuronal pathways subserved by inhibitory neurotransmitters. The important question is what these inhibitory neurotransmitter systems are. Possible links between ESM and GABA and/or dopamine were mentioned earlier, but much more data on this subject are needed before any definite conclusion can be reached.

In this review we have not considered mechanisms of action of other succinimide derivatives that are used as antiepileptic drugs, e.g., methsuximide and phensuximide, since there is very little available data on their basic pharmacological properties. It is know that these drugs have effects on clinical and experimental seizures that are similar to those of ESM; however, methsuximide and phensuximide are also capable of preventing maximal electroshock seizures and other experimental and clinical seizures that are not affected by ESM. This suggests that methsuximide and phensuximide have actions in addition to or different from those of ESM. Obviously, additional research is needed to establish the similarities and differences between the mechanism of action of ESM and those of other anticonvulsant succinimides.

In summary it should be apparent that the limited amount of data on the basic pharmacological effects of ESM only permits speculative conclusions about its antiepileptic mechanism of action. Although several mechanisms are possible, in this review we favor the concept that ESM enhances inhibitory processes in brain, perhaps by some effect on specific inhibitory neurotransmitter systems. This explanation is necessarily oversimplistic; however, it may provide some direction for future research on ESM as well as on certain seizure disorders.

REFERENCES

1. Adler, M. W. (1972): The effect of single and multiple lesions of the limbic system on cerebral excitability. *Psychopharmacologia,* 24:218–230.
2. Browne, T. R., Dreifuss, F. E., Dyken, P. R., Goode, D. J., Penry, J. K., Porter, R. J., White, B. G., and White, P. T. (1975): Ethosuximide in the treatment of absence (petit mal) seizures. *Neurology (Minneap.),* 25:515–524.
3. Čapek, R., and Esplin, B. (1977): Effects of ethosuximide on transmission of repetitive impulses and apparent rates of transmitter turnover in the spinal monosynaptic pathway. *J. Pharmacol. Exp. Ther.,* 201:320–325.
4. Chen, G., Weston, J. K., and Bratton, A. C., Jr. (1963): Anticonvulsant activity and toxicity of phensuximide, methsuximide, and ethosuximide. *Epilepsia,* 4:66–76.
5. Davis, H. L., Johnson, D. D., and Crawford, R. D. (1978): Epileptiform seizures in domestic fowl. IX. Implications of the absence of anticonvulsant activity of ethosuximide in a pharmacological model of epilepsy. *Can. J. Physiol. Pharmacol.,* 56:893–896.
6. Dow, R. C., Forfar, J. C., and McQueen, J. K. (1973): The effects of some anticonvulsant drugs on cobalt-induced epilepsy. *Epilepsia,* 14:203–212.
7. Englander, R. N., Johnson, R. N., Brickley, J. J., and Hanna, G. R. (1977): Effects of anticonvulsant drugs on thalamocortical excitability. *Neurology (Minneap.),* 27:1134–1139.
8. Erwin, V. G., and Deitrich, R. A. (1973): Inhibition of bovine brain aldehyde reductase by anticonvulsant compounds. *Biochem. Pharmacol.,* 2:2615–2624.
9. Ferrendelli, J. A., and Kinscherf, D. A. (1979): Inhibitory effects of anticonvulsant drugs on cyclic nucleotide accumulation in brain. *Ann. Neurol.,* 5:533–538.
10. Fromm, G. H., and Kohli, C. M. (1972): The role of inhibitory pathways in petit mal epilepsy. *Neurology, (Minneap.),* 22:1012–1020.
11. Gilbert, J. C., Scott, A. K., and Wyllie, M. G. (1974): Effects of ethosuximide on adenosine triphosphatase activities of some subcellular fractions prepared from rat cerebral cortex. *Br. J. Pharmacol.,* 50:452P–453P.
12. Gilbert, J. C., and Wyllie, M. G. (1974): The effects of the anticonvulsant ethosuximide on adenosine triphosphatase activities of synaptosomes prepared from rat cerebral cortex. *Br. J. Pharmacol.,* 52:139P–140P.
13. Godschalk, M., Džoljić, M. R., and Bonta, I. L. (1976): Antagonism of gamma-hydroxybutyrate-induced hypersynchronization in the ECoG of the rat by anti-petit mal drugs. *Neurosci. Lett.,* 3:145–150.
14. Gray, P., and Gilbert, J. C. (1970): Anticonvulsant drugs and xylose uptake by cerebral slices. *Biochem. J.,* 120:27P–28P.
15. Guberman, A. G., Gloor, P., and Sherwin, A. L. (1975): Response of generalized penicillin epilepsy in the cat to ethosuximide and diphenylhydantoin. *Neurology (Minneap.),* 25:758–764.
16. Julien, R. M., Fowler, G. W., and Danielson, M. G. (1975): The effect of antiepileptic drugs on estrogen-induced electrographic spike-wave discharges. *J. Pharmacol. Exp. Ther.,* 193:647–656.
17. Kastner, I., Klingberg, F., and Muller, M. (1970): Zur Wirkung des Ethosuximids auf die Kobalt-induzierte "Epilepsie" der Ratte. *Arch. Int. Pharmacodyn. Ther.,* 186:220–226.
18. Kastner, I., and Rougerie, A. (1978): Photisch ausgelöste Potentialfolgen nach lokaler Applikation von Ethosuximid ins Corpus geniculatum laterale. *Acta Biol. Med. Germ.,* 37:677–679.
19. Klunk, W. E., and Ferrendelli, J. A. (1980): Reversal of the anticonvulsant action of ethosuximide by drugs that diminish CNS dopaminergic neurotransmission. *Neurology (Minneap.),* 30:421.
20. Kobayashi, K., Shirakabe, T., Kishikawa, H., and Mori, A. (1976): Catecholamine levels in penicillin-induced epileptic focus of the cat cerebral cortex. *Acta Neurochir. [Suppl.],* 23:93–100.
21. Leznicki, A., and Dymecki, J. (1974): The effect of certain anticonvulsants *in vitro* and *in vivo* on enzyme activities in rat brain. *Neurol. Neurochir. Pol.,* 24:413–419.
22. Lockard, J. S., Levy, R. H., Congdon, W. C., DuCharme, L. L., and Patel, I. H. (1977): Efficacy testing of valproic acid compared to ethosuximide in monkey model: II. Seizure, EEG, and diurnal variations. *Epilepsia,* 18:205–224.
23. Lust, W. D., Kupferberg, H. J., Yonekawa, W. D., Penry, J. K., Passonneau, J. V., and Wheaton, A. B. (1978): Changes in brain metabolites induced by convulsants or electroshock: Effects of anticonvulsant agents. *Mol. Pharmacol.,* 14:347–356.
24. Meldrum, B. S., Horton, R. W., and Toseland, P. A. (1975): A primate model for testing anticonvulsant drugs. *Arch. Neurol.,* 32:289–294.
25. Nahorski, S. R. (1972): Biochemical effects of the

anticonvulsants trimethadione, ethosuximide, and chlordiazepoxide in rat brain. *J. Neurochem.*, 19:1937–1946.

26. Norton, P. R. E. (1970): The effect of drugs on barbiturate withdrawal convulsions in the rat. *J. Pharm. Pharmacol.*, 22:763–766.

27. Nowack, W. J., Johnson, R. N., Englander, R. N., and Hanna, G. R. (1979): Effects of valproate and ethosuximide on thalamocortical excitability. *Neurology (Minneap.)*, 29:96–99.

28. Roth, R. H., Walters, J. R., and Aghajanian, G. K. (1973): Effect of impulse flow on the release and synthesis of dopamine in the rat striatum. In: *Frontiers in Catecholamine Research,* edited by E. Udsin and S. H. Snyder, pp. 567–574. Pergamon Press, Oxford.

29. Sawaya, M. C. B., Horton, R. W., and Meldrom, B. S. (1975): Effects of anticonvulsant drugs on the cerebral enzymes metabolizing GABA. *Epilepsia,* 16:549–655.

30. Schettini, A., and Wilder, B. J. (1974): Effects of anticonvulsant drugs on enflurane cortical dysrhythmias. *Anesth. Analg. (Cleve.),* 53:951–962.

31. Scuvee-Moreau, J., Lepot, M., Brotchi, J., Gerebtzott, M. A., and Dresse, A. (1977): Action of phenytoin, ethosuximide, and of the carbidopa–L-dopa association in semi-chronic cobalt-induced epilepsy in the rat. *Arch. Int. Pharmacodyn. Ther.,* 230:92–99.

32. Snead, O. C. (1978): Gammahydroxybutyrate in the monkey: II. Effect of chronic oral anticonvulsant drugs. *Neurology (Minneap.),* 28:643–648.

33. Snead, O. C. (1978): Gammahydroxybutyrate in the monkey: III. Effect of intravenous anticonvulsant drugs. *Neurology (Minneap.),* 28:1173–1178.

34. Snead, O. C., Bearden, L. J., and Pegram, V. (1980): Effect of acute and chronic anticonvulsant administration on endogenous γ-hydroxybutyrate in rat brain. *Neuropharmacology,* 19:47–52.

35. Sohn, R. S., and Ferrendelli, J. A. (1976): Anticonvulsant drug mechanisms phenytoin, phenobarbital, and ethosuximide and Ca^{+2} flux in isolated presynaptic endings. *Arch. Neurol.,* 33:626–629.

36. Tabakoff, B., and von Wartburg, J. P. (1975): Separation of aldehyde reductases and alcohol dehydrogenase from brain by affinity chromatography: Metabolism of succinic semialdehyde and ethanol. *Biochem. Biophys. Res. Commun.,* 63:957–966.

37. Wenzel, J., Krueger, E., and Mueller, M. (1971): Hemmung Pentetrazol-induzierter hypersynchroner Aktivität im thalamokortikalen System durch Ethosuximid. *Acta Biol. Med. Germ.,* 26:567–572.

38. Winters, W. D., and Spooner, C. E. (1965): A neurophysiological comparison of gamma-hydroxybutyrate with pentobarbital in cats. *Electroencephalogr. Clin. Neurophysiol.,* 18:287–296.

39. Woodbury, D. M. (1980): Phenytoin: Proposed mechanisms of anticonvulsant action. In: *Antiepileptic Drugs: Mechanisms of Action,* edited by G. H. Glaser, J. K. Penry, and D. M. Woodbury, pp. 447–471. Raven Press, New York.

Antiepileptic Drugs, edited by D. M. Woodbury, J. K. Penry, and C. E. Pippenger. Raven Press, New York © 1982.

57

Other Succinimides

Methsuximide and Phensuximide

Roger J. Porter and Harvey J. Kupferberg

After Miller and Long (27) observed the structural similarity and heterocyclic nature of the available antiepileptic drugs—phenytoin, mephenytoin, trimethadione, phenobarbital, and phenacemide—many similar compounds were tested (49), but only the succinimides proved effective and nontoxic enough to be added to the antiepileptic armamentarium. Two of these are methsuximide (*N*,2-dimethyl-2-phenyl-succinimide, Celontin®) and phensuximide *N*-methyl-2-phenylsuccinimide, Milontin®) (Fig. 1).

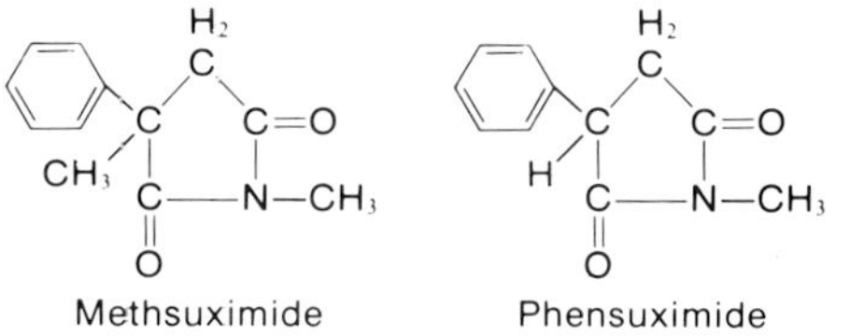

FIG. 1. Structures of methsuximide and phensuximide.

CHEMISTRY AND METHODS OF DETERMINATION

Chemistry

Methsuximide has a molecular weight of 203.23 and a melting point of 52°C. The molecular weight of phensuximide is 189.21, and its melting point is 72°C. Methsuximide is prepared by the action of methylamine on methylphenylsuccinic acid, and phensuximide is prepared by the action of methylamine on phenylsuccinic acid. Each of the compounds is marketed in the United States as both 150- and 300-mg capsules.

Methods of Analysis

Colorimetric and gas–liquid chromatographic methods have been used for the determination of both methsuximide and phensuximide in body fluids (17). The sensitivity of these procedures, however, is not sufficient to define the pharmacokinetics of the drug. Strong et al. (43) demonstrated that the levels of methsuximide are of the order of 50 ng/ml, well below the detectability of the earlier methods. They also noted that the *N*-demethylated product is found in microgram levels. They used electron impact selected ion monitoring to quantitate the parent drug and its metabolite. Kupferberg et al. (23) used a similar technique to determine the pharmacokinetics of methsuximide and phensuximide in epileptic patients. Parent drugs and *N*-demethylated metabolites were both determined. This method differed from that of Strong et al. (43) in that the *N*-butyl derivatives of the metabolites were made by a method similar to that of Greely (19) following extraction from plasma. The sensitivity of these methods is in the submicrogram range.

ABSORPTION, DISTRIBUTION, AND EXCRETION

The absorption of methsuximide was studied in rats by Nicholls and Orton (31) who evaluated the pattern of disappearance of [^{14}C]methsuximide from the small intestine and stomach. After 10 to 15 min, the disappearance was first order, with more rapid absorption from the small intestine (elimination half-life, 17 min) than from the stomach (elimination half-life, 52 min). After 6 hr 87% had been absorbed from the entire gastrointestinal tract. Glazko and Dill (17) found peak plasma methsuximide levels at 4 hr after oral administration of the drug to two dogs. The levels were 26 and 36 μg/ml, but it is possible that it was the desmethylmethsuximide that was actually measured.

Absorption studies of phensuximide in rats given oral doses of 100 mg/kg showed maximum plasma levels of the drug in 1 to 2 hr (17). In humans, peak plasma phensuximide levels of 10.3 and 19.3 μg/ml occurred 1 to 4 hr after dosing (17).

The distribution of methsuximide in rats was measured by Nicholls and Orton (31). Using an oral dose of 100 mg/kg of [^{14}C]methsuximide, they demonstrated rapid distribution in all eight tissues examined and noted that the lipophilic compound was especially concentrated in fat. Greater persistence of activity was also noted in the kidneys, liver, and adrenal glands. The high concentration of the drug in fat was noted earlier by Glazko and Dill (17) who used a colorimetric procedure. (Distribution of methsuximide in humans is discussed in the section on Biotransformation.)

The distribution of phensuximide in rats was also found to be rather uniform. Glazko and Dill (17) observed that the concentration in rat brain was similar to that in other tissues. Also, most of the activity was attributed to metabolites, not unchanged drug. Similar results have been obtained in the dog (18).

Dudley et al. (12) reported that methsuximide was excreted primarily as conjugated metabolites, especially α-(*p*-hydroxyphenyl)-α-methylsuccinimide and *N*-methyl-α-(*p*-hydroxyphenyl)-α-methylsuccinimide, in the dog. They found no unchanged methsuximide in a 48-hr urine specimen. In humans, less than 1% of methsuximide is excreted unchanged (17).

Glazko et al. (18) observed that excretion of ^{14}C-labeled metabolites of phensuximide in rat urine peaked 6 to 13 hr after dosing. In humans, the hydroxyphenyl metabolite of phensuximide has been shown to account for 27% of the dose (17).

BIOTRANSFORMATION

The metabolic patterns of phensuximide and methsuximide are useful in understanding the differences in antiepileptic potency of these two drugs. Glazko et al. (18) were the first to study the clinical pharmacology of phensuximide. Blood levels of the drug reached a maximum 1 to 2 hr after a single oral dose and were not detectable 24 hr later. Dudley et al. (13) demonstrated that in the dog phensuximide is initially metabolized to 2-phenylsuccinimide which is rapidly converted to 2-phenylsuccinamic acid by the liver enzyme dihydropyrimidinase. The 2-phenylsuccinamic acid is the primary metabolite in the dog and most likely in humans. Other metabolites of phensuximide have been identified. For example, Horning et al. (20) described several hydroxylated metabolites of phensuximide in the urine of epileptic patients receiving the drug. *p*-Hydroxyphenylphensuximide and *m*-hydroxyphenylphensuximide were two of several hydroxylated metabolites identified but not quantitated.

The metabolite of methsuximide, 2-methyl-2-phenylsuccinimide, was shown to be active (6) and was briefly tested in 36 patients (49).

Later, Nicholls and Orton (30,31) described the *N*-demethylation of methsuximide to 2-methyl-2-phenylsuccinimide in the rat. The rapid disappearance of the parent drug and the accumulation of the desmethyl metabolite led them to postulate that the metabolite might be the active agent. Other investigators have demonstrated the accumulation of this metabolite (22,43). The chemical structure of the *N*-demethylated product was established by Muni et al. (29).

The metabolic pathway of methsuximide appears to be similar to that of phensuximide. Many of the corresponding hydroxylated metabolites, e.g., *p*-hydroxymethsuximide, are found in the urine of patients receiving methsuximide (20). The major difference in metabolism of the two drugs lies in the fact that dihydropyrimidinase does not hydrolytically open the ring of 2-methyl-2-phenylsuccinimide (Fig. 2A) as it does with 2-phenylsuccinimide (Fig. 2B). Dihydropyrimidinase preferentially causes ring cleavage of monosubstituted ring structures such as 2-phenylsuccinimide and 5-phenylhydantoin. Because of this enzyme, the plasma levels of phensuximide and desmethylphensuximide have a different relationship to each other than does meth-

suximide with its demethylated metabolite. This point is well illustrated in Figs. 3 and 4.

The plasma levels of phensuximide and its demethylated metabolite following the oral administration of 1,500 mg of phensuximide to an epileptic patient are shown in Fig. 3. The levels of the parent drug always exceeded those of the metabolite, although the rates of disappearance were similar. The plasma half-life of each compound ranged from 4.5 to 12 hr (mean, 7.8 hr). The steady-state trough plasma concentrations following a daily dose of 3,000 mg averaged 5.7 μg/ml for phensuximide and 1.7 μg/ml for desmethylphensuximide. The mean ratio of desmethylphensuximide to phensuximide was 0.31.

The plasma levels of methsuximide and its *N*-demethylated product following the oral administration of 1,200 mg of methsuximide to an epileptic patient are shown in Fig. 4. In this case, the plasma levels of the metabolite, desmethylmethsuximide, exceeded those of the parent drug. The plasma half-life of methsuximide averaged 1.4 hr, whereas the *N*-demethylated product had a relatively long half-life, averaging 38 hr. The steady-state trough plasma concentrations of the

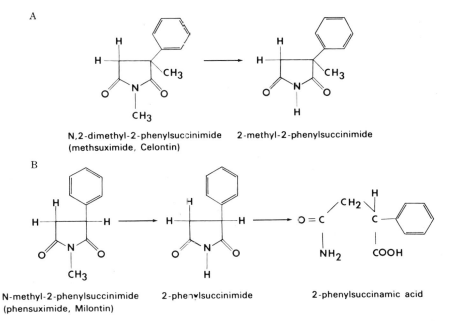

FIG. 2. *N*-Demethylation of methsuximide (**A**) and phensuximide (**B**).

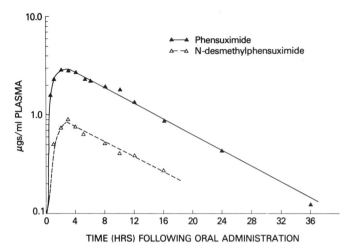

FIG. 3. Typical plasma concentration time course for phensuximide and its demethylated metabolite after a single 1,500-mg dose of phensuximide. (From Porter et al., ref. 33, with permission.)

parent drug and metabolite reflected the difference in their rates of metabolism. The mean plasma levels were 0.037 µg/ml and 28 µg/ml for methsuximide and desmethylmethsuximide, respectively. The mean ratio of desmethylmeth-

suximide to methsuximide was 675. These findings are similar to those of Strong et al. (43).

The differences between methsuximide and phensuximide in metabolism and accumulation of the drug or its further metabolism most likely

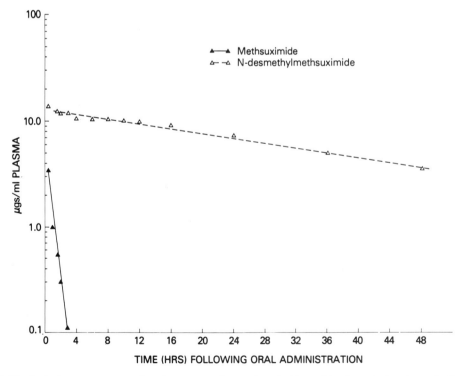

FIG. 4. Typical plasma concentration time course for methsuximide and its demethylated metabolite after a single 1,200-mg dose of methsuximide. (From Porter et al, ref. 33, with permission.)

account for the differences in their antiepileptic potency in patients. Although methsuximide is rapidly metabolized, its metabolite accumulates and has intrinsic anticonvulsant activity, whereas neither phensuximide nor its metabolite accumulate to any large extent when administered chronically.

RELATIONSHIP OF PLASMA CONCENTRATION TO SEIZURE CONTROL

The measurement of plasma methsuximide and phensuximide concentrations is not particularly useful because of the rapid N-demethylation of these drugs. The level of N-desmethylmethsuximide needed for seizure control was estimated to be greater than 10 μg/ml but less than 40 μg/ml in a series of 17 patients (43). This is in agreement with the findings from five of our patients, in whom the level of the metabolite varied from 20 to 40 μg/ml (mean, 28 μg/ml) (33). Seizure control could not be attained with the use of phensuximide.

DOSE-RELATED SIDE EFFECTS

Little is known about the correlation of dose-related side effects of phensuximide and methsuximide with blood levels of the drugs or their metabolites. In a case of combined overdosage with primidone and methsuximide, N-desmethylmethsuximide peaked at 125 mg/liter (21). An overdose of nearly 10 g of methsuximide alone was characterized by gradual onset of coma, including impairment of brainstem reflexes, with gradual improvement over several days (22); other similar cases have been reported (16,37). In some cases, there appeared to be a bimodal depression of consciousness or at least a prolonged delay in the appearance of coma; this may be related to the prolonged conversion of the drug to the metabolite or to delayed absorption. All patients recovered, apparently without sequelae, except one who had an early respiratory arrest (21). No overdose of phensuximide has been reported; its rapid clearance may preclude the potential of a severe effect from an overdose.

Drowsiness, nausea, anorexia, headaches, hiccoughs, and dizziness have been reported in epileptic patients routinely taking either drug (5,8–10,15,36,50–52). A curious observation of hematuria or proteinuria with phensuximide use has also been reported (28).

IDIOSYNCRATIC TOXICITY

There is little description of idiosyncratic toxicity from the succinimides. Buchanan (4) has summarized the data on ethosuximide toxicity up to 1972, but only a few reports on the adverse effects of methsuximide are available, and even fewer on phensuximide. A case of neonatal hemorrhage after maternal methsuximide therapy has been reported; the mother was also taking metharbital (3). A case of megaloblastic anemia occurred during combined phensuximide and phenobarbital therapy, but when the patient recovered, she resumed her previous treatment with the same drugs without ill effect (9a). Severe osteomalacia was reversed on removal of methsuximide (1); no other drugs were being used. Interestingly, methsuximide may be porphyrinogenic (2) and ethosuximide nonporphyrinogenic (32).

In addition to these cases, other possible serious side effects such as leukopenia, pancytopenia, and Stevens–Johnson syndrome have been reported, but they are presumably rare.

MECHANISM OF ACTION

The mechanism of action of the succinimides is unknown. According to Ferrendelli and Kupferberg (14), "there are not even any serious speculations."

THERAPEUTIC USE

Of the many α-phenyl succinimide derivatives evaluated by Chen et al. (6), phensuximide was the first to be tested clinically. Unfortunately, reports of its efficacy were conflicting. In 50 patients with "petit mal" epilepsy (some had "akinetic and myoclonic" attacks, and not all had confirmed spike-wave discharge), the seizures were completely controlled in 30% and suppressed by 78% in an additional 30% (48). Complete seizure control was reported in 26% of 20 "unselected cases" (28). However, it effected only partial control of seizures in 21 patients who met relatively strict criteria for classification of absence seizures (11). The combination of phensuximide and trimethadione, considered more effective than either drug alone in some patients, was beneficial in 15 patients, most of whom had absence seizures (5). In 200 patients, phensuximide brought about complete seizure control in 22% and more than 80% control in 29% (50,51).

Other investigators found phensuximide useful in many cases (9,40,41). In a study of 249 patients, phensuximide was observed to be less toxic than trimethadione and to work well in some patients, although the latter drug was thought more likely to be effective (34). Sato et al. (35) found 80% seizure control in two-thirds of their patients; however, the seizure type was not well delineated. Variable results with phensuximide were reported by other investigators (24,25,46).

In the mid-1950s, reports on phensuximide declined as the use of methsuximide increased. Zimmerman (49,51), who introduced methsuximide, used it to treat 25 patients and obtained complete seizure control in 10% and more than 80% control in half. Although the seizure type was not well defined in most studies, some investigators thought that methsuximide was useful in treating "psychomotor seizures" (8). Others observed a prominent effect in both "petit mal" and "psychomotor" seizures (15). In 100 cases of relatively well-documented "petit mal" seizures treated with methsuximide, 31% of the patients experienced complete seizure relief, and 13% had more than 80% control (52). The drug was noted to be both more efficacious and more toxic than phensuximide. Other investigators found methsuximide useful for the treatment of partial seizures (10) or a variety of partial and generalized seizures (36).

The confusion regarding the efficacy of phensuximide and methsuximide was partly explained when Chen et al. (7) demonstrated in mice that both drugs were effective against ex-

perimental electroshock seizures; ethosuximide was much less so. In contrast, all three succinimides were effective against pentylenetetrazol-induced seizures. Since antipentylenetetrazol activity has some correlation with protection against absence attacks in humans, ethosuximide was thought of as a relatively "pure" antiabsence medication. Conversely, methsuximide and, to a lesser extent, phensuximide were purported to have a broader spectrum of antiepileptic activity.

Of our five patients, none responded to phensuximide, but two showed considerable improvement with methsuximide (33). The large number of abnormal paroxysmal bursts on the 6-hr telemetered EEG during chronic phensuximide administration confirmed clinical observations that this drug had no effect on the seizures, whereas the two patients who responded to methsuximide showed a dramatic reduction in seizure frequency (Fig. 5). One of these pa-

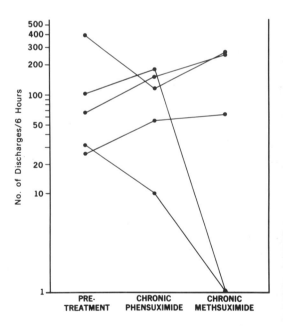

FIG. 5. Abnormal paroxysmal discharges on 6-hr telemetered EEG in five patients before treatment with phensuximide and methsuximide and during the chronic administration of each. (From Porter et al., ref. 33, with permission.)

tients had absence seizures, and the other, my-oclonic–atonic attacks.

It appears, therefore, that methsuximide is rapidly converted to desmethylmethsuximide which is slowly metabolized and exerts the major antiepileptic effect. Phensuximide, however, is converted to desmethylphensuximide which rapidly undergoes ring opening to α-phenylsuccinamic acid, a compound that almost certainly lacks antiepileptic activity. The failure of phensuximide or its desmethyl metabolite to accumulate to the extent of the desmethylmethsuximide after long-term administration probably explains why the antiepileptic effects of phensuximide are weaker than those of methsuximide.

One implication of this study may affect seizure therapy. Because phensuximide is metabolized to a compound that may be devoid of antiepileptic activity and because the half-life of the parent compound is brief, the drug is likely to be generally ineffective. This pharmacokinetic observation confirms the clinical opinions about phensuximide and probably explains its lack of popularity. The question that remains unanswered is whether some of the patients who are well managed on phensuximide would not do even better on other medications that have a more rational therapeutic basis.

OTHER SUCCINIMIDES

Another succinimide manufactured in Budapest but not marketed in the United States has been used clinically. This compound is α-methyl, α-phenyl-N-morpholinyl-methylene succinimide (Morpholep®). Early reports suggested efficacy against complex partial and absence seizures (26), absence attacks only (42), "minor and major" seizures (38,39), and primarily absence seizures (37). Some investigators found the medication effective for "resistant" absence seizures (44) and other refractory seizure types (45). One group suggested that this compound may be superior to the other succinimides (47). Many other succinimides have had trials in animals but no extensive use clinically.

CONVERSION

Methsuximide

Conversion factor:
$$CF = \frac{1000}{mol. \ wt.} = \frac{1000}{203.23} = 4.92$$
Conversion:
$$(\mu g/ml) \times 4.92 = (\mu moles/liter)$$
$$(\mu moles/liter) \div 4.92 = (\mu g/ml)$$

Phensuximide

Conversion factor:
$$CF = \frac{1000}{mol. \ wt.} = \frac{1000}{189.21} = 5.29$$
Conversion:
$$(\mu g/ml) \times 5.29 = (\mu moles/liter)$$
$$(\mu moles/liter) \div 5.29 = (\mu g/ml)$$

REFERENCES

1. Aponte, C. J., and Petrelli, M. P. (1973): Anticonvulsants and vitamin D metabolism. *J.A.M.A.*, 225:1248.
2. Birchfield, R. I., and Cowger, M. L. (1966): Acute intermittent porphyria with seizures. *Am. J. Dis. Child.*, 112:561–565.
3. Bleyer, W. A., and Skinner, A. L. (1976): Fatal neonatal hemorrhage after maternal anticonvulsant therapy. *J.A.M.A.*, 235:626–627.
4. Buchanan, R. A. (1972): Ethosuximide. Toxicity. In: *Antiepileptic Drugs*, edited by D. M. Woodbury, J. K. Penry, and R. P. Schmidt, pp. 449–454. Raven Press, New York.
5. Chao, D., and Fields, W. S. (1954): Combined drug therapy in petit mal epilepsy. *J. Pediatr.*, 45:293–296.
6. Chen, G., Portman, R., Ensor, C. R., and Bratton, A. C., Jr. (1951): The anticonvulsant activity of σ-phenyl succinimides. *J. Pharmacol. Exp. Ther.*, 103:54–61.
7. Chen, G. Weston, J. K., and Bratton, A. C., Jr. (1963): Anticonvulsant activity and toxicity of phensuximide, methsuximide and ethosuximide. *Epilepsia*, 4:66–76.
8. Cordoba, E. F., and Strobos, R. R. J. (1956): N-Methyl-α,α-methylphenylsuccinimide in psychomotor epilepsy. *Dis. Nerv. Syst.*, 17:383–385.
9. Davidson, D. T., Lombroso, C., and Markham, C. H. (1955): Methylphenylsuccinimide (Milontin) in epilepsy. *N. Engl. J. Med.*, 253:173–175.
9a. Doig, A., and Stanton, J. B. (1961): Megaloblastic anaemia during combined phensuximide and phenobarbitone therapy. *Br. Med. J.*, 5258:998–999.
10. Dow, R. S., Macfarlane, J. P., and Stevens, J. R.

(1958): Celontin in patients with refractory epilepsy. *J. Lancet,* 78:201–204.

11. Doyle, P. J., Livingston, S., and Pearson, P. H. (1953): Use of Milontin in the treatment of petit mal epilepsy (three per second spike and wave dysrhythmia). *J. Pediatr.,* 43:164–166.

12. Dudley, K. H., Bius, D. L., and Waldrop, C. D. (1974): Urinary metabolites of N-methyl-α-methyl-α-phenylsuccinimide (methsuximide) in the dog. *Drug Metab. Dispos.,* 2:113–122.

13. Dudley, K. H., Butler, T. C., and Bius, D. L. (1974): The role of dihydropyrimidinase in the metabolism of some hydantoin and succinimide drugs. *Drug Metab. Dispos.,* 2:103–112.

14. Ferrendelli, J. A., and Kupferberg, H. J. (1980): Antiepileptic drugs. Succinimides. In: *Antiepileptic Drugs: Mechanisms of Action,* edited by G. H. Glaser, J. K. Penry, and D. M. Woodbury, pp. 587–596. Raven Press, New York.

15. French, E. G., Rey-Bellet, J., and Lennox, W. G. (1958): Methsuximide in psychomotor and petit-mal seizures. *N. Engl. J. Med.,* 258:892–894.

16. Gellman, V. (1965): A case of accidental methsuximide (Celontin) ingestion. *Manitoba Med. Rev.,* 45:141–143.

17. Glazko, A. J., and Dill, W. A. (1972): Other succinimides. Methsuximide and phensuximide. In: *Antiepileptic Drugs,* edited by D. M. Woodbury, J. K. Penry, and R. P. Schmidt, pp. 455–464. Raven Press, New York.

18. Glazko, A. J., Dill, W. A., Wolf, L. M., and Miller, C. A. (1954): The determination and physiological disposition of Milontin (N-methyl-α-phenylsuccinimide). *J. Pharmacol. Exp. Ther.,* 111:113–424.

19. Greeley, R. H. (1974): New approach to derivatization and gas chromatographic analysis of barbiturates. *Clin. Chem.,* 20:192–194.

20. Horning, M. G., Butler, C. M., Lertratanangkoon, K., Hill, R. M., Zion, T. E., and Kellaway, P. (1976): Gas chromatography–mass spectrometry–computer studies of the metabolism of anticonvulsant drugs. In: *Quantitative Analytic Studies in Epilepsy,* edited by P. Kellaway and I. Petersén, pp. 95–114. Raven Press, New York.

21. Johnson, G. F., Least, C. J., Jr., Serum, J. W., Solow, E. B., and Solomon, H. M. (1976): Monitoring drug concentrations in a case of combined overdosage with primidone and methsuximide. *Clin. Chem.,* 22:915–921.

22. Karch, S. B. (1973): Methsuximide overdose. Delayed onset of profound coma. *J.A.M.A.,* 223:1463–1465.

23. Kupferberg, H. J., Yonekawa, W. D., Lacy, J. R., Porter, R. J., and Penry, J. K. (1977): Comparison of methsuximide and phensuximide metabolism in epileptic patients. In: *Antiepileptic Drug Monitoring,* edited by C. Gardner-Thorpe, D. Janz, H. Meinardi, and C. E. Pippenger, pp. 173–180. Pitman Medical, Tunbridge Wells.

24. Lange, E. Fuchs, R., and Kummer, M. (1966): On succinimide therapy—experiences gained using epimide "Spofa." *Psychiatr. Neurol. Med. Psychol. (Leipz.),* 18:109–114.

25. Lereboullet, J., Pluvinage, R., Vidart, L., and Thomas, J. (1953): Treatment of petit mal with phensuximide. *Bull. Soc. Anthrop. Hop. Paris,* 69:87–92.

26. Magyar, I., and Walsa, R. (1966): Antiepileptic value of succinimide derivatives. *Ther. Hung.,* 14:97–107.

27. Miller, C. A., and Long, L. M. (1951): Anticonvulsants. I. An investigation of N-R-α-R₁-α-phenylsuccinimides. *J. Am. Chem. Soc.,* 73:4895–4898.

28. Millichap, J. G. (1952): Milontin: A new drug in the treatment of petit mal. *Lancet,* 2:907–910.

29. Muni, I. A., Altshuler, C. H., and Neicheril, J. C. (1973): Identification of a blood metabolite of methsuximide by GLC–mass spectrometry. *J. Pharm. Sci.,* 62:1820–1823.

30. Nicholls, P. J., and Orton, T. C. (1971): Absorption, distribution and excretion of methsuximide in male rats. *Br. J. Pharmacol.,* 43:459P–460P.

31. Nicholls, P. J., and Orton, T. C. (1972): The physiological disposition of ^{14}C-methsuximide in the rat. *Br. J. Pharmacol.,* 45:48–59.

32. Orton, T. C., and Nicholls, P. J. (1972): Effect in rats of subacute administration of ethosuximide, methsuximide and phensuximide on hepatic microsomal enzymes and porphyrin turnover. *Biochem. Pharmacol.,* 21:2253–2261.

33. Porter, R. J., Penry, J. K., Lacy, J. R., Newmark, M. E., and Kupferberg, H. J. (1979): Plasma concentrations of phensuximide, methsuximide, and their metabolites in relation to clinical efficacy. *Neurology (Minneap.),* 29:1509–1513.

34. Rey-Bellet, J., and Lennox, W. G. (1957): Long-term effects of phensuximide (Milontin). *Arch. Neurol. Psychiatry,* 77:23–27.

35. Sato, T., Asano, S., Yasuda, T., Yamamoto, T., and Kato, M. (1959): Experience with Milontin in the treatment of petit mal seizures. *Jpn. J. Pediatr.,* 12:1120–1131.

36. Scholl, M. L., Abbott, J. A., and Schwab, R. S. (1959): Celontin—a new anticonvulsant. *Epilepsia,* 1:105–109.

37. Schulte, C. J. A., and Good, T. A. (1966): Acute intoxication due to methsuximide and diphenylhydantoin. *J. Pediatr.,* 68:635–637.

38. Schulz, H., and Schulze, H. A. F. (1969): Evaluation of the antiepileptic drug Morfolep on clinical and electroencephalographic basis. *Ther. Hung.,* 17:169–180.

39. Simonyi, J., and Bálint, S. (1968): Use of Morfolep for the treatment of epilepsy. *Ther. Hung.,* 16:159–163.

40. Smith, B., and Forster, F. M. (1953): The role of some experimental anticonvulsants, Mysoline, Milontin, and 1461L. *Med. Ann. D.C.,* 22:279–282,337.

41. Smith, B., and Forster, F. M. (1954): Mysoline and Milontin. Two new medicines for epilepsy. *Neurology (Minneap.),* 4:137–142.

42. Sörgl, H. J. (1967): Treatment of petit mal with Morfolep. *Ther. Hung.,* 15:18–19.

43. Strong, J. M., Abe, T., Gibbs, E. L., and Atkinson, A. J., Jr. (1974): Plasma levels of methsuximide and N-desmethylmethsuximide during methsuximide therapy. *Neurology (Minneap.),* 24:250–255.

44. Volanschi, D., and Florescu, D. (1969): Results of

the treatment with Morfolep in epilepsy. Clinical and electroencephalographic research. *Stud. Cercet Neurol.*, 14:443–457.

45. Volanschi, D., Florescu, D., and Tudor, S. (1971): Results in the treatment of epilepsy with Morfolep. The effects of Morfolep on partial seizures and generalized convulsive seizures. *Rev. Roum. Neurol.*, 8:361–389.

46. Vossen, R. (1958): Anticonvulsant effect of succinimides. *Dtsch. Med. Wochenschr.*, 83:1227–1230.

47. Vurdelja, N., Nikolić, V., Majstorović, M., and Popov, I. (1973): Morfolep in treatment of epilepsy in children. *Neuropsihijatrija*, 19:229–232.

48. Zimmerman, F. T. (1951): Use of methylphenylsuc-

cinimide in treatment of petit mal epilepsy. *Arch. Neurol. Psychiatry*, 66:156–162.

49. Zimmerman, F. T. (1953): New drugs in the treatment of petit mal epilepsy. *Am. J. Psychiatry*, 109:767–773.

50. Zimmerman, F. T. (1954): Milontin® and other new drugs in the treatment of petit mal epilepsy. *South. Med. J.*, 47:929–935.

51. Zimmerman, F. T. (1955): Milontin in the treatment of epilepsy. *N.Y. State J. Med.*, 55:2338–2342.

52. Zimmerman, F. T. (1956): Evaluation of N-methyl-α, α-methylphenyl succinimide in the treatment of petit mal epilepsy. *N.Y. State J. Med.*, 56:1460–1465.

Antiepileptic Drugs, edited by D. M. Woodbury, J. K. Penry, and C. E. Pippenger. Raven Press, New York © 1982.

58

Trimethadione

Chemistry and Methods of Determination

Kenneth H. Dudley, Daniel L. Bius, and Betsy T. King

Trimethadione (TMO) is at present little employed in antiepileptic therapy, its usefulness in the management of absence seizures having been overshadowed by clinical application of ethosuximide (ESM) and valproic acid (VPA) (25). Trimethadione is 3,5,5-trimethyloxazolidine-2,4-dione (Fig. 1), and, as with the other antiepileptics having *N*-alkyl substituents, the drug is extensively degraded by a metabolic *N*-dealkylation reaction (4,11,12,29). The product of trimethadione metabolism is 5,5-dimethyloxazolidine-2,4-dione (DMO, Fig. 1) (4). All present evidence points to the view that chronically administered TMO results in accumulation of DMO in body tissues and that this latter *N*-demethylated metabolite is the agent primarily responsible for the antiepileptic effect of TMO (14,34). This chapter will deal with the chemistry, properties, and methods of determination of both TMO and DMO and will include aspects not described in the previous review (2).

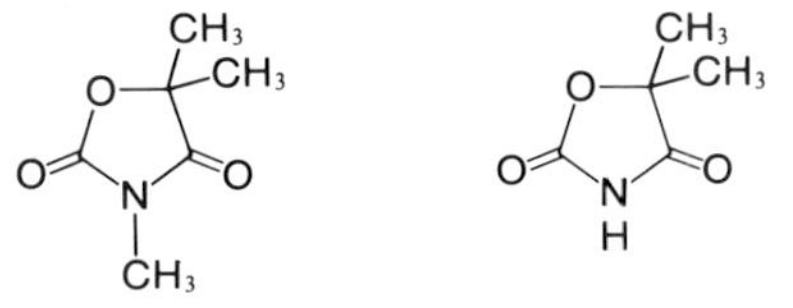

FIG. 1. Structures of trimethadione (TMO) and dimethadione (DMO).

PHYSICAL AND CHEMICAL PROPERTIES

As with most oxazolidine-2,4-diones having simple aliphatic substituents, TMO and DMO are white crystalline solids with low melting points and some degree of solubility in water (Table 1). Dimethadione, which contains the unsubstituted imide group (-CONHCO-), is a weak monobasic acid of pK_a 6.13 (9,35) and is largely ionized at a physiological pH of 7.4. As a general rule (15), the oxazolidine-2,4-diones form stable salts with metal ions, e.g., sodium, potassium, calcium, magnesium, zinc, copper, mercury, and silver. The silver salts are sparingly soluble. The sodium salt of an oxazolidine-2,4-dione is normally quite soluble and stable in aqueous solution, and this property permits quantitative estimations to be made by titrimetry (i.e., titration of the imide function) with dilute sodium hydroxide solution (21,30,31). As an example of salt formation with organic bases, the brucine salt of 5-ethyl-5-methyloxazolidine-2,4-dione (EMO) may be cited for its use in the resolution of the enantiomers of EMO (7).

Oxazolidine-2,4-diones such as DMO are stable in boiling water or dilute mineral acid. Although the sodium salts of oxazolidine-2,4-diones are stable in aqueous solution at ambient

TABLE 1. *Some physical properties of 3,5,5-trimethyloxazolidine-2,4-dione (TMO) and 5,5-dimethyloxazolidine-2,4-dione (DMO)*

Property	TMO	DMO
Molecular weight	143.14	129.11
Melting point (°C)	46[a]	76–77[b]
Boiling point (°C)	78–80/5 mm	—
pK'_a	—	6.13[c,d]
% ionized at pH 7.4	0	94
Solubility in water (w/v)	~5%	>50%
λ_{max} (ϵ)	—	208 (16,900)[e]
I.R.	[f]	[f]

[a]See ref. 30.

[b]See ref. 31.

[c]By radiochemical method at 37°C; ionic strength, 0.16; see ref. 9.

[d]By spectrophotometric method at 37°C; ionic strength, 0.16; see ref. 35.

[e]In 0.1 M phosphate buffer of pH 8 (T. C. Butler, *unpublished results*).

[f]Oxazolidine-2,4-diones show two υCO absorptions at 1828–1812 cm^{-1} (assigned to the 2-oxo group) and 1754–1730 cm^{-1} (assigned to the 4-oxo group). Spectra were determined in CHBr$_3$ solution; see ref. 26.

temperature, prolonged boiling of such solutions or an excess of alkali causes hydrolytic degradation (15). The 3-alkyloxazolidine-2,4-diones, an example being TMO, are moderately stable in dilute mineral acid, but such compounds are rapidly degraded by aqueous alkali (15). Trimethadione can be quantitated by addition of standard 0.1 N sodium hydroxide and back titration with standard acid to the endpoint of phenolphthalein indicator (30). Because of the structural features of the oxazolidine-2,4-dione system, it is possible that as many as three degradation products can be formed by the action of dilute alkali (15). In the cases of TMO and DMO, careful studies have been made of the structures and compositions of the degradation products, but many examples exist in which the structures of the degradation products have been accepted without rigorous proof (15).

Since DMO is the agent that accumulates in plasma and is primarily responsible for the antiepileptic effect in patients receiving chronic TMO therapy, knowledge of the solvent partitioning properties of DMO can be helpful in un-

derstanding and designing reliable analytic methodologies. Some partition ratios of DMO between organic solvents and aqueous 0.2 M potassium dihydrogen phosphate solution are summarized in Table 2.

A unique method based on the relationship of the solvent partitioning of a weak acid with buffers of different pH enables direct identification of suspected DMO in plasma (4). The method is based on equation 1, which was derived by assuming that the ionic form of the compound is confined entirely to the aqueous phase and that the undissociated form is distributed between the organic and aqueous phases with a constant partition coefficient.

$$\log(C_a/C_o - 1) = pH - pK' \qquad [1]$$

where C_a is the partition coefficient of the undissociated form of the acid between the organic and aqueous phases, and C_o is the observed partition ratio for the distribution of total acid, i.e., C_o is a ratio of the concentration of undissociated acid in the organic phase to the total concentration of the acid (ionized and undissociated) in the aqueous phase. Measurement of C_o at two or more values of pH permits calculation of C_a and pK'. One is able to test whether the experimental values of C_o conform

TABLE 2. *Partition ratios (K') of 5,5-dimethyloxazolidine-2,4-dione (DMO) between organic solvents and aqueous 0.2 M potassium dihydrogen phosphate solution*[a]

Organic phase	K'
Heptane	0
Carbon tetrachloride	0.006
Benzene	0.10
1,2-Dichloroethane	0.45
Chloroform	0.53
Ether	1.67
n-Butanol	3.1
Ethyl acetate	5.3

[a]Dimethadione concentrations in the aqueous phases were determined by the spectrophotometric method of Butler (4), and partition ratios were calculated from the formula,

$$K' = \frac{\text{DMO concentration in organic phase}}{\text{DMO concentration in aqueous phase}}$$

with the theoretical relationship to pH. The method has been applied to the identification of other antiepileptic drugs and metabolites in biological fluids (5–7,10).

SYNTHESIS

Several types of methods are available for the synthesis of oxazolidine-2,4-diones (15). The oxazolidine-2,4-diones can be prepared by hydrolytic reactions of heterocyclic intermediates, for example, by hydrolytic reactions of 2-thio-4-oxazolidones, 2-imino-4-oxazolidones, or dialuric acids. Only the routes involving the 2-thio- and 2-imino-4-oxazolidones can provide 5,5-disubstituted oxazolidine-2,4-diones; in those studies in which DMO and/or TMO were prepared by these routes, the yields were acceptable.

Oxazolidine-2,4-diones can also be prepared directly from acyclic intermediates, and these synthetic routes are generally regarded as more satisfactory. Such direct methods for construction of the 5,5-disubstituted oxazolidine-2,4-dione system include condensation of esters of α-hydroxy acids with urea, condensation of amides of α-hydroxy acids with alkyl carbonates or chloroformates, and cyclodehydration of urethans of α-hydroxy acids and their esters. Both ^{14}C-TMO and ^{14}C-DMO, with the ^{14}C label of both compounds being at the 2 position of the oxazolidine-2,4-dione system, have been prepared (9,13). The ^{14}C-DMO was prepared from a reaction of ^{14}C-urea with *n*-butyl-2-methyllactate in a sodium butylate–butanol solution (9). The ^{14}C-TMO was prepared by reaction of ^{14}C-DMO with dimethylsulfate in sodium ethylate–ethanol solution (13). Both of the labeled compounds have been utilized in studies of the metabolism and disposition of TMO (13), and ^{14}C-DMO has been widely employed as the analytical tool in studies of intracellular pH (8,33,35).

METHODS FOR DETERMINATION OF TMO AND DMO

Methods for the determination of TMO and/or DMO have been reviewed by Booker (2) and are summarized in Table 3. A method not cited in Booker's review (2) was the radiochemical technique of Butler et al. (13), a methodology that was developed to study the *N*-demethylation of ^{14}C-TMO by rat liver microsomes. An interesting outcome of this study was the demonstration of competition between TMO and metharbital in the *N*-demethylation reaction, a finding that suggested that these two drugs may be acted on by the same enzymes or, at least, may compete for the same active sites. Since Booker's review (2), the only developments made in the analytical methodology of TMO and DMO have centered on modifications of the gas chromatographic (GC) technique.

In the first GC method reported for TMO (19), serum samples of 5 μl were injected directly onto a 6-ft column of 10% Carbowax-Chromosorb® WAW maintained at an isothermal oven temperature of 140°C. The peak observed for TMO was well-defined and had a retention time of 1.5 min. Under the same conditions, the peak observed for DMO was "broad and not well reproducible," with a retention time of about 30 min. The internal standard method (17) was not employed. Quantitation of TMO was achieved by predetermination of the relationship of the peak area under the TMO peak to the concentration in standard samples. The investigators employed the spectrophotometric method of Butler (4) for the determination of DMO.

With the advent of the method of Booker and

TABLE 3. *Summary of methodologies (1941–1971) used for the detection and determination of 3,5,5-trimethyloxazolidine-2,4-dione (TMO) and of 5,5-dimethyloxazolidine-2,4-dione (DMO)*

Methodology	Compound	References
X-ray diffraction	TMO	24,27
Manometry	TMO	32
Titrimetry	TMO	30
	DMO	31
Radiometry	DMO	13
Spectrophotometry	DMO	4,35
Thin-layer chromatography	TMO	28,36
Gas–liquid chromatography	TMO	19
	TMO,DMO	3

Darcey (3), simultaneous determination of TMO and DMO in the same plasma sample became possible. In that method, a serum sample (2 ml) was acidified with 0.67 N sulfuric acid (1 ml), and 10% sodium tungstate solution (1 ml) was added to precipitate protein. After centrifugation, the protein-free supernatant (2 ml) was transferred and mixed with 0.66 N sulfuric acid (0.1 ml), sodium sulfate (1.5 g), and magnesium sulfate (1.5 g). A chloroform solution (1 ml) containing the internal standard 3-methyl-5-ethyl-5-methyloxazolidine-2,4-dione (para-methadione, PMO) was added, and an extraction was performed. A small volume (5 µl) of the chloroform phase was injected on a 4-ft glass column packed with 3% OV 17 on Gas Chrom Q®. An isothermal oven temperature of 100°C provided excellent base-line resolution of TMO, PMO, and DMO, with all substances being eluted from the column within a 7-min time frame. Midha et al. (23) applied the method to measurements of TMO and DMO in urine and homogenates of various tissues. A major modification of the extraction procedure included "fixing" of the internal standard/drug(s) ratio at the first step of the assay. A solvent evaporation step was also incorporated. The use of a glass column packed with a mixture of 15% Apiezon®-L and 5% OV 225 on Chromosorb® W was found best for the resolution and simultaneous determination of TMO and DMO as isolated in the extracts of tissue homogenates and urine.

Methods capable of determining DMO and/or TMO simultaneously with other antiepileptic agents have been reported. The underivatized method of Griffiths et al. (20) was designed for TMO and 10 other antiepileptic drugs. The procedure entailed extraction of plasma with a 10-fold volume of chloroform, evaporation of the organic extract by impingement with a stream of nitrogen at 25°C, and reconstitution of the dry drug extract in a small volume of methanol containing the internal standard. Methyl myristate was employed as a single internal standard for quantitation of all drugs. Gas chromatography was performed on a 6-ft column packed with 3% OV 17 on Chromosorb® W, and the condi-

tions involved a temperature program. Most of the drugs for which this procedure was designed are known to undergo extensive metabolic conversions to active metabolites. Unfortunately, the procedure does not allow for the determination of the important active metabolites, nor does it even allow for determination of such important drugs as phenytoin (PHT), phenobarbital (PB), and carbamazepine (CBZ). In addition, the overall method and quantitation step are complicated by the fact that calibration of the assay was not performed under the same procedural steps used for unknown samples.

Cremers and Verheesen (16) reported a similar method for the simultaneous determination of TMO and other antiepileptics including the major agents, PHT, PB, and CBZ. The method employed a single 3% OV 225 on Gas Chrom® Q column, but three sets of extraction procedures and GC conditions, with and without on-column methylation for derivatization, were devised in order to deal with the different chemical and chromatographic properties of the drugs. Unfortunately, the method did not entail a capability for determination of DMO or other active metabolites, and it failed to offer compensation for the degradation of PB and CBZ in the on-column methylation reaction (17). For reasons not explained, the authors discouraged the use of the internal standard method.

Löscher and Göbel (22) reported an extraction method that permitted fractionation of TMO, DMO, and seven other antiepileptic agents. The method required a total volume of 1.2 ml of serum and utilized six appropriate internal standards. Selections between two columns packed with 3% OV 17 on Gas Chrom® Q but differing in length and among different oven temperature programs were made depending on which drugs were present in a patient's serum sample. Trimethadione and DMO were isolated in the same extract of serum and were quantitated simultaneously by use of α-methyl-α-propylsuccinimide as the internal standard. The major drugs PHT, PB, CBZ, primidone (PRM), ESM, and VPA, as well as 2-ethyl-2-phenylmalondiamide, the ring-cleaved metabolite of PRM, could also be quantitated.

Certain comments are warranted as regards the current state of the art of GC methods for TMO and DMO. Methods that overlook or disclaim the usefulness of the internal standard method should be given cautious consideration, if not avoided, before adoption in therapeutic monitoring programs. Any method that utilizes an internal standard in the determination of unknown drug concentration but depends on measurement of an absolute parameter for calibration of an assay, should as well be cautiously employed. Such a method has inherent complications and potential pitfalls in the calculation of accurate analytical results, although these are problems that could be eliminated entirely by adherence to recommended guidelines of the internal standard method (17).

Another aspect deserving of comment regards the "recovery yield of DMO" and recent modifications that make use of solvent evaporation steps as a means to concentrate final organic extracts of DMO and TMO. Booker and Darcey (3) recognized that the chloroform extraction step of their procedure provided a low recovery of DMO, and they took appropriate measures, avoiding solvent evaporation, to increase recovery yield. They added dry quantities of certain inorganic sulfates to the aqueous phase as a means of "salting out" the metabolite. By consideration of the partition ratio (K') of DMO between chloroform and dihydrogen phosphate solution (Table 2) and of the procedural steps of the Booker and Darcey method (3), the theoretical calculation (18) can be made that the final chloroform extract, in the absence of inorganic sulfates in the aqueous phase, should contain about 20% of the initial amount of DMO in a 1-ml plasma sample. Booker and Darcey (3) determined experimentally that the recovery of DMO was 15% in the absence of added sulfates but 88% in the presence of saturating quantities of both sodium and magnesium sulfate at pH 3 or less.

However, the more recent attempts to improve methodologies for TMO and DMO by incorporation of solvent-evaporation steps (16,20,23) now raise a question concerned with the validity of such procedures. The practice of vacuum drying of drug extracts containing the oxazolidine-2,4-dione drugs has been generally avoided, since the volatility of these substances results in considerable loss. Some investigators, however, have relied on the practice of impingement with air or nitrogen at temperatures less than 50°C to concentrate organic solutions of these drug extracts. Controlled studies in our laboratory have shown that such "impingement methods" also result in considerable loss of either TMO or DMO. For example, triplicate samples containing 54 μg of TMO and 700 μg of DMO were made up in 5 ml of a 3 : 1 methylene chloride–diethyl ether solvent system. When the series of samples was taken to dryness by impingement with nitrogen at 25°C, about 49% of the TMO and 21% of the DMO were lost. When the same experiment was carried out on a Buchler Vortex-Evaporator® (vacuum drying without heat), about 89% of the TMO and 20% of the DMO were lost.

In a method developed recently in our laboratory primarily for simultaneous determination of TMO and DMO, solvent-evaporation steps of any type were avoided. Partition ratio (K') data were considered as a technical aid (18) to optimize drug recoveries in order to eliminate the necessity of adding weighed amounts of dry inorganic salts to plasma samples, i.e., to avoid cumbersome manipulations required for "salting out" DMO. In addition, calibration of the assay and determination of unknown samples were performed by the same procedural steps in adherence to guidelines of the internal standard method (17).

In this method (1), plasma (1 ml) and 1 N sulfuric acid (0.5 ml) containing internal standards (125 μg of PMO for quantitation of TMO and 400 μg of α,α,β-trimethylsuccinimide for quantitation of DMO) were added to a 10-ml centrifuge tube. With vortexing, a 10% sodium tungstate solution (0.5 ml) was added drop by drop to precipitate protein, and the mixture was allowed to stand (25°C, 15 min) and centrifuged. As much as possible of the supernatant liquid was transferred to a clean centrifuge tube, a 0.5-ml volume of methylene chloride : diethyl ether (3 : 1) was added, and an

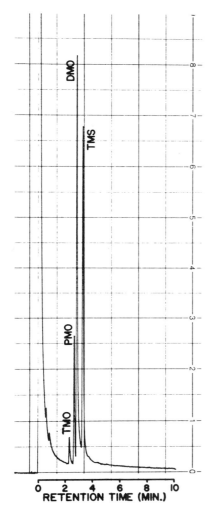

FIG. 2. Gas chromatogram of final extract from acidified human plasma spiked with TMO (36 µg/ml), DMO (1,200 µg/ml), PMO (125 µg/ml), and TMS (400 µg/ml). Abbreviations are explained in text.

extraction was performed. A 1-µl sample of the organic phase was removed for GC analysis. Chromatography was performed on a 1.8 m × 2 mm (i.d.) glass column packed with 3% DC-LSX-3-0295 on Gas Chrom® Q (120–140 mesh). An oven temperature program was employed. The initial temperature was 100°C (zero hold time), the rate of temperature rise was 16°/min, and the final temperature was 200°C (zero hold time). Calibration samples were constituted in blank human plasma to enable determination of

TMO in the range of 6 to 54 µg/ml and DMO in the range of 200 to 1,800 µg/ml. The recovery of TMO was essentially quantitative; DMO, 74%. A typical chromatogram is shown in Fig. 2.

CONVERSION

Trimethadione

Conversion factor:

$$CF = \frac{1000}{\text{mol. wt.}} = \frac{1000}{143.1} = 6.99$$

Conversion:

$$(\mu g/ml) \times 6.99 = (\mu moles/liter)$$
$$(\mu moles/liter) \div 6.99 = (\mu g/ml)$$

Dimethadione

Conversion factor:

$$CF = \frac{1000}{\text{mol. wt.}} = \frac{1000}{129.1} = 7.75$$

Conversion:

$$(\mu g/ml) \times 7.75 = (\mu moles/liter)$$
$$(\mu moles/liter) \div 7.75 = (\mu g/ml)$$

ACKNOWLEDGMENT

Support by U.S. Public Health Service Research Grant NS 12791 from the National Institute of Neurological and Communicative Disorders and Stroke is gratefully acknowledged.

REFERENCES

1. Bius, D. L., Teague, B. L., and Dudley, K. H. (1979): Simultaneous gas chromatographic determination of trimethadione and dimethadione in human plasma. *Ther. Drug Monitor.*, 1:495–505.
2. Booker, H. E. (1972): Trimethadione and other oxazolidinediones: Chemistry and methods for determination. In: *Antiepileptic Drugs*, edited by D. M. Woodbury, J. K. Penry, and R. P. Schmidt, pp. 385–393. Raven Press, New York.
3. Booker, H. E., and Darcey, B. (1971): Simultaneous determination of trimethadione and its metabolite, dimethadione, by gas–liquid chromatography. *Clin. Chem.*, 17:607–609.

4. Butler, T. C. (1953): Quantitative studies of the demethylation of trimethadione (Tridione). *J. Pharmacol. Exp. Ther.*, 108:11–17.

5. Butler, T. C. (1953): Quantitative studies of the demethylation of *N*-methyl barbital (metharbital, Gemonil). *J. Pharmacol. Exp. Ther.*, 108:474–480.

6. Butler, T. C. (1953): Quantitative studies of the physiological disposition of 3-methyl-5-ethyl-5-phenylhydantoin (Mesantoin) and 5-ethyl-5-phenylhydantoin (Nirvanol). *J. Pharmacol. Exp. Ther.*, 109:340–345.

7. Butler, T. C. (1955): Metabolic demethylation of 3,5-dimethyl-5-ethyl-2,4-oxazolidinedione (paramethadione, Paradione). *J. Pharmacol. Exp. Ther.*, 113:178–185.

8. Butler, T. C. (1965): The use of DMO-2-^{14}C (5,5-dimethyl-2,4-oxazolidinedione-2-^{14}C) and inulin-carboxyl-^{14}C for measurement of intracellular pH. In: *Advances in Tracer Methodology*, edited by S. Rothchild, pp. 189–192. Plenum Press, New York.

9. Butler, T. C., and Davidson, J. D. (1963): Synthesis of 5,5-dimethyl-2,4-oxazolidine-2-^{14}C (DMO-2-^{14}C). *J. Pharm. Sci.*, 52:1110–1111.

10. Butler, T. C., Mahaffee, C., and Waddell, W. J. (1954): Phenobarbital: Studies of elimination, accumulation, tolerance, and dosage schedules. *J. Pharmacol. Exp. Ther.*, 111:425–435.

11. Butler, T. C., Mahaffee, D., and Mahaffee, C. (1952): Metabolic demethylation of 3,5,5-trimethyl-2,4-oxazolidinedione (trimethadione, Tridione). *Proc. Soc. Exp. Biol. Med.*, 81:450–452.

12. Butler, T. C., and Waddell, W. J. (1954): The role of the liver in the demethylation of *N*-methyl derivatives of hydantoin and of 2,4-oxazolidinedione. *J. Pharmacol. Exp. Ther.*, 110:241–243.

13. Butler, T. C., Waddell, W. J., and Poole, D. T. (1965): Demethylation of trimethadione and metharbital by rat liver microsomal enzymes: Substrate concentration–yield relationships and competition between substrates. *Biochem. Pharmacol.*, 14:937–942.

14. Chamberlin, H. R., Waddell, W. J., and Butler, T. C. (1965): A study of the product of demethylation of trimethadione in the control of petit mal epilepsy. *Neurology (Minneap.)*, 15:449–454.

15. Clark-Lewis, J. W. (1958): 2,4-Oxazolidinediones. *Chem. Rev.*, 58:63–99.

16. Cremers, H. M. H. G., and Verheesen, P. E. (1973): A rapid method for the estimation of anti-epileptic drugs in blood serum by gas–liquid chromatography. *Clin. Chim. Acta*, 48:413–420.

17. Dudley, K. H. (1978): Internal standards in gas–liquid chromatographic determination of antiepileptic drugs. In: *Antiepileptic Drugs: Quantitative Analysis and Interpretation*, edited by C. E. Pippenger, J. K. Penry, and H. Kutt, pp. 19–34. Raven Press, New York.

18. Dudley, K. H. (1978): Use of the partition ratio in studies of antiepileptic drugs. In: *Antiepileptic Drugs: Quantitative Analysis and Interpretation*, edited by C. E. Pippenger, J. K. Penry, and H. Kutt, pp. 43–54. Raven Press, New York.

19. Frey, H.-H., and Schulz, R. (1970): Time course of the demethylation of trimethadione. *Acta Pharmacol. Toxicol. (Kbh.)*, 28:477–483.

20. Griffiths, W. C., Oleksyk, S. K., Dextraze, P., and

21. Diamond, I. (1973): The gas chromatographic determination of anticonvulsant drugs in serum. *Ann. Clin. Lab. Sci.*, 3:369–373.

21. King, F. E., and Clark-Lewis, J. W. (1951): The structure of some supposed azetid-2:4-diones. Part II. Derivatives of tartronic acid. *J. Chem. Soc.*, 3077–3079.

22. Löscher, W., and Göbel, W. (1978): Consecutive gas chromatographic determination of phenytoin, phenobarbital, primidone, phenylethylmalondiamide, carbamazepine, trimethadione, dimethadione, ethosuximide, and valproate from the same serum specimen. *Epilepsia*, 19:463–473.

23. Midha, K. K., Buttar, H. S., Rowe, H., and Dupuis, I. (1979): Metabolism and disposition of trimethadione in pregnant rats. *Epilepsia*, 20:417–423.

24. Penprase, W. G., and Biles, J. A. (1958): Microscopic and X-ray diffraction methods for the identification of sedatives and anticonvulsants. *J. Am. Pharm. Assoc.*, 47:523–528.

25. Penry, J. K., and Newmark, M. E. (1979): The use of antiepileptic drugs. *Ann. Intern. Med.*, 90:207–218.

26. Pianka, M., and Polton, D. J. (1960): Preparation of 3-substituted oxazolid-2,4-diones by cyclisation of *N*-substituted *N*-chloracylcarbamates. *J. Chem. Soc.*, 983–989.

27. Roy, J., Gadret, M., and Bregere, C. (1964): Analytical application of X-ray diffraction. VII. Diffraction spectra of some ursides, hydantoins, and barbiturate analogs. *Bull. Soc. Pharm. Bordeaux*, 103:3–8.

28. Sarsunova, M., and Tran-Thi-Hoang-Ba (1966): Separation of some drugs from the hypnotic and antiepileptic groups on poured layers of aluminum oxide. IX. *Cesk. Farm.*, 15:522–525.

29. Smith, J. A., Waddell, W. J., and Butler, T. C. (1963): Demethylation of *N*-methyl derivatives of barbituric acid, hydantoin, and 2,4-oxazolidinedione by rat liver microsomes. *Life Sci.*, 2:486–492.

30. Spielman, M. A. (1944): Some analgesic agents derived from oxazolidine-2,4-dione. *J. Am. Chem. Soc.*, 66:1244–1245.

31. Stoughton, R. W. (1941): 5,5-Dialkyl-2,4-oxazolidinediones. *J. Am. Chem. Soc.*, 63:2376–2379.

32. Taylor, J. D., and Bertcher, E. L. (1952): The determination and distribution of trimethadione (Tridione) in animal tissues. *J. Pharmacol. Exp. Ther.*, 106:277–285.

33. Waddell, W. J., and Bates, R. G. (1969): Intracellular pH. *Physiol. Rev.*, 49:285–329.

34. Waddell, W. J., and Butler, T. C. (1958): *N*-Methylated derivatives of barbituric acid, hydantoin, and oxazolidinedione used in the treatment of epilepsy. *Neurology (Minneap.)*, 8(Suppl. 1):106–112.

35. Waddell, W. J., and Butler, T. C. (1959): Calculation of intracellular pH from the distribution of 5,5-dimethyl-2,4-oxazolidinedione (DMO). Application to skeletal muscle of dog. *J. Clin. Invest.*, 38:720–729.

36. Yamamoto, J., Suzuki, M., and Okuo, S. (1965): Separation and quantitative analysis of pharmaceuticals. I. Identification and determination of anticonvulsive agents by thin-layer chromatography. *Yakuzaigaku*, 25:23–26.

Antiepileptic Drugs, edited by D. M. Woodbury, J. K. Penry, and C. E. Pippenger. Raven Press, New York © 1982.

59

Trimethadione

Absorption, Distribution, and Excretion

C. D. Withrow

Trimethadione (TMO) is rapidly and almost completely converted *in vivo* to dimethadione (DMO). Dimethadione is not further degraded and accumulates in large quantities when TMO is administered chronically for the treatment of epilepsy. Although the parent drug, TMO, can protect against seizures, it is now well established that DMO has anticonvulsant properties and that the accumulation of this active metabolite accounts for most of the antiseizure effects resulting from TMO treatment. (See Chapter 64 for references.) The pharmacokinetics and pharmacodynamics of DMO are therefore discussed here and in Chapters 60, 61, and 64 with the intent that the pharmacology of TMO will be better understood and placed in its proper therapeutic perspective. Included for completeness is a brief discussion of the pharmacology of paramethadione (PMO), the only other oxazolidinedione anticonvulsant drug available in the United States today.

TRIMETHADIONE

Absorption

Direct measurements of the rate of absorption of TMO after oral administration have been made in a single animal experiment. By use of a new gas chromatographic method for TMO analysis,

Frey and Schulz (16) showed that after the oral administration of single doses of TMO to three dogs, the concentration of TMO in serum rose rapidly, the maximal concentrations being reached after 1 hr in two animals and after 3 hr in the third.

In normal human volunteers, Booker (1) found that peak serum levels of TMO occurred 30 min after oral TMO administration. Other studies of the oral absorption of TMO in humans have involved measurement of the appearance of the demethylated metabolite, DMO, in plasma after oral administration of TMO (2,8,18). Although these experiments clearly indicate that TMO is absorbed when given orally, the observations are difficult to interpret quantitatively, since DMO accumulates in serum (8,18).

Numerous animal experiments have indicated directly and indirectly that TMO is rapidly absorbed from various sites. Taylor and Bertcher (34) found that blood levels of TMO were maximal 15 min after intraperitoneal injection. These results are in agreement with those of Theuson et al. (35) who showed that TMO rapidly appeared in plasma after intraperitoneal administration of radioactive TMO to rats. Chen et al. (9) reported significant protection of TMO-treated rats against pentylenetetrazol-induced seizures 30 min after oral administration of the drug. Ferngren (14) demonstrated that TMO injected subcutaneously gives significant protection against pentylenetetrazol when tested 30 min later. Swinyard et al. (32) showed that the time of peak anticonvulsant effects of TMO is 1½ hr and 1 hr after subcutaneous injection in rats and mice, respectively. Other reports have concluded that TMO given intraperitoneally is an effective anticonvulsant (17,39). However, the use of an anticonvulsant end point to estimate TMO concentrations can be misleading because TMO is rapidly demethylated to DMO, a compound that has anticonvulsant properties of its own (8,39). Richards and Everett (27) found that there was little difference between the doses of TMO necessary to cause ataxia when the drug was injected intravenously, intraperitoneally, or subcutaneously. An ataxia-producing dose given orally to mice showed its effects in 2 to 3 min. Tying the pylorus delayed this action for about 25 min, a finding that suggests that TMO is absorbed slowly from the stomach.

Distribution

The distribution of TMO has been studied directly in experimental animals. Trimethadione dispersed into a volume approximately equal to 60% of the body weight of mice (16). The apparent volume of distribution of TMO was found to be about 60% of body weight, a value approximately equal to total body water, in a single dog (16). In the same experiments, however, the volume of distribution of TMO was calculated to be about 90% of body weight in two other dogs. Theuson et al. (35) observed that TMO given intraperitoneally had an apparent volume of distribution of 82% of body weight.

In humans, the volume of distribution of TMO was found to be 60% of body weight (1).

Taylor and Bertcher (34) developed a manometric analytical method for TMO and determined the concentration–time relationship in the major organs of the mouse and also the distribution of the drug within the various anatomical regions of rabbit brain. Thirty minutes after it was injected into the peritoneal cavity of mice,

TMO was found in blood, brain, muscle, kidney, and liver. At 30 min, tissue/blood ratios were 0.61, 0.75, 0.94, and 0.62 for brain, kidney, muscle, and liver, respectively. The concentration of TMO decreased rapidly in blood and brain but declined more slowly in kidney. Brain-to-blood ratios, however, remained constant from 15 min to 3 hr after injection. Muscle concentrations of TMO remained stable for 6 hr, then declined. Liver concentrations of TMO increased after injection, reaching a maximum 2 hr later, and then declined slowly. Trimethadione could be detected in muscle and liver 10 and 12 hr, respectively, after administration. No significant differences in the concentrations of TMO in the cortex, white matter, and cerebellum of the rabbit brain were found 30 min after the intraperitoneal injection of the drug. Theuson et al. (35) synthesized radioactive TMO and carefully determined its uptake into several tissues of the rat after intraperitoneal injection. Trimethadione was passively distributed within 1 hr in cerebrospinal fluid and in the tissue water of the cerebral cortex, skeletal muscle, and the gastrointestinal tract. Trimethadione tissue-to-plasma ratios in liver, cardiac muscle, and salivary gland were 7 to 11% higher than ratios predicted from the water content of these tissues and of plasma, a finding perhaps attributable to contamination with bile and blood, blood, and saliva, respectively.

The disposition of TMO has been studied in the pregnant rat by Midha et al. (23). A single dose of TMO was given by gavage to pregnant animals during days 6 through 15 of gestation. Trimethadione concentrations in several fluids and tissues were measured 6, 12, and 24 hr after the last daily treatment. Small amounts of TMO were found in plasma, liver, brain, placenta, and the whole fetus 6 hr after the last TMO dose. Within 24 hr, TMO levels in plasma, placenta, and the whole fetus had decreased to trace amounts, but TMO concentrations in liver and brain declined more slowly. Trimethadione appears to reach effective concentrations rapidly in immature mouse brain, since subcutaneous injection of the drug protects mice against electroshock and chemical challenges 30 min later (14,15).

The binding of TMO to serum albumin in humans and dogs has been reported to be 8 to 11% and 6.5 to 9%, respectively (21). The binding of TMO to tissue and proteins has not been studied. However, tissue-to-blood ratios of 0.61 to 0.94, with wide variation, suggest that TMO is not significantly bound or actively transported in any of the tissues studied. Volumes of distribution of TMO of approximately 60% of body weight indicate that TMO is not bound and is passively distributed. There is no clear explanation of the reported volumes of distribution of TMO that exceed total body water.

Excretion

Several experiments have shown directly that only small amounts of unchanged TMO—less than 3%—are excreted by the rat (34,35). In humans, Richards and Everett (27) found that only about 50 mg of unchanged TMO was recovered in the urine 8 hr after the administration of 2.0 g of the drug. Booker (1) has reported that approximately 4% of the daily dose of TMO is excreted unchanged in the urine of patients on continuous TMO dosage. Swinyard et al. (33) provided indirect evidence that little unmetabolized TMO or its active metabolite is excreted by the kidney, since bilateral nephrectomy had no effect on the duration or potency of the anticonvulsant effects of TMO in rats. The data of Richards and Everett (27) vary somewhat from those of Swinyard and co-workers in that bilateral nephrectomy slightly prolonged the anticonvulsant effects of TMO in mice and markedly prolonged the hypnotic effects in rats. It should be emphasized again, however, that TMO is converted to an active anticonvulsant, DMO. Since this compound (DMO) is excreted unchanged by the kidney (4,37), interpretation of nephrectomy experiments must be made cautiously. Withrow et al. (39) have suggested a possible enterohepatic biliary circulation of TMO, but this has not been verified by direct

observations (35). Essentially nothing is known about the excretion of TMO by other routes.

DIMETHADIONE

Although DMO has been shown to have anticonvulsant properties in humans (8) and in experimental animals (39), it is not an official drug. The inclusion of a discussion of the pharmacology of DMO here and in Chapters 60, 61, and 64 is justified by the intimate relationships between TMO and DMO mentioned earlier. It is not possible to understand fully the pharmacodynamics of TMO without an appreciation of the pharmacodynamics of DMO.

Absorption

Dimethadione is a weak acid with a pK_a of 6.13 at 37°C. Absorption of the un-ionized form from the stomach, with a low pH, would therefore be expected to be rapid, but absorption should be expected to be less efficient from the more alkaline small intestine. In experimental animals, rapid absorption after intraperitoneal injection is shown by the quick onset of anticonvulsant effects (39). In humans, anticonvulsant effects after single doses are not reliable indicators of absorption because even complete absorption of a single dose of DMO used in drug trials would not give blood levels of the drug sufficient to affect seizures predictably.

Distribution

The distribution of DMO has been studied in detail because of the extensive use of this agent to measure intracellular pH (36,38) and because specific analytical methods exist for its determination. The volume of distribution of DMO is about 40% of body weight, a space value somewhere between extracellular fluid and total body water volumes. The distribution of DMO is not affected by binding to either plasma or tissue (12,21,38), but it is affected by changes in extracellular or intracellular acid–base values (38). It is rapidly taken up in every tissue studied, including mitochondria (36). In the experiments of Theuson et al. (35), DMO derived from the biotransformation of TMO was found within 1 hr in all tissues and fluids studied—cerebral cortex, cerebrospinal fluid, liver, cardiac muscle, salivary gland, skeletal muscle, and gastrointestinal tract plus contents. Midha et al. (23) found that the treatment of pregnant rats with TMO for several days of gestation resulted in the accumulation of large quantities of DMO in the placenta as well as in fetal liver and brain. Whole-body pH measurements in humans have used a 240-min equilibration period (22). In brain and cerebrospinal fluid (CSF), constant plasma-to-tissue or plasma-to-CSF ratios have been observed in 1 to 4 hr after intravenous injection (20,29,30).

Active transport of DMO by rat intestine (13) and by isolated rumen epithelium (31) has been reported. Active transport of DMO did not occur in skeletal muscle, Ehrlich ascites tumor cells, platelets, or beef heart mitochondria (7). Rollins and Reed (29) have shown that DMO is transported out of CSF in rats, but Kaplan and Pollay (19) did not find active transport of DMO out of this fluid. It is clear, however, that DMO levels in CSF are lower than those predicted from the pH gradient between blood and CSF (11,26,30). Thus, DMO may not be suitable for estimation of CSF pH. The precise effects that the low CSF values of DMO have on brain-cell pH estimates have not been established. The important point is that the CSF transport system for DMO has only slight effects on brain total DMO levels, at least in acute, single-dose experiments (29). Indirect evidence that DMO rapidly reaches effective concentrations in the brain of immature mice is provided by the experiments of Ferngren (14) and Ferngren and Paalzow (15). These workers showed that DMO prevents electroshock- and pentylenetetrazol-induced seizures in newborn and maturing mice between 1 and 21 days of age just 30 min after subcutaneous injection. Roos (30) did not find regional differences in DMO distribution in brain, since intracellular pH calculated by the DMO method was the same in cerebral cortex, cere-bellum, floor of the fourth ventricle, caudate nucleus, and cerebral white matter.

Excretion

Dimethadione is excreted unchanged by the kidney (37), but excretion is very slow. In dogs and humans, about 6% of the compound is excreted daily (6,16,18). Increased plasma levels and residual drug effects have been detected days or weeks after discontinuation of the drug. In normal male rats given tracer doses of TMO, 8% of the administered dose of TMO was recovered as DMO in urine collected for 24 hr after drug treatment (35). Dimethadione excretion in the pregnant rat appears to be faster than in male rats, since between 60 and 80% of an oral TMO dose was excreted in urine as DMO in 24 hr (23). Alkalinization of the urine with sodium bicarbonate or with acetazolamide treatment enhanced the excretion of DMO in humans and dogs (18,37). Since the amount of undissociated DMO is decreased in alkaline urine, and only this form undergoes tubular reabsorption, the urinary excretion of DMO is increased.

Dimethadione appeared promptly in pancreatic juice and bile when it was injected intravenously into dogs in which pancreatic juice production and bile flow were being stimulated with the continuous infusion of secretin (25). Furthermore, single injections of secretin enhanced DMO excretion in pancreatic juice and bile in dogs treated 90 min earlier with DMO (25). Treatment with secretin and cholecystokinin caused an increase in DMO excretion by the pancreas of normal humans treated with TMO for 3 days prior to testing (24). The excretion of DMO by other routes has not been studied.

The very slow renal excretion of DMO coupled with the lack of metabolism of DMO (see Chapter 60) has two consequences. First, since the usual daily anticonvulsant doses of TMO or DMO do not yield maximally effective blood levels of the drugs until several days after treatment begins, it is not surprising that it takes a few days for the antiseizure effects of TMO or

DMO to become evident (8,17). For example, Chamberlin et al. (8) have calculated that DMO will accumulate in the body until the total amount is 14.3 times the daily dose and that 90% of the equilibrium value is reached in 30 days. Second, the cessation of TMO or DMO treatment does not result in immediate increased seizure activity since the blood concentrations of the drugs decrease slowly. This observation has been made in humans treated with TMO and DMO (17). The short duration (several hours) of DMO anticonvulsant effects in rats after a single dose of the drug may result from redistribution, since significant excretion of DMO takes several days (16,18). The brief duration of analgesia in humans after one dose of TMO (28) could be the result of either redistribution of TMO or its conversion to DMO.

PARAMETHADIONE

Absorption

Swinyard et al. (33) have found that the time of peak anticonvulsant effects of PMO after subcutaneous injection is 1½ and 1 hr in mice and rats, respectively. These times are identical to those reported for TMO and indicate rapid absorption of the drug.

Distribution

The distribution of unmetabolized PMO has not been studied. Constant (11), however, has demonstrated that demethylated PMO levels in the posterior and anterior chambers of the eye exceed those in plasma but that less drug is found in CSF than in plasma. The total distribution of demethylated PMO was about 37% of body weight in mice (5) and 39 and 49% in two men given the drug orally (3).

Excretion

Only indirect information is available concerning the excretion of PMO. Swinyard et al. (33) found that bilateral nephrectomy increased

both the potency and the duration of the anticonvulsant effects of PMO. This suggests that either PMO or an active metabolite is excreted by the kidney. Butler (3) later showed that demethylated PMO is excreted by the kidney. In dogs, the rate of renal excretion of demethylated PMO is slower than that of DMO, but the rate of disappearance of demethylated PMO from the plasma of humans (25 to 45% per week) is comparable to that of DMO in humans (35% per week) (3). The effects of urinary pH on demethylated PMO excretion have not been determined. However, since the pK_a of this compound is 5.9 (10), alkalinization of the urine would be expected to increase its renal excretion. The demethylated product is excreted more rapidly in mice than in dogs (5).

SUMMARY

Trimethadione and PMO are rapidly absorbed from the gastrointestinal tract and other sites. They are distributed evenly in body water and do not appear to be bound or actively transported. The two drugs are demethylated by liver microsomes to DMO and the corresponding metabolite of PMO. Almost no unmetabolized TMO or PMO is excreted. Both metabolites are active anticonvulsants and contribute to the total effects of the parent drugs. The N-demethylated compounds are not distributed evenly in body water since their distribution is affected by pH gradients and, perhaps in some instances, by active transport mechanisms. Dimethadione has been found not to bind to plasma or muscle protein. The most remarkable fact concerning the absorption, distribution, and excretion of the oxazolidinediones is the persistence of DMO and N-desmethyl-PMO. The rate of disappearance of these two compounds is 35 to 40% per week.

ACKNOWLEDGMENTS

Supported in part by a U.S. Public Health Service Program Project Grant I-POI-NS-15767 from the National Institute of Neurological and

Communicative Disorders and Stroke. The expert secretarial assistance of Mrs. C. Bawden is greatly appreciated.

REFERENCES

1. Booker, H. E. (1972): Trimethadione and other oxazolidinediones. Relation of plasma levels to clinical control. In: *Antiepileptic Drugs*, edited by D. M. Woodbury, J. K. Penry, and R. P. Schmidt, pp. 403–407. Raven Press, New York.
2. Butler, T. C. (1953): Quantitative studies of the demethylation of trimethadione (Tridione®). *J. Pharmacol. Exp. Ther.*, 108:11–17.
3. Butler, T. C. (1955): Metabolic demethylation of 3,5-dimethyl-5-ethyl-2,4-oxazolidinedione (paramethadione, Paradione®). *J. Pharmacol. Exp. Ther.*, 113:178–185.
4. Butler, T. C., Mahaffee, D., and Mahaffee, C. (1952): Metabolic demethylation of 3,5,5-trimethyl-2,4-oxazolidinedione (trimethadione, Tridione®). *Proc. Soc. Exp. Biol. Med.*, 81:450–452.
5. Butler, T. C., and Waddell, W. J. (1955): A pharmacological comparison of the optical isomers of 5-ethyl-5-methyl-2,4-oxazolidinedione and of 3,5-dimethyl-5-ethyl-2,4-oxazolidinedione (paramethadione, Paradione®). *J. Pharmacol. Exp. Ther.*, 113:238–240.
6. Butler, T. C., and Waddell, W. J. (1958): *N*-Methylated derivatives of barbituric acid, hydantoin and oxazolidinedione used in the treatment of epilepsy. *Neurology (Minneap.)*, 8:106–112.
7. Butler, T. C., Waddell, W. J., and Poole, D. T. (1967): Intracellular pH based on the distribution of weak electrolytes. *Fed. Proc.*, 26:1327–1332.
8. Chamberlin, H. R., Waddell, W. J., and Butler, T. C. (1965): A study of the product of demethylation of trimethadione in the control of petit mal epilepsy. *Neurology (Minneap.)*, 15:449–454.
9. Chen, G., Ensor, C. R., and Clarke, I. G. (1951): Central nervous action of hydantoins, oxazolidinediones and thiazolidones. *Arch. Neurol. Psychiatry*, 66:329–337.
10. Clark-Lewis, J. W. (1958): 2,4-Oxazolidinediones. *Chem. Rev.*, 48:63–99.
11. Constant, M. A. (1961): The distribution of 5,5-dimethyl-2,4-oxazolidinedione (DMO) in ocular and cerebrospinal fluids. *Am. J. Ophthalmol.*, 51:969–976.
12. Constant, M. A. (1962): The distribution of 5,5-dimethyl-2,4-oxazolidinedione (DMO). II. Studies on the effect of carbonic anhydrase inhibitors and of plasma levels. *Invest. Ophthalmol.*, 1:609–617.
13. Dietschy, J. M., and Carter, N. W. (1965): Active transport of 5,5-dimethyl-2,4-oxazolidinedione. *Science*, 150:1294–1296.
14. Ferngren, H. (1968): Further studies on chemically induced seizures and their antagonism by anticonvulsants during postnatal development in the mouse. *Acta Pharmacol. Toxicol. (Kbh.)*, 26:177–188.
15. Ferngren, H., and Paalzow, L. (1969): High frequency electroshock seizures and their antagonism during postnatal development in the mouse. II. Effects of phenobarbital, sodium mephobarbital, trimethadione, dimethadione, ethosuximide and acetazolamide. *Acta Pharmacol. Toxicol. (Kbh.)*, 27:249–261.
16. Frey, H.-H., and Schulz, R. (1970): Time course of the demethylation of trimethadione. *Acta Pharmacol. Toxicol. (Kbh.)*, 28:477–483.
17. Goodman, L. S., Toman, J. E. P., and Swinyard, E. A. (1946): The anticonvulsant properties of Tridione®. *Am. J. Med.*, 1:213–288.
18. Jensen, B. N. (1962): Trimethadione in serum of patients with petit mal epilepsy. *Dan. Med. Bull.*, 9:74–79.
19. Kaplan, R. J., and Pollay, M. (1970): The movement of 5,5-dimethyl-2,4-oxazolidimedione (DMO) between CSF and plasma. *Life Sci.*, 9:625–629.
20. Kibler, R. F., O'Neill, R. P., and Robin, E. D. (1964): Intracellular acid–base relations of dog brain with reference to the brain extracellular volume. *J. Clin. Invest.*, 43:431–443.
21. Loscher, W. (1979): A comparative study of the protein binding of anticonvulsant drugs in serum of dog and man. *J. Pharmacol. Exp. Ther.*, 208:429–435.
22. Manfredi, F. (1963): Calculation of total body intracellular pH in normal human subjects from the distribution of 5,5-dimethyl-2,4-oxazolidinedione (DMO). *J. Lab. Clin. Med.*, 61:1005–1014.
23. Midha, K. K., Buttar, H. S., Rowe, M., and Dupuis, I. (1979): Metabolism and disposition of trimethadione in pregnant rats. *Epilepsia*, 20:417–423.
24. Noda, A., Hayakawa, T., Nakajima, S., Suzuki, T., and Toda, Y. (1975): Pancreatic excretion of 5,5-dimethyl-2,4-oxazolidinedione in normal subjects. *Dig. Dis.*, 20:1011–1018.
25. Noda, A., Toda, Y., Hayakawa, T., and Nakajima, S. (1973): The excretion of 5,5-dimethyl-2,4-oxazolidinedione from the canine pancreas and liver. *Dig. Dis.*, 18:498–505.
26. Reed, D. J., Withrow, C. D., and Woodbury, D. M. (1967): Electrolyte and acid-base parameters of rat cerebrospinal fluid. *Exp. Brain Res.*, 3:212–219.
27. Richards, R. K., and Everett, G. M. (1946): Tridione®: A new anticonvulsant drug. *J. Lab. Clin. Med.*, 31:1330–1336.
28. Richards, R. K., Everett, G. M., and Pickrell, K. L. (1946): Pharmacological and clinical studies of Tridione® with special reference to its analgesic action. *Anesth. Analg. (Cleve.)*, 25:147–151.
29. Rollins, D. E., and Reed, D. J. (1970): Transport of DMO out of cerebrospinal fluid of rats. *Am. J. Physiol.*, 219:1200–1204.
30. Roos, A. (1965): Intracellular pH and intracellular buffering power of the cat brain. *Am. J. Physiol.*, 209:1233–1246.
31. Stevens, C. E., Dobson, A., and Mammano, J. H. (1969): A transepithelial pump for weak electrolytes. *Am. J. Physiol.*, 216:983–987.
32. Swinyard, E. A., Brown, W. C., and Goodman, L. S. (1952): Comparative assays of antiepileptic drugs in mice and rats. *J. Pharmacol. Exp. Ther.*, 106:319–330.

33. Swinyard, E. A., Schiffman, D. O., and Goodman, L. S. (1952): Effects of liver injury and nephrectomy on the anticonvulsant activity of oxazolidine-2,4-diones. *J. Pharmacol. Exp. Ther.*, 105:365–370.

34. Taylor, J. D., and Bertcher, E. L. (1952): The determination and distribution of trimethadione (Tridione®) in animal tissues. *J. Pharmacol. Exp. Ther.*, 106:277–285.

35. Theuson, D. O., Withrow, C. D., Giam, C. S., and Woodbury, D. M. (1974): Uptake, distribution, metabolism, and excretion of trimethadione in rats. *Epilepsia*, 15:563–578.

36. Waddell, W. J., and Bates, R. G. (1969): Intracellular pH. *Physiol. Rev.*, 49:285–329.

37. Waddell, W. J., and Butler, T. C. (1957): Renal excretion of 5,5-dimethyl-2,4-oxazolidinedione (product of demethylation of trimethadione). *Proc. Soc. Exp. Biol. Med.*, 96:563–565.

38. Waddell, W. J., and Butler, T. C. (1959): Calculation of intracellular pH from the distribution of 5,5-dimethyl-2,4-oxazolidinedione (DMO). Application to skeletal muscle of the dog. *J. Clin. Invest.*, 38:720–729.

39. Withrow, C. D., Stout, R. J., Barton, L. J., Beacham, W. S., and Woodbury, D. M. (1968): Anticonvulsant effects of 5,5-dimethyl-2,4-oxazolidinedione (DMO). *J. Pharmacol. Exp. Ther.*, 161:335–341.

Antiepileptic Drugs, edited by D. M. Woodbury, J. K. Penry, and C. E. Pippenger. Raven Press, New York © 1982.

60

Trimethadione

Biotransformation

C. D. Withrow

Trimethadione (TMO) is converted to dimethadione (DMO) by rats (16,25), mice (13), humans (1,2,14), dogs (2,13), epileptic fowl (15), and chick embryos older than 8 days postfertilization (19).

Butler and co-workers have shown that TMO is quantitatively demethylated to dimethyloxazolidinedione (DMO) in dogs and humans (2), that the liver is important for the demethylation (5), and that the liver microsomal fraction is responsible for the demethylation (8). No products of ring cleavage of TMO have been isolated *in vivo* (24), an observation that supports the notion that DMO is the only important metabolic product of TMO.

The importance of the liver in the metabolic transformation of TMO has been supported by the experiments of Swinyard and co-workers. They reported that carbon tetrachloride-induced liver damage significantly increased the potency and duration of TMO and suggested that the liver is important for the degradation of TMO into substances with less anticonvulsant activity (23). Furthermore, they demonstrated that the effects of TMO were prolonged and that its potency increased in rats treated with β-diethylaminoethyldiphenylpropylacetate hydrochloride (SKF 525-A), a drug that inhibits many liver metabolic reactions (22).

Other tissues can also convert TMO to DMO.

Taylor and Bertcher (24) found that in rat tissue slices incubated 5 hr *in vitro* with TMO, the drug was altered in the following order of decreasing effectiveness: intestinal mucosa > kidney > liver = muscle > brain. The findings of Richards and Everett (17) that mice with livers damaged by carbon tetrachloride did not have prolonged protection against pentylenetetrazol convulsant effects also indicate indirectly that tissues other than liver are important for the degradation of TMO.

The rate of demethylation has been studied directly in mice and dogs (13). Trimethadione half-life was 46 min in mice and 8 hr in dogs. It was suggested that the longer half-life in dogs was the result of demethylating enzyme inhibition by high initial concentrations of TMO (see below). In chronic experiments, the same workers found that plasma concentrations of TMO were maximal 2 to 4 hr after oral ingestion of a daily dose of TMO. Theuson et al. (25) found that the half-life of the demethylation of TMO to DMO was 2.7 hr in rats. The half-life of TMO disappearance from the serum of human volunteers given TMO orally was 16 hr (1). Indirect approximations of TMO transformation to DMO have shown that a single dose of TMO was converted to DMO in 4 to 6 hr (12).

Trimethadione can compete with the microsomal demethylation of metharbital and inhibit its conversion to barbital, even though TMO has a lower affinity for the demethylating enzyme (8). Dimethadione, the demethylation product of TMO, can also inhibit the demethylation of metharbital and TMO. The possibility that high doses of TMO can inhibit its own metabolism was suggested by Conney (11) and was used by Frey and Schulz (13) to explain their observation that serum TMO levels in dogs remained constant for 60 to 90 min after intravenous injection of TMO and thus resulted in a serum half-life of 8 hr. It does not appear that TMO can induce liver microsomal enzymes (11,21).

When injected *in vivo* in 17-day-old chick embryos, TMO increased the hepatic activity of δ-aminolevulinic acid synthetase and inhibited cytochrome P-450 and aminopyrine demethylase (18).

DIMETHADIONE

Waddell and Butler (26) have shown that DMO in urine collected over a 2-day period accounted for 99% of the administered dose. Thus, DMO probably is not transformed further into additional metabolic products. Because DMO is metabolized and excreted very slowly, the administration of TMO or DMO in usual daily anticonvulsant doses results in the gradual accumulation of DMO in serum (14,16). Since DMO has anticonvulsant effects (9,28), the question arises as to the relative contributions of TMO and DMO to the total anticonvulsant effects observed after TMO administration. By use of a TMO-to-DMO anticonvulsant ratio of 1.25 measured in mice (12), as well as plasma TMO and DMO levels determined in dogs treated chronically with TMO, Frey and Schulz (13) concluded that unmetabolized TMO does not contribute more than 15% to the total anticonvulsant effects of TMO therapy.

PARAMETHADIONE

The metabolism of paramethadione (PMO) has been studied in detail by Butler (3). His results show that PMO is completely *N*-demethylated to 5-ethyl-5-methyl-2,4-oxazolidinedione in dogs

and humans and that this metabolite of PMO is excreted very slowly. Butler and Waddell (6) found that 33 to 38% of PMO was demethylated in mice in 2 hr, a rate more rapid than that observed in the dog (3). Daily doses of PMO given to humans resulted in a gradual rise in plasma demethylated PMO concentrations over a period of 2 weeks (3). The role of the metabolite of PMO in the total anticonvulsant effects of PMO has not been determined. However, these data for PMO are analogous to those given above for TMO and DMO. It is interesting to repeat the speculation of Butler (3,4) that demethylated PMO is of importance in this regard.

It has been reported that PMO treatment can induce liver enzymes (11).

SUMMARY

N-Demethylation of oxazolidinediones results in important differences in drug properties. These have been discussed by Butler and Waddell (4,7) and are summarized here for convenience.

The most obvious physical alteration of TMO and PMO brought about by demethylation is a change from drugs that do not ionize into compounds that do ionize in the range of physiologic pH. Dimethadione has a pK_a of 6.13 at 37°C, and PMO has a pK_a of 5.9 (10). Since most of the demethylated drugs would therefore exist at body pH primarily in the ionized form, the solubility in water increases, and lipid solubility decreases.

One consequence of the demethylation of TMO to DMO is that the volume of distribution of TMO is probably reduced from about 60% (12) to about 40% for DMO (27). A reduced fat solubility could account for these observations. It has been shown, however, that pH gradients also affect the distribution of DMO (27). The volume of distribution of demethylated PMO is about the same as that of DMO (3), but the distribution volume of PMO has not been measured.

A second consequence of the loss of an *N*-methyl group is that the rate of penetration and accumulation in specific tissues would be slowed. In the case of brain, DMO (20) and TMO (24,25) both appear to reach high levels rapidly. This is substantiated by the observations of Butler (4) who found that the methylation of DMO to TMO had little effect on either the delay of the onset of anesthesia or on the total dose of the compounds necessary to anesthetize mice. Seizure experiments showed, however, that TMO is a more potent anticonvulsant than equimolar DMO (13), although this may not be true when brain levels are taken into consideration (25). Testing of PMO and its metabolite as an anesthetic in mice revealed that the parent compound was about twice as potent as the demethylated product (6), an expected result if more PMO accumulates in brain.

Finally, *N*-demethylation of the oxazolidinediones should result in increased renal clearance because of increased polarization. Dimethadione and demethylated PMO are, nevertheless, among the most persistent compounds known (2–4).

ACKNOWLEDGMENTS

Supported in part by a U.S. Public Health Service Program Project Grant I-POI-NS-15767 from the National Institute of Neurological and Communicative Disorders and Stroke. The expert secretarial assistance of Mrs. C. Bawden is greatly appreciated.

REFERENCES

1. Booker, H. E. (1972): Trimethadione and other oxazolidinediones. Relation of plasma levels to clinical control. In: *Antiepileptic Drugs,* edited by D. M. Woodbury, J. K. Penry, and R. P. Schmidt, pp. 403–407. Raven Press, New York.
2. Butler, T. C. (1953): Quantitative studies of the demthylation of trimethadione (Tridione®). *J. Pharmacol. Exp. Ther.,* 108:11–17.
3. Butler, T. C. (1955): Metabolic demethylation of 3,5-dimethyl-5-ethyl-2,4-oxazolidinedione (paramethadione Paradione®). *J. Pharmacol. Exp. Ther.,* 113:178–185.
4. Butler, T. C. (1955): The effects of *N*-methylation in 5,5-disubstituted derivatives of barbituric acid, hydantoin, and 2,4-oxazolidinedione. *J. Am. Pharm. Assoc.,* 44:367–370.
5. Butler, T. C., and Waddell, W. J. (1954): The role of the liver in the demethylation of *N*-methyl derivatives of hydantoin and of 2,4-oxazolidinedione. *J. Pharmacol. Exp. Ther.,* 110:241–243.
6. Butler, T. C., and Waddell, W. J. (1955): A pharmacological comparison of the optical isomers of 5-ethyl-5-methyl-2,4-oxazolidinedione and 3,5-dimethyl-5-ethyl-2,4-oxazolidinedione (paramethadione, Paradione®). *J. Pharmacol. Exp. Ther.,* 113:238–240.
7. Butler, T. C., and Waddell, W. J. (1958): *N*-Methylated derivatives of barbituric acid, hydantoin and oxazolidinedione used in the treatment of epilepsy. *Neurology (Minneap.),* 8:106–112.
8. Butler, T. C., Waddell, W. J., and Poole, D. T. (1965): Demethylation of trimethadione and metharbital by rat liver microsomal enzymes: Substrate concentration–yield relationships and competition between substrates. *Biochem. Pharmacol.,* 14:937–942.
9. Chamberlin, H. R., Waddell, W. J., and Butler, T. C. (1965): A study of the product of demethylation of trimethadione in the control of petit mal epilepsy. *Neurology (Minneap.),* 15:449–454.
10. Clark-Lewis, J. W. (1958): 2,4-Oxazolidinediones. *Chem. Rev.,* 58:63–99.
11. Conney, A. H. (1967): Pharmacological implications of microsomal enzyme induction. *Pharmacol. Rev.,* 19:317–366.
12. Frey, H.-H. (1969): Determination of the anticonvulsant potency of unmetabolized trimethadione. *Acta Pharmacol. Toxicol. (Kbh.),* 27:295–300.
13. Frey, H.-H., and Schulz, R. (1970): Time course of the demethylation of trimethadione. *Acta Pharmacol. Toxicol. (Kbh.),* 28:477–483.
14. Jensen, B N. (1962): Trimethadione in serum of patients with petit mal epilepsy. *Dan. Med. Bull.,* 9:74–79.
15. Johnson, D. D., Davis, H. L., and Crawford, R. D. (1979): Pharmacological and biochemical studies in epileptic fowl. *Fed. Proc.,* 38:2417–2423.
16. Midha, K. K., Buttar, H. S., Rowe, M., and Dupuis, I. (1979): Metabolism and disposition of trimethadione in pregnant rats. *Epilepsia,* 20:417–423.
17. Richards, R. K., and Everett, G. M. (1946): Tridione®: A new anticonvulsant drug. *J. Lab. Clin. Med.,* 31:1330–1336.
18. Rifkind, A. B. (1972): Trimethadione inhibition of drug metabolism. Possible role in teratogenesis. *Pediatr. Res.,* 6:335.
19. Rifkind, A. B. (1974): Teratogenic effects of trimethadione and dimethadione in the chick embryo. *Toxicol. Appl. Pharmacol.,* 30:452–457.
20. Rollins, D. E., and Reed, D. J. (1970): Transport of DMO out of cerebrospinal fluid of rats. *Am. J. Physiol.,* 219:1200–1204.
21. Stevenson, I. H., O'Malley, K., and Shepherd, A. M. M. (1976): Relative induction potency of anticonvulsant drugs. *Study Group Inst. Res. Mult. Ment. Handicap,* 9:37–46.
22. Swinyard, E. A., Madsen, J. A., and Goodman, L. S. (1954): The effect of β-diethylaminoethyl-diphenylpropylacetate (SKF No. 525-A) on the anticonvulsant properties of antiepileptic drugs. *J. Pharmacol. Exp. Ther.,* 111:54–63.
23. Swinyard, E. A., Schiffman, D. O., and Goodman, L. S. (1952): Effects of liver injury and nephrectomy on the anticonvulsant activity of oxazolidine-2,4-diones. *J. Pharmacol. Exp. Ther.,* 105:365–370.

24. Taylor, J. D., and Bertcher, E. L. (1952): The deter-
    mination and distribution of trimethadione (Tri-
    dione®) in animal tissues. *J. Pharmacol. Exp. Ther.,*
    106:277–285.
25. Theuson, D. O., Withrow, C. D., Giam, C. S., and
    Woodbury, D. M. (1974): Uptake, distribution, me-
    tabolism and excretion of trimethadione in rats. *Epi-
    lepsia,* 15:563–578.
26. Waddell, W. J., and Butler, T. C. (1957): Renal ex-
    cretion of 5,5-dimethyl-2,4-oxazolidinedione (prod-
    uct of demethylation of trimethadione). *Proc. Soc. Exp.
    Biol. Med.,* 96:563–565.
27. Waddell, W. J., and Butler, T. C. (1959): Calculation
    of intracellular pH from the distribution of 5,5-di-
    methyl-2,4-oxazolidinedione (DMO). Application to
    skeletal muscle of the dog. *J. Clin. Invest.,* 38:720–
    729.
28. Withrow, C. D., Stout, R. J., Barton, L. J., Beach-
    am, W. S., and Woodbury, D. M. (1968): Anticon-
    vulsant effects of 5,5-dimethyl-2,4-oxazolidinedione
    (DMO). *J. Pharmacol. Exp. Ther.,* 161:335–341.

Antiepileptic Drugs, edited by D. M. Woodbury, J. K. Penry, and C. E. Pippenger. Raven Press, New York © 1982.

61

Trimethadione

Interactions with Other Drugs

C. D. Withrow

Although trimethadione (TMO) and paramethadione (PMO) have been in clinical use for many years, illustrations of important interactions with other drugs are scarce. The discussion that follows is, of necessity, limited.

ANTICONVULSANT EFFECTS

It has been reported that tricyclic antidepressant drugs may produce seizures in susceptible persons (8). This drug effect has been cited as a possible cause of decreased control in epileptic patients on TMO therapy (12), but this drug interaction has not been carefully documented. Consroe and Wolkin (4) have found that cannabidiol reduced the anticonvulsant potency of TMO in rats susceptible to audiogenic seizures.

OTHER CENTRAL NERVOUS SYSTEM EFFECTS

Trimethadione, dimethadione (DMO), PMO, and demethylated PMO all produce central nervous system (CNS) depression. The oxazolidinediones were found to be analgesic (17) and to have depressant effects on the CNS, such as ataxia, sedation, and sleep (16,17), especially when given in large doses. There is, then, the possibility that interactions with other CNS depressants can occur.

TRIMETHADIONE– PENTYLENETETRAZOL ANTAGONISM

The remarkable antagonism of pentylenetetrazol-induced seizures by TMO is well known. The isobol experiments of Loewe et al. (14) showed that TMO counteracted pentylenetetrazol-induced seizures, ejaculation, and death, whereas TMO-induced neurotoxicity was not antagonized by pentylenetetrazol. DeBonnevaux et al. (9) reported that pentylenetetrazol-induced stimulation of autonomic nervous centers, as manifested by miosis, hypertension, and hyperglycemia, was not prevented by TMO. The findings of Esplin and Curto (10) revealed that TMO and pentylenetetrazol antagonized each other's effects on synaptic transmission in the spinal cord. Goodman et al. (11) found that TMO not only prevented pentylenetetrazol-induced seizures but also completely suppressed pentylenetetrazol-caused EEG dysrhythmias in patients with absence seizures and in rabbits given subconvulsant doses of pentylenetetrazol. The TMO–pentylenetetrazol interaction is not of obvious clinical significance, but it does illustrate how drug interactions can be used to learn more about basic mechanisms of drug action.

DEMETHYLATION AND ENZYME INDUCTION

Trimethadione and metharbital interfere with the demethylation of each other by liver microsomes (2). Also, DMO, the product of demethylation of TMO, inhibits the demethylation of TMO and metharbital (2). It is conceivable, therefore, that other drugs that are N-demethylated by liver microsomes, or their products, could interfere with the demethylation of TMO, or vice versa.

It has been reported that PMO induces liver enzymes and that TMO does not (3,20). The importance of the effects of other enzyme inducers on TMO and PMO metabolism and anticonvulsant effects remains to be established. Trimethadione increased the hepatic activity of δ-aminolevulinic acid synthetase and inhibited cytochrome P-450 and amimopyrine demethylase activities in the chick embryo (18). The clinical significance of the effects of the oxazolidinediones on the liver needs additional study.

ACID-BASE EFFECTS OF DMO

The weakly acidic DMO largely exists as an anion at physiologic pH and must be excreted as such. If large concentrations of the anion are added to body fluids as a result of huge single doses of the drug or of accumulation during chronic treatment, extracellular metabolic acidosis occurs in rats (1) and in humans (1,15). This acidosis appears to be caused entirely by displacement of bicarbonate by DMO anions. In rats, acidosis has also been detected in muscle intracellular fluid (1).

Dimethadione also accumulates in the plasma of patients treated chronically with TMO. Thus, it is not surprising that Butler et al. (1) found an extracellular acidosis in two patients treated with TMO and showed that DMO anions can account for the observed decrease in plasma bicarbonate concentrations. It would be expected that the accumulation of demethylated PMO would also cause acid-base distortions during PMO administration, but this has not been studied.

A DMO-induced metabolic acidosis antagonized partial neuromuscular blockades with succinylcholine and decamethonium both *in vivo* and *in vitro,* but pancuronium bromide neuromuscular blocking effects were potentiated by the acidosis caused by DMO (7).

It is not clear if the acidosis, and in particular the intracellular acidosis, caused by DMO is responsible for the anticonvulsant effects of DMO or TMO. If it is important, however, drug treatment and physiologic distortions, e.g., salicylate therapy or hydration, that change cell pH might affect the response of a patient to the oxazolidinediones. Acid-base distortions caused by the oxazolidinediones could also conceivably cause changes in the absorption, distribution, or excretion of other drugs given concurrently and thus modify their therapeutic effectiveness. Finally, acid-base distortions caused by other agents, e.g., ammonium chloride, acetazolamide, and sodium bicarbonate, can affect the distribution (21) or excretion of DMO (13) and thereby possibly have effects on the anticonvulsant effect of either TMO or DMO.

An interesting aspect of possible interactions is the speculation of Constant (5,6) that the toxic effects of TMO on the eye could be accentuated by carbonic anhydrase inhibitor treatment or systemic acidosis, since she observed that DMO increased in vitreous humor in both situations.

OTHER INTERACTIONS

The levels of DMO in the CSF of rats and rabbits are increased by treatment with probenecid (6,19). Rollins and Reed (19), however, found that brain DMO space was increased only slightly by probenecid administration in acute experiments. Although it is possible that chronic experiments would yield different results, it does not seem likely that anticonvulsant effects of TMO or PMO would be affected by concurrent probenecid treatment.

An interesting interaction of TMO and desoxycorticosterone in chronic experiments has been described by Woodbury (22). Doses of TMO that had no effect on electroshock seizure threshold potentiated the effects of desoxycorticosterone on this threshold for 5 days after concurrent treatment was started. After that time, the potentiation decreased until it reversed into a desoxycorticosterone antagonism 19 days after the beginning of the experiment. No explanation for the biphasic effect of TMO is known.

ACKNOWLEDGMENTS

Supported in part by a U.S. Public Health Service Program Project Grant I-POI-NS-15767 from the National Institute of Neurological and Communicative Disorders and Stroke.

The expert secretarial assistance of Mrs. C. Bawden is greatly appreciated.

REFERENCES

1. Butler, T. C., Kurolwa, Y., Waddell, W. J., and Poole, D. T. (1966): Effects of 5,5-dimethyl-2,4-oxazolidinedione (DMO) on acid–base and electrolyte equilibria. *J. Pharmacol. Exp. Ther.*, 152:62–66.
2. Butler, T. C., Waddell, W. J., and Poole, D. T. (1965): Demethylation of trimethadone and metharbital by rat liver microsomal enzymes: Substrate concentration–yield relationships and competition between substrates. *Biochem. Pharmacol.*, 14:937–942.
3. Conney, A. H. (1967): Pharmacological implications of microsomal enzyme inductions. *Pharmacol. Rev.*, 19:317–366.
4. Consroe, P., and Wolkin, A. (1976): Cannabidiol–antiepileptic drug comparisons and interactions in experimentally induced seizures in rats. *J. Pharmacol. Exp. Ther.*, 201:26–32.
5. Constant, M. A. (1962): The distribution of 5,5-dimethyl-2,4-oxazolidinedione (DMO). II. Studies of the effect of carbonic anhydrase inhibitors and of plasma levels. *Invest. Ophthalmol.*, 1:609–617.
6. Constant, M. A. (1967): Distribution of 5,5-dimethyl-2,4-oxazolidinedione (DMO) in intraocular and cerebral fluids of rabbits. III. Effect of ammonium chloride and probenecid. *Invest. Ophthalmol.*, 6:484–491.
7. Crul-Sluijter, E. J., and Crul, J. F. (1974): Acidosis and neuromuscular blockade. *Acta Anaesthesicl. Scand.*, 18:224–236.
8. Dallos, V., and Heathfield, K. (1969): Iatrogenic epilepsy due to antidepressant drugs. *Br. Med. J.*, 4:80–82.

9. DeBonnevaux, S. C., Diez Altares, M. C., and Carrillo, L. (1968): Autonomic response to pentamethylenetetrazol following trimethadione and benzodiazepine administration. *Arch. Int. Pharmacodyn. Ther.*, 173:34–43.
10. Esplin, D. W., and Curto, E. M. (1957): Effects of trimethadione on synaptic transmission in the spinal cord. Antagonism of trimethadione and pentylenetetrazol. *J. Pharmacol. Exp. Ther.*, 121:457–467.
11. Goodman, L. S., Toman, J. E. P., and Swinyard, E. A. (1946): The anticonvulsant properties of Tridione®. *Am. J. Med.*, 1:213–228.
12. James, J. D., Braustein, M. L., Karis, A. W., and Hartshorn, E. A. (1978): *A Guide to Drug Interactions*, p. 310. McGraw-Hill, New York.
13. Jensen, B. N. (1962): Trimethadione in serum of patients with petit mal epilepsy. *Dan. Med. Bull*, 9:74–79.
14. Loewe, S., Aldous, R. A., Fox, R. S., Johnson, D. G., and Perkins, W. (1955): Isobols of dose–effect relations in the combination of pentylenetetrazole and trimethadione. *J. Pharmacol. Exp. Ther.*, 113:475–480.
15. Manfredi, F. (1963): Calculation of total body intracellular pH in normal human subjects from the distribution of 5,5-dimethyl-2,4-oxazolidinedione (DMO). *J. Lab. Clin. Med.*, 61:1005–1014.
16. Richards, R. K., and Everett, G. M. (1946): Tridione®: A new anticonvulsant drug. *J. Lab. Clin. Med.*, 31:1330–1336.
17. Richards, R. K., Everett, G. M., and Pickrell, K. L. (1946): Pharmacological and clinical studies of Tridione® with special reference to its analgesic action. *Anesth. Analg. (Cleve.)*, 25:147–151.
18. Rifkind, A. B. (1972): Trimethadione inhibition of drug metabolism. Possible role in teratogenesis. *Pediatr. Res.*, 6:335.
19. Rollins, D. E., and Reed, D. J. (1970): Transport of DMO out of cerebrospinal fluid of rats. *Am. J. Physiol.*, 219:1200–1204.
20. Stevenson, I. H., O'Malley, K., and Shepherd, A. M. M. (1976): Relative induction potency of anticonvulsant drugs. *Study Group Inst. Res. Ment. Mult. Handicap.*, 9:37–46.
21. Waddell, W. J., and Butler, T. C. (1959): Calculation of intracellular pH from the distribution of 5,5-dimethyl-2,4-oxazolidinedione (DMO). Application to skeletal muscle of the dog. *J. Clin. Invest.*, 38:720–729.
22. Woodbury, D. M. (1952): Effect of chronic administration of anticonvulsant drugs, alone and in combination with desoxycorticosterone, on electroshock seizure threshold and tissue electrolytes. *J. Pharmacol. Exp. Ther.*, 105:46–57.

Antiepileptic Drugs, edited by D. M. Woodbury, J. K. Penry, and C. E. Pippenger. Raven Press, New York © 1982.

62

Trimethadione

Relation of Plasma Concentration to Seizure Control

Harold E. Booker

Following the initial clinical reports of its efficacy in the late 1940s (3,5,7), trimethadione rapidly became the drug of choice, if not the only really effective drug then available, for the control of primary generalized seizures of the absence, akinetic, and myoclonic types (9). It is less effective when such attacks are of a secondary generalized nature and is generally ineffective in partial seizures and generalized tonic–clonic convulsions. There is even some evidence that it may aggravate the latter (6).

The close, almost one-to-one relationship of absence attacks to the occurrence of generalized 3- to 4-Hz spike-and-wave paroxysms in the EEG and the frequency of their occurrence in individual patients are conditions that seem ideal for establishing the relationship between plasma levels of trimethadione and clinical effect. This relationship is complicated, however, by the role of the only known metabolite, dimethadione, because it has antiepileptic effects that are at least as potent as those of trimethadione itself (8). Although methods for determining dimethadione concentrations in tissue and plasma have been available for some time, determining the kinetics of trimethadione itself and the relative contributions of trimethadione and dimethadione to clinical response awaited the introduction in the early 1970s of relatively simple methods of measuring trimethadione concentrations.

In addition, because of the efficacy and apparently greater safety of more recently introduced drugs, trimethadione no longer is the drug of choice for absence attacks. As this trend was established before the general advent of drug concentration monitoring, less information is available for trimethadione and dimethadione than for many other antiepileptic drugs.

RELATION OF DOSE TO PLASMA LEVEL

Our own data on the absorption of trimethadione and the relationship between dose and plasma levels were reported in detail in the first edition of *Antiepileptic Drugs* and will be briefly summarized here.

Trimethadione was rapidly absorbed by normal adult volunteers, with peak levels found at 30 min to 1 hr after a single oral dose. Plasma clearance stabilized rapidly, with an average half-life of 16 hr. The half-life of dimethadione in man is not known with accuracy but is quite long; from Jensen's data, it can be estimated at around 10 days or more (4). As would be expected from the differences in half-lives, trimethadione levels show more daily fluctuation than do dimethadione levels. In hospitalized subjects receiving three or four daily doses, early morning trimethadione levels were 70% of the peak level found in the evening, whereas dimethadione levels were very stable throughout the day.

In institutionalized subjects at steady state, trimethadione and dimethadione levels were highly correlated with trimethadione doses. Each mg/kg of daily trimethadione dose gave an average plasma trimethadione level of 0.6 μg/ml. Dimethadione levels averaged 20 times the trimethadione levels. The findings were similar but less consistent in ambulatory subjects, and the average ratio of the levels of dimethadione to trimethadione was 23.

Because of the long half-life of dimethadione, and because it appears to be the major therapeutic agent, a single daily dose of trimethadione should be adequate. However, there are no reported clinical trials of such a schedule, and trimethadione is by tradition prescribed in divided daily doses. Whether a single large daily dose would cause gastrointestinal disturbance or other problems is unknown, although Wells reported the use of rather heroic doses in three patients without apparent problems (9). At any rate, dose schedules can be flexible. It should be unnecessary to prescribe a dose to be taken during school hours, for instance. Most children find this objectionable and, consequently, many do not comply.

RELATION OF PLASMA LEVEL TO CONTROL OF SEIZURES

Chamberlin et al. (2) monitored dimethadione levels and correlated them with control of seizures in patients treated separately with dimethadione and trimethadione. The results show that treatment with dimethadione alone was as effective as treatment with trimethadione. Control of seizures was associated with comparable dimethadione levels regardless of the source of the dimethadione. Delay in clinical response, often of two weeks or more, paralleled the dimethadione levels. These results confirmed predictions that dimethadione is responsible for the

therapeutic effects of trimethadione (1,4), although they did not clearly establish the therapeutic range. Jensen had previously reported (4) that control was present in 8 of 10 patients whose dimethadione levels were above 700 μg/ml, whereas only 14 of 27 subjects were controlled when levels were below 700 μg/ml. Although the data as reported by Chamberlin et al. (2) are not as clear in this regard, significant improvement in seizure control appeared to be associated with dimethadione levels of the same order.

Thus, at steady state, control of seizures in these studies was associated with plasma dimethadione levels in the range of 700 μg/ml. Trimethadione doses of 50 mg/kg per 24 hr are needed to produce such dimethadione levels and will produce trimethadione levels in the range of 35 μg/ml. Our own data, as reported in detail in the first edition of *Antiepileptic Drugs,* are in good agreement. Reduction of seizures by 75% or more was associated with average trimethadione and dimethadione levels of 20.5 and 765 μg/ml, respectively. Dimethadione levels ranged from 470 to 1,200 μg/ml. The average levels in subjects with uncontrolled seizures were 40.2 μg/ml of trimethadione and 450 μg/ml of dimethadione (range, 130 to 690 μg/ml).

The doses in the subjects in our study were comparable, so that the finding of higher trimethadione and lower dimethadione levels in the uncontrolled as compared to the controlled subjects is interesting but unexplained. It could result from inefficient metabolism of trimethadione to dimethadione and thus be one reason for lack of efficacy in some subjects. However, little is known about individual differences in the rate of hepatic demethylation of trimethadione to dimethadione in man. An alternate explanation would be that compliance was better in the controlled subjects. Because of the differences in half-life, plasma dimethadione levels reflect trimethadione intake over the past 1 to 2 weeks or more, whereas trimethadione levels reflect drug intake over the previous 24 to 72 hr. Degree of compliance in many subjects improves as a function of the nearness of the next scheduled clinic visit, particularly when they know that plasma drug levels will be routinely monitored. This is the situation in our clinic, and our findings can be explained if we assume that the uncontrolled subjects had poor compliance generally but that it improved the day or so before their clinic visits. Under these conditions, one would expect lower levels of the metabolite and higher levels of parent drug. If so, it would be another argument for the value of frequent clinic visits and routine monitoring of plasma drug levels. It also illustrates the advantage of determining the levels of both the parent drug and the principal metabolite, particularly when the latter is also an active therapeutic or toxic agent.

SUMMARY

Although no longer the drug of choice, trimethadione remains an effective drug for control of primary generalized seizures of the absence type associated with 3- to 4-Hz spike-and-wave discharges in the EEG. It may also be effective in closely related seizure types (akinetic and myoclonic attacks). Because of the efficacy and apparent greater safety of ethosuximide and valproic acid, it should be reserved for patients who do not respond to or cannot safely take these other drugs. The therapeutic effect is caused by its only known metabolite, dimethadione, and seizure control is associated with dimethadione levels generally in the range of 700 μg/ml. Because of major differences in half-lives, plasma

trimethadione levels will reach a plateau at steady state long before the dimethadione levels do. This explains the delay in response, often of 2 weeks or more, frequently seen when treatment with trimethadione is started, dosage is changed, or the drug is withdrawn completely. It also probably explains the occasional observation that, once control has been obtained, the dose of trimethadione can be lowered without loss of control.

REFERENCES

1. Butler, T., and Waddell, W. (1958): N-Methylated derivatives of barbituric acid, hydantoin and oxazolidinedione used in the treatment of epilepsy. *Neurology (Minneap.),* 8:106–112.
2. Chamberlin, H., Waddell, W., and Butler, T. (1965): A study of the product of demethylation of trimethadione in the control of petit mal epilepsy. *Neurology (Minneap.),* 15:449–454.
3. Goodman, L., Toman, J., and Swinyard, E. (1946): The anticonvulsant properties of Tridione®; laboratory and clinical investigations. *Am. J. Med.,* 1:213–228.
4. Jensen, B. (1962): Trimethadione in the serum of patients with petit mal. *Dan. Med. Bull.,* 9:74–79.
5. Lennox, W. (1945): The petit mal epilepsies. Their treatment with Tridione®. *J.A.M.A.,* 129:1069–1075.
6. Lennox, W. (1947): Tridione® in the treatment of epilepsy. *J.A.M.A.,* 134:138–143.
7. Perlstein, M., and Andelman, M. (1946): Tridione®; its use in convulsive and related disorders. *J. Pediatr.,* 29:20–40.
8. Thueson, D., Withrow, C., Giam, C., and Woodbury, D. (1974): Uptake, distribution, metabolism and excretion of trimethadione in rats. *Epilepsia,* 15:563–578.
9. Wells, C. (1957): Trimethadione: Its dosage and toxicity. *Arch. Neurol. Psychiatry,* 77:140–155.

Antiepileptic Drugs, edited by D. M. Woodbury, J. K. Penry, and C. E. Pippenger. Raven Press, New York © 1982.

63

Trimethadione

Toxicity

Harold E. Booker

In 1957, Wells summarized the clinical features of trimethadione, including an extensive review of the then known complications (11). Little has been added since then other than the recognition of the potential for human teratogenesis and the description of a myasthenic syndrome associated with its use.

Most of the adverse effects of trimethadione on the nervous system are dose dependent and can be expected in the majority of patients if the dose is high enough. As they are not associated with any known histological changes, they are generally reversible. They probably result from the direct pharmacological effects of the drug, although it is unclear whether they are caused by trimethadione itself or by its only known metabolite, dimethadione. Given the relative therapeutic potencies and the preponderance of dimethadione in plasma (10), it is reasonable to assume a major role for the metabolite. The ability of trimethadione to aggravate generalized convulsions (7) can be considered an adverse effect, although this finding has not been universal.

Hemeralopia (day blindness) and photophobia are the most prevalent side effects, occurring in up to 30% of patients. These are felt to be retinal effects in which brightness discrimination is impaired (9). Visual acuity is decreased as background illumination is increased, and patients complain of a bothersome white glare in the visual fields. Thus, they shun bright lights and often wear dark glasses. No changes are apparent on external or ophthalmoscopic examination. Although there are no data relating the effects to plasma drug levels, they are dose dependent and reversible. Tolerance to these effects often develops, and they can usually be managed by dosage adjustment and/or the wearing of dark glasses. Photophobia in one patient treated with dimethadione alone suggests that it rather than trimethadione is the offender (3).

Although the mechanism of action is unknown, it is reasonable to assume that trimethadione and dimethadione alter the excitability of central neuronal networks in some way. Thus, it is not surprising that a variety of effects on arousal, mood, and cognition occasionally occur. Sedation, fatigue, lack of concentration, dizziness, and ataxia have been noted. Alternatively, insomnia, restlessness, confusion, and even hallucinatory psychoses have been reported (11). These reactions, particularly the milder ones, can usually be controlled by lowering the dose, although there are no data relating them directly to plasma levels.

Dermatological reactions are very common, but most are benign morbilliform or acneform rashes (11). More serious reactions include erythema multiforme and exfoliative dermatitis. They are not dose related and usually occur early in therapy.

The most common serious reactions involve depression of the bone marrow. They range from a benign, nonprogressive depression of the absolute neutrophil count in the peripheral blood to a fulminant pancytopenia (1). Although periodic routine peripheral counts are recommended, their value has been questioned, as the peripheral count is not an accurate or sensitive indicator of the state of the bone marrow. As megakaryocytes are frequently the earliest cell line to be affected, Denhoff and Laufler (4) have recommended frequent examination of the peripheral blood for platelets and megakaryocytes as well as clot retraction time. As with the skin reactions, complete withdrawal from trimethadione is indicated in all but the most benign forms, and even then the patient must be followed closely.

A nephrotic syndrome occurs but is usually reversible if the drug is withdrawn (11). Although rare, its occurrence raises the question of an autoimmune reaction. That trimethadione or dimethadione may be capable of initiating or inducing such reactions is supported by reports of a myasthenic syndrome associated with its use (2,8). Although extremely rare, such reactions can be serious, as a profound myasthenic crisis with apnea followed a generalized convulsion in one case (2). The patients responded to anticholinesterases, and the syndrome remitted in several months following drug withdrawal.

Maternal ingestion of trimethadione may have serious consequences for the fetus. Although it has not been specifically implicated in producing hemorrhagic disease of the newborn, fetal malformations appear to be common (5,6,12). They are felt by some to be so characteristic that the term ''fetal trimethadione syndrome'' has been applied. Malformed or low-set ears, cleft lip and palate, delayed mental development, speech impairment, urogenital malformations, skeletal malformations, and cardiac defects are the more common features. In addition, the rate of spontaneous abortion is high. Although the mother was taking other drugs in most of the reported cases, the evidence implicating trimethadione appears to be strong enough that its use during pregnancy cannot be recommended.

SUMMARY

Trimethadione is a potentially toxic drug. Reversible but troublesome adverse effects on the nervous system include hemeralopia and sedation. Bone marrow depression is the most frequent serious complication, followed by skin reactions and nephrosis. The potential for teratogenesis is so great that the use of trimethadione in pregnancy cannot be recommended. There are no data relating the adverse effects to plasma levels to serve as a guideline in management, and the more serious reactions are usually not dose related. It is unknown whether the major toxicity is caused by the drug or its only metabolite, dimethadione.

Despite the potential toxicity, trimethadione remains an effective drug for the control of primary generalized seizures of the absence, akinetic, and myoclonic types. It is indicated primarily when such seizures cannot be controlled by, or the patient cannot safely take, other apparently safer drugs. When trimethadione is used, an appreciation of the possible complications and careful observation of the patient can minimize the potential for toxicity.

REFERENCES

1. Abbott, I., and Schwab, R. (1950): The serious side effects of the newer antiepileptic drugs: Their control and prevention. *N. Engl. J. Med.*, 242:943–949.
2. Booker, H., Chun, R., and Sanguino, M. (1970): Myasthenia gravis syndrome associated with trimethadione. *J.A.M.A.*, 212:2262–2263.
3. Chamberlin, H., Waddell, W., and Butler, T. (1965): A study of the product of demethylation of trimethadione in the control of petit mal epilepsy. *Neurology (Minneap.)*, 15:449–454.
4. Denhoff, E., and Laufler, M. (1950): Clinical studies of the effects of 3,5,5-trimethyloxazolidine-2,4-dione (Tridione®) on the hematopoietic system, liver and kidney. *Pediatrics*, 5:695–707.

5. Feldman, G., Weaver, D., and Lovrien, E. (1977): The fetal trimethadione syndrome: Report of an additional family and further delineation of their syndrome. *Am. J. Dis. Child.*, 131:1389–1392.

6. German, J., Kowal, A., and Ehlers, K. (1970): Trimethadione and human teratogenesis. *Teratology*, 3:349–361.

7. Lennox, W. (1947): Tridione® in the treatment of epilepsy. *J.A.M.A.*, 134:138–143.

8. Peterson, H. (1966): Association of trimethadione therapy and myasthenia gravis. *N. Engl. J. Med.*, 274:506–507.

9. Sloan, L., and Gilger, A. (1947): Visual effects of Tridione®. *Am. J. Ophthalmol.*, 30:1387–1405.

10. Thueson, D., Withrow, C., Giam, C., and Woodbury, D. (1974): Uptake, distribution, metabolism, and excretion of trimethadione in rats. *Epilepsia*, 15:563–578.

11. Wells, C. (1957): Trimethadione: Its dosage and toxicity. *Arch. Neurol. Psychiatry*, 77:140–155.

12. Zackai, E., Mellman, W., Neiderer, B, and Hanson, J. (1975): The fetal trimethadione syndrome. *J. Pediatr.*, 87:280–284.

Antiepileptic Drugs, edited by D. M. Woodbury, J. K. Penry, and C. E. Pippenger. Raven Press, New York © 1982.

64

Trimethadione

Mechanisms of Action

C. D. Withrow

Although trimethadione (TMO) and other oxazolidinediones are no longer the drugs of choice for the treatment of absence seizures, research continues into how these agents exert their therapeutic effects. Investigations take such multiple approaches as studies of drug effects in experimental models, inquiries into neurophysiological and biochemical mechanisms concerned with central nervous system functions, and examinations of the pathological features of epilepsy. This chapter summarizes and integrates diverse findings with the hope that a better understanding of the mechanisms of action of TMO will emerge from the effort.

The pharmacology and the mechanisms of anticonvulsant action of TMO and other oxazolidinediones have been reviewed elsewhere (1,32,33). These discussions are recommended for detailed information about most older investigations concerned with many experimental and clinical effects of these drugs. The following discussion consists mostly of experiments reported since the most recent review (32), but some older studies not cited previously are included for completeness.

PHARMACOLOGICAL, PHYSIOLOGICAL, AND BIOCHEMICAL EFFECTS

Faingold and Berry (7) studied TMO and pentylenetetrazol (PTZ) interactions on the electroencephalogram (EEG) of the cat with computer-aided EEG analysis. They found that TMO effectively increased the dose of PTZ necessary to induce paroxysmal activity.

Tannhauser and Izquierdo (29) found that epileptogenic stimulation of the fornix caused a fall in hippocampal ribonucleic acid (RNA) concentrations in urethane-anesthetized rats. This decrease in RNA levels was prevented by pretreatment with TMO, phenytoin, cannabidiol, and phenobarbital; treatment of awake, unstimulated rats with these drugs had no effect on either hippocampal or neocortical RNA concentrations. Seizures provoked by PTZ injection, maximal electroshock, or hyponatremia had no effect on hippocampal or neocortical RNA levels.

Trimethadione increased survival time and delayed the time of the onset of seizures and NADH oxidation–reduction cycles in rats subjected to hyperbaric oxygen (17). Trimethadione had no effect on the initial oxidation of NADH or on the oxidation levels of NADH during the oxidation cycles. Because TMO did not change brain energy metabolism, it was concluded that TMO modifies seizures induced by high-pressure oxygen exposure through other mechanisms.

Trimethadione prevented most of the grand mal-type seizures caused by high doses of methadone in mice (24). However, TMO neither changed the LD_{50} of methadone nor added to effects of naloxone, a drug that did increase the methadone LD_{50} in mice.

Ito et al. (14) showed that a small dose of PTZ given daily for several days resulted in a progressive increase in seizure severity. Doses of TMO that prevented seizures in rats given only a single dose of PTZ did not suppress either the seizures or the increased electroencephalographic activity caused by daily multiple doses of PTZ; higher doses of TMO were more effective.

Trimethadione, phenobarbital, and urethane effectively reduced PTZ-induced cortical release of acetylcholine, whereas phenytoin enhanced the PTZ effect (11). Only TMO decreased cortical acetylcholine release in doses that did not cause general central nervous system depression.

In rats, TMO caused a marked depression of afterdischarge activity evoked with visual stimuli (25,31).

In barbiturate-dependent cats, many of the motor, autonomic, and behavioral signs precipitated by barbiturate withdrawal were reversed by TMO (21). Dimethyloxazolidinedione (DMO) was less effective and more toxic in this seizure model.

Veratridine depolarized cells in mouse cortical brain slices and caused marked accumulation of adenosine $3',5'$-monophosphate (cyclic AMP) and guanosine $3',5'$-monophosphate (cyclic GMP) in the tissue (9). Trimethadione, as well as other drugs effective against PTZ-induced seizures and absence seizures, did not prevent the veratridine-induced accumulation of cyclic AMP or cyclic GMP. Drugs that preferentially antagonize tonic–clonic seizures inhibited cyclic AMP and cyclic GMP accumulations caused by veratridine. These results were interpreted to indicate that TMO affects seizures by altering neurotransmission rather than by a direct effect on cellular membranes in the central nervous system.

Trimethadione given alone had no effects on cat brain monoamine metabolism (18). The drug did not change concentrations of 5-hydroxytryptamine, dopamine, or norepinephrine metabolites in cerebrospinal fluid except for a transient decrease in homovanillic acid, the major metabolite of dopamine. However, TMO did partially antagonize the increases in monoamine metabolites induced by convulsant doses of PTZ.

In studies on neuron R_{15} of the *Aplysia californica* abdominal ganglion, TMO treatment caused hyperpolarization of the bursting pacemaker potential and complete blockade of bursting (15).

Convulsant doses of PTZ induced an increase in prostaglandins and a thromboxane-like material in mouse brain tissue (27). Trimethadione in anticonvulsant doses prevented the rise in brain arachidonic acid metabolites. However, TMO had no effects on prostaglandin synthesis in *in vitro* synaptosomal preparations. It was therefore concluded that the PTZ-induced rise in brain prostaglandins and thromboxanes was the result of convulsions caused by PTZ and that TMO reduced this increase by decreasing seizure severity rather than by a direct effect on arachidonic acid metabolism.

The paroxysmal electrical and behavioral effects produced by leucine enkephalin were reduced or attenuated by single doses of TMO and other anticonvulsant drugs effective in absence seizures (26). Trimethadione given for 7 days appeared to be more effective than a single injection of the drug.

MECHANISMS OF ACTION

Before drug mechanisms of action are discussed, some cautions about interpretation of experimental results related to the oxazolidinediones should be listed.

Many studies of the antiseizure properties of the oxazolidinediones have been done with TMO, although almost all of the clinical anticonvulsant effects of TMO result from the accumulation of its major metabolite, DMO. It is not clear that TMO and DMO have identical antiepileptic properties (21,32); it is clear that TMO and DMO have quite different pharmacokinetic and physicochemical characteristics (32).

Most experiments reported are acute, single-dose studies with either TMO or DMO. The treatment of absence seizures requires drug administration for years.

Investigations of TMO mechanisms have primarily used PTZ-induced convulsions as an experimental model for absence seizures. It has not been proven conclusively that findings derived from TMO antagonism of the neurophysiological and biochemical effects caused by PTZ can be extrapolated to human epilepsy therapy.

The common pharmacological caveat related to dosage may apply. Some drug effects reported have been obtained with excessive doses of drugs and therefore may not be reliable indicators of drug mechanisms of action in the treatment of human epilepsy.

With these cautions in mind, we may now ask which of the many reported drug effects are most pertinent to understanding the antiseizure actions of TMO and related agents.

Trimethadione has several well-defined neurophysiological effects. In the spinal cord, the drug blocks repetitive transmission (5), prolongs postictal depression (6), and enhances presynaptic inhibition (19). The oxazolidinediones elevate seizure thresholds (28) and attenuate a kindling-like effect of chronic PTZ administration (14). Photically evoked afterdischarges were also blocked by TMO (25,31). Quantitative evaluations of PTZ–TMO interactions on the EEG of the cat were suggested to indicate that TMO prevented the buildup of a critical mass of foci necessary for PTZ to cause a generalized seizure (7). In some experiments, TMO seems to affect subcortical structures more than it does the cerebral cortex (3,20,23), but the clinical significance of this is not clear (12). Trimethadione has been reported to activate synaptic inputs with tonic inhibitory effects in abdominal ganglia of *Aplysia californica* (15).

The biochemical effects of TMO and related drugs have been studied in many *in vivo* and *in vitro* models. Trimethadione has no effect on acetylcholine synthesis or destruction (30). Pentylenetetrazol-induced acetylcholine release in the cortex was reduced by TMO, but this effect was not thought to be a direct action of the drug on acetylcholine discharge (11). Trimethadione does not change dopamine or norepinephrine levels in brain (18). Its effects on brain 5-hydroxytryptamine concentrations are conflicting (4,18) and not striking in any case. Trimethadione had no effect on GABA levels in rat brain (8), but a modification in GABA metabolism has been reported in other experiments (16). The effects of TMO on brain energy and carbohydrate metabolism do not give any obvious clues to its mechanism of action (32).

The experiments of Gross and Woodbury (13) with the toad bladder showed conclusively that TMO decreased potassium permeability in this preparation when potassium permeability was increased with PTZ. Mayevsky (17) has postulated that the anticonvulsant effects of TMO against seizures induced by high-pressure oxygen can be explained by prevention of potassium accumulation in the extracellular space of brain. On the other hand, TMO does not affect potassium release in the hippocampus (29).

Chronic TMO therapy results in the accumulation of large amounts of DMO anion in brain cells (32).

What do these observations concerning TMO's anticonvulsant effects mean when reviewed together? First, the neurophysiological effects of TMO account for, at least at the functional level, some of the antiepileptic properties of the drug. In particular, the enhancement of presynaptic and postsynaptic inhibition and the blockade of repetitive stimulation would decrease the severity of absence seizures. Further, the recruitment of inhibition (15) would also help to reduce convulsive activity.

Second, although enhancement of inhibition appears to be a prominent effect of TMO, GABA accumulation or alterations in GABA metabolism do not appear to be responsible. In fact, no putative neurotransmitters are affected by TMO. Whether or not modifications of potassium permeability are responsible for synaptic drug effects is not known, but it is reasonable to assume some relationship.

Third, the presence of large (10 mM or greater) amounts of DMO anion in brain cells during chronic TMO therapy must affect neuronal function in some important way. Dimethyloxazolidinedione has been reported to cause an intracellular acidosis in muscle (2), although others report no effect on intracellular pH (22). Acidosis, if it does occur, would change extracellular–intracellular potassium ratios, modify cellular enzyme activities, alter cellular transport and metabolic functions, and vary calcium ionization. But evidence supporting changes in potassium balance, cell metabolism, or other functions caused by DMO-induced acidosis is minimal. It is therefore possible that the effects of DMO anion accumulation are entirely unrelated to its alterations of acid–base balance; for example, DMO anion could have important effects on glial anion transport systems (34).

CONCLUSION

Flower (10) has stated that a discovery becomes dogma when nobody any longer refers to the initial papers. Since most of the citations included here are to original work, this can mean that there are as yet few dogma in understanding how TMO and related drugs exert their antiepileptic actions. No definitive, unifying explanation is possible at present. Lest pessimism prevail, however, we know a great deal about what the drugs do and don't do, and we know several fruitful areas of research to pursue. Progress is being made.

ACKNOWLEDGMENTS

Supported in part by a U. S. Public Health Service Program Project Grant 1-P01-NS-15767 from the National Institute of Neurological and Communicative Disorders and Stroke.

The expert secretarial assistance of Mrs. C. Bawden is appreciated.

REFERENCES

1. Aird, R. B., and Woodbury, D. M. (1974): *The Management of Epilepsy.* Charles C Thomas, Springfield, Illinois.
2. Butler, T. C., Kuroiwa, Y., Waddell, W. J., and Poole, D. T. (1966): Effects of 5,5-dimethyl-2,4-oxazolidinedione (DMO) on acid–base and electrolyte equilibria. *J. Pharmacol. Exp. Ther.,* 152:62–66.
3. Delgado, J. M. R., and Mihailevic, L. (1956): Use of intracerebral electrodes to evaluate drugs that act on the central nervous system. *Ann. N.Y. Acad. Sci.,* 64:644–666.
4. Diaz, P. M. (1974): Interaction of pentylenetetrazol and trimethadione on the metabolism of serotonin in brain and its relation to the anticonvulsant action of trimethadione. *Neuropharmacology,* 13:615–621.
5. Esplin, D. W., and Curto, E. M. (1957): Effects of

6. Esplin, D. W., and Freston, J. W. (1960): Physiological and pharmacological analysis of spinal cord convulsions. *J. Pharmacol. Exp. Ther.,* 130:68–80.
7. Faingold, C. L., and Berry, C. A. (1973): Quantitative evaluation of the pentylenetetrazol–anticonvulsant interaction of the EEG of the cat. *Eur. J. Pharmacol.,* 24:381–388.
8. Ferrari, R. A., and Arnold, A. (1961): The effect of central nervous system agents on rat-brain gamma-aminobutyric acid level. *Biochim. Biophys. Acta,* 52:361–367.
9. Ferrendelli, J. A., and Kinscherf, D. A. (1978): Inhibitory effects of anticonvulsant drugs on cyclic nucleotide accumulation in brain. *Ann. Neurol.,* 5:533–538.
10. Flower, R. (1981): Glucocorticoids, phospholipase A$_2$ and inflammation. *Trends Pharmacol. Sci.,* 2:186–189.
11. Gardner, C. R., and Webster, R. A. (1977): Convulsant–anticonvulsant interactions on seizure activity and cortical acetylcholine release. *Eur. J. Pharmacol.,* 42:247–256.
12. Glaser, G. H. (1980): Mechanisms of antiepileptic drug action: Clinical indicators. In: *Antiepileptic Drugs: Mechanisms of Action,* edited by G. H. Glaser, J. K. Penry, and D. M. Woodbury, pp. 11–20. Raven Press, New York.
13. Gross, G. J., and Woodbury, D. M. (1972): Effects of pentylenetetrazol on ion transport in the isolated toad bladder. *J. Pharmacol. Exp. Ther.,* 181:257–272.
14. Ito, T., Hori, M., Yoshida, K., and Shimizu, M. (1977): Effect of anticonvulsants on seizures developing in the course of daily administration of pentetrazol to rats. *Eur. J. Pharmacol.,* 45:165–172.
15. Kreisman, N. R., Murphy, M. F., and King, W. M. (1978): Effects of the anticonvulsant, trimethadione, on bursting pacemaker activity and recruitment of inhibition in the abdominal ganglion of *Aplysia californica. Comp. Biochem. Physiol.,* 60C:145–154.
16. Loscher, W., and Frey, H.-H. (1977): Effect of convulsant and anticonvulsant agents on level and metabolism of gamma-aminobutyric acid in mouse brain. *Naunyn Schmiedebergs Arch. Pharmacol.,* 296:263–269.
17. Mayevsky, A. (1975): The effects of trimethadione on brain energy metabolism and EEG activity of the conscious rat exposed to HPO. *J. Neurosci. Res.,* 1:131–142.
18. McMillen, B. A., and Isaac, L. (1978): Effects of pentylenetetrazol and trimethadione on feline brain monoamine metabolism. *Biochem. Pharmacol.,* 27:1815–1820.
19. Miyahara, J. T., Esplin, D. W., and Zablocka, B. (1966): Differential effects of depressant drugs on presynaptic inhibition. *J. Pharmacol. Exp. Ther.,* 154:118–127.
20. Morrell, F., Bradley, W., and Ptashne, M. (1959): Effect of drugs on discharge characteristics of chronic epileptogenic lesions. *Neurology (Minneap),* 9:492–498.
21. Okamoto, M., Rosenberg, H. C., and Boisse, N. R.

trimethadione on synaptic transmission in the spinal cord; antagonism of trimethadione and pentylenetetrazol. *J. Pharmacol. Exp. Ther.,* 121:457–467.

(1977): Evaluation of anticonvulsants in barbiturate withdrawal. *J. Pharmacol. Exp. Ther.*, 202:479–489.

22. Roos, A. (1975): Intercellular pH and distribution of weak acids across cell membranes. A study of D- and L-lactate and of DMO in rat diaphragm. *J. Physiol. (Lond.)*, 249:1–25.

23. Schallek, W., and Kuehn, A. (1963): Effects of trimethadione, diphenylhydantoin and chlordiazepoxide on after-discharges in the brain of the cat. *Proc. Soc. Exp. Biol. Med.*, 112:813–817.

24. Shannon, H. E., and Holtzman, S. G. (1976): Blockade of the specific lethal effects of narcotic analgesics in the mouse. *Eur. J. Pharmacol.*, 39:295–303.

25. Shearer, D. E., Fleming, D. E., and Bigler, E. D. (1976): The photically evoked afterdischarge; a model for the study of drugs useful in the treatment of petit mal epilepsy. *Epilepsia*, 17:429–435.

26. Snead, O. C., III, and Bearden, L. J. (1980): Anticonvulsants specific for petit mal antagonize epileptogenic effect of leucine enkephalin. *Science*, 210:1031–1033.

27. Steinhauer, H. B., Anhut, H., and Hertting, G. (1979): The synthesis of prostaglandins and thromboxane in the mouse brain in vivo: Influence of drug induced convulsions, hypoxia, and the anticonvulsants trimethadione and diazepam. *Naunyn Schmiedebergs Arch. Pharmacol.*, 310:53–58.

28. Swinyard, E. A. (1949): Laboratory assay of clinically effective antiepileptic drugs. *J. Am. Pharm. Assoc. Sci. Ed.*, 38:201–204.

29. Tannhauser, M., Izquierdo, I. (1974): Effect of seizures and anticonvulsant agents on hippocampal RNA concentration. *Pharmacology*, 11:139–145.

30. Torda, C., and Wolff, H. G. (1947): Effect of convulsant and anticonvulsant agents on acetylcholine metabolism (activity of choline acetylase, cholinesterase) and on sensitivity to acetylcholine of effector organs. *Am. J. Physiol.*, 151:345–354.

31. Turkanis, S. A., Chiu, P., Borys, H. K., and Karler, R. (1977): Influence of delta-9-tetrahydrocannabinol and cannabidiol on photically evoked after-discharge potentials. *Psychopharmacology*, 52:207–212.

32. Withrow, C. D. (1980): Oxazolidinediones. In: *Antiepileptic Drugs: Mechanisms of Action*, edited by G. H. Glaser, J. K. Penry, and D. M. Woodbury, pp. 577–586. Raven Press, New York.

33. Woodbury, D. M. (1969): Mechanisms of action of anticonvulsants. In: *Basic Mechanisms of the Epilepsies*, edited by H. H. Jasper, A. A. Ward, Jr., and A. Pope, pp. 647–681. Little, Brown, Boston.

34. Woodbury, D. M., and Kemp, J. K. (1977): Basic mechanisms of seizures: Neurophysiological and biochemical etiology. In: *Psychopathology and Brain Dysfunction*, edited by C. Shagass, S. Gershon, and A. J. Friedhoff, pp. 169–182. Raven Press, New York.

Antiepileptic Drugs, edited by D. M. Woodbury,
J. K. Penry, and C. E. Pippenger. Raven Press,
New York © 1982.

65

Benzodiazepines

Diazepam

Dieter Schmidt

Diazepam rapidly became a drug of first choice for the treatment of status epilepticus after its intravenous use was introduced 15 years ago (12,59). It has never gained comparable significance as an oral antiepileptic agent in contrast to its most widespread use as a minor tranquilizer. The clinical pharmacokinetics of diazepam and its therapeutic use in epilepsy have been reviewed by Mandelli et al. (137), Morselli (150), Browne and Penry (27), and Mattson (143). This chapter will review selected aspects of the clinical pharmacology of diazepam as related to its therapeutic use and toxic effects in the treatment of epilepsy.

CHEMISTRY AND METHODS OF DETERMINATION

Diazepam is a yellowish crystalline substance with a melting point of 125 to 126°C and a bitter taste. Its chemical name is 7-chloro-1,3-dihydro-1-methyl-5-phenyl-2H-1, 4-benzodiazepin-2-one with a sum formula of $C_{16}H_{13}ClN_2O$. The structural formula is shown in Fig. 3. The molecular weight is 284.8. The pK_a is 3.4. Diazepam is soluble in chloroform, ethanol, dioxane, and dilute hydrochloric acid. It is not soluble in water (20). The parenteral solution (Valium®) is therefore dissolved in 40% propylene glycol, 10% ethyl alcohol, and a so-

dium benzoate/benzoic acid buffer or in cremophor EL (Stesolid®). The synthesis of the substance was described by Sternbach and Reeder (194). A study of the structure–activity relationship indicates that substitutions on position 7 in the six-membered A ring influence antiepileptic activity and selectivity (197).

Methods of Determination

Various analytical procedures are available for the quantitative determination of diazepam and its major metabolites, N-desmethyldiazepam, oxazepam, and N-methyloxazepam, as extensively reviewed by Clifford and Smyth (33) and Hailey (75). Gas–liquid chromatography (GC) is the most widely used procedure. Electron-capture detectors are most suitable for direct determination of the 1,4-benzodiazepines or measurement of their benzophenone derivatives. This is mainly because of the electronegative chloride substituent in the 7 position of the molecule and the high resonance energy of the conjugated aromatic system (40). The GC methods differ with respect to internal standards and temperature conditions, and most require extensive cleaning of the extract. However, simple, direct, and readily automatable assays are available for therapeutic drug monitoring. The current GC procedures with electron-capture detector have a sensitivity of 1 to 10 ng of the compound per ml plasma and require only 100 μl to 2 ml of plasma (9,40,66,71,75, 102,213). A number of additional procedures with similar sensitivity and volume requirements include GC with nitrogen detectors (42), high-pressure liquid chromatography (132,160), and radioimmunoassays or radioreceptor assays (23,158,161). The combination of GC with sophisticated mass spectrometer systems is most suitable for metabolic studies and other research purposes (89). Gas–liquid chromatography with flame ionization detectors is mainly employed for toxicology and drug abuse detection (75). Less often used methods are thin-layer chromatography (196), cathode ray polarographic determination (18), and fluorometric screening (207).

Clorazepate can be determined directly (75) or by measurement of *N*-desmethyldiazepam to which it is decarboxylated in acid solutions (67,211).

ABSORPTION, DISTRIBUTION, AND EXCRETION

Absorption

Oral Administration

Following a single oral dose of 5, 10, or 20 mg of diazepam, mean peak plasma concentrations of 145 ng/ml (110–180 ng/ml), 216 ng/ml (130–300 ng/ml), and 370 ng/ml (300–500 ng/ml), respectively, were obtained, mostly within 30 to 90 min, indicating a rather rapid absorption (Fig. 1) (10,40,53,86,96,119). Absorption seemed complete in one study, as indicated by similar areas under the oral and the intravenous plasma concentration curves (102). The bioavailability of Valium® tablets was 75% in two volunteers (112). Chronic alcoholism (184) or the administration of morphine, pethidine, or atropine (55) will impair the absorption. Antacids or a standard meal may influence the rate of absorption of diazepam, but the extent of ab-

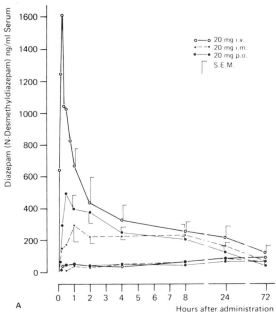

FIG. 1. Serum concentrations of diazepam and *N*-desmethyldiazepam following a single intravenous, intramuscular, or oral dose (**A**), a multiple oral dose (**B**), a single rectal dose (**C**), and a single intramuscular dose (**D**). (**A** and **B** from Hillestad et al., refs. 85, 86, and **C** and **D** from Meberg et al., ref. 144, with permission.)

(*Figure continues on facing page.*)

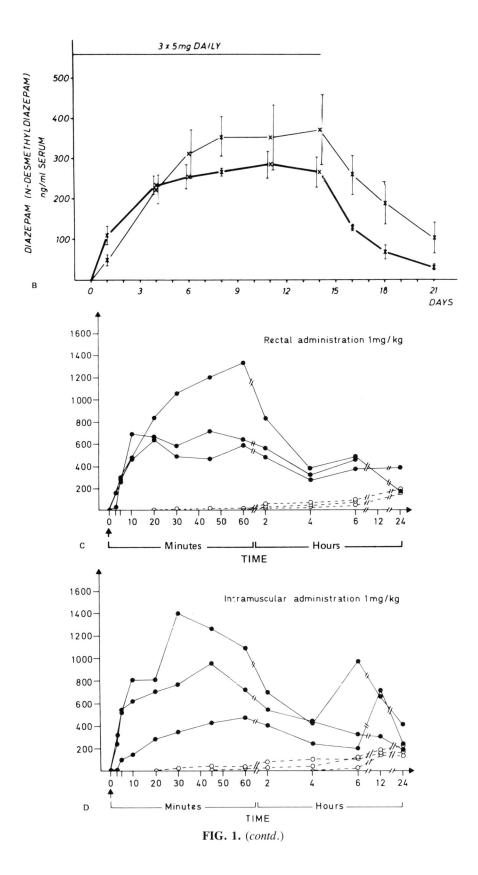

FIG. 1. (*contd.*)

sorption remains unaffected (67). Ingestion of metoclopramide (152) and possibly alcohol (80,128) may enhance the absorption. In children compared with adults and the elderly, an earlier peak (30 min) is observed (57). Clorazepate, a prodrug for *N*-desmethyldiazepam, results in peak concentrations of 479 ng/ml (318–611 ng/ml) of *N*-desmethyldiazepam in about 1 hr after a brief lag in absorption (215). The effect of antacids on the absorption of clorazepate is controversial (31,185).

Intravenous Administration

Following an intravenous dose of 10 or 20 mg of diazepam, peak plasma concentrations of about 700 to 800 ng/ml and 1,100 to 1,607 ng/ml, respectively, are reached within 3 to 15 min in volunteers (Fig. 1) (10,86). Haram et al. (77) studied the plasma concentration shortly after intravenous administration of 30 mg of diazepam during labor. After 55 sec, a plasma concentration of 1,047 ng/ml was recorded; at 135 sec after injection, a mean plasma concentration of 991 ng/ml was reached. These data indicate a most rapid increase in plasma concentration, surpassing the 500 ng/ml level that is minimally required for seizure control in less than 1 min. At doses of about 0.2 mg/kg, peak concentrations of approximately 500 ng/ml can be expected in children (4,100). In two newborns, peak concentrations of 5,775 to 10,800 ng/ml and 2,750 to 6,450 ng/ml were recorded 5 min after administration of 1 mg/kg or 0.5 mg/kg, respectively (126). Precipitation may occur when the intravenous diazepam solution is mixed with saline solutions (93). Adsorption of diazepam to the plastic tubing during infusion is possible (131).

Intramuscular Administration

After the intramuscular administration of 10 or 20 mg of diazepam, peak plasma concentrations of 35 to 300 ng/ml and 300 ng/ml, respectively, can be expected in adults within 30 to 60 min (Fig. 1) (11,13,86,121). The rather wide variation of plasma concentrations quite possi-

ble below 500 ng/ml and the late peak do not encourage the use of intramuscular administration in adults. The sources of variation include the site and the depth of the injection, the need to avoid injection into adipose tissue, the needle size, and the expertise of the person who performs the injection (53). In newborns and children up to 12 years, the intramuscular administration gave less erratic results and produced plasma concentrations above 500 ng/ml within the first 10 min. Peak concentrations of 206 to 1,400 ng/ml were recorded at 10 to 60 min after administration of 0.24 to 1 mg/kg (Fig. 1) (4,126,144).

Rectal Administration

Administration of 0.5 mg/kg or 1 mg/kg of diazepam solution in rectioles (rectal tube) resulted in peak plasma concentrations of 300 to 800 ng/ml within 4 to 45 min or of 600 to 1,400 ng/ml within 10 to 60 min. Plasma concentrations of 500 ng/ml required for acute seizure control are reached in infants and children under 11 years within 2 to 6 min (Fig. 1) (4,45,114,126,144). In contrast, suppositories are not suitable for acute treatment of a seizure in children (4,114) or in adults (121,177) because of delayed peaks and low plasma concentrations.

Distribution

After the peak concentration has been reached, a mostly biexponential decline of the plasma concentration can be observed; correspondingly, an open two-compartment model is usually employed. A short distribution half-life ($t_{1/2}\alpha$) of about 1 hr determines the rapid initial decline. Correspondingly, the plasma concentration may drop below therapeutic values (200 ng/ml) within 15 to 20 min after intravenous injection, depending on the initial peak concentration (Fig. 1). The subsequent slower decline results mainly from the elimination of the drug; its slope determines the apparent plasma elimination half-life ($t_{1/2}\beta$) (Table 1). A less frequently preferred three-compartment model with an additional deep compartment has been proposed by Kaplan et al. (102). A second smaller peak of the plasma concentration may occur after a meal. The mechanism of the redistribution is unclear; a change in plasma protein binding by food intake (118) and an enterohepatic circulation have been excluded.

Tissue Distribution

As a result of its low pK_a and its lipophilic character, diazepam distributes quickly in lipoid tissues and rapidly crosses the blood–brain barrier. In rats, diazepam is found in liver, kidneys, heart, lungs, spleen, testes, and muscular and perirenal adipose tissue in higher concentrations than in plasma 1 hr after intraperitoneal

administration of 0.6 mg/kg [³H]diazepam (178). In human scapular adipose tissue, diazepam accumulates moderately at 30 to 60 min after intravenous administration (139). After intravenous administration in mice, N^{14}-CH₃-diazepam is seen in brain within 18 sec by whole-body autoradiography (208). Based on its most rapid antiepileptic effect, sometimes observed within seconds after intravenous administration (Fig. 2), a very rapid penetration of diazepam into the human brain may be assumed. The subsequent decline and selective binding in different brain regions are rather difficult to predict from animal data. The decline probably begins within minutes after administration and is likely to differ for various brain regions. In addition, redistribution into the brain may also occur.

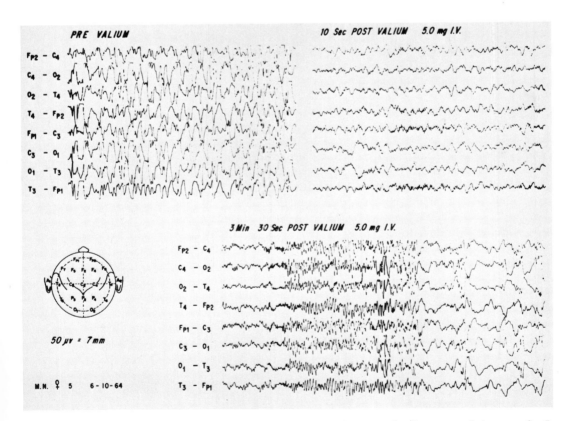

FIG. 2. Ten seconds after intravenous administration of 5 mg diazepam, the electroencephalogram of a 5-year-old girl in status epilepticus is completely free of polyspikes, which return 3½ min later, although there were no clinical signs. (From Lombroso, ref. 129, with permission.)

TABLE 1. *Pharmacokinetics of diazepam, N-desmethyldiazepam, and oxazepam*[a]

	Diazepam	Ref.	N-Desmethyl-diazepam	Ref.	Oxazepam	Ref.
Apparent volume of distribution (liter/kg)						
Volunteers	0.95–2.0	7,24,92,102,109,112	0.64–1.11 / 1.58[b]; 1.63[c]	111,203 / 215	0.7 (47.7–61.2 liters)	106,188
Epileptic patients						
Premature newborns	1.8 ± 0.3	150				
Infants	1.3 ± 0.2	150				
Children	2.6 ± 0.5	150				
Elderly (over 60 yr)	0.8–2.2	112	0.85 ± 0.14	113		
Liver disease	0.59–1.74	24,112	0.63 ± 0.12	111	(52–61 liters)	188
Species differences						
Dog	5.6	109				
Rabbit	5.5	109				
Guinea pig	2.5	109				
Rat	4.5	109				
Plasma protein binding (%)						
Volunteers	96–97	109,208	96.6	106	87–89	188
Fetus, newborn	84	97				
Liver disease	95.3 ± 1.8	112			86–87	188
Renal insufficiency	92.0 ± 7.7	95	94.5 ± 2.8	95		
Chronic alcoholism	97.8 ± 1.2	201				
Species differences						
Dog	96.0	109	95.9	109		
Rabbit	89.9	109	94.7	109		
Guinea pig	91.3	109	78.6	109		
Rat	86.3	109	90.5	109		
Distribution half-life ($t_{1/2}\alpha$, hr)						
Volunteers	0.96–2.2	102,109	0.17–0.78	65,111		
	1.1 ± 0.3[b]	108				
	4.2 ± 2.3[c]	108				
Epileptic patients			1.28 ± 0.44	215		
Apparent elimination half-life ($t_{1/2}\beta$, hr)						
Volunteers or psychiatric patients	32–36[b]	7,108	51 ± 6.2; 48–55[b]	111,113	5.1–5.6[b]	188
	28–54[c]	9,17,24,85,102,109,208	92; 51 ± 7[c]	85,203		
Epileptic patients	36.4 ± 4.9	82	39.2 ± 14.3[b]	215		
			40.4 ± 6.0[c]	215		

Premature newborns	75 ± 35	150				
Full-term newborns	31 ± 2	150				
Diazepam pretreated	18 ± 1	150				
Barbiturate, pretreated	29 ± 1	150				
Infants	10 ± 2	150				
Children	17 ± 3[b]	150				
Elderly (over 60–65 yr)	80–100	106	151 ± 60	113		
Liver disease	59–116	24,82,111,112	108.2 ± 40.3	111	5.3–5.8	188
Renal insufficiency						
Pregnancy	65 ± 29	148				
Species differences						
Dog	7.6	109	9	208		
Rabbit	2.7	109				
Guinea pig	2.4	109				
Rat	1.1	109	4	208		
Mouse						
Plasma clearance (ml/min)						
Volunteers or psychiatric patients	15–35	7,82,109,208	7.4–11.3	111,113	113–136	188
	26.0 ± 10.8[b]	108	16.73 ± 2[d]	203		
Epileptic patients	18.2 ± 7.0[c]	108				
	18.7 ± 2.3[e]	82	35.8 + 7.4[b]	215		
			34.6 ± 8.1[c]	215		
Liver disease	8–24	82,111,112	4.6	111	137–155	188
Elderly (over 60 yr)	10–32	112	4.3 ± 1.5	113		
Pregnancy	28 ± 10	148				

[a] Data are given as mean ± S.D. or the range of values.
[b] Single dose.
[c] Multiple dose.
[d] Total body clearance.
[e] Metabolic clearance rate.

Plasma and Tissue Protein Binding

The apparent volume of distribution of diazepam in volunteers ranges from 1 to 2 liter/kg (Table 1). It is higher in children or the elderly and increases in liver cirrhosis or hepatitis because of a lower protein binding (Table 1). Simultaneous ingestion of ethanol may decrease the volume of distribution (133), which is not affected by alcohol withdrawal (162).

Diazepam and N-desmethyldiazepam are both strongly bound to plasma proteins, mainly albumin, over the therapeutic range (Table 1). The apparent association constant K_{app} is 1.3 $M^{-1}10^{-4}$ for normal serum (116). The high protein binding is responsible for the fact that diazepam distributes only very little into red blood cells, resulting in a blood/plasma concentration ratio of 0.58 ± 0.15 (112), or into saliva (2–3.5%) and CSF, representing the free fraction of diazepam (43,81,100). Protein binding is unaffected by age or food intake (110) but is impaired *in vitro* by oleic acid (191), in liver disease, or in uremia, resulting in lower K_{app} of 0.9 and 0.2 $M^{-1}10^{-4}$, respectively, probably because of inhibitors of binding in serum (116,117). A lower protein binding increases the plasma clearance in man, as only the free fraction is extracted by the liver, independent of liver blood flow, but significant species differences are obvious, both in percentage of bound diazepam and in the fact that metabolism in dog, rabbit, and rat is affected by liver blood flow (109).

Excretion

In volunteers, the apparent elimination half-life of diazepam is about 1 to 2 days (Table 1). In patients with epilepsy chronically treated with enzyme-inducing antiepileptic drugs, the elimination half-life is about 30% shorter, corresponding to a higher metabolic clearance rate (Table 1) (82). The elimination is independent of the dose, with no evidence for zero-order kinetics (108), and is unaffected by the route of administration (86).

When single and multiple administrations were compared in humans, a similar or even a longer elimination half-life was seen with multiple administration, which indicates that diazepam does not induce its own metabolism in man (102,108) despite earlier suggestions (183). During chronic administration of diazepam to volunteers or psychiatric patients (15–20 mg daily), mean steady-state plasma concentrations of 200 to 1,000 ng/ml of diazepam and 120 to 1,070 ng/ml of N-desmethyldiazepam can be expected within 1 to 2 weeks (Fig. 1) (17, 39,85,102,208). Plasma concentrations of 100 to 500 ng/ml were determined in patients with epilepsy who were receiving additional antiepileptic drugs (21,42).

The elimination rate is age dependent. Premature newborns have a longer elimination half-life than full-term newborns (Table 1) who have an elimination half-life similar to that of adults. In contrast, infants and children have a shorter elimination half-life, which is probably the result of increased plasma clearance (Table 1). Comedication may also shorten the elimination half-life in newborns. The elderly show a longer elimination half-life, mostly because of a change in the volume of distribution (Table 1). Liver disease may decrease the clearance and enlarge the volume of distribution and thus produce a twofold to fivefold longer elimination half-life (Table 1) (68), whereas chronic alcohol intake without significant liver disease accelerates the elimination of diazepam (182).

N-Desmethyldiazepam is formed as long as diazepam is returning from the peripheral to the central compartment, which explains why the N-desmethyldiazepam elimination half-life tends to be longer when diazepam is given instead of N-desmethyldiazepam itself or clorazepate, its prodrug (Table 1). N-Desmethyldiazepam has a longer elimination half-life than diazepam (Table 1). With chronic treatment, N-desmethyldiazepam will accumulate more than diazepam in plasma and CSF, resulting in two to five times higher plasma concentrations when compared with single administration (Fig. 1) (54,85,108). In patients with liver disease, the plasma clearance of N-desmethyldiazepam is decreased (Table 1). Oxazepam has a very short elimination half-life because of its high plasma clearance which is independent of age and liver disease (Table 1).

Routes of Excretion

Man excretes 62 to 73% of the administered dose of diazepam in the urine and approximately 10% in the feces (178). The main urinary metabolites of diazepam are conjugated oxazepam and conjugated N-desmethyldiazepam, whereas conjugated N-methyloxazepam and free N-desmethyldiazepam or diazepam are of minor significance. During the first 24 hr, about 7 to 11% of the dose is excreted in the urine. With higher doses, e.g., in intoxication, a higher relative amount of the hydroxylated metabolites is excreted (101).

Diazepam or a diazepam metabolite may pass through the intestinal wall into the gut lumen, as about 5 to 18% of the administered [^{14}C]diazepam appears in stool despite the absence of significant biliary excretion of diazepam, which is less than 0.1% of the dose excreted (82,112). Consequently, there is no sound evidence for a significant enterohepatic circulation in man despite earlier suggestions (180,181). There are species differences in the relative amounts excreted in urine and in the feces (178).

BIOTRANSFORMATION

Demethylation of diazepam at N-1 to N-desmethyldiazepam, which is further metabolized by oxidation at C-3 to oxazepam, and direct oxidation of diazepam at C-3 to N-methyloxazepam are the major steps in the biotransformation of diazepam in man (Fig. 3). Oxidation of diazepam and N-desmethyldiazepam, N-methyloxazepam, and oxazepam at C-4 were described in different animal species (see Fig. 3) (5,178). The principal site of biotransformation is in the liver microsomes (2). Whereas the N-demethylation is rather rapid, as indicated by the appearance of N-desmethyldiazepam about 20 min after a single dose, the oxidation steps are slower (105).

The rapid antiepileptic effect shortly after intravenous administration and before N-des-

methyldiazepam concentrations are reached indicates that diazepam per se possesses antiepileptic activity. N-Desmethyldiazepam is a significant metabolite, since it possesses antiepileptic, sedative, hypnotic, and anxiolytic properties (39,203). In mice, N-desmethyldiazepam, oxazepam, and N-methyloxazepam have antipentylenetetrazol activity comparable to that of diazepam. At the ED_{50}, the therapeutic brain concentration is 100 ng/g for the three compounds. Oxazepam has the best therapeutic index of the three drugs (142). The antiepileptic activity of clorazepate, which is rapidly decarboxylated to N-desmethyldiazepam in the stomach, is currently being investigated in man (205,215). Oxazepam also has significant antiepileptic properties in man (130). Because of their low plasma concentrations, oxazepam and N-methyloxazepam do not significantly contribute to the antiepileptic effect of diazepam treatment.

The biotransformation of diazepam is age dependent. It is metabolized *in vitro* as early as the 13th week of pregnancy by human fetal liver microsomes to N-desmethyldiazepam and N-methyloxazepam but at a lower rate than by adult liver microsomes (2). In the first days after delivery, a limited *in vivo* capacity to form hydroxylated and demethylated metabolites and a lower glucuronizing capacity have been revealed (150,151). During the first years of life, the relative share of hydroxylated metabolites will continue to increase (150). Phenobarbital treatment during intrauterine life or after delivery will lead to increased biotransformation, resulting in more hydroxylated metabolites in the newborn (150).

There are significant species differences in biotransformation. Rats have a lower formation rate for N-desmethyldiazepam and a higher elimination rate for oxazepam compared with mice (Table 1). This explains why the effects of diazepam are longer lasting in mice than in rats; retention time of both metabolites, both active anticonvulsants, is longer in mice (141). The effect of phenobarbital on the *in vitro* metabolism of diazepam by liver microsomes indicated species differences. It led to more hy-

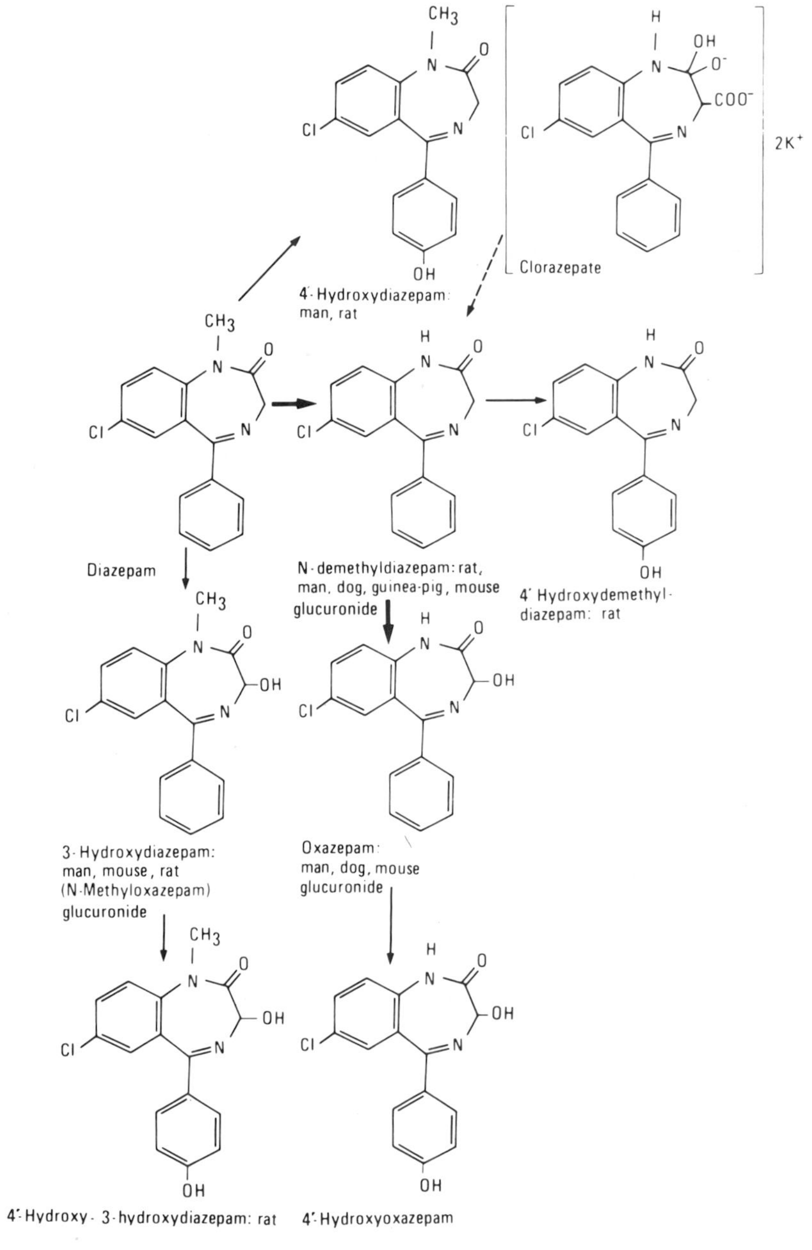

FIG. 3. Biotransformation of diazepam. Major steps are indicated by *thick arrows*. Note that the Cl at the 7 position remains intact. Clorazepate is decarboxylated to *N*-desmethyldiazepam. (Modified from Alvin and Bush, ref. 5, with permission.)

droxylated metabolites in mice and to more hydroxylated, *N*-demethylated, and polar metabolites (179) in rats, whereas in guinea pigs, only *N*-demethylated metabolites were increased (140).

INTERACTIONS WITH OTHER DRUGS

Diazepam rarely influences the pharmacokinetics of other drugs. It does not increase the urinary excretion of 6-β-hydroxycortisol, indicating that it is, if at all, not a potent enzyme inducer in man, nor does it influence the plasma levels of warfarin (156), ethanol, or tricyclic antidepressants (189). It does not displace phenytoin from its plasma protein binding sites (87). Whether it has an effect on the bilirubin-binding capacity of serum in newborns is controversial (3,217). Diazepam does not interfere with measurements of adrenal hormones in urine (36), nor does it affect the metabolic clearance rate of methylprednisolone and its sodium succinate (195). The influence of diazepam on the plasma concentration of phenytoin is controversial; both lower and higher plasma phenytoin levels have been reported after addition of diazepam (90,167,190,206). Diazepam may accelerate the elimination of phenobarbital in man and in the rat (84).

Diazepam pharmacokinetics are not significantly influenced by oral steroids (192). Whether phenobarbital or phenytoin influences the plasma concentration of diazepam is controversial (114,210). Disulfiram reduces the plasma clearance of diazepam and N-desmethyldiazepam, whereas oxazepam is not affected (134). Cimetidine lowers both the plasma clearance of diazepam and the apparent volume of distribution, which may lead to higher plasma levels of diazepam (107). With combined treatment with lithium carbonate and diazepam, but on neither drug alone, severe hypothermia has been described in one case (153). The mechanism of the interaction remains unclear. From a clinical perspective, apart from the obvious additional sedative effect when combined with sedative or hypnotic drugs or ethanol (149), diazepam is rarely involved in a drug interaction of clinical significance.

RELATION OF PLASMA CONCENTRATION TO SEIZURE CONTROL

The Relation of Dose to Plasma Concentration

The available clinical evidence suggests that diazepam plasma concentrations differ widely, up to 10-fold after a single oral dose (41,53,

137,165,218) and up to threefold with chronic treatment (17,54,208). Intramuscular injection leads to as much as 10-fold differences in plasma diazepam concentrations and to as much as fourfold differences in the CSF concentrations of diazepam and N-desmethyldiazepam (10,53, 81,99,121). Severalfold differences in plasma diazepam concentrations were reported following intravenous (21,24,61) and rectal (4) administration. Experimentally, over 10-fold differences in whole-brain concentration have been shown after intravenous administration of oxazepam (142). In conclusion, the poor correlation between dose and concentration in plasma and CSF (and probably in brain) makes it very difficult to predict the actual concentration correctly from the administered dose, regardless of the mode of administration.

Therapeutic Plasma Concentration

Sound clinical evidence for a relationship between plasma concentration and seizure control is based on prospective trials in which the plasma concentration is monitored before and during seizure control or at recurrence of a seizure. Unfortunately, only a few such studies are available (220). One report indicated that plasma concentrations of 300 to 700 ng/ml were needed for initial control of focal seizures after intravenous administration of 0.14 to 0.34 mg/kg of diazepam in three children aged 4, 5, and 15 years. Seizure control could be maintained with plasma diazepam concentrations of more than 130 to 180 ng/ml (49). In a second study, the individual therapeutic plasma concentrations were not given, but rectal administration (0.12–0.45 mg/kg) produced seizure control in two children with plasma concentrations of 183 to 1,135 ng/ml 10 min after administration (4). Two other children required 330 ng/ml and 250 ng/ml, respectively, for seizure control (4,210). Knudsen (114) noted that one child had febrile convulsions despite a plasma diazepam level of 1,185 ng/ml after rectal administration of 0.7 mg/kg of the drug.

The clinical evidence in adults is limited to plasma concentrations of diazepam associated with the suppression of EEG discharges. Matt-

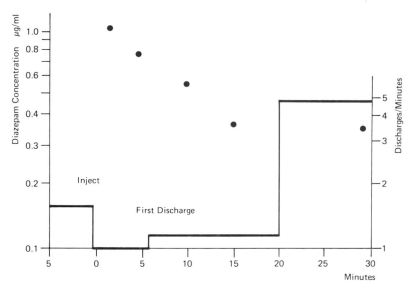

FIG. 4. The effect of intravenous administration of diazepam on 3- to 4-Hz spike-and-wave complexes. Discharges are suppressed at peak concentrations of about 1,000 ng/ml; suppression is maintained for 6 min until the plasma concentration falls below 700 ng/ml. Discharge frequency is indicated by a *bar graph*, scale on right. Diazepam concentrations are indicated by *filled circles*, scale on left. (From Booker and Celesia, ref. 21, with permission. Copyright © 1973, American Medical Association.)

son (143) noted persistent spiking in the EEG of a 52-year-old confused man despite plasma diazepam concentrations of 220 ng/ml. In another case, paroxysmal spiking with photic stimulation disappeared after 10 mg of diazepam was given intravenously and remained controlled at 110 ng/ml. Booker and Celesia (21) found a significant correlation between the suppression of interictal specific paroxysmal discharges in the EEG and the serum concentration of diazepam (Fig. 4). A plasma concentration of 1,300 ng/ml (600–2,000 ng/ml) was necessary in photosensitive patients for protection against stroboscopic stimulation. The suppression was maintained by plasma concentrations of about 500 ng/ml (100–500 ng/ml). In nonphotosensitive patients, the initial concentration for suppression of specific paroxysmal discharges was 1,800 ng/ml (600 –1,800 ng/ml). Discharges returned at 800 ng/ml (500–1,400 ng/ml). No suppression effect was observed in either group below 430 ng/ml (300–700 ng/ml).

Dasberg et al. (39) found that a minimal steady-state plasma concentration of 400 ng/ml was necessary for the anxiolytic effect of di-

azepam. A combination of the anxiolytic and the antiepileptic effect of diazepam has elegantly been demonstrated by Mattson (143) who described a 40-year-old man with anxiety-provoked hyperventilation which led to myoclonic seizures. Diazepam at plasma concentrations of 270 ng/ml relieved the anxiety, the emotional stimulus apparently was suppressed, and the spiking of the EEG and the seizures improved. Blood levels of more than 100 ng/ml were associated with an increase in β activity and a decrease in α activity in the EEGs of volunteers (50), as frequently seen with diazepam treatment (see 27,103).

Variation of Therapeutic Concentrations

When diazepam is given to a patient for acute seizure control, clinical and electroencephalographic evidence, reviewed above, indicates that the concentration required for initial control of the seizure or suppression of the EEG discharge is higher than the concentration needed to maintain the desired therapeutic effect. It is tempting to assume that a rapidly occuring change in the ''severity'' from the ictal to the postictal state is responsible for the lower plasma concentration requirements (176). Age or additional disease, as in hepatic encephalopathy, increases the sensitivity to the muscle-relaxant and depressant effects of diazepam (24,62,91,165).

The severalfold difference in therapeutic concentrations between patients may be the result of differences in the type or the "severity" of the epilepsy, or both. For the treatment of status epilepticus, a long duration of the status and acute underlying brain disease are significantly related to poor prognosis of treatment, which may be expected to require higher therapeutic concentrations if control can be achieved at all. Maintenance of suppression of specific focal or generalized discharges requires higher concentrations than does suppression of photosensitivity (21). Generalized EEG discharges are more readily suppressed by diazepam than are focal abnormalities (123,154). This suggests, if extrapolation from EEG data to clinical seizures is allowed, that primary generalized and focal epilepsies may possibly require different therapeutic concentrations for acute or chronic treatment.

Toxic Effects Related to Plasma Concentration

Side effects such as drowsiness, ataxia, and feelings of dizziness mostly occur at the beginning of treatment in up to an estimated 10 to 40% of patients (27) and disappear with reduction of the dose. Irritability, inattention, sedation, and hypotonia are more common in children (4) and may partly be related to the accumulation of *N*-desmethyldiazepam (114). Diazepam produced little change in REM sleep but a marked decrease in stage 4 sleep during short-term and subchronic oral administration and during withdrawal (94). The dose-related side effects tend to lessen or disappear with the duration of treatment because of the development of tolerance.

There seems to be a good correlation between the plasma concentration of diazepam and sedative effects after single-dose studies (86,96). At about 200 ng/ml, subjects tended to become slightly tired and drowsy (119). Most subjects were fast asleep at plasma concentrations of 1,600 ng/ml within 15 min after the intravenous administration. A transient deficiency in mental arithmetic, blurred vision, and amnesia persisted during the first 2 hr until the plasma concentration returned below 450 ng/ml (86,119). After intramuscular administration of 10 mg of diazepam, coordinative and reactive skills were impaired for as long as 5 hr at plasma concentrations exceeding 180 ng/ml (120). In other studies of mood ratings, mental and psychomotor tests, or measures of clinical sedation, the correlation to the plasma concentration was weak (61,98). According to Morselli (150), the appearance of disturbing side effects such as marked drowsiness, vertigo, ataxia, and impairment of performance is usually associated with plasma concentrations over 900 to 1,000 ng/ml. With chronic treatment, the correlation becomes more difficult because of the development of tolerance (85).

The most serious side effects after intravenous administration are the rare development of apnea, hypotension, cardiac arrest, or obtundation. After intravenous administration for status epilepticus, mild to severe hypotension or respiratory depression occurred in 5.2% of 246 patients, including one fatal case (0.4%), with additional sedative drug treatment (175). In otherwise apparently healthy patients with epilepsy, slow intravenous administration usually produces no clinically significant hypotension or hypoventilation (154). As a precaution, however, equipment and personnel trained in cardiopulmonary resuscitation should be available when diazepam is administered intravenously.

The reason for the hypotensive and respiratory depressant action of diazepam is not clear and may involve the propylene glycol solvent (see 143). Risk factors leading to these rare life-threatening side effects include combination with sedative drugs such as barbiturates (15,163,172), lidocaine/epinephrine (187), methaqualone (44), chlordiazepoxide, or amobarbital (69), and use of a rapid (bolus) injection of even as little as 2.5 or 5 mg (26,76). Additional risk factors include higher age (62,165) and decompensated liver disease; both increase the sensitivity to diazepam and slow the elimination half-life

(24,70,91). A low serum albumin possibly with a higher free fraction and advanced heart or lung disease or any other severe disease are additional risks (22).

Newborns, especially premature newborns, may develop transient side effects after the transplacental transfer of maternal diazepam. Transient respiratory depression, muscular hypotonia, and absence of primitive reflex action up to several days were seen when more than 175 mg of diazepam was administered to the mother in the 24 hr prior to delivery (6). A transient floppy infant syndrome (63), poor sucking, transient hypothermia (157), loss of beat-to-beat variation in the fetal heart immediately following the intravenous administration (174), occasional slight hyperbilirubinemia (168), and slightly lower Apgar scores in some (46,168) but not all studies (56,78) have been reported.

An apparently rare lethal intoxication by diazepam in combination with other drugs has been described in an addict (29). Massive oral overdose may lead to cardiac arrest (16), hypotension, apnea, and coma (71). Patients intoxicated with plasma concentrations of 20,000 ng/ml of diazepam and 5,000 ng/ml of N-desmethyldiazepam and concentrations of oxazepam and N-methyloxazepam above 1,000 ng/ml have survived. Rapid clinical recovery from diazepam overdose does not result from rapid elimination, as both N-desmethyldiazepam and and N-methyloxazepam have a long elimination half-life, but is more likely the result of tolerance to the depressant effect of the drug. Patients were fully alert at plasma concentrations of 1,800 to 7,000 ng/ml of diazepam and 600 to 5,000 ng/ml of N-desmethyldiazepam 1 or 2 days after a massive overdose (16). In a diazepam-induced coma, bullous skin lesions and exocrine sweat gland necrosis may occur (209). Apart from standard intensive care treatment, exchange transfusion (200) and physostigmine (127) have been employed in diazepam intoxications.

Tolerance

The development of tolerance may be the result of CNS adaptation to the effect of diazepam or of a decline in plasma concentration, or both. Experimental data have indicated increasing dose requirements with subsequent seizures in the same animal (186), but plasma or brain concentrations were not determined. Chronic treatment in the baboon, *Papio papio,* suggested a possibly dose-dependent development of tolerance to the effect of diazepam on epileptic seizures and measures of electrical activity of the brain (103). The evidence is not conclusive, but several clinical reports suggest that diazepam may lose some of its antiepileptic effect in about 40% of all cases within 4 to 6 months of treatment; plasma concentrations were not recorded, and fluctuation of disease may have occurred independently of drug intake (27,58,204). Diazepam has been shown to be less effective in acute treatment of a recurrent seizure than in the initial seizure (49). In cats, acute tolerance develops to inhibitory effects of diazepam (14). There is suggestive evidence in man that a degree of tolerance develops to the sedative effects of diazepam during multiple administration or during intoxication (71,85).

Habituation

Whether habituation or dependence develops among patients with epilepsy chronically treated with diazepam is not known. The addiction potential of diazepam in the general population is beyond the scope of this chapter (see 135). In newborns exposed to mostly long-term intrauterine diazepam, tremor, irritability and hypertonicity, poor weight gain, and vigorous sucking may occur after delivery and are thought of as a neonatal withdrawal syndrome (166). In adults, agitation, anxiety, insomnia, tremor, hallucinosis, and generalized tonic–clonic seizures have been seen in relation to the withdrawal of diazepam in single case reports (see 135).

Pharmacological Aspects of Clinical Use

Emergency Treatment

Our knowledge of therapeutic plasma concentrations of diazepam is based on rather few data with considerable individual variation. These preliminary data indicate that 500 to 700 ng/ml are rapidly needed as a minimum for acute seizure control and that more than 150 to 200 ng/ml are necessary for maintenance of seizure control. If the plasma concentrations following different routes of administration are compared with these requirements in mind (Fig. 1), the intravenous administration is preferable to other routes as it most rapidly produces therapeutic plasma concentrations. An initial dose of 0.2 to 0.3 mg/kg i.v. is slowly (1–5 mg/min) injected in children and adults until the seizure stops or serious side effects occur. When the initial administration produces no or only short-lasting seizure control, which may happen in about every third case, a second or third intravenous injection may be effective. An interval between injections of 20 to 30 min and a total dose of less that 100 mg in 24 hr are recommended.

During emergency treatment, drug monitoring is not necessary as the intravenous dose is titrated directly against the therapeutic or toxic effect of the drug during the injection. For newborns and infants, administration of 0.5 to 1 mg/kg of diazepam in rectiole results in therapeutic concentrations within minutes which are maintained for about 1 hr. The rectiole, a rectal tube containing a solution of the drug for application through a 4-cm tube inserted in the rectum, can be used quickly by informed parents. When it is squeezed until it is withdrawn, backflow of the solution into the container can be avoided. Intramuscular administration (0.5–1 mg/kg) is about as effective as rectal administration in children; in adults, however, it cannot be recommended because of erratic and often subtherapeutic concentrations with delayed peaks. Suppositories or oral treatment with diazepam are not suitable for acute treatment of a seizure because of late peaks and inadequately low concentrations in plasma.

Oral Treatment

Oral diazepam therapy is mainly used for associated psychiatric disease in epileptic patients and only rarely as an antiepileptic adjunct in patients with persistent seizures. The recommended therapeutic dose is 0.2 to 0.4 mg/kg for adults. Steady-state plasma concentrations of diazepam and N-desmethyldiazepam are reached within 5 to 10 days and 10 to 15 days after treatment, respectively. This interval will pass before the full therapeutic or toxic response of a dosage change can be anticipated. During chronic administration of diazepam, plasma N-desmethyldiazepam concentrations will be at least similar to or even higher than the plasma diazepam concentrations. For each 1 mg/kg per day, steady-state concentrations of about 100 ng/ml of diazepam and 200 ng/ml of N-desmethyldiazepam may be expected.

Premature newborns, patients with advanced liver disease, and the elderly have a longer elimination half-life, requiring a lower dose not only for pharmacokinetic reasons but also because the sensitivity to diazepam may be higher in all three patient groups. In contrast, infants or children have a shorter elimination half-life than full-term newborns or adults, who have a similar elimination half-life. The relative ineffectiveness of oral diazepam treatment may reflect the development of tolerance within the first months or subtherapeutic plasma concentrations of less than 500 ng/ml, or both. This suggests that therapeutic drug monitoring is helpful when the desired therapeutic effect is not obtained during chronic treatment or when side effects occur. The toxic plasma concentration ranges above 1,000 ng/ml of diazepam and 2,000 ng/ml of N-desmethyldiazepam, even though only preliminary data are available.

Pregnancy

Pregnancy prolongs the elimination half-life to about 2 to 3 days because of a change in the volume of distribution (Table 1). Cord blood concentrations are similar to or even higher than maternal blood concentrations (48). After repeated administration, accumulation of diazepam and N-desmethyldiazepam occurs in the fetus (78,136). After delivery, diazepam and N-desmethyldiazepam will remain in neonatal plasma for several days, causing mostly sedative side effects, especially in premature newborns, and possibly a neonatal withdrawal syndrome. Diazepam and *N*-desmethyldiazepam are found in breast milk in a concentration 4 to 10 times lower than in plasma (25,34,47) but may result in neonatal plasma concentrations in the range of 30 to 75% of the maternal concentration. The possible teratogenic effect and the development of side effects in the neonate suggest a critical benefit/risk evaluation prior to the use of diazepam during pregnancy or in nursing mothers.

Teratogenesis

The possible teratogenic effect of diazepam is difficult to assess because of chance correlations and confounding factors, e.g., maternal illness, familiary association to cleft lip and cleft palate (51), and consumption of other drugs (173). No definite causal relationship has been established, even though suggestive retrospective evidence on the association between the first trimester intake of benzodiazepines and oral clefts has been presented (1,169,170,173) but not always confirmed (38). If a teratogenic effect of diazepam exists in fact, it may induce a fourfold increase in relative risk; this implies an actual risk of 0.4% for having a child with cleft lip and cleft palate (170).

TOXICITY

Diazepam-induced disease seems to be exceptionally rare. Apart from transient and mostly mild dose-related neurological side effects, an aggravation of tonic or tonic–clonic seizures may rarely occur, especially in secondary generalized epilepsy (164,199). There is no sound evidence for hematological, hepatic, or renal toxicity. There are two reports of leucopenia (28,74) and one case of acute hepatic necrosis (37) in doubtful relation to diazepam in combination with antibiotics or amitryptiline. The drug is not an enzyme inducer of significance in man (156) but increases the smooth endoplasmic reticulum in human hepatocytes (155). In volunteers, a transient decrease in renal PAH and inulin clearance without clinical symptoms has been reported after its intravenous admin-

istration (202). Furthermore, diazepam does not significantly alter thyroid function (171) or tests of thyroid function (32), pituitary function, urinary excretion of catecholamines (79), prolactin levels, or blood sugar levels (145,216). It may increase growth hormone (122) and testosterone levels (8) and may have a varying influence on appetite and weight (27). After intramuscular injection, a transient rise of the serum creatine phosphokinase can be expected (13). Diazepam induces a number of electromyographic changes of no clinical relevance on motor nerves and skeletal muscle (88). Hypersensitivity reactions to diazepam are exceptionally rare (147). Whether diazepam inflicts damage to chromosomes is controversial (214). Diazepam may induce a brown coloration of the ocular lens after chronic intake (159). Usually mild thrombophlebitis occurs in about 3 to 7% of all patients after intravenous administration, especially when diazepam is rapidly administered or injected in a small vein or precipitates develop because of mixture with saline solution (124,125). Accidental intraarterial administration may lead to painful extensive limb tissue necrosis (64).

PHARMACODYNAMICS

The current state of knowledge of the possible mechanisms of the anticonvulsant action of diazepam has been extensively reviewed by Killam and Suria (104). This chapter can only briefly summarize some of the neurophysiological and neurochemical effects of diazepam and their possible relationship to the proposed mechanism of action, with special emphasis on the putative neurotransmitter γ-aminobutyric acid (GABA).

Neurophysiological Data

The spectrum of anticonvulsant action of diazepam on experimental seizures in animals has been repeatedly reviewed (27,143,198). Diazepam is most effective in the prevention of pentylenetetrazol-induced seizures and other experimental models of primary generalized epilepsy. In animal models of partial epilepsy, diazepam depresses but does not abolish abnormal discharges at the site of the cortical lesion but prevents the spread of the abnormal activity. It may further suppress the limbic system component of partial seizures regardless of whether the limbic activity is primarily or secondarily involved in the development of the seizures (27).

Further experimental and clinical studies after parenteral administration of diazepam have confirmed the suppression of secondary epileptiform activity and the impairment of the spread of primary epileptiform discharges without significant influence on the activity of the epileptogenic lesion itself (72).

The facilitatory action of diazepam in various mammalian GABAergic synapses has been reviewed by Haefely et al. (73). Diazepam enhances presynaptic inhibition in the spinal cord, the cuneate nucleus, and the cuneothalamic relay cells and reduces the firing rate of single Purkinje cells. Collateral inhibition of cortical pyramidal tract cells by the GABAergic basket cell and the recurrent inhibition of hippocampal pyramidal cells are intensified by benzodiazepines. There seems to be ample experimental evidence, then, that benzodiazepines facilitate GABAergic synaptic transmission and that this may be the only relevant synaptic action by benzodiazepines (73). In addition, benzodiazepines also enhance GABAergic transmission at nigral dopamine neurons (73). The mechanism of facilitation of GABAergic transmission by diazepam is not yet clear (146). At the postsynaptic site, a GABAmimetic action, potentiation of exogeneous GABA action, postsynaptic reversal of bicuculline antagonism, and changes in chloride conductance and the affinity of GABA for its receptor have been suggested (73). The presynaptic site may involve uptake and release of GABA (73).

Neurochemical Data

Neurochemical studies have shown that benzodiazepines bind with high affinity and specificity to proteins in synaptic membranes of the CNS *in vivo* and *in vitro* (73). These binding sites may partly represent the pharmacological receptors that benzodiazepines have to interact with in order to produce their effect (73). Studies on the neurochemical effects of the benzodiazepines, especially diazepam, show influence on a number of putative neurotransmitters such as the catecholamines, serotonin, acetylcholine, and glycine, as reviewed by Bertilsson (19). There is evidence that some of the effects of diazepam on these neurotransmitters may be secondary to the GABAmimetic effect of diazepam (52,193). In recent years, the major interest has been focused on the inhibitory transmitter GABA (19). Benzodiazepines are potent inhibitors of seizures, especially those provoked by a decrease of the activity in GABAergic neurons. Further, diazepam can modify changes in cerebellar cyclic GMP which, in turn, are associated with changes of the inhibitory GABA system. The GABA agonist muscimol and diazepam decrease GABA turnover in *N. caudatus* and *N. accumbens* (138). These experimental studies indicate that diazepam influences GABA neurons as would a GABA agonist (19,35). There is, then, evidence to believe that diazepam enhances GABA-mediated inhibition and that the facilitation of GABAergic transmission may be related to the neurochemical mechanism of action of diazepam (219).

THERAPEUTIC USE

Emergency Treatment

Diazepam is a drug of first choice for the treatment of status epilepticus or an ongoing epileptic seizure independent of the etiology or the type of seizure involved (Table 2). Seizure control may be difficult or impossible in patients with acute underlying brain injury, additional severe disease (e.g., coma of various etiology, metabolic acidosis) or a long duration of the status (12,212). Clonazepam is sometimes effective in cases where diazepam is not. The prophylactic use of diazepam rectioles in febrile episodes to prevent febrile convulsions is currently being evaluated and compared with chronic phenobarbital prophylaxis (115). The

TABLE 2. *Therapeutic effect of diazepam in various types of status epilepticus*[a]

Type of status epilepticus	Seizure-free patients		Number of studies
	N	%	
Grand mal status	177/224	79	10
Petit mal status			
Infantile spasms	6/13	46	3
Myoclonic–astatic seizures	26/43	60	3
Absence seizures	12/16	75	4
Status of partial seizures	59/67	88	6

[a]In many cases, multiple injections were required for lasting seizure control, and most patients received additional sedative or antiepileptic drugs (175).

drug has further been employed for control of other paroxysmal clinical events, e.g., action myoclonus, Ramsay–Hunt syndrome, and symptoms of withdrawal from alcohol or drugs.

Based on the pharmacokinetic considerations described above, intravenous injection is preferable to other routes of administration for emergency treatment. With slow intravenous administration, side effects are rare, and 70 to 80% of all seizures are stopped (Table 2). Resuscitation because of apnea or hypotension may rarely become necessary, but it should be considered when risk factors are present. These include old age, advanced heart, lung, or liver disease, previous sedative drug treatment, and rapid bolus injection.

Oral Treatment

Oral diazepam, 10 to 20 mg daily for adults, is used to treat psychiatric problems of the epileptic patient, e.g., anxiety or psychotic episodes with insomnia and tenseness or belligerence. As an antiepileptic adjunct, oral diazepam is reserved, if used at all, for rare drug-resistant cases after individual consideration of benefit versus risk. In uncontrolled studies, diazepam was more effective as an antiepileptic adjunct in absence seizures (60) or in myoclonic seizures or partial seizures, as reviewed by Browne and Penry (27).

Controlled studies indicate that diazepam is less effective than phenytoin or phenobarbital for treatment of generalized tonic–clonic seizures (30) and about as effective as pheneturide in control of partial seizures (83). Oxazepam has produced very good results in the only controlled trial for treatment of partial seizures (130). In a double-blind study, clorazepate was about as effective an adjunct as phenobarbital when added to phenytoin treatment of therapy-resistant patients with partial seizures (205). The relative ineffectiveness of oral diazepam treatment may be related to the development of tolerance within the first few months and may also be the result of subtherapeutic plasma concentrations (less than 500 ng/ml), suggesting that therapeutic monitoring is desirable with chronic oral treatment.

Accumulation of both diazepam and its metabolite *N*-desmethyldiazepam occurs with multiple administration. The combination of diazepam and other sedative drugs has additional sedative effects; otherwise, diazepam rarely shows clinically significant drug interactions. Premature newborns, patients with liver disease, and the elderly are at risk for toxicity because of a prolonged elimination half-life and increased drug sensitivity that require lower dosage and careful monitoring for toxicity. Diazepam-induced toxicity is exceptionally rare. Side effects are mostly dose related at plasma concentrations of around 1,000 ng/ml and overcome by dose reduction or development of tolerance. Therapeutic drug monitoring may be useful when unusual diazepam toxicity is suspected during chronic treatment.

SUMMARY AND OUTLOOK

Diazepam is a drug of first choice for the treatment of status epilepticus because of its rapid penetration into the brain, its prompt therapeutic action in a majority of cases, and its rare toxicity. For pharmacokinetic reasons, intravenous or rectal administration is preferable to other routes. From a clinical perspective, the oral use of diazepam is not well justified because of the development of tolerance and the uncertainty whether therapeutic concentrations are reached at all.

Areas of further interest are the factors regulating the relationship of the plasma concentration to the clinical effect, especially the development of tolerance, and the curious increase in sensitivity in the elderly or in patients with liver disease. The clinical and pharmacological reasons for individual variations in therapeutic concentration await further investigations. Promising data suggest the existence of diazepam receptors possibly linked with the mechanism(s) of action of the drug. The role of putative neurotransmitters, primarily γ-aminobutyric acid, in the proposed mechanism of action requires further studies, which may lead to insight into the role of neurotransmitters in the epileptic process in general.

CONVERSION

Conversion factor:

$$CF = \frac{1000}{\text{mol. wt.}} = \frac{1000}{284.8} = 3.51$$

Conversion:

$$(\mu g/ml) \times 3.51 = (\mu moles/liter)$$

$$(\mu moles/liter) \div 3.51 = (\mu g/ml)$$

REFERENCES

1. Aarskog, D. (1975): Association between maternal intake of diazepam and oral clefts. *Lancet*, 2:921.
2. Ackermann, E., and Richter, K. (1977): Diazepam metabolism in human foetal and adult liver. *Eur. J. Clin. Pharmacol.*, 11:43–49.
3. Adoni, A., Kapitulnik, J., Kaufmann, N.A., Ron, M., and Blondheim, S. H. (1973): Effect of maternal administration of diazepam on the bilirubin-binding capacity of cord blood serum. *Am. J. Obstet. Gynecol.*, 115:577–579.
4. Agurell, S., Berlin, A., Ferngren, H., and Hellström, B. (1975): Plasma levels of diazepam after parenteral and rectal administration in children. *Epilepsia*, 16:277–283.
5. Alvin, J. D., and Bush, M. T. (1977): Physiological disposition of anticonvulsants. The benzodiazepines. In: *Anticonvulsants*, edited by J. A. Vida, pp. 140–144. Academic Press, New York.
6. André, M., Sibout, M., Petry, J.-M., and Vert, P. (1973): Dépression respiratoire et neurologique chez le prématuré nouveau-né de mère traitée par Diazépam. *J. Gynecol. Obstet. Biol. Reprod. (Paris)*, 2:357–366.
7. Andreasen, P. B., Hendel, J., Greisen, G., and Hvidberg, E. F. (1976): Pharmacokinetics of diazepam in disordered liver function. *Eur. J. Clin. Pharmacol.*, 10:115–120.
8. Argüelles, A. E., and Rosner, J. (1975): Diazepam and plasma testosterone levels. *Lancet*, 2:607.
9. Arnold, E. (1975): A simple method for determining diazepam and its major metabolites in biological fluids: Application in bioavailability studies. *Acta Pharmacol. Toxicol. (Kbh.)*, 36:335–352.
10. Baird, E. S., and Hailey, D. M. (1972): Delayed recovery from a sedative: Correlation of the plasma levels of diazepam with clinical effects after oral and intravenous administration. *Br. J. Anaesthesiol.*, 44:803–808.
11. Baird, E. S., and Hailey, D. M. (1973): Plasma levels of diazepam and its major metabolite following intramuscular administration. *Br. J. Anaesthesiol.*, 45:546–548.
12. Bamberger, P., and Matthes, A. (1966): Eine neue Therapiemöglichkeit des Status epilepticus im Kindesalter mit Valium i.v. *Z. Kinderheilkd.*, 95:155–163.
13. Bank-Mikkelsen, O. K., Steiness, E., Arnold, E., Hansen, T., Sobye, M., and Lunding, M. (1978): Serum diazepam and serum creatine kinase after intra-muscular injection of diazepam in two different vehicles. *Acta Anaesthesiol. Scand. [Suppl.]*, 67:91–95.
14. Barnett, A., and Fiore, J. W. (1973): Acute tolerance to diazepam in cats. In: *The Benzodiazepines*, edited by S. Garattini, E. Mussini, and L. O. Randall, pp. 545–557. Raven Press, New York.
15. Bell, D. S. (1969): Dangers of treatment of status epilepticus with diazepam. *Br. Med. J.*, 1:159–161.
16. Berger, R., Green, G., and Melnick, A. (1975): Cardiac arrest caused by oral diazepam intoxication. *Clin. Pediatr.*, 14:842–844.
17. Berlin, A., Siwers, B., Agurell, S., Hiort, A., Sjöqvist, F., and Ström, S. (1972): Determination of bioavailability of diazepam in various formulations from steady state plasma concentration data. *Clin. Pharmacol. Ther.*, 13:733–744.
18. Berry, D. J. (1971): The cathode-ray polarographic determination of diazepam, 7-chloro-1,3-dihydro-1-methyl-5-phenyl-2H-1,4-benzodiazepine-2-one, in human plasma. *Clin. Chim. Acta*, 32:235–241.
19. Bertilsson, L. (1978): Mechanism of action of benzodiazepines—the GABA hypothesis. *Acta Psychiatr. Scand. [Suppl.]*, 274:19–26.
20. Beyer, K.-H., and Sadée, W. (1969): Analytische Daten von vier 5-Phenyl-1,4-benzodiazepinderivaten in Monographien. 6.Mitteilung zur Chemie und Analytik von Benzodiazepinderivaten. *Dtsch. Apoth. Z.* 109:312–314.
21. Booker, H. E., and Celesia, G. G. (1973): Serum concentrations of diazepam in subjects with epilepsy. *Arch. Neurol.*, 29:191–194.
22. Boston Collaborative Drug Surveillance Program (1973): Clinical depression of the central nervous system due to diazepam and chlordiazepoxide in re-

lation to cigarette smoking and age. *N. Engl. J. Med.*, 288:277–280.

23. Bourne, R. C., Robinson, J. D., and Teale, J. D. (1978): A simple radioimmunoassay for plasma diazepam and its application to single dose studies in man. *Br. J. Pharmacol.*, 63:371P.

24. Branch, R. A., Morgan, M. H., James, J., and Read, A. E. (1976): Intravenous administration of diazepam in patients with chronic liver disease. *Gut*, 17:975–983.

25. Brandt, R. (1976): Passage of diazepam and desmethyldiazepam into breast milk. *Arzneim. Forsch.*, 26:454–457.

26. Brauninger, G., and Ravin, M. (1974): Respiratory arrest following intravenous Valium. *Ann. Ophthalmol.*, 6:805–806.

27. Browne, T. R., and Penry, J. K. (1973): Benzodiazepines in the treatment of epilepsy. *Epilepsia*, 14:277–310.

28. Bussien, R. (1974): Granulocytopénie aiguë après administration simultanée de gentamicine et diazépam. *Nouv. Presse Méd.*, 3:1236.

29. Cardauns, H., and Iffland, R. (1973): Über eine tödliche Diazepam (Valium®) Vergiftung bei einem drogenabhängigen Jugendlichen. *Arch. Toxikol.*, 31:147–151.

30. Chien, C., and Keegan, D. (1972): Diazepam as an oral long-term anticonvulsant for epileptic mental patients. *Dis. Nerv. Syst.*, 33:100–104.

31. Chun, A. H. C., Carrigan, P. J., Hoffman, D. J., Kershner, R. P., and Stuart, J. D. (1977): Effect of antacids on absorption of clorazepate. *Clin. Pharmacol. Ther.*, 22:329–335.

32. Clark, F., Hall, R., and Ormston, B. J. (1971): Diazepam and tests of thyroid function. *Br. Med. J.*, 1:585–586.

33. Clifford, J. M., and Smyth, W. F. (1974): The determination of some 1,4-benzodiazepines and their metabolites in body fluids. A review. *Analyst*, 99:241–272.

34. Cole, A. P., and Hailey, D. M. (1975): Diazepam and active metabolite in breast milk and their transfer to the neonate. *Arch. Dis. Child.*, 50:741–742.

35. Costa, E., and Greengard, P., editors (1975): *Advances in Biochemical Psychopharmacology, Vol. 14: Mechanism of Action of Benzodiazepines*. Raven Press, New York.

36. Cryer, P. E., and Sode, J. (1971): Drug interference with measurement of adrenal hormones in urine: Analgesics and tranquilizer–sedatives. *Ann. Intern. Med.*, 75:697–702.

37. Cunningham, M. L. (1965): Acute hepatic necrosis following treatment with amitriptyline and diazepam. *Br. J. Psychiatry*, 111:1107–1109.

38. Czeizel, A. (1976): Diazepam, phenytoin, and aetiology of cleft lip and/or cleft palate. *Lancet*, 1:810.

39. Dasberg, H. H., Van der Kleijn, E., Guelen, P. J. R., and Van Praag, H. M. (1974): Plasma concentrations of diazepam and of its metabolite *N*-desmethyldiazepam in relation to anxiolytic effect. *Clin. Pharmacol. Ther.*, 15:473–483.

40. De Silva, J. A. F. (1978): Electron capture–GLC in the quantitation of 1,4-benzodiazepines. In: *Antiepileptic Drugs: Quantitative Analysis and Interpre-*

tation, edited by C. E. Pippenger, J. K. Penry, and H. Kutt, pp. 111–138. Raven Press, New York.

41. De Silva, J. A. F., Bekersky, I., Puglisi, C. V., Brooks, M. A., and Weinfeld, R. E. (1976): Determination of 1,4-benzodiazepines and -diazepin-2-ones in blood by electron-capture gas–liquid chromatography. *Anal. Chem.*, 48:10–19.

42. Dhar, A. K., and Kutt, H. (1979): Monitoring diazepam and desmethyldiazepam concentrations in plasma by gas–liquid chromatography, with use of a nitrogen-sensitive detector. *Clin. Chem.*, 25:137–140.

43. DiGregorio, G. J., Piraino, A. J., and Ruch, E. (1978): Diazepam concentrations in parotid saliva, mixed saliva, and plasma. *Clin. Pharmacol. Ther.*, 24:720–725.

44. Doughty, A. (1970): Unexpected danger of diazepam. *Br. Med. J.*, 2:239.

45. Dulac, O., Aicardi, J., Rey, E., and Olive, G. (1978): Blood levels of diazepam after single rectal administration in infants and children. *J. Pediatr.*, 93:1039–1041.

46. Erkkola, R., Kangas, L., and Pekkarinen, A. (1973): The transfer of diazepam across the placenta during labour. *Acta Obstet. Gynaecol. Scand.*, 52:167–170.

47. Erkkola, R., and Kanto, J. (1972): Diazepam and breast-feeding. *Lancet*, 1:1235–1236.

48. Erkkola, R., Kanto, J., and Sellman, R. (1974): Diazepam in early human pregnancy. *Acta Obstet. Gynaecol. Scand.*, 53:135–138.

49. Ferngren, H. G. (1974): Diazepam treatment for acute convulsions in children. *Epilepsia*, 15:27–37.

50. Fink, M., Irwin, P., Weinfeld, R. E., Schwartz, M. A., and Conney, A. H. (1976): Blood levels and electroencephalographic effects of diazepam and bromazepam. *Clin. Pharmacol. Ther.*, 20:184–191.

51. Friis, M. L. (1979): Epilepsy among parents of children with facial clefts. *Epilepsia*, 20:69–76.

52. Fuxe, K., Agnati, L. F., Bolme, P., Hökfelt, T., Lidbrink, P., Ljongdal, A., Perez de la Mora, M., and Ögren, S. O. (1975): The possible involvement of GABA mechanisms in the action of benzodiazepines on central catecholamine neurons. *Adv. Biochem. Psychopharmacol.*, 14:45–61.

53. Gamble, J. A. S., Dundee, J. W., and Assaf, R. A. E. (1975): Plasma diazepam levels after single dose oral and intramuscular administration. *Anaesthesia*, 30:164–169.

54. Gamble, J. A. S., Dundee, J. W., and Gray, R. C. (1976): Plasma diazepam concentrations following prolonged administration. *Br. J. Anaesth.*, 48:1087–1090.

55. Gamble, J. A. S., Gaston, J. H., Nair, S. G., and Dundee, J. W. (1976): Some pharmacological factors influencing the absorption of diazepam following oral administration. *Br. J. Anaesth.*, 48:1181–1185.

56. Gamble, J. A. S., Moore, J., Lamki, H., and Howard, P. J. (1977): A study of plasma diazepam levels in mother and infant. *Br. J. Obstet. Gynaecol.*, 84:588–591.

57. Garattini, S., Marcucci, F., Morselli, P. L., and Mussini, E. (1973): The significance of measuring blood levels of benzodiazepines. In: *Biological Ef-*

fects of Drugs in Relation to Their Plasma Concentrations, edited by D. S. Davies and B. N. C. Prichard, pp. 211–226, Macmillan, London.

58. Gastaut, H., Roger, J., and Lob, H. (1973): Medical treatment of epilepsy. In: *Anticonvulsant Drugs, Vol. II,* edited by J. Mercier, pp. 535–598. Pergamon Press, Oxford.

59. Gastaut, H., Roger, J., Soulayrol, R., Lob, H., and Tassinari, C. A. (1965): L'action du diazepam (Valium®) dans le traitement des formes non convulsives de l'épilepsie généralisée. *Rev. Neurol.,* 112:99–118.

60. Geller, M., and Christoff, N. (1971): Diazepam in the treatment of childhood epilepsy. *J.A.M.A.,* 215:2087–2090.

61. Ghoneim, M. M., Mewaldt, S. P., and Ambre, J. (1975): Plasma levels of diazepam and mood ratings. *Anesth. Analg. (Cleve.),* 54:173–177.

62. Giles, H. G., MacLeod, S. M., Wright, J. R., and Sellers, E. M. (1978): Influence of age and previous use on diazepam dosage required for endoscopy. *Can. Med. Assoc. J.,* 118:513–514.

63. Gillberg, C. (1977): "Floppy infant syndrome" and maternal diazepam. *Lancet,* 2:244.

64. Gould, J. D. M., and Lingam, S. (1977): Hazards of intraarterial diazepam. *Br. Med. J.,* 2:298–299.

65. Greenblatt, D. J. (1978): Determination of desmethyldiazepam in plasma by electron-capture GLC: Application to pharmacokinetic studies of clorazepate. *J. Pharm. Sci.,* 67:427–429.

66. Greenblatt, D. J. (1978): Simultaneous gas-chromatographic analysis for diazepam and its major metabolite, desmethyldiazepam, with use of double internal standardization. *Clin. Chem.,* 24:1838–1841.

67. Greenblatt, D. J., Allen, M. D., MacLaughlin, D. S., Harmatz, J. S., and Shader, R. I. (1978): Diazepam absorption: Effect of antacids and food. *Clin. Pharmacol. Ther.,* 24:600–609.

68. Greenblatt, D. J., Harmatz, J. S., and Shader, R. I. (1978): Factors influencing diazepam pharmacokinetics: Age, sex, and liver disease. *Int. J. Clin. Pharmacol.,* 16:177–179.

69. Greenblatt, D. J., and Koch-Weser, J. (1973): Adverse reactions to intravenous diazepam: A report from the Boston Collaborative Drug Surveillance Program. *Am. J. Med. Sci.,* 266:261–266.

70. Greenblatt, D. J., and Koch-Weser, J. (1974): Clinical toxicity of chlordiazepoxide and diazepam in relation to serum albumin concentration: A report from the Boston Collaborative Drug Surveillance Program. *Eur. J. Clin. Pharmacol.,* 7:259–262.

71. Greenblatt, D. J., Woo, E., Allen, M. D., Orsulak, P. J., and Shader, R. I. (1978): Rapid recovery from massive diazepam overdose. *J.A.M.A.,* 240:1872–1874.

72. Guerrero-Figueroa, R., Gallant, D. M., Guerrero-Figueroa, C., and Gallant, J. (1973): Electrophysiological analysis of the action of four benzodiazepine derivatives on the central nervous system. In *The Benzodiazepines,* edited by S. Garattini, E. Mussini, and L. O. Randall, pp. 489–511. Raven Press, New York.

73. Haefely, W., Polc, P., Schaffner, R., Keller, H. H., Pieri, L., and Möhler, H. (1978): Facilitation of GABA-ergic transmission by drugs. In: *GABA-Neu-*

rotransmitters, Alfred Benzon Symposium 12, pp. 357–375. Munksgaard, Copenhagen.

74. Haerten, K., and Pöttgen, W. (1975): Leukopenie nach Benzodiazepin-Derivaten. *Med. Welt.,* 26:1712–1714.

75. Hailey, D. M. (1974): Chromatography of the 1,4-benzodiazepines. *J. Chromatogr.,* 98:527–568.

76. Hall, S. C., and Ovassapian, A. (1977): Apnea after intravenous diazepam therapy. *J.A.M.A.,* 238:1052.

77. Haram, K., Bakke, O. M., Johannessen, K. H., and Lund, T. (1978): Transplacental passage of diazepam during labor: Influence of uterine contractions. *Clin. Pharmacol. Ther.,* 24:590–599.

78. Haram, K., Sagen, N., and Brandt, R. D. (1976): Transplacental passage of diazepam following intravenous injection immediately prior to operative vaginal delivery. *Int. J. Gynaecol. Obstet.,* 14:545–549.

79. Havard, C. W. H., Saldanha, V. F., Bird, R., and Gardner, R. (1972): The effect of diazepam on pituitary function in man. *J. Endocrinol.,* 52:79–85.

80. Hayes, S. L., Pablo, G., Radomski, T., and Palmer, R. F. (1977): Ethanol and oral diazepam absorption. *N. Engl. J. Med.,* 296:186–189.

81. Hendel, J. (1975): Cumulation in cerebrospinal fluid of the *N*-desmethyl metabolite after long-term treatment with diazepam in man. *Acta Pharmacol. Toxicol. (Kbh.),* 37:17–22.

82. Hepner, G. W., Vesell, E. S., Lipton, A., Harvey, H. A., Wilkinson, G. R., and Schenker, S. (1977): Disposition of aminopyrine, antipyrine, diazepam, and indocyanine green in patients with liver disease or on anticonvulsant drug therapy: Diazepam breath test and correlations in drug elimination. *J. Lab. Clin. Med.,* 90:440–456.

83. Hershon, H. I., and Parsonage, M. (1969): Comparative trial of diazepam and pheneturide in treatment of epilepsy. *Lancet,* 2:859–862.

84. Heubel, F., and Frank, R. (1970): Zur induktiven Wirkung von Diazepam. *Arzneim. Forsch.,* 20:1706–1708.

85. Hillestad, L., Hansen, T., and Melsom, H. (1974): Diazepam metabolism in normal man. II. Serum concentration and clinical effect after oral administration and cumulation. *Clin. Pharmacol. Ther.,* 16:485–489

86. Hillestad, L., Hansen, T., Melsom, H., and Drivenes, A. (1974): Diazepam metabolism in normal man. I. Serum concentrations and clinical effects after intravenous, intramuscular, and oral administration. *Clin. Pharmacol. Ther.,* 16:479–484.

87. Hooper, W. D., Sutherland, J. M., Bochner, F., Tyrer, J. H., and Eadie, M. J. (1973): The effect of certain drugs on the plasma protein binding of phenytoin. *Aust. N.Z.J. Med.,* 3:377–381.

88. Hopf, H. C., and Billmann, F. (1973): The effect of diazepam on motor nerves and skeletal muscle. *J. Neurol.,* 204:255–262.

89. Horning, M. G., Nowlin, J., Butler, C. M., Lertratanangkoon, K., Sommer, K., and Hill, R. M. (1975): Clinical applications of gas chromatography/mass spectrometer/computer systems. *Clin. Chem.,* 21:1282–1287.

90. Houghton, G. W., and Richens, A. (1974): The effect of benzodiazepines and pheneturide on phe-

nytoin metabolism in man. *Br. J. Clin. Pharmacol.*, 1:344–345.

91. Hoyumpa, A. M., Jr. (1978): Disposition and elimination of minor tranquilizers in the aged and in patients with liver disease. *South. Med. J.*, 71 (Suppl. 2):23–28.

92. Hvidberg, E. F., and Dam, M. (1976): Clinical pharmacokinetics of anticonvulsants. *Clin. Pharmacokinet.*, 1:161–188.

93. Jusko, W. J., Gretch, M., and Gassett, R. (1973): Precipitation of diazepam from intravenous preparations. *J.A.M.A.*, 225:176.

94. Kales, A., and Scharf, M. B. (1973): Sleep laboratory and clinical studies of the effects of benzodiazepines on sleep: Flurazepam, diazepam, chlordiazepoxide, and RO 5-4200. In: *The Benzodiazepines,* edited by S. Garattini, E. Mussini, and L. O. Randall, pp. 577–598. Raven Press, New York.

95. Kangas, L., Kanto, J., Forsström, J., and Iisalo, E. (1976): The protein binding of diazepam and *N*-desmethyldiazepam in patients with poor renal function. *Clin. Nephrol.*, 5:114–118.

96. Kanto, J. (1975): Plasma concentrations of diazepam and its metabolites after peroral, intramuscular, and rectal administration. *Int. J. Clin. Pharmacol.*, 12:427–432.

97. Kanto, J., Erkkola, R., and Sellman, R. (1973): Accumulation of diazepam and *N*-desmethyldiazepam in the fetal blood during the labour. *Ann. Clin. Res.*, 5:375–379.

98. Kanto, J., Iisalo, E. U. M., Hovi-Viander, M., and Kangas, L. (1979): A comparative study on the clinical effects of oxazepam and diazepam. Relationship between plasma level and effect. *Int. J. Clin. Pharmacol. Biopharm.*, 17:26–31.

99. Kanto, J., Kangas, L., and Siirtola, T. (1975): Cerebrospinal-fluid concentrations of diazepam and its metabolites in man. *Acta Pharmacol. Toxicol. (Kbh.)*, 36:328–334.

100. Kanto, J. H., Pihlajamaki, K. K., and Iisalo, E. U. M. (1974): Concentrations of diazepam in adipose tissue of children. *Br. J. Anaesth.*, 46:168.

101. Kanto, J., Sellman, R., Haataja, M., and Hurme, P. (1978): Plasma and urine concentrations of diazepam and its metabolites in children, adults and in diazepam-intoxicated patients. *Int. J. Clin. Pharmacol.*, 16:258–264.

102. Kaplan, S. A., Jack, M. L., Alexander, K., and Weinfeld, R. E. (1973): Pharmacokinetic profile of diazepam in man following single intravenous and oral and chronic oral administrations. *J. Pharm. Sci.*, 62:1789–1796.

103. Killam, E. K., Matsuzaki, M., and Killam, K. F. (1973): Effects of chronic administration of benzodiazepines on epileptic seizures and brain electrical activity in *Papio papio*. In: *The Benzodiazepines,* edited by S. Garattini, E. Mussini, and L. O. Randall, pp. 443–460. Raven Press, New York.

104. Killam, E. K., and Suria, A. (1980): Antiepileptic drugs—benzodiazepines. In: *Antiepileptic Drugs: Mechanisms of Action,* edited by G. H. Glaser, J. K. Penry, and D. M. Woodbury, pp. 597–615. Raven Press, New York.

105. Klotz, U. (1977): Wichtige Faktoren, die beim Menschen die Verteilung und Elimination von Diazepam beeinflussen. *Fortschr. Med.*, 95:1958–1964.

106. Klotz, U. (1978): Klinische Pharmakokinetik von Diazepam und seinen biologisch aktiven Metaboliten. *Klin. Wochenschr.*, 56:895–904.

107. Klotz, U., Anttila, V.-J., and Reimann, I. (1979): Cimetidine/diazepam interaction. *Lancet*, 2:699.

108. Klotz, U., Antonin, K. H., and Bieck, P. R. (1976): Comparison of the pharmacokinetics of diazepam after single and subchronic doses. *Eur. J. Clin. Pharmacol.*, 10:121–126.

109. Klotz, U., Antonin, K. H., and Bieck, P. R. (1976): Pharmacokinetics and plasma binding of diazepam in man, dog, rabbit, guinea pig and rat. *J. Pharmacol. Exp. Ther.*, 199:67–73.

110. Klotz, U., Antonin, K. H., and Bieck, P. (1977): Food intake and plasma binding of diazepam. *Br. J. Clin. Pharmacol.*, 4:85–86.

111. Klotz, U., Antonin, K. H., Brügel, H., and Bieck, P. R. (1977): Disposition of diazepam and its major metabolite desmethyldiazepam in patients with liver disease. *Clin. Pharmacol. Ther.*, 21:430–436.

112. Klotz, U., Avant, G. R., Hoyumpa, A., Schenker, S., and Wilkinson, G. R. (1975): The effects of age and liver disease on the disposition and elimination of diazepam in adult man. *J. Clin. Invest.*, 55:347–359.

113. Klotz, U., and Müller-Seydlitz, P. (1979): Altered elimination of desmethyldiazepam in the elderly. *Br. J. Clin. Pharmacol.*, 7:119–120.

114. Knudsen, F. U. (1977): Plasma-diazepam in infants after rectal administration in solution and by suppository. *Acta Paediatr. Scand.*, 66:563–567.

115. Knudsen, F. U., and Vestermark, S. (1978): Prophylactic diazepam or phenobarbitone in febrile convulsions: A prospective, controlled study. *Arch. Dis. Child.*, 53:660–663.

116. Kober, A., Jenner, Å, Sjöholm, I., Borgå, O., and Odar-Cederlöf, I. (1978): Differentiated effects of liver cirrhosis on the albumin binding sites for diazepam, salicylic acid and warfarin. *Biochem. Pharmacol.*, 27:2729–2735.

117. Kober, A., Sjöholm, I., Borgå, O., and Odar-Cederlöf, I. (1979): Protein binding of diazepam and digitoxin in uremic and normal serum. *Biochem. Pharmacol.*, 28:1037–1042.

118. Korttila, K., and Kangas, L. (1977): Unchanged protein binding and the increase of serum diazepam levels after food intake. *Acta Pharmacol. Toxicol. (Kbh.)*, 40:241–246.

119. Korttila, K., and Linnoila, M. (1975): Absorption and sedative effects of diazepam after oral administration and intramuscular administration into the vastus lateralis muscle and the deltoid muscle. *Br. J. Anaesth.*, 47:857–862.

120. Korttila, K., and Linnoila, M. (1975): Psychomotor skills related to driving after intramuscular administration of diazepam and meperidine. *Anesthesiology*, 42:685–691.

121. Korttila, K., Sothman, A., and Andersson, P. (1976): Polyethylene glycol as a solvent for diazepam: Bioavailability and clinical effects after intramuscular

administration, comparison of oral, intramuscular and rectal administration, and precipitation from intravenous solutions. *Acta Pharmacol. Toxicol. (Kbh.),* 39:104–117.

122. Koulu, M., Lammintausta, R., Kangas, L., and Dahlström, S. (1979): The effect of methysergide, pimozide, and sodium valproate on the diazepam-stimulated growth hormone secretion in man. *J. Clin. Endocrinol. Metab.,* 48:119–122.

123. Laguna, J. F., and Korein, J. (1972): Diagnostic value of diazepam in electroencephalography. *Arch. Neurol.,* 26:265–272.

124. Langdon, D. E. (1973): Thrombophlebitis following diazepam. *J.A.M.A.,* 225:1389.

125. Langdon, D. E., Harlan, J. R., and Bailey, R. L. (1973): Thrombophlebitis with diazepam used intravenously. *J.A.M.A.,* 223:184–185.

126. Langslet, A., Meberg, A., Bredesen, J. E., and Lunde, P. K. M. (1978): Plasma concentrations of diazepam and N-desmethyldiazepam in newborn infants after intravenous, intramuscular, rectal and oral administration. *Acta Paediatr. Scand.,* 67:699–704.

127. Larson, G. F., Hurlbert, B. J., and Wingard, D. W. (1977): Physostigmine reversal of diazepam-induced depression. *Anesth. Analg. (Cleve.),* 56:348–351.

128. Linnoila, M., Otterström, S., and Anttila, M. (1974): Serum chlordiazepoxide, diazepam and thioridazine concentrations after the simultaneous ingestion of alcohol or placebo drink. *Ann. Clin. Res.,* 6:4–6.

129. Lombroso, C. T. (1966): Treatment of status epilepticus with diazepam. *Neurology (Minneap.),* 16:629–634.

130. Lou, H. O. C. (1968): Oxazepam in the treatment of psychomotor epilepsy. *Neurology (Minneap.),* 18:986–990.

131. MacKichan, J., Duffner, P. K., and Cohen, M. E. (1979): Adsorption of diazepam to plastic tubing. *N. Engl. J. Med.,* 301:332–333.

132. MacKichan, J. J., Jusko, W. J., Duffner, P. K., and Cohen, M. E. (1979): Liquid-chromatographic assay of diazepam and its major metabolites in plasma. *Clin. Chem.,* 25:856–859.

133. MacLeod, S. M., Giles, H. G., Patzalek, G., Thiessen, J. J., and Sellers, E. M. (1977): Diazepam actions and plasma concentrations following ethanol ingestion. *Eur. J. Clin. Pharmacol.,* 11:345–349.

134. MacLeod, S. M., Sellers, E. M., Giles, H. G., Billings, B. J., Martin, P. R., Greenblatt, D. J., and Marshman, J. A. (1978): Interaction of disulfiram with benzodiazepines. *Clin. Pharmacol. Ther.,* 24:583–589.

135. Maletzky, B. M., and Klotter, J. (1976): Addiction to diazepam. *Int. J. Addict.,* 11:95–115.

136. Mandelli, M., Morselli, P. L., Nordio, S., Pardi, G., Principi, N., Sereni, F., and Tognoni, G. (1975): Placental transfer of diazepam and its disposition in the newborn. *Clin. Pharmacol. Ther.,* 17:564–572.

137. Mandelli, M., Tognoni, G., and Garattini, S. (1978): Clinical pharmacokinetics of diazepam. *Clin. Pharmacokinet.,* 3:72–91.

138. Mao, C. C., Marco, E., Revuelta, A., Bertilsson, L., and Costa, E. (1977): The turnover rate of γ-aminobutyric acid in the nuclei of telencephalon: Implications in the pharmacology of antipsychotics and

of a minor tranquilizer. *Biol. Psychiatry,* 12:359–371.

139. Marcucci, F., Fanelli, R., Frova, M., and Morselli, P. L. (1968): Levels of diazepam in adipose tissue of rats, mice and man. *Eur. J. Pharmacol.,* 4:464–466.

140. Marcucci, F., Fanelli, R., Mussini, E., and Garattini, S. (1970): Effect of phenobarbital on the *in vitro* metabolism of diazepam in several animal species. *Biochem. Pharmacol.,* 19:1771–1776.

141. Marcucci, F., Mussini, E., Fanelli, R., and Garattini, S. (1970): Species differences in diazepam metabolism. I. Metabolism of diazepam metabolites. *Biochem. Pharmacol.,* 19:1847–1851.

142. Marcucci, F., Mussini, E., Guaitani, A., Fanelli, R., and Garattini, S. (1971): Anticonvulsant activity and brain levels of diazepam and its metabolites in mice. *Eur. J. Pharmacol.,* 16:311–314.

143. Mattson, R. H. (1972): The benzodiazepines. In: *Antiepileptic Drugs,* edited by D. M. Woodbury, J. K. Penry, and R. P. Schmidt, pp. 497–516. Raven Press, New York.

144. Meberg, A., Langslet, A., Bredesen, J. E., and Lunde, P. K. M. (1978): Plasma concentration of diazepam and N-desmethyldiazepam in children after a single rectal or intramuscular dose of diazepam. *Eur. J. Clin. Pharmacol.,* 14:273–276.

145. Mehta, S. (1971): The influence of premedication with diazepam on the blood sugar level. *Anaesthesia,* 26:468–472.

146. Meldrum, B. (1978): Convulsant drugs, anticonvulsants and GABA-mediated neuronal inhibition. In: *GABA-Neurotransmitters, Alfred Benzon Symposium 12,* pp. 390–405. Munksgaard, Copenhagen.

147. Milner, L. (1977): Allergy to diazepam. *Br. Med. J.,* 1:144.

148. Moore, R. G., and McBride, W. G. (1978): The disposition kinetics of diazepam in pregnant women at parturition. *Eur. J. Clin. Pharmacol.,* 13:275–284.

149. Morland, J., Setekleiv, J., Haffner, J. F. W., Stromsaether, C. E., Danielsen, A., and Wethe, G. H. (1974): Combined effects of diazepam and ethanol on mental and psychomotor functions. *Acta Pharmacol. Toxicol. (Kbh.),* 34:5–15.

150. Morselli, P. L. (1977): Psychotropic drugs—benzodiazepines. In: *Drug Disposition During Development,* edited by P. L. Morselli, pp. 449–459. Spectrum Publications, New York.

151. Morselli, P. L., Principi, N., Tognoni, G., Reali, E., Belvedere, G., Standen, S. M., and Sereni, F. (1973): Diazepam elimination in premature and full term infants, and children. *J. Perinat. Med.,* 1:133–141.

152. Nair, S. G., Gamble, J. A. S., Dundee, J. W., and Howard, P. J. (1976): The influence of three antacids on the absorption and clinical action of oral diazepam. *Br. J. Anaesth.,* 48:1175–1180.

153. Naylor, G. J., and McHarg, A. (1977): Profound hypothermia on combined lithium carbonate and diazepam treatment. *Br. Med. J.,* 2:22.

154. Niedermeyer, E. (1970): Intravenous diazepam and its anticonvulsive action. *Johns Hopkins Med. J.,* 127:79–96.

155. Orlandi, F., Bamonti, F., Dini, M., Koch, M., and Jezequel, A. M. (1975): Hepatic cholesterol synthesis in man: Effect of diazepam and other drugs. *Eur. J. Clin. Invest.*, 5:139–146.

156. Orme, M., Breckenridge, A., and Brooks, R. V. (1972): Interactions on benzodiazepines with warfarin. *Br. Med. J.*, 3:611–614.

157. Owen, J. R., Irani, S. F., and Blair, A. W. (1972): Effect of diazepam administered to mothers during labour on temperature regulation of neonate. *Arch. Dis. Child.*, 47:107–110.

158. Owen, F., Lofthouse, R., and Bourne, R. C. (1979): A radioreceptor assay for diazepam and its metabolites in serum. *Clin. Chim. Acta*, 93:305–310.

159. Pau, H. (1974): Braune Einlagerungen in die Linse nach Diazepam-(Valium®-)Gaben. *Klin. Monatsbl. Augenheilkd.*, 164:446–448.

160. Perchalski, R. J., and Wilder, B. J. (1978): Determination of benzodiazepine anticonvulsants in plasma by high-performance liquid chromatography. *Anal. Chem.*, 50:554–557.

161. Peskar, B., and Spector, S. (1973): Quantitative determination of diazepam in blood by radioimmunoassay. *J. Pharmacol. Exp. Ther.*, 186:167–172.

162. Pond, S. M., Phillips, M., Benowitz, N. L., Galinsky, R. E., Tong, T. G., and Becker, C. E. (1979): Diazepam kinetics in acute alcohol withdrawal. *Clin. Pharmacol. Ther.*, 25:832–836.

163. Prensky, A. L., Raff, M. C., Moore, M. J., and Schwab, R. S. (1967): Intravenous diazepam in the treatment of prolonged seizure activity. *N. Engl. J. Med.*, 276:779–784.

164. Prior, P. F., Maclaine, G. N., Scott, D. F., and Laurance, B. M. (1971): Intravenous diazepam. *Lancet*, 2:434–435.

165. Reidenberg, M. M., Levy, M., Warner, H., Coutinho, C. B., Schwartz, M. A., Yu, G., and Cheripko, J. (1978): Relationship between diazepam dose, plasma level, age, and central nervous system depression. *Clin. Pharmacol. Ther.*, 23:371–374.

166. Rementeria, J. L., and Bhatt, K. (1977): Withdrawal symptoms in neonates from intrauterine exposure to diazepam. *J. Pediatr.*, 90:123–126.

167. Rogers, H. J., Haslam, R. A., Longstreth, J., and Lietman, P. S. (1977): Phenytoin intoxication during concurrent diazepam therapy. *J. Neurol. Neurosurg. Psychiatry*, 40:890–895.

168. Rosanelli, K. (1970): Über die Wirkung von pränatal verabreichtem Diazepam auf das Frühgeborene. *Geburtshilfe Frauenheilkd.*, 30:713–724.

169. Safra, M. J., and Oakley, G. P., Jr. (1975): Association between cleft lip with or without cleft palate and prenatal exposure to diazepam. *Lancet*, 2:478–480.

170. Safra, M. J., and Oakley, G. P., Jr. (1976): Valium: An oral cleft teratogen? *Cleft Palate J.*, 13:198–200.

171. Saldanha, V. F., Bird, R., and Havard, C. W. H. (1971): Effect of diazepam (Valium®) on dialysable thyroxine. *Postgrad. Med. J.*, 47:326–328.

172. Sawyer, G. T., Webster, D. D., and Schut, L. J. (1968): Treatment of uncontrolled seizure activity with diazepam. *J.A.M.A.*, 203:913–918.

173. Saxen, I., and Saxen, L. (1975): Association between maternal intake of diazepam and oral clefts. *Lancet*, 2:498.

174. Scher, J., Hailey, D. M., and Beard, R. W. (1972): The effects of diazepam on the fetus. *J. Obstet. Gynaecol. Brit. Commonw.*, 79:635–638.

175. Schmidt, D. (1981): *Behandlung der Epilepsien.* Thieme Verlag, Stuttgart.

176. Schmidt, D., and Janz, D. (1977): Therapeutic plasma concentrations of phenytoin and phenobarbitone. In: *Antiepileptic Drug Monitoring*, edited by C. Gardner-Thorpe, D. Janz, H. Meinardi, and C. E. Pippenger, pp. 214–225. Pitman Medical, Tunbridge Wells, Kent.

177. Schwartz, D. E., Vecchi, M., Ronco, A., and Kaiser, K. (1966): Blood levels after administration of 7-chloro-1,3-dihydro-1-methyl-5-phenyl-2H-1,4-benzodiazepine-2-one (Diazepam) in various forms. *Arzneim. Forsch.*, 16:1109–1110.

178. Schwartz, M. A., Koechlin, B. A., Postma, E., Palmer, S., and Krol, G. (1965): Metabolism of diazepam in rat, dog, and man. *J. Pharmacol. Exp. Ther.*, 149:423–435.

179. Schwartz, M. A., and Postma, E. (1968): Metabolism of diazepam *in vitro*. *Biochem. Pharmacol.*, 17:2443–2449.

180. Sellman, R., Hurme, M., and Kanto, J. (1977): Biliary excretion of diazepam and its metabolites in man after repeated oral doses. *Eur. J. Clin. Pharmacol.*, 12:209–212.

181. Sellman, R., Kanto, J., and Pekkarinen, J. (1975): Biliary excretion of diazepam and its metabolites in man. *Acta Pharmacol. Toxicol. (Kbh.)*, 37:242–249.

182. Sellman, R., Kanto, J., Raijola, E., and Pekkarinen, A. (1975): Human and animal study on elimination from plasma and metabolism of diazepam after chronic alcohol intake. *Acta Pharmacol. Toxicol. (Kbh.)*, 36:33–38.

183. Sellman, R., Kanto, J., Raijola, E., and Pekkarinen, A. (1975): Induction effect of diazepam on its own metabolism. *Acta Pharmacol. Toxicol. (Kbh.)*, 37:345–351.

184. Sellman, R., Pekkarinen, A., Kangas, L., and Raijola, E. (1975): Reduced concentrations of plasma diazepam in chronic alcoholic patients following an oral administration of diazepam. *Acta Pharmacol. Toxicol. (Kbh.)*, 36:25–32.

185. Shader, R. I., Georgotas, A., Greenblatt, D. J., Harmatz, J. S., and Allen, M. D. (1978): Impaired absorption of desmethyldiazepam from clorazepate by magnesium aluminum hydroxide. *Clin. Pharmacol. Ther.*, 24:308–315.

186. Sharer, L., and Kutt, H. (1971): Intravenous administration of diazepam. Effects on penicillin-induced focal seizures in the cat. *Arch. Neurol.*, 24:169–175.

187. Sherman, P. M. (1974): Cardiac arrest with diazepam. *J. Oral Surg.*, 32:567.

188. Shull, H. J., Wilkinson, G. R., Johnson, R., and Schenker, S. (1976): Normal disposition of oxazepam in acute viral hepatitis and cirrhosis. *Ann. Intern. Med.*, 84:420–425.

189. Silverman, G., and Braithwaite, R. A. (1973): Benzodiazepines and tricyclic antidepressant plasma levels. *Br. Med. J.*, 3:18–20.

190. Siris, J. H., Pippenger, C. E., Werner, W. L., and Masland, R. L. (1974): Anticonvulsant drug-serum levels in psychiatric patients with seizure disorders. *N.Y. State J. Med.*, 74:1554–1556.

191. Sjödin, T. (1977): Circular dichroism studies on the inhibiting effect of oleic acid on the binding of di-

azepam to human serum albumin. *Biochem. Pharmacol., 26:*2157–2161.

192. Sonnenberg, A., Koelz, H. R., Herz, R., Benes, I., and Blum, A. L. (1978): Der Einfluss oraler Kontrazeptiva auf die Demethylierung von Diazepam und Dimethyl-*N*-Aminoantipyrin. *Verh. Deutsch. Ges. Inn. Med.,* 84:1485–1488.

193. Stein, L., Wise, C. D., and Belluzzi, J. D. (1975): Effects of benzodiazepines on central serotonergic mechanisms. *Adv. Biochem. Psychopharmccol.,* 14:29–44.

194. Sternbach, L. H., and Reeder, E. (1961): Quinazolines and 1,4-benzodiazepines. IV. Transformations of 7-chloro-2-methylamino-5-phenyl-3H-1,4-benzodiazepine-4-oxide. *J. Org. Chem.,* 26:4936–4941.

195. Stjernholm, M. R., and Katz, F. H. (1975): Effects of diphenylhydantoin, phenobarbital, and diazepam on the metabolism of methylprednisolone and its sodium succinate. *J. Clin. Endocrinol. Metab.,* 41:887–893.

196. Sun, S.-R. (1978): Fluorescence–TLC densitometric determination of diazepam and other 1,4-benzodiazepines in serum. *J. Pharm. Sci.,* 67:1413–14.5.

197. Swinyard, E. A. (1969): Laboratory evaluation of antiepileptic drugs. Review of laboratory methods. *Epilepsia,* 10:107–119.

198. Swinyard, E. A., and Castellion, A. W. (1966): Anticonvulsant properties of some benzodiazepines. *J. Pharmacol. Exp. Ther.,* 151:369–375.

199. Tassinari, C. A., Gastaut, H., Dravet, C. and Roger, J. (1971): A paradoxical effect: Status epilepticus induced by benzodiazepines. *Electroencephalogr. Clin. Neurophysiol.,* 31:182.

200. Thearle, M. J., Dunn, P. M., and Hailey, D. M. (1973): Exchange transfusion for diazepam intoxication at birth followed by jejunal stenosis. *Proc. R. Soc. Med.,* 66:349–350.

201. Thiessen, J. J., Sellers, E. M., Denbeigh, P., and Dolman, L. (1976): Plasma protein binding of diazepam and tolbutamide in chronic alcoholics. *J. Clin. Pharmacol.,* 16:345–351.

202. Thompson, W. L. (1978): Management of alcohol withdrawal syndromes. *Arch. Intern. Med.,* 138:278–283.

203. Tognoni, G., Gomeni, R., De Maio, D., Albert, G. G., Franciosi, P., and Scieghi, G. (1975): Pharmacokinetics of *N*-demethyldiazepam in patients suffering from insomnia and treated with nortriptyline. *Br. J. Clin. Pharmacol.,* 2:227–232.

204. Trolle, E. (1965): Diazepam (Valium®) in the treatment of epilepsy. *Acta Neurol. Scand. [Suppl],* 13:535–539.

205. Troupin, A. S., Wilensky, A. J., Friel, P., Leal K., and Ojemann, L. M. (1980): Clorazepate as an anticonvulsant. In: *Antiepileptic Therapy: Advances in Drug Monitoring,* edited by S. I. Johannessen, P. L. Morselli, C. E. Pippenger, A. Richens, D. Schmidt, and H. Meinardi, pp. 291–298. Raven Press, New York.

206. Vajda, F. J. E., Prineas, R. J., and Lovell, R. R. H. (1971): Interaction between phenytoin and the benzodiazepines. *Br. Med. J.,* 1:346.

207. Valentour, J. C., Monforte, J. R., Lorenzo, B., and Sunshine, I. (1975): Fluorometric screening method for detecting benzodiazepines in blood and urine. *Clin. Chem.,* 21:1976–1979.

208. Van der Kleijn, E., Van Rossum, J. M., Muskens, E. T. J. M., and Rijntjes, N. V. M. (1971): Pharmacokinetics of diazepam in dogs, mice and humans. *Acta Pharmacol. Toxicol. [Suppl.] (Kbh.),* 3:109–127.

209. Varma, A. J., Fisher, B. K., and Sarin, M. K. (1977): Diazepam-induced coma with bullae and eccrine sweat gland necrosis. *Arch. Intern. Med.,* 137:1207–1210.

210. Viala, A., Cano, J. P., Dravet, C., Tassinari, C. A., and Roger, J. (1971): Blood levels of diazepam (Valium) and *N*-desmethyldiazepam in the epileptic child. *Psychiatr. Neurol. Neurochir.,* 74:153–158.

211. Viala, A., Cano, J.-P., Reynier, J.-F., and Rispe, R. (1978): Determination of *N*-desmethyldiazepam in plasma by gas chromatography with an internal standard. *J. Chromatogr.,* 147:349–357.

212. Wallis, W., Kutt, H., and McDowell, F. (1968): Intravenous diphenylhydantoin in the treatment of acute repetitive seizures. *Neurology (Minneap.),* 18:513–525.

213. Weinfeld, R. E., Posmanter, H. N., Khoo, K.-C., and Puglisi, C. V. (1977): Rapid determination of diazepam and nordiazepam in plasma by electron capture gas–liquid chromatography. *J. Chromatogr.,* 143:581–595.

214. White, B. J., Driscoll, E. J., Tjio, J.-H., and Smilack, Z. H. (1974): Chromosomal aberration rates and intravenously given diazepam. A negative study. *J.A.M.A.,* 230:414–417.

215. Wilensky, A. J., Levy, R. H., Troupin, A. S., Moretti-Ojemann, L., and Friel, P. (1978): Clorazepate kinetics in treated epileptics. *Clin. Pharmacol. Ther.,* 24:22–30.

216. Wilson, J. D., King, D. J., and Sheridan, B. (1979): Tranquillisers and plasma prolactin. *Br. Med. J.,* 1:123–124.

217. Windorfer, A., Jr. (1973): Untersuchungen über die Steigerung der Albumin-Bilirubin-Dissoz ation durch Medikamente *in vitro* und *in vivo. Monatsschr. Kinderheilkd.,* 121:469–470.

218. Zingales, I. A. (1973): Diazepam metabolism during chronic medication. Unbound fraction in plasma, erythrocytes and urine. *J. Chromatogr.,* 75:55–78.

219. Guidotti, A., and Ebstein, B. (1981): Role of GABA-benzo-diazepine receptor complex in epilepsy. In: *Neurotransmitters, Seizures, and Epilepsy,* edited by P. L. Morselli, K. G. Lloyd, W. Löscher, B. Meldrum, and E. H. Reynolds, pp. 85–91. Raven Press, New York.

220. Milligan, N., Dhillon, S., Richens, A., and Oxley, J. (1981): Rectal diazepam in the treatment of absence status: A Pharmacodynamic study. *J. Neurol. Neurosurg. Psychiatry,* 44:914-917.

Antiepileptic Drugs, edited by D. M. Woodbury, J. K. Penry, and C. E. Pippenger. Raven Press, New York © 1982.

66

Benzodiazepines

Clonazepam

F. E. Dreifuss and Susumu Sato

Clonazepam, 5-(2-chlorophenol)-1,3-dihydro-7-nitro-2H-1,4-benzodiazepine-2-one, a chlorinated derivative of nitrazepam, was approved for use as an antiepileptic drug by the United States Food and Drug Administration in 1975. The use of clonazepam (Clonopin®) in the treatment of epilepsy has been reviewed extensively (24,26,137,138).

Benzodiazepines were first synthesized by Dziewónski and Sternbach in 1933 (153), and in 1966 clonazepam was evaluated as one of the antiepileptic benzodiazepines by Swinyard and Castellion (154). The clinical application of this compound was not undertaken until the early 1970s. Clonazepam has the chemical structure shown in Fig. 1.

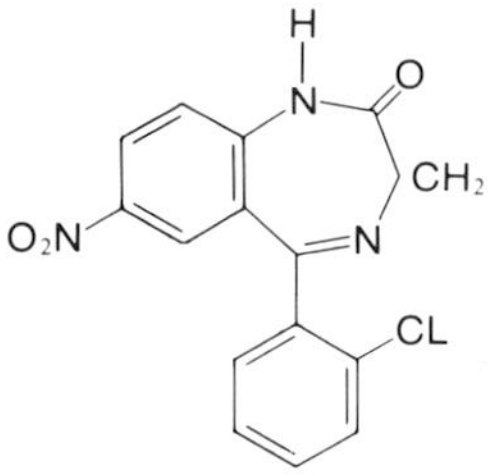

CHEMISTRY

Benzodiazepines are a class of heterocyclic six-membered-ring compounds transformed into seven-membered novel hetero-ring compounds. Substituents in the 7 position of ring A with the electron-withdrawing properties of heavier halogens, particularly with some nitro and trifluoromethyl groups, increase biological potency, e.g., activity against pentylenetetrazol-induced seizures. It has also been found that fluorine, chlorine, or two halogens at the *ortho* position of ring C have potent effects. Clonazepam has a nitro substitution at the 7 position of ring A and a chlorine at the *ortho* position of ring C.

Clonazepam is a light yellow crystalline powder with a molecular weight of 315.7. It shows pK_a values of 1.5 and 10.5. The pK_a of 1.5 corresponds to the removal of the proton of the protonated nitrogen in the 4 position of the molecule, and the pK_a of 10.5 corresponds to the deprotonation of the nitrogen in the 1 position. Thus, the compound is virtually undissociated throughout the physiological pH range (89).

METHODS OF DETERMINATION

In 1973, Naestoft et al. (129) described an electron-capture gas chromatographic assay for

CLONAZEPAM

FIG. 1. Structure of clonazepam.

clonazepam. In 1974 and 1976, de Silva et al. (42,43) reported an electron capture gas–liquid chromatographic assay for the determination of clonazepam in blood and urine. The original method required repeated extraction procedures and acid hydrolysis prior to the electron capture GLC analysis, a time-consuming technique. Since then, the extraction procedure has been improved, with the omission of acid hydrolysis (64,128,134). A gas chromatographic–mass spectrometric assay for clonazepam using positive ion chemical ionization with ammonia was described in 1977 and 1978 (121,122) and was subsequently modified to employ negative chemical ionization using methane as both the gas chromatographic carrier gas and the chemical ionization reagent gas (61). The sensitivity of this technique is considerably greater (61). Other modifications of GLC techniques have been reported (29,30,41,50,59,150). High-performance liquid chromatography (136,160) and thin-layer chromatography (156,164) have also been used.

A simple and specific radioimmunoassay technique for detection of clonazepam in plasma without extraction can be used with antibodies to clonazepam produced in rabbits and exhibiting a high degree of specificity for clonazepam (44,45). When [^{3}H]iodine is used as a tracer, the radioimmunoassay has a limited sensitivity of 5 ng/ml. A more rapid and less costly technique utilizes a radioimmunoassay with ^{125}I (44).

ABSORPTION AND DISTRIBUTION

Clonazepam appears to be well absorbed, and the peak plasma level occurs within 1 to 4 hr after oral administration, but it may occur as late as 8 hr (15,49,79,89). In dogs, a micronized preparation was rapidly and completely absorbed, but nonmicronized drug in a gelatin capsule was slowly and incompletely absorbed (89). Clonazepam administered orally in a solution of propylene glycol was absorbed completely. Micronization of clonazepam overcomes the dissolution rate-limiting characteristics of the compound in the overall absorption of the drug (89). After a single dose of 1.5 mg of

[2-^{14}C]clonazepam (55), the absorption rate ranged from 81.2 to 98.1% of the dose, calculated from total radioactivity and concentration mean values of the radioactive compound from the plasma. The distribution is rapid because of its high lipid solubility (97). Clonazepam is 47% protein bound (26). The volume of distribution (V_d) ranged from 1.5 to 4.4 liter/kg in eight healthy adult volunteers (17). Following intravenous administration of clonazepam to sheep, there was rapid equilibration of CSF and unbound serum concentrations of the drug, and the large volume of distribution suggested tissue binding (133).

PLASMA LEVEL AND HALF-LIFE

The mean plasma concentration was 5.0 to 7.8 ng/ml and 3.7 to 5.9 ng/ml, respectively, after intravenous and oral administration of 1.5 mg of clonazepam to four male patients (55). The half-lives ranged from 30.5 to 40.3 hr after 1.5 mg intravenously and from 26.5 to 49.2 hr after 1.5 mg orally. Oral administration of 9 mg gave similar half-lives of 26.8 to 32.5 hr in four patients. Ten adult males given a single 2-mg oral dose showed blood clonazepam levels of 6.5 to 13 ng/ml, and the corresponding half-lives ranged from 18.7 to 39.0 hr (mean, 26.4 hr) (89). In the latter study, five patients received 0.5 mg of clonazepam twice a day for 15 days and developed steady-state plasma clonazepam levels of 4.6 to 12.0 ng/ml, with plasma half-lives of 31 to 42 hr. These findings were similar to the single-dose studies, implying an absence of liver enzyme induction (15).

Ten children with absence seizures received clonazepam in daily doses ranging from 0.029 to 0.111 mg/kg for 8 weeks and reached steady-state plasma levels of the drug of 13 to 72 ng/ml and plasma half-lives between 22 and 33 hr (46) (Fig. 2). The relationship between serum clonazepam levels and dosage was more (46, 129,148) or less (9) linear (Fig. 3). Children have a considerably lower mean ratio of plasma level to oral dose (9) and a higher relative clearance value (96) than adults, implying that they require a higher dose to reach and maintain the same concentration. In children, who rapidly

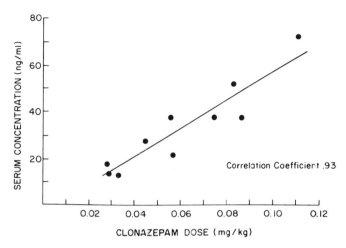

FIG. 2. Relationship of serum clonazepam concentration (ng/ml) to dose (mg/kg) in 10 children. (From Dreifuss et al., ref. 46, with permission.)

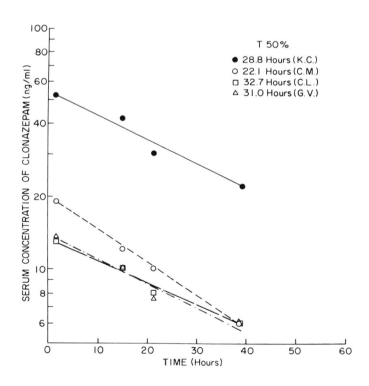

FIG. 3. Serum half-life (hr) of clonazepam in four children. Four serum clonazepam concentrations were determined for each patient within a 40-hr period while the dosage of clonazepam was delayed. (From Dreifuss et al., ref. 46, with permission.)

absorb and eliminate the drug, the daily oral dose should be divided into three administrations.

Clonazepam appears to be effective in reducing the frequency of absence seizures at serum levels of 13 to 72 ng/ml (9,46,96).

EXCRETION

Less than 0.5% of clonazepam was recovered unchanged in the urine in a 24-hr period (89, 148), indicating extensive biotransformation and/ or an alternative route of excretion. Total excretion of clonazepam and unconjugated 7-amino-clonazepam and 7-acetamino-clonazepam amounted to 5 to 20% of the dose given. The 3-hydroxy derivatives of all three compounds were detected only in trace amounts in the urine (148).

METABOLISM AND BIOTRANSFORMATION

The following metabolic products of clonazepam have been demonstrated in man (55): free compounds, including unaltered clonazepam; 7-amino derivative as the principal metabolite; 7-acetamido derivative; 3-hydroxy-7-amino derivative; and 3-hydroxy-7-acetamido derivative in small quantities. Conjugate compounds include the 7-amino derivative and the 7-aminophenol derivative (99). In 27 patients, a daily dose of 6 mg of clonazepam yielded plasma levels of both clonazepam and its principal metabolite, the 7-amino derivative, in the range of 30 to 80 ng/ml (mean, 50 ng/ml).

The pharmacokinetic behavior of the 7-amino metabolite of clonazepam administered exogenously and formed endogenously from the parent drug was studied in a group of Rhesus monkeys, using constant-rate venous infusions. The biological half-life of the 7-amino metabolite was shorter than that of clonazepam (104). The average peak concentration of metabolite occurred at approximately the same time as that of the parent compound, and the ratio between them varied between 1 to 3 and 3 to 1 (148). The nitro compounds are pharmacologically active, whereas the amino compounds are not. However, the plasma level of the 3-hydroxy-7-nitro metabolite appears to contribute insignificantly to the pharmacological effect of clonazepam itself (60,96).

THE RELATION OF PLASMA LEVEL TO SEIZURE CONTROL

There is no correlation between antiepileptic efficacy and plasma clonazepam levels (S. Sato, J. K. Penry, F. E. Dreifuss, and P. R. Dyken, *unpublished data*), although the range of plasma levels coinciding with excellent seizure control was similar in several studies (9, 46,96). Patients with absence seizures who showed no generalized spike-wave discharges on the 12-hr telemetered EEG had clonazepam levels of 8.6 to 19.4 ng/ml during the first week of treatment and 18.4 to 42.5 ng/ml during the eighth and 17th treatment weeks (S. Sato, J. K. Penry, F. E. Dreifuss, and P. R. Dyken, *unpublished data*). Patients with high levels of phenobarbital who showed clonazepam levels of less than 10 ng/ml were those who responded poorly to the addition of clonazepam (130).

Abrupt discontinuation of clonazepam should be avoided because of the possibility of generalized tonic–clonic seizures or status epilepticus (26).

PHARMACODYNAMICS

Mechanisms of Action

Although clonazepam induces a moderate elevation of whole brain serotonin, its effect on the physiological activity of serotonin is uncertain (168). In mice, the increase in serotonin and 5-hydroxyindoleacetic acid observed on acute administration of clonazepam was not seen following chronic administration of high doses for 8 days (84,85). In the mouse, clonazepam elevates brain tryptophan levels, although this is not because of altered serotonin synthesis, decreases serotonin utilization, and blocks the egress of 5-hydroxyindoleacetic acid from the brain (86). Some suggest that clonazepam influences central dopaminergic systems through a direct effect on dopaminergic presynaptic mechanisms (167). The observation that benzodiazepines potentiated the dopamine–GABA-dependent stereotyped gnawing behavior in mice suggested that the benzodiazepines may act by sensitizing GABA receptors to the action of GABA (4). Stimulation of benzodiazepine receptor binding may involve a novel type of GABA receptor (91). In monkeys, clonazepam abolished γ-hydroxybutyrate-induced EEG changes but exacerbated myoclonic jerks (149).

The recent discovery of specific benzodiazepine receptors in rat brain (23,124,125) led to the description of [^{3}H]diazepam binding sites in human brains. In the human brain, the cerebral and cerebellar cortical regions contain the highest densities of [^{3}H]diazepam binding sites. Clonazepam and diazepam have higher affinities for these binding sites in all human brain regions than do other benzodiazepines. The ability of benzodiazepines to displace [^{3}H]diazepam from the receptors is thought to correlate with the recommended daily clinical doses and clinical effects (22,124,125). The use of [^{3}H]fluoronitrazepam showed specific benzodiazepine binding sites in mouse and human brain identical to those found with [^{3}H]diazepam (38,152). Both presynaptic and postsynaptic GABA-mediated inhibition appear to be facilitated by benzodiazepines. It may be that the benzodiazepines somehow increase the potency or effectiveness of the inhibitory neurotransmitter, and, although the regulation of the function of GABA receptors may be quite complex, it would seem that the anticonvulsant actions of benzodiazepines, barbiturates, and valproate may, in part, involve similar mechanisms. It has also been suggested that the benzodiazepines may exert their pharmacological effects by mimicking the effects of glycine at its central nervous system receptor sites (175).

Clonazepam is effective against generalized tonic–clonic seizures induced in rats by ouabain (40) and in mice and rats by pentylenetetrazol (173). It has a very potent inhibitory effect on convulsions induced by maximal electroshock, strychnine, and picrotoxin (173). Clonazepam protects dogs against tonic–clonic seizures induced by amygdala kindling (166).

However, it has little effect on afterdischarges in the electroencephalogram induced by stimulation of the cerebral cortex in cats (173). It is very effective against photically induced epilepsy in *Papio papio* (116) but is ineffective against febrile convulsions in mice subjected to microwave diathermy (88). The articonvulsant activity of clonazepam experimentally appears to be at least partially mediated by inhibition of synaptic recovery and the enhancement of presynaptic inhibition (173). Clonazepam shortens the duration of primary epileptiform discharge and prolongs the intermittent interval in cortical, amygdaloid, and intralaminar thalamic epileptic foci induced by a high concentration of penicillin G in cats. The anticonvulsant effects of clonazepam may result from blockade of neuronal pathways that spread the discharge from the site of origin to the effector organ and from the elevation of seizure threshold (158).

Electroencephalographic studies have shown that clonazepam is particularly effective in suppressing generalized discharge such as the 3-per-sec spike and wave of absence seizures, the slow spike and wave of atypical absence, and the generalized polyspike and wave discharge frequently associated with generalized tonic–clonic seizures or myoclonic seizures. It also appears to be effective in suppressing the discharge of reflex epilepsies, particularly photic-induced seizures (13,20,26,36,46,62,63,77, 112). The effect on hypsarrhythmia is less striking but may be quite marked (48,112,162,169). Focal epileptic discharge is less consistently abolished; thus, it may be decreased (2,57, 71,80), unchanged (132), or increased (77). However, clonazepam does appear to prevent the propagation of seizures. Both intravenous and oral clonazepam may produce rapid beta rhythms (16 to 30 Hz) (26,77).

EFFECT OF CLONAZEPAM ON SPECIFIC SEIZURE TYPES

Clinical Trials

Most therapeutic trials are conducted on patients with refractory seizures by the addition of the drug under study. "Add-on" studies have two major drawbacks. One is the bias introduced by the placebo effect of a new drug. The second is that the most refractory patients may give no indication of how effective the drug will be in previously untreated patients. Controlled trials render the most objective, rapid, and definitive answers to questions of efficacy.

Absence Seizures

Reports on the effectiveness of clonazepam in absence seizures have included open (14, 20,58,106,107,111,132,159) and controlled (36,46,119,130,159) studies. In all studies, clonazepam was extremely effective in the control of absence seizures. In the study in which clonazepam was compared with ethosuximide (46), clonazepam was superior to ethosuximide in the normalization of the EEG, but adverse side effects and the development of tolerance greatly reduced this advantage (S. Sato, J. K. Penry, F. E. Dreifuss, and P. R. Dyken, *unpublished data*).

Tonic–Clonic Seizures

In general, phenytoin, phenobarbital, primidone, and carbamazepine are drugs of choice in the treatment of generalized tonic–clonic seizures. Clonazepam is effective and may completely control seizures in some 10 to 70% of patients   (8,14,16,18,33,52,78,100,109,118, 127,140). Many reports have indicated that generalized tonic–clonic seizures are exacerbated by the addition of clonazepam to the therapeutic regimen (20,111,127,139–141). In other series (100,132), the drug has been found to be ineffective in this seizure type. When given intravenously, clonazepam suppresses the EEG abnormality and abolishes generalized tonic–clonic status epilepticus.

Complex Partial Seizures

Although phenytoin, carbamazepine, primidone, and phenobarbital are all more effective in protecting experimental animals against maximal electroshock seizures than is clonazepam, this drug has been found effective in several series, both controlled (17,77,111) and uncontrolled or open (14,58,78,92,93,95,106,107, 109,111,118,132,145) studies. The development of tolerance or decreasing efficacy on long-term administration has been noted several times (1,58,111,113,118). Some reports, however, have specifically stated that efficacy was not decreased over time (36,145).

Simple Partial Seizures

In general, clonazepam is less effective than phenytoin, primidone, or carbamazepine in simple partial seizures, but it has been shown to be effective in controlled trials (52,120) and in some uncontrolled studies (1,70,111,132,145). The latter studies suggest that the drug is effective even in epilepsia partialis continua. Clonazepam seems to be more effective in partial than in generalized tonic–clonic seizures, and it has been noted that secondary generalization has not been facilitated by the administration of clonazepam (62). The drug's effectiveness in epilepsia partialis continua (78,145) is achieved despite persistence of the electroencephalographic focus.

Atypical Absence (Lennox–Gastaut Syndrome)

The Lennox–Gastaut syndrome is one of the most severe forms of childhood epilepsy. It is a chronic encephalopathy characterized electroencephalographically by slow spikes and waves and often by focal abnormalities with a shifting hemisphere emphasis. It is manifested in a variety of seizures, the most severe of which is the drop attack, in which injuries frequently occur.

The benzodiazepines, and particularly clonazepam, have been found to have beneficial effects in many children with this syndrome, and these have been observed in both controlled (125,166) and uncontrolled (8,14,20,48,70, 72,77,82,98,100,131,132,142–144,162) studies. The results were frequently better at the beginning of treatment than later, and this may have been because of the development of tolerance or the rather variable natural history of the condition. On occasion, treatment failures may respond to corticotropin (ACTH) or hydrocortisone (48) when added to the treatment regimen. Since its introduction, valproic acid has virtually superseded clonazepam in the treatment of the Lennox–Gastaut syndrome and is considerably more effective.

Massive Infantile Spasms

Infantile spasms consist of a heterogeneous group of seizure disorders usually characterized by massive flexion myoclonic spasms, at times by extensor spasms, and frequently associated with a hypsarrhythmic EEG pattern, intractability to treatment, and mental retardation. Others are phenotypically similar but date from birth and are associated with severe neurological abnormalities. Treatment of choice has been the administration of corticosteroids. The effects of benzodiazepines are highlighted by the good results obtained with nitrazepam. The results with clonazepam appear to be disappointing, but they vary widely; some authors have found that the drug is ineffective (70,72,77,127), whereas others have met with more success (48,62,112,162,169). Vassella et al. (162) reported control of infantile spasms in about one-third of the patients treated. The limiting factor appeared to be increased bronchial secretions.

Myoclonic Seizures

There are several syndromes described under the rubric of myoclonic epilepsy. These include bilateral massive epileptic myoclonus (juvenile myoclonic epilepsy), a relatively benign seizure form frequently accompanied by generalized tonic–clonic seizures. In this condition, clonazepam has been found to be quite effective in both controlled and uncontrolled studies (58,62,111,119,127,132,137). Other forms of myoclonic epilepsy have also benefited significantly (7,52,72,77,78,100,107,123). In progressive hereditary myoclonic epilepsy and the

Ramsay–Hunt syndrome, clonazepam has been of significant benefit (14,62,105).

The intention myoclonus seen in postencephalitic and postanoxic states has been quite successfully treated with clonazepam (21,31, 35,56,65,75,123). Chadwick et al. (34,35) suggested that the protective effect of clonazepam in myoclonic seizures may be the result of increased cerebral serotonin concentrations; it is not surprising, therefore, that the myoclonic seizures responding to clonazepam are those that benefit from 5-hydroxytryptophan. Myoclonus associated with methyl bromide poisoning has been successfully treated with clonazepam (67,157).

Photosensitive Seizures

Clonazepam is a potent anticonvulsant in *Papio papio,* a model of light-sensitive epilepsy. Of all the medications tested in this model, clonazepam had the greatest protective effect. Photosensitive seizures are of great interest as a form of reflex epilepsy. A large portion of the population is affected by the photomyoclonic and photoconvulsive epilepsies as well as a variety of self-induced photosensitive seizures. Clonazepam is effective not only in reducing the response to photic stimulation but also in alleviating the desire for self-induction of seizures (3,20,70,78,93,139).

Miscellaneous Paroxysmal Conditions

Clonazepam has been administered with some success in a large number of paroxysmal disorders. Successes have been claimed for it in eclamptic convulsive attacks (11), in Gilles de la Tourette syndrome (66), in trigeminal neuralgia (28,37,39), in the stiff man syndrome (162,171), in chorea (135), in blepharospasm (117), in restless legs (115), and in tardive dyskinesia (146).

Status Epilepticus

Clonazepam has been effective in controlling various forms of status epilepticus, generalized tonic–clonic seizures, absence seizures, partial seizures with complex symptomatology, simple partial seizures, clonic seizures, tonic seizures, myoclonic seizures, and epilepsia partialis continua (27,47,70,90,94,126,161). A single dose of 1 to 4 mg of clonazepam is usually sufficient to abolish status epilepticus and to ameliorate paroxysmal activity in the EEG. In this use, clonazepam is usually more effective than diazepam. Whereas intravenous diazepam has been associated with the precipitation of a tonic status (155), this effect has not been reported with clonazepam. A transitory increase in myoclonic jerks and in EEG paroxysmal activity has been described in a case of status with the Ramsay–Hunt syndrome (14).

Clonazepam is not available in the United States for intravenous use, and in this country diazepam is still the drug of choice for status epilepticus.

SIDE EFFECTS

In seven controlled studies (12,17,36,52, 113,119,159), side effects of clonazepam were observed in 16 to 90% (median, 67%) of patients, and these led to eventual discontinuation of the drug in 10 to 36%. In other series, side effects in 30 to 82% of patients caused eventual termination of the drug in 12 to 18% (78,107,130). Table 1 shows the side effects of clonazepam in our double-blind study of clonazepam versus ethosuximide (S. Sato, J. K. Penry, F. E. Dreifuss, and P. R. Dyken, *unpublished data*). Side effects in 34 (92%) of 37 children with absence seizures required eventual discontinuation of clonazepam in 27% of the patients.

The common side effects of clonazepam include drowsiness, ataxia, and behavioral and personality changes. Drowsiness and ataxia usually appear a few hours after the first days of clonazepam therapy and improve with adjustment of the dosage. Drowsiness occurs in 10 to 85% (median, 62%) of patients and ataxia in 7 to 43% (median, 12%). Significant behavioral and personality changes, such as hyperactivity, restlessness, short attention span, ir-

ritability, disruptiveness, and aggressiveness, are seen commonly in children and occasionally in adults and occur in 2 to 51% (median, 12%) of patients.

Other neurological side effects of clonazepam include, rather commonly, nystagmus, dizziness, dysarthria, and hypotonia and, less commonly, blurred vision, diplopia (13,51), and psychotic reactions (6,107,113). Increased frequency of various types of seizures has been reported (5,25,127,144). Different varieties of seizures may emerge (5,73,112,113,174). Slight weight gain (less than 10% within 17 weeks) was a fairly common problem in our series (S. Sato, J. K. Penry, F. E. Dreifuss, and P. R. Dyken, *unpublished data*). Occasionally, nausea has been reported (13,36). Hypersecretion and hypersalivation may be troublesome in children and infants (138,169).

Hematological side effects have been rarely reported. Leukopenia has occasionally occurred (19), and thrombocytopenic purpura has been documented (113,163).

Dermatological side effects include skin pigmentation (78), transient hair loss (130), and an extensive rash (69). Hepatic or renal complications have not been observed.

Reasons for withdrawing clonazepam have included freedom from seizures, lack of clinical effect, intolerable behavior, personality changes, psychotic reactions, persistent drowsiness, leukopenia, increase of seizure frequency, and the development of other types of seizures. There is no correlation between the dose of clonazepam and the occurrence of side effects (109), but this has been disputed (76). However, the rate of dosage increase has been thought to be significant in the development of side effects (54). There is no relationship between side effects and plasma concentration of the drug (9,148). However, drowsiness, dysarthria, irritability, and hypotonia have occurred when plasma clonazepam concentrations have ranged between 22 and 81 ng/ml. In four patients, seizures became more frequent when plasma levels of the drug exceeded 100 ng/ml, and in two patients, status epilepticus was observed when the concentration exceeded 180 ng/ml (9). Se-

TABLE 1. *Side effects of clonazepam in 37 children with absence seizures*

No.	Age	Sex	Drowsiness	Ataxia	Nystagmus	Hyperactivity	Personality change	Increased seizures	Change in seizure type	Weight gain >10%	Leukopenia	Did not complete trial	None	Phenobarbital	Metharbital	Primidone	Phenytoin	Acetazolamide
Untreated																		
1	12	M	×	×	×									×				
2	9	F											×					
3	12	F	×		×								×					
4	13	M			×	×				×						×		
5	6	F		×		×				×			×					
6	12	F	×				×					×	×					
7	9	F	×	×	×					×				×				
8	7	M	×	×		×		×				×		×				
9	8	M	×			×						×		×				
10	9	M				×	×			×				×				
11	5	M		×		×	×					×		×				
12	15	M	×						×							×	×	
13	7	F	×					×				×					×	
14	9	M	×	×				×				×		×				
15	13	F	×						×						×		×	
16	7	M	×	×		×	×						×					
17	11	M											×					
18	8	F												×				
19	6	F				×				×			×					
20	12	F	×											×			×	
Refractory																		
21	5	F	×															
22	9	F			×												×	×
23	11	F	×		×	×				×			×					
24	11	F	×	×	×	×												
25	12	F		×										×				
26	14	F		×	×									×				
27	13	M		×							×	×						
28	10	M	×	×														×
29	9	M	×	×	×					×							×	
30	9	M	×	×			×			×				×				
31	13	F	×											×			×	
32	6	F	×	×						×							×	
33	14	F				×	×	×				×					×	
34	8	F					×	×				×				×		
35	12	F				×				×				×				
36	9	M							×	×				×				
37	7	M	×	×				×				×						
Total			21	16	9	12	7	6	3	11	1	10						

rious dysphoria appeared to be associated with an elevated level of clonazepam in some cases, and the upper limit of drug level was thought to be about 70 ng/ml before this toxic effect appeared (148). The main metabolite, 7-amino-clonazepam, was found in much higher concentration in patients suffering from withdrawal symptoms (pronounced dysphoria, irritability, restlessness, sleeplessness, and tremor of the hands) than in those who had no such reactions (148).

A febrile reaction in a severely retarded 18-year-old man who had been taking clonazepam for some 6 months abated within 2 days of discontinuing the drug (68). Anticonvulsant drugs may depress cellular immunity regardless of the drug, the dose, the duration of treatment, or the age when treatment was started (114). A 4-year-old child who ingested a large amount of clonazepam had a plasma level of 69 ng/ml and experienced seven episodes of coma interspersed with alert agitation during the first 24 hr; during the coma his pupils were pinpoint (170).

Clonazepam does not exacerbate porphyria and has been used to treat seizures in this condition (108).

DRUG INTERACTIONS

The potential problem of drug interactions occurs whenever multiple drugs are administered. Clonazepam appears to be relatively inert in this regard. It has been given together with most other antiepileptic drugs, usually without untoward effects. The drug interactions that have been observed appear be inconstant; thus, serum phenytoin levels after the administration of clonazepam have been noted either to rise (53,78,81) or to fall (12). In the case of the latter, there was a concomitant increase in phenytoin metabolites, suggesting an increase in metabolism. The administration of phenytoin has led to a diminution in blood levels of clonazepam and levels of its 7-amino-clonazepam metabolite (148); similar effects have been observed with other antiepileptic drugs (147).

In other cases, the addition of clonazepam

has had no effect on blood levels of phenytoin or carbamazepine (110). Lai et al. (101–103) noted that carbamazepine infusion led to diminution in clonazepam levels. They attributed this finding to enzyme induction, with an increase in D-glucaric acid which characterizes such activity. Benetello et al. (12) reported diminished phenobarbital levels, Bekersky et al. (10) found an increased plasma clearance of clonazepam with the addition of phenobarbital, and Nanda et al. (130) observed lower blood clonazepam levels with the addition of phenobarbital. These reports noted no interaction between clonazepam and the other antiepileptic drugs. Windorfer and Sauer (172) found that serum levels of phenytoin and primidone increased on administration of clonazepam, but Johannessen et al. (87) could find no effect on the levels of phenytoin, phenobarbital, or carbamazepine.

It is generally recommended that amphetamines or methylphenidate not be administered together with clonazepam because of the danger of producing nervous system depression and respiratory irregularities (32). The simultaneous administration of clonazepam and valproate carries the danger of exacerbating absence attacks with the possibility of continuous absence seizures (petit mal status) (74,83,151,165). Although some patients tolerate and benefit from this combination of drugs, this hazard has to be borne in mind when its use is considered.

TERATOGENICITY

The anticonvulsant drugs most often implicated in teratogenicity are phenytoin, phenobarbital, and trimethadione. Although now rarely used, trimethadione carries the greatest risk of teratogenicity. There is at the present time no evidence that clonazepam is significantly teratogenic.

SUMMARY

Clonazepam is a potent benzodiazepine anticonvulsant with activity against the various types of seizures. It is generally most effective in the treatment of absence seizures, the Lennox–Gastaut syndrome, and the myoclonic epilepsies. It is less useful in infantile spasms and in partial seizures, although complex partial seizures may be alleviated to some extent. Reflex epilepsies, including photic-sensitive epilepsy, respond well to clonazepam. Administration of the drug may lead to the emergence of other seizure types. Initial success may be followed by the development of tolerance.

Side effects are common, and most patients experience drowsiness and some ataxia and changes in mood. Severe toxicity is rare, and apart from possible adverse reactions to simultaneous administration of clonazepam and valproate, there is little evidence for clinically significant drug interaction.

The drug may exert its effect, at least in part, through modification of GABA-mediated synaptic systems and has an effect on serotonin metabolism. It is well absorbed after oral administration: blood concentration is usually maximal within 2 to 4 hr. Metabolism occurs principally by formation of an inactive 7-amino derivative, and less than 5% of the drug is recovered in the urine unchanged.

CONVERSION

Conversion factor:

$$CF = \frac{1000}{mol.\ wt.} = \frac{1000}{315.5} = 3.17$$

Conversion:

$$(\mu g/ml) \times 3.17 = (\mu moles/liter)$$

$$(\mu moles/liter) \div 3.17 = (\mu g/ml)$$

REFERENCES

1. Aarli, J. A. (1973): Effect of clonazepam (Ro 5-4023) on epileptic seizures. *Acta Neurol. Scand.*, 49:11–17.
2. Ahmad, S., Perucca, E., and Richens, A. (1977): Effect of frusemide, mexiletine, (+)-propranolol and three benzodiazepine drugs on interictal spike discharges in the electroencephalogram. *Br. J. Clin. Pharmacol.*, 4:683–688.
3. Ames, F. F., and Enderstein, O. (1976): Clinical and EEG response to clonazepam in four patients with self induced photosensitive epilepsy. *S. Afr. Med. J.*, 50:1432–1434.
4. Arnt, J., Christensen, A. V., and Scheel-Krueger, J. (1979): Benzodiazepines potentiate GABA–dopamine-dependent stereotyped gnawing in mice. *J. Pharm. Pharmacol.*, 31:56–58.
5. Bang, F., Birket-Smith, E., and Mikkelsen, B. (1976): Clonazepam in the treatment of epilepsy. A clinical long-term follow-up study. *Epilepsia*, 17:323–324.
6. Barfod, S., and Wendelboe, J. (1977): Severe psychiatric side effects of clonazepam treatment. 2 cases. *Ugeskr. Laeger*, 139:2450.
7. Bark, N. (1977): Clonazepam in the treatment of epilepsy in handicapped patients. *Br. J. Ment. Subnorm.*, 23:84–87.
8. Barnett, A. M. (1973): Treatment of epilepsy with clonazepam (Ro 5-4023). *S. Afr. Med. J.*, 47:1683–1686.
9. Baruzzi, A., Bordo, B., Bossi, L., Castelli, D., Gerna, M., Tognoni, G., and Zagnoni, P. (1977): Plasma levels of di-*n*-propylacetate and clonazepam in epilepsy patients. *Int. J. Clin. Pharmacol. Biopharm.*, 15:403–408.
10. Bekersky, I., Maggio, A. C., Mattaliano, V. J., Boxenbaum, H. G., Maynard, D. C., Cohen, P. D., and Kaplan, S. A. (1977): Influence of phenobarbital on the disposition of clonazepam and antipyrine in the dog. *J. Pharmacokinet. Biopharm.*, 5:507–512.
11. Beltrami, M., Mangaldo, R., and Frassineti, E. (1978): Clonazepam in the treatment of eclamptic convulsive attacks. *Minerva Anestesiol.*, 44:257–261.
12. Benetello, P., Furlanut, M., Testa, G., and Santi, R. (1977): Effect of benzodiazepines on serum levels of phenobarbital and diphenylhydantoin. *Riv. Farmacol. Ter.*, 8:109–112.
13. Bensch, J., Blennow, G., Ferngren, H., Gamstorp, I., Herrlin, K. M., Kubista, J., Arvidsson, A., and Dahlström, H. (1977): A double-blind study of clonazepam in the treatment of therapy resistant epilepsy in children. *Dev. Med. Child Neurol.*, 19:335–342.
14. Bergamini. L., Mutani, R., and Liboni, W. (1970): Elektroenczephalographische under klinische Bewertung des neuen Benzodiazepin Ro 5/4023. *Electroencephalogr. Electromyogr.*, 1:182–188.
15. Berlin, A., and Dahlström, H. (1975): Pharmacokinetics of the anticonvulsant drug clonazepam evaluated from single oral and intravenous doses and by repeated oral administration. *Eur. J. Clin. Pharmacol.*, 9:155–159.
16. Bielman, P., Levoc, T., and Gagnon, M. A. (1978): Clonazepam: Its efficacy in association with phenytoin and phenobarbital in mental patients with generalized major motor seizures. *Int. J. Clin. Pharmacol. Biopharm.*, 16:268–273.
17. Birket-Smith, E., Lund, M., Mikkelsen, B., Vestermark, S., Zander Olsen, P., and Holm, P. (1973): A controlled trial on Ro 5-4023 (clonazepam) in the treatment of psychomotor epilepsy. *Acta Neurol. Scand.*, 49:18–25.

18. Birket-Smith, E., and Mikkelsen, B. (1972): Preliminary observations on the effect of a new benzodiazepine (Ro 5-4023) in epilepsy. *Acta Neurol. Scand.*, 48:385–389.

19. Bittner-Manicka, M., and Wasilewski, R. (1976): Preliminary clinical evaluation of Rivotril in epilepsy. *Neurol. Neurochir. Pol.*, 26:519–525.

20. Bladin, P. F. (1973): The use of clonazepam as an anticonvulsant—clinical evaluation. *Med. J. Aust.*, 1:683–688.

21. Boudouresques, J., Roger, J., Khalil, R., Vigouroux, R. A., Gossett, A., Pellisier, J. F., and Tassinari, C. A. (1971): A propos de deux observationes de syndrome de Lance et Adams: Effet therapeutique de Ro5-4023. *Rev. Neurol.*, 125:306–309.

22. Braestrup, C., Albrechtsen, R., and Squires, R. F. (1977): High densities of benzodiazepine receptors in human cortical areas. *Nature*, 269:702–704.

23. Braestrup, C., and Squires, R. F. (1977): Specific benzodiazepine receptors in rat brain characterized by high-affinity ^{3}H-diazepam binding. *Proc. Natl. Acad. Sci. U.S.A.*, 74:3805–3809.

24. Browne, T. R. (1976): Clonazepam: A review of a new anticonvulsant drug. *Arch. Neurol.*, 33:326–332.

25. Browne, T. R. (1978): Clonazepam. *N. Engl. J. Med.*, 299:812–816.

26. Browne, T. R., and Penry, J. K. (1973): Benzodiazepines in the treatment of epilepsy. *Epilepsia*, 15:277–310.

27. Bücking, P. H. (1977): Electroclinical correlations during anticonvulsive therapy of status epilepticus and chronic focal epilepsies using clonazepam. *Schweiz. Arch. Neurol. Neurochir. Psychiatr.*, 121:187–205.

28. Caccia, M. R. (1975): Clonazepam in facial neuralgia and cluster headache. *Eur. Neurol.*, 13:560–563.

29. Cano, J. P., Catalin, J., Viala, A., Roger, J., Tassinari, C. A., Dravet, C., and Gastaut, H. (1976): Determination of clonazepam ("Rivotril" or "Ro 5-4023") in plasma by gas chromatography using an internal standard. *Eur. J. Toxicol. Environ. Hyg.*, 9:213–225.

30. Cano, J. P., Guintrand, J., Aubert, C., Viala, A., and Covo, J. (1977): Determination of flunitrazepam, desmethylflunitrazepam and clonazepam in plasma by gas liquid chromatography with an internal standard. *Arzneim. Forsch.*, 27:338–342.

31. Carroll, W. M., and Walsh, P. J. (1978): Functional independence in postanoxic myoclonus: Contribution of L-5-HTP, sodium valproate and clonazepam. *Br. Med. J.*, 2:1612.

32. Carson, J. J., and Gilden, C. (1975): Treatment of minor motor seizures with clonazepam. *Dev. Med. Child Neurol.*, 17:306–310.

33. Caso, A., Raphael-Fernandez, G., Romo, A., Martinez, C., Garibay, E., and Padilla, J. (1973): Evaluacion neuropsiquiatrica del clonazepam (Ro 5-4023) en pacientes epilepticos. *Gac. Med. Mex.*, 106:385–392.

34. Chadwick, D., and French, A. T. (1979): Uremic myoclonus: An example of reticular reflex myoclonus? *J. Neurol. Neurosurg. Psychiatry*, 42:52–55.

35. Chadwick, D., Hallett, M., Harris, R., Jenner, P., Reynolds, E. H., and Marsden, C. D. (1977): Clinical, biochemical and physiological features distinguishing myoclonus responsive to 5-hydroxytryptophan, tryptophan with a monoamine oxidase inhibitor, and clonazepam. *Brain*, 100:455–487.

36. Chandra, B. (1973): Clonazepam in the treatment of petit mal. *Asian J. Med.*, 9:433–436.

37. Chandra, B. (1976): The use of clonazepam in the treatment of tic douloureux (a preliminary report). *Proc. Aust. Assoc. Neurol.*, 13:119–122.

38. Chang, R. S. L., and Snyder, S. H. (1978): Benzodiazepine receptors: Labeling in intact animals with ^{3}H-flunitrazepam. *Eur. J. Pharmacol.*, 48:213–218.

39. Court, J. E., and Kase, C. S. (1976): Treatment of tic douloureux with a new anticonvulsant (clonazepam). *J. Neurol. Neurosurg. Psychiatry*, 39:297–299.

40. Davidson, D. L., Tsukada, Y., and Barbeau, A. (1978): Ouabain induced seizures: Site of production and response to anticonvulsants. *Can. J. Neurol. Sci.*, 5:405–411.

41. De Boer, A. B., Roest-Kaiser, J., Bracht, H., and Breimer, D. D. (1978): Assay of underivated nitrazepam and clonazepam in plasma by capillary gas chromatography applied to pharmacokinetic and bioavailability studies in humans. *J. Chromatogr.*, 145:105–114.

42. de Silva, J. A. F., Bekersky, I., Puglisi, C. V., Brooks, M. A., and Weinfeld, R. E. (1976): Determination of 1,4-benzodiazepines and -diazepine-2-ones in blood by electron-capture gas–liquid chromatography. *Anal. Chem.*, 48:10–19.

43. de Silva, J. A. F., Puglisi, C. V., and Munno, N. (1974): Determination of clonazepam and flunitrazepam in blood and urine by electron-capture GLC. *J. Pharm. Sci.*, 63:520–527.

44. Dixon, R., and Crews, T. (1977): An iodine-125 radioimmune assay for the determination of the anticonvulsant agent clonazepam directly in plasma. *Res. Commun. Chem. Pathol. Pharmacol.*, 18:477–486.

45. Dixon, W. R., Young, R. L., Ning, R., and Liebman, A. (1977): Radioimmunoassay of the anticonvulsant agent clonazepam. *J. Pharm. Sci.*, 66:235–237.

46. Dreifuss, F. E., Penry, J. K., Rose, S. W., Kupferberg, H. J., Dyken, P., and Sato, S. (1975): Serum clonazepam concentrations in children with absence seizures. *Neurology (Minneap.)*, 23:255–258.

47. *Drug and Therapeutics Bulletin* (1976): Drugs for status epilepticus. *Drug Ther. Bull.*, 14:89–91.

48. Dumermuth, G., and Kovacs, E. (1973): The effect of clonazepam (Ro 5-4023) in the syndrome of infantile spasms with hypsarrhythmias and in petit mal variant or Lennox syndrome. *Acta Neurol. Scand.*, 49:26–28.

49. Eadie, M. J., Tyrer, J. H., Smith, G. A., and McKauge, L. (1977): Pharmacokinetics of drugs used for petit mal absence epilepsy. *Proc. Aust. Assoc. Neurol.*, 14:172–183.

50. Edelbrook, P. M., and De Wolff, F. A. (1978): Improved micromethod for determination of underivated clonazepam in serum by gas chromatography. *Clin. Chem.*, 24:774–777.

51. Edwards, V. E. (1974): Side effects of clonazepam therapy. *Proc. Aust. Assoc. Neurol.*, 11:199–202.

52. Edwards, V. E., and Eadie, M. J. (1973): Clonazepam—a clinical study of its effectiveness as an anticonvulsant. *Proc. Aust. Assoc. Neurol.*, 10:61–66.

53. Eeg-Olofsson, O. (1973): Experiences with Rivotril in treatment with epilepsy—particularly minor motor epilepsy—in mentally retarded children. *Acta Neurol. Scand.*, 49:29–31.

54. Elian, M., Lund, M., and Melsen, S. (1973): The rate of dosage increase of clonazepam. *Acta Neurol. Scand.*, 49:32–35.

55. Eschenhof, E. (1973): Untersuchung über das Schicksal des Antikonvulsivums Clonazepam in Organismus der Ratte, des Hundes und des Menschen. *Arzneim. Forsch.*, 23:390–400.

56. Fahn, S. (1978): Postanoxic action myoclonus: Improvement with valproic acid. *N. Engl. J. Med.*, 299:313–314.

57. Fariello, R., and Mutani, R. (1970): Valutazione sperimentale dell'efficacia del nuovo farmaco anticomiziale Ro 5-4023. *Riv. Neurol. Clin.*, 40:174–183.

58. Fazio, C., Manfredi, M., and Piccinelli, A. (1975): Treatment of epileptic seizures with clonazepam. *Arch. Neurol.*, 32:304–307.

59. Ferguson, J. L., and Couri, D. (1977): Electron capture gas chromatography determination of benzodiazepines and metabolites. *J. Anal. Toxicol.*, 1:171–174.

60. Fukushima, H., Nakamura, M., and Matsumoto, T. (1977): Pharmacological studies of clonazepam and its metabolites in mice. *Oyo Yakuri*, 14:357–361.

61. Garland, W. A., and Min, B. H. (1979): Determination of clonazepam in human plasma by gas chromatography—negative ion chemical ionization mass spectrometry. *J. Chromatogr.*, 172:279–286.

62. Gastaut, H. (1970): Proprietes anti-epileptiques exceptionneles d'une benzodiazepine nouvelle le Ro 05-4023. *Vie Med.*, 51:517.

63. Gastaut, H., Courjon, J., Poire, R., and Weber, M. (1971): Treatment of status epilepticus with a new benzodiazepine more active than diazepam. *Epilepsia*, 12:197–214.

64. Gerna, M., and Morselli, P. L. (1976): A simple and sensitive gas chromatographic method for the determination of clonazepam in human plasma. *J. Chromatogr.*, 115:445–450.

65. Goldberg, M. A., and Dorman, J. D. (1976): Intention myoclonus: Successful treatment with clonazepam. *Neurology (Minneap.)*, 26:24–26.

66. Gonce, M., and Barbeau, A. (1977): Seven cases of Gilles de la Tourette's syndrome: Partial relief with clonazepam: A pilot study. *Can. J. Neurol. Sci.*, 4:279–283.

67. Goulon, M., Nouailhat, F., Escourolle, R., and Zaranz-Imirizaldu, J. J. (1975): Methyl bromide poisoning. Report of 3 cases with one death. Anatom-ical study in one case of stupor and myoclonus with a 5 years' survey. *Rev. Neurol.*, 131:445–468.

68. Gray, R., and Folkerts, L. N. (1977): Drug fever due to clonazepam. *Drug. Intell. Clin. Pharm.*, 11:367.

69. Gregoriades, A. D., and Franges, E. G. (1977): Clinical observation on clonazepam in intractable epilepsy. In: *Epilepsy: The Eighth International Symposium*, edited by J. K. Penry, pp. 169–175. Raven Press, New York.

70. Groh, C., and Rosenmayr, F. W. (1973): Orale Dauertherapie mit Clonazepam (Ro 05-4023) bei Epilepsien des Kindes und Jugendalters. *Acta Neurol. Scand.*, 49:36–43.

71. Häkkinen, V. (1973): Effect of clonazepam (Ro 5-4023) on interictal EEG abnormalities. *Acta Neurol. Scand.*, 49:44.

72. Hanson, R. A., and Menkes, J. M. (1972): A new anticonvulsant in the management of minor motor seizures. *Dev. Med. Child Neurol.*, 14:3–14.

73. Hansson, O., and Tonnby, B. (1976): Serious psychological symptoms caused by clonazepam. *Lakartidningen*, 73:1209–1210.

74. Hildebrandt, W. K. (1979): Concomitant use of clonazepam and valproic acid in treatment of epileptic seizures (letter). *Am. J. Hosp. Pharm.*, 36:22.

75. Hoehn, M. M., and Cherington, M. (1977): Spinal myoclonus. *Neurology (Minneap.)*, 27 942–946.

76. Hollister, L. E. (1975): Dose-ranging studies of clonazepam in man. *Psychopharmacol. Commun.*, 1:89–92.

77. Hooshmand, H. (1972): Intractable seizures. Treatment with a new benzodiazepine anticonvulsant. *Arch. Neurol.*, 27:205–208.

78. Huang, C. Y., McLeod, J. G., Sampson, D., and Hensley, W. J. (1974): Clonazepam in the treatment of epilepsy. *Med. J. Aust.*, 2:5–8.

79. Hvidberg, E. F., and Sjö, O. (1975): Clinical pharmacokinetic experiences with clonazepam. In: *Clinical Pharmacology of Anti-Epileptic Drugs*, edited by H. Schneider, D. Janz, C. Gardner-Thorpe, H. Meinardi, and A. L. Sherwin, pp. 242–246. Springer-Verlag, Berlin.

80. Iinuma, K., Tamahashi, S., Otomo, H., Onuma, A., and Takamatsu, N. (1978): Immediate changes of the electroencephalograms after intravenous injection of clonazepam and their relation to its effect on clinical fits in children with minor seizures. *Tohoku J. Exp. Med.*, 125:223–231.

81. Inami, M., and Hara, T. (1977): The effects of clonazepam on the plasma diphenylhydantoin level in epileptic patients. *Electroencephalogr. Clin. Neurophysiol.*, 43:497.

82. Jeavons, P. (1977): Management of childhood epilepsy. *Br. Med. J.*, 1:986.

83. Jeavons, R. M., Clark, J. E., and Maheshwari, M. C. (1977): Treatment of generalized epilepsies of childhood and adolescence with sodium valproate ("Epilim"). *Dev. Med. Child Neurol.*, 19:9–25.

84. Jenner, P., Chadwick, D., Reynolds, E. H., and Marsden, C. D. (1975): Altered 5-HT metabolism with clonazepam, diazepam and diphenyhydantoin. *J. Pharm. Pharmacol.*, 27:707–710.

85. Jenner, P., Chadwick, D., Reynolds, E. H., and Marsden, C. D. (1975): Clonazepam-induced changes in 5-hydroxytryptamine metabolism in animals and man. *J. Pharm. Pharmacol.*, 27:38P.

86. Jenner, P., Marsden, C. D., Pratt, J., and Reynolds, E. H. (1978): Altered serotoninergic activity in mouse brain induced by clonazepam. *Br. J. Pharmacol.*, 64:432.

87. Johannessen, S. I., Strandjord, R. E., and Munthe-Kaas, A. W. (1977): Lack of effort of clonazepam on serum levels of diphenylhydantoin, phenobarbital, and carbamazepine. *Acta Neurol. Scand.*, 55:506–512.

88. Julien, R. M., and Fowler, G. W. (1977): A comparative study of the efficacy of newer antiepileptic drugs on experimentally-induced febrile convulsions. *Neuropharmacology*, 16:719–724.

89. Kaplan, S. A., Alexander, K., Jack, M. L., Puglisi, C. V., deSilva, J. A. F., Lee, T. L., and Weinfeld, R. E. (1974): Pharmacokinetic profiles of clonazepam in dog and humans and of flunitrazepam in dog. *J. Pharm. Sci.*, 63:527–532.

90. Karbowski, K. (1976): Der Petit-mal Status. *Schweiz. Med. Wochenschr.*, 29:973–981.

91. Karobath, M., and Sperk, B. (1979): Stimulation of benzodiazepine receptor binding of gamma-aminobutyric acid. *Proc. Natl. Acad. Sci. U.S.A.*, 76:1004–1006.

92. Kato, H., and Mori, T. (1977): A clinical and electroencephalographic study on antiepileptic activity of clonazepam. Relationship between clinical effects of oral administration and electroencephalographic effects of intravenous administration. *Folia Psychiatr. Neurol. Jpn.*, 31:183–194.

93. Kato, H., Mori, T., Moriuchi, I., Yoshimura, T., and Iwata, T. (1976): Antiepileptic activity of clonazepam—an antiepileptic benzodiazepine derivative. *Brain Nerve (Tokyo)*, 28:565–577.

94. Ketz, E., Bernomiti, C., and Siegfried, J. (1973): Clinical and EEG study of clonazepam (Ro 5-4023) with particular reference to status epilepticus. *Acta Neurol. Scand.*, 49:47–53.

95. Kick, H., and Dreyer, R. (1973): Klinische Erfahrungen mit Clonazepam unter besonderer Berucksightigung psychomotorische Anfalle. *Acta Neurol. Scand.*, 49:54–59.

96. Knop, H. J., Edmunds, L. C., Blom, G. F., Bruens, J. H., Bongers, E., Meinardi, H., Meijer, J. W. A., Guelen, P. J. M., and van der Kleijn, E. (1977): Clonazepam: A clinical trial. Pharmacokinetic and clinical aspects. In: *Antiepileptic Drug Monitoring*, edited by C. Gardner-Thorpe, D. Janz, H. Meinardi, and C. E. Pippenger, pp. 226–263. Pitman Medical, Tunbridge Wells, Kent.

97. Knop, H. J., van der Kleijn, E., and Edmunds, L. C. (1975): Pharmacokinetics of clonazepam in man and laboratory animals. In: *Clinical Pharmacology of Antiepileptic Drugs*, edited by H. Schneider, D. Janz, C. Gardner-Thorpe, H. Meinardi, and A. L. Sherwin, pp. 247–260. Springer-Verlag, Berlin.

98. Kohler, C., Clere, J., and Girtanner, B. (1975): Interet du clonazepam dans le traitement des manifestations convulsives avec encephalopathie chez l'enfant. *Rev. Neuropsychiatr. Infant.*, 23:381–387.

99. Krugers Dagneaux, P. G. L., and Klein Elhorst, J. T. (1975): Qualitative analysis of clonazepam and its metabolites in urine and plasma. *Pharm. Weekbl.*, 110:1137–1142.

100. Kruse, R., and Blankenhorn, V. (1973): Zusammenfassender Erfahrungsbericht über die klinische Anwendung und Wirksamkeit von Ro 5-4023 (Clonazepam) auf verschiedene Formen epileptischer Anfalle. *Acta Neurol. Scand.*, 49:60–71.

101. Lai, A. A. (1978): Investigations of the pharmacokinetics of clonazepam and its interaction with carbamazepine in monkeys and humans. *Diss. Abstr. Int. B. 1978*, 39:669.

102. Lai, A. A., and Levy, R. H. (1979): Pharmacokinetic description of drug interactions by induction: Carbamazepine–clonazepam in monkeys. *J. Pharm. Sci.*, 68:416–421.

103. Lai, A. A., Levy, R. H., and Cutler, R. E. (1978): Time-course of interaction between carbamazepine and clonazepam in normal man. *Clin. Pharmacol. Ther.*, 24:316–323.

104. Lai, A. A., Min, B. H., Garland, W. A., and Levy, R. H. (1979): Kinetics of biotransformation of clonazepam to its 7-amino metabolite in monkey. *J. Pharmacokinet. Biopharm.*, 7:87–95.

105. Laitinen, L., and Toivakka, E. (1973): Clonazepam (Ro 5-4023) in the treatment of myoclonus epilepsy. *Acta Neurol. Scand.*, 49:72–76.

106. Lance, J. W., and Anthony, M. (1977): Sodium valproate and clonazepam in the treatment of intractable epilepsy. *Proc. Aust. Assoc. Neurol.*, 12:55–60.

107. Lance, J. W., and Anthony, M. (1977): Sodium valproate and clonazepam in the treatment of intractable epilepsy. *Arch. Neurol.*, 34:14–17.

108. Larson, A. W., Wasserstrom, W. R., Felsher, B. F., and Chih, J. C. (1978): Posttraumatic epilepsy and acute intermittent porphyria: Effects of phenytoin, carbamazepine and clonazepam. *Neurology (Minneap.)*, 28:824–828.

109. Lehtovaara, R. (1973): A clinical trial with clonazepam. *Acta Neurol. Scand.*, 49:77–81.

110. Lehtovaara, R., Bardy, A., Hari, R., and Majuri, H. (1978): Sodium valproate and clonazepam interactions with phenytoin and carbamazepine. In: *Advances in Epileptology, 1977: Psychology, Pharmacotherapy, and New Diagnostic Approaches*, edited by H. Meinardi and A. J. Rowan, pp. 269–270. Swets and Zeitlinger, Amsterdam.

111. Lund, M., and Trolle, E. (1973): Clonazepam in the treatment of epilepsy. *Acta Neurol. Scand.*, 49:82–90.

112. Martin, D., and Hirt, H. R. (1973): Klinische Erfahrungen mit Clonazepam (Rivotril) in der Epilepsiebehandlung bei Kindern. *Neuropaediatrie*, 4:245–266.

113. Masland, R. L. (1975): A controlled trial of clonazepam in temporal lobe epilepsy. *Acta Neurol. Scand.*, 51:49–54.

114. Massimo, L., Pasino, M., Rosanda-Vadala, C., Tonini, G. P., De Negri, M., and Saccomani, L. (1976): Immunological side effects of anticonvulsants. *Lancet*, 1:860.

115. Matthews, W. B. (1979): Treatment of the restless

legs syndrome with clonazepam (letter). *Br. Med. J.*, 1:751.

116. Meldrum, B. S., Anlezark, G., Balzamo, E., Horton, R. W., and Trimble, M. (1975): Photically induced epilepsy in *Papio papio* as a model for drug studies. *Adv. Neurol.*, 10:119–132.

117. Merikangas, J. R., and Reynolds, C. F. (1979): Blepharospasm: Successful treatment with clonazepam. *Ann. Neurol.*, 5:401–402.

118. Mikkelsen, B., and Birket-Smith, E. (1973): A clinical study of the benzodiazepine Ro 5-4023 (clonazepam) in the treatment of epilepsy. *Acta Neurol. Scand.*, 49:91–96.

119. Mikkelsen, B., Birket-Smith, E., Brandt, S., Holm, P., Lund, M., Thorn, I., Vestermark, S., and Zander Olsen, P. (1976): Clonazepam in the treatment of epilepsy. A controlled clinical trial in simple absences, bilateral massive epileptic myoclonus, and atonic seizures. *Arch. Neurol.*, 33:322–325.

120. Mikkelsen, B., Birket-Smith, E., Holm, P., Lund, M., Vestermark, S., and Zander Olsen, P. (1975): A controlled trial on clonazepam (Ro 5-4023), Rivotril) in the treatment of focal epilepsy and secondary generalized grand mal epilepsy. *Acta Neurol. Scand.*, 51:55–61.

121. Min, B. H., and Garland, W. A. (1977): Determination of clonazepam and its 7-amino metabolite in plasma and blood by gas chromatographic–chemical ionization mass spectrometry. *J. Chromatogr.*, 139:121–133.

122. Min, B. H., Garland, W. A., Khoo, K.-C., and Torres, G. S. (1978): Determination of clonazepam and its amino and acetamido metabolites in human plasma by combined gas chromatography chemical ionization mass spectrometry and selected ion monitoring. *Biomed. Mass Spectrom.*, 5:692–698.

123. Minoli, G., and Tredici, G. (1974): Levodopa in treatment of myoclonus. *Lancet*, 2:472.

124. Moehler, H., and Okada, T. (1977): Benzodiazepine receptor: Demonstration in the central nervous system. *Science*, 198:849–851.

125. Moehler, H., Okada, T., Heitz, P., and Ulrich, J. (1978): Biochemical identification of the site of action of benzodiazepines in human brain by ^{3}H-diazepam binding. *Life Sci.*, 22:985–995.

126. Mori, T., Kato, H., Ikeda, S., and Morizaki, I. (1977): Antiepileptic activity of clonazepam: A benzodiazepine antiepileptic. II. Effects of intravenous injection of clonazepam. *Brain Nerve (Tokyo)*, 29:171–180.

127. Munthe-Kaas, A. W., and Strandjord, R. E. (1973): Clonazepam in the treatment of epileptic seizures. *Acta Neurol. Scand.*, 49:97–102.

128. Naestoft, J., and Larsen, N. E. (1974): Quantitative determination of clonazepam and its metabolites in human plasma by gas chromatography. *J. Chromatogr.*, 93:113–122.

129. Naestoft, J., Lund, M., Larsen, N. E., and Hvidberg, E. (1973): Assay and pharmacokinetics of clonazepam in humans. *Acta Neurol. Scand.*, 49:103–108.

130. Nanda, R. N., Johnson, R. H., Keogh, H. J., Lambie, D. G., and Melville, I. D. (1977): Treatment of epilepsy with clonazepam and its effect on other anticonvulsants. *J. Neurol. Neurosurg. Psychiatry*, 40:538–543.

131. Nogen, A. B. (1978): The utility of clonazepam in epilepsy of various types. Observations with 22 childhood cases. *Clin. Pediatr.*, 17:71–74.

132. Oller-Daurella, L. (1969): Resultados obtenidos con nuevos derivados benzodiazepinicos en el tratamiento la epilepsia. *Ciencias Neurol.*, 3:3.

133. Parry, G. G. (1977): Concentration of clonazepam in serum and cerebrospinal fluid of the sheep. *Pharmacology*, 15:318–323.

134. Parry, G. G., and Ferry. D. B. (1976): Rapid gas chromatographic method for the determination of clonazepam in serum and cerebrospinal fluid. *J. Chromatogr.*, 128:166–168.

135. Peiris, J. B., Boralessa, H., and Lionel, N. D. W. (1976): Clonazepam in the treatment of choreiform activity. *Med. J. Aust.*, 1:225–227.

136. Perchalski, R. J., and Wilder, B. J. (1978): Determination of benzodiazepine anticonvulsants in plasma by high performance liquid chromatography. *Anal. Chem.*, 59:554–557.

137. Pinder, R. M., Brogden, R. N., Speight, T. M., and Avery, G. S. (1976): Clonazepam: A review of its pharmacological properties and therapeutic efficacy in epilepsy. *Drugs*, 12:321–361.

138. Pinder, R. M., Brogden, R. N., Speight, T. M., and Avery, G. S. (1977): Clonazepam (Rivotril–Roche): An independent report. *Curr. Ther. Res.*, 18:25–32.

139. Rail, L. R. (1973): The treatment of self-induced photic epilepsy. *Proc. Aust. Assoc. Neurol.*, 9:121–123.

140. Rett, A. (1973): Zwei Jahre Erfahrungen mit Clonazepam bei zerebralen Krampfanfallen im Kindesalter. *Acta Neurol. Scand.*, 49:109–116.

141. Rosenmayr, F. W., and Groh, C. (1973): Wirkung von Clonazepam auf das EEG von Kindern und Jugendlichen. *Acta Neurol. Scand.*, 49:117–123.

142. Roussounis, S. H., and Rudolf, N. M. (1977): A long term electroclinical study of clonazepam in children with intractable seizures. *Electroencephalogr. Clin. Neurophysiol.*, 43:528–529.

143. Roussounis, S. H., and Rudolf, N. (1977): Clonazepam in the treatment of children with intractable seizures. *Dev. Med. Child Neurol.*, 19:326–334.

144. Sato, S., Penry, J. K., Dreifuss, F. E., and Dyken, P. R. (1977). Clonazepam in the treatment of absence seizures. *Neurology (Minneap.)*, 27:371.

145. Scollo-Lavizzari, G., Pralle, W., and de la Cruz, N. (1974): Clinical experience with clonazepam (Rivotril) in the treatment of epilepsy in adults. *Eur. Neurol.*, 11:340–344.

146. Sedman, G. (1976): Clonazepam in treatment of tardive oral dyskinesia. *Br. Med. J.*, 2:583.

147. Shakir, R., Nanda, R. N., Lambie, D. G., and Johnson, R. H. (1979): Comparative trial of valproate and clonazepam in chronic epilepsy. *Arch. Neurol.*, 36:301–304.

148. Sjö, O., Hvidberg, E. F., Naestoft, J., and Lund, M. (1975): Pharmacokinetics and side effects of clonazepam and its 7-amino-metabolite in man. *Eur. J. Clin. Pharmacol.*, 8:249–254.

149. Snead, O. C., III. (1978): Gamma hydroxybutyrate

in the monkey. III. Effect of intravenous drugs. *Neurology (Minneap.)*, 28:1173–1178.

150. Solow, E. B., and Kenfield, C. D. (1977): A micromethod for the determination of clonazepam in serum by electron-capture gas–liquid chromatography. *J. Anal. Toxicol.*, 1:155–157.

151. Sommerbeck, K. W., Theilgaard, A., and Rasmussen, K. E. (1977): Valproate sodium: Evaluation of so called psychotropic effect. A controlled study. *Epilepsia*, 18:159–167.

152. Speth, R. C., Wastek, G. J., Johnson, P. G., and Yamamura, H. I. (1978): Benzodiazepine binding in human brain: Characterization using ^{3}H-flunitrazepam. *Life Sci.*, 22:859–866.

153. Sternbach, L. H. (1973): Chemistry of 1,4-benzodiazepines and some aspects of the structure–activity relationship. In: *The Benzodiazepines*, edited by S. Garattini, E. Mussini, and L. O. Randall, pp. 1–26. Raven Press, New York.

154. Swinyard, E. A., and Castellion, A. W. (1966): Anticonvulsant properties of some benzodiazepines. *J. Pharmacol. Exp. Ther.*, 151:369–375.

155. Tassinari, C. A., Dravet, C., Roger, J., Cano, J. P., and Gastaut, H. (1972): Tonic status epilepticus precipitated by intravenous benzodiazepine in five patients with Lennox–Gastaut syndrome. *Epilepsia*, 13:421–435.

156. Tewari, S. N., and Shukla, S. K. (1977): Separation and indentification of 1,4-benzodiazepine drugs present in the biological fluids by two dimensional TLC. *Pharmazie*, 32:536.

157. Toyonaga, K., and Tokuda, S. (1976): Physiological examination and treatment by clonazepam of action myoclonus due to methyl bromide intoxication. *Clin. Neurol. (Tokyo)*, 16:830–831.

158. Tsuchiya, T., Fukushima, H., and Kitagawa, S. (1976): Effects of benzodiazepines on penicillin-induced epileptic discharges. *Nippon Acta Radiol.*, 72:861–877.

159. Turner, M., Cordero Funes, J. R., Aspinwall, R., Cantlon, B., Fejerman, N., and Loñ, J. C. (1970): Ensayo de valoracion clinicoelectroen–cefalographica de un nuevo derivado benzodiazepinico (Ro 05-4023) por administracion oral en pacientes epilepticos con tecnica de doble ceguera. *Acta Neurol. Lat. Am.*, 16:158–163.

160. Uges, D. R. A., and Bouma, P. (1978): An improved determination of clonazepam in serum by HPLC. *Pharm. Weekbl.*, 113:1156–1158.

161. Van Huffelen, A. C., and Magnus, O. (1976): The treatment of status epilepticus with clonazepam. *Ned. Tijdschr. Geneeskd.*, 120:1734–1738.

162. Vassella, F., Pavlincova, E., Schneider, H. J., Ru-

din, H. J., and Karbowski, K. (1973): Treatment of infantile spasms and Lennox–Gastaut syndrome with clonazepam. *Epilepsia*, 14:165–175.

163. Veall, R. M., and Hogarth, H. C. (1975): Thrombocytopenia during treatment with clonazepam. *Br. Med. J.*, 4:462.

164. Wad, N. T., and Hanfli, E. J. (1977): Simplified thin layer chromatographic method for the simultaneous determination of clonazepam, diazepam and their metabolites in serum. *J. Chromatogr.*, 143:214–218.

165. Watson, W. A. (1979): Interaction between clonazepam and sodium valproate. *N. Engl. J. Med.*, 300:678–679.

166. Wauquier, A., Ashton, D., and Melis, W. (1979): Behavioral analysis of amygdaloid kindling in beagle dogs and effects of clonazepam, diazepam, phenobarbital, diphenylhydantoin, and flunarizine on seizure manifestation. *Exp. Neurol.*, 64:579–586.

167. Weiner, W. J., Goetz, C., Nausieda, P. A., and Klawans, H. L. (1977): Clonazepam and dopamine-related stereotyped behavior. *Life Sci.*, 21:901–905.

168. Weiner, W. J., Goetz, C., Nausieda, P. A., and Kalwans, H. L. (1977): Clonazepam and 5-hydroxy-tryptophan-induced myoclonic stereotypy. *Eur. J. Pharmacol.*, 46:21–24.

169. Weinmann, H. M., and Willms, E. (1973): Kurzer Erfahrungsbericht uber die Wirksamkeit des antikonvulsivums Ro 5-4023 (Clonazepam) auf verschiedene Epilepsieforme. *Acta Neurol. Scand.*, 49:124–132.

170. Welch, T. E., Rumack, B. H., and Hammond, K. (1977): Clonazepam overdose resulting in cyclic coma. *Clin. Toxicol.*, 10:433–436.

171. Westblom, U. (1977): Stiff man syndrome and clonazepam. *J.A.M.A.*, 237:1930.

172. Windorfer, A., Jr., and Sauer, W. (1977): Drug interactions during anticonvulsant therapy in childhood: Diphenylhydantoin, primidone, phenobarbitone, clonazepam, nitrazepam, carbamazepine and dipropylacetate. *Neuropaediatrie*, 8:29–41.

173. Yajima, T., Uritani, K., Aoki, R., Suzuki, T., and Nakamura, K. (1976): Anticonvulsant activity of clonozepam in experimental animals. *Nippon Acta Radiol.*, 72:763–794.

174. Yamauchi, T., Hirabayashi, Y., and Kataoka, N. (1978): A clinical study of clonazepam in the treatment of epilepsy. *Brain Nerve (Tokyo)*, 30:107–116.

175. Young, A. B., Zukin, S. R., and Snyder, S. H. (1974): Interaction of benzodiazepines with central nervous glycine receptors: Possible mechanism of action. *Proc. Natl. Acad. Sci. U.S.A.*, 71:2246–2250.

Antiepileptic Drugs, edited by D. M. Woodbury, J. K. Penry, and C. E. Pippenger. Raven Press, New York © 1982.

67

Benzodiazepines

Nitrazepam

Agostino Baruzzi, Roberto Michelucci, and Carlo Alberto Tassinari

Nitrazepam was synthesized by Sternback, Fryer, Keller, Metlesics, Sach, and Steiger in 1963 (112). Since then, it has gained widespread fame as a potent and relatively nontoxic sleep-inducing agent. In addition to being effective for the treatment of insomnia, nitrazepam has also been used as an oral antiepileptic drug in some countries, where it is still utilized in the treatment of a few selected forms of epilepsy.

CHEMISTRY AND METHODS OF DETERMINATION

Chemistry

Nitrazepam is a yellow, odorless, tasteless crystalline powder with a melting point of 226 to 229°C. Its chemical name is 1,3-dihydro-7-nitro-5-phenyl-2H-1,4-benzodiazepine-2-one with a sum formula of $C_{15}H_{11}N_3O_3$. The structural formula is shown in Fig. 1. Its molecular weight is 281.3.

Nitrazepam shows pK_a values of 3.2 and 10.8; the drug is practically insoluble in water but soluble in chloroform, ethanol, ether, and diluted inorganic acids.

The most important structure–activity relationship for the 1,4-benzodiazepines involves the character of the substituent at position 7 in the A ring. Electron withdrawing substituents generally increase the activity, with Cl, as in diazepam, imparting broad anticonvulsant efficacy, and NO_2, as in nitrazepam, being more selective for antipentylenetetrazol activity (116).

Methods of Determination

The quantitative determination of nitrazepam in biological fluids can be performed with various methods. Gas–liquid chromatographic (GLC), spectrophotometric, thin-layer chromatographic, and ^{14}C-labeling techniques developed before 1973 were reviewed by Browne and Penry (17). The thin-layer chromatographic and photometric methods are not sufficiently specific or sensitive for clinical monitoring or pharmacokinetic studies, and the ^{14}C-labeling method is not applicable to the detection of plasma nitrazepam concentrations after administration of commercial nitrazepam preparations.

Since 1973, fluorometric, GLC, high-pressure liquid chromatographic, radioimmunoassay, and radioreceptor techniques have been developed. The fluorometric technique is able to detect nitrazepam and the sum of 7-amino and

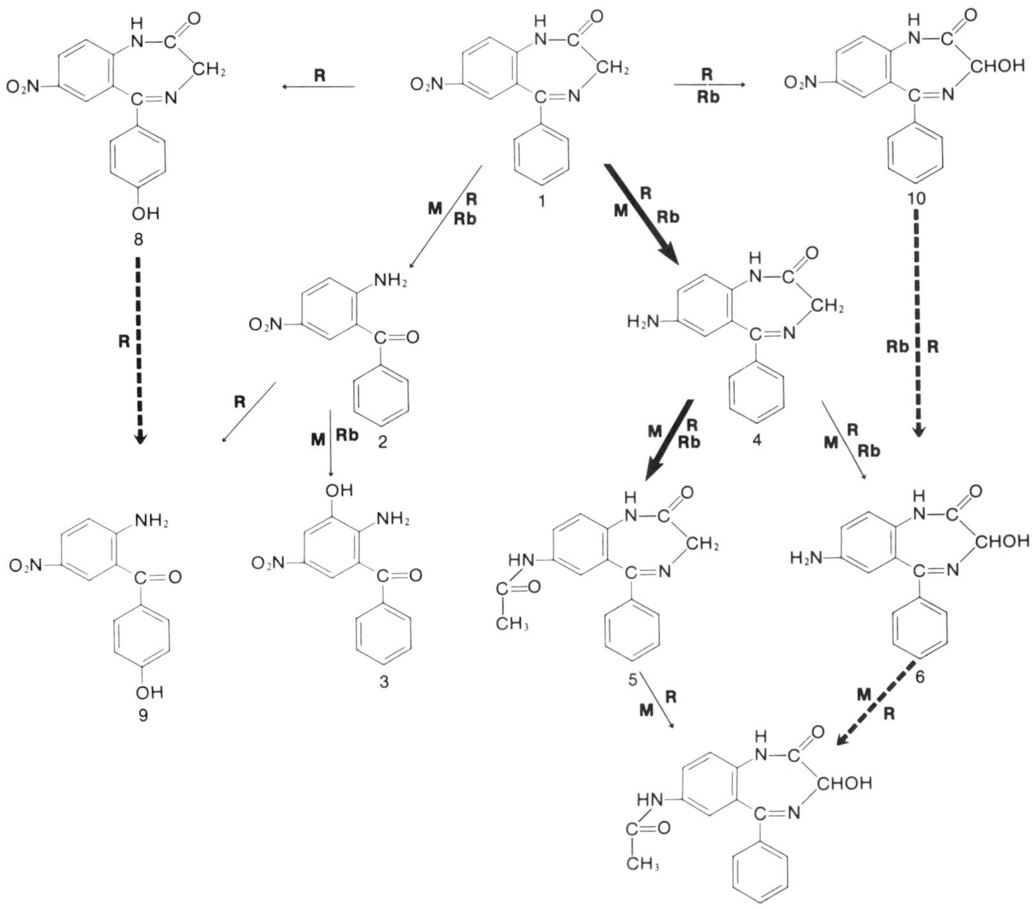

FIG. 1. Proposed metabolic pathways of nitrazepam in humans, rat, and rabbit (102,105,123). **1,** nitrazepam; **2,** 2-amino-5-nitrobenzophenone; **3,** 2-amino-3-hydroxy-5-nitrobenzophenone; **4,** 7-aminonitrazepam; **5,** 7-acetamidonitrazepam; **6,** 3-hydroxy-7-aminonitrazepam; **7,** 3-hydroxy-7-acetamidonitrazepam; **8,** 4′-hydroxynitrazepam; **9,** 2-amino-4′-hydroxy-5-nitrobenzophenone; **10,** 3-hydroxynitrazepam; **M,** takes place in humans; **R,** takes place in rat; **Rb,** takes place in rabbit. Major metabolic steps are indicated by *thick arrows; dashed arrows* represent uncertain pathways.

7-acetamido metabolites at plasma concentrations over 10 ng/ml after selective extractions of the compounds (100,101). The radioimmunoassay has a limit of sensitivity of 4 ng/ml using 10 μl of plasma. Because of its rapidity and simplicity, it is suitable for clinical monitoring of nitrazepam in epileptic patients and for pharmacokinetics and bioavailability studies that require small-volume samples; the limit is represented by a cross-reactivity with some other benzodiazepines (29). The high affinity that benzodiazepines show for the receptor and the

specificity of binding have been utilized for a radioreceptor assay (47).

Gas–liquid chromatography is the most widely used procedure. Nitrazepam can be measured with good sensitivity by a direct method (27,54,55) or after an acid hydrolysis (54,86) utilizing electron capture detectors (ECD); after derivatization (methyl derivative), it has been measured either by ECD or nitrogen-selective detectors (8,28,30).

In the clinical monitoring of nitrazepam in plasma, the direct method is preferred because it is fairly rapid and simple, even though it requires thorough inactivation of the column. The acid hydrolysis and derivatization techniques require more complex extraction and purification procedures (54).

The GLC methods described, which differ in their internal standards and stationary phases, have a sensitivity of 0.2 to 5 ng/ml of plasma and require 0.5 to 1 ml of plasma.

In the main metabolic step nitrazepam loses the electrophilic 7-nitro group, yielding compounds not detectable using an ECD. The 7-amino and 7-acetamido metabolites, however, can be measured in the urine, with a detection limit of 50 ng/ml, utilizing a nitrogen-selective detector (55).

Nitrazepam, 7-aminonitrazepam, and 7-acetamidonitrazepam have also been analyzed in the urine by high-pressure liquid chromatography on a column packed with an anion exchange resin (89). The method seems applicable only to the analysis of relatively high levels of nitrazepam in urine.

ABSORPTION, DISTRIBUTION, AND EXCRETION

Absorption

After a single oral dose of 5 or 10 mg of nitrazepam, mean peak plasma concentrations of 35 to 47 ng/ml and 83 to 84 ng/ml, respectively, were found in different studies, mostly in young healthy volunteers (14,16,27,48, 57–59,63, 86,102). In elderly patients suffering from various debilitating diseases, a mean peak plasma concentration of 22 ng/ml was observed after a single oral dose of 5 mg of nitrazepam (48,59). Generally, peak absorption occurred within 2 to 3 hr, but in a few cases relatively fast (30 min) or slow (4 hr) absorption was reported (16,27).

The absolute bioavailability of this drug was determined in six healthy adult volunteers who first received an intravenous injection of 10 mg of nitrazepam base dissolved in 2 ml of glycerolformal and, 2 weeks later, an equal oral dose of a commercially prepared formulation (102). Despite considerable interindividual variation,

ranging from 53 to 94% of the dose, an average of 78% of the unchanged drug was absorbed. One partial explanation for the reduced extent of bioavailability of nitrazepam may be the formation of 2-amino-5-nitrobenzophenone caused by acid hydrolysis in the stomach (102).

Subsequent studies compared the relative bioavailability of different oral preparations. Møller Jensen (86) observed identical serum curves for two brands of nitrazepam, and De Boer et al. (27) showed evidence of significant differences with respect to peak level times. It was suggested, however, that the differences found among the various brands of nitrazepam with regard to peak level times or extent of absorption are probably not important in practice (15).

Distribution

The disposition of nitrazepam may be described in terms of a two-compartment open model. In fact, a biexponential decline of the plasma concentration is observed either after i.v. administration or after the peak concentration has been reached for oral administration. The initial rapid decrease of plasma nitrazepam concentrations is determined by a short distribution half-life ($T_{1/2}\alpha \sim 2$ hr), but this phase was not observed in single cases where absorption was very slow (16,27,58). The subsequent slower decrease, mainly reflecting the elimination of the drug, is consistent with the apparent elimination half-life ($T_{1/2}\beta$).

A second small increase in plasma concentration has been observed between 4 and 8 hr following oral nitrazepam administration (16,27) (Fig. 2). This second peak concentration in serum is reasonably explained by an enterohepatic recycling of nitrazepam, which seems to be enhanced by food intake (16,27). This latter hypothesis could not be confirmed by Kangas et al. (58) who failed to find a second peak concentration in serum following oral nitrazepam administration, but most of his patients had not eaten or had taken only little food.

The apparent volume of distribution of nitrazepam, calculated during the β elimination phase

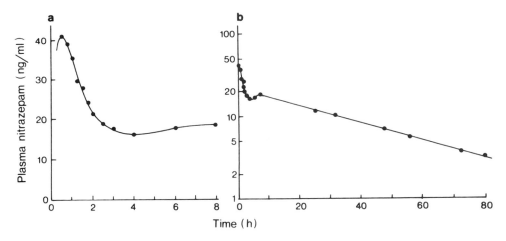

FIG. 2. Plasma concentration curve of unchanged nitrazepam on linear scale (**a**) and on log scale (**b**) following oral administration of a 5-mg dose in a single subject. (From Breimer et al., ref. 16, with permission.)

after i.v. injection of 10 mg of the drug, was found to vary in six young healthy volunteers from 1.50 to 2.76 liter/kg, with a mean of 1.95 liter/kg (101). After oral administration, Kangas et al. (59) reported mean volumes of distribution (calculated on the assumption that bioavailability was complete) of 2.4 ± 0.8 and 4.8 ± 1.7 liter/kg, respectively, in groups of 25 young volunteers and of 12 old patients. This study showed a good positive correlation of elimination half-life and apparent volume of distribution in young and old subjects, although total clearance was not significantly different in the two groups (4.1 ± 2.0 and 4.7 ± 1.5 liter/hr). The authors suggested that at steady state a greater amount of the administered dose will be present in aged subjects at receptor sites in the central nervous system and that the increased sensitivity to nitrazepam in the elderly could possibly result from the increased volume of distribution. Similar results for the apparent volume of distribution were reported by the same authors in a different group of 12 young volunteers (58).

The percentage of the non-protein-bound fraction of nitrazepam at different concentrations has been shown *in vitro* to range from 13.2 to 14.2% (102). Similar findings of 12.0 and 13% in four healthy volunteers (58), of 9.6

to 15.6% (mean, 11.9 ± 2.1) in 10 women at the end of the pregnancy, and of 8.6 to 14.1% (mean, 12.0 ± 1.8) in their 10 newborns (60) were reported. The extent of protein binding in old age and in disease states has not been reported.

The high protein binding and the liposolubility of nitrazepam are responsible for the fact that the drug distributes with only a small fraction in liquid body compartments. After i.p. administration of [^{14}C]nitrazepam (40 mg/kg) to "young" and "old" rats, the tissue distribution of radioactivity was found to be higher in kidney and liver, followed by spleen, heart, and lung, than in plasma between 2 and 6 hr after injection (45). The brain-to-plasma ratio was consistently lower in "young" rats than in "old" rats, suggesting a different distribution pattern (45). After i.v. injection of [^{14}C]nitrazepam (5 mg/kg) in rats, a brain-to-plasma concentration ratio of 0.60 was observed between 15 and 30 min after administration (117). After a 5-mg single oral dose in 38 patients with neurological disorders, the percentage ratio between the mean cerebrospinal fluid (CSF) and plasma concentrations increased from 8% at 2 hr to 15.6% at 36 hr (62). Although it was suggested that the CSF concentration can reflect the non-protein-bound fraction in the plasma, the time dependence of the CSF-to-plasma ratio indicates that factors other than simple protein binding determine equilibrium of nitrazepam between CSF and plasma. Moreover, these observations suggest a slow equilibration of nitrazepam between plasma and the CSF (62).

A similar time-dependent ratio between saliva and serum concentration was observed. Nevertheless, the salivary concentrations were very low and did not reflect the non-protein-bound fraction in serum. A possible explanation, given by the authors, for the low levels in saliva is that a tight adsorption of nitrazepam to the insoluble particles of saliva may occur (58).

Transfer of nitrazepam across the human placenta has been documented both at the beginning of the second trimester and during the last weeks of pregnancy (60). In early pregnancy, the concentration of nitrazepam in umbilical circulation and amniotic fluid was significantly lower than that in maternal plasma (60), but in late pregnancy an equilibrium between fetal and maternal tissues was observed (60,102). Nitrazepam is poorly excreted in the milk of lactating mothers; it seems unlikely that the very small quantities of the drug can produce any pharmacological or toxic effects in the child (102).

Excretion

In young, healthy volunteers, the apparent plasma elimination half-life ($T_{1/2}\beta$) of nitrazepam ranged from a mean of 25 to 30.6 hr after a 5-mg single oral dose (16,27,48,58,59,63,86). Similar values were reported after a single oral dose of 10 mg of nitrazepam (63,102). Furthermore, in six healthy subjects the elimination half-lives varied from 17.8 to 24.0 hr after a single intravenous injection of 10 mg of the drug. (102). In a group of 12 geriatric patients (66–89 years) affected by various disabling diseases and on multidrug therapy, a $T_{1/2}\beta$ of 40.4 ± 16.2 hr was reported (48,59). After the end of 2 weeks of continuous nitrazepam treatment in a group of 11 young volunteers and 2 months in a group of 10 old patients, apparent plasma half-lives were 24.2 ± 4.9 and

39.6 ± 13.8 hr, respectively (59). There was no significant change in the elimination half-life of the drug after 24 days of treatment in four healthy subjects (102). The present findings suggest that the elimination of nitrazepam is independent of the dose and route of administration. The unchanged half-life of nitrazepam in the acute and long-term studies in both young and old subjects suggests that nitrazepam does not induce its own metabolism.

According to published results, the elimination rate of nitrazepam seems to be age dependent. Nevertheless, Castelden et al. (20), studying the half-life of nitrazepam in two groups of young (under 40 years; mean, 25.3) and old (over 68 years; mean, 74.7) subjects, failed to confirm any age-related difference in pharmacokinetics. It is noteworthy that the old patients were self-sufficient and living in the community and none had seen his or her general practitioner within a year of the study. In this respect, they differed from the elderly in the study of Kangas et al. (59), whose patients were cared for in medical wards and were partly or totally bedridden.

During prolonged treatment with nitrazepam, the time required to reach a steady-state level was about 3.5 days and 7.5 days in young volunteers and old patients, respectively, in accordance with the corresponding half-life values. Steady-state levels, calculated as a mean of repeated follow-up individual samples, were, respectively, 57 ± 17 and 45 ± 12 ng/ml for daily oral nitrazepam doses of 75.3 ± 2.1 and 86.6 ± 9.0 μg/kg (59).

Routes of Excretion

Nitrazepam and its metabolites are mainly excreted in the urine in humans. In six healthy adults, following a single oral administration of 5 mg of nitrazepam labeled with ^{14}C, urinary excretion 144 hr after dosage varied from 45 to 65% of the total radioactivity introduced with the dose (102). In another subject, who had received a single oral dose of 10 mg of ^{14}C-labeled nitrazepam and, three months later, an equal dose of the same preparation by intravenous injection, the total renal excretion determined during the first 120 hr was 71% and 93%, respectively (102). It was suggested that the lower percentage after oral administration is explained by incomplete absorption.

Similar results were obtained in 15 healthy volunteers after a single 5-mg tablet of nitrazepam. The mean total 7-day excretion of nitrazepam and its main metabolites in the urine was approximately 50% of the administered dose (56), with a large interindividual variation. With regard to the proportions of the various excretion products of nitrazepam appearing in the urine, it was found that unchanged nitrazepam is excreted in small amounts via the kidneys (1%), whereas its main metabolites (7-acetamidonitrazepam and 7-aminonitrazepam) are excreted to a larger extent (21 and 31%, respectively) both as free and conjugated metabolites (56).

Fecal excretion of nitrazepam was studied in four healthy adults following the oral or i.v. administration of a 30-mg dose of [2-^{14}C]nitrazepam. At 144 hr after administration, the cumulative fecal excretion of nitrazepam or its metabolites varied from 8 to 13% of the dose when the drug was injected i.v. and 14 to 20% when it was given orally (102). The rest of the dose, incomplete absorption of the drug apart, may be bound to tissues or to deep compartments from where it is very slowly eliminated, or it may be excreted as metabolites not measurable by the available methods [e.g., 3-hydroxynitrazepam, benzophenones (56)].

The possibility of biliary excretion of nitrazepam has been mentioned (56).

Some species variations do exist in the excretory route of most of the benzodiazepines. In rats, fecal excretion is the major route of elimination of nitrazepam, and an enterohepatic cycling of the biliary metabolites of nitrazepam has been established following [^{14}C]nitrazepam intravenous injection (117).

BIOTRANSFORMATION

Rieder and Wendt (102) reviewed the metabolism of nitrazepam in humans and the rat in 1973. Since then, not much additional information has been gained. The main line of metabolism in humans and the rat begins with the reduction of the nitro group to the corresponding amine (7-aminonitrazepam); this latter compound is then acetylated to the 7-acetamido derivative, which is the prevailing metabolite (see Fig. 1). A small proportion of these two metabolites is then hydroxylated in position 3, yielding the 3-OH derivatives. Intestinal microflora and/or intestinal tissue enzymes as well as hepatic enzymes play an important role in the first of these metabolic steps (nitroreduction) (46), whereas the acetylation and hydroxylation are performed in the liver (5,6,64). It has been found that the acetylation of 7-aminonitrazepam is achieved by genetically controlled polymorphic acetylation (64), but there is no evidence that acetylation phenotype may be important in connection with nitrazepam therapy (74).

A secondary line of metabolism involves the formation of benzophenones: 2-amino-5-nitrobenzophenone and relative hydroxylated compounds (2-amino-3-hydroxy-5-nitrobenzophenone in humans and 2-amino-4'-hydroxy-5-nitrobenzophenone in the rat) (102). There are significant species differences in biotransformation. Sawada and Hara (105) have shown that 2-amino-3-hydroxy-5-nitrobenzophenone was the major metabolite excreted, mainly as the conjugated form, in the urine of rabbits fed nitrazepam. Additional pathways of nitrazepam metabolism in rats, consisting of 3-hydroxylation and 4'-hydroxylation of nitrazepam, have also been described (35,102,123).

INTERACTION WITH OTHER DRUGS

Nitrazepam is probably ineffective in altering the rate of metabolism of concomitantly administered drugs. Stevenson (113) and Stevenson et al. (114) observed no significant change in plasma test drug (antipyrine and phenylbutazone) half-lives or in the urinary output of 6β-hydroxycortisol after nitrazepam treatment. Consistent with these results, nitrazepam does not influence the plasma levels and effects of warfarin (92), phenprocoumon (9), or tricyclic antidepressants (88,108) in humans. Nevertheless, a possible interference of nitrazepam with the anticoagulant effects of phenprocoumon was shown in rats (67), and Ballinger et al. (3) observed a mild and insignificant influence of nitrazepam on plasma imipramine levels in humans.

Benzodiazepines are known to potentiate the action of CNS depressant drugs such as ethanol or barbiturates. Chambers and Jefferson (21) showed that intraperitoneal nitrazepam was, among five benzodiazepines tested (chlordiazepoxide, diazepam, medazepam, nitrazepam, and oxazepam), one of the most effective compounds in increasing the duration of pentobarbital sodium-induced sleeping times in mice.

No further data are available in the literature about possible interactions of clinical significance between nitrazepam and other antiepileptic drugs.

RELATION OF PLASMA CONCENTRATION TO CLINICAL EFFECTS

Kangas et al. (59) studied plasma nitrazepam levels in a group of 44 children affected by different types of epilepsy. All subjects were on chronic treatment with nitrazepam at a daily oral dose of 280 ± 110 µg/kg. Blood samples were taken 8 to 14 hr after the preceding dose. In 95% of the plasma samples studied, the concentrations of nitrazepam were between 40 and 180 ng/ml (mean, 114 ng/ml); a significant correlation was found between the daily dose and the plasma concentration (Fig. 3). Most children had a successful clinical response, but, because all of the patients were on combined anticonvulsant therapy, no desirable "therapeutic" plasma level of the drug could be defined. However, the authors suggested an upper "therapeutic" level of about 200 to 220 ng/ml, because when higher plasma concentrations of nitrazepam (>200 ng/ml) were reached, toxic effects (e.g., sedation) developed (Fig. 4).

Kangas et al. (61) observed, in 61 patients receiving a single oral 5-mg dose of nitrazepam

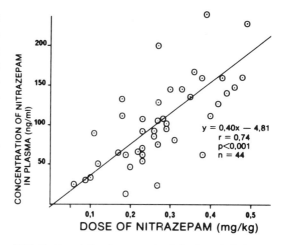

FIG. 3. Correlation between the daily dose and plasma concentration of nitrazepam in epileptic children during continuous treatment with nitrazepam. (From Kangas et al., ref. 59, with permission.)

for premedication in minor surgery, a significant correlation between the subjective sedative effect and plasma concentration of the drug during the period of increasing plasma concentrations. Similar results have been obtained in other studies. Grundström et al. (41), using the critical flicker fusion method, estimated the sedative–hypnotic effects of diazepam and nitrazepam in eight healthy volunteers. The peak effects of sedation occurred 1.5 hr after nitrazepam intake, whereas the peak plasma concentration usually occurred after 3 to 4 hr. Furthermore, the sedative effects had almost disappeared 6 hr after intake of nitrazepam, while the drug concentrations were still significantly high.

Kangas et al. (63) also showed, in 10 healthy volunteers given a single oral dose of nitrazepam, a significant positive correlation between the subjective sedative effects and the magnitude of the peak nitrazepam concentrations in plasma, especially when the plasma levels of nitrazepam were rising.

Tolerance

The development of tolerance to the anticonvulsant effects of nitrazepam has been reported

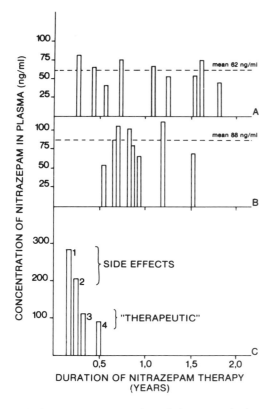

FIG. 4. Plasma concentration of nitrazepam in three epileptic children during continuous therapy. No evidence of enzyme induction causing a decrease in the concentration during long-term treatment was found (note the unchanged daily dose in growing children). **A:** 6- to 8-year-old boy receiving nitrazepam, 3.75 mg/day; mean steady-state concentration, 62 ng/ml. **B:** 8- to 9-year-old girl given nitrazepam, 12.5 mg/ day; mean steady-state concentration, 88 ng/ml. **C:** An example of titration of nitrazepam from "toxic" to "therapeutic" level in a 1- to 1.5-year-old boy. The doses of nitrazepam were: **1,** 4.5 mg/day; **2,** 3.75 mg/day; **3,** 3.0 mg/day (2.5 hr after the preceding dose); and **4,** 3.0 mg/day (8.5 hr after the preceding dose). (From Kangas et al., ref. 59, with permission.)

(36,42–44,84). It is probably caused by a decreased response of the central nervous system to a constant plasma concentration of nitrazepam, since there is no evidence that nitrazepam induces liver microsomal enzymes (91,92,114) and thereby stimulates its own metabolism during long-term treatment (59,102) (Fig. 4).

Dependence

The development of dependence of the barbiturate–alcohol type after prolonged use of nitrazepam is possible but rare. Darcy (26) described a delirium-tremens-like syndrome after discontinuation of nitrazepam in a 51-year-old man who had been taking nitrazepam (20 mg) nightly for years. Rebound insomnia is a more important effect after discontinuation of the drug. Adam et al. (1) and Kales et al. (52,53) observed a significant worsening of sleep on withdrawal from nitrazepam. Kales et al. (52) hypothesize, on the basis of the demonstration of benzodiazepine receptors in the brain, that the abrupt withdrawal of benzodiazepine drugs with a short duration of action, such as nitrazepam, results in an intensive form of rebound insomnia because of a lag in the production and replacement of endogenous benzodiazepine-like substances whose production decreases if active benzodiazepine drugs are introduced exogenously. The poor sleep caused by withdrawal of nitrazepam is a further reminder of how such drugs create conditions that lead to perpetuation of intake.

TOXICITY

The most common side effects related to long-term nitrazepam administration include symptoms of CNS depression (drowsiness, ataxia, incoordination) which may be minimized by beginning with a low dose of nitrazepam and slowly increasing the dose (17). These adverse reactions are probably more frequent in the elderly (38) and are dose related in frequency. On the other hand, symptoms of CNS stimulation such as nightmares, insomnia, and agitation have been reported, but to a lesser extent (37,38,119). Other relatively common side effects are dizziness, inattention, hypotonia, and muscle weakness.

In children, increased salivation and hypersecretion of the tracheobronchial tree have been noted by several investigators (42,43,84,122); in adults, such effects were less frequent or negligible (73). There is some evidence

(22,34,85,97,103) that nitrazepam may produce respiratory depression and subsequent CO_2 narcosis when given to patients with chronic obstructive bronchitis and ventilatory failure.

Several studies have shown that the administration of nitrazepam may impair human performance on the subsequent day (10,76,94,95). Of particular interest are the data concerning the residual effects of nitrazepam on the performance of skills related to driving or other usual activities (71,104). Lahtinen et al. (69) observed in 32 healthy young volunteers 8 hr after 5- or 10-mg oral doses of nitrazepam an impairment of psychomotor skills which was dose related. It was suggested that precautions must be taken when prescribing large doses (over 5 mg) of nitrazepam as a hypnotic to subjects needing their normal skills in daily work.

Nitrazepam has rarely been shown to increase seizure frequency. Martin (78) reported the occurrence of tonic seizures after an intravenous injection of nitrazepam in a patient with petit mal status, and, as described by Peterson (96), six out of 108 epileptic patients treated with oral nitrazepam had an exacerbation of seizures. Gibbs and Anderson (36) observed 14 patients who experienced increased frequency and severity of grand mal seizures. In a 12-year-old boy affected by Lennox–Gastaut syndrome, parenteral administration of 15 mg of nitrazepam caused tonic status epilepticus 11 min after injection (118).

Miscellaneous Side Effects

MacLean (75) described the case of a 55-year-old woman who developed acroparesthesias after receiving 10-mg doses of nitrazepam as long-term therapy. Hypothermia occurred in an elderly patient following the administration of 5 mg of nitrazepam (49), and a 40-year-old man with a history of gout had acute attacks after taking 10 mg of nitrazepam (70).

A case of leukopenia has been reported to be caused by nitrazepam (96), and of interest are some cutaneous reactions attributed to nitrazepam in the studies of Greenblatt and Allen (38)

and Arndt and Jick (2). Generalized urticaria (77), opisthotonus with dystonia (77), headache (96), and anorexia (36) have been reported in single cases.

Nitrazepam and the Elderly

Nitrazepam may be dangerous to the elderly. Evans and Jarvis (31) reported a syndrome characterized by mental confusion, disorientation, ataxia, postural hypotension, and incontinence occurring in old people taking 5 mg of nitrazepam at night. During chronic use in psychogeriatric inpatients, nitrazepam (10 mg) produced impairment of many functions such as ability to move and memory and caused fecal and urinary incontinence, excessive muscle relaxation, and persistent sedation and drowsiness (72). Castelden et al. (20) observed an increased sensitivity to a dose of 10 mg of nitrazepam in old age. Since elderly patients are readily susceptible to excessive CNS depression at high drug doses, Greenblatt and Allen (38) suggest that for hypnotic use there is little reason to exceed 5-mg doses of nitrazepam for most old patients.

Overdose

Nitrazepam is rarely fatal in overdosage. Out of 1,176 hypnotic drug overdosages, 102 involved nitrazepam; only six patients were deeply comatose, and these nevertheless recovered uneventfully in 12 hr (80,81). Bardhan (4) described a case of a 23-year-old man who developed a cerebellar syndrome (nystagmus, ataxia, dysarthria) after taking 180 mg of nitrazepam. Ridley (99) reported the occurrence of bullous lesions of the type sometimes seen with barbiturate overdosage in a 24-year-old woman who was comatose for 36 hr after ingesting 100 tablets of nitrazepam.

Nitrazepam overdosage has been implicated in a comatose patient whose EEG was composed of activity in the alpha frequency range (18,19). The point of major practical importance is that "alpha coma" has been seen mainly in cases of pontomesencephalic infarction or diffuse posthypoxic cerebral cortical necrosis, and in such cases it has usually carried a poor prognosis. It is suggested that when patients in coma exhibit generalized nonreactive alpha activity, a pharmacological intoxication should be considered, and, if this is confirmed, a complete recovery should be expected.

Teratogenicity

We have been unable to find any published data concerning a possible teratogenic effect of nitrazepam. Only Saxen and Saxen (106) suggested evidence of a correlation between the first-trimester maternal intake of benzodiazepines (diazepam, oxazepam, nitrazepam, chlordiazepoxide) and the occurrence of oral clefts (especially cleft palate) in newborns.

PHARMACODYNAMICS

Mechanisms of action

Anticonvulsant activity of nitrazepam has been evaluated against a wide variety of experimental seizure models. Benzodiazepines, notably nitrazepam, have been shown to be most effective in preventing pentylenetetrazol-induced seizures in both mice and rats (12,68,83,116). A much greater dose is needed to raise the threshold at which maximal electroshock induces seizures in the same animals (83,116). Nitrazepam appeared to be between diazepam and clonazepam in potency and duration of action in the maximal electroshock seizure test (83,116).

In a study to determine whether benzodiazepines preferentially antagonize seizures induced by chemical convulsants acting on the GABA system, such as 3-mercaptopropionic acid (3-MP), bicuculline and picrotoxin, nitrazepam seemed to be more effective against pentylenetetrazol than against 3-MP (115). Furthermore, nitrazepam prevents, as do other benzodiazepines, photically induced seizures in the baboon *Papio papio* (65), which may correlate

well with the effectiveness of this drug in reducing photosensitivity in humans (32).

With respect to models of partial epilepsy, many studies have detailed the action of benzodiazepines on experimentally induced cortical foci. Benzodiazepines prevent the motor manifestations of focal seizure discharges and depress the spread of abnormal electrical activity from the site of the lesion (17).

Electroencephalographic studies in humans have shown that nitrazepam, consistent with the action of other benzodiazepines, may produce an increase in low-voltage fast activity and a decrease of alpha frequency, especially in frontal areas (79,87). It has been shown that nitrazepam has a suppressive effect in humans in regard to the photosensitive response in the EEG (32).

Nitrazepam has characteristic effects on sleep stages. As do other benzodiazepines, it reduces the time spent in drowsiness during the night (stage 1), increases the total time in stage 2 sleep, and decreases the time spent in slow-wave sleep (stages 3 and 4); also, the time spent in the paradoxical or rapid eye movement phase is usually shortened (93).

Responses evoked in cortical and subcortical areas by local or sensory inputs have been shown to be altered by benzodiazepines. In the baboon, evoked potential studies showed nitrazepam-induced changes in evoked responses in the occipital regions that paralleled seizure control (65).

In experimental animals, benzodiazepines have various pharmacological effects on limbic system structures. Shalleck et al. (107) found that nitrazepam increased the afterdischarge threshold of the amygdala in cats, and Morillo (90) showed that nitrazepam exerts strong inhibitory actions on the response of the hippocampus to stimulation of the ipsilateral amygdala in cats.

Data documenting significant participation of GABA in the action of benzodiazepines have been extensively reviewed by Killam and Suria (66). Benzodiazepines exert GABAmimetic actions wherever these occur. Benzodiazepines enhance presynaptic inhibition in some regions of the CNS such as the spinal cord and caudate nucleus where GABA is the presumed mediator of presynaptic inhibition (66). At the same time, benzodiazepines probably increase postsynaptic inhibition whenever it is mediated by GABA (66). Benzodiazepines appear to act indirectly on GABA mechanisms. Costa and Guidotti (25) hypothesize that benzodiazepines are not direct GABA receptor agonists but that they bind to specific benzodiazepine receptors in the brain.

The effectiveness of various benzodiazepines in displacing [^{3}H]diazepam binding to rat brain membranes correlates well with their affinity for the specific receptors. With respect to this action, nitrazepam has been found to be a compound of intermediate potency, as have diazepam or chlorazepate (13,121). Secondary to a primary action on GABA mechanisms, other neurotransmitters may play minor roles in the action of benzodiazepines.

Many authors have shown that chlordiazepoxide, diazepam, and nitrazepam in fairly high doses (10 mg/kg) may decrease the turnover rate of norepinephrine and dopamine in some regions of the rat brain (24,120). Stein et al. (111) reported that benzodiazepines may impair serotonin turnover rate and suggested that such effects could explain their anxiolytic actions.

Even the cholinergic system may be involved in the action of benzodiazepines. Consolo et al. (23) have found evidence that not only diazepam but nitrazepam and lorazepam as well are effective in increasing rat hemispheric acetylcholine levels, perhaps by blocking the release of acetylcholine from nerve terminals. It has been suggested that benzodiazepines indirectly alter the turnover rate of catecholamines, serotonin, and acetylcholine, but that the primary action of benzodiazepines is on the GABA system which, in turn, may affect or alter monoamine function in the brain (23,33,111).

Nitrazepam, as well as diazepam and other benzodiazepines, is a very potent agent in displacing radiolabeled strychnine, a glycine antagonist, from the glycine receptors, an ability that correlates well with affinity for this receptor site (110). It is suggested that benzodiazepines mimic the neurophysiological actions of glycine, a prominent inhibitory transmitter in the brainstem and spinal cord; this action would account for the antianxiety and muscle relaxant effects of benzodiazepines (110).

THERAPEUTIC USE

Reports on the efficacy of nitrazepam in chronic oral treatment of epilepsy start in 1964, peak in the 1967–1968 period, and then progressively decrease.

Effective daily doses of nitrazepam range from 0.25 mg to 3 mg/kg, the highest being used in children mainly suffering from hypsarrhythmia. Mean daily doses vary from 0.5 mg/kg in adults to 1 mg/kg in children. Therapeutic plasma levels are quite variable and consequently are considered of little relevance in clinical practice (50).

Nitrazepam has been found effective in a variety of seizures occurring in different forms of epilepsy (17). Most reports, however, seem to indicate that nitrazepam is chiefly useful in the treatment of infantile spasms with hypsarrhythmia (or West syndrome) and in the so-called infantile myoclonic seizures (the two conditions often being reported under the same heading of myoclonic seizures) (82).

We have reviewed 81 cases of West syndrome (infantile spasms with hypsarrhythmic records occurring mainly in the first 2 years of life), and 55 of these responded satisfactorily to nitrazepam treatment (7,11,36,39,51,77,109,122). Gibbs and Anderson (36), however, included under the heading of infantile spasms with hypsarrhythmia subjects up to 12 years of age who could be considered as having a Lennox–Gastaut syndrome. Curiously, Jong (51) considered nitrazepam effective in all cases of epilepsy except hypsarrhythmia, since he did not observe significant effects in his four cases.

Volzke et al. (122) studied 24 children treated with oral nitrazepam in doses ranging from 0.7 to 2 mg/kg (mean, 1 mg/kg) and observed beneficial results in 13 patients (54%) with a follow-up varying from 2 to 17 months. From the study of Borselli et al. (11), it would seem that patients with symptomatic West syndrome (11 cases) are less likely to respond well (3 out of 11) to nitrazepam treatment, and understandably so. These findings, however, must be considered from the viewpoint of the great heterogeneity of the reported cases, probably related to such significant factors as the age of the patients, the etiology of the syndrome, the duration of the follow-up, and criteria for the definition of improvement. When the problem was first considered (17,40), it was not clear whether ACTH or nitrazepam was the most useful treatment of infantile spasms; this is still an unanswered question.

In myoclonic seizures occurring mainly in children later in the life, as compared to hypsarrhythmia, nitrazepam was also found effective. Such cases can be found particularly in the reports of Millichap and Ortiz (84), Benedetti et al. (7), Snyder (109), and Lundberg and Stalberg (73). According to Jeavons (50), nitrazepam is likely to be one of the most effective benzodiazepines for the control of myoclonic seizures.

More than 50 cases have been reported under the specific heading of "myoclonic seizures" or "myoclonic epilepsy" but it is quite difficult to determine from these reports precisely if and what kind of "myoclonic seizures" responded best to nitrazepam and for how long the improvement was maintained. Patients with myoclonic or absence seizures or both, are particularly likely to display photosensitivity, and there is evidence that benzodiazepines, notably nitrazepam, can block paroxysmal responses in both types of seizures (32,98). Nitrazepam was also found effective in some patients with "minor motor seizures" (96), a term that unfortunately covers a wide range of different seizures and forms of epilepsy. Similarly, "astatic seizures" benefited as well from therapy with nitrazepam.

A number of cases of what could be referred to as Lennox–Gastaut syndrome were classified under different labels in the literature. We found reports of approximately 50 patients affected by such a syndrome (36,39,51) who benefited to some extent from treatment with nitrazepam. In

an unpublished study, nitrazepam was added to previous treatment in 50 children aged 2 to 12 years with a Lennox–Gastaut syndrome (C. Dravet, J. Roger, C. A. Tassinari, *unpublished data,* 1968). Dosages varied from 15 to 30 mg, with a maximum daily dose of 50 to 75 mg. A very significant clinical and electroencephalographic improvement was observed in 27 children. It was noted that nitrazepam could significantly control the atypical absences and that tonic seizures persisted as the sole symptomatology. The positive effects, however, disappeared or significantly decreased over a follow-up period ranging from 8 days to 3 months in 13 patients. The treatment was stopped in five patients because of side effects. Good results persisted for up to 3 months in seven patients and up to 2 years in two others. Nineteen children had only a mild clinical improvement, and four were unhelped by nitrazepam.

The main side effects observed in eight patients were hypotonia, drowsiness, and, in children under 3 years of age, disturbances of swallowing. Interestingly, 25 out of the 27 patients who showed good improvement with nitrazepam therapy had previously been treated with diazepam; 10 of them had more or less transitory good results, and nine did not respond at all. The conclusions were that in the Lennox–Gastaut syndrome nitrazepam was more useful than diazepam, particularly in control of atypical absences.

With regard to primary generalized epilepsy (typical absences of petit mal and tonic–clonic seizures), we found reports of 48 patients mainly affected by typical absences, of whom 18 significantly improved after nitrazepam treatment (39,51,73,77,96). Of 27 patients only or mainly suffering from tonic–clonic seizures, nine had a significant improvement following nitrazepam therapy (11,51,77).

Nitrazepam has also been found effective in partial seizures. Of 110 patients with partial seizures reported by various authors, 77 had complex symptomatology, mostly of "psychomotor" type (or "temporal lobe" seizures). Clinically significant improvement or, rarely, complete seizure control was observed in 19 out of 35 patients with various partial seizures and in 17 out of 62 patients with psychomotor seizures (7,51,77). To the previously reported cases we should add those of Lundberg and Stalberg (73) who observed in 21 adult patients (15 with psychomotor epilepsy and 6 with partial attacks of other types) in whom other therapy had been unsuccessful that nitrazepam effected excellent control of the seizures in 20 cases with a follow-up of 3 years.

Parenteral Nitrazepam in Treatment of Status Epilepticus

From the reports of Martin (78), Oller-Daurella (*personal communication,* 1968: 14 cases), and Lison and Fassoni (*personal communication,* 1968: 20 cases), as well as from unpublished data from the Center St. Paul, Marseilles, it was concluded that nitrazepam is, by slow injection, as effective as clonazepam in the control of status epilepticus (unilateral, partial, and generalized with or without convulsions). Martin (78) and Tassinari et al. (118), however, have observed—as with other benzodiazepines—instances of status epilepticus paradoxically induced by i.v. injection of nitrazepam in cases of Lennox–Gastaut syndrome.

SUMMARY

Nitrazepam is a widely used and safe hypnotic drug. The compound is effective in the treatment of various types of epilepsy, primarily infantile spasms, myoclonic seizures, and Lennox–Gastaut syndrome. Reflex epilepsies, including photosensitive epilepsy, respond well to nitrazepam. Initial success, however, may be followed by the development of tolerance.

Side effects are common but mild: most patients experience drowsiness, ataxia, and, for hypnotic use, impairment of psychomotor skills the morning following oral administration. Also, after chronic treatment in children, hypotonia and increased salivary and bronchial secretion may often occur. The drug is safe in overdosage.

Nitrazepam probably does not alter the rate of metabolism of concomitantly administered drugs.

Some neurotransmitters, GABA in particular, play an important role in the action of nitrazepam.

The compound is well absorbed after oral administration, and peak plasma concentrations occur within 2 to 3 hr. The main metabolic pathway leads, by reduction of the nitro group, to the corresponding amine and, by acetylation of the latter, to the 7-acetamido derivative which is the prevailing but inactive metabolite.

CONVERSION

Conversion factor:

$$CF = \frac{1000}{mol.\ wt.} = \frac{1000}{281.26} = 3.56$$

Conversion:

$$(\mu g/ml) \times 3.56 = (\mu moles/liter)$$

$$(\mu moles/liter) \div 3.56 = (\mu g/ml)$$

REFERENCES

1. Adam, K., Adamson, L., Březinová, V., Hunter, W. M., and Oswald, I. (1976): Nitrazepam: Lastingly effective but trouble on withdrawal. *Br. Med. J.,* 1:1558–1560.
2. Arndt, K. A.. and Jick, H. (1976): Rates of cutaneous reactions to drugs: A report from the Boston Collaborative Drug Surveillance Program. *Drug Intel. Clin. Pharmacol.,* 9:648–654.
3. Ballinger, B. R., Presly, A., Raid, A. H.. and Stevenson, I. H. (1974): The effects of hypnotics on imipramine treatment. *Psychopharmacologia,* 39:267–274.
4. Bardhan, K. D. (1969): Cerebellar syndrome after nitrazepam overdosage. *Lancet,* 1:1319–1320.
5. Bartosek, I., Kvetina, J., Guaiani, A., and Garattini, S. (1970): Comparative study of nitrazepam metabolism in perfused isolated liver laboratory animals. *Eur. J. Pharmacol.,* 11:378–382.
6. Bartosek, I., Mussini, E., Saronio, C., and Garattini, S. (1970): Studies on nitrazepam reduction in vitro. *Eur. J. Pharmacol.,* 11:249–253.
7. Benedetti, P., Ammaniti, M., and Cogliati Dezza, G. (1967): L'impiego del Ro-4-5360 nell'epilessia infantile, contributo clinico. *Infanzia Anormale (Roma),* 75:287–296.
8. Bente, H. B. (1978): Nitrogen-selective detectors: Application to quantitation of antiepileptic drugs: In: *Antiepileptic Drugs: Quantitative Analysis and In-*

terpretation, edited by C. E. Pippenger, J. K. Penry, and H. Kutt, pp. 139–145. Raven Press, New York.

9. Bieger, R., de Jonge, H., and Loeliger, E. A. (1972): Influence of nitrazepam on oral anticoagulation with phenprocoumon. *Clin. Pharmacol. Ther.,* 13:361–365.

10. Borland, R. G., and Nicholson, A. N. (1975): Comparison of the residual effects of two benzodiazepines (nitrazepam and flurazepam hydrochloride) and pentobarbitone sodium on human performance. *Br. J. Clin. Pharmacol.,* 2:9–17.

11. Borselli, L., Corvaglia, E., and Falchi, G. (1967): L'impiego di un nuovo nitroderivato del clordiazepossido (1,3 diidro-7-nitro-5-fenil-2H-1,4-benzodiazepin-2-one o Mogadon) nella terapia dell'epilessia infantile. *Riv. Clin. Pediatr.,* 2:450–456.

12. Boyer, P. A. (1966): Anticonvulsant properties of benzodiazepines. *Dis. Nerv. Syst.,* 27:35–42.

13. Braestrup, C., and Squires, R. F. (1978): Pharmacological characterization of benzodiazepine receptors in the brain. *Eur. J. Pharmacol.,* 48:263–270.

14. Breimer, D. D. (1977): Clinical pharmacokinetics of hypnotics. *Clin. Pharmacokinet.,* 2:93–109.

15. Breimer, D. D. (1979): Clinical pharmacokinetic and biopharmaceutical aspects of hypnotic drug therapy. In: *Sleep Research,* edited by R. G. Priest, A. Pletscher, and J. Ward, pp. 63–81. MTP Press, Lancaster.

16. Breimer, D. D., Bracht, H., and De Boer, A. G. (1977): Plasma level profile of nitrazepam (Mogadon) following oral administration. *Br. J. Clin. Pharmacol.,* 4:709–711.

17. Browne, I. R., and Penry, J. K. (1973): Benzodiazepines in the treatment of epilepsy. *Epilepsia,* 14:277–310.

18. Carroll, W. M., and Mastaglia, F. L. (1977): Alpha and beta coma in drug intoxication. *Br. Med. J.,* 2:1518–1519.

19. Carroll, W. M., and Mastaglia, F. L. (1979): Alpha and beta coma in drug intoxication uncomplicated by cerebral hypoxia. *Electroencephalogr. Clin. Neurophysiol.,* 46:95–105.

20. Castelden, C. M., George, C. F., Marcer, D., and Hallet, C. (1977): Increased sensitivity to nitrazepam in old age. *Br. Med. J.,* 1:10–12.

21. Chambers, D. M., and Jefferson, G. C. (1977): Some observations of the mechanism of benzodiazepine–barbiturate interactions in the mouse. *Br. J. Pharmacol.,* 60:393–399.

22. Clark, T. J. H., Collins, J. V., and Tong, D. (1971): Respiratory depression caused by nitrazepam in patients with respiratory failure. *Lancet,* 2:737–738.

23. Consolo, S., Garattini, S., and Ladinsky, H. (1975): Action of the benzodiazepines on the cholinergic system. *Adv. Biochem. Psychopharmacol.,* 14:63–80.

24. Corrodi, H., Fuxe, K., Lidbrink, P., and Olson, L. (1971): Minor tranquillizers, stress and central catecholamine neurons. *Brain Res.,* 29:1–16.

25. Costa, E., and Guidotti, A. (1979): Molecular mechanisms in the receptor action of benzodiazepines. *Annu. Rev. Pharmacol. Toxicol.,* 19:531–545.

26. Darcy, L. (1972): Delirium tremens following withdrawal of nitrazepam. *Med. J. Aust.,* 2:450.

27. De Boer, A. G., Röst-Kaiser, J., Bracht, H., and Breimer, D. D. (1978): Assay of underivatized nitrazepam and clonazepam in plasma by capillary gas chromatography applied to pharmacokinetic and bioavailability studies in humans. *J. Chromatogr.,* 145:105–114.

28. De Silva, J. A. F. (1978): Electron capture-GLC in the quantitation of 1,4-benzodiazepines. In: *Antiepileptic Drugs: Quantitative Analysis and Interpretation,* edited by C. E. Pippenger, J. K. Penry, and H. Kutt, pp. 111–138. Raven Press, New York.

29. Dixon, R., Lucek, R., Young, R., Ning, R., and Darragh, A. (1979): Radioimmunoassay for nitrazepam in plasma. *Life Sci.,* 25:311–316.

30. Ehrsson, M., and Tilly, A. (1973): Electron capture gas chromatography of nitrazepam in human plasma as methyl derivatives. *Anal. Lett.,* 6:197–210.

31. Evans, J. G., and Jarvis, E. H. (1972): Nitrazepam and the elderly. *Br. Med. J.,* 4:487.

32. Friedel, B., and Kunath, J. (1970): Anderung der photosensiblen Reizschwelle in EEG durch Nitrazepam. *Arzneim. Forsch.,* 6:168–177.

33. Fuxe, K., Agnati, L. F., Bolme, P., Hökfelt, T., Lidbrink, P., Ljungdahl, A., de la Mora, M. P., and Ögren, S. (1975): The possible involvement of GABA mechanisms in the action of benzodiazepines on central catecholamine neurons. *Adv. Biochem. Psychopharmacol.,* 14:45–61.

34. Gaddie, J., Legge, J. S., Palmer, K. N. V., Petrie, J. C., and Wood, R. A. (1972): Effect of nitrazepam in chronic obstructive bronchitis. *Br. Med. J.,* 2:688–689.

35. Garattini, S., Marcucci, F., and Mussini, E. (1977): The metabolism and pharmacokinetics of selected benzodiazepines. In: *Psychotherapeutic Drugs,* edited by E. Usdin and I. S. Forrest, pp. 1039–1087. Marcel Dekker, Basel, New York.

36. Gibbs, F. A., and Anderson, E. M. (1965): Treatment of hypsarrhythmia and infantile spasms with a Librium analogue. *Neurology (Minneap.),* 15:1173–1176.

37. Girdwood, R. H. (1973): Nitrazepam nightmares. *Br. Med. J.,* 1:353.

38. Greenblatt, D. J., and Allen, M. D. (1978): Toxicity of nitrazepam in the elderly: A report from the Boston Collaborative Drug Surveillance Program. *Br. J. Clin. Pharmacol.,* 5:407–413.

39. Grossi-Bianchi, M. L., and Pistone, F. M. (1967): Effetto ipnogeno ed effetto anticomiziale del nitrazepam nei bambini. *Minerva Pediatr.,* 19:1073–1082.

40. Grossi-Bianchi, M. L., and Pistone, F. M. (1968): Comparison of treatment with ACTH and nitrazepam in some forms of infantile convulsive syndromes. *Riv. Clin. Pediatr.,* 81:233–234.

41. Grundström, R., Holmberg, G., and Hansen, T. (1978): Degree of sedation obtained with various doses of diazepam and nitrazepam. *Acta Pharmacol. Toxicol. (Kbh.),* 43:13–18.

42. Hagberg, B. (1967): The Librium-analogue Mogadon in the treatment of epilepsy in children. *Acta Neurol. Scand. [Suppl.],* 31:167.

43. Hagberg, B. (1968): The chlordiazepoxide HCl (Librium) analogue nitrazepam (Mogadon) in the

treatment of epilepsy in children. *Dev. Med. Child. Neurol.*, 10:302–308.

44. Hambert, O., and Petersen, J. W. (1970): Clinical, electroencephalographical and neuropharmacological studies in syndromes of progressive myoclonus epilepsy. *Acta Neurol. Scand.*, 46:149–186.

45. Hewick, D. S., and Shaw, V. (1978): Tissue distribution of radioactivity after injection of [^{14}C]nitrazepam in young and old rats. *J. Pharm. Pharmacol.*, 30:318–319.

46. Hewick, D. S., and Shaw, V. (1978): The importance of the intestinal microflora in nitrazepam metabolism in the rat. *Br. J. Pharmacol.*, 62:427.

47. Hunt, P., Husson, J. M., and Raynaud, J. P. (1979): A radioreceptor assay for benzodiazepines. *J. Pharm. Pharmacol.*, 31:448–451.

48. Lisalo, E., Kangas, L., and Ruikka, I. (1977): Pharmacokinetics of nitrazepam in young volunteers and aged patients. *Br. J. Clin. Pharmacol.*, 4:646–647.

49. Impallomeni, M., and Ezzat, R. (1976): Hypothermia associated with nitrazepam administration. *Br. Med. J.*, 1:223–224.

50. Jeavons, P. M. (1977): Choice of drug therapy in epilepsy. *Practitioner*, 219:542–556.

51. Jong, T. H. (1964): Klinische Erfahrungen mit dem Benzodiazepinderivat Ro-4-5360 bei der Behandlung der Epilepsie. *Schweiz. Med. Wochenschr.*, 94:730–733.

52. Kales, A., Scharf, M. B., and Kales, J. D. (1978): Rebound insomnia: A new clinical syndrome. *Science*, 201:1039–1041.

53. Kales, A., Scharf, M. B., Kales, J. D., and Soldatos, C. R. (1979): Rebound insomnia. A potential hazard following withdrawal of certain benzodiazepines. *J.A.M.A.*, 241:1692–1695.

54. Kangas, L. (1977): Comparison of two gas–liquid chromatographic methods for the determination of nitrazepam in plasma. *J. Chromatogr.*, 136:259–270.

55. Kangas, L. (1979): Determination of nitrazepam and its main metabolites in urine by gas–liquid chromatography: Use of electron capture and nitrogen-selective detectors. *J. Chromatogr.*, 172:273–278.

56. Kangas, L. (1979): Urinary elimination of nitrazepam and its main metabolites. *Acta Pharmacol. Toxicol. (Kbh.)*, 45:16–19.

57. Kangas, L., Allonen, H., Lammintausta, R., Pynnönen, S., and Salonen, M. (1977): Pharmacokinetics of nitrazepam in human plasma and saliva. *Acta Pharmacol. Toxicol. (Kbh.)*, 41:56.

58. Kangas, L., Allonen, H., Lammintausta, R., Salonen, M., and Pekkarinen, A. (1979): Pharmacokinetics of nitrazepam in saliva and serum after a single oral dose. *Acta Pharmacol. Toxicol. (Kbh.)*, 45:20–24.

59. Kangas, L., Iisalo, E., Kanto, J., Lehtinen, V., Pynnönen, S., Ruikka, I., Salminen, J., Sillanpää, M., and Syvälahti, E. (1979): Human pharmacokinetics of nitrazepam: Effect of age and diseases. *Eur. J. Clin. Pharmacol.*, 15:163–170.

60. Kangas, L., Kanto, J., and Erkkola, R. (1977): Transfer of nitrazepam across the human placenta. *Eur. J. Clin. Pharmacol.*, 12:355–357.

61. Kangas, L., Kanto, J., and Mansikka, M. (1977):

Nitrazepam premedication for minor surgery. *Br. J. Anaesth.*, 49:1153–1157.

62. Kangas, L., Kanto, J., Siirtola, T., and Pekkarinen, A. (1977): Cerebrospinal-fluid concentrations of nitrazepam in man. *Acta Pharmacol. Toxicol. (Kbh.)*, 41:74–79.

63. Kangas, L., Kanto, J., and Syvälahti, E. (1977): Plasma nitrazepam concentrations after an acute intake and their correlation to sedation and serum growth hormone levels. *Acta Pharmacol. Toxicol. (Kbh.)*, 41:65–73.

64. Karim, A. K. M. B., and Price Evans, D. A. (1976): Polymorphic acetylation of nitrazepam. *J. Med. Genet.*, 13:17–19.

65. Killam, E. K., Matsuzaki, M., and Killam, K. F. (1973): Effects of chronic administration of benzodiazepines on epileptic seizures and brain electrical activity in *Papio papio*. In: *The Benzodiazepines*, edited by S. Garattini, E. Mussini, and L. O. Randall, pp. 443–460. Raven Press, New York.

66. Killam, E. K., and Suria, A. (1980): Antiepileptic drugs—benzodiazepines. In: *Antiepileptic Drugs: Mechanisms of Action*, edited by G. H. Glaser, J. K. Penry, and D. M. Woodbury, pp. 597–615. Raven Press, New York.

67. Kinawi, A., and Teller, C. (1978): Zur Interaktion von Phenprocoumon mit Diazepam und Nitrazepam. *J. Clin. Chem. Clin. Biochem.*, 16:313–314.

68. Krall, R. L., Penry, J. K., White, B. G., Kupferberg, H. J., and Swinyard, E. A. (1978): Antiepileptic drug development: II. Anticonvulsant drug screening. *Epilepsia*, 19:409–428.

69. Lahtinen, U., Lahtinen, A., and Pekkola, P. (1978): The effect of nitrazepam on manual skill, grip strength, and reaction time with special reference to subjective evaluation of effects on sleep. *Acta Pharmacol. Toxicol. (Kbh.)*, 42:130–134.

70. Leng, C. O. (1975): Drug-precipitated acute attacks of gout. *Br. Med. J.*, 2:561.

71. Linnoila, M. (1973): Drug interaction on psychomotor skills related to driving: Hypnotics and alcohol. *Ann. Med. Exp. Biol. Fenn.*, 51:118–124.

72. Linnoila, M. and Viukari, M. (1976): Efficacy and side effects of nitrazepam and thioridazine as sleeping aids in psychogeriatric in-patients. *Br. J. Psychiatry*, 128:566–569.

73. Lundberg, P. O., and Stalberg, E. (1971): Mogadon in der Behandlung von Epilepsie bei Erwachsenen. *Arch. Psychiatr. Nervenkr.*, 214:46–55.

74. Lunde, P. K. M., Frislid, K., and Hansteen, V. (1977): Disease and acetylation polymorphism. *Clin. Pharmacokinet.*, 2:182–197.

75. MacLean, H. (1973): Nitrazepam: Another interesting syndrome. *Br. Med. J.*, 1:488.

76. Malpas, A., Rowan, A. J., Joyce, C. R. B., and Scott, D. F. (1970): Persistent behavioural and encephalographic changes after single doses of nitrazepam and amylobarbitone sodium. *Br. Med. J.*, 2:762–764.

77. Markham, C. H. (1964): The treatment of myoclonic seizures of infancy and childhood with LA-I. *Pediatrics*, 34:511–518.

78. Martin, D. (1970): Intravenous nitrazepam in the treatment of epilepsy. *Neuropaediatrie*, 2:27–37.

79. Matthes, A. (1965): 1,3-Dihydro-7-nitro-5-phenyl-2H-1,4-benzodiazepin-2-on als Schlafmittel im Kindesalter. *Arzneim. Forsch.,* 15:1157–1158.

80. Matthew, H., Proudfoot, A. T., Aitken, R. C. B., Raeburn, J. A., and Wright, N. (1969): Nitrazepam—a safe hypnotic. *Br. Med. J.,* 3:23–25.

81. Matthew, H., Roscoe, P., and Wright, N. (1972): Acute poisoning. A comparison of hypnotic drugs. *Practitioner,* 208:254–258.

82. Mattson, R. M. (1972): The benzodiazepines. In: *Antiepileptic Drugs,* edited by D. M. Woodbury, J. K. Penry, and R. P. Schmidt, pp. 497–518. Raven Press, New York.

83. Millichap, J. G. (1969): Relation of laboratory evaluation to clinical effectiveness of antiepileptic drugs. *Epilepsia,* 10:315–328.

84. Millichap, J. G., and Ortiz, W. R. (1966): Nitrazepam in myoclonic epilepsies. *Am. J. Dis. Child.,* 112:242–248.

85. Model, D. G. (1973): Nitrazepam induced respiratory depression in chronic obstructive lung disease. *Br. J. Dis. Chest,* 67:128–130.

86. Møller Jensen, K. (1975): Determination of nitrazepam in serum by gas–liquid chromatography. *J. Chromatogr.,* 111:389–396.

87. Montagu, J. D. (1971): Effects of quinalbarbitone (secobarbital) and nitrazepam on the EEG in man. Quantitative investigations. *Eur. J. Pharmacol.,* 14:238–249.

88. Moody, J. P., Whyte, S. F., Mac Donald, A. J., and Naylor, G. J. (1977): Pharmacokinetic aspects of protriptyline plasma levels. *Eur. J. Clin. Pharmacol.,* 11:51–56.

89. Moore, B., Nickless, G., Hallett, C., and Howard, A. G. (1977): Analysis of nitrazepam and its metabolites by high-pressure liquid chromatography. *J. Chromatogr.,* 137:215–217.

90. Morillo, A. (1962): Effects of benzodiazepines upon amygdala and hyppocampus of the cat. *Int. J. Neuropharmacol.,* 1:353–359.

91. O'Malley, K. (1971): Safety of hypnotics. *Br. Med. J.,* 1:729.

92. Orme, M., Breckenridge, A., and Brooks, R. V. (1972): Interactions of benzodiazepines with warfarin. *Br. Med. J.,* 3:611–614.

93. Oswald, I., Lewis, S. A., Tagney, J., Firth, H., and Haider, I. (1973): Benzodiazepines and human sleep. In: *The Benzodiazepines,* edited by S. Garattini, E. Mussini, and L. O. Randall, pp. 613–625. Raven Press, New York.

94. Peck, A. W., Adams, R., Bye, C., and Wilkinson, R. T. (1976): Residual effects of hypnotic drugs: Evidence for individual differences on vigilance. *Psychopharmacology,* 47:213–216.

95. Peck, A. W., Bye, C. E., and Claridge, R. (1977): Differences between light and sound sleepers in the residual effects of nitrazepam. *Br. J. Clin. Pharmacol.,* 4:101–108.

96. Peterson, W. G. (1967): Clinical study of Mogadon, a new anticonvulsant. *Neurology (Minneap.),* 17:878–880.

97. Pines, A. (1972): Nitrazepam in chronic obstructive bronchitis. *Br. Med. J.,* 3:352.

98. Poiré, R., and Royer, J. (1968): Comparative experimental electrographic study of anticonvulsant properties of a new derivative of the benzodiazepines Ro 5-4023. *Electroencephalogr. Clin. Neurophysiol.,* 27:106.

99. Ridley, C. M. (1971): Bullous lesions in nitrazepam overdosage. *Br. Med. J.,* 3:28.

100. Rieder, J. (1973): A fluorimetric method for determining nitrazepam and the sum of its main metabolites in plasma and urine. *Arzneim. Forsch.,* 23:207–211.

101. Rieder, J. (1973): Plasma levels and derived pharmacokinetic characteristics of unchanged nitrazepam in man. *Arzneim. Forsch.,* 23:212–218.

102. Rieder, J., and Wendt, G. (1973): Pharmacokinetics and metabolism of the hypnotic nitrazepam. In: *The Benzodiazepines,* edited by S. Garattini, E. Mussini, and L. O. Randall, pp. 99–127. Raven Press, New York.

103. Rudolf, M., Geddes, D. M., Turner, J. A., and Saunders, K. B. (1978): Depression of central respiratory drive by nitrazepam. *Thorax,* 33:97–100.

104. Saario, I., Linnoila, M., and Maki, M. (1975): Interaction of drugs with alcohol on human psychomotor skills related to driving: Effect of sleep deprivation or two weeks' treatment with hypnotics. *J. Clin. Pharmacol.,* 15:52–59.

105. Sawada, H., and Hara, A. (1976): Novel metabolite of nitrazepam in the rabbit urine. *Experientia,* 32:987–988.

106. Saxén, I., and Saxén, L. (1975): Association between maternal intake of diazepam and oral clefts. *Lancet,* 2:498.

107. Shalleck, W., Thomas, J., Kuehn, A., and Zabransky, F. (1965): Effects of Mogadon on responses to stimulation of sciatic nerve, amygdala and hypothalamus of cat. *Int. J. Neuropharmacol.,* 4:317–326.

108. Silverman, G., and Braithwaite, R. A. (1973): Benzodiazepines and tricyclic antidepressant plasma levels. *Br. Med. J.,* 3:18–20.

109. Snyder, C. H. (1968): Myoclonic epilepsy in children: Short-term comparative study of two benzodiazepine derivatives in treatment. *South Med. J.,* 61:17–20.

110. Snyder, S. H., and Enna, S. J. (1975): The role of central glycine receptors in the pharmacologic actions of benzodiazepines. *Adv. Biochem. Psychopharmacol.,* 14:81–91.

111. Stein, L., Wise, C. D., and Belluzzi, J. D. (1975): Effects of benzodiazepines on central serotonergic mechanisms. *Adv. Biochem. Psychopharmacol.,* 14:29–44.

112. Sternbach, L. H., Fryer, R. I., Keller, O., Metlesics, W., Sach, G., and Steiger, N. (1963): Quinazolines and 1-4 benzodiazepines. X. Nitro-substituted 5-phenyl-1,4-benzodiazepine derivatives. *J. Med. Pharm. Chem.,* 6:261–265.

113. Stevenson, I. H., (1977): Factors influencing antipyrine elimination. *Br. J. Clin. Pharmacol.,* 4:261–265.

114. Stevenson, I. H., Browning, M., Crooks, J., and O'Malley, K. (1972): Changes in human drug me-

tabolism after long-term exposure to hypnotics. *Br. Med. J.*, 4:322–324.

115. Stone, W. E., and Javid, M. J. (1978): Benzodiazepines and phenobarbital as antagonists of dissimilar chemical convulsants. *Epilepsia*, 19:361–368.

116. Swinyard, A., and Castellion, A. W. (1966): Anticonvulsant properties of some benzodiazepines. *J. Pharmacol. Exp. Ther.*, 151:369–375.

117. Tanayama, S., Momose, S., and Kanai, Y. (1974): Comparative studies on the metabolic disposition of 8-chloro-6-phenyl-4H-S-triazolo[4,3-*a*][1,4] benzodiazepine (D-40TA) and nitrazepam after single and repeated administration in rats. *Xenobiotica*, 4:229–236.

118. Tassinari, C. A., Dravet, C., Roger J., Cano, J. P., and Gastaut, H. (1972): Tonic status epilepticus precipitated by intravenous benzodiazepine in five patients with Lennox–Gastaut syndrome. *Epilepsia*, 13:421–435.

119. Taylor, F. (1973): Nitrazepam and the elderly. *Br. Med. J.*, 1:113–114.

120. Taylor, K. M., and Laverty, R. (1969): The effect of chlordiazepoxide, diazepam and nitrazepam on catecholamine metabolism in regions of the rat brain. *Eur. J. Pharmacol.*, 8:296–301.

121. Valli, M., and Pringuey, D. (1980): Actualités concernant le mechanisme d'action biochimique des benzodiazépines. *Therapie*, 35:561–569.

122. Volzke, E., Doose, H., and Stephan, E. (1967): The treatment of infantile spasms and hypsarrhythmia with Mogadon. *Epilepsia*, 8:64–70.

123. Yanagi, Y., Haga, F., Endo, M., and Kitagawa, S. (1975): Comparative metabolic study of nimetazepam and its desmethyl derivative (nitrazepam) in rats. *Xenobiotica*, 5:245–257.

Antiepileptic Drugs, edited by D. M. Woodbury, J. K. Penry, and C. E. Pippenger. Raven Press, New York © 1982.

68

Other Antiepileptic Drugs

Sulfonamides and Derivatives: Acetazolamide

Dixon M. Woodbury and John W. Kemp

The group of unsubstituted sulfonamides that inhibit the enzyme carbonic anhydrase has been shown to have anticonvulsant properties in experimental animals and to include useful antiepileptics in humans. These agents include acetazolamide (5-acetamido-1,3,4-thiadiazole-2-sulfonamide, Diamox®), the most extensively studied drug of this group, and methazolamide (Neptazone®), an agent little used at present. The usefulness of these agents is limited because of the rapid development of tolerance to their anticonvulsant effects. Their only well-documented biochemical effect is inhibition of carbonic anhydrase. Consequently, the anticonvulsant effect is thought to be mediated through inhibition of this enzyme, mainly in brain. Since this enzyme, which catalyzes the hydration and dehydration of carbon dioxide, is found in many tissues other than brain, inhibition of carbonic anhydrase in these tissues by acetazolamide causes disturbances of their function and thereby can cause side effects; it also can alter the distribution of acetazolamide and other drugs in the body.

It is important, therefore, to summarize the absorption, distribution, biotransformation, excretion, toxicity, mechanism of action, and therapeutic uses of acetazolamide and methazolamide. Maren (31) has written a comprehensive review of carbonic anhydrase and its inhibition by drugs, and Woodbury (58) has reviewed the mechanism of the antiepileptic action of acetazolamide. Excellent discussions of carbonic anhydrase (CA) are found in the reviews by Carter (6) and Lindskog et al. (27) and of its reactions with sulfonamides by Coleman (9).

CHEMISTRY AND METHODS OF DETERMINATION

The structures of acetazolamide and methazolamide are shown in Fig. 1.

Acetazolamide is an unsubstituted sulfonamide with a pK_a of 7.4. The structure–activity relationships of the carbonic anhydrase inhibitors have been described by Maren (33). All unsubstituted aromatic sulfonamides (aryl–SO_2NH_2) inhibit CA, and no other class of organic compounds approaches these in activity. The K_I for inhibition of CA in red cells and brain for acetazolamide is in the range of 1 to 6×10^{-8} M. Ability to inhibit CA also increases, in a homologous series, with lipid solubility of the undissociated sulfonamide molecule. Alkyl substitution in the SO_2NH_2 group confers only weak inhibitory activity to the molecule, whereas aromatic substitution yields high inhibitory activity, and resonating heterocyclic structures (e.g., acetazolamide, ethoxzolamide, benzolamide) confer very high activity on the SO_2NH_2 group. In benzene sulfonamides, ester or amide substitution in the *para* position yields far more active

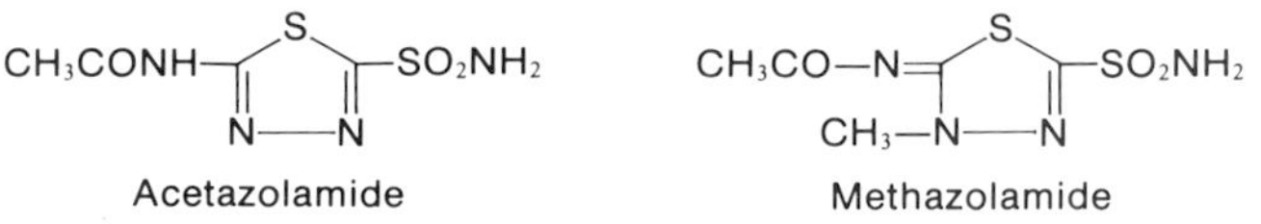

FIG. 1. Structures of acetazolamide and methazolamide.

compounds than *ortho* or *meta* substitution. Very large or bulky fused-ring systems with multiple substituents seem to repress activity. Also, introduction of an acidic group appears to increase inhibitory activity in a degree relative to the strength of the acid group.

Methods for quantifying the concentrations of acetazolamide in body fluids utilize the carbonic anhydrase inhibition method of Maren et al. (34; see 19 for application of this method to epileptics), GLC with electron capture (54), and HPLC (3). Earlier workers (18) used a modification of the colorimetric procedure of Bratten and Marshall, but this is much less sensitive than the enzyme inhibition, GLC, or HPLC procedures. The GLC method is able to detect 10 ng/ sample, the HPLC method is sensitive to 25 ng/ ml plasma, and the enzyme assay 200 ng/ml. The molecular weight of acetazolamide is 222.

ABSORPTION

Acetazolamide is present in gastric juice (pH 2.0) predominantly in the un-ionized form. Since this form is adequately soluble in gastric juice, it is absorbed from the stomach to some extent. However, absorption occurs mainly in the duodenum and upper jejunum where the surface area is larger, the pH higher, and the solubility of the drug greater. The factors that affect the absorption of most weak acids also influence the absorption of acetazolamide, namely, pH, lipid and water solubility, and concentration in the gastrointestinal fluids.

Absorption is rapid, and peak levels in the plasma are reached 2 to 4 hr after oral ingestion of a single dose. In humans, oral doses in the range of 5 to 10 mg/kg appear to be completely absorbed (35), but at high doses, absorption is erratic and results in variable levels in the plasma (36). Absorption is complete within 2 hr in the dog (35). Bayne et al. (3) found in humans that

a single oral dose of 500 mg in the form of a tablet was absorbed more rapidly, reached a higher level (26 μg/ml), and fell off more rapidly than did a 500-mg timed-release formulation. The peak time of absorption of the regular tablet was 3.5 hr, whereas for the timed-released preparation, the plateau was reached at 3.5 hr but maintained a value of about 10 μg/ ml until 10 hr. However, after this time, the plasma concentration fell off very slowly and at the same rate as that of the regular tablet, and at 45 hr after ingestion, significant levels were still present in the plasma.

DISTRIBUTION

Plasma Binding

Following absorption, acetazolamide is bound to plasma proteins to the extent of about 60 to 70% in rats, 50 to 60% in cats, 45 to 60% in dogs, and 90 to 95% in humans (Table 1). Thus, the unbound levels are about 30 to 40% of the total except in humans in whom the value is 10% or less. The nature of the forces involved in the binding and the proteins to which the drug is bound have not been elucidated. Also, it is not known if other drugs compete with acetazolamide for binding to the protein. The percentage of acetazolamide bound is dose dependent (Table 1). This is evidence for saturation of the acetazolamide-binding proteins in plasma. The increased free levels at higher doses result in an increase in the rate of excretion in the urine and a decrease in the plasma half-life of acetazolamide. Since the pK_a of acetazolamide is 7.4, at the pH of blood (7.4), half of the free level exists as the un-ionized, freely diffusible molecule. It is this molecule that penetrates into tissues and is available for binding to and subsequent inhibition of carbonic anhydrase (see below).

Plasma Half-Life and Volume of Distribution

The plasma half-life of acetazolamide varies markedly with the species (Table 1). The decay time, when plotted on semilogarithmic paper, has two components: a very rapid one, the half-lives of which for various species are shown in Table 1, and a slow one. The rapid component represents movement of unbound diffusible acetazolamide into the total body water (36). After penetrating the cells, the drug also binds to the carbonic anhydrase present in tissues, including erythrocytes, renal cortex and medulla, stomach, salivary glands, pancreas, and brain. The slow component of the plasma decay curve, therefore, represents both the very low dissociation constant of the enzyme–inhibitor complex [EI] in the enzyme-containing tissues and the rate of renal excretion of acetazolamide that shifts the equilibrium, $[E_{FREE}] + [I_{FREE}] \rightleftarrows [EI]$, to the left by removing free drug. The half-life of the slow component in the dog, for example, is about 2 days. This is in contrast to the half-life of the fast or mobile component of about 100 min (Table 1). After 24 hr, 90% of the drug in the body is bound to carbonic anhydrase in the various tissues as the enzyme–inhibitor [EI] complex. Of this amount, most is found in erythrocytes, kidney, and stomach, which contain very high concentrations of this enzyme. As seen in Fig. 2, erythrocytes contain very high concentrations of [3H]acetazolamide as compared to other tissues (see also 19,54).

In a dog given 5 mg/kg (22 μmoles/kg) of acetazolamide, it was observed (30,31) that in the rapid phase of the plasma decay curve, 95% of the drug exists in the free form. Only 1.14 μmoles/kg were present as [EI], and this was mostly in red cells (1 μmole/kg), kidneys (0.1 μmole/kg), and stomach (0.04 μmole/kg); the amounts in the other carbonic anhydrase-containing tissues were negligible. The free level declined rapidly by first-order kinetics with a half-life of 100 min. The concentration of free acetazolamide was sufficiently high for 4 hr that more than 99.5% of the enzyme was inhibited. This is an amount sufficient to produce a thera-peutic effect, e.g., prevention of seizures in epileptics, blockade of experimentally induced seizures in animals (see 43, for example). By 8 hr, the free concentration in plasma was small, and the therapeutic effect was finished. At this time, of the 22 μmoles/kg injected into the animal, less than 1 μmole was free drug, and all of the remaining drug was bound to carbonic anhydrase. The total molar concentration of acetazolamide found in the tissues 24 to 48 hr after ingestion of the drug was found to be a measure of the molar concentration of carbonic anhydrase, because it was almost all bound as [EI] (30,31).

The apparent volumes of distribution of acetazolamide in humans and in dogs in doses from 5 to 20 mg/kg are shown in Table 1. In humans, the value based on total plasma concentration is 0.2 liter/kg (20%) (36), and in the dog, 0.4 liter/kg (40%) (37). The difference between human and dog results mainly from differences in plasma binding of these two species (Table 1). If the volume of distribution in humans is calculated from the free level in the plasma, it is 1.8 liter/kg (180%), a value that indicates accumulation or binding in tissues even during the early phase of the distribution of acetazolamide in the body. Most of the excess over the amount in total body water is bound to erythrocyte carbonic anhydrase, as described above. The volume of distribution in dogs based on the free plasma level is also greater than can be accounted for in total body water (1.0 liter/kg).

Distribution into Tissues and Transcellular Fluids

As just described, acetazolamide rapidly diffuses into tissue water as the free form and then binds to tissue carbonic anhydrase. In these tissues, its concentration is higher than in plasma. Thus, in the rat (Fig. 2), the concentration of [3H]acetazolamide is higher in erythrocytes, salivary glands, liver, and thyroid gland than the total concentration in plasma and considerably higher than the concentration of the free drug in plasma. The highest concentration is

TABLE 1. *Plasma binding, plasma total and free levels, brain levels, volume of distribution, and plasma half-life of acetazolamide in various species*

Species	Ref.	Dose (mg/kg) and route	% Bound in plasma	Plasma Total	Plasma Free	Brain	RBC	Muscle	Saliva	CSF	Volume of distribution (liter/kg)	Plasma half-life (hr)
Man												
Child	36	14 i.v.	90	46	4.6					0.6	0.2^a, 1.8^b	1.6 (fast phase)
Adult	31,36		95	10–20	0.5–1.0					0.1–0.2		
			90	25–50	2.5–5.0					0.3–0.5		
			83	75	13							
Adult	19	1.5 oral		6–9			22–29					10–12 (2nd phase)
		2.5 oral		12–16			26–39					
		5.0 oral		20–30			30–52					
Adult epileptics	19	9.1–11.1 oral (250 mg bid)		30 (plateau)			52					ca. 15
		4 days		19								
		1–2 wk		13			51–53					
		1 mo		11								
		2–8 mo										
	54,3,6	(250 mg) oral	94	14(10–18 at 1–3 hr)	0.6–1.1	18(13–29) (2–7 h)			0.1–0.18			2 (fast phase) 13 (slow phase)
	3	7.2 (500 mg) oral	—	26(3.5 hr)								

Species/Age		Dose & route									
Dog											
Adult	37	5 i.v.	60	12	4.8					0.4[a],1.0[b]	1.7 (fast phase)
	31		60	2.3	0.8–1.2			0.1–0.15			48 (slow phase)
			45	10–20	5.5–11.0			0.5–1.0			
			33	15–50	16–33			1.25–2.5			
Cat											
Adult	31	i.v.	63	2–3	0.7–1.1			0.2–0.3			2
	39		51	10–20	4.9–9.8			1–2			
Rat											
Adult	31	i.v.	69	2–3							1.1
	31		67	10–20							
			60	25–50							
			36	70–100							
			24	260–350							
	31	20 oral	67	101(0.5hr)	33	4.8	112	56			
			65	32(2.0hr)	11	3.5	101	42			
	19	20 i.p.		11(3hr)		12(3hr)	40(3 hr)				
Mouse											
Adult	31	i.p.	16	2–3							0.2
	31		5	10–20							

[a] Volume of distribution based on total concentration of acetazolamide in plasma early after administration.

[b] Volume of distribution based on unbound concentration of acetazolamide in plasma early after administration.

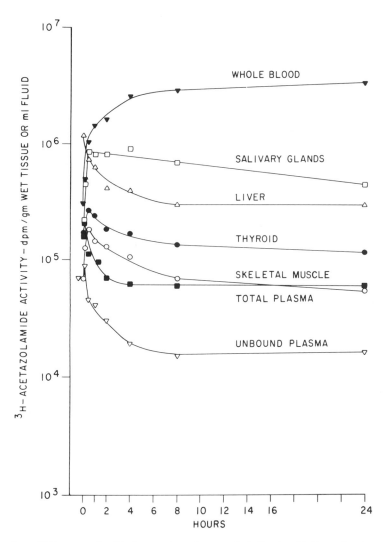

FIG. 2. Distribution of ^{3}H-acetazolamide into various tissues of adult rats with time after i.p. administration.

found in erythrocytes which also contain the most carbonic anhydrase. These tissues are carbonic anhydrase-containing tissues, and the high concentrations undoubtedly reflect the high affinity of acetazolamide for this enzyme.

It has also been shown (see 31 for a summary) that the concentration of the drug is higher in stomach, kidney, cortex and medulla, pancreas, choroid plexus, ciliary process, and inner ear tissues, all of which are secretory organs in which carbonic anhydrase is present and involved in the secretory process. The concentration of the drug in non-carbonic anhydrase-con-

taining tissues such as smooth muscle and heart is about the same as that of the free drug in the plasma.

The concentration of acetazolamide in various tissues of 3-day-old rats has also been assessed. The concentration relative to plasma is lower than in the same tissues in adult rats with the exception of muscle in which the concentration is the same as the free level in plasma. These tissues (liver, salivary glands, thyroid, erythrocytes) in 3-day-old rats have a lower concentration of carbonic anhydrase than do the corresponding adult tissues and, consequently, a lower concentration of acetazolamide. This is further evidence that the binding involves carbonic anhydrase.

Acetazolamide penetrates into all transcellular fluids (31). The levels in cerebrospinal fluid (CSF), aqueous humor, saliva (54), and gastric juice are generally lower than the free level in plasma. The level in bile is higher than the free level in plasma, and acetazolamide is probably actively excreted in bile, as are many other drugs that are weak acids. The concentration in milk also appears to be higher than that in plasma (35); further experimentation should reveal if acetazolamide is actively secreted into this fluid. The low level in saliva relative to the free drug concentration in plasma suggests that this drug may be actively reabsorbed across the ducts of the salivary gland. Acetazolamide crosses the placenta and enters the fetal bloodstream and tissues; large doses cause teratogenic effects.

CSF and Brain Distribution

The concentration of acetazolamide in the CSF in various species of animals (humans, dog, cat) is lower than the free level in the plasma. This can be explained either by removal of the drug by bulk flow of CSF, similar to the process by which inulin is removed, by active secretion out of the CSF across the choroid plexus, or by both processes, after its slow entrance into the CSF via the cerebral capillaries across the blood–brain barrier. Since the concentration of acetazolamide in CSF can be increased by large doses of acetazolamide to a greater extent than the increase in plasma concentration, it appears that the drug obeys saturation kinetics in its movement across the choroid plexus. This suggests that it is actively transported out of the CSF and that saturation of the transport system blocks this transport and increases CSF (and brain) levels of the drug (see 59 for a summary). Further evidence for active transport out of CSF could be obtained by determining if the concentration in the CSF is increased by probenecid, a drug that blocks the transport of weak acids out of CSF. In the adult rat, the CSF distribution of [³H]acetazolamide (Fig. 3) is lower than the

concentration in the total plasma but is the same as the concentration of the free drug in plasma after equilibration has occurred. This requires about 24 hr. Why the drug concentration in the CSF of rats is the same as that of the free drug in plasma—which is not the case for the other species that have been examined—is a problem that requires further investigation.

The concentration of acetazolamide in brain of adult rats is lower than the total concentration in plasma but higher than that of CSF; however, in 3-day-old rats the CSF concentration is higher than that of brain (see Fig. 3 and Table 1). When the brain concentration in adult rats is compared with that in the CSF (or free plasma concentration since it is the same as that in CSF), the concentration is much higher in brain (Fig. 4). This is to be expected since glial cells in brain contain carbonic anhydrase and since CSF is in equilibrium with the interstitial fluid of the brain and serves as the source of drug for this tissue. The brain/CSF ratio for [³H]acetazolamide in adult rats at equilibrium (24 hr) is 2.0, and in 3-day-old rats it is 1.1 (Fig. 4). The concentration of acetazolamide starts to increase in the brain relative to the CSF and approaches the adult values about the 10th day after birth, a time when glial cells begin to proliferate in the brain. Since glial cells are the main carbonic anhydrase-containing cells in the brain (12), it is likely that the acetazolamide found in the brain is localized to these cells.

Studies on the subcellular distribution of carbonic anhydrase in brain have demonstrated that the drug is found predominately (75 to 80%) in the cytoplasm (supernatant fraction) and in crude mitochondria (20 to 25%) (20). However, the crude mitochondrial fraction in brain contains synaptosomes and myelin, as well as mitochondria. Subsequent studies (5,50–52,67) have demonstrated that carbonic anhydrase is also found in myelin and cell membranes. Its presence in mitochondria is still debatable, although data from this laboratory (J. W. Kemp and D. M. Woodbury, *unpublished observations*) have demonstrated its presence in these subcellular organelles. Since low doses of acetazolamide inhibit the enzyme in the cytoplasm but not that

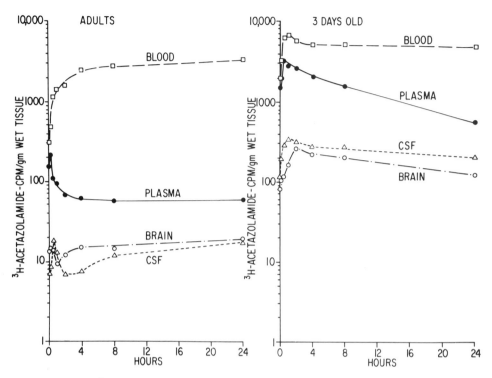

FIG. 3. Distribution of ^{3}H-acetazolamide into erythrocytes, plasma, brain, and CSF of adult and 3-day-old rats with time after i.p. administration.

in the crude mitochondria, it is evident that the drug does not readily penetrate the mitochondria or other constituents of this fraction (61). This suggests that its anticonvulsant effect is mediated through an action on the enzyme in the cytoplasm (see 61,62 for further discussion of this hypothesis).

The concentration of acetazolamide in brain and CSF can be influenced by many factors. In anticonvulsant doses, the carbonic anhydrase in the choroid plexus is inhibited and its activity reduced. This results in a reduction of CSF production and flow. Since some of the drug in the CSF of humans is undoubtedly removed by bulk flow of CSF, the reduced CSF flow produced by acetazolamide will decrease its outflow and thereby increase the concentration of this drug in the CSF and in the brain. This will result in increased inhibition of the brain enzyme. Drugs such as digitalis glycosides, the high-ceiling

saluretics, ethacrynic acid, and furosemide that inhibit CSF production and decrease flow can also increase the concentration of acetazolamide in CSF and brain. Also, drugs such as probenecid that inhibit active transport of drugs out of CSF could also increase the level of acetazolamide in CSF and brain by blocking its transport out of CSF.

The acid–base status of the patient can also alter the distribution of acetazolamide in the body and in the CSF and brain. Since it is a weak acid with a pK_a of 7.4, alteration of pH of the extracellular or cellular fluids affects the percentage of drug in the un-ionized form. It is in this form that the drug freely diffuses across cell membranes. The potentiation by CO_2 and ammonium chloride of the inhibitory effect of acetazolamide on experimental seizures in animals can be explained, at least in part, as a result of the acidosis produced by these agents increas-

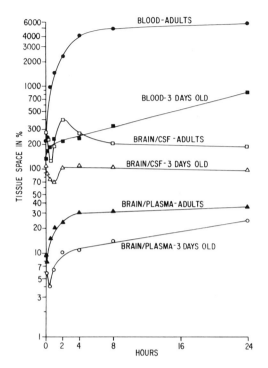

FIG. 4. Tissue/plasma and tissue/CSF ratio in percent of ³H-acetazolamide in adult and 3-day-old rats. Note that there are higher spaces of blood, brain/plasma, and brain/CSF in adult than in 3-day-old rats.

ing the concentration of un-ionized drug in the plasma (13,42,65). This would increase the level of drug in the brain and hence its anticonvulsant effect.

BIOTRANSFORMATION

In humans, 100% of a single orally administered dose of acetazolamide is recovered in the urine in 24 hr (31); there is no evidence that it is metabolized to another substance in the liver (31). In dogs, the average total amount recovered in the urine is 70%, all present as acetazolamide. Some is secreted in the bile and lost in feces, but the fate of the remainder is not known (31). In rats, only 30% of acetazolamide is recovered as such in urine, but a large fraction is excreted in the bile and presumably in the feces (31). No evidence has been found that metabolism of the drug occurs in rats. Only un-

changed drug is found in the urine of cats; hence, it is also not metabolized in this species (1).

EXCRETION

As is the case with certain other sulfonamides that are acetylated on the amino nitrogen, acetazolamide is secreted by renal tubular cells in humans (31,36); about 80% of the drug is excreted by tubular secretion. In the dog, clearance of unbound acetazolamide is equal to or slightly below that of creatinine (35); however, Weiner et al. (56) have shown that probenecid decreases this clearance, a fact suggesting that, in addition to reabsorption, tubular secretion also occurs in this species. Thus, as for many weak acids, the excretion of acetazolamide is dependent both on passive tubular reabsorption as the un-ionized molecule and on tubular secretion as the anionic species.

High doses of the drug inhibit renal carbonic anhydrase which results in increased urinary excretion of bicarbonate and alkalinization of the urine. This results in systemic metabolic acidosis. The increased pH of the urine decreases the percentage of the drug in the un-ionized form. This, therefore, decreases the amount reabsorbed and increases urinary excretion. However, the systemic metabolic acidosis decreases the amount in the ionized form, and hence, less is available for tubular secretion, but more of the un-ionized species is available for penetration into cells. The net effect of the high doses, therefore, depends on which of these processes predominates when the pH is changed and on what happens to intracellular pH in renal tubule cells as compared with cells in other tissues.

INTERACTIONS WITH OTHER DRUGS

Since acetazolamide is not metabolized by the liver, its level in the body cannot be affected by drugs that either induce or inhibit the drug-metabolizing enzymes in the liver. However, it is actively excreted in the bile and in the feces. Consequently, drugs that either decrease or accelerate bile flow or inhibit the transport of weak acids into bile can alter the level of the drug in the plasma. Although no such effects have been reported in humans, such changes are theoretically possible and should be kept in mind.

The absorption of drugs from the intestinal tract is also altered by acetazolamide (53). This effect appears to be related to inhibition of carbonic anhydrase in isolated loops of duodenum and ileum in rats. For example, Schnell and Miya (53) found that the absorption in the ileum of d-amphetamine was decreased and that of salicylic acid was increased by acetazolamide. Plasma levels reflected the effect on absorption; the pH of the ileal contents was decreased. In the duodenum, acetazolamide increased the absorption of d-amphetamine and decreased that of salicylic acid; the pH of the contents was not changed. It has not been determined if this drug affects absorption of other drugs from the intestinal tract in humans, but this remains a real possibility.

Probenecid, which blocks renal tubular secretion of acids, has been shown to decrease the excretion of acetazolamide in urine. This increases the level in the plasma and also in the CSF and brain and thereby can affect its anticonvulsant activity.

The interaction of acetazolamide with drugs that affect CSF production and with factors that alter acid–base balance in the body are discussed in a previous section. In rats, acetazolamide has been shown to enhance the degree of central depression produced by pentobarbital (46), to increase the duration of pentobarbital-induced sleep time, and to increase the brain pentobarbital space (45). This last effect is probably a result of the ability of acetazolamide to decrease CSF flow and thereby decrease the bulk removal of pentobarbital from the brain. It is likely that this effect occurs in humans not only for pentobarbital but also for other sedatives and anticonvulsants.

Since acetazolamide is bound to plasma proteins to an extent greater than 90% in humans, it is likely that many drugs that are bound to the same proteins can compete with this drug for the binding sites. Although this has not been demonstrated clinically, it, too, remains a the-

oretical possibility. However, Inui et al. (19) found that phenytoin, phenobarbital, primidone, carbamazepine, and ethosuximide given in various combinations with acetazolamide did not alter the plasma concentrations of acetazolamide in epileptic patients.

Acetazolamide also influences the activity of other drugs because of the many effects in the body that result from inhibition of carbonic anhydrase. Thus, alkalinization of urine and production of a saluresis, production of a systemic acidosis, inhibition of CSF production, decreased secretion of ocular fluids, and other changes that result from carbonic anhydrase inhibition can all produce effects on the penetration of other drugs into various fluids and tissues and on the level of other drugs in the plasma. Most of the effects are in the direction of increasing the concentration of weak acids in the tissues. In the case of anticonvulsants, most of which are weak acids, this would be an advantage, because adequate concentrations of the anticonvulsant in brain could be obtained with lower doses, with the consequent reduction in side effects caused by the anticonvulsant. It would seem reasonable, therefore, to use acetazolamide in combination with other anticonvulsants, particularly in patients refractory to these drugs and in those in whom side effects may be troublesome.

PHARMACOLOGICAL EFFECTS

Acetazolamide is a potent anticonvulsant agent in both laboratory animals and epileptic patients (2,11,28,29,38,43,60,61,66). In experimental animals, it abolishes the tonic extensor component of the maximal electroshock seizure, as does CO_2, and it potentiates this effect of CO_2 on seizure pattern (60,61). The anticonvulsant action of acetazolamide is not abolished by nephrectomy; hence, this action is independent of the systemic acidosis it produces from inhibition of renal CA.

Falbriard and Gangloff (11) noted that acetazolamide slightly increased the threshold voltage for stimulation of the cortex and markedly increased the threshold of the diencephalon. This drug also obtunds audiogenic seizures. It protects against seizures produced by inhalation of 30% CO_2 or by withdrawal from 50% CO_2 (65). In addition, acetazolamide protects against seizures evoked by various pharmacological agents. It reduces the intensity of spinal discharges induced by convulsive doses of strychnine, and it antagonizes pentylenetetrazole- and picrotoxin-induced seizures, but in doses higher than those necessary to protect against MES seizures. It thus possesses, as does CO_2, a wide spectrum of anticonvulsant action. Also, as is the case with CO_2, acetazolamide selectively depresses monosynaptic pathways in the spinal cord without affecting synaptic recovery or posttetanic potentiation (see 60 for summary). Thus, both acetazolamide and CO_2 have the same spectrum of effects on the nervous system and probably act in the same manner, by causing an accumulation of CO_2 in the brain, as discussed below.

These data have been interpreted to mean that acetazolamide and CO_2 affect some neuronal process that is more critically concerned in the spinal cord monosynaptic pathway than in polysynaptic circuits. The most outstanding difference between the component synapses of these two systems is that the safety factor with which transmission occurs is lower for monosynaptic than for polysynaptic pathways. It is suggested, therefore, that acetazolamide and CO_2 decrease the safety factor of transmission and that depression is produced by the drug at all synapses in which the safety factor is low, as in the spinal monosynaptic pathways.

Further evidence that carbonic anhydrase is involved in the spread of discharges was presented by Davenport (10) who observed that in rabbits treated with a carbonic anhydrase inhibitor, thiophene-2-sulfonamide, local stimulation of the cerebral cortex did not affect the general electrical activity of the stimulated area.

Carbonic anhydrase inhibitors other than acetazolamide have also been shown to affect the nervous system. Sulfanilamide abolishes the tonic extensor component of the MES in experimental animals and possesses a weak antiepileptic effect in man. Methazolamide and ethoxzolamide, congeners of acetazolamide, also exhibit anticonvulsant activity in experimental animals (15,16).

Millichap and co-workers (39–41) have presented convincing evidence that carbonic anhydrase is of functional significance in the development of the electroshock seizure pattern in maturing rats and guinea pigs. They suggest that this enzyme is important in the development of the ability to exhibit maximal tonic convulsions, in which a generalized spread of the seizure discharge is probably involved, but that the enzyme probably is not involved in the capacity to exhibit clonic seizures, which involves localized neuronal discharges. This suggestion is supported by their observations that the hyperkinetic behavior induced by electroshock in rats not over 10 days old is refractory to acetazolamide, that the clonic seizures induced by electroshock in 10- to 20-day-old rats were abolished only by very large doses of this drug, and that the tonic type of seizures seen in 21-day or older rats was abolished by low doses of acetazolamide.

There is much experimental and clinical evidence (see 61 for summary) that tolerance develops to the anticonvulsant effects of acetazolamide. If the anticonvulsant activity of acetazolamide results from a localized increase in P_{CO_2} in neuronal cells, it follows logically that the tolerance that is known to develop to the anticonvulsant effect of acetazolamide should be accompanied by tolerance to the anticonvulsant effect of CO_2. That this assumption is correct was demonstrated by Koch and Woodbury (23) who found that tolerance developed to the repeated administration of acetazolamide and that cross tolerance concurrently developed to CO_2. These data provide further strong evidence for a common mode of action of CO_2 and acetazolamide.

MECHANISM OF ACTION OF ACETAZOLAMIDE

Since the only well-documented biochemical effect of acetazolamide is inhibition of carbonic anhydrase, it has been demonstrated that the mechanism of its anticonvulsant action (as well as the other sulfonamide CA inhibitors) is through inhibition of this enzyme in the brain (15,16,43). The consequence of inhibition of brain carbonic anhydrase is CO_2 accumulation, which appears to cause the anticonvulsant effect of this drug, and, as mentioned above, acetazolamide and CO_2 have identical actions as far as their effects on the central nervous system are concerned. However, in higher doses, acetazolamide produces a greater effect on the brain by causing a retention of CO_2 in the body secondary to inhibition of red cell carbonic anhydrase (see summary in 31).

Summaries of the mechanism of action of this drug on the CNS have been provided by Woodbury and colleagues (57,58,60–63).

Because the primary anticonvulsant effect of acetazolamide is mediated through an effect on brain carbonic anhydrase, it is pertinent to discuss the distribution of this enzyme in brain. Studies originally carried out by Giacobini (12) and subsequently by other investigators (21,49,50,55) have demonstrated that carbonic anhydrase is located in the glial cells of the brain and also appears to be located in the glial product, myelin (5,21,50–52,67). Roussel et al. (50) have demonstrated by the indirect immunoperoxidase technique that the carbonic anhydrase C(CAC) isoenzyme is specifically localized in the cytoplasm of oligodendrocytes and astrocytes and that it is also present in the cytoplasmic areas of the myelin sheath but does not appear in the compact myelin. No reaction was found in neuronal cell bodies. These workers also noted a strong positive reaction to the antiserum in the choroid plexus. Subcellular distribution studies show that the enzyme is located in the cytosolic, membrane (mitochondria, microsomes), and myelin fractions of brain cells, predominantly glia, as discussed above.

The role of carbonic anhydrase in myelin is not clear, but it may be concerned with enhancing CO_2 transfer across the myelin sheath or in formation of myelin, since the carboxylation of acetyl CoA to malonyl CoA by the biotin-requiring enzyme acetyl CoA carboxylase requires HCO_3^- and not CO_2 as one of its substrates. Whether acetazolamide inhibits formation of myelin has not been ascertained, but data in this laboratory have demonstrated that in rat cerebral cortex, the fixation of $^{14}CO_2$ into the acid-soluble and combined protein and lipid fractions is inhibited by acetazolamide. Which of the various enzymatic pathways for CO_2 fixation in the brain is inhibited by acetazolamide awaits further experimentation. Also, whether the decreased incorporation of CO_2 into various substrates is related to the anticonvulsant effects of the carbonic anhydrase inhibitors is not known. Further work is obviously necessary.

When acetazolamide is given, the carbonic anhydrase in the brain is inhibited to the extent of $>99.0\%$. This results in an accumulation of total CO_2 in the brain (24,48,61). This CO_2 accumulation is sufficient to account for the prevention of the tonic extensor component of the MES, since the effects on the brain of CO_2 itself are identical to those of acetazolamide (60,61). In high doses, acetazolamide inhibits erythrocyte carbonic anhydrase (see below) and causes some CO_2 accumulation which may contribute to the anti-MES effect of the drug (15,16). The mechanism of the increase in total CO_2 in the brain is not completely known, but some unpublished data from studies in this laboratory suggest that glial cell carbonic anhydrase plays a role in the transfer of H^+ and/or HCO_3^- from neurons to glial cells and that interference with this process by acetazolamide causes CO_2 to back up in neurons in sufficient amounts to block the spread of a seizure discharge and so result in an anticonvulsant effect. Thus, glial cells, in addition to their role in maintaining K^+ homeostasis in the interstitial fluid of the brain, also regulate acid–base balance in the brain, a process that requires carbonic anhydrase.

Other evidence for a role of glial cell carbonic anhydrase in the regulation of brain excitability comes from studies on cobalt-induced focal epileptogenic lesions in the frontal cortex of rats (J. K. McQueen and D. M. Woodbury, *unpublished observations;* see 58,63,64 for summaries). Such lesions caused an increase in glial cell carbonic anhydrase in the regions of increased polyspike activity in the EEG (around primary focus in frontal cortex, secondary focus on opposite side, parietal cortex) but not in areas in which polyspike activity was not present (occipital cortex). The increase in carbonic anhydrase was accompanied by a decrease in total brain CO_2 and an increase in CO_2 fixation. These effects are opposite to those produced by acetazolamide and suggest that the glial carbonic anhydrase response to increased neuronal activity enhances the ability of these cells to handle the greater metabolic production of CO_2 caused by the increased neuronal activity. Since acetazolamide given either acutely or chronically to cobalt-implanted rats inhibits carbonic anhydrase in the glial cells, increases polyspike activity on the electroencephalogram, and enhances clinical seizure activity in such rats, it is evident that this glial enzyme response is a protective mechanism to the increased neuronal activity that, by maintaining K^+ and acid–base homeostasis, delimits the spread of seizure activity. Thus, acetazolamide has two effects on seizure properties: (a) the anti-MES effect, which measures spread of seizure activity and effectiveness against generalized tonic–clonic seizures in epileptic patients and appears to be directly related to CO_2 accumulation as a result of inhibition of carbonic anhydrase, and (b) an excitatory effect (decrease in electroshock seizure threshold and enhanced seizure and polyspike activity), generally with higher doses, which appears to be related to blockade of a glial anion (Cl^-, HCO_3^-) transport system that requires this enzyme.

As mentioned below, experimental animals develop tolerance to the anti-MES effects of chronically administered acetazolamide (23). Epileptic patients also develop tolerance with long-term treatment (2,19,28,29,38). The development of tolerance to the anticonvulsant effects of acetazolamide results from both the induction of increased enzyme in glial cells and the production of more glial cells. Thus, the glial cells play an active role mediated via carbonic anhydrase in regulating excitability of the brain as well as in maintaining anion homeostasis. The development of tolerance to acetazolamide, which is the main cause of its limited use in epileptic patients, is thus the result of induction of carbonic anhydrase in glial cells and proliferation of glia. Therefore, a higher dose of acetazolamide is required to produce the same degree of inhibition achieved initially.

These data support a fundamental role of carbonic anhydrase in glial cell metabolism such that any drug, hormone, injury, or other insult that compromises the rate at which this enzyme can catalyze the hydration of CO_2 to form HCO_3^- for anion transport into glial cells and for CO_2 fixation reactions involving synthesis of fatty acids for myelin formation, synthesis of neurotransmitters, synthesis of carbamyl phosphate for pyrimidine synthesis or urea cycle amino acids, and formation of oxalacetate for utilization in the Krebs cycle will immediately set in motion the machinery for synthesis of new carbonic anhydrase to relieve these compromised vital functions of the cell.

In addition to the carbonic anhydrase inhibitor drugs and cobalt implantation, as described above, increases of carbonic anhydrase activity in glial cells can be observed during maturation and aging (26,39–41,64), in audiogenic seizure mice (64), in mice given several subconvulsive doses of strychnine, which also induces tolerance to the convulsant effects of this drug, and in animals subjected to multiple electroshock seizures (*unpublished observations*).

The induction of carbonic anhydrase activity in glial cells by acetazolamide is probably through enhanced protein synthesis and appears to be regulated by cyclic AMP which, in turn, is regulated by norepinephrine. It is of particular interest that Kimelberg and colleagues (8,22,44) have shown *in vitro* that both norepinephrine and dibutyryl cyclic AMP induce an increase in the carbonic anhydrase activity found in the soluble but not in the membrane fraction of cultured astrocytes obtained from 1- to 3-day-old rat brains and that this increase parallels the rate of process extension of these astrocytes. There was also an induced increase in Na^+,K^+-ATPase, but the increase did not parallel growth of the fibers. The stimulation by norepinephrine was blocked by propanolol. Norepinephrine also increased the phosphorylation of carbonic anhydrase, an effect also blocked by propanolol. Thus, the norepinephrine-induced increase in cyclic AMP levels in brain results in activation of astroglial carbonic anhydrase because of cyclic AMP-stimulated phosphorylation of the enzyme (8). Such experiments provide direct evidence for a role of adrenergic stimulation and cyclic AMP in regulation carbonic anhydrase activity and growth of glial cells and presumably in regulation of brain excitability.

The regulation of excitability may be due to the transmitter-induced increase in carbonic anhydrase as a normal response. Thus, Church et al. (8) have proposed that the activation of astroglial carbonic anhydrase by putative transmitters may be involved in specific ion-transport responses of these cells, which, under certain conditions, can lead to astroglial swelling. Further evidence is that the anticonvulsant effect of acetazolamide is blocked by reserpine which depletes biogenic amines, particularly the catecholamines (17,25). How or whether this is related to effects on carbonic anhydrase is still unclear.

Effects of acetazolamide and other inhibitors of this enzyme on neurotransmitters have been little studied (see 57 for summary). Acetazolamide, similarly to CO_2, increases GABA levels in the brain (60), which may account for some of its anticonvulsant effects. Whether this is related to its inhibition of carbonic anhydrase is not known. Effects on other neurotransmitters are also unknown.

CLINICAL USE

Many reports attest to the efficacy of acetazolamide and other sulfonamide carbonic anhydrase inhibitors against various types of epilepsy. Acetazolamide was first introduced for the therapy of epilepsy by Bergstrom et al. (4), and subsequent reports (2,14,19,28,29,38) confirmed its effectiveness in most types of epilepsy (generalized tonic–clonic, absence, and complex partial seizures). However, the value of these carbonic anhydrase inhibitors is limited because of the rapid development of tolerance to their anticonvulsant effects (2,28,29,38). This shortens their effectiveness to a time period of rarely longer than 3 to 6 months. They are, however, useful for longer periods of time when used as adjuncts to primary antiepileptic drugs such as ethosuximide or phenytoin. Once tolerance has developed, withdrawal of the drugs for a period of time restores susceptibility to their antiepileptic effects. Acetazolamide has also proved of value as an adjunct drug, used intermittently, in the therapy of catamenial epilepsy. In such patients, water retention occurs, and this drug causes a saluretic effect. Hydrochlorothiazide is also used but does not have an antiepileptic effect. Hence, it is not known whether the antiepileptic effect of acetazolamide also contributes to the control of seizures in such patients. Acetazolamide is probably most useful in absence attacks (14), particularly in combination with ethosuximide. Tolerance development, however, limits its period of usefulness even in this condition.

Toxicity, as described below, is particularly low and is mainly related to tingling of hands and feet, an effect that disappears in a few days. Transient somnolence also is occasionally present.

Onset of the antiepileptic effect of acetazolamide is rapid, and seizures in patients with absences may cease within 3 to 4 hr. However, recurrence may also occur within 24 hr of cessation of administration of the drug. Since the half-life is 10 to 12 hr in humans, steady-state plasma levels are reached only after 40 to 48 hr. The usual dose is 250 mg given 1 to 3 times a day (250 to 750 mg/day). Doses larger than this do not produce any greater effects, since inhibition of brain carbonic anhydrase has occurred to the maximal extent possible. High doses increase erythrocyte drug levels to about 50 μg/ml (19), a level sufficient to cause the side effects discussed above which appear to result from CO_2 retention as a result of inhibition of CO_2 exchange across the erythrocyte membrane. Hence, erythrocyte levels of acetazolamide appear to be a better indicator of toxicity than do plasma levels (19).

Relation of Plasma Acetazolamide Levels to Therapeutic Effect

The plasma levels of acetazolamide in humans in effective antiepileptic doses (250 mg three times daily or about 10 mg/kg per day) are 10 to 14 μg/ml. Inui et al. (19) found that four of eight patients given 500 mg/day (250 mg twice daily) were free of focal motor or generalized tonic–clonic seizures when their plasma acetazolamide concentrations reached 8 to 14 μg/ml; the other four had reduced frequencies of attacks at plasma concentrations in the same range. Erythrocyte concentrations in these patients ranged from 49 to 53 μg/ml. Except for brain, the levels of acetazolamide in carbonic anhydrase-containing tissues, as discussed above, are considerably higher than those in the plasma. In muscle, which contains a carbonic anhydrase that is resistant to inhibition by acetazolamide and does not bind this drug (47), the concentration in the blood-free tissue is nearly the same as in an ultrafiltrate of plasma and varies with the plasma concentration.

Development of Tolerance

Tolerance to the anticonvulsant effects of acetazolamide develops with long-term administration to animals (23,61,65) or humans (2,19,28,29,38). This is the main limitation to its therapeutic use. Inui et al. (19) showed that with long-term use of the drug, the initially high plasma levels (see Table 1) decrease after 1 to 2 months to a plateau value about 60% of the initial steady-state concentration. This is paralleled by a tolerance to its anticonvulsant effects, and an increased dose is required to obtain the same effect. The decrease in plasma level is not accompanied by a decrease in the concentration of acetazolamide in the erythrocytes, an observation that suggests that the drug in the plasma has moved into the erythrocytes and other carbonic anhydrase-containing tissues, including brain, because its presence in the body has induced the synthesis of more carbonic anhydrase to combat the inhibition imposed by the drug. The increased amount of carbonic anhydrase would then allow more binding of acetazolamide as the [EI] complex. The only source of the drug to move into the cells is the plasma. Data from the effects of chronic acetazolamide treatment of rats with cobalt-induced focal epileptogenic lesions support this postulate, since this drug increased activity of this enzyme in the primary and secondary focal areas of such rats, and this was accompanied by tolerance to the effects of the acetazolamide (see 63,64 for summary).

Toxicity

Very large doses of acetazolamide can be tolerated without significant side effects. In fact, it is one of the least toxic of the antiepileptic drugs. All effects would seem to be related to inhibition of carbonic anhydrase with the exception of the hypersensitivity reactions. Several subjective complaints have been noted, such as drowsiness and paresthesias. The most severe objective reactions are skin rashes, abdominal distention, and cyanosis. Reactions similar to those produced by other sulfonamides have also been reported (see 7 for summary).

Inui et al. (19) have described the time sequence of the appearance of side effects with acetazolamide on administration of 5 mg/kg to four healthy adults, correlated with the concentration of the drug in the erythrocytes. In these four subjects, the concentration of acetazolamide in the erythrocytes rapidly rose to values greater than 40 μg/ml, and all four developed symptoms attributable to the drug as follows: 1 hr after administration, face paresthesia, numbness of the extremities, hyperpnea, all of which lasted for 24 hr; 3 to 4 hr, dizziness, nausea, and perspiration; 6 hr, weakness of hands, numbness of fingers, and pallakisuria. Most symptoms disappeared in 8 to 24 hr. In hepatic cirrhosis, episodes of disorientation may be induced by acetazolamide. It has been postulated that alkalinization of the urine diverts ammonia of renal origin from the urine into the systemic circulation and produces the disorientation. Calculus formation and ureteral colic have been attributed to the marked reduction in urinary citrate produced by acetazolamide and associated with either no change or even a rise in urinary calcium.

Teratogenic effects of acetazolamide have been described in experimental animals, and it is recommended that this drug not be given to women in early pregnancy (32).

METHAZOLAMIDE

Methazolamide has a pK_a of 7.2 and, like acetazolamide, is a weak acid whose movement across cells is dependent on the un-ionized form; hence, it is pH dependent. It is similar to acetazolamide in many respects but is more readily diffusible into tissues, and the free levels in the tissues are the same as the free levels in plasma. The pertinent data for this drug are summarized in Table 2. Plasma binding is approximately equal in all species (55 to 70%) except the mouse. Brain and CSF levels are generally higher relative to plasma than with acetazolamide, and the drug penetrates into brain much faster than does acetazolamide. The CSF/plasma ratio is 0.15 for methazolamide.

In humans, after an oral dose, the plasma half-life is as long as 10 hr. Excretion in the urine of the unchanged drug is by glomerular filtration and tubular reabsorption. In humans, about 20 to 30% of methazolamide is removed as such in urine; the remainder of 70 to 80% is metabolized to an as yet unknown compound.

Functionally, a lower dose of methazolamide than of acetazolamide is required to inhibit carbonic anhydrase because higher levels in the tissues can be obtained for the same dose.

As with acetazolamide, binding of methazolamide to tissue carbonic anhydrase does occur. The pharmacology of this drug is summarized elsewhere by Maren (31). Its pharmacological effects and mechanism of action are like those of acetazolamide, as discussed above.

SUMMARY

Acetazolamide is rapidly absorbed, becomes effective within hours, and is rapidly eliminated in the urine as the unchanged drug. Metabolism by the liver does not occur. Binding to plasma proteins is high (90% in humans), and only the free form is available for diffusion into tissues. This process is pH dependent. Soon after administration, the drug is present in total body water as the free drug, which is present in sufficient concentrations to inhibit carbonic anhydrase in brain and other tissues and to produce its anticonvulsant and other effects. Binding occurs to tissue carbonic anhydrase to form the enzyme–inhibitor complex [EI], and after 24 hr, almost all of the drug is present in tissue in this form. This complex has a low dissociation constant; hence, the drug is released from the tissues only slowly as it is excreted in the urine. This is a slow process with a half-life of several days.

Acetazolamide penetrates into the brain and CSF slowly and reaches a concentration much

TABLE 2. *Plasma binding, plasma total and free levels, brain levels, and plasma half-life of methazolamide in various species[a]*

Species (adult)	Dose (mg/kg) and route	% Bound in plasma	Plasma Total	Plasma Free	Brain	RBC	Muscle	CSF	Plasma half-life (min)
Man	oral	55	2–50	2.9–23				0.3–7.5	300
Dog	i.v.	55	2–50						150
Cat	i.v.	68	2–50						180
Rat	20 oral	55	103	46	20	110	35		—
			76	34	3	120	45		
Mouse	i.v.	5	2–50						66

[a]Compiled from Maren (31).

lower than the total level in the plasma. The concentration in the brain, however, is higher than that in the CSF, and the brain level is dependent on its concentration in this fluid. The concentration in brain and CSF is dependent on many factors such as the rate of CSF flow, the rate of transport of the drug out of the CSF, and the permeability of the blood–brain barrier. Most of the bound drug in the body is found in the erythrocytes which contain a high concentration of carbonic anhydrase.

Renal excretion of acetazolamide is by tubular reabsorption and secretion. Biliary excretion of the drug also occurs, particularly in dogs and rats.

Few drug interactions with acetazolamide have been described, but many theoretical possibilities for interaction exist.

The toxicity of acetazolamide is low, and generally minor side effects result from its use.

Acetazolamide exerts its anticonvulsant action by inhibiting carbonic anhydrase in glial cells of brain. This results in CO_2 accumulation in brain, an effect that blocks spread of seizure activity.

CONVERSION

Acetazolamide

Conversion factor:

$$CF = \frac{1000}{\text{mol. wt.}} = \frac{1000}{222} = 4.50$$

Conversion:

$(\mu g/ml) \times 4.50 = (\mu moles/liter)$
$(\mu moles/liter) \div 4.50 = (\mu g/ml)$

ACKNOWLEDGMENTS

This work was supported in part by U.S. Public Health Service Program–Project Grant 5-PO1-NS-15767 from the National Institute of Neurological and Communicative Disorders and Stroke. D.M. Woodbury is a Research Career Awardee (5-K6-NS-13-838) of the N.I.N.C.D.S.

REFERENCES

1. Achor, L. B., and Roth, L. J. (1957): Metabolic fate of acetazolamide-S^{35} (Diamox) in the cat. *Fed. Proc.*, 16:277.
2. Ansell, B., and Clarke, E. (1956): Acetazolamide in treatment of epilepsy. *Br. Med. J.*, 1:650–661.
3. Bayne, W. F., Rogers, G., and Crisologo, N. (1975): Assay for acetazolamide in plasma. *J. Pharm. Sci.*, 64:402–404.
4. Bergstrom, W. H., Garzoli, R. F., Lombroso, C., Davidson, D. T., and Wallace W. M. (1952): Observations on metabolic and clinical effects of carbonic anhydrase inhibitors in epileptics. *Am. J. Dis. Child.*, 84:71–73.
5. Cammer, W., Fredman, T., Rose, A. L., and Norton, W. T. (1976): Brain carbonic anhydrase: Activity in isolated myelin and the effect of hexachlorophene. *J. Neurochem.*, 27:165–171.
6. Carter, M. J. (1972): Carbonic anhydrase: Isoenzymes, properties, distribution, and functional significance. *Biol. Rev.*, 47:465–513.
7. Chao, D. H. C., and Plumb, R. L. (1961): Diamox in epilepsy: A critical review of 178 cases. *J. Pediatr.*, 58:211–228.
8. Church, G. A., Kimelberg, H. K., and Sapirstein, V. S. (1980): Stimulation of carbonic anhydrase activity and phosphorylation in primary astroglial cultures by norepinephrine. *J. Neurochem.*, 34:873–879.
9. Coleman, J. E. (1975): Chemical reactions of sulfonamides with carbonic anhydrase. *Annu. Rev. Pharmacol.*, 15:221–242.
10. Davenport, H. W. (1946): Carbonic anhydrase in the nervous system. *J. Neurophysiol.*, 9:41–46.
11. Falbriard, A., and Gangloff, H. (1955): Action d'un inhibiteur de la carboanhydrase l'acetazolamide, sur l'excitabilite du cortex, du thalamus et du rhinencephale. *Experientia*, 11:234–235.
12. Giacobini, E. (1962): A cytochemical study of the localization of carbonic anhydrase in the nervous system. *J. Neurochem.*, 9:169–177.
13. Goldberg, M. A., Barlow, C. F., and Roth, L. J. (1961): The effects of carbon dioxide on the entry and accumulation of drugs in the central nervous system. *J. Pharmacol. Exp. Ther.*, 131:308–318.
14. Golla, F. L., and Sessions, H. R. (1957): Control of petit mal by acetazolamide. *J. Ment. Sci.*, 103:214–217.
15. Gray, W. D., Maren, T. H., Sisson, G. M., and Smith, F. H. (1957): Carbonic anhydrase inhibition VII. Carbonic anhydrase inhibition and anticonvulsant effect. *J. Pharmacol. Exp. Ther.*, 121:160–170.
16. Gray, W. D., and Rauh, C. E. (1967): The anticonvulsant action of inhibitors of carbonic anhydrase: Site and mode of action in rats and mice. *J. Pharmacol. Exp. Ther.*, 156:383–396.
17. Gray, W. D., and Rauh, C. E. (1971): The relation between monoamines in brain and the anticonvulsant action of inhibitors of carbonic anhydrase. *J. Pharmacol. Exp. Ther.*, 177:206–218.
18. Harke, W., Schirren, C., and Wehrmann, R. (1959): Experimentelle Untersuchungen zur Bestimmung der Acetazolamid-Ausscheidung im menschlichen Harn

mittels eines Diazotier- und Kupplungsverfahrens. *Klin. Wochenschr.*, 37:1040–1044.

19. Inui, M., Azuma, H., Yorifuji, K., Nishimura, T., and Hatada, N. (1982): A study on the concentration of an antiepileptic-acetazolamide-in blood. *Epilepsia (in press).*

20. Karler, R., and Woodbury, D. M. (1960): Intracellular distribution of carbonic anhydrase. *Biochem. J.,* 75:538–543.

21. Kimelberg, H. K., Biddlecome, S., Narumi, S., and Bourke, R. S. (1978): ATPase and carbonic anhydrase activities of bulk-isolated neuron, glia, and synaptosome fractions from rat brain. *Brain Res.,* 141:305–323.

22. Kimelberg, H. K., Narumi, S., Biddlecome, S., and Bourke, R. S. (1978): (Na$^+$ + K$^+$)ATPase, ^{86}Rb$^+$ transport and carbonic anhydrase activity in isolated brain cells and cultured astrocytes. In: *Dynamic Properties of Glia Cells,* edited by E. Schoffeniels, G. Franck, L. Hertz, and D. B. Tower, pp. 347–357. Pergamon Press, Oxford.

23. Koch, A., and Woodbury, D. M. (1958): Effects of carbonic anhydrase inhibition on brain excitability. *J. Pharmacol. Exp. Ther.,* 122:335–342.

24. Koch, A., and Woodbury, D. M. (1960): Carbonic anhydrase inhibition and brain electrolyte composition. *Am. J. Physiol.,* 198:434–440.

25. Koslow, S. H., and Roth, L. J. (1971): Reserpine and acetazolamide in maximum electroshock seizure in the rat. *J. Pharmacol. Exp. Ther.,* 176:711–717.

26. Koul, O., and Konungo, M. S. (1975): Alterations in carbonic anhydrase of the brain of rats as a function of age. *Exp. Gerontol.,* 10:273–278.

27. Lindskog, S., Henderson, L. E., Kannan, K. K., Liljas, A., Nyman, P. O., and Strandberg, B. (1971): Carbonic anhydrase. In: *The Enzymes, Vol. 5.,* Third Edition, edited by P. D. Boyer, pp. 587–665. Academic Press, New York.

28. Lombroso, C. T., Davidson, D. T., Jr., and Gross-Bianchi, M. L. (1956): Further evaluation of acetazolamide (Diamox) in treatment of epilepsy. *J.A.M.A.,* 160:268–272.

29. Lombroso, C. T., and Forsythe, I. (1960): A long-term follow-up of acetazolamide (Diamox) in the treatment of epilepsy. *Epilepsia,* 1:493–500.

30. Maren, T. H. (1963): The binding of inhibitors to carbonic anhydrase *in vivo:* Drugs as markers for enzyme. In: *Proc. 1st International Pharmacology Meeting,* pp. 39–48. Pergamon Press, New York.

31. Maren, T. H. (1967): Carbonic anhydrase: Chemistry, physiology, and inhibition. *Physiol. Rev.,* 47:595–781.

32. Maren, T. H. (1971): Editorial. Teratology and carbonic anhydrase inhibition. *Arch. Ophthalmol.,* 85:1–2.

33. Maren, T. H. (1976): Relations between structure and biological activity of sulfonamides. *Annu. Rev. Pharmacol. Toxicol.,* 16:309–327.

34. Maren, T. H., Ash, V. I., and Bailey, E. M. (1954): Carbonic anhydrase inhibition. II. A method for determination of carbonic anhydrase inhibitors, particularly of Diamox. *Bull. Johns Hopkins Hosp.,* 95:244–249.

35. Maren, T. H., Mayer, E., and Wadsworth, B. C. (1954): Carbonic anhydrase inhibition. I. The pharmacology of Diamox (2-acetylamino-1,3,4-thiadiazole-5-sulfonamide). *Bull. Johns Hopkins Hosp.,* 95:199–243.

36. Maren, T. H., and Robinson, B. (1960): The pharmacology of acetazolamide as related to cerebrospinal fluid and the treatment of hydrocephalus. *Bull. Johns Hopkins Hosp.,* 106:1–24.

37. Maren, T. H., Wadsworth, B. C., Yale, E. K., and Alonso, L. G. (1954): Carbonic anhydrase inhibition. III. Effects of Diamox on electrolyte metabolism. *Bull. Johns Hopkins Hosp.,* 95:277–321.

38. Millichap, J. G. (1956): Anticonvulsant action of Diamox in children. *Neurology (Minneap.),* 6:552–559.

39. Millichap, J. G. (1957): Development of seizure patterns in newborn animals. Significance of brain carbonic anhydrase. *Proc. Soc. Exp. Biol. Med.,* 96:125–129.

40. Millichap, J. G. (1958): Seizure patterns in young animals. II. Significance of brain carbonic anhydrase. *Proc. Soc. Exp. Biol. Med.,* 97:606–611.

41. Millichap, J. G., Balter, M., and Hernandez, P. (1958): Development of susceptibility to seizures in young animals. III. Brain water, electrolyte and acid–base metabolism. *Proc. Soc. Exp. Biol. Med.,* 99:6–11.

42. Millichap, J. G., Thatcher, L. D., and Williams, P. M. (1955): Anticonvulsant action of acetazolamide, alone and in combination with ammonium chloride. *Fed. Proc.* 14:370.

43. Millichap, J. G., Woodbury, D. M., and Goodman, L. S. (1955): Mechanism of the anticonvulsant action of acetazolamide, a carbonic anhydrase inhibitor. *J. Pharmacol. Exp. Ther.,* 115:251–258.

44. Narumi, S., Kimelberg, H. K., and Bourke, R. S. (1978): Effects of norepinephrine on the morphology and some enzyme activities of primary monolayer cultures from rat brain. *J. Neurochem.,* 31:1479–1490.

45. Reed, D. J. (1968): The effects of acetazolamide on pentobarbital sleep-time and cerebrospinal fluid flow of rats. *Arch. Int. Pharmacodyn. Ther.,* 171:206–215.

46. Reed, D. J., and Woodbury, D. M. (1962): Effect of urea and acetazolamide on brain volume and cerebrospinal fluid pressure. *J. Physiol. (Lond),* 164:265–273.

47. Register, A. M., Koester, M. K., and Noltman, E. A. (1978): Discovery of carbonic anhydrase in rabbit skeletal muscle and evidence for its identity with "basic muscle protein." *J. Biol. Chem.,* 253:4143–4152.

48. Rollins, D. E., Withrow, C. D., and Woodbury, D. M. (1970): Tissue acid–base balance in acetazolamide-treated rats. *J. Pharmacol. Exp. Ther.,* 174:535–540.

49. Rose, S. P. R., and Sinha, A. K. (1971): Bulk separation of neurones and glia: A comparison of techniques. *Brain Res.,* 33:205–217.

50. Roussel, G., Delaunoy, J. P., Nussbaum, J.-L., and Mandel, P. (1979): Demonstration of a specific localization of carbonic anhydrase C in the glial cells of rat CNS by an immunohistochemical method. *Brain Res.,* 160:47–55.

51. Sapirstein, V. S., and Lees, M. B. (1978): Purifica-

tion of myelin carbonic anhydrase. *J. Neurochem.*, 31:505–511.

52. Sapirstein, V. S., Lees, M. B., and Trachtenberg, M. C. (1978): Soluble and membrane bound carbonic anhydrases from rat CNS: Regional development. *J. Neurochem.*, 31:283–287.

53. Schnell, R. C., and Miya, T. S. (1970): Altered absorption of drugs from the rat small intestine by carbonic anhydrase inhibition. *J. Pharmacol. Exp. Ther.*, 174:177–184.

54. Sylvia, M. W., Vinod, P. S., and Sidney, E. (1977): GLC analysis of acetazolamide in blood, plasma, and saliva following oral administration to normal subjects. *J. Pharm. Sci.*, 66:527–530.

55. Tower, D. B., and Young, G. M. (1973): The activities of butyrylcholinesterase and carbonic anhydrase, the rate of anaerobic glycolysis, and the question of a constant density of glial cells in cerebral cortices of various mammalian species from mouse to whale. *J. Neurochem.*, 20:269–278.

56. Weiner, I. M., Washington, J. A., and Mudge, G. H. (1959): Studies on the renal excretion of salicylate in the dog. *Bull. Johns Hopkins Hosp.*, 105:284–297.

57. Woodbury, D. M. (1977): Pharmacology and mechanisms of action of antiepileptic drugs. In: *Scientific Approaches to Clinical Neurology,* edited by E. S. Goldensohn and S. H. Appel, pp. 693–726. Lea and Febiger, Philadelphia.

58. Woodbury, D. M. (1980): Carbonic anhydrase inhibitors. *Adv. Neurol.*, 27:617–633.

59. Woodbury, D. M. (1981): Pharmacology of anticonvulsant drugs in CSF. In: *Neurobiology of Cerebrospinal Fluid, Vol. II.,* edited by J. Wood. Plenum Press, New York (*in press*).

60. Woodbury, D. M., and Esplin, D. W. (1969): Neuropharmacology and neurochemistry of anticonvulsant drugs. *Proc. Assoc. Res. Nerv. Ment. Dis.*, 37:24–56.

61. Woodbury, D. M., and Karler, R. (1960): The role of carbon dioxide in the nervous system. *Anesthesiology,* 21:686–703.

62. Woodbury, D. M., and Kemp, J. W. (1970): Some possible mechanisms of action of antiepileptic drugs. *Pharmakopsychiatr. Neuropsychopharmakol.,* 3:201–226.

63. Woodbury, D. M., and Kemp, J. W. (1977): Basic mechanisms of seizures: Neurophysiological and biochemical etiology. In: *Psychopathology and Brain Dysfunction,* edited by C. Shagass, S. Gershon, and A. J. Friedhoff, pp. 149–182. Raven Press, New York.

64. Woodbury, D. M., and Kemp, J. W. (1979): Initiation, propagation and arrest of seizures. In: *Pathophysiology of Cerebral Energy Metabolism,* edited by B. B. Mrsulja, L. M. Rakic, I. Klatzo, and M. Spatz, pp. 313–351. Plenum Press, New York.

65. Woodbury, D. M., and Rollins, L. T. (1954): Anticonvulsant effects of acetazolamide, alone and in combination with CO_2, on experimental seizures in mice. *Fed. Proc.,* 13:418.

66. Woodbury, D. M., Rollins, L. T., Gardner, M. D., Hirschi, W. L., Hogan, J. R., Rallison, M. L., Tanner, G. S., and Brodie, D. A. (1958): Effects of carbon dioxide on brain excitability and electrolytes. *Am. J. Physiol.,* 192:79–90.

67. Yandrasitz, J. R., Ernst, S. A., and Salganicoff, L. (1976): The subcellular distribution of carbonic anhydrase in homogenates of perfused rat brain. *J. Neurochem.,* 27:707–715.

Antiepileptic Drugs, edited by D. M. Woodbury, J. K. Penry, and C. E. Pippenger. Raven Press, New York © 1982.

69

Other Antiepileptic Drugs

Bromides

Dixon M. Woodbury and C. E. Pippenger

Bromide was the first of the modern antiepileptic drugs. Its introduction by Locock in 1857 (14) for the treatment of catamenial seizures marked a sharp historical break from earlier inadequate methods of treatment. The clinical use of bromide preparations became popular within a short time after this and introduced an era in which the greatest emphasis was placed on the use of sedative drugs. Although it has been progressively superseded by phenobarbital since 1912 and eclipsed by phenytoin since 1938 and by other drugs since then, bromide continues to find some useful application in the treatment of generalized tonic–clonic seizures unassociated with other seizure types. The main disadvantage is the low ratio between the therapeutically effective dose and its toxicity, manifested mostly as sedation and psychic disturbances.

Bromide is chiefly of interest because it is a simple inorganic ion with anticonvulsant activity, although its mechanisms of action are not known despite its use for more than a century. Because of the low therapeutic ratio of bromide, it is important to understand its absorption, distribution, and excretion for its rational use.

Excellent reviews of the historical discussions of the clinical application of the bromides in the management of seizure disorders by Sir Charles Locock have been published by Lennox (12) and Joynt (10).

ABSORPTION

Following oral ingestion by humans, bromide is rapidly absorbed from the intestinal tract in a manner similar to that of chloride. Chloride is actively transported across the intestinal mucosal cells, but it is not known with certainty that bromide is actively transported across these cells. Since no bromide is excreted in the feces (20), all of an orally administered dose is absorbed into the bloodstream.

Radiobromide, when introduced into the stomach in which the pylorus is ligated, is not absorbed into the circulation (20). Thus, absorption is from the small intestine.

DISTRIBUTION

Volume of Distribution, Plasma Half-Life, and Distribution into Cells and Intracellular Fluids

After absorption, the bromide ion rapidly distributes, as does chloride, throughout the extracellular space and into cells. The volume of distribution is the same as that of chloride in most species except humans, where it is very slightly higher (4). Since chloride is distributed passively across most cell membranes according to the transmembrane potential, it is likely that bromide distributes in the same manner. Thus, the concentration in the cells of tissues with high transmembrane potentials, such as muscle, is low, whereas in the cells of tissues with low potentials, such as erythrocytes, smooth muscle, and liver, the concentrations are high. For example, the ratio between the concentration of bromide in red cells and plasma is 0.45 (22); the corresponding ratio for chloride is 0.67. On the basis of passive distribution, this would yield a potential difference across the red cell membrane of -20 mV, as calculated from the Nernst equation. This is a higher potential than that calculated from the chloride distribution ratio (-10 mV); it is also higher than the potential difference (-10 mV) measured in the red cells of *Amphiuma* by a glass ultramicroelectrode. These calculations suggest that bromide is actively transported out of red blood cells, but this conclusion must await further data and measurement of the red blood cell-to-plasma ratio of chloride simultaneously with that of bromide. It is of interest, however, that Weir and Hastings (25) found the red blood cell-to-serum ratio of bromide to be 0.75, whereas Gamble et al. (5) observed that it was 0.55. Hence, the reported ratios are variable, and it is, therefore, not settled whether bromide is passively or actively distributed across the red blood cell membrane. Still, the concentration in the red cells (about half the plasma concentration), with a low potential difference (-10 mV), is considerably higher than that of muscle (about one-eighth the plasma concentration), with a high potential difference (-90 mV). As the bromide level is increased in the body, the concentration of chloride is decreased in direct proportion to the increase in bromide. With large doses of bromide, as much as 45% of the total chloride in the body may be replaced.

All the drug entering the extracellular fluid is freely diffusible, because no binding to plasma proteins occurs (9,22). With the exception of gastric juice, brain, and teeth, into which entrance is slow, bromide rapidly reaches a steady state in most organs in 10 min. The volume of distribution in humans usually ranges from 0.23 to 0.29 liter/kg (23 to 29% of body weight), the same as that of chloride; in one study, however, the volume of distribution was higher (0.42 liter/kg) (9) (Table 1). Some differential distribution of bromide as compared to chloride does occur. For example, the ratio of the concentration of bromide in gastric mucosa, gastric juice, saliva, and possibly the thyroid to that in plasma is higher than the chloride ratio in these same tissues and fluids (8,21).

The plasma half-life of bromide in humans is long (9,22); by use of radioactive bromide ([82]Br), it was found to be 12 days. In this study, the bromide was not incorporated in fat or bound to plasma proteins. Thus, the rate of elimination of bromide is slow, and its rate of absorption from the intestinal tract rapid. As a consequence, when therapy is first initiated, the levels of the drug build up rapidly in the body at the expense of chloride, which is more readily excreted by the kidney than bromide. Even in mice, in which drugs are generally excreted rapidly, the excretion of bromide is slow; the plasma half-life in mice is 1.5 days (20). When radiobromide is ingested in humans, the steady-state level in the plasma is reached about 2 to 3 hr after oral administration (22). In rats, the time of peak effect for elevation of the electroshock seizure threshold by a dose of 2 g/kg (20 meq/kg) is 4 hr, and the elevated threshold stays at the peak level for 24 hr; by 96 hr, the threshold has returned to normal.

Bromide is present in all transcellular fluids. Its concentration in saliva is 1.5 times that in plasma (21). The bromide in the swallowed saliva is reabsorbed into the gastroenteric circulation. The high concentration of bromide in saliva suggests an active secretory process for this anion, like that of chloride, in salivary glands. Similarly, bromide is concentrated by the gastric mucosa and secreted into the lumen of the stomach in the gastric juices (8). This process is also active, as is the secretion of chloride. However, bromide is in a relatively higher concentration in gastric juices than is chloride. The bromide secreted into the gastric secretion is

TABLE 1. Concentration of bromide ion in various tissues and fluids and its volume of distribution and half-life in the body of various species

Species	Ref.	Dose (g/kg) and route	Dose (mmoles/kg)	Time after administration (hr)	Concentration (meq/liter)				Brain/plasma	CSF/plasma	Muscle/plasma	Volume of distribution (liter/kg)[c]	Plasma half-life (days)
					Plasma	Brain	CSF	Muscle					
Man Adult	9	0.1 oral	1.0	14	2.70		0.69			0.25		0.42	
				36	2.94		0.91			0.31			
	4			60	2.35		0.65			0.28			
	22											0.23–0.29	
	1	[82]Br		6[a]	19.60							0.24	12
				24[a]	13.50							0.24	
				48[a]	9.60							0.26	
				82[a]	8.20							0.26	
Dog Adult	23,24	11.8 oral		24	28.4	8.20	21.5		0.29				
Rabbit Adult	17	[82]Br		24	0.77	0.14	0.61		0.19	0.79			
					5.64	1.16	4.51		0.21	0.80			
					16.20	4.06	14.70		0.25	0.91			
					21.30	6.33	21.80		0.30	1.00			
Rat Adult	4	[82]Br											
	[b]	2 i.p.	20										
	[b]	1.2 i.p.	11	8	24.20	3.35	—	2.66	0.14	—	0.11		0.8
	[b]	[82]Br							0.15				
	[b]	[82]Br							0.22				
Immature (8 day old)	20												
Mouse	7	0.9	9.0	5	29								1.5
		1.26	12.5	5	39								
		1.85	18.0	5	55								
		2.13	21.0	5	59								
		2.7	26.0	5	69								

[a] Chronic abuse, time after [82]Br administration.
[b] Unpublished observations from this laboratory.
[c] The ratio between the volume of distribution of bromide and that of chloride for various species is as follows (4): man, 1.02 to 1.07; dog, 1.05; rat, 1.00.

reabsorbed into the circulation when it enters the small intestine. Bromide also enters the cerebrospinal fluid (CSF), but in this case its concentration is lower than that of plasma. The explanation for this is considered below. Some bromide also enters bile and reaches the intestinal tract, where reabsorption into blood must occur, since no bromide is found in feces.

The bromide space of immature animals is larger than that of the adult, just as the chloride space is larger. Most of this is distributed in the large extracellular spaces in the tissues of immature animals.

Brain and CSF Distribution

Unlike tissues in which the tissue-to-plasma bromide concentration ratios are either equal to or higher than those of chloride, the ratios of the concentration of bromide to plasma in brain and CSF are lower than the corresponding ratios for chloride. For example, the brain-to-plasma ratio of bromide in rabbits is 0.19, and the CSF-to-plasma ratio is 0.79 (Table 1), whereas the brain-to-plasma ratio of chloride is 0.28 to 0.32, and the CSF-to-plasma ratio is 1.2. Previous data have shown that bromide is removed from the CSF by two processes, as are other inorganic monovalent anions such as iodide, perchlorate, and thiocyanate that have lower concentrations in the CSF and brain than in plasma: (a) bulk flow of CSF via the arachnoid villi and (b) active transport out of the CSF across the choroid plexus (19,26).

Active transport across the choroid plexus appears to be the more important process. This is demonstrated by the fact that inhibitors of CSF production and flow have less effect on the concentration of monovalent inorganic anions in the CSF and brain than do agents that inhibit their transport out of the CSF (large loads of these same anions). Figure 1 shows the effects of large loads of the same monovalent anions on the distribution of radioactive iodide, thiocyanate, perchlorate, and bromide between brain and plasma and between CSF and plasma. It can be seen that a large load (generally 5 meq/kg) of each anion increases its own concentration in

both CSF and brain. Thus, as shown by Pollay (17) and depicted for two dose levels in Fig. 1 and summarized for four dose levels in Table 1, increasing the level of bromide in the plasma progressively increases the brain-to-plasma ratio of ^{82}Br in rabbits from 0.19 to 0.3 (58% increase) and the CSF-to-plasma ratio from 0.79 to 1.0 (28% increase). The concentration ratios in brain and CSF of the other radioactive anions were also increased by loading the animals with their same nonradioactive anion. The large load of bromide saturates the carrier system that transports bromide out of the CSF across the choroid plexus and inhibits this process. All of these monovalent anions compete for this transport system and inhibit each other's removal from the CSF. Since bromide entering the brain and CSF from the blood cannot be removed from the CSF by transport across the choroid plexus, its concentration in the CSF increases. Also, since the CSF is in rapid and complete equilibrium with the interstitial space of the brain, the increased level in the CSF resulting from inhibition of its removal by various large doses of bromide also increases the brain level.

The dose of bromide used is in the range of anticonvulsant activity in rats and other species, and it is likely that part of its anticonvulsant effect is mediated through an effect on CSF transport. Certainly, self-blockade of this transport system results in an increased level of bromide in the brain. The extracellular space of adult rat brain is 14% as measured by inulin (31). Since the concentration of bromide in the CSF is closer to the concentration of bromide in the interstitial space of the brain, the more meaningful bromide space to calculate is the brain-to-CSF ratio. From the data in Table 1, this value is 0.19/0.79 = 0.23 for the nonloaded animals and 0.3/1.00 = 0.3 for the animals receiving the largest load of bromide. This latter figure is equal to the chloride space of the brain in these animals and is larger than the extracellular space (14%), as is the 23% space in the nonloaded animals. These data show that bromide is present in brain cells and that the concentration there is lower in the nonloaded than in the loaded animals. Since the ratio of bromide concentration

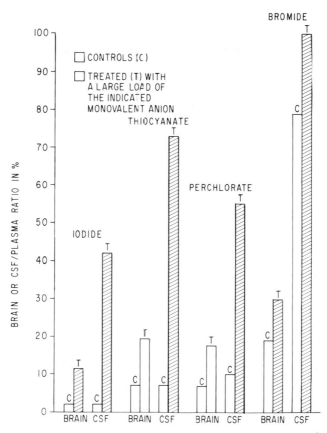

FIG. 1. The effect of a large load, usually 5 meq/kg, of the indicated monovalent anion on the distribution of radioactive iodide, thiocyanate, perchlorate, and bromide between brain and plasma and between CSF and plasma. The iodide data were plotted from the results of Reed et al. (19); thiocyanate from Pollay (16); perchlorate from the unpublished observations of Woodbury; and bromide from Pollay (17). See text for discussion. (From Woodbury, ref. 28, with permission.)

in cells to that in CSF (extracellular) fluid is lower than the chloride ratio in the nonloaded animals and the same as that of chloride in the loaded animals, it appears likely that bromide is transported across brain cells and that anticonvulsant doses of the drug block this transport. When transport is blocked, bromide distributes like chloride. The mechanisms of action of bromide are probably related to inhibition of this transport process.

As shown in Table 1, the CSF-to-plasma ratio of bromide in humans (0.31) is lower than that in rabbits (0.79) and in dogs (0.76). This low ratio suggests that in humans as well as the animals this anion is actively transported out of the CSF. Evidence for this is provided by the fact that a large load of bromide increases the CSF-to-plasma ratio of bromide, as it does in animals; the effect is dose dependent.

That bromide is present in brain cells is demonstrated by the experiments of Kuriyama (11) who found that this anion was present in synaptosomes and mitochondria of mouse brain. The synaptosomal uptake of bromide was energy independent and was inhibited by other monovalent inorganic anions such as nitrate and iodide and by monovalent organic anions such as pyruvate and lactate. The accumulation (or binding) of bromide by mitochondria was much less than that by synaptosomes. The uptake appears to resemble an anion-exchange process. Chlorpromazine inhibited the synaptosomal binding of bromide.

BIOTRANSFORMATION

Bromide is not metabolized by the body; it enters and leaves the body only as the monovalent anion.

EXCRETION

In humans, the bromide ion is slowly, but almost completely, excreted in the urine. Most of the amount that enters saliva, bile, and gastric juice is reabsorbed from the small intestine and excreted in the urine, since none is excreted in the feces. Excretion of small amounts of bromide may occur in skin, in nasal and conjunctival secretions, and in saliva not swallowed. The half-life of ^{82}Br in urine of humans is the same as that in plasma, 12 days (21). This is a reflection of a urinary excretion of about 5% of the body bromide per day. The concentration of ^{82}Br in urine is 1.5 times that in plasma.

Söremark (21) observed that a diurnal variation exists for the excretion of bromide. During sleep, negligible quantities of bromide were excreted in urine. In subjects not allowed to sleep, the rate of bromide excretion did not fall. This interesting phenomenon has not been explained.

The amount of bromide excreted is related to the total halide concentration in the body and also to the bromide-to-halide ratio in plasma (2). The kidney functions to maintain the total halide content of the extracellular fluid at a normal value, but it somewhat preferentially reabsorbs bromide and excretes chloride. Thus, the ratio of bromide to total halide in urine is slightly lower than the corresponding ratio in plasma. The preferential chloride excretion becomes less marked at high plasma bromide levels. This suggests that bromide may be actively reabsorbed by the renal tubular cells and that high loads of bromide saturate the carrier system and thereby decrease bromide reabsorption.

Large loads of chloride, whether administered as sodium chloride or ammonium chloride, and drugs, such as the mercurials, that induce chloruresis hasten the excretion of bromide by reducing its reabsorption and thereby increase the ratio of bromide to total halide in the urine. Treatment of bromide intoxication is accomplished by this procedure.

Bromide is also excreted at a much slower rate than is the iodide ion. In equivalent amounts, 21% of a bromide dose is excreted in 76 hr, whereas 98% of an iodide dose is excreted in 24 hr (8). Iodide and bromide probably compete for reabsorption across the renal tubular cells.

INTERACTIONS WITH OTHER DRUGS

Since bromide is a central nervous system depressant, it would be expected to enhance the effects of other depressant drugs. This has been shown to occur in experimental animals. For example, bromide increases the chlorpromazine-induced sleeping time in mice (15). Such an effect probably also occurs in humans.

There is no evidence that bromide induces or inhibits the activity of drug-metabolizing enzymes in the liver. Nor does it compete for binding sites on plasma proteins, since it is not bound to these proteins.

It has not been determined whether large doses of bromide block the active exit of organic anions out of CSF, as does probenecid. However, since bromide is actively transported out of the CSF, this remains a theoretical possibility that deserves exploration. It is possible that the organic and inorganic transport systems in the choroid plexus use the same carrier system.

PHARMACOLOGICAL EFFECTS

In mice, bromide is most effective in blocking seizures induced by pentylenetetrazol (ED_{50}, 900 mg/kg or 9 mmoles/kg) (7). It also blocks the tonic extensor component of the tonic–clonic pattern induced by intravenous pentylenetetrazol (ED_{50}, 1,250 mg/kg or 12.5 mmoles/kg) or maximal electrical stimulation (ED_{50}, 2,800 mg/kg or 28 mmoles/kg) (7). In addition, bromide raises the minimal electroshock seizure threshold (ED_{50}, 1,800 mg/kg or 18.0 mmoles/kg). However, the blockage of tonic extensor seizures in the MES test is achieved only in toxic doses (TD_{50}, 2,200 mg/kg or 22 mmoles/kg). Bromide also blocks seizures induced by strychnine and by withdrawal from high concentrations of CO_2 in rats (ED_{50}, 2,880 mg/kg or 28.6 mmoles/kg) (30).

The effects of bromide on various neurophysiological parameters such as posttetanic potentiation or blockade of repetitive discharge in the spinal cord, evoked afterdischarge in the brain, and epileptogenic foci induced by penicillin, cobalt, or alumina gel have not been elucidated. Neither have its effects in kindled animals.

Even less information has been obtained on its neurochemical effects. N. K. Chakravarty and D. M. Woodbury (*unpublished observations*) have shown that a dose of 2,000 mg/kg (20 mmoles/kg) of bromide decreased intracellular sodium and caused an intracellular acidosis in brain cells of rats 24 hr after injection, a time when it had increased minimal electroshock threshold maximally. These data would suggest that bromide acts by altering membrane permeability and/or transport processes. In anticonvulsant doses Kemp and Woodbury (29; J. W. Kemp and D. M. Woodbury, *unpublished observations*) have shown that bromide also inhibits the activities of carbonic anhydrase and HCO_3^--ATPase in homogenates of rat brain tested *in vitro*. Gill et al. (6) have demonstrated that bromide (1×10^{-2}M) inhibits active chloride transport in isolated glial cells from rat brain. In large doses it inhibits oxidative metabolism of brain slices. See Woodbury (27) for an earlier review of the pharmalogical effects and mechanisms of action of bromide.

MECHANISMS OF ACTION

It is evident from the neurochemical data that bromide has marked actions on glial cells. This conclusion is derived from the fact that it inhibits carbonic anhydrase, also a glial enzyme, and blocks active Cl^- transport, also a glial process. Since the inhibition of carbonic anhydrase occurs at a lower dose than its inhibition of HCO_3^--ATPase, it is likely that at least some of its anticonvulsant effects result from inhibition of carbonic anhydrase. Both carbonic

anhydrase and HCO_3^--ATPase appear to be involved in active Cl^- transport by glial cells [see review by Woodbury and Kemp (29)], and bromide inhibition of these two enzymes as well as of Cl^- transport may contribute to its anticonvulsant action and also to the intracellular acidosis it produces, which probably occurs in glial cells. Since Cl^- transport into glial cells appears to be coupled to HCO_3^- transport, inhibition of this process by bromide would cause marked changes in acid–base status of the interstitial and intracellular fluids in the brain. The nature of these changes is yet to be elucidated.

In addition to effects on active transport across glial cell membranes, there is evidence that bromide affects passive movements of ions across brain cell membranes (see 27 for review). Thus, since bromide has a smaller hydrated diameter than chloride, its passive movement across cell membranes is faster than chloride; hence, in the large doses necessary to exert an anticonvulsant effect, bromide competes with chloride for anion channels in postsynaptic membranes that are activated by inhibitory neurotransmitters. Consequently, the faster movement of bromide would hyperpolarize the membrane and thus prevent spread of an epileptic discharge.

CLINICAL USE

The clinical management of seizure disorders by bromide has been reviewed by Carter (3) and Livingston and Pearson (13). Bromide is an effective agent in the management of certain intractable seizure disorders. Bromide has been reported to be effective in the management of major motor seizures, minor motor seizures, and focal seizures. However, the severe side effects of this agent, particularly the development of psychotic behavior that is associated with chronic bromide therapy, requires that it be administered with caution.

The optimal serum concentration of bromide necessary to achieve seizure control ranges from 10 to 20 mM. At serum concentrations about 15 mM, toxic symptoms frequently develop. Therefore, as serum bromide concentrations approach 10 mM, dosage increments should be small, and the patient's clinical course followed carefully. It is to be emphasized that the half-life of bromide is 12 days. Therefore, following any dosage change, the time required to reach a new steady state is 60 days. If a patient develops clinical symptoms of bromide intoxication, the medication should be discontinued until clinical improvement is clearly evident. Because of the slow elimination of bromide from the body, clinical signs of drug intoxication may persist for several days or weeks after discontinuation of therapy.

Relation of Plasma Bromide Levels to Therapeutic and Toxic Effect

A correlation among anticonvulsant activity, toxicity, log dose of administered sodium bromide, and the plasma concentration of bromide has been shown in mice by Grewal et al. (7). The results of this study are depicted in Fig. 2.

The relationship between the log dose of sodium bromide and the concentration of plasma bromide is linear. In mice, bromide is most effective against pentylenetetrazol-induced seizures and least effective in abolishing the tonic extensor phase of maximal electroshock seizures. The toxic dose (TD_{50}) lies between these two values. The data suggest that the efficacy of bromide can be determined by the concentration of the drug in the plasma. Brain and CSF levels also correlate with the plasma bromide levels.

In humans, there is also a reasonably good correlation between the therapeutic and toxic doses and the plasma bromide levels. The usual therapeutic dose of bromide in the treatment of generalized tonic–clonic seizures is 1 g three times daily, but this may be increased slowly to a maximum of 2 g three times daily. This dose generally produces plasma bromide levels

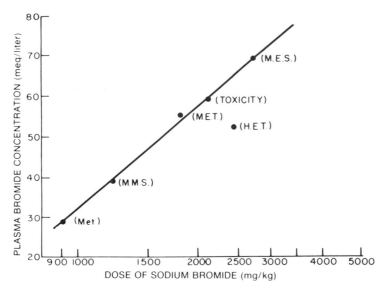

FIG. 2. Correlation between the dose of sodium bromide and the plasma bromide concentration in mice. The regression line was fitted to the plotted points by the method of least squares. The letters in parentheses indicate the ED_{50} or TD_{50} for various anticonvulsant and toxicity assay tests used to assess the correlation among dose, anticonvulsant or toxic effects, and plasma bromide level. Met, pentylenetetrazol test—elevation of threshold for minimal seizures induced by pentylenetetrazol; M.M.S., maximal pentylenetetrazol seizures test—ability of bromide to modify pattern of tonic–clonic seizures evoked by intravenous pentylenetetrazol; M.E.T., minimal electroshock seizure test—elevation of threshold for 60-cycle alternating current; H.E.T., hyponatremic electroshock threshold test—elevation of alternating current electroshock threshold in hyponatremic animals; M.E.S., maximal electroshock seizure test—modification of tonic–clonic pattern induced by supramaximal electrical stimulation; TOXICITY, TD_{50} for minimal overt signs of neurological deficit (From Grewal et al. ref. 7, with permission.)

of 10 to 20 meq/liter (1,000 to 2,000 μg/ml sodium bromide), which is the effective blood level range for the treatment of epilepsy. Toxic symptoms usually develop with levels of 15 meq/liter (1,500 μg/ml or greater). Therefore, in patients in whom the dose has to be raised to attain seizure control, toxic levels are necessary, and seizure control can be gained only at the expense of sedation and other toxic effects of the drug. The correlation between severity of bromide intoxication and plasma bromide levels is not perfect, however; patients in poor physical condition may show signs of severe intoxication with relatively low concentrations of the drug. Since the therapeutic and toxic doses overlap to some extent, careful adjustment of the daily bromide intake is essential to control the seizures. This requires an awareness of the factors that affect the plasma bromide levels, such as the physical condition of the patient, food, salt intake, dehydration, vomiting, diarrhea, and impaired renal function.

It is of interest that bromide was the first antiepileptic drug for which it was suggested that a correlation existed between serum concentration and clinical toxicity (32).

Toxicity

Acute bromide intoxication is rare because the drug irritates the gastrointestinal tract, and it is difficult to ingest and retain a sufficient amount to elevate plasma and brain bromide to a toxic level without vomiting. Chronic toxicity, however, does occur readily because bromide is very slowly excreted by the kidney, with a half-life of 12 days. Consequently, it tends to accumulate if taken daily, and a toxic level may be attained over a period of weeks.

The chronic state of bromide intoxication is called bromism (see 18). The signs and symptoms are referable to the nervous system, skin, glandular secretions, and gastrointestinal tract. The central nervous system effects are most common and dangerous. Mental disturbances consist of impaired thought and memory, drowsiness, dizziness, irritability, and emotional distortions. In higher doses, delirium, de-

lusions, hallucinations, mania, lethargy, or coma may occur. Electroencephalographic changes also appear at high plasma bromide levels. Neurological disturbances are also present and are generally characterized by motor incoordination.

The skin manifestations are reflected in a dermatitis known as a bromide rash. Other types of rashes occur more rarely. The respiratory, lacrimal, and exocrine glands are also affected. A mild conjunctivitis may occur. In the gastrointestinal tract, irritation by bromide produces many side effects such as anorexia, constipation, and gastric distress.

Large doses may cause emaciation as a result of weight loss and depletion of extracellular fluid.

Treatment of bromide intoxication involves hastening the excretion of bromide by administration of large quantities of sodium chloride and a chloruretic agent (see Excretion).

SUMMARY

Bromide is rapidly and completely absorbed from the fluid in the small intestine and distributed in the body generally in the same volume as chloride. The plasma half-life of the drug in humans is 12 days. Preferential accumulation occurs in gastric juice, saliva, and possibly the thyroid. Red cells have high concentrations of bromide because the transmembrane potential is low and the drug is probably passively distributed across the membranes of these cells. Bromide is distributed in muscle, as are chloride and iodide. Therapeutic doses of bromide (1 to 2 g three times a day) give plasma levels of 10 to 20 mM. Toxic manifestations appear at levels greater than 15 mM. No plasma binding or biotransformation of bromide occurs.

Bromide concentrations in CSF and brain are lower than in plasma. In humans, the CSF-to-plasma ratio is 0.3. The brain bromide space is less than the chloride space, even when based on CSF levels. Large loads of bromide increase the CSF and brain levels relative to the plasma. The evidence suggests that this monovalent inorganic anion is actively transported out of the CSF across the choroid plexus, as are iodide, thiocyanate, and perchlorate anions. Active transport across brain cells is also thought to occur, and this is blocked by anticonvulsant doses of the drug. The mechanisms of action of bromide as an antiepileptic agent is probably related to the inhibition of the transport of bromide out of the CSF and across brain cells.

Bromide is excreted slowly in the urine in competition with chloride. Reabsorption of these two anions occurs in the renal tubular cells, but bromide is preferentially reabsorbed. Large loads of chloride, however, can increase the excretion of bromide, as can chloruretic agents. This is the basis for treatment of chronic bromide intoxication (bromism). Bromism is characterized by side effects referable to the central nervous system, skin, exocrine glands, and the gastrointestinal tract.

ACKNOWLEDGMENTS

This work was supported by U. S. Public Health Service Program Project Grant 5-PO1-NS-15767 from the National Institute of Neurological and Communicative Disorders and Stroke. Dr. Woodbury is a Research Career Awardee (5-K6-NS-13838) of the NINCDS.

REFERENCES

1. Blumberg, A., and Nelp, W. B. (1966): Total body bromide excretion in a case of prolonged bromide intoxication. *Helv. Med. Acta,* 33:330–333.
2. Bodansky, O., and Modell, W. J. (1941): The differential excretion of bromide and chloride ions and its role in bromide retention. *J. Pharmacol. Exp. Ther.,* 73:51–65.
3. Carter, S. (1951): Use of anticonvulsant drugs. *Gen. Practitioner,* 4:41–46.
4. Cotlove, E., and Hogben, C. A. M. (1962): Chloride. In: *Mineral Metabolism. An Advanced Treatise.* Vol. II, Part B, *The Elements,* edited by C. L. Comar and F. Bronner, pp. 109–173. Academic Press, New York.
5. Gamble, J. J., Jr., Robertson, J. S., Hannigan, C. A., Foster, C. G., and Farr, L. E. (1953): Chloride, bromide, sodium, and sucrose spaces in man. *J. Clin. Invest.,* 32:483–489.
6. Gill, T. H., Young, O. M., and Tower, D. B. (1974): The uptake of ^{36}Cl into astrocytes in tissue culture by potassium-dependent, saturable process. *J. Neurochem.,* 23:1011–1018.
7. Grewal, M. S., Swinyard, E. A., Jensen, H. V., and

Goodman, L. S. (1954): Correlation between anticonvulsant activity and plasma concentration of bromide. *J. Pharmacol. Exp. Ther.,* 112:109–115.
8. Gross, J. (1962): Iodine and bromide. In: *Mineral Metabolism. An Advanced Treatise.* Vol. II, Part B. *The Elements,* edited by C. L. Comar and F. Bronner, pp. 221–285. Academic Press, New York.
9. Haerer, A. F., Tourtellotte, W. W., Richard, K. A., Gustafson, G. M., and Bryan, E. R. (1964): A study of the blood–cerebrospinal fluid–brain barrier in multiple sclerosis. I. Blood–cerebrospinal fluid barrier to sodium bromide. *Neurology (Minneap.),* 14:345–354.
10. Joynt, R. J. (1974): The use of bromides for epilepsy. *Am. J. Dis. Child.,* 128:362–363.
11. Kuriyama, K. (1970): Association of bromide with the synaptosomal fraction of mouse brain. *Life Sci.,* 9:1371–1380.
12. Lennox, W. G., (1957): The centenary of bromides. *N. Engl. J. Med.,* 265:887–890.
13. Livingston, S., and Pearson, P. H. (1953): Bromides and the treatment of epilepsy in children. *Am. J. Dis. Child.,* 86:717–720.
14. Locock, C. (1857): Discussion of paper by E. H. Sieveking: Analysis of 52 cases of epilepsy observed by author. *Lancet,* 1:527.
15. Norden, L. G., and Plaa, G. L. (1963): Interaction between sodium bromide and chlorpromazine. *Toxicol. Appl. Pharmacol.,* 5:437–444.
16. Pollay, M. (1966): Cerebrospinal fluid transport and the thiocyanate space of the brain. *Am. J. Physiol.,* 210:275–279.
17. Pollay, M. (1967): The processes affecting the distribution of bromide in blood, brain, and cerebrospinal fluid. *Exp. Neurol.,* 17:74–85.
18. Pozuelo-Utonda, J., Crawford, D. C., and Anderson, J. C. (1966): Bromism and epilepsy. *Int. J. Neuropsychiatry,* 2:90–97.
19. Reed, D. J., Woodbury, D. M., Jacobs, L., and Squires, R. (1965): Factors affecting the distribution of iodide in brain and cerebrospinal fluid. *Am. J. Physiol.,* 209:757–764.
20. Söremark, R. (1960): Distribution and kinetics of bromide ions in the mammalian body. Some experimental investigations using Br^{80m} and Br^{82}. *Acta Radiol. [Suppl.] (Stockh.),* 190:1–114.
21. Söremark, R. (1960): Excretion of bromide ions by human urine. *Acta Physiol. Scand.,* 50:306–310.
22. Söremark, R. (1960): The biological half-life of bromide ions in human blood. *Acta Physiol. Scand.,* 50:119–123.
23. Wallace, G. B., and Brodie, B. B. (1939): The distribution of iodide, thiocyanate, bromide, and chloride in the central nervous system and spinal fluid. *J. Pharmacol. Exp. Ther.,* 65:220–226.
24. Wallace, G. B., and Brodie, B. B. (1940): The passage of bromide, iodide and thiocyanate into and out of the cerebrospinal fluid. *J. Pharmacol. Exp. Ther.,* 68:50–55.
25. Weir, E. G., and Hastings, A. B. (1939): The distribution of bromide and chloride in tissues and body fluids. *J. Biol. Chem.,* 129:547–558.
26. Woodbury, D. M. (1967): Distribution of nonelectro-

lytes and electrolytes in the brain as affected by alterations in cerebrospinal fluid secretion. *Prog. Brain Res.*, 29:297–313.

27. Woodbury, D. M. (1969): Mechanisms of action of anticonvulsants. In: *Basic Mechanisms of the Epilepsies,* edited by H. H. Jasper, A. A. Ward, and A. Pope, pp. 647–681. Little, Brown, Boston.

28. Woodbury, D. M. (1969): Role of pharmacological factors in the evaluation of anticonvulsant drugs. *Epilepsia,* 10:121–144.

29. Woodbury, D. M., and Kemp, J. W. (1977): Basic mechanisms of seizures: Neurophysiological and biochemical etiology. In: *Psychopathology and Brain Dysfunction,* edited by C. Shagass, S. Gershon, and A. J. Friedhoff, pp. 149–182. Raven Press, New York.

30. Woodbury, D. M., Rollins, L. T., Gardner, M. D., Hirschi, W. C., Hogan, J. R., Rallison, M. L., Tanner, G. S., and Brodie, D. A. (1958): Effects of carbon dioxide on brain excitability and electrolytes. *Am. J. Physiol.,* 192:79–90.

31. Woodward, D. L., Reed, D. J., and Woodbury, D. M. (1967): Extracellular space of rat cerebral cortex. *Am. J. Physiol.,* 212:367–370.

32. Wuth, O. (1927): Rational bromide treatment; new methods for its control. *J.A.M.A.,* 88:2013–2017.

Antiepileptic Drugs, edited by D. M. Woodbury,
J. K. Penry, and C E. Pippenger. Raven Press,
New York © 1982.

70

Potential Antiepileptic Drugs

Eterobarb: Absorption, Distribution, Biotransformation, and Excretion

Mark A. Goldberg

Eterobarb, or dimethoxymethylphenobarbital (DMMP), has been reported to be an effective anticonvulsant in animals and man. Although it has not been as extensively studied as many of the older anticonvulsants, the available information concerning its distribution and biotransformation exceeds, in many respects, that of several of these agents and permits a relatively good understanding of its clinical pharmacokinetics.

CHEMISTRY AND METHODS OF DETERMINATION

Eterobarb, or 1,3-bis(methoxymethyl)-5-ethyl-5-phenylbarbituric acid (Fig. 1), is one of a series of alkoxymethyl derivatives of barbituric acid synthesized by Samour et al. (12) by condensation with various alkyl halomethyl ethers. Preliminary anticonvulsant screening of the series showed DMMP to be the most active in protecting mice from maximal electroshock seizures. The compound has a molecular weight of 320 and is soluble in acetone, dichloroethane, and chloroform. It is a much weaker acid than phenobarbital, and, although it can be extracted from acidified aqueous solutions with organic solvents, back extraction into alkaline solutions is incomplete.

Thin-Layer Chromatography

Eterobarb and its metabolites (following extraction from serum) can be separated by thin-layer chromatography (TLC), although spot recognition and quantitation are difficult. Alvin and Bush (1) employed ChromAR-1000 plates developed with chloroform–acetone (9 : 1) in a descending system and found R_f values of 0.83 to 0.86 for DMMP as compared with 0.47 to 0.51 for phenobarbital (PB) and 0.74 to 0.77 for methoxymethylphenobarbital (MMP). Ascending TLC on silicagel plates developed with iso-octane–glacial acetic acid–acetone (15 : 3 : 1) has also provided adequate separation with R_f values of 0.64 for DMMP, 0.29 for MMP, and 0.20 for PB (9). Spots may be visualized by UV, and the plate scraped; scrapings may be extracted and quantitated by standard methods for the determination of barbiturates (Chapter 21).

Eterobarb can be isolated and purified by the countercurrent distribution technique. Alvin and Bush (1) employed a 4 × 4 system with iso-

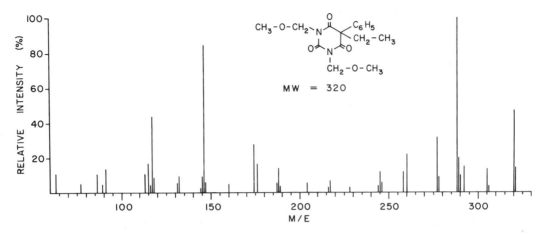

FIG. 1. The mass spectrum and structural formula of unlabeled dimethyoxymethylphenobarbital, [²H₀]DMMP. (From Goldberg et al., ref. 6, with permission.)

octane versus 0.1 M borate buffer, pH 10. They also described appropriate solvents for the separation of the metabolites of the parent compound by this method.

Gas–Liquid Chromatography

Eterobarb can be measured by gas–liquid chromatography (GLC) following extraction from serum or tissue without prior derivatization. Goldberg et al. (6) used 1 m × 2 mm silanized glass columns packed with 2% OV-101 on GasChrom Q at 185°C with helium as the carrier gas (34 ml/min). Under these conditions, retention time was only 80 sec. Three percent OV-17 at 215°C has been used for measurement of DMMP with a longer retention time (4.3 min) (11). Phenobarbital and MMP, the major metabolites of DMMP, have also been determined with GLC by using standard methods of detecting barbiturates. These compounds may be methylated with trimethylphenylammonium or diazomethane prior to separation on 3% OV-17 GasChrom Q (3). Appropriate internal standards must be used as with all GLC techniques.

Gas Chromotography–Mass Spectrometry

Gas chromatography–mass spectrometry (GC/MS) is one of the newer analytical techniques in clinical pharmacology and has been em-

ployed to evaluate the metabolism of DMMP. For this reason, a brief description of this method follows. Several reviews are available (7,8).

The metabolism of DMMP has been investigated in man both after a single dose and during chronic administration, employing an integrated GC/MS system (6). Gas chromatography is an excellent separative technique but provides little or no information about the identity of the components measured. Mass spectrometry yields a great deal of information about the structure of a pure compound, which is often sufficient for its identification. Coupling the two instruments results in an extremely sensitive analytical method that is well suited to problems in clinical pharmacology. With the use of a multiple-ion monitoring device or an interactive computer to control the system as well as store information, an even more versatile instrument is available. Recently, the use of compounds labeled with stable isotopes has increased the precision and reproducibility of the method and permitted experiments in man that were previously unsafe or impossible. The use of stable isotopes such as ²H, ¹³C, ¹⁵N, and ¹⁸O carries negligible risk, as these isotopes occur naturally, and additional tracer doses do not add appreciably to the body's burden.

The output of a mass spectrometer consists of a highly characteristic pattern of fragments into which a molecule splits when it is ionized. Un-

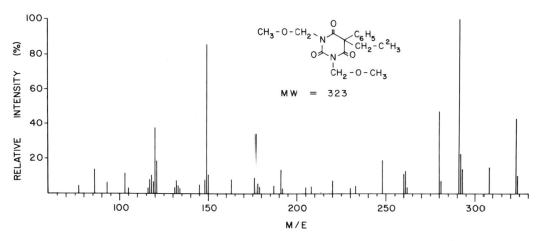

FIG.2. The mass spectrum and structural formula of dimethoxymethylphenobarbital labeled with three atoms of deuterium, [$^2H_3$]DMMP. (From Goldberg et al., ref. 6, with permission.)

der constant conditions both the masses of these fragments and their relative abundance are characteristic of a particular molecule. These data constitute a mass spectrum and are generally represented as a bar graph normalized so that the most abundant ion has a relative abundance of 100%. Figure 1 illustrates the mass spectrum of DMMP. The abscissa is the mass/charge ratio (m/e), and because the charge is usually unity, this normally corresponds to the mass of the fragment. The most abundant ion has a mass of 288, with a second peak at 146, representing a relative abundance of 84.63 as compared with 100.00 for the largest peak. Figure 2 is the mass

spectrum of DMMP synthesized with three atoms of deuterium on the ethyl group, [$^2H_3$]DMMP. The largest peak has been shifted up 3 mass units to 291, and the second largest to 149. If a mixture of unlabeled and labeled drug were analyzed, both sets of spectra would be obtained, with each pair of peaks separated by 3 mass units. Such pairs are termed doublets, and the relative heights of each peak within such doublets is a measure of the relative proportion of labeled and unlabeled material in the original mixture. Figures 3 and 4 are the mass spectra of the *N*-methyl derivatives of MMP and phenobarbital with most abundant ions at 247 and 233, respectively. In

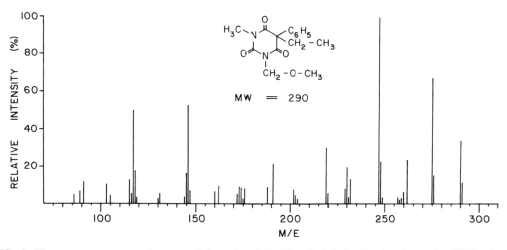

FIG. 3. The mass spectrum and structural formula of the *N*-methyl derivative (made on the GLC column) of monomethoxymethylphenobarbital, [$^2H_0$]MMP.

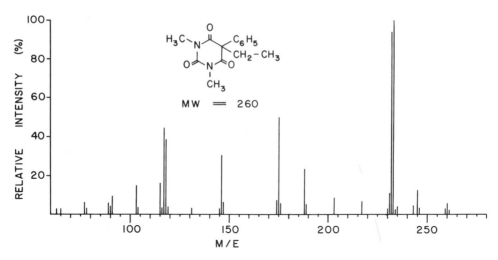

FIG. 4. The mass spectrum and structural formula of the *N*-methyl derivative (made on the GLC column) of phenobarbital.

general, the most abundant peak is monitored for quantitative studies, but smaller peaks may be used if necessary, particularly for purposes of identification.

Gal et al. (3) monitored masses 288, 291, and 294 in their study of DMMP and masses 275, 278, and 235 to measure MMP.

BIOTRANSFORMATION, DISTRIBUTION, AND EXCRETION

Reports of the effectiveness of DMMP as an anticonvulsant in experimental animals and in patients with epilepsy stimulated considerable interest in the biotransformation of this compound. Examination of its structure (Fig. 1) suggests a number of possible metabolites, and it was thought that these metabolites may contribute to the anticonvulsant activity of the compound in a manner analogous to the case of primidone. A number of reports describing its metabolic fate have appeared.

Animal Studies

Alvin and Bush (1) investigated the biotransformation of [^{14}C]DMMP by a 9000 × *g* supernatant of rat liver homogenate. After 8 min of incubation, 44% of the DMMP in the incubation mix had undergone biotransformation. Nearly all of the metabolites (96%) were found to be indistinguishable from reference MMP by several methods. The remainder were made up of a small amount of PB and an unidentified metabolite. Methoxymethylphenobarbital was then isolated and incubated with fresh supernatant and underwent almost quantitative transformation to PB, but at a much slower rate. Again, a small amount of an unidentified metabolite was noted. They subsequently administered [^{14}C]-DMMP to rats and found only PB and *p*-hydroxyphenobarbital and its conjugates in the urine of these animals over a 4-day period.

Baumel et al. (2) undertook a more extensive investigation of the metabolism and distribution of MMP in the rat. Thirty minutes after intraperitoneal administration of [^{14}C]DMMP, the parent compound accounted for less than 3% of plasma radioactivity, whereas MMP was 76% and PB 12% of the activity. Plasma MMP increased for 1 hr and then decreased with a half-life of 0.8 hr. A small amount of another metabolite, which they suggested might be mephobarbital, was detected at the early time intervals. When MMP was administered orally to rats, peak serum levels were obtained in 30 to 60 min and then rapidly declined. When the hepatic microsome enzyme inhibitor SKF-525A was administered prior to DMMP, there was a marked reduction in serum MMP levels, a corresponding increase in serum DMMP levels, and a decline in serum PB levels, thus confirming the hepatic microsomal enzymes as the site of biotransformation of this compound. Gal et al. (3), using GC/MS, found that DMMP peaked in the serum approximately 20 min after intravenous injection, with a rapid decline to almost undetectable levels at 2 hr. They too reported detecting high levels of MMP within the first 40 min after administration of the parent compound. In contrast to the above studies, Rapport and Kupferberg (11) were unable to detect MMP in the serum of mice unless very large doses of DMMP or a metabolic inhibitor were administered. It appears likely that their failure to detect MMP was a consequence of the extraction method employed. The same authors also compared serum levels of PB derived from DMMP to serum PB levels from directly administered PB. They reported that within 2 hr, equivalent doses resulted in almost identical serum levels of PB regardless of the drug administered. They were unable to detect any other metabolites of DMMP in mice.

Tissue Distribution

As would be expected, tissue levels generally reflect serum concentrations of DMMP and its metabolites. Only minute amounts of DMMP have been found in the brains of experimental animals after i.p. or i.v. administration. Gal et al. (3), using the most sensitive technique, GC/MS, were able to detect a peak value of about 10 μmole/g at 10 min after i.v. administration of 6 mg/kg to the rat. These levels then fell with a half-life of approximately 5 min. Maximum levels of MMP have been found in brain at 40 to 60 min after administration of DMMP either by i.v. or i.p. routes. Following the administration of MMP orally, peak brain levels occurred at about 1 hr and subsequently declined (2). In all studies, PB accumulated over time following a single dose, with maximum levels occurring at 4 hr, which is the longest duration of any of the studies in animals.

The relatively slow penetration of MMP into brain as compared with phenobarbital may be a reflection of the greater protein binding of the former. In any related series of barbiturates, greater lipid solubility is associated with increased plasma protein binding (5). Eterobarb has a greater lipid solubility than its metabolites and therefore should have the greatest penetration into brain. The plasma levels achieved are so low, however, that this is rarely demonstrated except in the first few minutes following i.v. administration (3). Under ordinary conditions, the high lipid solubility of DMMP permits its rapid entry into hepatic cells where it can then undergo metabolic degradation by the microsomal enzyme systems more rapidly. This rapid degradation by the liver, when associated with oral administration, has been referred to as the "first pass" effect.

In summary, the preclinical studies indicated that DMMP was rapidly metabolized by hepatic microsomal enzymes to MMP, which was subsequently broken down to PB. Tissue levels of the two metabolites generally reflected the serum levels, and a small amount of an unidentified third metabolite was noted by several, but not all, investigators. The primary question then facing clinical investigators related to the accumulation of the metabolites of the parent compound as well as specific differences in metabolism by humans.

Clinical Pharmacology

Single-Dose Pharmacokinetics

A total of 10 patients have been evaluated in studies using labeled DMMP. Matsumoto and Gallagher (9) administered [14C]DMMP to four patients orally. They were unable to detect unchanged DMMP in the serum or urine of any of the patients over a 5-day study period. Both [14C]MMP and [14C]PB appeared in the serum within 5 min after administration. The MMP peaked at 30 min and declined with a half-life of 4 to 6 hr. Phenobarbital reached maximum concentration several hours after administration and then demonstrated its usual long half-life.

Examination of the urine for metabolites revealed that 27% of the administered drug was excreted in the first 24 hr. The urine contained unchanged PB and trace amounts of MMP and three polar metabolites. One of these was *p*-hydroxyphenobarbital. All three of the metabolites were in part conjugated as glucuronides. In addition, a large percentage of the radioactivity in the urine was unextractable with ether.

Goldberg et al. (6) administered deuterated DMMP to six patients who had not received PB or a related barbiturate. All subjects were given 120 mg of eterobarb in a capsule that contained an equimolar mixture of unlabeled drug, [$^2H_0$]DMMP, and drug labeled with three atoms of deuterium, [$^2H_3$]DMMP. This served to facilitate the study of single-dose pharmacokinetics of the parent compound and known metabolites in blood and saliva and enabled a search for additional metabolites in urine.

No unchanged DMMP was found in any of the samples of serum, saliva, or urine of any subject at any time following oral administra-tion despite a detection level of 50 pmole/ml. This was consistent with the rapid decline seen in the animal experiments and indicated a prominent "first pass" effect. Serum levels of MMP and phenobarbital in a patient are shown in Fig. 5; MMP was detected in serum within 30 min and usually reached a peak within 90 min. In five of six patients, a peak level averaging 1.96 nmole/ml (0.46 μg/ml) was reached in an average of 1.3 hr. Following the peak, serum levels of MMP fell rapidly with a half-life of approximately 3.3 hr. Phenobarbital was detectable early, usually within 15 min after oral administration of DMMP, and rose to an average maximum of 4.90 nmole/ml (1.37 μg/ml) in 12 to 24 hr. As expected, serum levels of PB fell slowly with a half-life of 4 to 7 days (6).

Because the drug was administered in a labeled form in which the isotopic label was metabolically stable, the metabolites were also labeled, and $^2H_0$ and $^2H_3$ variants of both MMP and PB could be measured separately. The levels of the two variants paralleled each other

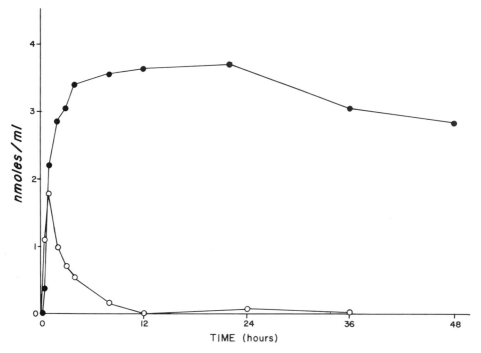

FIG. 5. Typical plasma concentrations for MMP (*open circles*) and PB (*closed circles*) following oral administration of single 12-mg dose of DMMP. (From Goldberg et al., ref. 6, with permission.)

closely for both compounds and showed no systematic deviation from equality, which would have suggested an isotope effect on metabolism. This parallelism is illustrated in Fig. 6.

Chronic Pharmacokinetics

All patients chronically treated with DMMP develop serum levels of PB that are within or above the usually accepted therapeutic range (4,6,10). In the study of Mattson et al. (10), patients receiving an average of 420 mg of DMMP per day (6.2 mg/kg) developed serum levels of 27 µg/ml. In the study of Gallagher et al. (4), patients receiving an average of 6.7 mg/kg of DMMP had a serum concentration of 43 µg/ml. Matsumoto and Gallagher (9) administered [14C]DMMP to two patients who had been chronically treated with unlabeled drug. One patient received the labeled compound orally, and the second received it intravenously. In the former patient, PB levels were slightly higher in the early time period following administration as compared with the pretreatment study. There was a concomitant decline in MMP levels in that patient, suggesting more rapid dealkylation after chronic administration. In the other patient, there was no difference between oral

and intravenous administration with the exception of the finding of very small amounts of unchanged DMMP in the early time periods following the i.v. dose.

Goldberg et al. (6) maintained two patients on 240 mg of DMMP daily for several months. They were then given a single dose of 100% [2H3]DMMP in place of the usual dose of unlabeled DMMP which was subsequently reinstituted. This interposed pulse of deuterated DMMP allowed measurement of single-dose pharmacokinetics in chronically treated patients, which was then compared with the study of the same patients prior to the initiation of chronic therapy.

Figure 7 shows the serum levels of [2H0]MMP and [2H3]MMP during the steady-state phase of the study following the pulse dose of deuterated drug in one of the chronically treated subjects. There appeared to be no effect of unlabeled MMP on the kinetics of elimination of [2H3]MMP. This indicates that the factors controlling distribution and elimination of MMP are linear and not subject to saturation under these conditions. A similar observation was made in the other patient.

Figure 8 compares the time course of plasma levels of MMP following the initial dose of

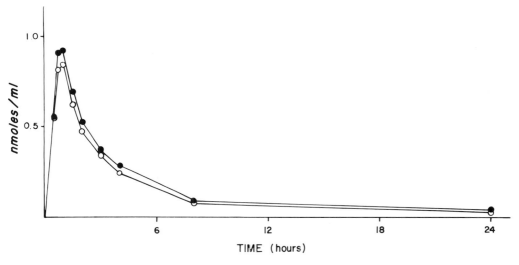

FIG. 6. Comparison of the time course of plasma levels of [2H0]MMP (*open circles*) and [2H3]MMP (*closed circles*) following a single oral dose of an equimolar mixture of [2H0]DMMP and [2H3]DMMP. The near identity of the two curves indicates that there is no difference in metabolism of the isotope-labeled compound.

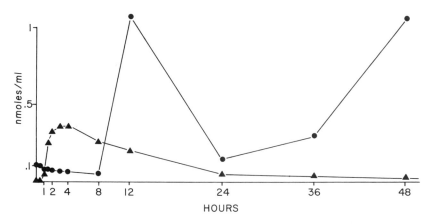

FIG. 7. Plasma levels of [$^2H_0$]MMP (*circles*) and [$^2H_3$]MMP (*triangles*) during steady-state treatment of a patient with [$^2H_0$]DMMP at zero time. Subsequent doses of [$^2H_0$]DMMP were given at 7, 33, and 48 hr. (From Goldberg et al., ref. 6, with permission.)

DMMP and an interposed dose of [$^2H_3$]DMMP during steady state. In both patients, the concentration of MMP rose to a higher peak and fell with a shorter time constant following the initial dose. This difference was not caused by an isotope effect in metabolism, as the time courses of [$^2H_0$]MMP and [$^2H_3$]MMP are virtually identical when administered simultaneously (see Fig. 6). It appears likely that it resulted from a difference in the pharmaceutical formulation between the two doses (6).

Urine from the initial study was analyzed for the presence of metabolites of DMMP by seeking doublets in the mass spectra that are separated by 1, 2, or 3 mass units. In order to monitor approximately 50 gas chromatographic peaks in each urine sample, the mass spectrometer scanned the output of the gas chromatograph through a mass range of 10 to 520 continuously every 2 sec under the control of a data system that also recorded all of the output data digitally on magnetic tape. The output from a single urine

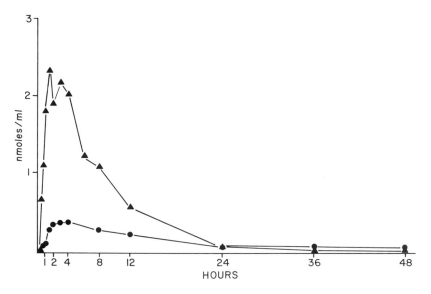

FIG. 8. Comparison of plasma concentration profiles of MMP after the initial single dose and an interposed dose of labeled DMMP. See text for explanation. (From Goldberg et al., ref. 6, with permission.)

sample resulted in a matrix of the order of 500 mass units $\times$ 500 scans or 250,000 data points for each of 25 samples. It was therefore impossible to seek out significant doublets manually. A program was developed (13) to conduct this search automatically using the data from the magnetic tape and an IBM 360/91 computer.

Doublet-containing spectra identified in most specimens were derived from PB and *p*-hydroxyphenobarbital. No DMMP or MMP were found in any sample. An additional doublet-containing spectrum was found consistently in five of six patients. This occurred in a peak eluting at 85 sec, and the doublet was separated by 1 mass unit (124–125). It was not present in urine from a patient receiving only PB and was quite variable in quantity and relationship to phenobarbital. The exact composition of this possible metabolite remains unknown, but it may be related to the unidentified metabolite described by others.

SUMMARY AND CONCLUSIONS

Eterobarb is rapidly absorbed following oral administration but undergoes rapid and complete metabolism in the liver, i.e., the first pass effect.

The initial metabolite is MMP which appears in the blood in very low concentration (0.5 µg/ml) and with a short half-life that precludes accumulation.

The major metabolite of DMMP is phenobarbital, which in usual dosages reaches high therapeutic concentrations in serum.

The anticonvulsant effects of DMMP can be completely explained by its conversion to phenobarbital.

Small amounts of as yet unidentified metabolites may occur, but these are present in very low concentration and appear to be polar compounds which would not be expected to cross the blood–brain barrier.

The reported decreased sedation that may occur in patients receiving DMMP cannot be explained by its biotransformation or pharmaco-kinetics and, in fact, is difficult to understand in the light of existing data on barbiturate pharmacology.

REFERENCES

1. Alvin, J., and Bush, M. (1974): The metabolic fate of *N,N*-dimethoxymethylphenobarbital in the rat. *J. Pharmacol. Exp. Ther.*, 188:8–14.
2. Baumel, I., Gallagher, B., DiMicco, J., and Dionne, R. (1976): Metabolism, distribution and anticonvulsant properties of *N,N*-dimethoxymethylphenobarbital in the rat. *J. Pharmacol. Exp. Ther.*, 196:180–187.
3. Gal, J., Hodshon, B., and Cho, A. (1975): Quantitative determination of phenobarbital derivatives by GC/MS. In: *Proceedings of the Second International Conference on Stable Isotopes*, edited by E. Klein and P. Klein, pp. 177–185. United States Atomic Energy Commission, Washington.
4. Gallagher, B., Baumel, I., Woodbury, S., and DiMicco, J. (1975): Clinical evaluation of eterobarb, a new anticonvulsant drug. *Neurology (Minneap.)*, 25:399–404.
5. Goldbaum, L. R., and Smith, P. K. (1954): The interaction of barbiturates with serum albumin and its possible relation to their disposition and pharmacological actions. *J. Pharmacol. Exp. Ther.*, 111:197–209.
6. Goldberg, M. A., Gal, J., Cho, A. K., and Jenden, D. J. (1979): Metabolism of dimethoxymethylphenobarbital (eterobarb) in patients with epilepsy. *Ann. Neurol.*, 5:121–126.
7. Jenden, D. J. (1978): Applications of GC/MS in psychopharmacology. In: *Psychopharmacology: A Generation of Progress*, edited by M. A. Lipton, A. DiMascio, and K. F. Killam, pp. 879–886. Raven Press, New York.
8. Jenden, D. J., and Cho, A. K. (1979): Selected ion monitoring in pharmacology. *Biochem. Pharmacol.*, 28:705–713.
9. Matsumoto, H., and Gallagher, B. (1976): Metabolism and excretion of ^{14}C eterobarb in epileptic patients. In: *Epileptology*, edited by D. Janz, pp. 122–129. Georg Thieme, Stuttgart.
10. Mattson, R., Williamson, M., and Hanahan, E. (1976): Eterobarb therapy in epilepsy. *Neurology (Minneap.)*, 26:1014–1017.
11. Rapport, R., and Kupferberg, H. (1973): Metabolism of dimethyoxymethylphenobarbital in mice. Relationship between brain phenobarbital levels and anticonvulsant activity. *J. Med. Chem.*, 16:599–602.
12. Samour, C., and Reinhard, V. J. (1971): Anticonvulsants 1. Alkoxymethyl derivatives of barbiturates and diphenylhydantoin. *J. Med. Chem.*, 14:187–189.
13. Steinborn, J. A., and Jenden, D. J. (1976): A method for the automatic detection of isotopic clusters in repetitive GC/MS scans. In: *Proceedings of the 24th Annual Conference on Mass Spectrometry and Allied Topics, San Diego*, pp. 172. American Society for Mass Spectrometry, San Diego, CA.

Antiepileptic Drugs, edited by D. M. Woodbury,
J. K. Penry, and C. E. Pippenger. Raven Press,
New York © 1982.

71

Potential Antiepileptic Drugs

Eterobarb: Clinical Aspects

Richard H. Mattson

Eterobarb (1,3-dimethoxymethylphenobarbital) was synthesized and tested for pharmacological properties by Samour et al. (11) in 1971. The development of this new antiepileptic drug represents the most recent effort in a 70-year search for an analog or derivative of phenobarbital possessing the same broad spectrum of efficacy and relative safety but with lesser hypnotic properties.

The initial animal studies by Samour et al. (11) gave promise that eterobarb indeed had antiepileptic properties comparable to those of phenobarbital but was without hypnotic effects. Subsequently, clinical studies were undertaken by Gallagher et al. (2) in 1972 to test the effect in human subjects. This open trial suggested that eterobarb possessed antiepileptic efficacy equal to or greater than phenobarbital and in many cases was associated with less sedative effect. Later clinical trials supported these findings (4,5,9, 12,14).

Pharmacological studies of eterobarb in both animals and humans have indicated a rapid biotransformation to phenobarbital and much lesser amounts of monomethoxymethylphenobarbital (1,6,8,10). Animal studies of monomethoxymethylphenobarbital have shown anticonvulsive potency comparable to or somewhat less than phenobarbital (1,10). Very small quantities of methyl- and dimethylphenobarbital have

also been found in animals by some investigators (1,8). Studies of urinary excretion in animals and humans have identified unmetabolized phenobarbital and conjugated hydroxyphenobarbital (1,6,8), although in humans other unidentified metabolites also have been detected (8,10).

EFFICACY

The initial clinical trials of eterobarb were carried out by Gallagher et al. (2,4) in 37 patients with intractable tonic–clonic and/or partial seizures. They reported a 47 to 70% decrease in seizures in 12 of 13 patients (93%) with tonic–clonic seizures and in 19 of 28 patients (67%) with partial seizures. Smith and Roomet (14) obtained comparable results in 20 patients. Smith (12) also tested eterobarb in 10 children with poorly controlled seizures and reported improvement in all patients. Seizures decreased a mean of 81%. Mattson et al. (9) carried out a controlled trial comparing the efficacy and toxicity of eterobarb and phenobarbital in a 3-month crossover study in which neither patients nor investigator were aware of which drug was being given. All patients were also receiving phenytoin, the levels of which were kept constant throughout the trial. Of the 21 patients completing the 6-month study (each drug was administered for 3 months), there was no significant difference in mean number of seizures occurring while on either drug. This indicated that eterobarb possessed equal efficacy to phenobarbital under the design of the trial.

It was noted that the mean phenobarbital levels in patients taking eterobarb were significantly higher than in those receiving phenobarbital (27 versus 22 μg/ml). The possibility that eterobarb in some way conferred greater efficacy was suggested by the observation that three patients were removed from the trial when status epilepticus developed during crossover from eterobarb to phenobarbital (Fig. 1). Interestingly, the phenobarbital and phenytoin levels remained unchanged at the time of the status epilepticus. Such a finding in three cases might have been coincidental, but it raised the possibility that some metabolite of eterobarb, such as monomethoxymethylphenobarbital, had disappeared during the crossover, resulting in the exacerbation of seizures.

Before the blind was broken, a drug of preference was selected by each of the 27 patients given both drugs; 12 selected eterobarb, 6 phenobarbital, and 9 had no preference. The patient's choice was based on overall benefit judged by better seizure control and/or reduction in side effects. A similar study of 18 patients was reported by Gallagher and Woodbury (5). Eight patients who had fewer seizures were receiving eterobarb, two had fewer attacks while on phenobarbital, and six had no significant difference in seizure frequency between the two drug treatment periods. Mean serum concentration of phenobarbital was 59 μg/ml during eterobarb treatment and 44 μg/ml while the patients were taking phenobarbital. Goldberg et al. (6) concluded that the superior efficacy found in patients receiving eterobarb could be explained as an expected consequence of the higher phenobarbital levels.

TOXICITY

Systemic side effects have not been found in any of the 126 patients reported in various clinical studies. Perhaps twice as many other pa-

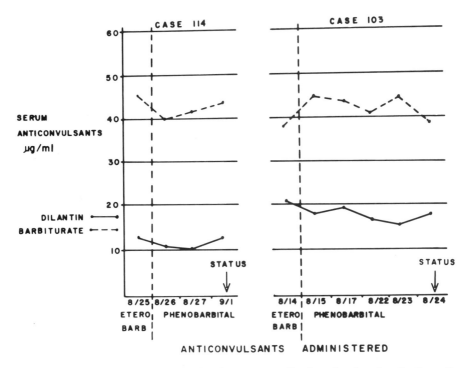

FIG. 1. Anticonvulsant levels in two patients in whom status epilepticus developed at the time of crossover from eterobarb to phenobarbital. (From ref. 9, with permission.)

tients have safely received the drug at some time. The absence of these side effects is not surprising, since those patients with a history of barbiturate sensitivity were excluded from most eterobarb trials. However, eterobarb or its metabolites have not produced changes in liver, kidney or other organ function. We have treated 57 patients with eterobarb over the past 9 years. The patients have received the drug for a mean of 3.5 years, and no systemic toxicity has been detected. Among these 57 patients was one woman who became pregnant while taking eterobarb and subsequently delivered a normal male child.

Neurotoxic side effects have been similar to those associated with the use of phenobarbital (Chapter 26). The initial animal studies (11) and open clinical trials (2,4) suggested that eterobarb produced much less sedation than phenobarbital while providing similar or superior seizure control. Smith et al. (13) found confirmatory evidence in a controlled study of volunteers. In this study, 40 subjects were divided into four groups and received either eterobarb, phenobarbital, placebo, or no treatment. Subjective and objective side effects as well as psychological test performance were measured over the next 14 weeks. Neurotoxicity appeared at lower blood levels of phenobarbital in those receiving phenobarbital than in those taking eterobarb. Interestingly, two student volunteers withdrew from the study because their ability to study was impaired. Both were subsequently found to be taking the placebo. Similarly, one patient in the controlled trial by Mattson et al. (9) became markedly sedated on beginning the unknown drug. Prior to this, she had been receiving eterobarb and tolerating it well with serum phenobarbital levels near 25 µg/ml. The appearance of side effects of sedation, dysarthria, and irritability forced withdrawal from the trial. Subsequent analysis revealed that she had been randomized to eterobarb, so, in fact, no change in medication had actually occurred, and her serum phenobarbital level similarly remained unchanged. These examples illustrate the powerful potential for placebo effect and difficulty in assessing side effects in uncontrolled trials. In the controlled studies by Mattson et al.

(9) and Gallagher and Woodbury (5), the side effects reported were similar in patients on eterobarb or phenobarbital. Since serum phenobarbital levels were higher when patients were receiving eterobarb than when receiving phenobarbital, it has been suggested that eterobarb therapy possesses a higher therapeutic index (sedative dose/effective dose) than phenobarbital.

In an unpublished study, we found no acute neurotoxicity in six barbiturate-naive patients when they were given 120 mg of eterobarb three times daily for 2 weeks. Sedation appeared only when metabolically derived phenobarbital accumulated in the blood. This finding indicates that eterobarb and its metabolites, including monomethoxymethylphenobarbital, are free of side effects in quantities found after administration of usual doses of eterobarb. This is in sharp contrast to the acute effect of primidone which often produces neurotoxicity before appreciable amounts of phenobarbital accumulate in the blood (3).

DISCUSSION

Clinical studies have consistently found that eterobarb therapy confers equal or greater seizure control than that obtained when the same patients received phenobarbital. Because only small quantities of the other active anticonvulsant metabolite, monomethoxymethylphenobarbital, have been found in the blood of epileptic patients treated with eterobarb, the greater efficacy of eterobarb may have resulted from higher blood phenobarbital levels. The reports of equal or lesser degrees of neurotoxicity in patients is more difficult to explain. We have suggested that some metabolite of eterobarb, possibly monomethoxyphenobarbital, may possess both agonist and antagonist properties to phenobarbital, blocking brain receptors for sedation while conferring antiepileptic effects. Such a pharmacodynamic interaction would be analogous to the effect of nalorphine on morphine (7). Goldberg et al. (6) correctly point out that no current data on barbiturate pharmacology support such a mechanism of action in eterobarb treatment.

CONCLUSION

The efficacy and safety of enterobarb seem well documented, albeit in a relatively small number of studies. Further pharmacological studies are needed to provide evidence of actions of enterobarb independent of or in addition to the metabolically derived phenobarbital.

REFERENCES

1. Baumel, I., Gallagher, B., DiMicco, J., and Dionne, R. (1976): Metabolism, distribution and anticonvulsant properties of *N,N*-dimethoxymethylphenobarbital in the rat. *J. Pharmacol. Exp. Ther.*, 196:180–187.
2. Gallagher, B. B., Baumel, I. P., and Mattson, R. H. (1973): Clinical evaluation of a new anticonvulsant: Dimethoxymethylphenobarbital. *Neurology (Minneap.)*, 25:405.
3. Gallagher, B. B., Baumel, I. P., Mattson, R. H., and Woodbury, S. G. (1973): Primidone, diphenylhydantoin, and phenobarbital: Aspects of acute and chronic toxicity. *Neurology (Minneap.)*, 23:145–149.
4. Gallagher, B. B., Baumel, I. P., Woodbury, S., and DiMicco, J. (1975): Clinical evaluation of eterobarb, a new anticonvulsant drug. *Neurology (Minneap.)*, 25:399–404.
5. Gallagher, B. B., and Woodbury, S. (1976): A double blind comparison of the anticonvulsants, eterobarb and phenobarbital. In: *Epileptology*, edited by D. Janz, Georg Thieme, Stuttgart.
6. Goldberg, M., Gal, J., Cho, A. K., and Jenden, D. J. (1979): Metabolism of dimethoxymethylphenobar-bital (Eterobarb) in patients with epilepsy. *Ann. Neurol.*, 5:121–126.
7. Martin, W. R., Eades, C. G., Thompson, J. A., Huppler, R. E., and Gilbert, P. E. (1976): The effect of morphine and nalorphine-like drugs in the non-dependent and morphine dependent chronic spinal dog. *J. Pharmacol. Exp. Ther.*, 197:517–532.
8. Matsumoto, H., and Gallagher, B. (1976): Metabolism and excretion of C eterobarb in epileptic patients. In: *Proceedings of the 7th International Symposium on Epilepsy*, edited by D. Janz, pp. 122–129. Littleton, Ma. Publishing Science Group.
9. Mattson, R. H., Williamson, P. D., and Hanahan, E. (1976): Eterobarb therapy in epilepsy. *Neurology (Minneap.)*, 26:1014–1017.
10. Rapport, R., and Kupferberg, H. (1973): Metabolism of dimethoxymethylphenobarbital in mice. Relationship between brain phenobarbital levels and anticonvulsant activity. *J. Med. Chem.*, 16:599–602.
11. Samour, C. M., Reinhard, J. R., and Vida, J. A. (1971): Anticonvulsants 1. Alkoxymethyl derivatives of barbiturates and dephenylhydantoin. *J. Med. Chem.*, 14:187–189.
12. Smith, D. (1977): A clinical evaluation of eterobarb in epileptic children: In: *Advances in Epileptology— 1977*, edited by H. Meinardi and A. J. Rowan, pp. 318–321. Swetz & Zeitlinger, Amsterdam.
13. Smith, D., Goldstein, S., and Roomet, A. (1975): A comparison of the hypnotic effects of the anticonvulsant dimethoxymethylphenobarbital and sodium phenobarbital in normal human volunteers. *Epilepsia*, 16:201.
14. Smith, D., and Roomet, A. (1975): A clinical and EEG evaluation of eterobarb vs. phenobarbital. The effect of eterobarb on the EEG of patients with uncontrolled epilepsy. *Electroencephalogr. Clin. Neurophysiol.*, 39:296.

Antiepileptic Drugs, edited by D. M. Woodbury,
J. K. Penry, and C. E. Pippenger. Raven Press,
New York © 1982.

72

Potential Antiepileptic Drugs

Cinromide

Robert J. Perchalski, Barry J. Karas, and B. J. Wilder

Cinnamamides have been studied for many years for their effects on the central nervous system. Lott and Christiansen (10) investigated numerous propenoic acid amides, including phenyl-substituted (cinnamamide) derivatives, as hypnotics. Parke, Davis and Company (11) patented various N-alkyl homologs and reported their effectiveness against convulsive doses of pentylenetetrazol (PTZ) in rats. More recently, Balsamo et al. (1,2) tested geometrical isomers of N-alkyl-α,β-dimethylcinnamamides and found that trans isomers acted as anticonvulsants and central nervous system depressants, whereas cis isomers acted as central nervous system stimulants. They also found increased anticonvulsant activity after substitution of halogens (Cl, Br) on the phenyl ring. Since 1978, cinromide (designated by Burroughs Wellcome Company as BW122U) has been undergoing clinical testing as a broad-spectrum anticonvulsant.

CHEMISTRY AND METHODS OF DETERMINATION

Cinromide (3-bromo-N-ethylcinnamamide; 3-(3-bromophenyl)-N-ethyl propenamide; Fig. 1) is a white crystalline substance with a molecular weight of 254.1. It is prepared from 3-bromocinnamic acid by synthesis of the acid chloride using thionyl chloride in benzene followed by

conversion to the amide with ethylamine (6). The pure compound (m.p. 87°–88.5°C) is insoluble in water but very soluble in organic solvents and propylene glycol.

The primary method of analysis of cinromide and its metabolites is liquid chromatography (HPLC and TLC) with ultraviolet absorbance detection. Gas–liquid chromatography is ill-suited to simultaneous analysis because of the wide range of concentrations that must be covered (10 ng/ml to 80 μg/ml) and the chemical and chromatographic differences in the three analytes (primary amide, secondary amide, and carboxylic acid). The high ultraviolet absorptivity of these compounds at 280 nm allows sensitive determination and elimination of interferences that are present at lower wavelengths.

Perchalski et al. (12) reported the simultaneous determination of cinromide (BEC), the dealkylated metabolite (3-bromocinnamamide, BC), the hydrolysis product (3-bromocinnamic

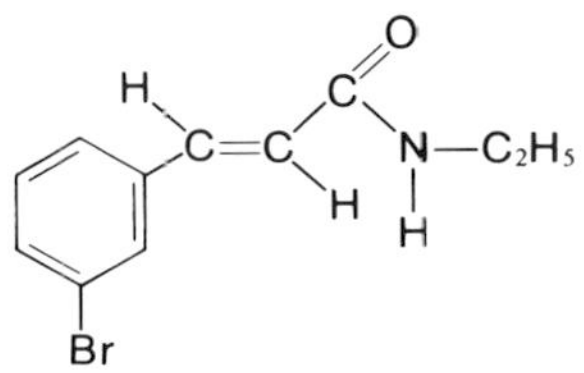

Fig. 1. Structure of cinromide.

acid, BCA), and carbamazepine (CBZ) by reversed-phase high-pressure liquid chromatography. The latter anticonvulsant was included because it is used widely and is chromatographically similar to BC. The retention of the ionizable metabolite, BCA, which normally elutes in the void volume of a reversed-phase system, was increased by addition of a buffer and ion-pairing reagent to the mobile phase, allowing determination of all compounds of interest in a single chromatographic run. An elevated column temperature was used to maximize resolution and minimize system pressure and retention time (13). An analog of cinromide, 3-bromo-N-isopropyl cinnamamide, was added as an internal standard. Figure 2 shows a diagram of the extraction procedure, and Fig. 3 shows typical chromatograms of plasma from a patient during and after the administration of cinromide, run under conditions currently in use in our laboratory.

A thin-layer chromatographic analysis of BEC, BC, and BCA has been published by DeAngelis et al. (5). This procedure involves a single extraction of 1 ml of acidified plasma with benzene, evaporation of a measured volume of the organic phase, application of the dissolved residue to a silica gel plate, and development with one of two mobile phases, depending on the analytes of interest (BEC and BC were estimated with one mobile phase; BCA was determined separately under different elution condi-

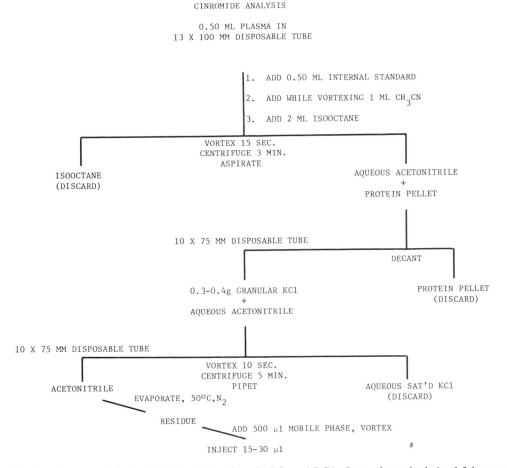

Fig. 2. Sample preparation for HPLC analysis of BEC, BC, and BCA. Internal standard: 1 ml 3-bromo-N-isopropylcinnamamide (75 μg/ml isopropanol) to 25 ml with 0.1 M ascorbic acid (aqueous).

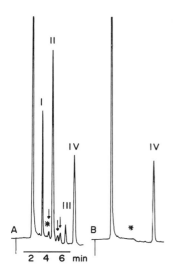

Fig. 3. Chromatograms of plasma extracts: (**A**) from patient taking cinromide; (**B**) from patient after withdrawal of cinromide. Column: 250 mm × 4.6 mm i.d. Spherisorb® ODS (5 μm); temperature, 52°C. Mobile phase: 0.03 M potassium phosphate (pH 6.0), 0.005 M tetrabutylammonium perchlorate in 55% methanol. Peaks are: I, 3-bromocinnamic acid; II, 3-bromocinnamamide; III, 3-bromo-*N*-ethylcinnamamide; IV, 3-bromo-*N*-isopropylcinnamamide (internal standard). Arrows show unidentified but probable metabolites. *Asterisk* indicates eightfold increase in sensitivity.

tions). No internal standard was used, and resolution of BC from CBZ was not verified. The method was applied to samples obtained from animals and humans known to be taking cinromide as sole medication.

ABSORPTION, DISTRIBUTION, BIOTRANSFORMATION, AND EXCRETION

Absorption

Although cinromide is rapidly absorbed, reaching peak concentrations in about 1 hr (12) in humans, significant levels of parent drug (>1 μg/ml) are not maintained. This is probably in part because of extensive first-pass hepatic biotransformation (9) which results in a rapid buildup of relatively high metabolite levels. However, the parent drug cannot be discounted, nor is it totally eliminated by first-pass metabolism, since peak levels of up to 8 μg/ml are obtained shortly after dosing in humans. This rapid appearance of parent drug in plasma has been linked with an immediate hypnotic and sedative effect in dogs and an anticonvulsant effect in rats (3).

Studies in dogs show that almost all of an oral dose of BEC is absorbed, with less than 2% appearing in the feces as parent drug (3). Similar absorption studies in humans have not been reported.

Distribution

Lane and Levy (7), in pharmacokinetic studies in rhesus monkeys, reported that a one-compartment model adequately described the relationship between BEC and BC, indicating that distribution is relatively uniform and rapid. Volumes of distribution for dogs and rats have been given as 1.9 liter/kg and 1.3 liter/kg, respectively (3). A later report by Welch et al. (15) gave the brain-to-plasma ratios of BEC and BC as about 2 at steady-state levels in rats. Our preliminary studies of protein binding by comparison of plasma and saliva concentrations show that 43%, 82%, and ≥99% of BEC, BC, and BCA, respectively, are bound in human plasma. Lockard et al. (9) have also observed this extensive (99%) binding of BCA in monkeys. The decreases in plasma levels of phenytoin (8–51%), valproic acid (30–51%), and carbamazepine (0–50%) (Burroughs Wellcome Company, *personal communication*) observed after administration of cinromide may be caused by displacement of these drugs from plasma protein by the high levels of BCA that accumulate during continuous dosing.

Biotransformation

The metabolic pattern of cinromide (3) as it is presently known is shown in Fig. 4. The only metabolites that are considered active and substantially present in plasma are the dealkylation (BC) and hydrolysis (BCA) products. In humans, steady-state plasma concentrations of BC are 5 to 10 times those of the parent drug, as

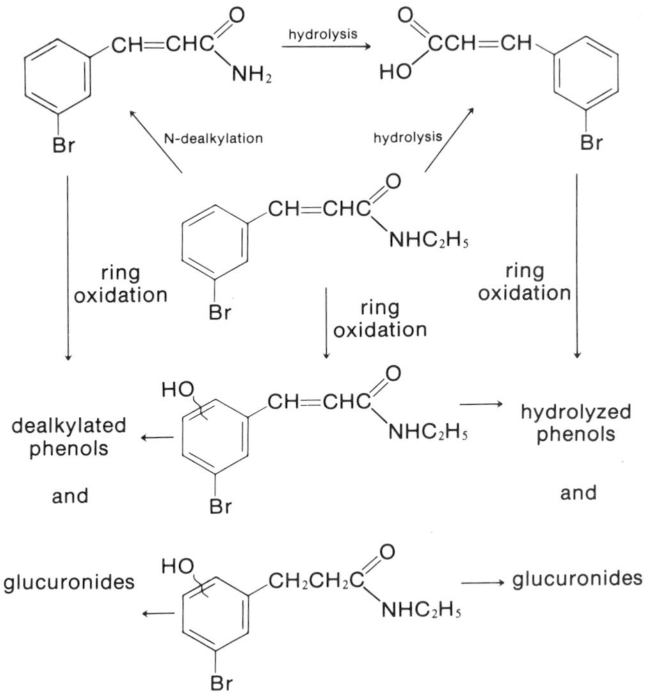

Fig. 4. Metabolism of cinromide.

are concentrations of BCA in relation to those of BC. The ranges of trough concentrations (just before dosing), therefore, are usually ≤ 1 $\mu g/ml$, 1 to 8 $\mu g/ml$, and 20 to 80 $\mu g/ml$ for BEC, BC, and BCA, respectively.

Excretion

Cinromide is eliminated primarily by hepatic biotransformation and renal excretion. Welch et al. (15) reported plasma half-lives of 0.5, 0.6, and 1 hr for cinromide in rats, dogs, and humans, respectively, and about 5 hr for BC in humans. The most recent data determined by this group for dogs shows half-lives of 1.1 hr, 1 hr, and 2.2 hr for BEC, BC, and BCA, respectively (5). Lane and Levy (7), in their work with monkeys, reported half-lives of 1.0 ± 0.1 hr for BEC and 4.6 ± 0.6 hr for BC, and total body clearances of 6.0 ± 2.1 liter/hr and 0.69 ± 0.11 liter/hr for the parent drug and amide, respectively.

Perchalski et al. (3) found half-lives of about 1 hr for BEC and 5 to 7 hr for BC in four epi-

leptic patients. Data obtained during the past year in our laboratory show that BCA has a half-life of about 11.5 hr in humans.

RELATION OF DOSAGE AND PLASMA CONCENTRATION TO SEIZURE CONTROL

Animal Studies

Early efficacy studies conducted by the Burroughs Wellcome Company (3,14) indicated that cinromide might serve as a broad-spectrum anticonvulsant. The parent drug was effective in preventing maximal electroshock seizures in mice at oral (p.o.) doses of 80 mg/kg (ED_{50}) and intraperitoneal (i.p.) doses of 60 mg/kg (ED_{50}), and in rats at 26 mg/kg, i.p. and 58 mg/kg, p.o. Pentylenetetrazol-induced convulsions were prevented at ED_{50} values of 300 mg/kg, p.o. and 90 mg/kg, i.p., and 600 mg/kg, p.o. and 58 mg/kg, i.p. in the mouse and rat, respectively. Cinromide elevated the PTZ threshold in the rat at 75 mg/kg, p.o., and gave 100% protection against low-frequency electroshock (psychomotor seizure test) in the mouse at 400 mg/kg, p.o. Maximal electroshock seizures were prevented in dogs at an ED_{50} of 300 mg/kg, p.o. Mice treated for 13 consecutive days with BEC did not develop tolerance when tested with maximal electroshock. Limited testing of the dealkylated metabolite (BC) in rats showed that it was equipotent with BEC against maximal electroshock but somewhat less potent against PTZ.

Lockard et al. have evaluated BEC and BC at steady-state concentrations in their alumina gel monkey model (focal and secondarily generalized tonic–clonic epilepsy) with respect to EEG (8) and clinical (9) effects. In the EEG study, a steady-state concentration of 7 to 14 μg/ml of BC obtained by constant intravenous infusion of BEC significantly reduced seizure frequency and duration and interictal bursting. In the clinical study, medication was administered by gastric bolus or continuous gastric infusion of BEC or synthetic BC, allowing evaluation of the anticonvulsant effects of the metabolite alone. Individual differences were noted among the animals, ranging from a significant reduction of seizures or alteration of seizure type to minimal effect. Plasma levels greater than 5 μg/ml of BC were linked with desirable effects. The authors recognized the importance of continued evaluation of BEC and BC with the inclusion of 3-bromocinnamic acid.

Human Studies

Investigation of the efficacy of cinromide in the treatment of human epilepsy began in 1978. In the initial phase of this study (Burroughs Wellcome Company, *personal communication*), 53 epileptic patients with histories of refractory partial seizures were evaluated during a 2-week initial period of hospitalization, during which time the daily dosage of cinromide, administered in four portions, was increased periodically from 1,200 to 4,800 mg or to the maximum tolerated dose. Patients were then followed as outpatients for 8 weeks after which the drug was discontinued over a 2- to 3-week

period. Seizures were decreased by ≥50% in 17% of the patients and by 20% in 50% of those evaluated ($N = 42$). Significant effects included decreases in seizure intensity or increases in seizure-free periods. Steady-state plasma levels for a dose of 35 mg/kg averaged 0.7 μg/ml, 2.4 μg/ml, and 33.0 μg/ml for BEC, BC, and BCA, respectively, but showed no correlation with efficacy or side effects.

Lockman et al. (L. A. Lockman, A. D. Rothner, G. Erenberg, F. S. Wright, G. Cloutier, and E. Geiger, *unpublished data*, 1980) used cinromide in the treatment of the Lennox–Gastaut syndrome in eight children. Oral doses of up to 100 mg/kg per day were well tolerated. One patient showed marked improvement, three showed moderate improvement, and the remainder showed slight improvement.

We have conducted a pilot study of cinromide in eight patients. The drug was discontinued in seven patients because of adverse side effects. One patient with a history of refractory complex partial seizures completed the 18-week study with a marked reduction in seizure frequency and has been continued on 450 mg of cinromide four times a day (24 mg/kg) for 2 years. Plasma levels of BEC, BC, and BCA determined in the last year for this patient averaged 0.41 ± 0.25 μg/ml, 3.1 ± 1.4 μg/ml, and 37 ± 10 μg/ml, respectively. During this study a dose–response relationship was determined for a 51.8-kg epileptic female (12). Midday trough levels of BEC and BC were recorded and averaged for 3-day constant-dosage intervals. Plots of average levels for each dosage interval against dose of BEC were linear, with correlation coefficients of 0.980 and 0.999 for BEC and BC, respectively. Slopes indicated plasma level changes of 0.00400 μg/ml of BEC per mg BEC/kg per day and 0.0617 μg/ml of BC per mg BEC/kg per day.

TOXICITY

The oral LD_{50} values of cinromide in rats and mice are 4.4 g/kg and 2.3 g/kg, respectively (3,14). Cloutier et al. (4) conducted a three-phase dose-tolerance study to determine the safety of acute, multiple, and prolonged dosage regimens in humans. In the acute study (single dose, 150 mg to 1,500 mg), subjects who received 1,200 to 1,500 mg reported mild to moderate drowsiness. No significant effects were reported by subjects who received 600 mg of cinromide every 6 hr for three doses. In the prolonged study, 16 normal volunteers were given up to 900 mg four times a day for 28 days. All experienced adverse side effects at doses above 1,800 mg/day, including drowsiness, dizziness, lightheadedness, nystagmus, and ataxia. Three subjects were dropped because of nausea and vomiting. Other side effects that have been reported include skin rash, neutropenia, and elevated liver isoenzymes (SGOT/SGPT). No clinically significant abnormalities have been observed in vital signs, electrocardiograms, or pituitary function (FSH/ LH), blood coagulation (PT, PTT, fibrinogen), or ophthalmologic tests. No teratogenic effects or fetal deaths were recorded for rats that received up to 1,500 mg/kg per day on days 6 through 15 of gestation (3).

SUMMARY

Cinromide (3-bromo-*N*-ethylcinnamamide, BEC) is currently under investigation as a broad-spectrum anticonvulsant. The parent drug and its deethylated metabolite, 3-bromocinnamamide (BC), exhibit protection against maximal electroshock and PTZ-induced and psychomotor convulsions. A second metabolite, 3-bromocinnamic acid (BCA), may also have antiepileptic properties. In adults, BEC has demonstrated activity when used as adjunctive therapy in patients with refractory partial seizures. Addition of cinromide to the therapeutic regimen of children with Lennox–Gastaut syndrome resulted in significant suppression of seizures. In humans, half-lives of BEC, BC, and BCA are 1 to 2 hr, 5 to 7 hr, and 11.5 hr, respectively. The drug is usually given in four daily doses to total 20 to 40 mg/kg per day in adults and up to 100 mg/kg per day in children. Steady-state plasma levels for a 35 mg/kg dose average 0.7 μg/ml, 2.4 μg/ml, and 33.0 μg/ml for parent drug and amide and acid metabolites, re-

spectively. Undesirable side effects include drowsiness, dizziness, lightheadedness, nystagmus, ataxia, nausea, vomiting, skin rashes, neutropenia, and hepatic enzyme abnormalities.

Further information is necessary to establish the time course of activity of the drug and its metabolites. Although the parent drug may be responsible for the initial effects, the short half-life and low steady-state plasma levels point to the more persistent, more concentrated metabolites as probable active agents.

CONVERSION

Conversion factor:

$$CF = \frac{1000}{mol.\ wt.} = \frac{1000}{254.1} = 3.94$$

Conversion:

$$(\mu g/ml) \times 3.94 = (\mu moles/liter)$$

$$(\mu moles/liter) \div 3.94 = (\mu g/ml)$$

ACKNOWLEDGMENT

This work was completed with the generous assistance of the Veterans Administration, the Epilepsy Research Foundation of Florida, Inc., and Burroughs Wellcome Company.

REFERENCES

1. Balsamo, A., Basili, P. L., Crotti, P., Macchia, B., Macchia, F., Cuttica, A., and Passerini, N. (1977): Structure activity relationships in cinnamamides. 2. Synthesis and pharmacological evaluation of some (*E*)- and (*Z*)-*N*-alkyl-α,β-dimethylcinnamamides substituted on the phenyl group. *J. Med. Chem.*, 20:48–53.
2. Balsamo, A., Basili, P. L., Crotti, P., Macchia, B., Macchia, F., Pecchia, A., Cuttica, A., and Passerini, N. (1975): Structure activity relationships in cinnamamides. 1. Synthesis and pharmacological evaluation of some (*E*)-and (*Z*)-*N*-alkyl-α,β-dimethylcinnamamides. *J. Med. Chem.*, 18:842–846.
3. Burroughs Wellcome Company (1975): *Report on the Pharmacology and Toxicology of B.W.122U.* Burroughs Wellcome, Research Triangle Park, North Carolina.
4. Cloutier, G., Gabriel, M., Geiger, E., Cook, L., Rogers, J., Cummings, W., and Cato, A. (1980): Cinromide: Phase I testing of a potential antiepileptic. In: *Advances in Epileptology: The Xth Epilepsy Inter-*

national Symposium, edited by J. A. Wada and J. K. Penry, p. 351. Raven Press, New York.

5. DeAngelis, R. L., Robinson, M. M., Brown, A. R., Johnson, T. E., and Welch, R. M. (1980): Quantitation of the anticonvulsant cinromide (3-bromo-*N*-ethyl-cinnamamide) and its major plasma metabolites by thin-layer chromatography. *J. Chromatogr.,* 221:353–360.

6. Grivsky, E. M. (1976): Substituted cinnamic acid amides. German Patent 2,535,599 (Wellcome Foundation Ltd.). *Chem. Abstr.* 84:164492X.

7. Lane, E. A., and Levy, R. H. (1980): The pharmacokinetics of cinromide and an active metabolite, *N*-deethylcinromide in the rhesus monkey. In: *Advances in Epileptology: The Xth Epilepsy International Symposium,* edited by J. A. Wada and J. K. Penny, p. 355. Raven Press, New York.

8. Lockard, J. S., Levy, R. H., DuCharme, L. L., and Congdon, W. C. (1979): Experimental anticonvulsant cinromide in monkey model: Preliminary efficacy. *Epilepsia,* 20:339–350.

9. Lockard, J. S., Levy, R. H., DuCharme, L. L., and Congdon, W. C. (1980): Cinromide's metabolite in monkey model: Gastric administration and seizure control. *Epilepsia,* 21:177–182.

10. Lott, W. A. and Christiansen, W. G. (1934): A study of acrylic amides and ureides as hypnotics. *J. Am. Pharm. Assoc.* 23:788–793.

11. Parke, Davis and Company (1952): *N*-Alkylcinnamamides. British Patent 663,903. *Chem. Abstr.* 46:6336.

12. Perchalski, R. J., Bruni, J., Wilder, B. J., and Willmore, L. J. (1979): Simultaneous determination of the anticonvulsants, cinromide (3-bromo-*N*-ethyl-cinnamamide), 3-bromocinnamamide and carbamazepine in plasma by high performance liquid chromatography. *J. Chromatogr.,* 163:187–193.

13. Perchalski, R. J., and Wilder, B. J. (1979): Reverse phase liquid chromatography at increased temperature. *Anal. Chem.,* 51:774–776.

14. Soroko, F. E., Grivsky, E. M., Kenney, B. T., Bache, R. E., and Maxwell, R. A. (1979): The anticonvulsant activity of cinromide. *Fed. Proc.,* 38:753.

15. Welch, R., Hsu, S., Grivsky, E., and Soroko, F. E. (1978): Anticonvulsant activity and metabolism of cinromide in animals and man. In: *Eleventh International Congress of Neuro-Psychopharmacology,* p. 383. Elsevier, Amsterdam.

Antiepileptic Drugs, edited by D. M. Woodbury, J. K. Penry, and C. E. Pippenger Raven Press, New York © 1982

73

Potential Antiepileptic Drugs

Mexiletine

James J. Cereghino

Mexiletine was synthesized in the chemical laboratories of C. H. Boehringer Sohn in Ingelheim, West Germany. A claims priority was filed in 1966 (F.R. 1,551,055), and a United States patent was obtained in 1972 (35). The development of mexiletine has been chronicled by Koppe (34). The search for nonaddicting anorectic compounds to replace phenmetrazine (Preludin®) led to the discovery of pronounced anticonvulsant activity and minimal side effects in a compound that was a structural variant of both phenmetrazine and β-blocking agents. That compound, originally designated Kö 1173, was later named mexiletine.

Subsequently, pharmacological studies in Britain indicated that mexiletine had a high degree of antiarrhythmic activity. The drug has been extensively studied and is marketed in Europe as an antiarrhythmic. The development of mexiletine as an antiepileptic drug has occurred chiefly in North America. Because use of the drug as an antiepileptic has often drawn from the cardiac experience, information from the latter will be presented when appropriate.

In March, 1970, at the request of Pharma-Research Canada, Ltd., the NINCDS Epilepsy Advisory Committee reviewed the pharmacological, toxicological, and teratological data from animal studies of mexiletine and recommended that the compound be tested in humans. A "Notice of Claimed Investigational Exemption for a New Drug'' (IND) for the testing of mexiletine as an antiepileptic drug was filed with the U.S. Food and Drug Administration by Pharma-Research, and clinical studies were initiated in 1970. The IND was transferred to Boehringer Ingelheim, Ltd., in 1976.

CHEMISTRY

The structural formula of mexiletine, 1-(2',6'-dimethyl)-phenoxy-2-aminopropane, is illustrated in Fig. 1. Replacement of the ether bridge by an -NH or carbonamide group, as in lidocaine or procainamide, does not increase the anticonvulsant activity of mexiletine (34). Mexiletine is commercially available as the hydrochloride. It is a slightly bitter, white crystalline powder with a molecular weight of 215.5. It is easily soluble in water. The melting point is approximately 199.2 to 201.8°C (Pharma-Research, *personal communication*). The pK_a of mexiletine has been reported as 8.4 at 25°C (4) and 8.75 (43).

METHODS OF DETERMINATION

The fluorometric method of determining the mexiletine concentration in body fluids is neither sensitive nor selective enough for use in

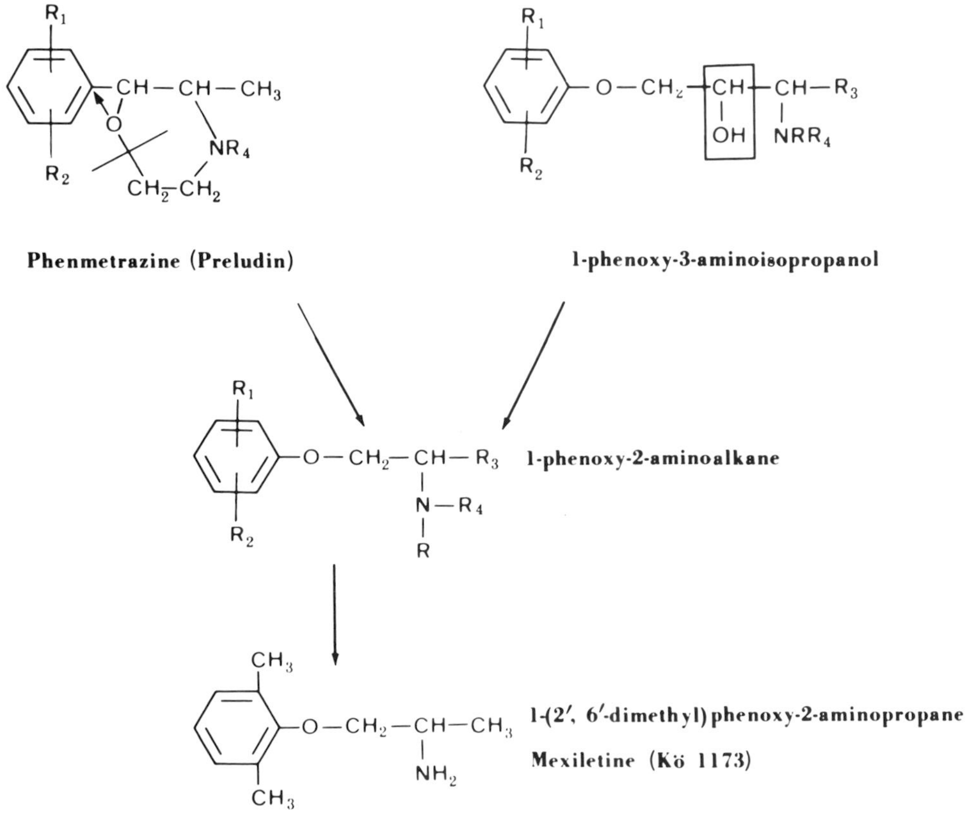

Fig. 1. Molecular variations of structure of phenmetrazine (an oxazine) and β blockers (1-phenoxy-3-aminoisopropanol, R = H) 1-phenoxy-2-aminoalkane and further variation to mexiletine (R_1, R_2, R_4 = H; R_3 = CH_3). Adapted from Koppe (34).

detailed investigations, and thus, gas–liquid chromatographic (GLC) methods are used (C. H. Boehringer Sohn, *personal communication*). Many GLC methods have been described for determination of mexiletine in plasma (8,22,23,28,29,33,47,48), urine (5,29,49), or saliva (4). These methods can detect plasma mexiletine levels of >100 ng/ml. The GLC method of Kelly et al. (29) is typical: mexiletine is extracted by organic solvent (diethyl ether) from samples made alkaline with sodium hydroxide; mexiletine may be chromatographed directly, but sensitivity and reproducibility are improved by converting the extracted mexiletine to the acetyl derivative by acetic anhydride. This derivative is then injected into a GLC us-

ing a nitrogen-sensitive flame ionization detector. Diphenhydramine is the internal standard.

The sensitivity of the GLC method can be increased by use of an electron-capture detector to measure levels as low as 10 ng/ml in plasma (15,21,40,56), urine, saliva, and bile (4,5, 49,56).

Kelly et al. (29), using duplicate plasma and urine specimens, compared the spectrophotofluorometric and GLC methods and found a coefficient of +0.99 between the methods. The coefficient between duplicate plasma samples determined by an electron-capture GLC method (15) and by a flame-ionization GLC method (40) was +0.92 from 30 min to 30 hr (15).

The method of determination will be referenced each time plasma concentrations are reported.

ABSORPTION

Prescott et al. (43) postulated that mexiletine is almost completely ionized in the acidic gastric contents and is thus presumably so poorly lipid soluble that absorption from the stomach is negligible. The pH is higher below the stomach, and the percentage of mexiletine in the unionized form is higher. Absorption is thought to occur almost totally in the upper part of the small intestine. As a result, the rate of gastric emptying is considered to be a major factor in controlling the rate of mexiletine absorption.

Mexiletine has been administered both orally and intravenously to presumably healthy volunteers. Six fasting volunteers, 30 to 39 years of age, received a 3 mg/kg dose of mexiletine in solution (18,19,50). Plasma concentrations determined by GLC (29) reached a maximum of 300 to 400 ng/ml (0.3–0.4 μg/ml) within 2 to 3 hr. Acidic urine was not maintained.

In a study by Prescott et al. (43), five presumably healthy fasting male volunteers, 28 to 42 years of age, received a single oral dose of 400 mg of mexiletine taken with 50 ml of water. Peak plasma concentrations determined by GLC (29) of 870 to 1,550 ng/ml (0.87–1.55 μg/ml) occurred within 2 to 4 hr (mean, 3 hr) of drug ingestion. At an unspecified time in relation to the above dose, these subjects also received a solution of 3 mg/kg of mexiletine in 200 ml of water; "similar" mean peak concentrations occurred at 2 hr. Acidic urine was not maintained.

Campbell et al. (10) studied five healthy male volunteers, 25 to 28 years of age, who were given 200 mg of mexiletine orally 1 to 2 hr after a light breakfast. Plasma concentrations determined by GLC (28) reached a peak 2 hr after administration. Acidic urine was not maintained.

To six healthy men, ages 27 to 47 years (mean, 33 years) and weighing 69 to 91 kg (mean, 81 kg), Häselbarth et al. (22) administered either 400 mg of mexiletine orally in capsule form or 432 mg of mexiletine hydrochloride in a sustained release form (hard gelatin capsule filled with six identical film tablets, each containing 72 mg of active substance, with controlled slow release obtained by specific coating of the nuclei). Peak plasma concentrations of 770 ng/ml (0.77 ± 0.13 μg/ml) were obtained an average of 2.2 hr after administration of the conventional capsules. With the slow release form, flat and delayed maximum plasma levels occurred between 7.8 and 11.1 hr (mean, 9.2 hr), with a peak concentration of 340 ng/ml (0.34 ± 0.12 μg/ml).

Pottage (42) and Prescott et al. (43) observed that absorption of mexiletine is impaired by myocardial infarction and narcotic analgesics (e.g., heroin or morphine) that inhibit gastric emptying. Long-term oral therapy in cardiac patients has revealed no problems with the absorption of mexiletine. Metoclopramide enhances and atropine decreases the rate of mexiletine absorption (57).

Cereghino et al. (15) studied eight men, ages 23 to 63 years, who were receiving various dosages of phenytoin, primidone, or phenobarbital for complex partial seizures. Two fasting patients each received a single oral dose of 100, 200, 300, or 400 mg of mexiletine. Plasma mexiletine concentrations, determined by GLC methods (15,40), ranged up to 795 ng/ml (0.7 μg/ml), with peak concentrations occurring from 1 to 3 hr after administration. The data suggested that peak concentrations were reached more rapidly with higher doses. The effect of the other antiepileptic drugs on gastric motility and therefore on plasma mexiletine concentrations is unknown. Acidic urine was not maintained.

A slow release formulation of mexiletine has been developed to maintain plasma concentration for 12 hr (7).

DISTRIBUTION

After a bolus intravenous injection of 100 mg of mexiletine over a 4-min period to four healthy male volunteers, plasma concentrations, determined by GLC (28), fell rapidly as a result of extensive uptake and distribution in tissues (43). The plasma concentration–time curve appeared to be the result of at least three simultaneous exponential processes representing fast and slow distribution phases with a much slower elimination phase. The total volume of distribution (VD_t) was 663 ± 238 liters. The volume of the central compartment (VD_c) was 185 ± 97 liters. Prescott et al. (43) interpreted these data as being consistent with a three-compartment model. The first or "central" compartment would consist of the blood volume and tissues such as myocardium, brain, liver, kidney, and lung which are rapidly equilibrating. The second and third compartments would consist of "deep" or "peripheral" tissue (skin, muscle, fat) which take up the drug more slowly.

Häselbarth et al. (22) intravenously administered 250 mg of mexiletine in 10 ml of solution to six healthy male volunteers (27–47 years of age, 69–91 kg) and calculated the kinetic microconstants only from the intravenous experimental results. The VD_c was 5.5 liter/kg.

The mean volume of distribution for 10 cardiac patients who received a single 200-mg dose of mexiletine intravenously over a 5-min period was 6.63 liter/kg or 464.01 liters for a 70-kg person (10).

The clinical effects of mexiletine presumably occur when the drug is in the target organ (myocardium or brain), and these effects are thought to correlate best with the amount of drug in the central compartment, as indicated by the plasma concentrations (43). No studies have yet reported brain concentrations of mexiletine.

The work by Talbot et al. (50), using an ultrafiltration technique, indicates plasma protein binding in adults to the extent of about 70% (2.5 µg/ml). Prescott et al. (43) believe the amount bound is insignificant in relation to the total amount of drug in the body, resulting in no risk of drug interaction caused by displacement of mexiletine from plasma proteins by other drugs. They estimate that less than 1% of the total amount of drug in the body is in the blood after distribution (43).

The concentration of mexiletine is about 15% higher in whole blood than in plasma (43).

The distribution of mexiletine has not been extensively studied in children. Two children who received doses of 8.6 mg/kg had low plasma concentrations, but doses to 15 and 25 mg/kg produced concentrations in the usual adult therapeutic range (24).

EXCRETION

There are large variations in plasma mexiletine concentrations among individuals regardless of dose, mode of administration, or state of health. Kaye et al. (27) and Kiddie and colleagues (30–32) postulated that this variation may in part be the result of fluctuations in urinary pH, with mexiletine being more rapidly eliminated from the body when the urine is acidic than when it is alkaline. Their studies involved four healthy volunteers who received two 100-mg mexiletine capsules orally on three separate occasions: when the urine was maintained at about pH 5 (by ammonium chloride ingestion), when it was maintained at about pH 8 (by sodium bicarbonate ingestion), and when the urinary pH was uncontrolled. A 200-mg dose of mexiletine was also given intravenously to four volunteers when the urine was maintained at about pH 5 and on another occasion when it was kept at about pH 8. The half-life of mexiletine after intravenous administration was 2.8 hr, and 48-hr urinary excretion was 57.5% of the dose at pH 5. At pH 8, the half-life increased to 8.6 hr, and 48-hr urinary excretion was 0.6% of the dose. Similar results were obtained with the oral route of administration. Buccal absorption, renal excretion, and plasma elimination half-life were thus shown to be dependent on urinary pH. The authors postulated that unless the urine stays within the range of pH 5 or 6, a given dose of mexiletine could be either ineffective or toxic.

Prescott et al. (43) found that the renal clearance of mexiletine at low urinary pH exceeded the normal glomerular filtration rate, and thus, mexiletine could be inferred to undergo active tubular secretion. They also found a highly significant inverse correlation between the logarithms of renal clearance and urinary pH. This group, unlike others (27,30,32), concluded that, despite the pH-dependent renal clearance, normal physiological variation in urinary pH seems unlikely to have a major effect on the half-life or steady-state plasma concentration of the drug.

Beckett and Chidomere (4) administered 200-mg doses of mexiletine orally to four healthy male volunteers with acidic urine (pH 5.0 ± 0.2) maintained by oral doses of ammonium chloride. Two subjects were also studied under "normal" urinary pH. The half-life was reduced from 9 ± 2 hr with uncontrolled urinary pH to 4.5 ± 1 hr with acidic urinary pH. Urinary excretion of unchanged mexiletine was 10 to 23% in 24 hr with uncontrolled urinary pH and increased to 30 to 55% in 24 hr with acidic urinary pH.

Johnston et al. (26) gave six healthy volunteers (three men and three women, 20–30 years of age, 57–78 kg) a loading dose of 400 mg of mexiletine orally followed by 150-mg oral doses at 4 p.m., 12 midnight, and 7 a.m. each day for 5 days. Blood samples were drawn daily at 4, 6, and 8 hr after the 7 a.m. dose. Urine was collected in 2-hr intervals from 3 to 9 hr after the 7 a.m. dose, with recording of volume and determination of pH within 5 min of micturition. The mean urinary pH was 5.71 and ranged between pH 5.04 and 7.86. Multiple regression analysis utilizing the variables of urine volume, urinary pH, urinary excretion of mexiletine, plasma mexiletine concentrations, renal clearance of mexiletine, sample time, and day of study, confirmed that at high urinary pH, excretion and clearance of mexiletine are low, whereas the plasma concentration is high. These findings, with spontaneous changes in urinary pH during chronic administration of subtherapeutic doses of mexiletine to healthy volunteers, suggest that the amount of plasma mexiletine could increase by more than 50% following a spontaneous rise in urinary pH. The authors postulated that spontaneous extremes of urinary pH may account for some cases of inefficacy of the drug or for the occurrence of side effects. They rec-

ommended that urinary pH be measured during mexiletine therapy and that attention be paid to factors likely to alter urinary pH such as diet or use of antacids.

Studies of mexiletine half-life have generally been performed under conditions of uncontrolled urinary pH. Table 1 indicates half-life values for populations of "normal" volunteers, cardiac patients, and epileptic patients with various dosages of mexiletine. The prolonged half-life in cardiac patients has been attributed to reduced hepatic blood flow and impaired drug metabolism. The half-life in epileptic patients (Table 1) would appear to be more rapid, although urinary pH was uncontrolled, making speculation tenuous. Because the drug is metabolized primarily by oxidative processes, Beckett and Chidomere (4) postulated that there may be a difference in the rate of metabolism in smokers and nonsmokers and that enzyme inducers such as phenobarbital may increase metabolism. Assuming a half-life of approximately 12 hr, 3 to 4 days would be required to reach steady state with an oral dose of 200 to 300 mg three times a day (6).

Prescott et al. (43), examining mean body clearance of mexiletine in healthy volunteers, found that a mean of 7.9% (range, 1.4–14.5%) of the administered dose was recovered unchanged in the urine in 3 days. The mean renal clearance was 49 ± 25 ml/min with a mean urinary pH of 6.17. Total body clearance was calculated as 751 ± 414 ml/min after intravenous administration and 681 ± 178 ml/min after oral administration. In cardiac patients, total body clearance was relatively decreased, a finding the authors attributed mainly to decreased metabolic clearance, possibly related to reduced hepatic flow, the effect of other drug therapy, accumulation of mexiletine metabolites, or decreased activity of hepatic drug-metabolizing enzymes in these older patients.

Campbell et al. (10) observed that in 156 cardiac patients 2 to 48% (mean, 14 ± 3%) of the daily dose was excreted in the urine during the 48 hr after the last dose. There was a significant linear correlation between recovery of

TABLE 1. *Plasma half-life of mexiletine (hr) following intravenous or oral administration of the drug to "normal" volunteers, cardiac patients, and epileptic patients* [a]

"Normal" volunteers		Cardiac patients		Epileptic patients		
Intravenous	Oral	Intravenous	Oral	Intravenous	Oral	Reference
11.5	10.2	18.6[b]	18.6[b]			18,19,50
(N = 6)	(N = 6)	(N = 11)	(N = 11)			
10.4	9.4	16.7	12.1			43
(N = 4)	(N = 0)	(N = 12)	(N = 6)			
11.77	11.40	13.24	11.31			10,11
(N = 5)	(N = 5)	(N = 10)	(N = 30)			
2.8[c]						30,32
8.6[d]						
(N = 4)						
	9[e]					4
	(N = 2)					
	4.5[c]					
	(N = 4)					
6.34 ± 1.48	"Similar"					22
(N = 6)						
					9–12	54
					(N = 18)	
					2.7–7.2	15
					(N = 8)	

[a]Dosages of mexiletine varied among the studies. Urinary pH was uncontrolled unless otherwise indicated.
[b]Intravenous and oral data combined.
[c]Urinary pH of 5.
[d]Urinary pH of 8.
[e]Normal urinary pH.

the unchanged drug in the urine and output of urine.

Renal insufficiency did not modify the rate of elimination of mexiletine after a single intravenous injection of 1.5 mg/kg to 11 patients with a creatinine clearance of 2 to 38 ml/min (2). Urinary acidity was not controlled.

After intravenous administration of 20 mg of tritium-labeled mexiletine to five women, aged 35 to 81 years, with cancer of the bladder (one case), uterus (one case), and uterine cervix (three cases), ^{3}H activity was eliminated from the serum with a mean half-life of 17.9 hr. After oral administration of 50 mg of tritium-labeled mexiletine to five men, aged 49 to 76 years, with Hodgkin's disease (one case), tonsillar cancer (one case), and bronchial cancer (three cases), ^{3}H activity was eliminated from the serum with a mean half-life of 20.7 hr. The maximum serum concentration of labeled drug was obtained 2 hr after administration (V. Häselbarth, *personal communication*). The relationship between half-

life of serum mexiletine concentration and half-life of ^{3}H activity is not known.

Mexiletine freely crosses the placenta, and concentrations in maternal and cord blood are equal. Mexiletine is excreted in breast milk but not in sufficient quantity to be measurable in the plasma of the breast-fed infant (52).

There appears to be a linear relationship between plasma and saliva concentration, with a salivary–plasma concentration ratio of 1.5 to 3 (3).

BIOTRANSFORMATION

Mexiletine is extensively metabolized by humans (Fig. 2). Scott et al. (45), utilizing a technique combining gas chromatography, chemical ionization and high-resolution electron mass spectrometry, and proton and ^{13}C nuclear magnetic resonance spectrometry, identified the drug and two major metabolites in urine. The identified metabolites were a glucuronide of the free base with a hydroxyl group para to the ether linkage (IV) and a free base with a methyl group replaced by a CH_2-OH group (VII). Anticonvulsant activity of both metabolites is suspected but has not been demonstrated (45).

Beckett and Chidomere (4,5) administered mexiletine to volunteers under conditions of controlled acidic urinary pH and reported on the alcohols of the two major metabolites (VIII and IX) and minor metabolic routes of *N*-oxidation (Va and Vb), deamination to the ketone (III) and reduction to the alcohol (IV), and *N*-methylation (II) (see Fig. 2).

MECHANISM OF ACTION

Mexiletine has been administered in various doses below the toxic range to multiple animal species (mice, rats, rabbits, cats, and dogs) with a resultant increase in vigilance, increased exploratory motor activity, and reduction in motor coordination (20; C. H. Boehringer Sohn, *personal communication*). In the toxic dose range, episodic cramps, mostly of the clonic type, were observed and were more pronounced in mice (57–84 mg/kg orally) than in rats (410–500 mg/ kg orally). To further delineate these effects, EEG studies were performed in encephale isole cats immobilized with gallamine triethyliodide and artificially ventilated. Intravenous doses of 1 to 3 mg/kg of mexiletine produced no clear-cut change in the cortical or subcortical EEG. After intravenous administration of 10 mg/kg, a "fleeting depression" of the EEG to the isoelectric baseline was recorded, but no signs of seizures were recorded. Afterdischarge was prolonged by 64% after an intravenous dose of 1 mg/kg, by 27% after a dose of 3 mg/kg, and was shortened after a dose of 10 mg/kg. These results thus suggest a central nervous system stimulant effect in the lower dose range and the opposite effect at the 10 mg/kg dose.

The ED_{50} for maximal extensor spasm in mice produced by electroshock 1 hr after oral administration of a mexiletine emulsion was 23 mg/ kg. Following intravenous injection in mice, mexiletine showed a dose-dependent anticonvulsant response to electroshock given 15 and 60 min after administration of the drug (C. H. Boehringer Sohn, *personal communication*).

Data from the Anticonvulsant Drug Screening Project of the Antiepileptic Drug Develop-

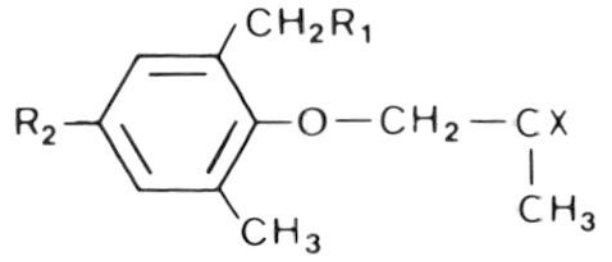

	R_1	R_2	X	
I	H	H	HNH_2	Mexiletine (1-(2', 6'-dimethyl)phenoxy-2-aminopropane)
II	H	H	$HNHCH_3$	N-Methylmexiletine
III	H	H	(=O)	1-(2', 6'-dimethyl)phenoxypropan-2-one
IV	H	H	HOH	1-(2', 6'-dimethyl)phenoxypropan-2-ol
Va	H	H	HNHOH	N-Hydroxymexiletine
Vb	H	H	(=NOH)	1-(2', 6'-dimethyl)phenoxypropan-2-one oxime
VI	H	OH	HNH_2	1-(4'-hydroxy,2',6'-dimethyl)phenoxy-2-aminopropane
VII	OH	H	HNH_2	1-(2'-hydroxymethyl, 6'-methyl)phenoxy-2-aminopropane
VIII	H	OH	HOH	1-(4'-hydroxy,2',6'-dimethyl)phenoxypropan-2-ol
IX	OH	H	HOH	1-(2'-hydroxymethyl, 6'-methyl)phenoxypropan-2-ol

Fig. 2. Structures of metabolic products of mexiletine (I). (From Beckett and Chidomere, ref. 5, with permission.)

ment Program (for procedures, see 36) on a racemic mixture of mexiletine hydrochloride with saline solvent produced an MES ED_{50} of 9.9 mg/kg (range, 7.1–11.7 mg/kg), scMET ED_{50} of >300 mg/kg and TD_{50} of 41.6 mg/kg (range, 35.7–53.0 mg/kg) (14).

E. A. Swinyard and H. J. Kupferberg (*personal communication*), examining the effect of mexiletine on pentylenetetrazole-induced seizures in mice, have shown that mexiletine may shorten the time to first twitch. This is in contrast to drugs that either increase (e.g., phenobarbital) or fail to alter (e.g., phenytoin) the time to first twitch.

An oral dose of 40 mg/kg of mexiletine in mice produced nearly a fourfold increase in the intravenous LD_{100} of pentylenetetrazole-induced seizures. Mexiletine exerted minimal to no effect on strychnine-induced seizures and tremorine-induced tremors in mice. It exerted slight analgesic effects and had no local anesthetic properties in mice. The drug has a temperature-reducing effect consistent with central nervous system depressant activity (C. H. Boehringer Sohn, *personal communication*).

Electrical stimulation of the amygdala in cats produces a psychomotor component and episodic cramps progressing to generalized tonic–clonic cramps. Intraperitoneal administration of 3 to 10 mg/kg of mexiletine inhibited the episodic cramps for a period of 1 to 4 hr (I. J. Kuhn, reported in 20). Kuhn, using chronic aluminum hydroxide implantation in the amygdala or caudate nucleus (animal unspecified but presumably cat), showed that intraperitoneal administration of 10 mg/kg of mexiletine prevented epileptiform episodes "in many cases, but the EEG abnormality was hardly affected."

Mitchell (reported in 20) found that rat cortex slices incubated with tritiated GABA and then continuously perfused with Krebs solution released tritiated GABA following electrical stimulation. When the slices were perfused with mexiletine (5×10^{-4} M), GABA uptake was reduced by 16% compared to controls. Phenytoin perfusion (concentration not specified) had no effect on the spontaneous or evoked release of tritiated GABA. This evidence suggests that the anticonvulsant mode of action might be to inhibit the reuptake of GABA as a central nervous system inhibitory transmitter.

Danneberg and Shelley (20) have summarized other neuropharmacological aspects of mexiletine as follows: mexiletine has no action on the autonomic nervous system, does not interfere with the function of biogenic amines, does not inhibit acetylcholine-induced spasm in the guinea pig rectum, and does not affect the vasodilating activity of acetylcholine. It does not modify the vascular effects of norepinephrine and epinephrine and has no α- or β-adrenergic blocking properties. Mexiletine does not inhibit the compulsive gnawing induced by apomorphine in rats, indicating that it has no action on dopaminergic terminals. Neither preganglionic nor postganglionic inhibitory effects have been demonstrated by electrical stimulation of the cervical sympathetic nerve to the nictitating membrane. The drug has no antihistaminic activity and does not show any characteristics of a neuroleptic agent (e.g., it does not alter amphetamine toxicity in mice and has no effect on the lethal dose of epinephrine).

Enantiomorphically pure $R(-)$- and $S(+)$-mexiletine have been synthesized from $R(-)$- and $S(+)$-alanine and subjected to neuropharmacological evaluation in mice. No stereoselectivity for the anticonvulsant activity or metabolic rate of the mexiletine isomers was demonstrated (41).

The antiarrhythmic mode of action has been studied in humans and in several *in vitro* and *in vivo* models. Mexiletine is a Class I antiarrhythmic with a strong local anesthetic effect on frog sciatic nerve, a direct cardiac membrane action reducing the entry of inward depolarizing current, and a shortening of action potential duration (46,53).

Mexiletine significantly increases oxygen consumption in homogenized slices of brain of Wistar rats and inhibits oxygen consumption in intact tissue (39).

CLINICAL TRIALS

Results from an uncontrolled study of 19 medically refractory adolescent and adult epileptic patients receiving 300 or 400 mg of mexiletine daily suggested that mexiletine was effective in the treatment of complex partial seizures but not effective for generalized tonic–clonic, absence, akinetic, or elementary partial seizures. The therapeutic plasma concentration appeared to be in the range of 400 to 700 ng/ml (0.4–0.7 μg/ml). Mild insomnia and transient mild anorexia were noted as side effects. Three patients were observed to have an increase in complex partial seizures (54,55).

In preparation for a prospective controlled study of mexiletine as an adjunct in the treatment of epilepsy, Cereghino et al. (13) performed a study with eight institutionalized men with uncontrolled seizures; their weights, medical regimens, and seizure types were similar. Two patients each received total daily dosages of 200, 400, 600, or 800 mg of mexiletine administered in capsules four times a day for 7 days in addition to their usual antiepileptic medication. After the first day, plasma mexiletine concentrations were significantly higher for the 600- and 800-mg dosages than for the 200- and 400-mg dosages. The differences in plasma concentrations between the 200- and 400-mg dosages and between the 600- and 800-mg dosages were not statistically significant. Plasma concentrations for the 200- and 400-mg dosages were generally below 400 ng/ml (0.4 μg/ml), whereas at dosages of 600 and 800 mg, the concentrations ranged from 400 to >1,100 ng/ml (0.4–1.1 μg/ml) after the first day. Based on plasma concentrations and clinical impressions of the ability of the patients to tolerate initiation of the drug, a dosage of 800 mg/day was selected for subsequent studies. Urinary acidity was not controlled.

A double-blind study with replicated Latin-square design was originally planned at the New Castle State Hospital (14; J. J. Cereghino, J. T. Brock, B. G. White, L. D. Smith, J. C. Van Meter and J. K. Penry, *unpublished data*). The 23-week study was to have consisted of four 21-day treatment periods with each period separated by 21 days of usual antiepileptic medications. Thirty-six patients (19 men and 17 women, ages 19–53 years) with multiple seizure types were divided into four groups by restrictive randomization, and each group was randomly assigned to one of four potential treatments: (a) mexiletine, 800 mg/day, plus phenobarbital, 300 mg/day, plus phenytoin placebo; (b) mexiletine, 800 mg/day, plus phenytoin, 300 mg/day, plus phenobarbital placebo; (c) phenytoin, 300 mg/day, plus phenobarbital, 300 mg/day, plus mexiletine placebo; or (d) mexiletine, 800 mg/day, plus phenytoin, 300 mg/day, plus phenobarbital, 300 mg/day. Criteria for removing a patient from a treatment for excess seizures or side effects were established in advance.

During the first treatment period, an increased frequency of seizures in all treatment groups caused clinical concern, and the study design was altered before the second treatment period. Table 2 illustrates the modified study design. Groups 3 and 4 continued to have medication administered in a blind fashion; physicians knew which drugs patients were receiving, but hospital staff and patients did not. Groups 1 and 2 received mexiletine in the same blind fashion but received their usual medications unblinded. Groups 1 and 2 formed a two-period changeover design, and groups 3 and 4 formed a three-period changeover design. For some individual patients, mexiletine appeared to be efficacious, but statistical comparisons demonstrated no effect of the drug on seizure frequency. Urinary acidity was not controlled.

A further double-blind crossover study was undertaken with the same patients (14, J. J. Cereghino et al., *unpublished data*). One group received their usual prestudy antiepileptic medications plus 800 mg of mexiletine daily, whereas the other group received their usual prestudy medications plus mexiletine placebo. The first treatment period was 12 weeks, and then crossover occurred for the second 12-week treatment period. There was no statistical difference in seizure frequency overall or for any specific seizure type between mexiletine or mexiletine placebo. Urinary acidity was not controlled.

Plasma concentrations of mexiletine in these studies ranged up to 3,000 ng/ml (3.0 μg/ml), with a mean of 893 ng/ml (0.8 μg/ml).

Cinca et al. (17) administered daily doses of 400 to 600 mg of mexiletine to 30 patients (18

TABLE 2. *Modified design of mexiletine study*[a]

	T_1[c]	T_2	T_3
		R-$T_1T_1T_1$-RRR[b]-$T_2T_2T_2$-RRR-$T_3T_3T_3$-R	
Group 1	MEX, 800 mg/day	R	R
	PB, 300 mg/day	MEX, placebo	MEX, 800 mg/day
	PHT, placebo		
Group 2	MEX, 800 mg/day	R	R
	PHT, 300 mg/day	MEX, 800 mg/day	MEX, placebo
	PB, placebo		
Group 3	PHT, 300 mg/day	MEX 800 mg/day	PHT, 300 mg/day
	PB, 300 mg/day	PHT, 300 mg/day	PB, 300 mg/day
	MEX, placebo	PB, 300 mg/day	MEX, placebo
Group 4	MEX, 800 mg/day	PHT, 300 mg/day	MEX, 800 mg/day
	PHT, 300 mg/day	PB, 300 mg/day	PHT, 300 mg/day
	PB, 300 mg/day	MEX, placebo	PB, 300 mg/day

[a] R, usual antiepileptic medications for 1 week; T_1, test drugs for 1 week of first treatment period; T_2, test drugs for 1 week of second treatment period; T_3, test drugs for 1 week of third treatment period.
[b] Study design modified.
[c] Initial study treatments.

with "grand mal," 2 with "petit mal," 5 with "temporal focal seizures," and 5 with several other seizure types). Plasma concentrations of the drug were not measured. Of the 30 patients, 23% showed "definite clinical improvement," 30% had no change in clinical condition, and 47% experienced "exacerbations of seizures." The authors concluded that the effectiveness of the agent remains doubtful.

Six epileptic patients with spontaneous frequent and persistent spike, polyspike, and spike-and-wave interictal EEG discharges received a single intravenous dose of 100 mg of mexiletine in a double-blind manner (1,44). Comparison of 10 min of control EEG with two 10-min periods of EEG after the injection showed no significant reduction in paroxysmal EEG discharges. There was no significant difference in the discharge count between mexiletine and saline injection, whereas injection of 5 mg of diazepam showed a significant decrease compared to saline.

The clinical studies of mexiletine as an antiepileptic drug may be summarized as follows:

1. There is no statistical evidence from controlled clinical trials that mexiletine is effective as either a primary or a supplemental antiepileptic drug.
2. There is no evidence that mexiletine normalizes the EEG.

3. Uncontrolled case reports indicate that mexiletine improves seizure control.
4. Case reports suggest that mexiletine precipitates seizures, but controlled clinical trials fail to substantiate this impression.

None of the clinical studies would suggest any reason for the failure of mexiletine to control seizures. The plasma concentration, when reported, has fallen in the range of 400 to 700 ng/ml (0.4–0.7 µg/ml), the suggested therapeutic range (54). The suggested cardiac therapeutic range is from 500 to 2,000 ng/ml (0.5 to 2.0 µg/ml), but the margin between therapeutic and toxic plasma concentrations is small (16). Many epileptic patients have actually been in the cardiac presumed therapeutic range.

The urinary pH has not been controlled in the antiepileptic drug studies, which may significantly alter the plasma mexiletine concentration. The cardiac studies have similarly not been performed under conditions of controlled urinary pH, and yet the efficacy of mexiletine has been apparent. A possible interaction of mexiletine with other antiepileptic drugs has not been clinically apparent. One study (J. J. Cereghino et al., *unpublished data*) found elevation of phenytoin concentrations when time series analysis was performed. It does not appear likely that an interaction could account for lack of antiepileptic efficacy of mexiletine.

Mexiletine effectively controls ventricular dysrhythmias with acute myocardial infarction. There is also evidence that long-term oral mexiletine therapy may be effective in controlling recurrent ventricular arrhythmias of ischemic heart disease without recurrent infarctions, and idiopathic arrhythmias. The usual regimen is an intravenous bolus injection to control the acute arrhythmia followed by an initially rapid, but gradually decreasing, rate of intravenous infusion, then continuous intravenous maintenance infusion, and ultimately, oral administration. The initial bolus injection is usually in the range of 150 to 250 mg administered over 2 to 5 min followed by a loading infusion of 250 mg in 30 min, then 250 mg in 2.5 hr and 500 mg in 8 hr. Twenty-four-hour maintenance infusion is 500 to 1,000 mg. A typical oral regimen would consist of a starting dose of 400 to 600 mg followed in 4 to 6 hr by a 150- to 350-mg maintenance dose which is then continued at 8-hr intervals (16,37,58).

TOXICITY

Nausea and vomiting are observed with initiation of mexiletine therapy in some patients. Hiccups and an unpleasant taste have also been noted (37; J. J. Cereghino et al., *unpublished data*). Toxicity is more frequently observed in acutely ill cardiac patients than in epileptic patients.

Mexiletine may cause a fine tremor of the hands which becomes more marked with increasing concentrations and is accompanied by dizziness, blurred vision, and, occasionally, nausea (51). Ataxia, increased somnolence, and confusion were observed in some patients in the New Castle studies (J. J. Cereghino et al., *unpublished data*), but mental and physical impairments prevented most patients from communicating the more subtle central nervous system symptoms.

Hypotension and bradycardia, particularly as a result of sinus arrest, have been observed in cardiac patients (16,37). No cardiac side effects have been observed in patients with epilepsy. Decreased platelet count and development of a positive antinuclear factor have been noted in one patient and may have been related to mexiletine use (12).

In a cardiac study, side effects were experienced by 73% of 83 patients (9). The incidence was to some extent, but not completely, dose related. The mean therapeutic concentration in 44 patients without side effects was 1,330 ng/ml (1.33 ± 1.0 μ/ml), whereas the mean concentration in 46 patients with side effects was 2,490 ng/ml (2.49 ± 0.24 μg/ml). Intolerable side effects occurred with a mean concentration of 3,330 ng/ml (3.3 ± 0.5 μg/ml), with a range of 500 to 6,000 ng/ml (0.5–6.0 μg/ml), but were tolerable with a mean concentration of 2,100 ng/ml (2.1 ± 0.2 μg/ml) with a range of 600 to 6,500 ng/ml (0.6–6.5 μg/ml).

OVERDOSAGE

One fatal case (25,38) of mexiletine overdosage has been reported. A 22-year-old non-epileptic man ingested 22 200-mg tablets which had been prescribed for his father. About 30 min after ingestion, nausea and parethesias of the tongue occurred. One hour later, he had a generalized tonic–clonic seizure that lasted about 5 min. He may have been hypoxic for 10 min before cardiac massage and ventilation were started. On arrival at the emergency room, he was "cyanosed, rigid, and convulsing." Pulse rate was 15/min, and blood pressure was unrecordable. The electrocardiogram showed complete heart block with a low escape rhythm, and within 5 min, ventricular asystole occurred with evidence of atrial activity. Resuscitation measures were discontinued 2 hr after admission. The plasma mexiletine concentration postmortem (not specified, but probably 3 to 4 hr after ingestion) was 34 to 37 μg/ml (approximately 30 times the therapeutic concentration).

SUMMARY

Mexiletine, 1 - (2′,6′-dimethyl) - phenoxy-2-aminopropine, is patented by C. H. Boehringer Sohn of Ingelheim, West Germany. It has been investigated as a cardiac antiarrhythmic and as an adjunct antiepileptic drug. The drug is commercially available as the hydrochloride, is easily soluble in water, and has a pK_a of 8.4 at 25°C.

Several gas chromatographic methods can detect plasma mexiletine levels of 100 ng/ml and above, which is an adequate range for clinical use. The sensitivity of the gas chromatographic methods can be increased by use of an electron capture detector; levels of about 10 ng/ml in serum, urine, saliva, and bile can be detected with this method.

Absorption of mexiletine occurs mainly in the upper part of the small intestine, and the gastric emptying rate may be a major controlling factor. Distribution would appear to be consistent with a three-compartment model. The drug behaves as a base, and renal clearance is pH dependent. Some authors postulate that spontaneous extremes of urinary pH may account for some cases of inefficacy of the drug or for occurrence of side effects, but interpretation of the data is inconsistent.

Mexiletine has numerous metabolites, and anticonvulsant activity of the major metabolites is suspected but has not been demonstrated. The mode of action is not certain. The anticonvulsant mode of action might be to inhibit reuptake of GABA as a central nervous system inhibitory transmitter.

There is no evidence from controlled clinical trials that mexiletine is effective as either a primary or supplemental antiepileptic medication. There are uncontrolled case reports that mexiletine has improved seizure control. Reported plasma concentrations have been in or exceeded the presumed therapeutic range of 400 to 700 ng/ml (0.4–0.7 μg/ml). The therapeutic steady-state plasma concentration in cardiac patients is presumed to be in the range of 500 to 2,000 ng/ml (0.5–2.0 μg/ml). Side effects are experienced at higher concentrations and limit the dosage.

Nausea and vomiting may be observed with initiation of therapy. A fine tremor of the hands, dizziness, blurred vision, ataxia, increased somnolence, and mental confusion have also been observed. The only reported fatality was a case of deliberate overdosage.

CONVERSION

Conversion factor:

$$CF = \frac{1000}{mol.\ wt.} = \frac{1000}{215.5} = 4.64$$

Conversion:

$$(\mu g/ml) \times 4.64 = (\mu moles/liter)$$
$$(\mu moles/liter) \div 4.64 = (\mu g/ml)$$

REFERENCES

1. Ahmad, S., Perucca, E., and Richens, A. (1977): The effect of frusemide, mexiletine, (+)-propanolol and three benzodiazepine drugs on interictal spike discharges in the electroencephalograms of epileptic patients. *Br. J. Clin. Pharmacol.*, 4:683–688.
2. Baudinet, G., Henrard, L., Quinaux, N., El Allaf, D., De Landsheere, C., Carlier, J., and Dresse, A. (1980): Pharmacokinetics of mexiletine in renal insufficiency. *Acta Cardiol. [Suppl.]*, 25:55–65.
3. Beckett, A. H., and Chidomere, E. C. (1976): The relationship between plasma levels, salivary concentrations and urinary excretion rates of mexiletine. *J. Pharm. Pharmacol. [Suppl.]*, 28:58P.
4. Beckett, A. H., and Chidomere, E. C. (1977): The distribution, metabolism and excretion of mexiletine in man. *Postgrad. Med. J.*, 53(Suppl. 1):60–66.
5. Beckett, A. H., and Chidomere, E. C. (1977): The identification and analysis of mexiletine and its metabolic products in man. *J. Pharm. Pharmacol.*, 29:281–285.
6. Bogaert, M. (1980): Adaptation of the dose of mexiletine according to pharmacokinetic data. *Acta Cardiol. [Suppl.]*, 25:67–73.
7. Boyle, D. McC., Chapman, C., Kinney, C., McIlmoyle, E. L., Salathia, K., and Shanks, R. G. (1980): A comparison of mexiletine and a slow release formulation of mexiletine in patients admitted to a coronary care unit. *Br. J. Clin. Pharmacol.*, 9:293P.
8. Bradbrook, I. D., James C., and Rogers, H. J. (1977): A rapid method for the determination of plasma mexiletine levels by gas chromatography. *Br. J. Clin. Pharmacol.*, 4:380–382.
9. Campbell, N. P. S., Chaturvedi, N. C., Kelly, J. G., Strong, J. E., Shanks, R. G., and Pantridge, J. F. (1973): Mexiletine (Kö 1173) in the management of ventricular dysrhythmias. *Lancet*, 2:404–407.
10. Campbell, N. P. S., Kelly, J. G., Adgey, A. A. J., and Shanks, R. G. (1978): The clinical pharmacology of mexiletine. *Br. J. Clin. Pharmacol.*, 6:103–108.
11. Campbell, N. P. S., Kelly, J. G., Adgey, A. A. J., and Shanks, R. G. (1978): Mexiletine in normal volunteers. *Br. J. Clin. Pharmacol.*, 6:372–373.
12. Campbell, N. P. S., Kelly, J. G., Shanks, R. G., and Adgey, A. A. J. (1977): Long term oral antiarrhythmic therapy with mexiletine. *Postgrad. Med. J.*, 53:143–145.
13. Cereghino, J. J., Brock, J. T., Van Meter, J. C., Penry, J. K., Kupferberg, H. J., Smith, L. D., and

White, B. G. (1975): A multiple-dose study of mexiletine (Kö 1173). *Epilepsia,* 16:673–677.

14. Cereghino, J. J., Penry, J. K., and Brock, J. T. (1977): A controlled prospective study of the use of mexiletine as an adjunct antiepileptic drug. In: *Excerpta Medica International Congress Series, No. 427. 11th World Congress of Neurology, Amsterdam, September 11–16, 1977,* edited by W. A. den Hartog Jager, G. W. Bruyn, and A. P. J. Heijstee, pp. 85–86. Excerpta Medica, Amsterdam.

15. Cereghino, J. J., Wilder, B. J., Kupferberg, H. J., Yonekawa, W. D., Perchalski, R. J., Ramsey, R. E., White, B. G., Penry, J. K., and Smith, L. D. (1975): A single-dose study of mexiletine (Kö 1173). *Epilepsia,* 16:665–672.

16. Chew, C. Y. C., Collett, J., and Singh, B. H. (1979): Mexiletine: A review of its pharmacological properties and therapeutic efficacy in arrhythmias. *Drugs,* 17:161–181.

17. Cinca, I., Ionescu, M., Dimitriu, R., Nicolae, I., Rusu, I., and Guguianu, S. (1975): Studii privind eficienta medicamentului Kö-1173 in epilepsie. *Neurol. Psihiatr. Neurochir.,* 20:209–214.

18. Clark, R. A., Julian, D. G., Nimmo, J., Prescott, L. F., and Talbot, R. (1973): Clinical pharmacological studies of Kö 1173—a new antiarrhythmic agent. *Br. J. Pharmacol.,* 47:622P–623P.

19. Clark, R. A., Talbot, R. G., Nimmo, J., Prescott, L. F., and Julian, D. G. (1973): Kö 1173—an effective new antiarrhythmic drug. *Br. Heart J.,* 35:558.

20. Danneberg, P. B., and Shelley, J. H. (1977): The pharmacology of mexiletine. *Postgrad. Med. J.,* 53(Suppl. 1):25–29.

21. Frydman, A., Lafarge, J. P., Vial, F., Rulliere, R., and Alexandre, J. M. (1978): New electron-capture gas–liquid chromatographic method for the determination of mexiletine plasma levels in man. *J. Chromatogr.,* 145:401–411.

22. Häselbarth, V., Deovendans, J. E., and Wolfe. M. (1981): Kinetics and bioavailability of mexiletine in healthy subjects. *Clin. Pharmacol. Ther.,* 29:729–736.

23. Holt, D. W., Flanagan, R. J., Hayler, A. M., and Loizou, M. (1979): Simple gas–liquid chromatographic method for the measurement of mexiletine and lignocaine in blood-plasma or serum. *J. Chromatogr.,* 169:295–301.

24. Holt, D. W., Walsh, A. C., Curry, P. V., and Tynan, M. (1979): Paediatric use of mexiletine and disopyramide. *Br. Med. J.,* 2:1476–1477.

25. Jequier, P., Jones, R., and Mackintosh, A. (1976): Fatal mexiletine overdose. *Lancet,* 1:429.

26. Johnston, A., Burgess, C. D., Warrington, S. J., Wadsworth, J., and Hamer, N. A. J. (1979): The effect of spontaneous changes in urinary pH on mexiletine plasma concentrations and excretion during chronic administration to healthy volunteers. *Br. J. Clin. Pharmacol.,* 8:349–352.

27. Kaye, C. M., Kiddie, M. A., and Turner, P. (1977): Variable pharmacokinetics of mexiletine. *Postgrad. Med. J.,* 53(Suppl. 1):56–58.

28. Kelly, J. G. (1977): Measurement of plasma mexiletine concentrations. *Postgrad. Med. J.,* 53(Suppl. 1):48–49.

29. Kelly, J. G., Nimmo, J., Rae, R., Shanks, R. G., and Prescott, L. F. (1973): Spectrophotofluorometric and gas–liquid chromatographic methods for the estimation of mexiletine (Kö 1173) in plasma and urine. *J. Pharm. Pharmacol.,* 25:550–553.

30. Kiddie, M. A., and Kaye, C. M. (1974): The renal excretion of mexiletine (Kö 1173) under controlled conditions of urine pH. *Br. J. Clin. Pharmacol.,* 1:86–87.

31. Kiddie, M. A., and Kaye, C. M. (1976): The influence of pH on the buccal absorption, and renal and plasma elimination of mexiletine and lignocaine. *Br. J. Clin. Pharmacol.,* 3:350P–352P.

32. Kiddie, M. A., Kaye, C. M., Turner, P., and Shaw, T. R. D. (1974): The influence of urinary pH on the elimination of mexiletine. *Br. J. Clin. Pharmacol.,* 1:229–232.

33. Kiddie, M. A., Royds, R. B., and Shaw, T. R. D. (1973): Preliminary studies on the pharmacology of an antidysrhythmic, Kö 1173, in man. *Br. J. Pharmacol.,* 47:674P–675P.

34. Koppe, H. G. (1977): The development of mexiletine. *Postgrad. Med. J.,* 53(Suppl. 1):22–25.

35. Koppe, H., Zeile, K., Kummer, W., Stahle, H., and Danneberg, P. (1972): Pharmaceutical compositions comprising certain 1-phenoxy-2-amino-alkanes. U.S. Patent 3,659,019, April 25, 1972.

36. Krall, R. L., Penry, J. K., White, B. G., Kupferberg, H. J., and Swinyard, E. A. (1978): Antiepileptic drug development: II. Anticonvulsant drug screening. *Epilepsia,* 19:409–428.

37. Kulbertus, H. E. (1980): Clinical antiarrhythmic efficacy of mexiletine: A review. *Acta Cardiol. [Suppl.],*25:111–120.

38. Mackintosh, A. F., and Jequier, P. (1977): Fatal mexiletine overdose. *Postgrad. Med. J.,* 53(Suppl. 1):134.

39. Moreno, A., Rabadan, F., and Hidalgo, A. (1979): Efectos de la mexiletina sobre el consumo de oxígeno y glucosa en cerebro, hígado y miocardio de rata *in vitro. Rev. Esp. Fisiol.,* 35:317–320.

40. Perchalski, R. J., Wilder, B. J., and Hammer, R. H. (1974): Flame-ionization and electron-capture GLC determination of 1-(2,6-dimethylphenoxy)-2-aminopropane in plasma. *J. Pharm. Sci.,* 63:1489–1491.

41. Porter, R. J., Kupferberg, H. J., and Riley, T. (1978): Anticonvulsant activity and disposition of the enantiomers $R(-)$ and $S(+)$ of mexiletine. In: *Abstracts 1306–2986, 7th International Congress of Pharmacology, Paris, July 16–21, 1978,* edited by J. R. Boisler, P. Lechart, and J. Fichelle, p. 818. Pergamon Press, Oxford.

42. Pottage, A. (1977): Oral dosage schedules for mexiletine. *Postgrad. Med. J.,* 53(Suppl. 1):155–157.

43. Prescott, L. F., Pottage, A., and Clements, J. A. (1977): Absorption, distribution and elimination of mexiletine. *Postgrad. Med. J.,* 53(Suppl. 1):50–55.

44. Richens, A. (1976): *Drug Treatment of Epilepsy,* pp. 162–163. Henry Kimpton, London.

45. Scott, K. N., Couch, M. W., Wilder, B. J., and Williams, C. M. (1973): The use of mass spectroscopy and ^{13}C and ^1H nuclear magnetic resonance in the characterization of 1-methyl-(2,6-xylyloxy) ethylamine metabolites. *Drug Metab. Dispos.,* 1:506–515.

46. Singh, B. N., and Vaughan Williams, E. M. (1972): Investigations of the mode of action of a new antidysrhythmic drug, Kö 1173. *Br. J. Pharmacol.,* 44:1–9.

47. Smith, K. J., and Meffin, P. J. (1980): Mexiletine analysis in blood and plasma using gas chromatography and nitrogen-selective detection. *J. Chromatogr.,* 181:469–472.

48. Stavenow, L., Hanson, A., and Johansson, B. W. (1979): Mexiletine in treatment of ventricular arrhythmias. *Acta Med. Scand.,* 205:411–415.

49. Szinai, N., Perchalski, R. J., Hammer, R. H., Wilder, B. J., and Streiff, R. R. (1973): GLC determination of 1-(2,6-dimethylphenoxy)-2-aminopropane in urine. *J. Pharm. Sci.,* 62:1376–1378.

50. Talbot, R. G., Clark, R. A., Nimmo, J., Neilson, J. M. M., Julian, D. G., and Prescott, L. F. (1973): Treatment of ventricular arrhythmias with mexiletine (Kö 1173). *Lancet,* 2:399–403.

51. Talbot, R. G., Julian, D. G., and Prescott, L. F. (1976): Long-term treatment of ventricular arrhythmias with oral mexiletine. *Am. Heart J.,* 91:58–65.

52. Timmis, A. D., Jackson, G., and Holt, D. W. (1980): Mexiletine for control of ventricular dysrhythmias in pregnancy. *Lancet,* 2:647–648.

53. Vaughan Williams, E. M. (1977): Mexiletine in isolated tissue models. *Postgrad. Med. J.,* 53(Suppl. 1):30–34.

54. Wilder, B. J. (1974): Kö 1173. Report of clinical and pharmacological study. (Experimental anticonvulsant drug). In: *Epilepsy Center Workshop,* pp. 6–7. V.A. Hospital and Yale University, New Haven.

55. Wilder, B. J., Lanlois, Y., and Hammer, R. H. (1973): Clinical and laboratory studies of a new anticonvulsant drug. *Epilepsia,* 14:102.

56. Willox, S., and Singh, B. N. (1976): Sensitive gas chromatographic method for the estimation of a new antiarrhythmic compound, mexiletine (Kö 1173), in biological fluids. *J. Chromatogr.,* 128:196–198.

57. Wing, L. M. H., Meffin, P. J., Grygiel, J. J., Smith, K. J., and Birkett, D. J. (1980): The effect of metoclopramide and atropine on the absorption of orally administered mexiletine. *Br. J. Clin. Pharmacol.,* 9:505–509.

58. Zipes, D. P., and Troup, P. J. (1978): New antiarrhythmic agents: Amiodarone, aprindine, disopyramide, ethmozin, mexiletine, tocainide, verapamil. *Am. J. Cardiol.,* 41:1005–1024.

Antiepileptic Drugs, edited by D. M. Woodbury,
J. K. Penry, and C. E. Pippenger. Raven Press,
New York © 1982

74

Potential Anticonvulsants

GABA Receptor Agonists

Kenneth G. Lloyd and Paolo L. Morselli

Over the past 10 years it often has been proposed that epilepsy is related to dysfunction of GABA neurons (53,69,70,72,86,98,101). Such a hypothesis was originally generated by the observations of Hayashi (40) in 1959 and Tower (100) in 1960 who demonstrated in both animals and man an anticonvulsant effect of GABA either topically applied or systemically administered at high doses (2,000 mg/day). The concomitant observations of Coursin (18,19) and later of Hennequet et al. (41) further strengthened the hypothesis that alterations in the functioning of the GABAergic system could have a bearing on convulsive states.

Today, the data supporting such a theory are numerous and consistent. Several authors have reported that brain material removed from an epileptic focus (of either animal models or epileptic patients) and CSF of epileptic patients are deficient in parameters related to GABAergic neurotransmission, e.g., GABA levels, glutamic acid decarboxylase (GAD) activity, and [^{3}H]GABA binding (53,68,76,85,101,103, 107).

Further support derives from the observation that impairment of GABA neuron function leads to seizures: this may arise from inhibition of GABA synthesis in both animals and man (10,60,98,101) or from blockade of GABA receptors or of the GABA-receptor-mediated increase in chloride conductance (25,45,64, 65,95). Thus, compounds such as isoniazide, allylglycine, and 3-mercaptopropionic acid, all potent inhibitors of GAD, induce severe convulsions, as do GABA receptor antagonists acting by blocking either the receptor sites (bicuculline) or the ionophore controlling the GABA-mediated chloride flux (picrotoxinin). This seizure activity is apparently related to reduction in the neurotransmitter action of GABA rather than to any metabolic action, as convulsions can be induced by inhibition of GAD even in the presence of elevated GABA levels (99, 106). Consistent with the hypothesis are the observations that reversal of the GABA deficit effectively antagonizes seizures. Thus, pyridoxal phosphate, the cofactor for GAD, immediately reverses vitamin B$_6$-dependent seizures in laboratory animals (43,61,69,88,98) and in epileptic patients (19,101). Furthermore, increasing GABA synaptic activity by inhibition of GABA transaminase (GABA-T) may have anticonvulsant effects (54,84,98). Similarly, several clinically used antiepileptic drugs (phenytoin and barbiturates) augment GABAergic transmission, suggesting an involvement of GABA neurons in the mechanism of action of these drugs (39,45,60,64,65,70).

With this background, it seems reasonable that direct-acting GABAmimetic agents (i.e., GABA receptor agonists) should be effective anticonvulsants and probably antiepileptics.

This hypothesis has not previously been amenable to direct testing in either man or animals, as the available GABA receptor agonists have been either toxic (muscimol) or so lipophobic that they scarcely entered into the brain (GABA, isoguvacine) or both (muscimol) (4,14,15, 48,66,101). However, nontoxic GABA agonists capable of crossing the blood–brain barrier have recently been synthesized (46,47). Thus, progabide, SL 75 102, and THIP (described below) are neurophysiologically defined as GABA receptor agonists (22,23) that displace [^{3}H]GABA from its binding sites on rat brain membranes (3,8,48). These compounds are structurally related to GABA, as are muscimol, isoguvacine, 3-aminopropanesulfonic acid and kojic amine (Fig. 1).

Another group of compounds that have been suggested to exert their anticonvulsant effect via

a GABA receptor-mediated event are the benzodiazepines. It has, in fact, been proposed that the benzodiazepine binding site modulates GABA receptor function by means of an as yet unidentified factor ("GABA-modulin"), increasing the affinity of the receptor for GABA (17,37). Although they are not GABA receptor agonists, the benzodiazepines can thus be considered to exert their action via the GABA receptor rather than by altering the available GABA levels (37,39). Barbiturates also may have a presynaptic effect on GABA-mediated inhibition, and this effect could involve GABA ionophores (45,64,65).

In this chapter, we review the available information related to those compounds that can be defined as true GABA receptor agonists and whose anticonvulsant effect has been clearly

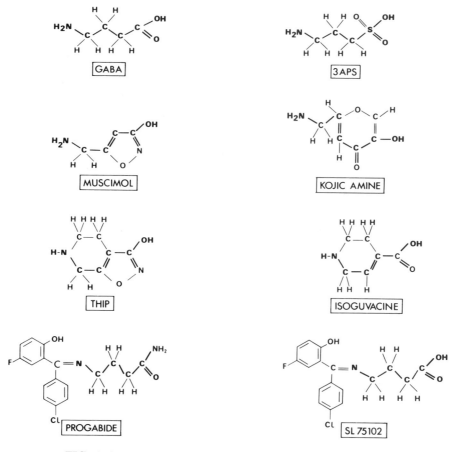

FIG. 1. Structural formulas of GABA and some GABA agonists.

documented. The benzodiazepines and barbiturates are treated in detail in Chapters 27 and 65–67.

CHEMISTRY AND METHODS
OF DETERMINATION

For most of the compounds considered in this chapter, the chemical information available in the literature is rather scarce and fragmentary; hence, a complete description of their physico-chemical properties is impossible.

Muscimol

Muscimol (agarin, pantherine, 5-aminomethyl-3-hydroxyisoxazole) is a naturally occurring compound which was first isolated from *Amanita stabiliformis* (94) and from *Amanita muscaria* (75). It can be obtained also from ibotenic acid by decarboxylation (82) or from γ-chloro-β,β-dimethoxybutyrohydroxylamic acid by cyclization in acid medium followed by a nucleophilic substitution of the chlorine by NH_3 (32). The compound ($C_4H_6N_2O_2$) has a molecular weight of 114.1, and it appears as pale yellow crystals, melting at 170°C. It is readily soluble in water, scarcely soluble in methanol and ethanol, and practically insoluble in organic solvents such as benzene, ethylacetate, chloroform, and hexane.

There are no methods described for the determination of concentrations of unlabeled muscimol in biological fluids and tissues; the methods available in the literature refer to the identification of the ^3H-labeled compounds. In general, they are based on the extraction of the radioactive species with either 5% trichloroacetic acid (TCA) or 0.4 N perchloric acid following homogenization and subsequent centrifugation. The acid supernatant is then loaded onto a Dowex-50® ion-exchange column. The unchanged muscimol can then be collected, after washing with water, by eluting the column with 2 N NH_4OH (4,66,93). A volatile radioactive fraction attributable to muscimol metabolites can be collected in the acidic and water fractions (4,66). Thin-layer chromatography systems described for verifying purity and identity of the eluted radioactive fraction include methanol : ammonia (24 : 1 v/v), methanol : water (7 : 3 v/v), and *n*-butanol : glacial acetic acid : water (5 : 1 : 2 v/v) (4,66,93).

Homotaurine

3-Aminopropanesulfonic acid (homotaurine) is a weak organic acid, being structurally related both to taurine and to GABA. 3-Aminopropanesulfonic acid ($H_{10}SNO_3$) has a molecular weight of 139.1; it melts at >250°C (with decomposition), and it is water soluble. There are no methods described for its determination or quantification in body fluids.

Isoguvacine

Isoguvacine (1,2,3,6-tetrahydropyridine-4-carboxylic acid) is a synthetic compound related to a constituent of the betel nut, and it can be regarded as a semirigid analog of *trans*-4-aminocrotonic acid (48). Isoguvacine ($C_6H_9O_2N$) has a molecular weight of 127.15 and a melting point >250°C. It appears as a white crystalline powder and is not light sensitive. It is stable in aqueous solution and has a water solubility of 6%. There are no methods described for its determination in body fluids.

THIP

THIP (4,5,6,7-tetrahydroisoxazolo-[5,4-*c*]-pyridin-3-ol) is an original synthetic compound which may be considered a bicyclic analog of muscimol (47). THIP ($C_6H_8N_2O_2$) has a molecular weight of 140.0 and melts at 242 to 244°C (with decomposition). It appears as colorless crystals and is water soluble. The maximum absorbance in the UV is observed at 212 nm. There are no described methods for its quantification in body fluids or tissues.

Progabide

Progabide (4-{[(4-chlorophenyl) (5-fluoro-2-hydroxy-phenyl)methylene]amino}-butamide) is a synthetic compound defined as the Schiff base obtained from γ-aminobutyramide and a substituted benzophenone (47).

Progabide ($C_{17}H_{16}ClFN_2O_2$) has a molecular weight of 334.78 and a melting point of 138 to 142°C. It appears as a nonhygroscopic microcrystalline yellow powder and is not light sensitive. The compound is easily soluble in alcohols, acetone, toluene, and chloroform, whereas its solubility is very limited in ether and water (<0.5%).

In solution in strongly acidic medium, the compound is relatively instable, whereas no degradation can be observed at neutral or basic pH.

The maximum of absorbance in the UV is observed at 332 nm. The determination of progabide in biological fluids and tissues can be performed by a GLC method as recently described (34).

To plasma samples or tissue homogenates 1 ml of 0.2 M acetate buffer (pH 4.7) is added together with 5 ml of toluene. Samples are then extracted for 30 min, and, following centrifugation, the organic phase is transferred to another tube and brought to dryness at 60°C under a gentle stream of nitrogen. The dry residue is then reacted with heptafluorobutyric anhydride (HFBA) for 20 min at 60°C and then brought again to dryness. After two washings with n-hexane, the dry residue is redissolved in 50 to 100 μl of n-hexane, and 1.2 μl of the solution is injected into a gas chromatograph equipped with a [63]Ni electron capture detector. Operating conditions are: oven temperature, 230°C; injection port, 250°C; detector temperature, 275°C; nitrogen gas flow, 40 ml/min. The column is glass tubing 2 m long, 2 mm ID, packed with OV-17 3% on GasChromQ® (80–100 mesh), conditioned for 1 hr at 270°C (nitrogen flow 40 ml/min), 4 hr at 320°C (no nitrogen flow), and 24 hr at 280°C (nitrogen flow 4 ml/min). (Chloro-4-phenylchloro-5-hydroxy-2-benzylidene)-amino-4-butyramide was used as internal standard. Under the conditions described, retention times are 3.4 min for progabide and 5.9 min for the internal standard. The minimal detectable amount (injected) is of the order of 10 pg, corresponding to a minimal sensitivity of 10 to 20 ng per sample.

SL 75 102

SL 75 102 (4{[(4-chlorophenyl) (5-fluoro-2-hydroxyphenyl) methylene]amino}butanoic acid) is the acid analog of progabide. As the monosodium salt ($C_{17}H_{14}ClFNO_3Na$), it has a molecular weight of 357.75 and a melting point of 231°C. It appears as a nonhygroscopic microcrystalline yellow powder and is not light sensitive. The compound is soluble in alcohol and water (>5%) as well as in less polar solvents. As is progabide, SL 75 102 is somewhat instable in acid solutions, slowly decomposing to yield GABA and ortho-benzophenone. The determination of SL 75 102 in biological fluids and tissues can be performed by HPLC or GLC with minor modifications of the method described for progabide (34).

Kojic Amine

Kojic amine [2-(aminomethyl)-5-hydroxy-4-H-pyran-4-one] is a synthetic cyclic analog of GABA also related to muscimol (3,105). Kojic amine ($C_6H_7NO_3$) has a molecular weight of 141.0 and melts at 180°C. The compound is soluble in water. There are no described methods for its determination in biological fluids.

ABSORPTION, DISTRIBUTION, AND EXCRETION

Muscimol

Very little is known about the pharmacokinetics of muscimol in either experimental animals or man. No systematic studies have been performed on its disposition, and the available data are mainly derived from studies using the ^{3}H-labeled compound, where the primary aim was not the definition of the kinetic profile of the molecule but its rate of penetration into the central nervous system (4,27,66,93).

No data are available on oral absorption of muscimol in the rat. Following its intravenous administration, plasma concentrations of the compound (tritium labeled in the methylene side chain) decay very rapidly, with an apparent blood half-life of about 20 min (4). Such a decay of [³H]muscimol concentrations in blood is paralleled by a rapid rise in levels of not yet identified volatile metabolites. Although measurable amounts of radioactivity are present in the mouse brain 1 min after intravenous administration (66), maximal brain concentrations of the order of 0.036 to 0.150 ng/g (equivalent to 0.02% of the administered dose) are reached in both mice and rats only after 30 to 45 min (4,66,93). It should be noted that, in studies with [³H]muscimol labeled in the methylene chain, about 90% of the brain radioactivity was represented by "volatile compounds," whereas in the case of [³H]muscimol labeled in the isoxazole ring, only 50% of the radioactivity present in the brain (which was only 30 to 40% of that observed with the tritium label in the side chain) was represented by unchanged muscimol (27,66).

The computed brain-to-blood or brain-to-plasma ratios in the rat suggest that muscimol as such penetrates the central nervous system in only very limited amounts, brain concentrations being 1,000 to 5,000 times smaller than the blood concentrations (4).

Muscimol apparently distributes rather unevenly in the rat brain. The data on its distribution in discrete rat brain regions are, however, rather contradictory, and further information is needed. According to Snodgrass (93), the highest levels may be observed in the cerebellum, hippocampus, and substantia nigra, but according to Baraldi et al. (4), the highest levels are found in the pituitary, colliculi, and substantia nigra, with the lowest concentrations being found in the cortex and cerebellum.

Higher blood and brain concentrations were observed after pretreatment with GABA-T inhibitors (4,27,66), and apparently such an increase in brain level of unchanged muscimol is accompanied by an increased protective activity against bicuculline-induced convulsions in mice (27).

Very limited data are available on muscimol excretion. According to Ott et al. (82), in the mouse, only a very small fraction of unchanged muscimol is excreted in the urine after intraperitoneal administration. There are no data on the kinetics of muscimol in man.

Progabide

In the rat, progabide administered by the intraperitoneal route is rapidly absorbed, with peak plasma levels being attained within 20 to 40 min. In the case of oral administration (suspension in polysorbate-80), maximal concentrations are also achieved within 30 to 40 min but are generally followed by a plateau, suggesting a relatively slow absorptive process.

Balance studies indicate that the molecule is nearly completely absorbed; however, it undergoes an extensive first-pass effect, and the estimated bioavailability in the rat is of the order of 10 to 15% (24). Autoradiographic and quantitative studies with [¹⁴C]progabide labeled either in the benzophenone nucleus or in the GABAmide chain have shown a rapid distribution of progabide and its metabolites to various organs and tissues as well as a rapid penetration of the unchanged molecule into the brain, brain-to-plasma ratios being constantly >1 over the 8 hr following drug administration (Fig. 2). After oral and intravenous administration of [¹⁴C]progabide labeled in the GABA-mide chain, about 50% of the label was recovered in the 72-hr urine, 9 to 10% was present in the 72-hr feces, and 25 to 30% in the expired air, 10 to 15% remaining in the carcass. Additional balance studies with the ¹⁴C label on the benzophenone showed an excellent recovery of total radioactivity over 72 to 96 hr. Specific studies on biliary excretion indicate that 77% of the labeled dose is eliminated in the bile in 7 hr with over one half of the dose being excreted within the first hour. This finding, together with the excretion in feces of 10% of the dose after intravenous administration, suggests the possibility of an extensive enterohepatic recycling. In the rat, the apparent plasma half-life of progabide after intravenous or peritoneal administration is 40 to 60 min, although it may be longer after oral administration.

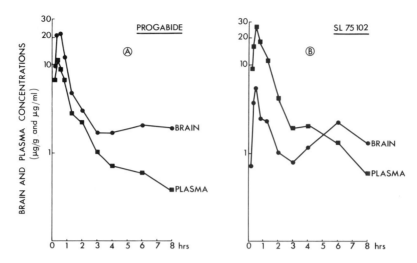

FIG. 2. Plasma and brain levels of progabide and SL 75 102 in the rat following administration of 100 mg/kg i.p. of either compound. The difference in the brain/plasma ratio between the two compounds is evident.

In dogs and cats, progabide is rapidly absorbed, with maximal plasma concentrations being attained between 1 and 3 hr. The computed plasma half-life is 2 to 3 hr in the dog and 3 to 4 hr in the cat.

The pharmacokinetic behavior of progabide in the monkey has recently been studied by Levy et al. (44). In the rhesus monkey, progabide administered at the dose of 50 mg/kg (dissolved in 100% PEG 400) is rapidly absorbed, with peak plasma levels attained 30 min after dosing and an estimated bioavailability of 29 to 69% (mean, 47%). Following intravenous administration, the rate of disappearance of progabide follows first-order kinetics, and it can be described by a one-compartment open model, suggesting a rapid distribution to various body organs and tissues. The apparent plasma half-life has been found to be of the order of 0.5 to 0.8 hr. The apparent volume of distribution is about 2 liter/kg, with a plasma clearance of 5 to 9 liter/hr, suggesting a high (>0.5) extraction ratio. Evaluation of plasma progabide levels during 7 days of constant-rate intravenous infusion indicates that steady-state plasma levels are rapidly attained and maintained during the 7-day treatment without modification of plasma clearance values. In all the species studied, progabide was found present as such in urine only in traces,

whereas free and conjugated benzophenones accounted for 8 to 10% of the excreted urinary material.

In man, peak plasma levels of progabide are usually attained 1 to 3 hr following oral intake (Fig. 3) and are proportional to the administered dose (11,13). Estimated bioavailability in man may range from 15 to 25% with coarse material to 50 to 65% with micronized preparations. With the use of gastro-resistant soft gelatine capsules containing progabide in oily suspension, peak plasma levels are attained 3 to 6 hr after dosing, with an estimated bioavailability of 22 to 42%. Studies with the ^{14}C-labeled compound have shown that in man 41.7% of administered radioactivity may be collected in the 48-hr urine, whereas 48.7% is present in the 96-hr feces. Preliminary observations on progabide CSF concentrations undergoing chronic treatment indicate that the plasma protein binding of progabide is of 94 to 98%. The apparent plasma half-life in healthy volunteers after a single dose may vary from 4 to 8 hr. Differences in either peak time or apparent plasma half-life could not be detected following repeated administration to healthy volunteers (11,13). Furthermore, progabide does not appear to modify the urinary D-glucaric acid excretion. Steady-state levels are reached in 2 to 4 days and maintained over the

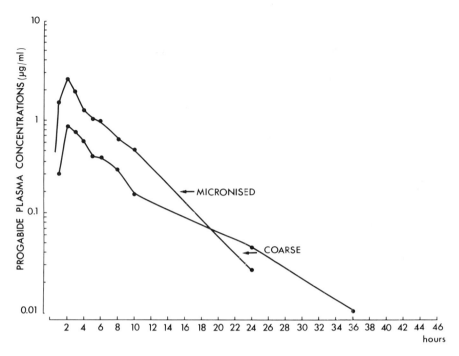

FIG. 3. Plasma levels of progabide in man following oral administration of 300 mg as either micronized or coarse material in hard gelatine capsules.

15-day observation period. Findings similar to those described for normal volunteers have also been obtained in epileptic patients.

Other GABA Agonists

No information is currently available on the pharmacokinetics of compounds such as THIP, isoguvacine, 3-aminopropanesulfonic acid, or kojic amine.

BIOTRANSFORMATION

Muscimol

Muscimol is rapidly degraded in both mice and rats. Possible major catabolic pathways could be represented by either oxidative deamination or transamination of the side chain (Fig. 4). Studies carried out after pretreating mice and rats with either GABA-T inhibitors such as aminooxyacetic acid (AOAA), ethanolamine sulfate (EOS), and γ-acetylenic GABA (GAG) or

a liver microsomal drug-metabolizing inhibitor such as SKF 525-A have shown that transamination of the side chain is very probably the major metabolic pathway. In fact, although no modification in either blood or brain levels of muscimol and its metabolites could be observed after SKF 525-A (4), a consistent rise (10-fold) in blood and brain muscimol concentrations was evident after pretreatment with GABA-T inhibitors in both mice and rats (4, 27,66). Such a rise in muscimol concentrations was furthermore accompanied by a reduction in volatile and nonvolatile metabolites (4,27,66). Another possible metabolic route could be represented by the cleavage of the oxygen–nitrogen bond in the isoxazole ring (66).

Progabide

Animal and human data indicate that progabide is extensively metabolized in the body. Only trace amounts of unchanged compound can be recovered in the urine of various animal spe-

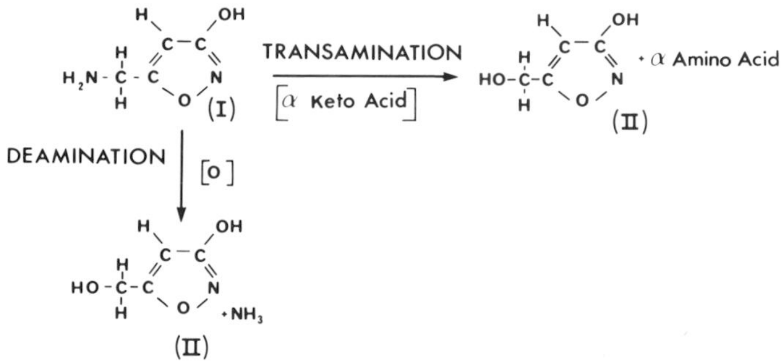

FIG. 4. Reported metabolic pathways for muscimol (4,66). I, muscimol; II, 3,5-dihydroxymethylisoxazole.

cies, and in man the amount of unmetabolized progabide found in urine was less than 2 to 3% of the administered dose. The possible metabolic pathways and the metabolites identified up to now are shown in Fig. 5. By oxidative deamination or transamination, progabide can yield the corresponding acid, SL 75 102, and by cleavage of the imine bond it gives rise to the *ortho*-hydroxybenzophenone and to GABAmide (8,11,24). GABA can subsequently be formed either by transamination or oxidative deamination of the GABAmide or by hydrolysis of SL 75 102.

The enzymatic systems responsible for the cleavage of the imine bond and of the likely transamination have not yet been identified. However, based on the available evidence, they are present in the brain, since both [^{14}C]-GABAmide and [^{14}C]GABA are found in the brain following systemic administration of [^{14}C]progabide (Fig. 6). In contrast, radioactivity could not be detected in the brain of rats receiving systemically equivalent doses of either ^{14}C-labeled GABAmide or GABA (24). It is noteworthy to mention that not only progabide but also SL 75 102 and GABAmide are active GABAmimetic agents (8). It may also be interesting to underline the fact that these four com-

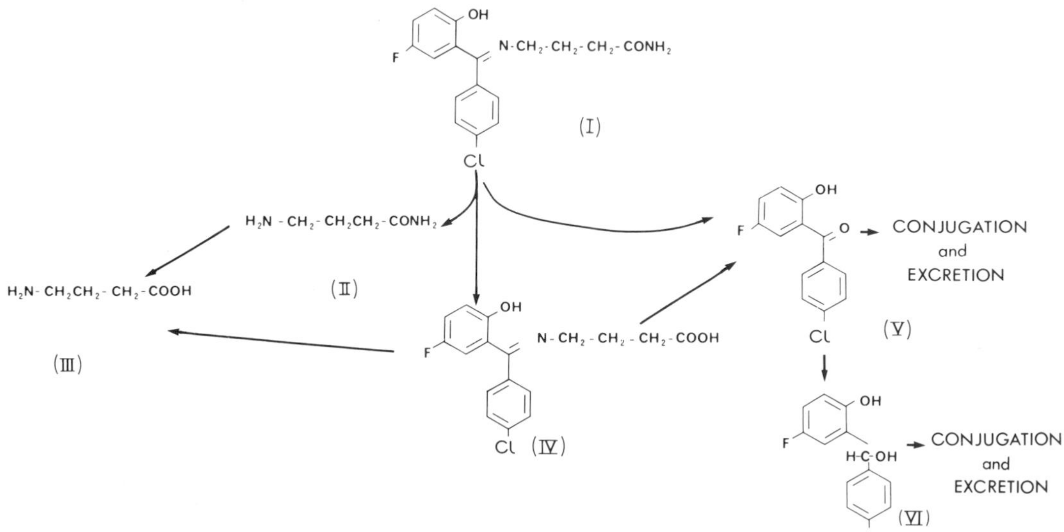

FIG. 5. Metabolic pathways of progabide: I, progabide; II, GABAmide; III, GABA; IV, SL 75 102; V, substituted *ortho*-hydroxybenzophenone; VI, substituted benzhydrol.

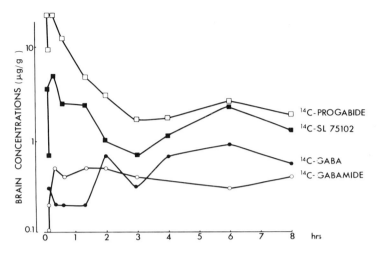

FIG. 6. Brain concentration of [^{14}C]progabide, [^{14}C]SL 75 102, [^{14}C]GABAmide, and [^{14}C]GABA in the rat following administration of [^{14}C]progabide, 100 mg/kg, i.p.

pounds give a full account of brain radioactivity after administration of [^{14}C]progabide labeled in the side chain. In contrast to this situation in the cerebral tissue, it is very likely that other compounds are formed in the periphery, since progabide and SL 75 102 could account for only 4% of the biliary radioactivity, the majority of the radioactivity being represented by very polar compounds (24).

The expiration of radioactive CO_2, which was observed in rats receiving progabide labeled in the side chain, probably results from peripheral oxidative deamination of GABA to succinic acid, which is subsequently oxidized via the Krebs tricarboxylic acid cycle to CO_2.

DRUG INTERACTIONS

No information is available on possible drug interactions for THIP, 3-aminopropanesulfonic acid, and isoguvacine. As mentioned before, the metabolic breakdown of muscimol can be inhibited by concomitant or previous administration of inhibitors of GABA-T. In the case of progabide at very high doses, the compound may show an inducing effect on hepatic microsomal mixed-function oxidases of the rat, as indicated by an enhanced activity of *p*-nitroanisol *o*-demethylation, aniline *p*-hydroxylation and amidopyrine *N*-demethylation (24). However, in

monkeys and man, the kinetics of progabide are not modified after repeated treatment with therapeutic doses, and chronic treatment with progabide did not modify D-glucaric acid excretion in healthy volunteers (11,13).

Moreover, in a group of epileptic patients, progabide did not seem to affect plasma levels of associated antiepileptic drugs such as phenobarbital and carbamazepine (9,57,73). Preliminary evidence, however, tends to suggest that an interaction is possible with phenytoin, since a modest increase in levels of phenytoin could be observed in 9 of 11 patients during concomitant treatment with phenytoin and progabide (102). Further studies are obviously needed to gain more precise information on the possible ''displacing'' effect of the acid metabolite as well as the possible competitive metabolic inhibition or induction exerted by other antiepileptic drugs on progabide and vice versa.

THERAPEUTIC LEVELS

During chronic administration of progabide to epileptic patients receiving associated drug treatment, morning plasma levels of progabide are apparently unrelated to the daily dose administered.

For an oral intake of 900 to 1800 mg/day, plasma levels of 0.2 to 2.0 µg/ml may be observed, with a fivefold or sixfold interindividual variability for the same dose expressed as mg/kg. Possible therapeutic plasma concentrations have not yet been determined. In patients responding favorably to the progabide treatment, monitored plasma levels ranged from 0.30 to 1.5 µg/ml. No information is available on the therapeutic levels of other GABA agonists.

TOXICITY

Laboratory Animals

Incidence

Few reports are available on the incidence of toxic effects of GABA agonists. Of the two drugs for which substantial information is available (muscimol and progabide), the acute toxicity is mainly related to central nervous system dysfunction (see below) and appears in a dose-dependent manner. For progabide, the "therapeutic ratio" is much more favorable than for muscimol. The toxic effects of progabide can be considered similar to those of the benzodiazepines, drugs that also are thought to act via GABA receptors.

Neurological Aspects of Toxicity

In rodents, the signs of acute toxicity common to all GABA receptor agonists are sedation and myorelaxation (Table 1). However, the induction of these effects in relation to their LD_{50} varies widely among compounds, with muscimol being the most sedative and myorelaxant. The benzodiazepines (e.g., chlordiazepoxide) and progabide are relatively much less myorelaxant or sedative. As both muscimol (4,66) and progabide (8,24) are extensively metabolized, it is not known to what extent the myorelaxation and sedation may be caused by metabolites not related to GABA agonist activity.

The GABAmimetics do not induce catalepsy in rats, although they greatly potentiate the cataleptic effects of cataleptogenic neuroleptics; with noncataleptogenic neuroleptics such as sulpiride, GABAmimetics do not induce a cataleptic state (6,7,54,55).

A worsening of the EEG pattern with appearance of paroxysmal features occasionally accompanied by irregular diffuse myoclonus and worsening of photosensitive seizures has been observed in man and the baboon following either muscimol or THIP administration (69–71,91). Whether these effects are related to the compounds themselves or to their metabolites is not currently known.

Chronic Aspects

Data from the pregnant rabbit indicate that progabide is well tolerated and devoid of any embryotoxic activity. In the rat, progabide in an oral dose of up to 1,000 mg/kg per day had no effect on either litter size or litter weight.

TABLE 1. *Biological activities of GABA receptor agonists*

Drug	Neurophysiological GABA agonist activity (bicuculline sensitive)[a]	Displacement of [³H]GABA binding (IC_{50}, µM)	Anticonvulsant effect (bicuculline) (ED_{50}, mg/kg, i.p.)
Progabide	Not tested	35 (8)	20 (54)
SL 75 102	+ + (23)	1.4 (8)	20[b]
Muscimol	+ + + (20)	0.009 (8)	0.25 (54)
THIP	+ + + (48)	0.13 (48)	0.80[b]
Isoguvacine	+ + + (48)	0.037 (48)	>60[b]
3-aminopropane sulfonic acid	+ + + (22)	0.083 (52)	—
GABA	+ + (20)	0.215 (52)	—
Kojic amine	+ (110)	4.0 (vs. [³H]muscimol) (110)	>30[b]

[a] +, weaker than GABA; + +, similar to GABA; + + +, more potent than GABA. References are in parentheses.
[b] P. Worms and K. G. Lloyd (*unpublished data*).

Information from chronic toxicity studies indicates that in rabbits and baboons the compound was devoid of toxicity over a 3-month treatment period in doses of up to 300 and 250 mg/kg, respectively. Similar results were obtained in dogs up to 240 mg/kg.

Neuroendocrine Effects

The available data on the neuroendocrine effects of GABA agonists are rather scarce and controversial. In the laboratory rat, muscimol, when injected intraventricularly, increases plasma prolactin levels (74). However, when it is administered systemically, a decrease in prolactin secretion, apparently independent of dopaminergic control, may be observed (74). Muscimol may also block the increase in prolactin associated with inhibition of dopamine synthesis or dopamine receptor blockade (31,74).

It has been reported (15,97) that in man plasma prolactin levels rose significantly in a dose-dependent manner within 120 min after a 5- to 9-mg oral dose of muscimol. In parallel, growth hormone rose modestly, while TSH and cortisol levels remained unchanged. A possible effect of GABA on prolactin has been hypothesized.

A point that we feel worthwhile to stress once again is that there is no evidence that these observed effects are caused by the intact muscimol rather than by one of its metabolites.

The effects of progabide on different hormone levels and responses to provocative stimuli (combined pituitary stimulation test) were evaluated in volunteers following treatment for 7 days with 1,200 mg/day. Progabide did not appear to modify any of the examined parameters, the only exception being the growth hormone response to hypoglycemia, which was inhibited by the compound. Parameters for which evidence of modifications could not be found were: T_4, T_3 uptake, FT_1, thyroxin-binding globulin, TSH (basal and after TRH), androgens, prolactin (basal and after TRH), FSH, LH (basal and after LHRH), and cortisol (basal and after hypoglycemia) (58,59).

The discrepancies between the observations with muscimol and those with progabide in man

seem to suggest that part of the effects observed after systemic administration of muscimol may be caused by the deaminated metabolite 3,5-dihydroxymethylisoxazole. This compound is, in fact, structurally very close to γ-hydroxybutyrate, a compound known to possess dopamine neuron-blocking properties (92).

PHARMACODYNAMICS

Pharmacological Effects

Neuropharmacological Data

Of the GABA agonists studied to date, a broad spectrum of anticonvulsant activity in different animal models has been observed (Table 2). Thus, muscimol reduces the seizures induced by bicuculline, picrotoxinin, pentylenetetrazol (PTZ), strychnine, sound (in sensitive mice), mercaptopropionic acid, allylglycine, and isoniazid (2,67,77,108; P. Worms and K. G. Lloyd, *unpublished data*). Although the data in Table 2 are representative of the anticonvulsant activity of muscimol, not all authors agree on the antistrychnine action of the compound (67,77,108). This is likely because of differences in the experimental techniques used. It should be noted that in spite of the anticonvulsant action of muscimol in many animal models, in the photosensitive baboon, muscimol (0.25–10 mg/kg i.v.) exacerbates the behavioral and EEG epileptic activity (83). Furthermore, muscimol is ineffective against electroshock-induced seizures.

THIP, a potent GABA receptor agonist as defined neurophysiologically and pharmacologically (Table 2), exerts an anticonvulsant effect against bicuculline convulsions but not mortality, picrotoxin, PTZ, strychnine, electroshock, and audiogenic stress (Table 2; K. G. Lloyd and P. Worms, *unpublished data*) as well as isoniazid (48). However, isoguvacine, another GABA receptor agonist (Table 1), is inactive as an anticonvulsant (bicuculline, audiogenic seizures) when administered systemically but is effective when injected intracerebral ventricularly (2) (Table 2).

TABLE 2. *Pharmacological effects of GABA receptor agonists in laboratory animals*

Test system	Muscimol	THIP	Progabide	APSA[a]	Chlordiazepoxide
Acute lethality, mouse					
LD$_{50}$ (mg/kg, i.p.)	12.5 (54)	80–160[b]	2,000 (54)	Not tested	270 (5)
Locomotor activity decrease,					
mouse, ED$_{50}$ (mg/kg, i.p.)	0.65 (54)	Not tested	120 (54)	Not tested	26 (54)
Decrease muscle strength,					
mouse, ED$_{50}$ (mg/kg, i.p.)	0.45 (54)	Not tested	200 (54)	Not tested	4.5 (54)
Anti-bicuculline convulsions,					
mouse, ED$_{50}$ (mg/kg, i.p.)	0.25 (54)	0.8[c]	20 (54)	Not tested	0.75 (54)
Anti-picrotoxinin convulsions,					
mouse ED$_{50}$ (mg/kg, i.p.)	1.1 (54)	20[c]	105 (54)	Not tested	3 (54)
Anti-pentylenetetrazole convulsions,					
mouse, ED$_{50}$ (mg/kg, i.p.)	0.6 (54)	2.0[c]	30 (54)	+[d] (1)	1.0 (54)
Anti-strychnine lethality,					
mouse, ED$_{50}$ (mg/kg, i.p.)	0.9 (54)	9.0[c]	75 (54)	Not tested	3.8 (54)
Anti-electroshock convulsions,					
mouse, ED$_{50}$ (mg/kg, i.p.)	2 (54)	>20[c]	75 (54)	Not tested	6.5 (54)
Penicillin-induced EEG focus,					
cat, ED$_{50}$ (mg/kg, i.v.)	Not tested	Not tested	5 (54)	5 (30)	Not tested
Photosensitive baboon	Exacerbates (83)	Exacerbates (71)	Antagonizes[e]	Not tested	Not tested
Therapeutic ratios					
LD$_{50}$/ED$_{50}$ (bicuc.)	50 (54)	27–54 (54)	100 (54)	—	360 (54)
ED$_{50}$ (locom)/ED$_{50}$ (bicuc.)	2–6 (54)	—	6 (54)	—	35 (54)
ED$_{50}$ (myorelax)/ED$_{50}$ (bicuc.)	1–8 (54)	—	10 (54)	—	6 (54)

[a]3-Aminopropanesulfonic acid.
[b]A. Christensen and A. Krogsgaard-Larsen *(personal communication)*.
[c]P. Worms and K. G. Lloyd *(unpublished data)*.
[d]Positive effect; no quantitation available.
[e]R. Naquet *(personal communication)*.

Progabide is a GABA receptor agonist and prodrug, slowly liberating GABA within the central nervous system (8). This latter effect may partially account for the duration of action of the drug, but it cannot explain the immediate onset of action (within 10 sec of injection). This anticonvulsant action appears to be caused by GABA receptor agonist properties of the drug (8; see below). Progabide exhibits an anticonvulsant action against audiogenic seizures, electroshock, strychnine, PTZ (convulsions or mortality), picrotoxin, picrotoxinin, bicuculline (convulsions or mortality), and allyglycine (Table 2; P. Worms and K. G. Lloyd, *unpublished data*). It also blocks the focal epilepsy induced by intracortical or intraamygdala injection of penicillin (K. G. Lloyd, *unpublished data*). This is in contrast to muscimol which is inactive against electroshock and the mortality induced by high doses of PTZ or bicuculline (108). Other

GABA prodrugs have been shown to exhibit anticonvulsant activity; thus, *N*-benzoyl-GABA and *N*-pivaloyl-GABA are effective against PTZ- or bicuculline-induced convulsions (33). Progabide has, in general, more favorable therapeutic ratios than the other GABA receptor agonists tested to date in this system (Table 2).

3-Aminopropanesulfonic acid (homotaurine) is a putative GABA agonist for which relatively few studies exist. It significantly delays the onset of convulsions caused by hyperbaric oxygen or cobalt application on the sensorimotor cortex (1). This compound is also effective against the focal epilepsy caused by penicillin or estrogen administration (29) but enhances the epileptogenic effects of systemically administered penicillin (30). This compound is ineffective against strychnine-induced convulsions (1).

Kojic amine is a new GABA analog which appears to be a GABA receptor agonist as defined either by displacement of [³H]GABA (3) or [³H]muscimol (110) binding and by neurophysiological experiments (bicuculline-sensitive inhibition of cerebellar Purkinje or cortex cells) (110). The compound may also interact with β-adrenergic receptors (105). The anticonvulsant spectrum of this compound has not been very thoroughly investigated; however, it is effective against mercaptopropionic acid-induced convulsions (3).

The benzodiazepines are well known for their broad spectrum of anticonvulsant properties (see Table 2 for chlordiazepoxide, for example). It has been suggested from both pharmacological (17) and neurophysiological (39) evidence that this activity is linked to a GABA receptor function (for further details, see below).

Neurophysiological Data

GABA receptor agonists, by definition, have the same neurophysiological effect as GABA itself in model systems for GABA receptors. Thus, microiontophoresis of muscimol induces a bicuculline-sensitive (strychnine-insensitive) decrease in the firing rate of cat spinal cord interneurons (20). Iontophoretically applied muscimol also depresses the firing rate of rat cortical neurons (109) and rat substantia nigra neurons (79). Intravenous muscimol decreases the firing rate of dorsal Deiters' neurons in the rat (108). Muscimol causes a bicuculline- and/or picrotoxin-sensitive increase in membrane conductance in the rat dorsal root ganglion (22) and the crayfish stretch receptor (42,81).

Progabide injected intravenously causes a potent reduction in the firing rate of neurons in the rat dorsal Deiters' nucleus. However, the low solubility of this compound does not allow it to be used in microiontophoresis. The acidic metabolite, SL 75 102, which has an anticonvulsant spectrum parallel to that of progabide (46) and is more potent in displacing [³H]-GABA from its binding sites on rat or human brain membranes (8), causes a depolarization associated with an increased chloride conductance in the rat dorsal root ganglion preparation. This effect is bicuculline- and picrotoxin-sensitive. Furthermore, SL 75 102 exerts a cross-desensitization with GABA and has the same reversal potential as the neurotransmitter (23).

3-Aminopropanesulfonic acid (APSA) depolarizes the rat dorsal root ganglion, increasing chloride conductance in a bicuculline- and picrotoxin-sensitive manner. Its action induces a cross-desensitization to that of GABA (22). Bowery and Brown (12) found APSA to be more potent than GABA on the GABA receptor of the rat superior cervical ganglion. Nistri and Corradetti (78) found that this compound induces a dorsal root depolarization in the frog spinal cord which was chloride dependent and inhibited by picrotoxin.

There is a lack of published information on the neurophysiological aspects of the newer "putative" GABA agonists such as THIP and isoguvacine. It is known (50) that both of these compounds produce a bicuculline-sensitive decrease in the firing rate of cat dorsal horn interneurons. In this aspect, isoguvacine appears to be two to four times more potent than THIP (which is equipotent to GABA). However, isoguvacine apparently does not easily cross the blood–brain barrier (48; A. Christensen and A. Krogsgaard-Larsen, *personal communication*).

Kojic amine inhibits the firing of spontaneously active or glutamate-activated cortical neurons, these effects being of slow onset and considerably longer duration than those of GABA (110). These effects on the cortical neurons are bicuculline sensitive and can be enhanced by diaminobutyric acid (DABA). Kojic amine may also inhibit the spontaneous firing of cerebellar Purkinje cells (110).

Although the benzodiazepines seem to lack a direct effect on the GABA receptor, they potentiate the dorsal root potential and presynaptic inhibition in the rat spinal cord and antagonize the effect of bicuculline on the striatonigral evoked potential, all of which are thought to be mediated by GABA (39). However, Curtis et al. (21) did not observe any effect of diazepam on the dorsal root potential. In cultured mouse fetal spinal cord neurons, iontophoresed diazepam or chlordiazepoxide potentiate the effects of GABA but not those of strychnine or glutamate (62).

Neurochemical Data

The GABA receptor agonists all have a similar profile in their actions on neurochemical parameters. Thus, all displace [³H]GABA or [³H]muscimol from its binding site(s) in rat (Table 2) or human (43,52) brain membrane preparations. The order of potency is: muscimol > APSA > THIP > GABA > SL 75 102 > kojic amine > progabide. At these concentrations, none of these compounds (except perhaps APSA, for which studies apparently have not been performed) inhibit GABA uptake, metabolism (via GABA-T), or synthesis (GAD activity) (8,45,49,110; B. Scatton, *personal communication*). It should be noted that muscimol is likely metabolized by GABA-T (4,27). Also, progabide and SL 75 102 are slowly metabolized to form GABA (8) which is then a substrate for GABA-T.

GABAmimetics also affect other neurotransmitter systems, although the results are not always clear as to whether these are direct or indirect effects, e.g., via interneurons. Thus, on systemic injection, GABA agonists decrease the biochemical indices of dopamine neuron activity and the activation of dopamine neurons induced by neuroleptics (55). However, when they are injected intranigrally, there is evidence that GABA receptor agonists induce biochemical indications of dopaminergic hyperactivity (16,89). *In vitro*, GABA agonists increase striatal dopamine synthesis and release (35). The effects of intranigral injection are likely to be at least partially mediated by interneurons, as it is known that GABA agonists iontophoresed in the substantia nigra decrease pars reticulata neuronal activity while increasing the pars compacta neuron firing rate (36). In spite of these divergent results, it would appear that the overall effect of systemic administration of GABA receptor agonists on nigrostriatal dopamine pathway function is one of inhibition (51,55).

Thus, in anticonvulsant doses, progabide or muscimol administered intraperitoneally, decrease stereotypies caused by dopamine receptor stimulation (8,108), decrease both basal and neuroleptic-induced striatal dopamine release (7,56), increase neuroleptic-induced catalepsy (54), and potentiate the antistereotypic effects of haloperidol (56).

The other well-studied neurochemical effect of GABA agonists is the interaction with striatal acetylcholine (ACh) systems. Thus, muscimol (87,90) and progabide (87) increase striatal ACh levels, an indication of a decrease in ACh turnover (38). [For further references on the topic, see Guyenet et al. (38).] Although this could be via an effect on dopaminergic neurons (51), it is more likely independent of the striatal dopamine nerve endings, since in rats with a 90% destruction of the nigrostriatal dopamine pathway, the effect of the GABA agonists on striatal ACh levels is maintained (87). It should be noted that this effect of GABA receptor agonists on striatal ACh neurons occurs at doses lower than the anticonvulsant doses. At the anticonvulsant doses, it seems that the effect on the dopamine system is predominant (6). It has been reported that muscimol stimulates striatal choline uptake, which has been interpreted as an indication of enhanced cholinergic activity (26). However, this situation could also be reflective of a feedback-regulated attempt to overcome the decreased acetylcholine release induced by the GABA agonist.

Proposed Mechanisms of Action

The proposed mechanism of anticonvulsant action of the GABA receptor agonists (muscimol, progabide, APSA, THIP, kojic amine) is via a direct stimulation of postsynaptic GABA receptors, which increases chloride conductance across the membrane. This leads to a diminution in cell firing and a decrease in the hyperexcitable state of the brain. The evidence (as reviewed above) is that all GABA receptor agonists displace [³H]GABA from its binding sites and exert bicuculline- and picrotoxin- (but not strychnine-) sensitive effects on cell firing. In addition, those GABA receptor agonists studied increase chloride conductance and have a cross-desensitization with GABA. Those GABA agonists known to enter into the brain display a broad anticonvulsant profile.

The benzodiazepines, although not fulfilling the strict requirements for GABA agonist activity, appear to exert their anticonvulsant effect via an action mediated by GABA receptors. Thus, the interaction of a benzodiazepine with its receptor induces a secondary alteration in the GABA receptor, enhancing its responsiveness to available GABA. This occurs via a change in the affinity for GABA as shown neurochemically (17,37) or neurophysiologically (63) and has been proposed to be via the removal of an inhibitor of GABA receptor function termed GABA-modulin (17,37).

Although we have not dealt with the barbiturates in this chapter, it is worth commenting on the possibility that these compounds act via the picrotoxinin-sensitive chloride ionophore, which is controlled by the GABA receptor. Thus, barbiturates displace [³H]dihydropicrotoxinin from its binding sites (80,81) and increase the synaptic responses to GABA (64,65). However, these drugs do not displace [³H]GABA from its binding site (28,52,81), indicating that their action is not via the primary GABA recognition site.

THERAPEUTIC USE

Since the early data of Tower (100) in 1960 and of Hennequet et al. (41) in 1961 on the effects of GABA in epileptic patients, no other data have been available until recently on the possible clinical effects of GABA receptor agonists in epilepsy. The only two compounds for which data in patients have appeared in the last 3 years are muscimol and progabide. However, the data on muscimol refer to various clinical situations other than epilepsy, and the available data on progabide appear to confirm the potential value of GABA receptor agonists for the treatment of epilepsy.

Muscimol

Given orally at doses of 5 to 10 mg, either to volunteers or to neuropsychiatric patients, muscimol manifests CNS activity, and the observed effects appear to be dose dependent (14,15,91,96,97,104). At doses less than 5 mg, muscimol appears to exert a certain tranquilizing effect, whereas at doses of 7 to 10 mg it may induce strong sedation, dizziness, mental confusion, vivid dreams, and exacerbation of psychotic manifestations such as hallucinations and delusional thinking (14,91,96,104).

This symptomatology may be accompanied by diffuse myoclonic twitching and paroxysmal slowing of the EEG (14,91,96). As in the case of neuroendocrine responses, most of the above-mentioned effects become manifest 60 to 120 min after drug intake, and the question of whether they are really caused by muscimol or by metabolites remains unanswered.

If we consider, however, that in man the effects of γ-hydroxybutyrate are very similar to those reported for muscimol and that, as in animals, the entry of unchanged muscimol into the brain is very likely to be minimal, the possibility that most of the reported symptomatology is caused by metabolites appears probable.

Progabide

In two open pilot studies of progabide on a total of 36 patients suffering from severe epilepsy and scarcely responding to the available antiepileptic drugs, a considerable reduction in seizure frequency (>50%) was observed in 47% of the cases (9,83). Progabide administered at doses of 900 to 2,400 mg/day (15–30 mg/kg) for 4 to 8 weeks was found effective in both partial and generalized seizures. It may be worthwhile to mention that two of four patients receiving progabide as monotherapy responded very favorably to the drug. General and biological tolerance were remarkably good, and, as already mentioned, plasma levels of associated drugs were not modified by the 4 to 8 week treatment with progabide.

A series of double-blind crossover trials are presently being done on a large number of patients with severe epilepsy. Preliminary data from the first two double-blind studies (57,102) on patients suffering from either partial seizures or primary and secondary generalized epilepsies seem to confirm that progabide has a significant antiepileptic efficacy. In these series of observations, sleepiness and mild hypotonia were the most frequently observed side effects; in no case, however, were they severe enough to necessitate drug withdrawal.

SUMMARY AND CONCLUSIONS

On consideration of the diverse chemical, pharmacological, biochemical, and clinical information reviewed above, it is evident that the concept that GABA receptor agonists may represent a useful alternative for improvement of the treatment of convulsive disorders has received validation both in experimental models and in preliminary clinical trials.

Although it is true that several of the presently available GABA agonists do not easily cross the blood–brain barrier, the use of carrier molecules and lipophilic GABA receptor agonists has been shown to be a valid approach.

Previous statements that a GABA receptor agonist would not be clinically useful (because of indiscriminate inhibition of cortical function) (70,86) have proved to be incorrect, probably for at least two reasons: (a) the reasoning was based on results obtained with compounds (such as muscimol) that are toxic, are very rapidly metabolized to yet unknown and possibly toxic metabolites, and can enter the brain to only a very limited extent; (b) the animal models used to predict the inefficacy of GABA receptor agonists cannot be considered representative of human epilepsy.

It would therefore appear that in order to reasonably predict the clinical efficacy (or lack thereof) of potential antiepileptic drugs, a variety of convulsive situations and models must be assessed.

On the basis of the available evidence (Tables 1 and 2), it appears that at least two or three new GABA receptor agonists are effective in several animal models, although they exacerbate the convulsive pattern in the photosensitive baboon. However, the fact that progabide is active in all models (baboon included) suggests that if they are devoid of toxic effects and have the desirable pharmacokinetic properties, GABA receptor agonists may be effective in all forms or models of experimental seizures. Such a broad spectrum of activity appears to be confirmed by preliminary results in epileptic patients.

One conclusion that can be drawn from the material reviewed is that the systemic administration (in both animals and man) of GABA receptor agonists capable of penetrating the CNS does not result in an "indiscriminate inhibition" of cortical function, but rather, it leads to a reestablishment of the compromised GABA transmission.

GABA receptor agonists thus appear to be a promising useful complement or alternative to the existing antiepileptic drugs.

The possible development of compounds with high affinity for the GABA receptors, acting through a physiological mechanism, and with fewer side effects appears to be a new trend toward the improvement of the treatment of the epileptic patient.

REFERENCES

1. Adembri, G., Bartolini, A., Bartolini, R., Giotti, A., and Zilletti, L. (1974): Anticonvulsive action of homotaurine and taurine. Br. J. Pharmacol., 52:439P–440P.
2. Anlezark, G., Collins, J., and Meldrum, B. S. (1977): GABA agonists and audiogenic seizures. Neurosci. Lett., 7:337–340.
3. Atkinson, J. G., Gérard, Y., Rokach, J., Rooney, C. S., McFarlane, C. S., Rackham, A., and Shave, N. N. (1979): Kojic amine—a novel GABA analog. J. Med. Chem., 22:99–106.
4. Baraldi, M., Grandison, L., and Guidotti, A. (1979): Distribution and metabolism of muscimol in the brain and other tissues of the rat. Neuropharmacology, 18:57–62.
5. Barnes, C. D., and Eltherington, L. G. (1973): Drug Dosage in Laboratory Animals. University of California Press, Los Angeles.
6. Bartholini, G. (1981): Neuronal network in the basal ganglia as related to extrapyramidal function. In: Advances in Experimental Medicine: Claude Bernard

Century Tribute, edited by S. Marazzato-Parvez and H. Parvez. Elsevier, Amsterdam (*in press*).

7. Bartholini, G., Lloyd, K. G., Worms, P., Constantinidis, J., and Tissot, R. (1979): GABA and GABAergic medication: Relation to striatal dopamine function and parkinsonism. In: *The Extrapyramidal System and Its Disorders,* edited by L. J. Poirier, T. L. Sourkes, and P. J. Bédard, pp. 253–257. Raven Press, New York.

8. Bartholini, G., Scatton, B., Zivkovic, B., and Lloyd, K. G. (1979): On the mode of action of SL 76002, a new GABA receptor agonist. In: *GABA-Neurotransmitters,* edited by P. Krogsgaard-Larsen, J. Scheel-Kruger, and H. Kofod, pp. 326–340. Munksgaard, Copenhagen.

9. Baruzzi, A., Pazzaglia, P., Loiseau, P., Cenraud, B., Zarifian, E., Mitchard, M., and Morselli, P. L. (1978): Preliminary observations on the effects of SL 76002, a new GABA agonist, in the epileptic patient. In: *X Epilepsy International Symposium,* pp. 199–200. Raven Press, New York.

10. Baxter, C. F., and Roberts, E. (1960): Demonstration of thiosemicarbazide-induced convulsions in rats with elevated brain levels of γ-aminobutyric acid. *Proc. Soc. Exp. Biol. Med.,* 104:426–427.

11. Bianchetti, G., Bossi, L., Braithwaite, R., Caqueret, H., London, D. R., and Morselli, P. L. (1982): Clinical pharmacokinetics of Progabide (SL 76002) a new GABA agonist. (*In preparation.*)

12. Bowery, N. G., and Brown, D. A. (1974): Depolarizing actions of γ-aminobutyric acid and related compounds on rat superior cervical ganglia *in vitro. Br. J. Pharmacol.,* 50:205–218.

13. Braithwaite, R. A., Bianchetti, G., Caqueret, H., Dubruc, C., and Morselli, P. L. (1980): The disposition of a new GABA mimetic drug in man—SL 76002. *Prog. Neuro-Psychopharmacol., Suppl. 1980,* p. 89.

14. Chase, T. N., and Tamminga, C. A. (1979): GABA system participation in human motor, cognitive and endocrine function. In: *GABA-Neurotransmitters,* edited by P. Krogsgaard-Larsen, J. Scheel-Kruger, and H. Kofod, pp. 283–294. Munksgaard, Copenhagen.

15. Chase, T. N., and Walters, J. R. (1976): Pharmacologic approaches to the manipulation of GABA-mediated synaptic function in man. In: *GABA in Nervous System Function,* edited by E. Roberts, T. N. Chase, and D. B. Tower, pp. 497–514. Raven Press, New York.

16. Cheramy, A., Nieoullon, A. and Glowinski, J. (1978): GABAergic processes involved in the control of dopamine release from nigrostriatal dopaminergic neurons in the cat. *Eur. J. Pharmacol.,* 48:281–295.

17. Costa, E., and Guidotti, A. (1979): Recent studies on the mechanism whereby benzodiazepines facilitate GABAergic transmission. In: *GABA-Biochemistry and CNS Functions,* edited by P. Mandel and F. V. De Feudis, pp. 371–378. Plenum Press, New York.

18. Coursin, D. B. (1954): Convulsive seizures in infants with pyridoxine deficient diet. *J.A.M.A.,* 154:406–408.

19. Coursin, D. B. (1955): Vitamin B_6 deficiency in infants: A follow-up study. *Am. J. Dis. Child.,* 90:344–348.

20. Curtis, D. R., Duggan, A. W., Felix, D., and Johnston, G. A. R. (1971): Bicuculline, an antagonist of GABA and synaptic inhibition in the spinal cord. *Brain Res.,* 32:69–96.

21. Curtis, D. R., Game, C. J. A., and Lodge, D. (1976): Benzodiazepines and central glycine receptors. *Br. J. Pharmacol.,* 56:307–311.

22. Desarmenien, M., Headley, P. M., Santangelo, F., and Feltz, P. (1980): The effects of various GABA-mimetics on dorsal root ganglion neurons *in vitro:* A physiological analysis. *Brain Res. Bull.,* 5(*Suppl.* 2):471–475.

23. Desarmenien, M., Feltz, P., Headley, P. M., and Santangelo, F. (1981): SL 75102 as an aminobutyric acid agonist: Experiments on dorsal root ganglion neurones *in vitro. Br. J. Pharmacol.,* 72:355–364.

24. Durand, A., Dring, G., Mas-Chamberlin, C., Gillette, G., Rouchouse, A., and Morselli, P. L. (1982): Autoradiographic and pharmacokinetic studies on Progabide (SL 76002) in the experimental animal. (*In preparation.*)

25. Enna, S. J. (1979): Biochemical pharmacology of GABAergic agonists. *Life Sci.,* 24:1727–1738.

26. Enna, S. J., Ferkany, J. W., and Butler, I. J. (1981): Chronology of neurochemical alterations induced by GABA agonist administration. In: *GABA and Benzodiazepine Receptors,* edited by E. Costa, G. DiChiara, and G. L. Gessa, pp. 181–189. Raven Press, New York.

27. Enna, S. J., Maggi, A., Worms, P., and Lloyd, K. G. (1980): Muscimol: Brain penetration and anticonvulsant potency following GABA-T inhibition. *Brain Res. Bull.* 5 (*Suppl.* 2):461–464.

28. Enna, S. J., and Snyder, S. H. (1975): Properties of γ-aminobutyric acid (GABA) receptor binding in rat brain synaptic membrane functions. *Brain Res.,* 100:81–97.

29. Fariello, R. G. (1980): Action of inhibitory amino acids on acute epileptic foci: An electrographic study. *Exp. Neurol.,* 66:55–63.

30. Fariello, R. G., and Golden, G. T. (1980): Homotaurine: A GABA agonist with anticonvulsant effects. *Biobehav. Rev.* (*in press*).

31. Fuxe, K., Andersson, K., Ogren, S. O., Perez de la Mora, M., Schwarcz, R., Hökfelt, T., Eneroth, P., Gustafsson, J. A., and Skett, P. (1979): GABA neurons and their interaction with monoamine neurons. An anatomical, pharmacological and functional analysis. In: *GABA-Neurotransmitters,* edited by P. Krogsgaard-Larsen, J. Scheel-Kruger, and H. Kofod, pp. 74–94. Munksgaard, Copenhagen.

32. Gagneux, A. R., Häflinger, F., Engster, C. H., and Good, R. (1965): Synthesis of Pantherine (Agarin). *Tetrahedron Lett.,* 25:2077–2079.

33. Galzigna, L., Garbin, L., Bianchi, M., and Marzotto, A. (1978): Properties of two derivatives of γ-aminobutyric acid (GABA) capable of abolishing cardiazol- and bicuculline-induced convulsions in the rat. *Arch. Int. Pharmacodyn.,* 253:73–85.

34. Gillette, G., Dring, G., and Fraisse, J. (1982): A gas chromatographic method for the determination

of Progabide in biological fluids and tissues. *J. Chromatogr.* (*in press*).

35. Giorguieff, M. F., Kemel, M. L., Besson, M. J., and Glowinski, J. (1977): Involvement of cholinergic and GABA-receptors in the control of dopamine release from rat striatal slices. In: *Parkinson's Disease—Concepts and Prospects*, edited by J. P. W. L. Lakke, J. Korf, and H. Wessling, pp. 31–52. Excerpta Medica, Amsterdam.

36. Grace, A., and Bunney, B. S. (1979): Paradoxical GABA excitation of nigral dopaminergic cells: Indirect mediation through reticulata inhibitory neurons. *Eur. J. Pharmacol.*, 59:211–218.

37. Guidotti, A., Baraldi, M., Schwartz, J. P., and Costa, E. (1979): Molecular mechanisms regulating the interactions between the benzodiazepines and GABA receptors in the central nervous system. *Pharmacol. Biochem. Behav.*, 10:803–807.

38. Guyenet, P., Javoy, F., Euvrard, C., and Glowinski, J. (1977): The effect of drugs on choline and acetylcholine content in the rat striatum following two methods of sacrifice. *Neuropharmacology*, 16:385–390.

39. Haefely, W., Kulcsar, A., Möhler, H., Pieri, L., Polc, P., and Schaffner, R. (1975): Possible involvement of GABA in the central actions of benzodiazepines. In: *Mechanism of Action of Benzodiazepines*, edited by E. Costa and P. Greengard, pp. 131–151. Raven Press, New York.

40. Hayashi, T. (1959): The inhibitory action of β-hydroxy-γ-aminobutyric acid upon the seizure following stimulation of the motor cortex of the dog. *J. Physiol. (Lond.)*, 145:570–578.

41. Hennequet, M. J., Lyon, A., Debris, P., and Laballe, J. C. (1961): La pyridoxino dépendance, maladie métabolique s'exprimant par des crises convulsives pyridoxino-sensibles (première observation familiale). *Rev. Neurol.*, 105:406–419.

42. Hori, N., Ikeda, K., and Roberts, E. (1978): Muscimol, GABA and picrotoxin: Effects on membrane conductance of a crustacean neuron. *Brain Res.*, 141:364–370.

43. Iversen, L. L. (1978): Biochemical psychopharmacology of GABA. In: *Psychopharmacology: A Generation of Progress*, edited by M. A. Lipton, A. Di Mascio, and K. F. Killam, pp. 24–38. Raven Press, New York.

44. Johno, I., Ludwick, B. T., and Levy, H. R. (1981): Pharmacokinetic of progabide profile (SL 76002) in the rhesus monkey. Epilepsy International Congress, Kyoto, September 1981, Abstr. FP4-5-18-1, p. 188.

45. Johnston, G. A. R. (1976): Physiologic pharmacology of GABA and its antagonists in the vertebrate nervous system. In: *GABA in Nervous System Function*, edited by E. Roberts, T. N. Chase, and D. B. Tower, pp. 395–412. Raven Press, New York.

46. Kaplan, J. P., Raizon, B. M., Desarmenien, M., Fletz, P., Headley, P. M., Worms, P., Lloyd, K. G., and Bartholini, G. (1980): New anticonvulsants: Schiff bases of GABA and GABAmide. *J. Med. Chem.*, 23:702–704.

47. Krogsgaard-Larsen, P. (1977): Muscimol analogues II. Synthesis of some bicyclic-3-isoxazolol zwitterions. *Acta Chem. Scand.*, 331:584–588.

48. Krogsgaard-Larsen, P., and Arnt, J. (1979): GABA receptor agonists: Relationship between structural and biological activity *in vivo* and *in vitro*. In: *GABA-Biochemistry and CNS Function*, edited by P. Mandel and F. V. De Feudis, pp. 303–321. Plenum Press, New York.

49. Krogsgaard-Larsen, P., Hjeds, H., Curtis, D. R., Lodge, D., and Johnston, G. A. R. (1979): Dihydromuscimol, thiomuscimol and related compounds as GABA analogues. *J. Neurochem.*, 32:1717–1724.

50. Krogsgaard-Larsen, P., Johnston, G. A. R., Lodge, D., and Curtis, D. R. (1977): A new class of GABA agonists. *Nature*, 268:53–55.

51. Lloyd, K. G. (1978): Neurotransmitter interactions related to central dopamine neurons. In: *Essays in Neurochemistry and Neuropharmacology*, Vol. 3, edited by M. B. H. Youdim, W. Lovenberg, D. F. Sharman, and J. R. Lagnado, pp. 129–207. John Wiley & Sons, New York.

52. Lloyd, K. G., and Dreksler, S. (1978): An analysis of (^{3}H)gamma-aminobutyric acid (GABA) binding in the human brain. *Brain Res.*, 163:77–87.

53. Lloyd, K. G., Munari, C., Worms, P., Bossi, L., Bancaud, J., Talairach, J., and Morselli, P. L. (1980): The role of GABA-mediated neurotransmission in convulsive states. In: *GABA and Benzodiazepine Receptors*, edited by E. Costa, G. DiChiara, and G. L. Gessa, pp. 199–206. Raven Press, New York.

54. Lloyd, K. G., Worms, P., Depoortere, H., and Bartholini, G. (1979): Pharmacological profile of SL 76002, a new GABA-mimetic drug. In: *GABA-Neurotransmitters*, edited by P. Krogsgaard-Larsen, J. Scheel-Kruger, and H. Kofod, pp. 308–325. Munksgaard, Copenhagen.

55. Lloyd, K. G., Worms, P., Scatton, B., Zivkovic, V., and Bartholini, G. (1979): The influence of GABA on dopamine neuron activity. In: *Presynaptic Receptors*, edited by S. Z. Langer, L. Starke, and M. L. Dubocovich, pp. 207–212. Pergamon Press, New York.

56. Lloyd, K. G., Worms, P., Zivkovic, B., Scatton, B., and Bartholini, G. (1980): Interaction of GABA mimetics with nigro-striatal dopamine neurons. *Brain Res. Bull.*, 5 *(Suppl. 2)*:439–445.

57. Loiseau, P., Cenraud, B., Bossi, L., and Morselli, P. L. (1981): A double blind controlled study versus placebo with progabide (SL 76002) in severe epilepsy. In: *Advances in Epileptology: XIIth Epilepsy International Symposium*, edited by M. Dam, L. Gram, and J. K. Penry, pp. 135–140. Raven Press, New York.

58. London, D. R., Kandell, F. Loizou, L. A., Butt, W. R., Morselli, P. L., Bossi, L., and Van Landeghem, V. (1981): The neuroendocrine effects of progabide in healthy male volunteers, Abs. FP-4-2. *Proceedings Epilepsy International Congress, Kyoto.*

59. London, D. R., Loizou, L. A., Butt, W. R., Rovei, V., Bianchetti, G., and Morselli, P. L. (1980): The effect of anticonvulsant drugs on hormonal responses in normal volunteers. In: *Antiepileptic Therapy: Advances in Drug Monitoring*, edited by S. J. Johannessen, P. L. Morselli, C. E. Pippenger, A. Richens, D. Schmidt, and H. Meinardi, pp. 405–411. Raven Press, New York.

60. Löscher, W., and Frey, H. J. (1977): Effect of convulsant and anticonvulsant agents on levels and metabolism of γ-aminobutyric acid in mouse brain. *Naunyn Schmiedebergs Arch. Pharmacol.,* 296:263–269.

61. Lott, I. T., Coulombe, T., Di Paolo, R. V., Richardson, E. P., and Levy, H. L. (1978): Vitamin of B_6-dependent seizures: Pathology and chemical findings in brain. *Neurology (Minneap.),* 28:47–54.

62. MacDonald, R. A., and Barker, J. L. (1978): Benzodiazepines specifically modulate GABA-mediated postsynaptic inhibition in cultured mammalian neurons. *Nature,* 271:263–564.

63. MacDonald, R. A., and Barker, J. L. (1978): Specific antagonism of GABA-mediated postsynaptic inhibition in cultured mammalian spinal cord neurons: A common mode of convulsant action. *Neurology (Minneap.),* 28:325–330.

64. MacDonald, R. A., and Barker, J. L. (1979): Anticonvulsant and anaesthetic barbiturates: Different postsynaptic actions in cultured mammalian neurons. *Neurology (Minneap.),* 29:432–447.

65. MacDonald, R. A., and Barker, J. L. (1979): Enhancement of GABA-mediated postsynaptic inhibition in cultured mammalian spinal cord neurons: A common mode of anticonvulsant action. *Brain Res.,* 167:323–336.

66. Maggi, A., and Enna, S. J. (1979): Characteristics of muscimol accumulation in mouse brain after systemic administration. *Neuropharmacology,* 18:361–366.

67. Matthews, W. D., and McCafferty, G. P. (1979): Anticonvulsant activity of muscimol against seizures induced by impairment of GABA-mediated transmission. *Neuropharmacology,* 18:885–889.

68. McGeer, P. L., McGeer, E. G., and Wada, J. A. (1971): Glutamic acid decarboxylase in Parkinson's disease and epilepsy. *Neurology (Minneap.),* 21:1000–1007.

69. Meldrum, B. S. (1975): Epilepsy and γ-aminobutyric acid-mediated inhibition. *Int. Rev. Neurobiol.,* 17:1–36.

70. Meldrum, B. S. (1978): Gamma-aminobutyric acid and the search for new anticonvulsant drugs. *Lancet,* 2:304–306.

71. Meldrum, B. S., and Horton, R. (1980): Effect of the bicyclic GABA agonist, THIP, on myoclonic seizure responses in mice and baboons with reflex epilepsy. *Eur. J. Pharmacol.,* 61:231–237.

72. Morselli, P. L., and Baruzzi, A. (1980): New antiepileptic drugs—New trends? In: *Advances in Epileptology: XIth Epilepsy International Symposium,* edited by R. Canger, F. Angeleri, and J. K. Penry, pp. 377–390. Raven Press, New York.

73. Morselli, P. L., Bossi, L., Henry, J. F., Zarifian, E., and Bartholini, G. (1980): On the therapeutic action of SL 76002, a new GABA mimetic agent: Preliminary observations in neuropsychiatric disorders. *Brain Res. Bull.,* 5 *(Suppl. 2):* 411–414.

74. Müller, E. E., Cocchi, D., Locatelli, V., Krogsgaard-Larsen, P., Bruno, F., and Racagni, G. (1979): GABAergic neurotransmission and the secretion of prolactin in the rat. In: *GABA-Neurotransmitters,* edited by P. Krogsgaard-Larsen, J. Scheel-Kruger, and H. Kofod, pp. 518–532. Munksgaard, Copenhagen.

75. Müller, G. F., and Eugster, C. H. (1965): Muscimol, ein pharmakodynamisch wirksamer Stoff aus *Amanita muscaria. Helv. Chim. Acta,* 48:910–926.

76. Munari, C., Rovei, V., Lloyd, K., Talairach J., Sanjuan, M., Vedrenne, C., Bancaud, J., and Morselli, P. L. (1979): Neuropharmacological and neurochemical observations in epileptic patients undergoing neurosurgery. In: *Abstracts, XI Epilepsy International Symposium,* Florence, Italy, p. 158.

77. Naik, S. R., Guidotti, A., and Costa, E. (1976): Central GABA receptor agonists: Comparison of muscimol and baclofen. *Neuropharmacology,* 15:479–484.

78. Nistri, A., and Corradetti, R. (1978): A comparison of the effects of GABA, 3-aminopropanesulfonic acid and imidazoleacetic acid on the frog spinal cord. *Neuropharmacology,* 17:13–19.

79. Olpe, H. R., and Koella, W. P. (1978): The action of muscimol on neurons of the substantia nigra in the rat. *Experientia,* 34:235.

80. Olsen, R. W., Ticku, M. K., Greenlee, D., and Van Ness, P. (1979): GABA receptor and ionophore binding sites: Interaction with various drugs. In: *GABA-Neurotransmitters,* edited by P. Krogsgaard-Larsen, J. Scheel-Kruger, and H. Kofod, pp. 165–178. Munksgaard, Copenhagen.

81. Olsen, R. W., Ticku, M. K., Van Ness, P., and Greenlee, D. (1979): Effects of drugs on γ-aminobutyric acid receptors, uptake, release and synthesis in vitro. *Brain Res.,* 139:277–294.

82. Ott, J., Wheaton, P. S., and Chilton, W. S. (1975): Fate of muscimol in the mouse. *Physiol. Chem. Phys.,* 7:381–384.

83. Pedley, T. A., Horton, R. W., and Meldrum, B. S. (1979): Electroencephalographic and behavioural effects of a GABA agonist (muscimol) on photosensitive epilepsy in the baboon, *Papio papio. Epilepsia,* 20:409–416.

84. Pinder, R., Brogden, R. N., Speight, T. M., and Avery, G. S. (1977): Sodium valproate: A review of its pharmacological properties and therapeutic efficacy in epilepsy. *Drugs,* 13:81–123.

85. Ribak, C. E., Harris, A. B., Vaughan, J. E., and Roberts, E. (1979): Inhibitory GABAergic nerve terminals decrease at sites of focal epilepsy. *Science,* 205:211–214.

86. Roberts, E. (1976): Disinhibition as an organizing principle in the nervous system. The role of the GABA system. Application to neurologic and psychiatric disorders. In: *GABA in Nervous System Function,* edited by E. Roberts, T. N. Chase, and D. B. Tower, pp. 515–539. Raven Press, New York.

87. Scatton, B., and Bartholini, G. (1979): Increase in striatal acetylcholine levels by GABA mimetic drugs: Lack of the involvement of the nigrostriatal dopaminergic neurons. *Eur. J. Pharmacol.,* 56:181–182.

88. Schechter, P. J., Tranier, Y., Jung, M. J., and Sjoerdsma, A. (1977): Antiseizure activity of γ-acetylenic-γ-aminobutyric acid: A catalytic irreversible inhibitor of γ-aminobutyric acid transaminase. *J. Pharmacol. Exp. Ther.,* 201:606–612.

89. Scheel-Kruger, J., Arnt, J., Braestrup, C., Chris-

tensen, A. V., Cools, A. R., and Magelund, G. (1978): GABA–dopamine interaction in substantia nigra and nucleus accumbens—relevance to behavioural stimulation and stereotyped behavior. In: *Dopamine*, edited by P. J. Roberts, G. N. Woodruff, and L. L. Iversen, pp. 343–347. Raven Press, New York.

90. Sethy, V. H. (1978): Dopaminergic, GABAergic and cholinergic interactions in the regulation of striatal acetylcholine concentrations. *Res. Commun. Chem. Pathol. Pharmacol.*, 21:359–362.

91. Shoulson, I., Goldblatt, D., Charlton, M., and Joynt, R. J. (1978): Huntington's disease: Treatment with muscimol, a GABA-mimetic drug. *Ann. Neurol.*, 4:279–284.

92. Snead, O. C. (1978): Gamma-hydroxybutyrate in the monkey. IV. Dopaminergic mechanisms. *Neurology, (Minneap.)* 28:1179–1182.

93. Snodgrass, S. R. (1978): Use of ^{3}H-muscimol for GABA receptor studies. *Nature*, 273:392–394.

94. Takemoto, T., Nakajima, T., and Sakuma, R. (1964): Isolation of aflycidal constituents "ibotonic acid" from *Amanita muscaria*. *J. Pharm. Soc. Jpn.*, 84:1233–1234.

95. Takeuchi, A. (1976): Studies on the inhibitory effects of GABA in invertebrate nervous systems. In: *GABA in Nervous System Function*, edited by E. Roberts, T. N. Chase, and D. B. Tower, pp. 255–268. Raven Press, New York.

96. Tamminga, C. A., Crayton, J. W., and Chase, T. N. (1978): Muscimol: GABA agonist therapy in schizophrenia. *Am. J. Psychiatry*, 135:746–747.

97. Tamminga, C. A., Neophytides, A., Chase, T. N., and Frohman, L. A. (1978): Stimulation of prolactine and growth hormone secretion by muscimol, a γ-aminobutyric acid agonist. *J. Clin. Endocrinol. Metab.*, 47:1348–1351.

98. Tapia, R. (1974): The role of γ-aminobutyric acid metabolism in the regulation of cerebral excitability. In: *Neurohumoral Coding of Brain Function*, edited by R. D. Myers and R. R. Drucker, pp. 3–26. Plenum Press, New York.

99. Tapia, R., and Covarrubias, M. (1978): Glutamate decarboxylase, properties and the synaptic function of GABA. In: *Amino Acids as Chemical Transmitters*, edited by F. Fonnum, pp. 431–438. Plenum Press, New York.

100. Tower, D. B. (1960): Administration of GABA to

man: Systemic effect and anticonvulsant action. In: *Inhibition in the Nervous System and GABA*, edited by E. Roberts, pp. 562–578. Pergamon Press, New York.

101. Tower, D. B. (1976): GABA and seizures: Clinical correlates in man. In: *GABA in Nervous System Function*, edited by E. Roberts, T. N. Chase, and D. B. Tower, pp. 461–478. Raven Press, New York.

102. Van Der Linden, G. J., Meinardi, H., Meijer, J. W. A., Bossi, L., and Gomeni, C. (1981): A double blind cross-over trial with SL 76002 against placebo in patients with secondary generalized epilepsy. In: *Advances in Epileptology: XIIth Epilepsy International Symposium*, edited by M. Dam, L. Gram, and J. K. Penry, pp. 135–140. Raven Press, New York.

103. Van Gelder, N. M., and Courtois, A. (1972): Close correlation between changing content of specific amino acids in epileptogenic cortex of cats, and severity of epilepsy. *Brain Res.*, 43:477–484.

104. Waser, P. B. (1967): The pharmacology of *Amanita muscaria*. In: *Ethnopharmacologic Search for Psycho-Active Drugs*, edited by D. Efron, B. Halin, and N. Kline, pp. 419–439. U.S. Public Health Service Publication N1645, Washington.

105. Williams, H. W. R. (1976): Synthesis of some 4-pyranones and 4-pyridines structurally related to isoproterenol. *Can. J. Chem.*, 54:3377–3382.

106. Wood, J. D., Kurylo, E., and Peesker, S. J. (1978): The possible involvement of GABA and its compartmentation in the mechanism of some convulsant and anticonvulsant agents. In: *Amino Acids as Chemical Transmitters*, edited by F. Fonnum, pp. 439–444. Plenum Press, New York.

107. Wood, J. H., Hare, J. A., Glaeser, B. S., Ballenger, J. C., and Post, R. M. (1979): Low cerebrospinal fluid γ-aminobutyric acid content in seizure patients. *Neurology (Minneap.)*, 29:1203–1208.

108. Worms, P., Depoortere, H., and Lloyd, K. G. (1979): Neuropharmacological spectrum of muscimol. *Life Sci.*, 25:607–614.

109. Yarbrough, G. G. (1978): Nipecotic acid and 2,4-diaminobutyric acid enhance the actions of muscimol on cerebral cortical neurons. *Can. J. Physiol. Pharmacol.*, 56:443–446.

110. Yarbrough, G. G., Williams, M., and Haubrich, D. R. (1979): The neuropharmacology of a novel γ-aminobutyric acid analog, kojic amine. *Arch. Int. Pharmacodyn.*, 241:266–279.

Author Index

Subject Index